CRANIAL
COMPUTED
TOMOGRAPHY
AND MRI

CRANIAL
COMPUTED
TOMOGRAPHY
AND MRI SECOND EDITION

Seungho Howard Lee, M.D.

Clinical Professor of Radiology
Robert Wood Johnson Medical School
University of Medicine and Dentistry of New Jersey
Neuroradiologist-in-Chief
Muhlenberg Regional Medical Center
Plainfield, New Jersey and
Somerset Medical Center
Somerville, New Jersey

Krishna C.V.G. Rao, M.D.

Clinical Professor of Radiology
University of Maryland School of Medicine
Chief, Department of Radiology
Prince George's General Hospital and Medical Center
Cheverly, Maryland

McGraw-Hill Book Company

New York   St. Louis   San Francisco   Auckland   Bogotá   Hamburg
Johannesburg   Lisbon   London   Madrid   Mexico   Milan   Montreal   New Delhi
Panama   Paris   San Juan   São Paulo   Singapore   Sydney   Tokyo   Toronto

Library of Congress Cataloging-in-Publication Data

Cranial computed tomography and MRI.

   Rev. ed. of: Cranial computed tomography. c1983.
   Includes bibliographies and index.
   1. Cranium—Radiography. 2. Head—Diseases—
Diagnosis. 3. Tomography. 4. Magnetic resonance
imaging. I. Lee, Seungho Howard. II. Rao,
Krishna C. V. G. III. Cranial computed tomography.
[DNLM: 1. Nuclear Magnetic Resonance—diagnostic use.
2. Skull—radiography. 3. Tomography, X-Ray Computed.
WE 705 C8893]
RC936.C717 1986   617'.5107572   86-21161
ISBN 0-07-037459-7

CRANIAL COMPUTED TOMOGRAPHY AND MRI

3 4 5 6 7 8 9 0 HD HD 8 9

ISBN 0-07-037459-7

This book was set in Palatino by Waldman Graphics, Inc; the editor was J. Dereck Jeffers; the production supervisor was Avé McCracken; the cover was designed by Edward R. Schultheis; project supervision was done by The Total Book.
The Maple–Vail Book Manufacturing Group was printer and binder.

To our wives, Taeja Kim and Kusuma, and
to our children, Michele, Jennifer, Anil, and Sudhir

Contents

List of Contributors

Scott W. Atlas, M.D.
Instructor of Radiology
University of Pennsylvania
School of Medicine and Hospital
Philadelphia, Pennsylvania

Larissa T. Bilaniuk, M.D.
Professor Radiology
University of Pennsylvania School of Medicine and
    Hospital
Philadelphia, Pennsylvania

William G. Bradley, Jr., M.D., Ph.D.
Associate Clinical Professor of Radiology
University of California, San Francisco
Director of MR Imaging Laboratory
Huntington Medical Research Institutes and Hospital
Pasadena, California

David L. Daniels, M.D.
Associate Professor of Radiology
Medical College of Wisconsin
Milwaukee, Wisconsin

Richard E. Fernandez, M.D.
Neuroradiologist
Kimball Medical Center
Lakewood, New Jersey

Charles R. Fitz, M.D.
Adjunct Professor of Radiology
George Washington University, Medical School
Chief of Neuroradiology
Children's Hospital
Washington, D.C.

Mokhtar H. Gado, M.D.
Professor of Radiology
Chief of Neuroradiology
Mallinckrodt Institute of Radiology and Washington
    University School of Medicine
St. Louis, Missouri

Herbert I. Goldberg, M.D.
Professor of Radiology
University of Pennsylvania School of Medicine and
    Hospital
Philadelphia, Pennsylvania

Kalyanmay Goshhajra, M.D.
Clinical Associate Professor of Radiology
University of Pittsburgh
Allegheny Valley General Hospital
Pittsburgh, Pennsylvania

Derek C. Harwood-Nash, M.D.
Professor and Chairman
Department of Radiology
Sick Children's Hospital
University of Toronto College of Medicine
Toronto, Canada

Victor M. Haughton, M.D.
Professor of Radiology
Director of Neuroradiological Research
Medical College of Wisconsin
Milwaukee, Wisconsin

Stephen A. Kieffer, M.D.
Professor and Chairman
Department of Radiology
State University of New York
Upstate Medical Center
Syracuse, New York

Pulla R. S. Kishore, M.D.
Professor and Chairman
Department of Radiology
Medical College of Virginia and Hospital
Richmond, Virginia

Keith E. Kortman, M.D.
Assistant Clinical Professor of Radiology
University of California, Los Angeles
Research Radiologist
Huntington Medical Research Institutes and Hospital
Pasadena, California

Seungho Howard Lee, M.D.
Clinical Professor of Radiology
Robert Wood Johnson Medical School
University of Medicine and Dentistry of New Jersey
Neuroradiologist–in–Chief
Muhlenberg Regional Medical Center
Plainfield, New Jersey and
Somerset Medical Center
Somerville, New Jersey

Maurice H. Lipper, M.B., Ch. B.
Associate Professor of Radiology
Medical College of Virginia and Hospital
McGuire Veterans Administration Medical Center
Richmond, Virginia

Gordon E. Melville, M.D.
Clinical Assistant Professor of Radiology
Robert Wood Johnson Medical School
University of Medicine and Dentistry of New Jersey
Muhlenberg Regional Medical Center
Plainfield, New Jersey
Somerset Medical Center
Somerville, New Jersey

Krishna C. V. G. Rao, M.D.
Clinical Professor of Radiology
University of Maryland Medical School
Chief of Radiology
Prince George's General Hospital and Medical Center
Cheverly, Maryland

Katherine A. Shaffer, M.D.
Associate Professor of Radiology
Medical College of Wisconsin
Milwaukee, Wisconsin

Karel G. TerBrugge, M.D.
Associate Professor of Radiology
University of Toronto College of Medicine
Toronto Western Hospital
Toronto, Canada

Theodore Villafana, Ph.D.
Professor of Radiology
Director of Diagnostic Physics
Temple University School of Medicine and Hospital
Philadelphia, Pennsylvania

J. Powell Williams, M.D.
Professor of Radiology
University of Southern Alabama School of Medicine and
    Hospital
Mobile, Alabama

Robert A. Zimmerman, M.D.
Professor of Radiology
University of Pennsylvania School of Medicine and
    Hospital
Philadelphia, Pennsylvania

Preface

Radiologic advancement is usually punctuated by new technological development. Since the first edition of this book, significant devlopment in neuroradiologic imaging has occurred due to faster CT scanners with better image resolution and the recent introduction of Magnetic Resonance Imaging into the medical field. Although considerable amounts of information on both technical and clinical application of MRI is rapidly accumulating, its exact impact on other neuroimaging diagnostic modality, in particular computed tomography, is not certain. We have attempted, in this second edition, to depict the current transformation status interfacing computed tomography and MRI in the practice of neurosciences. This is reflected in the change of title of the book.

The editors are deeply grateful to all the coauthors of the present work and to our clinical colleagues who have contributed much of the interesting material. We are extremely thankful to the editors at McGraw-Hill; Avé McCracken, Annette Bodzin, Robert McGrath, J. Derek Jeffers, and B. J. Clark for their consistent help. Special thanks to our colleagues in the department of radiology, University of Maryland Hospital, Prince George's Hospital, Somerset Medical Center and Muhlenberg Regional Medical Center, and especially the staff in The Warren Imaging Center. Special thanks, also, to Al Lavitola and Tom Bland for photography and Sue Janho and Catherine Gonzalez for typing the manuscripts.

S. Howard Lee
Krishna C.V.G. Rao

CRANIAL
COMPUTED
TOMOGRAPHY
AND MRI

1

PHYSICS AND INSTRUMENTATION: CT AND MRI

Theodore Villafana

SECTION A: COMPUTED TOMOGRAPHY

INTRODUCTION

Few innovations in radiology have fomented as much excitement and fundamental change as has computed, or computerized, tomography (CT). It turns out that a wealth of radiological information had been overlooked in classical radiology and tomography (Ter-Pogossian 1974). In fact, even now, computed tomography as we know it is probably just the beginning of what may come. Radiologists, of course, have been caught up in this imaging revolution. They must become increasingly familiar with the physical principles, instrumentation, and tech-

nical limitations of computed tomography in order to make accurate and precise diagnostic interpretations. The purpose of this chapter is to provide a fuller understanding of the basic CT scanning principles of direct importance to the clinician. The presentation here consists, first, of a brief review of the basis and the limitations of classical radiographic imaging. Second, classical tomography, as an attempt to overcome some of the problems of classical radiography, is also briefly discussed. Finally, computed tomography and its limitations are discussed fully.

Basic X-Ray Image Formation

The basic aim of diagnostic radiology is to record on a film (or display on a monitor) a pattern of densities

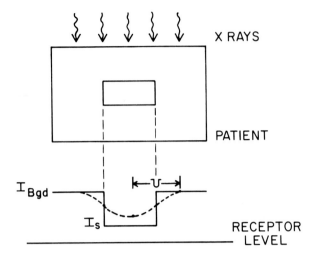

Figure 1-1 An intensity profile of the x-ray beam as it emerges from the patient. Here a hypothetical square anatomical structure ideally casts a shadow (I_s) relative to the adjoining background tissue (I_{Bgd}). The relative depth of the shadow or subject contrast, C_s, depends on the difference in attenuation between the two areas. Factors such as scatter, motion, and focal spot size tend to degrade both subject contrast and the edge character of the pattern (dashed curve). *U* is the resulting unsharpness or distance over which edge is blurred.

(or illumination levels on a monitor) which corresponds to and conveys diagnostic information on the size, shape, and distribution of the anatomic tissues within a patient. For instance, in Figure 1-1, we see a beam of x-rays penetrating a "simplified patient" consisting simply of a square block of tissue surrounded by a different but uniform tissue background. As the x-rays pass through the patient they are attenuated; that is, they are both absorbed and scattered within the patient. Attentuation, however, will depend on the type of tissues present and on the x-ray beam energy. Finally, the x-rays emerge from the patient and arrive at the image receptor level, where they are detected or recorded.

Figure 1-1 depicts one particular x-ray intensity profile. It is important to realize that this x-ray intensity profile is the sum total of the transmitted primary beam and the scattered radiation reaching the receptor level. Each point along the final profile thus depends on the x-ray attenuation which occurred along each ray-path within the patient, as well as the scatter generated. Note also that the final

two-dimensional image is composed of the collection of all such intensity profiles within the patient for the entire exposed field.

Let us study further the representation of radiographic images by intensity profiles, as this is the key to understanding CT technology. Referring again to Figure 1-1, we see that if x-rays penetrate a square object, a square x-ray profile is expected. This profile exhibits a certain depth (subject shadow) as well as a certain edge character. It should be clear that if the anatomic square structure under study had been more similar in atomic number and density to the background medium, the pattern depth or shadow would have been diminished and visualization would have been poorer. The relative x-ray intensity difference between the background and the anatomic structure of interest is referred to as the *relative subject contrast* (C_s).

$$C_s = \frac{I_{Bgd} - I_s}{I_{Bgd}} \tag{1}$$

Subject contrast depends on a number of factors, of which the beam energy is one of the most important. Beam energy in turn is governed by the operating kilovoltage and the beam filtration present in the beam. The second factor is the atomic number difference between the background and the anatomic structure in question. Figure 1-2 plots subject contrast as a function of beam energy for various combinations of anatomic tissues. Note that subject contrast diminishes as beam energy increases and as tissues become more similar. The practical importance of the C_s measure and how it limits routine radiography can be illustrated by the case of blood vessels within soft-tissue surrounds. Visualization of brain or renal vasculature, for instance, is extremely poor even under the most advantageous circumstance. However, introduction of contrast media into the blood vessel drastically increases its attenuation properties as compared to the surrounding tissues, and the blood vessels "light up." Introducing contrast media greatly increases subject contrast, and visualization is then markedly improved.

In addition to subject contrast, a second important aspect of the x-ray image is its edge character.

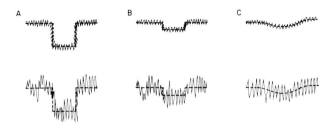

Figure 1-3 The effects of x-ray noise (quantum mottle) on x-ray intensity profiles. **A.** Ideal intensity profile with relatively high subject contrast (depth of shadow). Increasing amounts of noise mask the x-ray image, but it may still be detected. **B.** Ideal profile with relatively low subject contrast. Increasing amounts of noise readily obscure pattern. **C.** Unsharp and low subject contrast pattern is also readily obscured by noise.

Figure 1-1 shows the ideal case, in which the x-ray image has exactly the same well-defined edges as the structure itself. In general, this is not the case; unsharp edges usually appear. Deviation from a well-defined edge is quantitated with the concept of *unsharpness* (or *blur*). Unsharpness represents the smear around the edge and is simply expressed as the distance from the point of maximum intensity to the point of minimum intensity. A number of factors affect unsharpness in the x-ray image. The most important of these are anatomic and patient motion, scatter, focal-spot size, relative geometry of the patient, and the x-ray source. The concept of unsharpness can be applied not only to the x-ray image but also to the final recorded and visible image by incorporating the recording-system image-degrading effects.

In addition to subject contrast and unsharpness, a third aspect of the x-ray image is *quantum mottle* (or *x-ray image noise*). Quantum mottle can be simply defined as the relative flucutation in photon number arriving at the image plane. Figure 1-3 illustrates how quantum mottle can seriously obscure both the

edge character and the depth character of a given image, especially for low subject contrast and small object sizes. Quantum mottle arises from the fact that there are random fluctuations in the x-ray emission spectrum of the x-ray source as well as in the interactions the x-rays undergo within the patient.

To minimize the effect of quantum mottle in the x-ray image, the overall number of photons utilized at the image plane must be increased. This can be accomplished by increases in x-ray tube current, or kilovoltage, or by a decrease in distance from the x-ray source to the image receptor. Attempts to decrease quantum mottle in such a manner, however, may result in increased radiation dose to the patient.

CLASSICAL RADIOGRAPHY

In classical radiography, one attempts to record directly the x-ray intensity profiles in the form of a density distribution on a film. This process, though simple and direct, forms the major limitation for classical radiography. The reason for this limitation is clear when one considers the fact that the patient is made up of a complex distribution of different tissues and structures. Any particular x-ray intensity profile emerging from the patient is thus the compounded sum of the attenuation which oc-

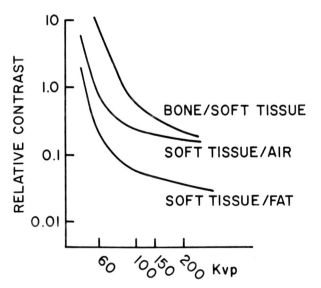

Figure 1-2 Plot of subject contrast between typical tissues as a function of energy. Note how subject contrast diminishes with increasing energy and with increasing similarity in tissue densities. (Adapted from Meredith and Massey 1972.)

curred in the patient along a particular ray-path (the superimposition effect). Under these conditions contour can interfere with contour and shadow with shadow. What will finally be most prominent in the recorded image is that anatomic structure with the greatest absorption. Thus lesions can be ''lost'' behind the ribs or the heart shadow or, in the skull, behind the fossa as well as along the base of the calvarium. In practice, this information loss is compensated for in part by obtaining two views perpendicular to each other, such as anterior-posterior and lateral views, or in obtaining oblique views.

Other limitations in classical radiography include the presence of scatter and the use of nonlinear receptors. Scatter is a major source of image degradation; hence scatter-eliminating grids are generally used. It is true that the use of high-ratio grids reduces scatter as much as 95 to 98 percent, depending on patient thickness and grid ratio. However, it is also true that the difference in subject contrast between such structures as gray matter and white matter is less than 1 percent. As a result, even a small percentage of scatter can obscure visualization of subtle tissue differences.

In the case of nonlinear receptors, the basic problem is the fact that at low subject- or tissue-contrast different structures may have densities falling in the nonlinear response region of the receptor. These nonlinear regions yield less film contrast. This can be seen in the H&D response curve and the corresponding film contrast curve illustrated in Figure 1-4. Here, film contrast is merely the slope of the H&D response curve and determines the actual density differences seen on the film. Note that the point of maximum film contrast occurs at about the middle of the linear region. This means that slight exposure or x-ray intensity differences at this level of the H&D curve result in the greatest displayed density differences. Film contrast progressively falls toward both the high-density and low-density sides of the linear region. Final displayed density difference is referred to as *image, radiographic,* or *broad-area contrast.*

Figure 1-4 illustrates these ideas graphically. Here a given slight exposure difference along *B* is finally displayed with a density difference of ΔB. If expo-

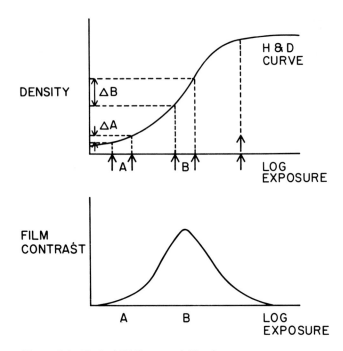

Figure 1-4 Typical H&D curve plotting log exposure versus resulting optical density. Nonlinearity of this curve results in a variable film contrast as seen in the lower figure where the film contrast at any point of the curve is plotted as merely the slope of the H&D curve at each point. Slight differences in exposure along *B* lying on the linear portion of the H&D curve are displayed with the greatest difference in densities or image contrast (ΔB) and thus are better visualized. Exposures at the lower densities (*A*) or at higher densities are visualized at lower image contrast (ΔA).

sures had been such that tissue structures of interest were in the low-density region, i.e., along *A*, then final displayed contrast would be ΔA, and the observed density difference would be less than that obtained along the center of the H&D curve. Radiographically, this can be seen in Figure 1-5*A*, where a bullet is not visible in an approximately correctly exposed chest film, which usually leaves the mediastinum area at relatively low densities and thus low display contrast. Figure 1-5*B* shows the same patient but with exposures sufficiently high so that structures of interest are displayed at higher densities and thus higher display contrast; presence of the bullet then becomes obvious.

One last observation should be made here, that even if the exposure factors (kilovoltage and mil-

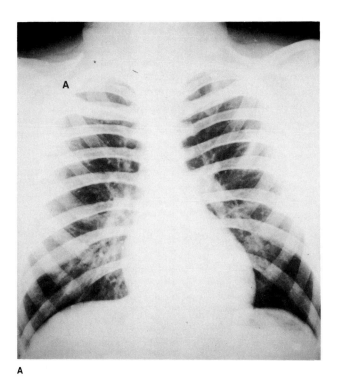

A

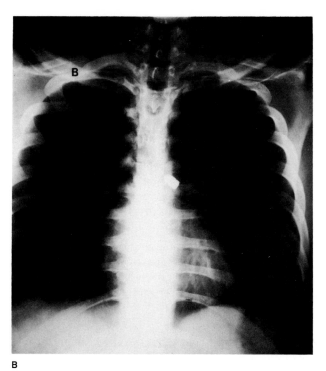

B

Figure 1-5 Example of loss of important image details in classical radiography as a function of density on the film. **A.** Correctly exposed chest film leaving heart shadow and mediastinum at low density and thus low image contrast. **B.** Bullet obviously present when film is exposed to higher density levels where image contrast is higher.

liamperage) are selected optimally for a given tissue or subject contrast, one may still be limited by a relatively small final display contrast. In CT scanning, under computer control one can increase and optimize the display contrast, utilizing the full black-and-white capability of modern cathode ray tube (CRT) monitors. This is referred to as *windowing*. For instance, exposures along *B* in Figure 1-4, rather than being displayed with display contrast ΔB, can be windowed in such a way that one can arbitrarily assign them any desired gray-scale values, including the full range of white to black. This important feature is discussed further in a subsequent section.

The following limiting factors of classical radiography as seen in this section can then be summarized:

1. Superimposition of three-dimensional informa-
tion onto two dimensions causes the loss of low-tissue-contrast anatomic structures.
2. Presence of scatter obscures low-tissue-contrast anatomic structures.
3. Presence of nonlinear film receptors limits display contrast at high and low densities, as well as the fact that display contrast is not adjustable on film.

CLASSICAL TOMOGRAPHY

Classical tomography was formulated in an attempt to minimize the problem of the superimposition of three-dimensional information onto two dimensions. It is based on moving the x-ray source and film cassette relative to each other in such a way that the recorded images of anatomic structures within the patient are blurred. However, one anatomic layer (referred to as the *focal, fulcrum,* or *pivot plane*) within the patient remains stationary relative to the film and is recorded unblurred. Thus the third dimension (patient thickness, or depth) is removed, and presumably only the specified or pivot layer is recorded at full contrast and sharpness. It is clear, however, that the scatter problem is still present, as well as the limitations of nonlinear film and screen systems.

Classical tomography has been reviewed in depth (Littleton 1976), and the reader is referred to a wealth of literature already available. What must be emphasized here is that tomography has certain inherent limitations which result in less than optimal information acquisition. These limitations can be summarized as follows:

1. There is incomplete tomographic blurring of the nonfocused planes. This means that obscuring anatomy is never completely and totally removed. The degree of blurring depends on distance from the focal plane. Therefore, structures near the focal plane affect the image to a greater extent than structures far from the focal plane.
2. Some blur occurs within the focal plane itself, obscuring the anatomy one desires to visualize, since theoretically only an infinitesimally thin plane is truly in focus. This may be overcome in part by scanning over wide-arc angles (thin-section tomography). Finally, some blur also may occur within the focal plane because of mechanical vibration of the moving apparatus.
3. Tomographic blur is dependent on the direction of motion relative to the shape of the anatomy to be blurred. For example, linear tomography does not blur structures whose boundaries are parallel to the direction of arc motion; rather, only structures whose margins are at an angle to the arc motion are blurred.
4. Even though unwanted structures are blurred, they contribute fog background density to the film, which lowers the relative contrast of the structures within the pivot plane.

COMPUTED TOMOGRAPHY

We now come to computed tomography (CT). CT has in great measure overcome the various limitations of both classical radiography and classical tomography. This has been accomplished by

1. Scanning only a thin, well-defined volume of interest, which serves to minimize the superimposition effect
2. Minimizing scatter by collimating down to relatively thin volumes
3. Using linear detectors with computerized windowing functions

The final success of the diagnostic task hinges on how well the image displays or conveys diagnostic information on the distribution of anatomic structures within the patient. In classical radiography the emerging x-ray beam is recorded directly, with an intensifying screen/film combination. The emerging beam, however, represents the total attenuation which occurred within the patient cross section, and as discussed previously the superimposition effect is present. Ideally, one would like to have displayed a point-by-point characterization of the anatomical cross section under study. The characterization presently most useful is that of x-ray attenuation in tissue. Recently a host of other characterizations and different radiation types have been proposed and studied with varying degrees of success. These include the atomic number and electron density (Phelps 1975; Rutherford 1976; Latchaw 1978), nuclear magnetic resonance properties (Hinshaw 1979; Moore 1980; Holland 1980; Partain 1980), ultrasound acoustic impedance (Carson 1977; Kak 1979), microwaves (Kak 1979; Maini 1980), neutrons (Koeppe 1981), protons (Cormack 1976), and isotopic emission (Emission Computed Tomography I, 1980; Emission Computed Tomography II, 1981). CT reconstructions based on fluoroscopic techniques have also been developed (Baily 1976; Kak 1977).

The computed tomography approach consists in isolating a specific planar volume within the patient. This plane, or slice, has a thickness z as seen in

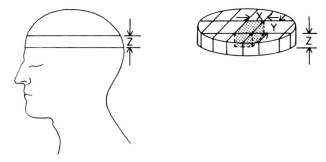

Figure 1-6 Cross-sectional slice across patient—the expanded view showing arrangement of pixels (or picture elements) of dimensions *x* by *y* in a grid array. Volume element (or voxel) is formed in a third dimension due to the finite slice thickness.

Figure 1-6. The x-ray beam to be utilized passes through only this volume; thus superimposition and scatter effects are greatly minimized but not totally eliminated. Final characterization of tissues within the scanned volume will be expressed and displayed for each element area given by *x* and *y* as seen in Figure 1-6. This element area is referred to as a *pixel* (*pi*cture *el*ement). The volume formed by virtue of the slice having some thickness *z* is referred to as a *voxel* (*vo*lume *el*ement). In practice, the whole patient part is arbitrarily broken down into a matrix array of such pixels. The pioneer EMI Mark I unit consisted of an 80 × 80 array in which each pixel corresponded to a 3 mm × 3 mm area within the patient and had a slice thickness of 13 mm. Matrix sizes of modern units are 256 × 256, 512 × 512, or even higher. Pixel sizes now correspond to 1 mm by 1 mm or an even smaller area within the patient. Different CT units have different pixel configurations. In most cases, however, the critical parameter is not the number of pixels but rather the area and volume they correspond to within the patient.

Attenuation Coefficients and Algorithms

The tissue type within each pixel is characterized by the tissue's property of x-ray attenuation, which is defined simply as the removal of x-ray photons from the beam. This removal can be accomplished either by absorption (energy deposited at or near the site of photon interaction) or scatter events (energy removed from the site of photon interaction). Tissues in general have different attenuation properties, depending on their atomic number and physical density and the incident photon energy. One can describe the attenutation of a material in terms of the *attenuation coefficient*, usually symbolized by the Greek letter μ and having units of cm^{-1}. The attenuation coefficient is quite familiar to radiological scientists and with the advent of CT scanning has taken on special importance to the clinical radiologist. Table 1-1 lists typical biological tissues of interest and their corresponding attenuation coefficients. Also shown is their representation on an arbitrary scale on which bone is specified as +1000, air as −1000, and water as zero. This scale is now usually referred to as the Hounsfield scale in honor of the inventor of computed tomography, Godfrey N. Hounsfield (1972). Formerly these numbers were referred to as EMI and Delta numbers by the early CT manufacturers. More commonly they are now simply referred to as *CT numbers*. (For extensive tabulation of attenuation coefficients and CT numbers, see Phelps 1975*b*, Rao 1975, and McCullough 1975.)

The decision to characterize tissue types by Hounsfield numbers and to specify an array of pixels within the patient still leaves the problem of actually determining the value of the CT number for each pixel within that patient. Figure 1-7 shows a

Table 1-1 Attenuation Coefficient and CT No. for Biological Tissues at 60 keV

Tissue	Attenuation coefficient μ (cm^{-1})	CT number
Bone	0.400	+1000
Blood	0.215	+100 (approx.)
Brain matter	0.210	+30 (approx.)
CSF	0.207	+5 (approx.)
Water	0.203	0
Fat	0.185	−100 (approx.)
Air	0.0002	−1000

Source: Adapted from Phelps et al. 1975*b*.

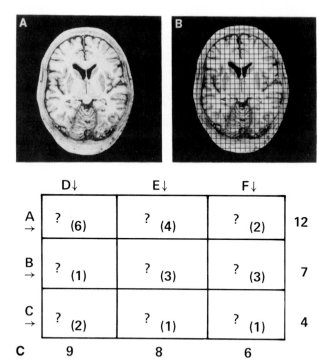

Figure 1-7   A Cross-sectional slice of brain showing structures to be imaged. **B.** Grid array of pixels superimposed over brain slice. The task in CT scanning is to determine tissue type within each pixel. **C.** As an example of how pixel values are determined, here is an unknown 3 × 3 array of pixels. Each pixel has some number value. Even though the interior values are unknown, the total exterior sums along the horizontal paths A, B, and C and vertical paths D, E, and F as well as along various angles can be determined (transmission values when using x-rays). Mathematical techniques (algorithms) are available to reconstruct the true interior values from this type of exterior data even for a very large number of pixels. (Solutions to pixel values are shown in parentheses.)

simplified 3 × 3 matrix array containing nine pixels, each having specific but unknown values of attenuation. The task is to determine the attenuation for each pixel. If x-rays are passed through ray-path *A*, a total attenuation corresponding to, for instance, 12 units is determined. This value is referred to as a *ray sum* and represents the total attenuation occurring from the sum of the attenuation in all the pixels along that ray. Likewise, ray-paths *B* and *C* yield totals of 7 and 4, respectively. The process is repeated from another angle perpendicular to the first (ray-paths *D, E,* and *F*), and ray sums of 9, 8, and 6 are found. Now the task is to assign or reconstruct values for each pixel which will conform

with ray sums experimentally found from the two angles used. One may, in fact, "play" with the numbers and finally arrive at the correct distribution, such as that indicated in Figure 1-6. In practice ray sums also have to be taken at various angles for accuracy.

In the case of matrix arrays which are, for instance, 512 × 512 in extent, one must determine ray scans over many different angles (from 180° to 360°), and the amount of data to be collected is formidable—so much so that a computer is necessary to keep track of the data and to perform the actual calculations necessary for a successful reconstruction. The model, or calculation sheme used for reconstruction, is referred to as an *algorithm*. The most popular algorithm for commercial scanners is the filtered back-projection algorithm. In this algorithm the ray sum for each row of pixels, for a first approximation, is assigned to each pixel along that row (this is called *back projection*). As each new set of data corresponding to a new angle of scan is determined, it is also back-projected and averaged into each pixel. Such a procedure, though not directly intuitive, does in fact, as seen in Figure 1-8, result in a successful image reconstruction. Note in Figure 1-8 that back projection is accomplished by linearly smearing (back-projecting) the image for a number of different angles, and the sum, or superimposition, of all the

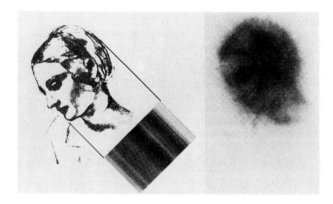

Figure 1-8   Example of back-projection technique using a pictorial view of a face. The value of the density along each line is given by the average along each line. In this particular case the average is obtained via a smearing motion (equivalent to back projection). When all such projections are summed, the original face is, surprisingly enough, reconstructed. (After Gordon 1975.)

views represents a reconstruction of the original image.

For CT images it is the computer which processes the ray sums and accomplishes the necessary back projections. In practice, before back projection is implemented, each intensity profile is modified or filtered to minimize starlike artifacts caused by use of a finite set of angular images made to correspond to a square pixel. A number of *filter functions* are incorporated in the algorithms which have been used or proposed, and the reader is referred to various reviews (Gordon 1974; Brooks 1975). These filter functions, which are sometimes called *kernels,* can also incorporate varying degrees of *smoothing.* Smoothing may sometimes be of value when noise limits the detail visible in the image (Joseph 1978*a*). Many CT units have a number of filter functions available, and the user should be aware of possible improvements in the images and the possibility of decreasing patient dose with their use. It should, however, also be realized that the smoothing operation degrades image resolution and thus limits the smallest sizes that can be displayed. It should be considered only as a noise suppressant in imaging relatively large structures.

Data-Collection Geometry

It is worth repeating that the reconstruction process involves the collection of x-ray transmission values outside the patient. These transmission values are an index of how much the radiation was attenuated in passage through the patient. The collection of such data from a number of different angles around the patient is used to calculate the attenuation occurring at each picture element within the patient. Various data-collection schemes have been employed for the acquisition of x-ray transmission data. All schemes involve some geometrical pattern of scanning around the patient coupled with use of a suitable radiation detector. The signal from the radiation detector is digitized by the use of an analog-to-digital (A/D) converter and passed onto the computer for processing. After the reconstruction is completed, the results are displayed on a video monitor. The images can be preserved for long-term storage either on discs or on magnetic tape. The overall layout is illustrated in Figure 1-9.

Translate/Rotate Geometry

The first successful clinical CT scanner was based on a translate/rotate gantry geometry. In this type of system the x-ray beam is collimated down to the desired slice thickness and to a narrow slit. The resulting x-ray pattern is referred to as a *pencil beam.* The pencil beam is then passed through the patient and is incident on a radiation detector, as seen in Figure 1-10. The quantity of radiation arriving at the detector for each ray-path will depend on the total

Figure 1-9 Block diagram of a typical CT system. After x-rays emerge from the patient they are detected, amplified, and digitized with an analog-to-digital (A/D) converter. After computer processing, the reconstruction results are assigned a gray scale and displayed on a CRT video monitor from which hard-copy views may be obtained. Since CRTs are analog devices the image data must be converted from digital form back to analog form. CT number data can also be outputted to a line printer for quantitative analysis. Normally a tape or disc system is also used for storage of data for later redisplay and/or image manipulation.

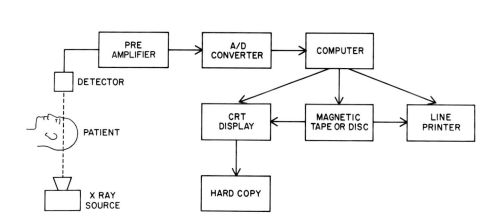

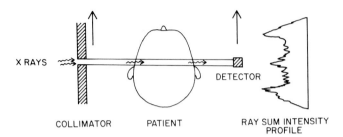

X RAYS

COLLIMATOR   PATIENT   DETECTOR   RAY SUM INTENSITY PROFILE

Figure 1-10 First-generation type CT configuration. A pencil beam is formed with a collimator and passed through the patient at a particular angle onto a detector traversing the patient along with the x-ray pencil beam. A ray sum intensity profile is thus detected and channeled to the computer for processing. The process is repeated at 1° intervals for 180°.

attenuation which occurred along the ray-path for each volume element (voxel) traversed.

In order to determine the ray-attenuation sums for each row of voxels, the pencil beam is made to linearly scan, or translate, across the patient. During the translate motion the detector, being rigidly connected to the x-ray tube, moves in such a manner that it always intercepts the x-ray pencil beam. The signals detected during the translation motion form a profile representing the ray sums along all voxel rows.

To determine the ray-sum profiles at different angles, the unit must sequentially rotate and perform a translation movement across the patient for each angle of rotation. The original EMI Mark I system rotated a total of 180° one degree at a time (the configuration usually referred to as *first-generation geometry*). These movements required a total of 5½ to 6 minutes to complete. Unfortunately, patient motion and resulting mismatch between patient position and pixel position resulted in severe image streaks. To reduce overall patient examination time, two detectors were placed side by side in the Z (or slice thickness) directions and the x-ray beam made wide enough to include both these detectors. This had the effect of providing two image slices simultaneously and shortening the overall time needed to obtain all the slices desired, as well as minimizing patient motion between slices.

Individual slice scan times may be reduced sig-

nificantly by providing for multiple pencil beams, with each beam directed at its own detector. This has the effect of obtaining ray sums from different angles on one translation (the configuration referred to as *second-generation geometry*). This is illustrated in Figure 1-11 for a three-pencil-beam system. Here the pencil beams are configured to be at a 1° angle to one another. Consequently, during one translation data are collected for three different angles, and the unit can be rotated 3° instead of 1° as for a single-pencil-beam configuration. Scan times can thus be reduced approximately three times, since the unit need complete only one-third the number of rotations and translations. (Sixty rotations at 3° increments will still provide for 180° around the patient and 180 ray-sum profiles.) Additionally, one may provide for a second bank of detectors identical to the first, to detect and process two slices simultaneously. To further reduce scan times one may incorporate even more pencil beams, each with its own detector. Thus 10 beams will require 10 detectors and only 18 rotations, 20 beams will require 9 rotations, etc. In fact, given sufficient beams and detectors, scan times can be effectively reduced to a few seconds. In this latter case, since scan times are relatively short, the second bank of detectors may be eliminated, for a considerable cost saving.

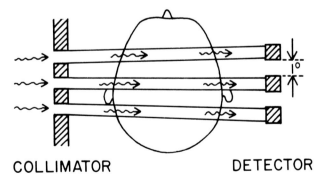

COLLIMATOR   DETECTOR

Figure 1-11 Configuration for second-generation gantry systems. A series of pencil beams pass through the patient at an angle, for instance, of 1° to one another. To obtain 180° of information the number of translations across the patient is then reduced by 180/*N* where *N* is the number of detectors. When possible another row of detectors is added to obtain a second slice simultaneously with the first slice.

Rotate-Only Geometry

The logical extension of using more and more pencil beams is to open up the x-ray beam in the transverse plane to produce a fan beam large enough to encompass the entire patient. This is the so-called *third-generation geometry.* This fan beam is incident on a whole array of detectors, which move along with the fan, as in Figure 1-12. In this process one eliminates entirely the time-consuming translation motion. Note that not only must detectors number at least 180 (one for each of the 180° of view), but actually one needs even more detectors, since the array must be large enough to include a wide range of patient diameters. It is also necessary to include additional detectors to serve as monitoring chambers to correct for any variations in x-ray output. Modern third-generation units use from 400 to over 600 detectors, with scan times of 2 to 10 seconds. At these scanning times it is not necessary to have a second array of detectors for simultaneous two-plane scanning, as was common with single-pencil and some multiple-pencil systems. This reduces the cost and complexity of the equipment considerably.

One problem, however, with third-generation configuration is related to the detector calibration problem. The reconstruction process requires extremely high precision, and slight variations (even less than 1 percent) in x-ray output or in detector electronics must be corrected for. Each individual detector must then be calibrated to assure constancy and uniformity of response as compared to adjacent detectors. In first- and second-generation systems, because of the translation motion, the detectors were out from behind the patient and were directly exposed through air to the x-ray beam at the extreme ends of their travel during each scan motion. They could thus be easily calibrated in air before traversing the patient. Third-generation systems preclude the possibility of frequent calibrations, in that detectors are always behind the patient and cannot be calibrated between individual scans. The result is the formation of artifactual ring structures, each ring corresponding to a drift in one or more detectors, as seen in Figure 1-13. Ring artifacts can be minimized with certain algorithm corrections; however, stability of detector system as well as uniformity of detector response are crucial. In fact, detector drifts of less than 1 percent can cause visible artifacts (Shepp 1977).

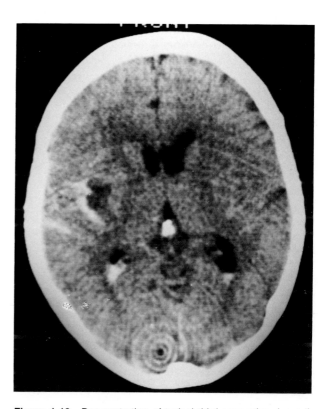

Figure 1-13 Demonstration of typical third-generation ring artifacts. These ring structures are caused by slight detector calibration drifts (typically less than 1 percent).

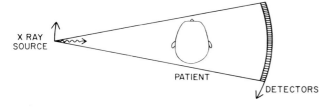

Figure 1-12 Configuration for a third-generation gantry system. Here an entire fan of x-rays is passed through the patient onto the array of detectors. Since all portions of the patient are viewed, translation motion across the patient is entirely eliminated.

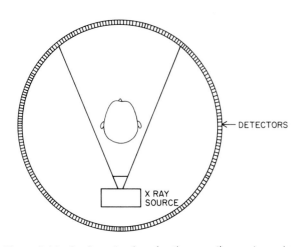

Figure 1-14   Configuration for a fourth-generation gantry system. Here detectors are fixed around the entire gantry and the x-ray tube rotates around the patient.

One possible method of avoiding detector-calibration problems, as found in third-generation configurations, is to use a ring of detectors fixed around the entire periphery of the gantry (*fourth-generation geometry*). This configuration is seen in Figures 1-14

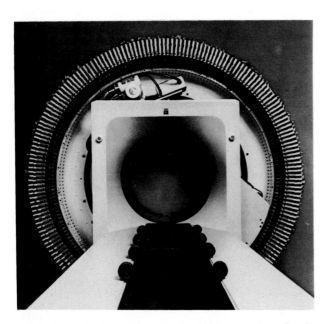

Figure 1-15   Photograph of detector configuration for a fourth-generation gantry system.

and 1-15. In such an arrangement the x-ray beam rotates around the patient and always radiates a freshly calibrated detector. The added complexity and cost of fixing detectors around the entire gantry periphery and the associated electronics are obvious. Recently, some modern CT designs have reverted back to third-generation configurations, especially in view of the fact that algorithms to minimize ring-artifact formation have been greatly improved. Variations on the fourth-generation configuration include putting the x-ray tube outside the detector array. This allows the use of a smaller detector ring as well as more closely packed detectors. In this configuration (which was pioneered by the EMI Corporation), provision is made for moving the detector ring out of the direct x-ray beam path—a motion called by the manufacturer *nutation*. Another variation, put forward by the Artronics Corporation (no longer in business), is the so-called "hula hoop" gantry. Here tube and detectors move around the patient in hula hoop fashion so that the x-ray beam is effectively parallel through the patient, allowing for more effective collimation. The reader is referred to a number of review papers for further discussion on geometries and CT scanning in general (Gordon 1975; Ter-Pogossian 1977; Brooks 1976b; Kak 1979).

ELECTRON SCAN GEOMETRY (CINE CT)

One gantry configuration which is being called by some a fifth-generation system consists of a stationary gantry/detector system with a moving electron beam sweeping across an extended anode target arranged semicircularly around the patient (Boyd 1982; Lipton 1985). In this approach there are actually multiple target layers so that electrons sequentially sweeping across each result in the formation of eight successive fan beams of x-rays. The result of all this is that one can acquire up to eight image slices within a very short period of time. This high-speed image acquisition (about 50 milliseconds per image) allows for cine-type scan sequences. Additionally, flow phenomena can also be studied. Though holding promise for neuro work, applications to date of this scanning concept have been limited to cardiac imaging (Brundage 1985; Lipton 1986).

Detectors

Let us now look at the various radiation detector types commonly used in CT scanning. Three general types of detection system have emerged: the scintillation detector/photomultiplier, the scintillation detector/photodiode multiplier, and the pressurized ionization chamber. Each of these is briefly discussed in turn.

Scintillation Detector/Photomultiplier

This type of detector package is most familiar to the clinician in that it is the type commonly used for nuclear medicine scans. It consists of a solid scintillation crystal such as NaI (Tl), which has the property of emitting light when x-ray or gamma photons are incident upon it. This emitted light falls upon a photocathode surface which converts the light to an electronic signal, which in turn is amplified within a photomultiplier. In CT scanning the signal is then digitized and transmitted to the computer for processing. Examples of typical scintillation crystals used in such configurations are seen in Table 1-2. Scintillation crystal/photomultiplier technology is well established and is used extensively in first- and second-generation CT units.

The photomultiplier itself is a configuration of surfaces called *dynodes,* arranged so that each electron emitted from the photocathode falling on such a surface knocks out three to ten electrons. These in turn are accelerated to another dynode surface, where each knocks out another three to ten electrons. This multiplication process continues for nine to ten dynode stages, and electron multiplication by millions is possible. Photomultiplier drift, a function of applied voltage and electronic stability, critically affects the multiplication process. In spite of this, systems of this type are very efficient and made the original CT scanners possible.

Scintillation Crystal/Photodiode Multiplier

There is at present a definite trend toward the use of solid-state photodiode-multiplier scintillation-crystal systems. Here, instead of coupling the emitted scintillation light to a photomultiplier, it is coupled to a silicon photodiode. Advantages include high stability, small size, and possible cost saving.

One solid-state variation on detector packages which is under development is the use of a semiconductor photoconductive crystal which produces an electric current directly when irradiated, without the intermediate step of light production. As for any other CT detector, sensitivity and stability as well as size must be evaluated.

Pressurized Ionization Chambers

One of the requirements for CT detectors is that they be small and capable of being configured very close to one another to provide for full capture of the incident radiation. The ionization chamber approach comes very close to providing these features. Such a chamber consists of one large assembly having very thin walls defining each small collection region as in Figure 1-16. This configuration yields a very high packing density of these small detectors. Additionally, xenon gas is perfused evenly throughout the assembly to assure uniformity of response. Some disadvantages include the fact that xenon gas

Table 1-2   CT Detectors

Detector types	Chemical form
Scintillation crystals + photomultiplier	Sodium iodide NaI (Tl)
	Calcium fluoride CaF_2
	Bismuth germanate $Bi_4Ge_3O_{12}$ (BGO)
Scintillation crystals + photodiode	Cadmium tungstate $CdWO_4$
	Cesium iodide CsI (Na)
Ionization chamber	Xenon (under pressure)

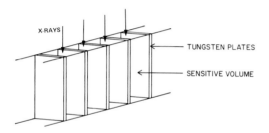

Figure 1-16 Close-up view of adjacent plates within a pressurized xenon gas detector. The small size of these detectors allows for very small data sampling distances; also, there is minimal information loss between detector cells (high capture ratio).

does not provide for as much absorption efficiency as solid state detectors. To compensate for these losses, ionization chambers are pressurized at 10 to 30 atm (providing more gas molecules for absorbing the x-ray beam) and are constructed with relatively great depths (providing greater path length for x-ray photons to be absorbed). Some attenuation loss is experienced within the relatively thick face plate needed to withstand the relatively high xenon gas pressure, and this serves to attenuate the x-ray beam.

Detector Requirements

Detectors, to be effective in CT scanning applications, should have the characteristics listed in Table 1-3. The need for *high absorption efficiency* is self-evident. This provides for maximum utilization of the photons incident on the face of the detector. Here the important factors are the physical density, atomic number, size, and thickness of the detector. *Conversion efficiency* relates to the ability of the detector to convert the absorbed x-ray energy to a usable

Table 1-3   Favorable Detector Characteristics

High absorption efficiency
High conversion efficiency
High capture efficiency
Good temporal response (little afterglow)
Wide dynamic range
High reproducibility and stability

electronic signal. *Capture efficiency* means that the size of the detector and the distance to adjacent detectors should be such that as many as possible of the photons passing through the patient are incident on (or captured by) the detector face. The total detector efficiency is merely the running product of these three individual efficiencies. Total detector efficiency is also referred to as "dose efficiency." Typical dose efficiencies fall between 50 and 60 percent. The *temporal response* of a detector should be as fast as possible in that in a scanning configuration each detector sees the radiation for a relatively short time measured in milliseconds. Within this time, the signal must be processed and the detector be ready for the next measurement. It is clear that the performance of a unit would be severely degraded if the detector had a significantly delayed response, sometimes referred to as *phosphorescence* or *afterglow*. With significant afterglow, correlation between the specific voxel the x-ray beam is traversing and the signal received by the computer would be lost. Afterglow would be especially limiting for fast, dynamic scanning. Because of the relatively poor temporal response of NaI (TI) and CaF_2, these crystals are no longer used in modern scanners. *Wide dynamic range* refers to the ability of the detector to respond linearly to a wide range of x-ray intensities. When scanning patients the x-ray beam is sometimes passing through air having negligible attenuation and consequently forming a very intense signal at the detector and may then traverse a thick patient or body part having a high beam attenuation. The x-ray signal formed at the detector would then be very low. Ideally a detector should respond linearly between these two extremes; a dynamic range of 10,000 to 1 should be minimal. Finally, *high reproducibility and stability* are required to avoid drift and the resultant detector fluctuation or noise.

CT Image Display and Recording

What the computer understands to be an image consists merely of an array of CT numbers, one number corresponding to each pixel. In order for the viewer to see a "real" image, this array of numbers must be displayed on a suitable medium such as a video monitor. Three considerations must be taken into account for the proper display and storage of CT images:

1. Adjustment of the video monitor display characteristics of brightness and display contrast, i.e., the video gray scale
2. Selection of settings (center and window) to optimize the display of anatomic tissues of interest within the given video gray scale
3. Recording of the image for long-term storage

Video Gray Scale

Every video device has its own gray scale. The gray scale refers to the manner in which the device goes from its darkest to its brightest illumination. The gray scale usually is displayed as a graded series of steps, that at one end representing the darkest and that at the other end the brightest illumination. Steps in between, therefore, have intermediate values of gray, and the rapidity with which they go from light to dark is the video monitor contrast. Rather than steps, some units have a continuous illumination strip. In any case the result is the same, namely, that one can observe the actual display brightness and contrast of the monitor. Adjustments can be made exactly as one controls monitor display characteristics during image-intensified fluoroscopy, ultrasound video, or home video viewing. These settings are usually chosen initially and remain fixed thereafter. The basis for actual settings varies for each individual viewer. Usually, however, the final gray scale should display both the very darkest and the very brightest that the monitor can display, as well as a relatively uniform gradation of gray between these two extremes. Most installations have a monitor for direct viewing and a monitor to obtain hard-copy films. In the latter case, the gray scale should be adjusted to match the needs of the film which will be used to record the image. Selection of film, as well as the monitor brightness and contrast used to record the film, are not trivial matters, and care must be taken to assure the best possible film image (Schwenker 1979).

Variations in window and center settings reported between CT sites are usually due in part to differences in initial gray-scale settings and differences in video monitor display characteristics.

Center and Window Settings

One of the biggest differences between radiographic film viewing and CT viewing is the ability in the latter to *window* the anatomic tissues of interest. By this is meant that one can optimize the viewing of particular tissues of interest by assigning to them the full range of blacks and whites available on the CRT monitor. For example, the center setting assigns the video mid-gray value to the CT number (or tissue) desired; the window setting defines the CT number range which will occupy the scale from black to white. To illustrate, consider a head CT scan viewed at a center of $+50$ and a window of 200 CT units. The $+50$ corresponds to the approximate CT number of gray and white matter, and it is these tissues that will be displayed with the mid-gray illumination. A window of 200 CT units implies that the range will be from $+150$ (100 above 50) to -50 (100 below 50). Consequently all tissues having CT numbers of 150 or above will be displayed as white, while all tissues at -50 and below will be displayed as black. On these settings, bone calcifications and blood pools will appear light and ventricular volumes will appear darker. The above settings may be ideal for a head scan, but different settings are needed for body scanning, since body scanning involves a greater range of tissue types, and a greater window must be selected.

The power of the windowing function will be appreciated when it is recalled that in film radiography one must accept whatever exposure was made and is limited to what is seen on the film. Film, however, is nonlinear and thus results in different image contrast, depending on the density. Additionally, films may be underexposed or overexposed. In either case, as discussed previously, information is lost at both the low- and high-density regions of the film. Figure 1-17 illustrates the role of windowing using linear detectors. If the full tissue range of -1000 to $+1000$ is displayed, note that the

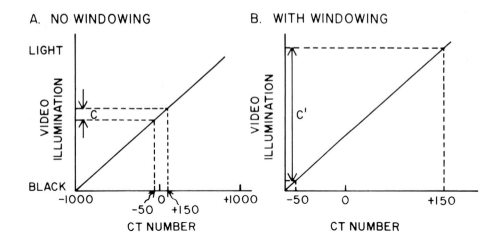

A. NO WINDOWING

LIGHT

VIDEO ILLUMINATION

C

BLACK

-1000   -50 +150   +1000

CT NUMBER

B. WITH WINDOWING

VIDEO ILLUMINATION

C'

-50   0   +150

CT NUMBER

Figure 1-17 On a scale of −1000 to +1000, if no windowing is available, a given CT number difference such as −50 to +150 is displayed with only a limited range of gray values (low image contrast *C*). With windowing invoked, the same CT number range can be displayed with up to the maximum video range from white to black (high image contrast *C*); thus, −50 can be assigned full dark and +150 is assigned full light.

particular tissues of interest in the previous example (−50 to +150) would be limited to a relatively small range of grays, and visualization would be poor. However, with windowing as in Figure 1-17, the full black-and-white range is assigned between the −50 and +150 CT values, and visualization of these particular tissues is optimum in that the greatest illumination difference results.

Long-Term Storage Media

It has always been necessary to record the final image for patient records and subsequent comparisons and for referring physicians. Such recording can be done on film as for classical radiography. However, it is advantageous to record the actual computer image, consisting of all the pixel values, since pixel values, if available, can allow for subsequent windowing and redisplay and for computer manipulations such as magnification, CT number, or tissue identification and various image-enhancement routines. Thus magnetic tape and magnetic disc systems are usually incorporated into the basic CT instrumentation. In fact, the basic image-recording configuration of a clinical scanner may consist of some or all of the items listed in Table 1-4.

FILM   Film continues to be the most popular and economic long-term storage medium. It should be realized that the films used in CT imaging are quite

different from the films used in radiography, inasmuch as one is recording an image off a video monitor. Consequently, the film usually consists of a single emulsion sensitive to the light-emission spectrum of the video-screen phosphor. Additionally, these nonscreen films tend to be linear. To facilitate film recording, multi-image-format cameras have been developed, consisting of a self-enclosed video monitor with independent access to the computer pixel image information. The arrangement is such that the camera exposes the film to the particular size format desired. For instance, both four views (or image slices) on an 8 × 10 film and nine views on a 14 × 17 film are quite popular.

Table 1-4   Storage Media

Medium	Pixels recoverable?	Comments
Polaroid film	No	Relatively expensive; relatively poor contrast scale
Film	No	Convenient, various sizes available
Magnetic tape	Yes	Access time long, good for long-term storage
Floppy disc	Yes	Convenient size and format; relatively expensive
Magnetic discs	Yes	Expensive but fast

Polaroid film originally had three drawbacks: limited film contrast range, expense, and the need for mounting for permanent records. To a lesser extent there was also the nuisance of paper wrappers, the wait for development, and the need for coating. Newer Polaroid film emulsions available have extended film contrast range and do not need coating. This form of image recording, however, will probably still remain limited to relatively low patient-volume sites where the capital cost of multi-image cameras or tape recorders is a factor and sites where rapid film processing equipment is not available.

MAGNETIC TAPE   Magnetic tape recording of computer outputs is a well-established technology. Pixel values, as well as patient identification data, can be readily recorded in relatively short times (a few seconds). This means that images can be redisplayed at any subsequent time, and different computer manipulations of the images, including windowing, are possible. Additionally, the fidelity of the images is excellent. A number of drawbacks exist, however. For example, storage space is limited to between 100 and 300 images per tape, depending on the number of pixels on the image. A 256×256 pixel array demands 4 times less tape space than a 512×512 pixel array. A few hundred images, in the case of a busy site, means that only one or two days' worth of patient images may be stored on one tape. In practice, this is a severe limitation, since accessing patient images on different tapes requires an inordinate amount of time, because of the need for loading and reloading tapes, as well as the relatively slow search times characteristic of magnetic tape systems. Finally, the number of tapes accumulated and the required floor storage space have dictated the recycling of tapes. Thus it is not uncommon to find tapes covering only 6 to 12 months, or even less, at a particular site.

DISC-BASED SYSTEMS   Two basic approaches to disc imaging have evolved. One approach uses so-called ''floppy'' discs. These discs are relatively small and flexible. In many cases a full patient examination or more can be recorded on one disc and can be conveniently transported to another room or site for image review at an independent viewing station. Disc search time is essentially negligible. However, the cost of each disc is such that many sites rely on magnetic tape recording for long-term storage and use floppy discs only for recent patients or for particularly interesting cases.

Another disc-based system consists of a bank of large discs capable of storing thousands of images. These are random-access devices, so that stepping through every image in the file to find the required one is not necessary and search and access times are minimal. Viewing at remote consoles is possible only via direct data-link connection to the computer. The overall costs of such a system are relatively high. Every CT scanner, however, is outfitted with discs for short-term storage of image data.

Artifacts in CT Scanning

CT scanning, like any imaging modality, has artifacts unique to it. Many artifacts have multiple causes, and their description requires rigorous mathematical techniques. Here we present a number of the more significant artifacts that the clinician should be aware of. Artifacts can manifest themselves either visibly in the form of streaks or quantitatively in the form of inaccurate CT numbers.

Streaks arise in general because there is an inconsistency in a particular ray-path through the patient. This inconsistency can be due either to an error along the ray or to inconsistencies between rays. Table 1-5 summarizes the various sources of artifacts. Classification of artifacts has been troublesome (Joseph 1981). For our purposes here we have classified artifacts according to what is happening to the data. Each of the artifacts listed in Table 1-5 is discussed in turn.

Data Formation

In this section we are concerned with how data are formed as the x-rays pass through the patient. As previously discussed, the transmitted x-ray beam detected in CT scanning is an index of the degree of attenuation which has occurred as the beam passed

Table 1-5   Sources of CT Artifacts

Source area	Cause
Data formation	Patient motion
	Polychromatic effects
	Equipment misalignment
	Faulty x-ray source
Data acquisition	Slice geometry
	Profile sampling
	Angular sampling
Data measurement	Detector imbalance
	Detector nonlinearity
	Scatter collimation
Data processing	Algorithm effects

through the patient. Reference to Figure 1-6 shows that the patient contour is arbitrarily divided up into pixels. To accomplish the CT scan process, ray-paths along different angles around the patient are obtained. Thus data are collected for the attenuation at each point in the field from different angles. If such ray-path data are inconsistent—that is, if the pixel does not contribute the same attenuation regardless of the particular angle of view—then streaks result. The most familiar example of data inconsistency is that caused by patient motion.

PATIENT MOTION   Motion has plagued CT scanning from the beginning (Alfidi 1976). The original CT scan units took up to 6 minutes of scan time. The inordinate amount of time allowed for considerable patient motion during the course of the examination. When such motion occurs during the scanning process, the computer has no means of keeping track of where the pixels are in space and which ray-path sums belong to which row and column. This inconsistency results in severe streaking and is especially aggravated by the presence of high-density structures. In early CT units, the relatively long scanning time necessary was so limiting that it provided the impetus to develop faster and faster scanners. Presently, modern scanners can routinely perform scans in less than 5 to 10 seconds.

It should be clear that motion not only introduces artifactual streaks but, as in classical radiography, may cause both a loss of *spatial resolution* (the ability to visualize fine spatial detail) and a loss of *tissue resolution* (the ability to visualize small differences in tissue densities), also called *density resolution*. These losses are usually minimal as compared to the presence of streaks. To minimize motion artifacts one may, in addition to scanning faster, provide for immobilization of the patient. Another approach used in earlier scanners involves overscanning. Here the patient was typically scanned 40° to 60° beyond the normal 180° or 360°, the rationale being that one is then collecting repeat, or redundant, views. For instance, if the patient has moved between the beginning of the scan and the end, there will be a discrepancy between the data collected on the 0° pass and the 180° pass. If the patient has not moved during the scan, these two views should be identical; any difference detected is entirely due to patient motion. Under computer control these differences can be averaged (or feathered) out. One obvious drawback to overscanning is the fact that scan times are longer, introducing the possibility of further motion artifacts. In spite of this, however, overscanning was shown to be useful in slower scanners.

POLYCHROMATIC EFFECTS   Probably the best-known polychromatic artifact referred to in clinical practice is the beam-hardening artifact. The basis for this artifact is the fact that in the reconstruction process one attempts to assign an attenuation coefficient value to each volume element (voxel) within the patient. However, attenuation coefficients are highly dependent on x-ray beam energy. Photons in x-ray beams do not have a unique energy but rather are polychromatic; that is, they are made up of photons having a wide distribution of energy. As the beam passes through the patient, the lower-energy photons are preferentially absorbed, and we say that the beam becomes harder. (This is similar to the rationale for the use of filters in diagnostic radiology to reduce the patient dose.) Any given voxel within the patient is, however, viewed along different ray-paths for each different angular projection. Consequently, the x-ray beam, having experienced different degrees of beam hardening, will have a different energy as it passes any particular voxel along these different ray-paths (see Fig. 1-18). The overall result will be a general decrease in the CT numbers, since higher energies imply lower attenuation coefficients. This effect is most notable along ray-paths containing thicker and denser bony structures, as along the orbit-base views. The visual result is dark streaks, since higher energies result in the display of CT numbers denoting less dense tissues. The best example of this effect is the interpetrous bone hypodensity streaks seen in Figure 1-19. This particular artifact is also caused in part by the nonlinear partial volume effect (Glover 1980).

Beam hardening also leads to a spillover effect near the interface of bony structures with adjoining softer tissues. This is evident at the edge of the skull and was originally interpreted as the cerebral cortex (Ambrose 1973). Its artifactual nature was demonstrated by Gado and Phelps (1975), and it is now referred to as the *pseudocortex.* The basis for this effect, which is also referred to as *cupping,* is illus-

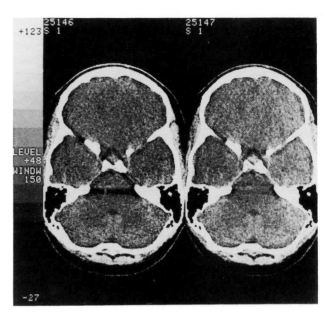

Figure 1-19 *Left:* Interpetrous bone artifact. *Right:* Same view after bone corrections are performed.

trated in Figure 1-18: rays passing through the periphery of a structure suffer less hardening than rays passing through the center of that structure. The central regions thus are displayed as having lower CT numbers and appear darker. A similar effect is seen in the apical artifact discussed in the CT number accuracy section and illustrated in Figure 1-26. The original water-bag systems circumvented many of these problems by providing for an essentially equal path length for all rays in all projections. Another approach to minimize beam-hardening effects is to add filtration to the beam or to add specially shaped compensating attenuators to the beam. These approaches will be discussed further under the section on CT number variations.

Beam hardening has been discussed at length and a number of algorithms have been proposed to correct for the beam-hardening artifact (Brooks 1976a; Duerinckx 1978; McDavid 1977a; Joseph 1978b). Typical CT scanners include within their reconstruction algorithm a so-called water correction based on the linearization of the data collected. However, a more complete correction usually involves off-line proces-

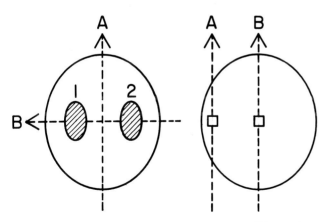

Figure 1-18 Demonstration of beam hardening in CT scanning. *Left:* Interpetrous bone hypodensity artifact. Ray *A* suffers a different degree of beam hardening from Ray *B*, which travels through bony structures 1 and 2. The result is an inconsistency in the CT numbers calculated, and streaks result between the bony structures. *Right:* Cupping artifact. Rays such as *A*, passing through the periphery of a uniform structure, suffer less attenuation than rays such as *B*, passing through the center of that structure. Result is an apparent cupping, or increase in tissue density toward the periphery.

ing which may take from seconds to minutes per image to perform. Algorithms of this kind are referred to as *bone* or *calcium correction algorithms* and, because of the necessity of off-line processing, are often implemented only for specially selected cases.

EQUIPMENT MISALIGNMENT Mechanical misalignment of the x-ray source and radiation detectors may lead to artifactual streak formation. The basic problem is that of isocenter location (Shepp 1977). If an aluminum pin is placed at the isocenter and scanned, its position will be isocentric for all views and projections. If a misalignment is present, an inconsistency results between angular views, and streaks sometimes referred to as "tuning fork" streaks result.

Another misalignment problem may occur for 180° dual-slice scanners. Hounsfield (1977) has described what happens when the central ray of the x-ray beam is not aligned perpendicular to the axis of the patient's head. Under these conditions a bony structure may be included within the collimated x-ray field in the Z direction for the 0° view but excluded from the 180° view. The result is a vertical streak along the edges of the bony object. One practical lesson from this is that when possible one should align the patient in such a way that bony structures fall along the 90° views and not along the 0° and 180° views. The petrous bones, for instance, satisfy this for scanners rotating 180° from the posterior to the anterior hemispheres. However, the eye lens is then exposed to the primary beam, and relatively high radiation dose results (McCullough 1980). Since the appearance of this artifact depends mainly on the 0° and 180° views, overscanning will serve to minimize it.

FAULTY X-RAY SOURCE If the x-ray output varies during the scan process, an obvious inconsistency in data immediately arises, since detectors cannot distinguish between increases or decreases in radiation level due to increases or decreases in x-ray output and those due to increased or decreased absorption along the ray-path. All CT units include reference detectors to detect output variations for the purposes of correcting for such changes. These corrections, however, are for data from a single an-

gular view. If variations are present between angular views, streaks crisscrossing the image field and forming moiré patterns result (Joseph 1981; Stockham 1979). These are assumed to be most likely related to the speed of anode rotation, which is also called *anode wobble*. Other possible x-ray source problems include momentary high-voltage arcing and fluctuations, which may reduce or increase instantaneous x-ray output. Again, such changes, though detected by reference chambers, still result in inconsistencies between angular views, and streaks result.

Data Acquisition

In this section, artifactual effects resulting from the manner in which the data are collected are studied.

SLICE GEOMETRY The thickness of the slice scanned determines a very significant though nonvisible artifact: the partial volume effect. To understand this effect and its significance in practice, remember that the pixel displayed represents a volume in the patient given by both the area size and the slice thickness (the voxel). The voxel representing some finite patient volume may contain more than one tissue type. What happens is that if tissues are relatively similar (small CT number differences), then the total contents of the voxel are in effect linearly averaged. It is this average CT number value which is assigned to the voxel. Figure 1-20 illustrates this effect. For

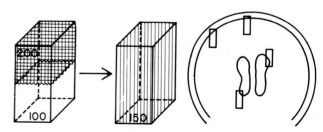

Figure 1-20 *Left:* Example of the partial volume artifact. Here, if a particular voxel contains different tissues, the final computed value will be characterized by some weighted average CT number. If the CT numbers are very different from each other, the summing average process is exponential and therefore nonlinear, and streaks may result. *Right:* Cross-sectional view of voxel positions at various levels within the skull, showing a varying degree of partial-volume averaging for different tissue-structure boundaries.

instance, if half of the pixel is filled with a tissue having a CT number of 100 and the other half with a tissue having a CT number of 200, the average of the two is 150, and this voxel will be displayed as if it were filled with a tissue type of CT number 150 which, in fact, is not present within the voxel.

This effect is significant for relatively small anatomic structure sizes or for tissue volumes which are rapidly changing in size. Examples are the orbital base level and regions near the calvarium. Additionally, vascular structures, blood clots (Lim 1977), and thin flat structures, as well as optic nerve visualization (Salvolini 1978), are subject to the partial volume effect. The result of the partial volume effect is the loss of tissue and spatial resolution and not necessarily streaks. In many instances, however, volume averaging is nonlinear in that tissue types within the voxel have widely different CT numbers. This, in turn, results in large exponential, nonlinear absorption differences. An example of this would be the bony structures of the petrous ridges and the adjacent brain matter. The result is the interpetrous ridge lucency artifact which has been discussed previously. At first this artifact was thought to be entirely due to beam-hardening effects. However, these artifacts were subsequently shown to be partly due to the nonlinear partial volume effect, which in turn is related to the sampling slice thickness (Glover 1980). Thus this artifact can be minimized by diminishing the slice thickness, although it cannot be eliminated entirely unless beam hardness is also corrected for.

The basis for the nonlinear partial volume effect is that the detector response varies nonlinearly with the degree of bony intrusion into any given volume element; that is, the net signal at the detectors depends on the relative amount of soft tissue and bony tissue within the voxel. However, this dependence does not vary linearly, since attenuation in each material is an exponential function. These nonlinearities result in an inconsistency in the data collected as the volume element is viewed from various angles around the patient, and it is this inconsistency that creates the streaks observed. These streaks appear not only across the petrous bones but also from the occipital protuberance and wherever there are

relatively large, abrupt variations in tissue or structure densities. To minimize this artifact, one merely reduces the slice thickness, in which case one must contend with more image noise because of fewer photons being detected. Alternatively, x-ray tube factors may be adjusted upward, resulting in a greater patient dose for the thinner slices.

Another slice-geometry artifact is that associated with the fact that the x-ray beam is diverging as it passes through the patent. This causes some interesting effects. For instance, where is the slice thickness indicated? Figure 1-21 shows that there is no unique slice thickness; thickness varies throughout the scanned volume! By convention, we specify the thickness at the center of rotation (isocenter) of the CT unit. If the scan is completely around the patient (360°), the volume actually being imaged is symmetrically depressed in the center. The consequences of this effect are:

1. Partial volume effects are then a function of position in the field, as well as whether 180° or 360° scans are obtained. As a result, greater spatial and tissue resolution will be found in the center than at the periphery.

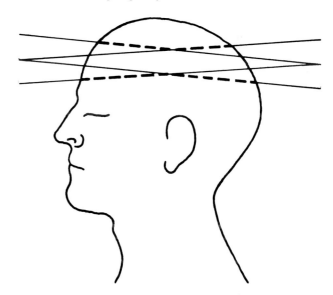

Figure 1-21 Beam diverges as it passes through patient. As beam rotates around patient it forms, not a parallel-sided slice, but rather a concave slice with center thinner than the periphery.

2. A missed volume may occur between slices, as with the EMI Mark I unit, where as much as 10 percent of the total scan volume could be missed (Goodenough 1975). These effects are minimized when patient scan volumes are relatively far from the x-ray source (less beam divergence) and when slices are exactly juxtaposed (or overlapped) at the center. Overlapping, of course, results in an increase in patient dose. The effect depends on exposure geometry; that is, there is less beam divergence for greater source to patient distance.

PROFILE SAMPLING   Figure 1-22 shows an intensity profile of the x-ray beam after it has emerged from the patient. This profile, together with all the other profiles taken at different angles or views around the patient, represents the total ray-sum information necessary for the reconstruction process. In third- and fourth-generation systems, this intensity profile is sampled by the detector array. Each detector intercepts and averages that portion of the profile which is incident over its face. This constitutes a sampling process. The sampled profile as it is transmitted to the computer is then seen to be not the exact replica of the incident profile but only a representation of

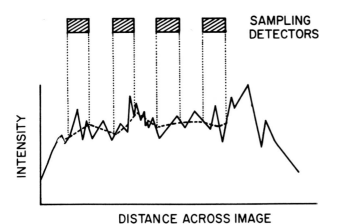

DISTANCE ACROSS IMAGE

Figure 1-22   Demonstration of how a series of finite-size detectors sample an x-ray intensity profile as it emerges from the patient. Each detector responds in proportion to the average intensity sampled. The discrete distribution processed by the computer is then given by the dashed curve. Note the loss of information at the peaks and valleys as well as in the voids between the detectors.

it, and in fact generally is degraded. This degradation takes the final form of decreased tissue and spatial resolution (note that valleys and peaks tend to flatten or smooth out). Additionally, information is lost between detectors. These effects are a function of how large the detectors are as well as the space between them. As either of these dimensions increases, progressive degradation occurs. First- and second-generation systems provide for continuous sampling along the scans, and no interdetector dead spaces exist.

From Figure 1-22 it can be seen that the sampled image has features in it that are not present in the original profile. These bogus features consist of valleys and peaks that do not match the original profiles. In general, low-frequency details* not present in the original image are introduced into the resulting data. This effect is referred to as *aliasing* and is characteristic of all digitizing and sampling systems. The aliasing effect is further illustrated in Figure 1-23. Here we have an elementary sinusoidal-type profile having some particular frequency. It is seen that if the profile is sampled over very short intervals (Fig. 1-23*A*), that profile is completely and accurately determined both in frequency and in amplitude. However, if sampling distances are relatively long, as in Figure 1-23*D*, the pattern resulting has totally different amplitudes and has a lower frequency than the original pattern. Thus a poorly sampled profile introduces patterns in the final result not present in the original.

If the pattern is sampled only once within each cycle, the response is flat, as in Figure 1-23*C*. Figure 1-23*B* shows that when the pattern is sampled at least twice in a cycle, the frequency recorded is identical to that of the original pattern. We refer to this sampling frequency as the *Nyquist frequency* (f_n). The Nyquist frequency is seen to be merely twice the maximum frequency (f_m) present in the x-ray profile:

$$f_n = 2f_m \qquad (2)$$

The maximum frequency associated with a structure

---

* By frequency is meant the rapidity with which profiles change; thus high frequency implies sharp edges or relatively small structures.

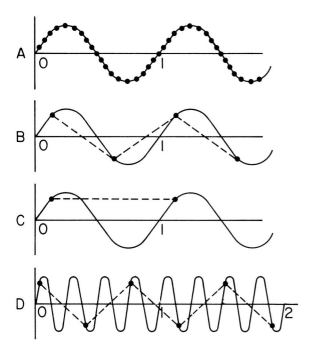

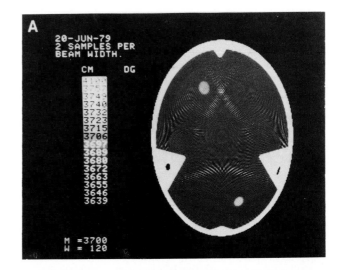

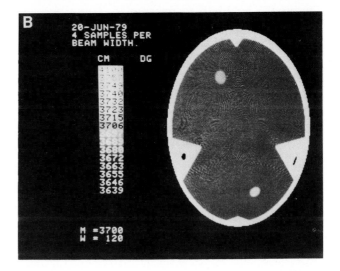

struction appear as shown for a computer simulation in Figure 1-24. Aliasing patterns serve to mask details in the clinical reconstruction. However, in practice their visibility may at times be suppressed by noise present in the image (Stockham 1979). Aliasing streaks can be serious. Examples are clip or

Figure 1-23 Demonstration of the aliasing effect with a pure sinusoidal profile distribution. *Curve A:* If samples are taken at rates much greater than the frequency of the information distribution being sampled, all the frequency as well as all the amplitude information is saved. *Curve B:* If samples are taken at twice the frequency of the distribution, as shown here, all the frequency information is saved (this is the Nyquist frequency). Note, however, that some amplitude information is still lost. *Curve C:* If samples are taken at a rate equal to the frequency of the information distribution, all the frequency and amplitude information will be lost; that is, a flat response results. *Curve D:* Aliasing occurs if sampling rate is less than twice the frequency of the information distribution. Information *not* present in the original is then produced. For example, if time distribution is 4 cycles per millimeter and a sample is obtained every 1½ cycles, as shown here, then the apparent frequency detected is approximately ¾ cycle per millimeter. In general, aliasing results in lower frequencies appearing. The result is streaks in the image.

of dimension d is $1/d$. Thus to sample at the Nyquist frequency the profile must be sampled at

$$f_n = \frac{2}{d} \qquad (3)$$

When sharp discontinuities are present in the scanned image, Equation (3) does not hold and aliasing artifacts appear in the reconstructed image.

Visually, aliasing artifacts for a complete recon-

Figure 1-24 Aliasing streaks due to undersampling. Overlapping streaks emanating over the periphery of the skull result in a moiré pattern. The lower figure shows a phantom simulation sampled at a rate twice that of the upper figure: 0.96 mm sample spacing versus 0.48 mm. (After Stockham 1979 and Joseph 1981.)

star artifacts, which usually consist of streaks emanating from small high-density structures within the patient such as a surgical clip or any metallic object. Similar artifacts can also be seen coming from tooth fillings, gas/liquid interfaces in the stomach, and bony protuberances in skull. It should also be noted that these streaks are also partly due to nonlinear partial volume effects, detector nonlinearity, and angular undersampling. One final artifact related to the presence of small or sharp high-contrast structure is that related to the presence of opaque markers such as catheters on the surface of patients to correlate anatomic level with radiographic views, as were commonly used for early scanners. It has been shown that the use of opaque catheters for this purpose does indeed generate artifacts (Villafana 1978b).

Since aliasing is due to insufficient sampling, an obvious solution is to sample at higher rates, taking readings closer together or using smaller detectors packed closer. The minimum rate to avoid aliasing effects as discussed above is the Nyquist rate, which is a function of the anatomic structure sizes and the presence of sharp discontinuities. Another method which can be used to minimize aliasing is to purposely smooth or eliminate sharp discontinuities in the profiles before they are sampled. This is accomplished by having a relatively wide sampling aperture. One drawback of this approach is that spatial and tissue resolution are sacrificed as well.

A third method to suppress aliasing, which has the advantage of not degrading resolution, is the one-quarter detector shift technique. This technique, which has been successfully applied to fan-beam third-generation geometry (Peters 1977; Brooks 1979), consists of offsetting the central detector by one-fourth of the detector dimensions. As a result, as the scanner obtains views around the patient, all the views from 180° to 360° are exactly interleaved with the views from 0° to 179°—that is, the view at 180° is interleaved with that from 0° and the 360° view is interleaved with that from 180°. The result is that each view is offset by one-half of the detector dimensions. The significance of this is that the highest frequency available at the detector is determined by the detector dimensions, and we thus need, according to Equation (3), to obtain two samples per

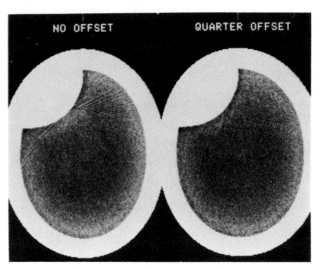

Figure 1-25 Verification of the removal of aliasing streaks seen on the left by quarter offset or shift of the central detector in a third-generation geometry array. (After Brooks 1979.)

detector width *d* (a frequency of 2/d); the quarter offset provides exactly this sampling interval, and aliasing streaks are markedly reduced, as seen in Figure 1-25.

ANGULAR SAMPLING Just as a particular profile can be undersampled as discussed above, the number of profiles or angular view samples around the patient can be deficient. Such angular undersampling also leads to the formation of streak artifacts. However, these streaks, although radiating from small, dense objects, always occur at some distance from the object. It has been shown that undersampling along the profile is more important and leads to more severe aliasing streaks as compared to undersampling the number of angular views around the patient (Brooks 1979; Schulz 1977). Streaks due to view undersampling usually lead to artifacts in the image emanating from the undersampled structure but first appear at some distance from that structure.

To summarize this section: Data acquisition or sampling schemes play a key role in the quality and accuracy of the final image. Sampling includes the thickness of the slice, the sampling along each profile, and the number of views around the patient. Effects can range from simple inaccuracies in the CT number to severe streaks obliterating the desired diagnostic information. Some of the ways to minimize aliasing streaks include thinner slices, closely packed small detectors, and quarter-shifted detector geometry.

Data Measurement

DETECTOR IMBALANCE We have already emphasized that detectors should have high efficiency and high reproducibility. Of importance also is that each detector in an array of detectors be matched in response as compared to the other detectors in the array. When an imbalance occurs, for instance, in a third-generation system, ring artifacts such as those in Figure 1-13 result. Imbalance may result from individual detector gain shifts. Shepp (1977) has shown that shifts as low as 0.1 percent can result in visible streaks. Furthermore, the appearance of streaks is more severe if detector error affects only one ray-path or a small group of ray-paths, as in first-, second-, and third-generation systems. Fourth-generation system detector errors affect the whole view (each detector sees the whole patient), and as a result, inconsistency is smoothed over the whole image and detector matching is not as critical.

When shifts occur they can be calibrated out. This calibration is performed whenever the detector is out from behind the patient. Calibration is automatic for first-, second-, and fourth-generation systems. Third-generation systems, however, present a problem in that the detectors are behind the patient throughout the examination. The resulting ring artifacts (Fig. 1-13) are particularly troublesome. To minimize these ring artifacts these units must be calibrated between patients typically every few hours especially for solid-state detector systems.

DETECTOR NONLINEARITIES Ideally, the response of a detector should be directly proportional to the quantity of radiation incident on it. In CT scanning, the range of x-ray intensities may be as high as 10,000 to 1 or even higher. The detector should have a dynamic range at least this high. Some factors contributing to detector nonlinearity (Joseph 1981) are dark current or leakage (current flow in the absence of radiation), saturation (detector output is at its maximum and higher intensities do not evoke higher output), and hysteresis (detector continues to respond after irradiation ends). One form of hysteresis is the afterglow of scintillation detectors. All these may lead to inconsistency in data and can result in streaks. The severity of these streaks is related to the contrast of the structure as well as the presence of abrupt discontinuities in its shape. One way to minimize the detector nonlinearity problem is to reduce the range of intensities arriving at the detector. This can be accomplished by placing the patient within a water box to provide equal ray-paths as was used in the original EMI Mark I system. A compensating wedge filter can also be used (see Fig. 1-27).

SCATTER COLLIMATION Scatter present at the detector plane is similar to that from leakage in the detector. This can be appreciated by considering a very dense object. The primary x-ray intensity behind this object is expected to be low; however, small amounts of scatter at the detector will indicate a higher than actual transmission. The resulting data are inconsistent with data from ray-paths not traversing the high-contrast object, and streaks can result. Scatter is less of a problem in first-, second-, and third-generation systems, where scatter-rejecting collimation can be incorporated into detectors. In fourth-generation systems, unlike the others, stationary detectors must accept radiation from a wide range of angles, and collimation cannot be used. Consequently these latter systems are more susceptible to scatter effects.

Data Processing

The final step to be considered here is how the data are processed within the computer. The specific algorithm used may introduce artifacts into the final image which are not due to sampling or measurement factors. Examples of this are the use of an edge-enhancement algorithm, which can result in a false subarachnoid space. Another example is that described by Hounsfield (1977), Stockham (1979), and Joseph (1981), involving scanning long, straight-edged, bony, or high-contrast structures. Approximations normally used in algorithms lead to the formation of streaks along the edge of such structures. These streaks can be minimized by using narrower collimators for first- and second-generation units and smaller detectors for third- and fourth-generation units. The use of hardened (filtered) x-ray beams also helps. Needless to say, algorithm-induced artifacts are mathematically complex, and further discussion is beyond our scope here.

CT Number Accuracy

In the previous section the factors resulting in mainly visible streak artifacts were studied. In this section the factors affecting actual accuracy of the CT numbers are considered.

A number of factors limiting the absolute accuracy of CT numbers are listed in Table 1-6. As discussed in an earlier section, the CT reconstruction process computes a value for the linear attenuation coefficient of each volume element within the patient scanned. In all CT designs, the computer then assigns to the attenuation coefficient a value based on the arbitrary -1000 for air to $+1000$ for bone scale. (Modern units are capable of accurately computing and displaying values up to $+3000$ and above.) These values (CT numbers or Hounsfield numbers) represent quantitative data from which tissue identification can be made. In general, they are related to the attenuation coefficient of water (μ_w) as follows:

$$\text{CT no.} = \frac{\mu - \mu_w}{\mu_w} \times 1000 \qquad (4)$$

Table 1-6 Factors Affecting CT Number Accuracy

X-ray beam kilovoltage and filtration
Patient thickness and shape
Tissue type and location
Partial volume effect
Algorithm and calibration shifts

where μ = the attenuation coefficient of the material the CT number is specified for. Table 1-1 gives a short list of CT numbers for typical tissues. All CT scanners have provision for determining the CT number for any specified point or region of points in the image field, either by direct interaction with the video display, using a region-of-interest (ROI) indicator, or by direct printout on a line printer.

Since CT numbers characterize the tissue or its chemical composition, it is no wonder that considerable effort has been expended to use these quantitative data. This involves not only identifying gross tissue type but, among other more sophisticated applications, the determination of bone mineral content (Weissberger 1978; Exner 1979; Revak 1980; Genant 1985) and the identification of calcified versus noncalcified pulmonary nodules (Siegelman 1980; Checkley 1984; Zerhouni 1982). In fact, CT scanning can be configured to determine directly the effective atomic numbers or electron densities (tomochemistry) instead of the attenuation coefficients (McDavid 1977b; Latchaw 1978).

The question of validity must be posed before undue reliance is placed on CT numbers. A number of factors affect the validity of correlating directly the CT number obtained from a particular CT machine and the tissue it is supposed to characterize (McCullough 1977; Levi 1982). Specific factors to be considered are given in Table 1-6, from which it is easy to see that one cannot in fact expect the CT numbers from one machine to match those from another exactly. One reason is that CT numbers are dependent on x-ray beam energy. Thus correlation cannot be rigorously exected between units operated at different kilovoltage (Ruegsegger 1978) or even between similar units operated at the same nominal kilovoltage, because of kilovoltage calibration inaccuracies. CT number anomalies can also occur for the same unit whenever the kilovoltage shifts. In general, the CT number of any material will shift as a function of the difference between the atomic number of that material and the atomic number of water: it will increase for materials with an atomic number less than water and decrease for materials with an atomic number greater than water (Zatz 1976). A tight quality-assurance program monitoring the constancy of CT numbers for a given unit is necessary as well as frequent system calibration by service engineers.

Beam filtration also affects the energy distibution of the x-ray beam. In general, the greater the filtration the harder the beam (or the greater the effective beam energy), and also the beam becomes more monochromatic and therefore less subject to further hardening. This means that CT numbers are subject to variation between units depending on the degree of beam filtration incorporated in each unit as well as the calibration and shift effects discussed above. It is also interesting to note that some CT units provide for two filtration modes, one for head scans and a relatively thicker filtration for body scans, the rationale being that the greater tissue-path lengths in bodies would produce greater beam hardening.

Greater initial filtration would then reduce this effect, in that the beam is prehardened via the additional filter and closer to a monochromatic beam before it enters the patient. Patient thickness is crucial in determining the CT numbers finally computed. Again, beam hardening is involved, in that different patient thicknesses yield different beam paths and different degrees of beam hardening. This is illustrated in Figure 1-26. It can also be seen that results will depend on the shape of the body parts. Figure 1-26 also illustrates the so-called apical artifact (DiChiro 1978), in which CT number variations occur between the slice levels scanned, owing to varying head thickness and thus different degrees of beam hardening.

It has already been noted that the original EMI Mark I unit provided a water box surrounding the patient's head. This meant that all ray-paths were more nearly equal, as seen in Figure 1-27, for any orientation around the head. With such a configuration beam hardening is minimal. Figure 1-27 also

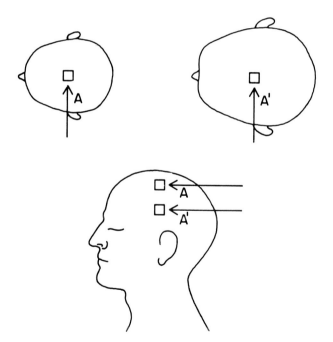

Figure 1-26 Different degrees of beam hardening yielded by different patient thicknesses and the effect on CT number accuracy. Ray-path A to any particular pixel is shorter in the smaller patient on the left than ray-path A' in the larger patient on the right. As shown in the lower figure, even in the same patient path length to any given pixel can differ dependng on slice level (apical artifact). All these effects are further compounded when the beam rotates around the patient and path length is a function of ray angle.

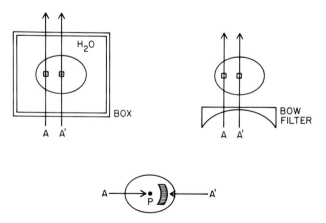

Figure 1-27 *Left:* In original CT units a water bath providing a fixed path length for any and all ray-paths, such as A and A', resulted in minimal beam-hardening effects on CT numbers. *Right:* In an attempt to equalize ray-paths A and A' without a water bath one can provide for a "bow tie" filter arrangement. Here varying filter thickness results in attenuation matching the curvature of the patient. *Bottom:* Presence of dense structures (shaded region) aggravates the beam-hardening problem between ray-paths A and A', since the beam through a point such as P suffers different beam hardening along the two paths indicated. This is particularly severe for ray-paths falling along the edges of the structures, and image streaks are usually formed.

shows one attempt to provide for a fixed path length by providing for a "bow tie" compensating filter. Here added filter thickness toward the periphery of the bow tie presumably compensates for decreased peripheral patient thickness. Patient centering here will obviously be important, and the configuration will not be as effective as a water box. Some advanced designs provide for varying the shape of this bow tie as a function of reconstruction field size to more accurately accomplish equalization of the ray-paths. Figure 1-27 also shows how the presence of dense structures adds to the beam-hardening problem. Discrepancies for ray-paths tangent to the edges of the structure in fact result in severe image streaking.

The partial volume effect also strongly influences CT number accuracy. This was discussed in the previous section and will not be discussed further here.

Finally, the question of algorithms must be addressed. Each CT manufacturer attempts to minimize the beam-hardening problem and to calibrate its CT number scale to maximize accuracy. Such algorithms vary between manufacturers, and the actual field calibrations on any given unit and at any given time will vary.

An additional application of the quantitative use of CT number data is in dynamic scanning. In this approach the absolute value of the CT number is unimportant; rather it is the relative change in the CT numbers at a point which is observed. Here a given tissue slice is repeatedly scanned while contrast is being administered. A region of interest (ROI) is defined and a plot of the average CT number within that ROI versus time is obtained. Note that beam hardening is not a problem since measurements are made within the same region. Presumably the CT number variation here is proportional to the time concentration of contrast within the ROI, which in turn is a function of the blood flow and vascularization properties of the tissue within that ROI (Michael 1985; Som 1986).

To accomplish dynamic scanning the CT x-ray tube must be capable of withstanding high heat loads due to the need for rapid successive scan acquisition. One software approach which extends capability for obtaining data at short time intervals is that of segmental scanning. That is, the data from a 360° scan, which normally produces only one image, are divided up and reallocated into a multiple number of overlapping shorter angular segment scans. Thus, for instance, one 360° scan can be reconstructed as three images (or more) at shorter intervals of time with data from one angular interval overlapping the other.

This section can be summarized simply by stating that great caution must be exercised in using CT numbers, not only between and within different manufacturers' models but also for one's own unit, as a function of the factors listed in Table 1-6.

CT Reconstruction Performance

As already seen, CT performance is a somewhat complex area of study. A number of different aspects of it require discussion, as seen in Table 1-7.

Table 1-7   Aspects of CT Reconstruction Performance

CT number performance
   CT number accuracy
   CT number linearity
   Spatial independence of CT numbers
   Sensitivity to artifactual effects
   Contrast scale
Geometrical and mechanical factors
   Divergence of beam
   Focal-spot penumbra
   Source and detector collimation and alignment
   Dual-slice effects
   Slice location and table incrementation
   Mechanical vibration
Imaging performance
   Spatial resolution
   Tissue resolution
   Noise characteristics
Patient dose
   Single-slice dose
   Multiple-slice dose
   Dose profile

The interested reader is also referred to a number of articles reviewing CT performance and comparisons between specific CT units (Weaver 1975; McCullough 1976; Bassano 1977; Cohen 1979*b*; McCullough 1980). Attention is also drawn to a very comprehensive but somewhat mathematical and technical text (Newton and Potts, 1981).

CT Number Performance

CT NUMBER ACCURACY CT numbers have been discussed at length in previous sections, especially as related to factors causing artifactual variations in their reproducibility and accuracy. To quantitate the accuracy of CT numbers one merely scans a collection of plastics having known attenuation coefficients (or CT numbers) in a water bath. The CT numbers computed are then compared to the known values. In addition, these data when plotted should form a straight line (CT number linearity). There is no generally accepted performance standard covering day-to-day variations in CT numbers; each site should set its own limits, taking into account the manufacturer's recommendations. Generally these variations should not exceed 10 to 20 percent. It should again be noted that CT numbers vary with beam energy. Thus kilovoltage and beam filtration as well as size of the phantom used will affect the CT number. Proper field service calibration of the unit, however, will assure that water gives a CT number of zero for a given reconstruction scan circle or field size and that the known plastics scanned also display their correct CT numbers.

SPATIAL INDEPENDENCE OF CT NUMBERS Clearly it is desirable for computed CT numbers to be independent of spatial position in the reconstruction field. Spatial independence or uniformity is readily measured by scanning a uniform water bath. Variations in CT numbers can be quantitated by computing the standard deviation. This computation is readily available on all commercial scanners, as is the selection of the region of interest over which such determinations are made. In general, for a water bath, the standard deviation in CT numbers in particular regions over the field should not be greater

than a factor of 2 as compared to the central region (McCullough 1976).

CONTRAST SCALE Reference is often made to the contrast scale, defined as the change in the linear attenuation coefficient per CT number (McCullough 1976). It specifies the range of attenuation coefficients which will appear as one CT number. Thus, if the manufacturer's specified performance is 0.5 percent accuracy, the contrast scale should be at least 0.5 percent per CT number. In general, the contrast scale is used to compare results between different CT units. It is necessary because different CT number normalizations may be incorporated in individual CT units. Examples of this would be, for instance, a scale of -500 to $+500$ as in early CT units as compared to the current -1000 to $+1000$ scale. Even if two units have the same nominal scale, there may still be differences. Thus, to make one's results independent of one's particular unit, one should specify the contrast scale. This would particularly apply in making statements pertaining to CT numbers and noise performance values.

It is relatively simple to determine the contrast scale (CS). It may be done by simply scanning Plexiglas in a water bath and using the following equation:

$$CS = \frac{\mu_{plex} - \mu_{H_2O}}{(CT\ no.)_{plex} - (CT\ no.)_{H_2O}} \frac{cm^{-1}}{CT\ no.} \quad (5)$$

In this equation the average linear attenuation coefficient difference between Plexiglas and water $(\mu_{plex} - \mu_{H_2O})$ is constant and is equal to 0.001 cm^{-1} for the range of 100 to 150 kV and for moderate beam filtration (AAPM, Report Number 1). $(CT\ no.)_{plex} - (CT\ no.)_{H_2O}$ is the actual measured CT number difference.

Geometrical and Mechanical Factors

A number of geometric and mechanical factors affect the performance of CT scanners. It has been shown, for instance, that the slice is not necessarily uniformly thick throughout the patient volume; also, all points within the defined slice volume do not contribute equally to the image (Goodenough 1977;

Brooks 1977). Six reasons for this effect are discussed in the following paragraphs.

DIVERGENCE OF BEAM The x-ray beam is not parallel but rather diverges as it passes through the patient (see Figure 1-21). If the beam is then made to rotate 180° or 360° around the patient, the actual volume scanned is depressed in the center. Slice width is defined at the center of rotation; therefore, this results in volume elements at the center contributing more to the CT response than those off the center. This is shown in Figure 1-28 (top), where a theoretical slice is shown. When the x-ray beam is superimposed, the voxels at the periphery intercept fewer x-rays than those at the center.

FOCAL-SPOT PENUMBRA As is true for classical radiography, finite size focal spots are utilized for CT scanning x-ray tubes; thus focal-spot effects are also expected. These effects take the form of the expected decrease in overall resolution as the focal spot size increases. Probably more important, however, is that the focal spot contributes to nonuniformity of the slice along the z direction. This nonuniformity in turn results in a nonuniform sensitivity response of the detector. This effect was particularly true for early dual-slice units utilizing relatively large focal-spot dimensions extending along the z direction.

SOURCE AND DETECTOR COLLIMATION Any given size focal spot will form some penumbral region at the detector. To reduce unnecessary dose to the patient, efforts at collimation or increasing detector size may be made. These efforts, however, add to the non-uniformity of the CT response, since the beam will then be even more divergent, because tighter source collimation provides for a smaller effective focal-spot size, and there is more divergence from a point source than from an extended source. Also, larger detector sizes result in larger beam diameter, which in turn results in more divergence; that is, the beam is parallel along the central ray and becomes less so for peripheral rays as the beam diameter increases.

Collimation, since it affects x-ray beam field size, obviously affects scatter degradation of the image and also contributes to the patient dose. First-, sec-

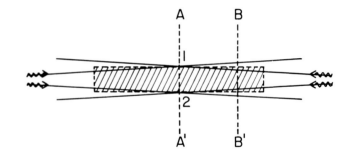

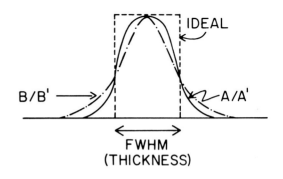

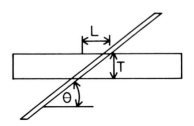

Figure 1-28 Determination of sensitivity profiles. *Top:* CT response varies along lines perpendicular to the slice plane such as *AA'* and *BB'* because of the divergent nature of beam. *Middle:* Curve *AA'*: sensitivity profile along the center defines the slice thickness as the full width of half maximum (*FWHM*). Curve *BB'*: sensitivity profile along a line closer to the periphery. Note the greater degree of flaring out in the tails and the decreased response within the slice thickness borders. The ideal sensitivity curve should be uniform within the confines of the slice and drop to zero response just outside the slice. *Bottom:* Slice thickness and sensitivity profiles may be determined by scanning an inclined ramp (usually made of a thin slice of aluminum). Thickness (*T*) is determined from length *L* measured on the CT scan. Slice thickness is computed from knowledge of the ramp angle (Θ) and simple trigonometry (e.g., $T = L$ tangent Θ).

ond-, and third-generation CT systems can easily incorporate collimation, but fourth-generation systems cannot, since detectors must view x-rays emerging from the patient from different angles. Self-collimation can be incorporated in xenon ionization chamber detector systems. Here the chamber walls, though thin, are made up of a highly absorbent material like tungsten arranged in relatively long channels. As a result, image scatter degradation is minimized.

Detector collimator alignment also presents a possible source of problems. This effect, as well as how to measure it on dual-slice units, has been described by Goodenough (1977).

DUAL-SLICE EFFECTS Units that scan two slices simultaneously inherently produce two partially overlapped and inclined beams, as seen in Figure 1-29. This effect may lead to asymmetric slice profiles. Hounsfield (1977) has described an additional consequence of this: the possibility of just including an object at the 0° view (clipping it) and missing it

at the 180° view; the resulting inconsistency in the data would lead to streaking, especially if the object was very dense, like bone. If one rotates over 360°, this inconsistency is minimized as is the resulting streaking. In fact, even rotating only an extra 30° to 60° may alleviate the clipping problem. Extra rotation also provides for the possibility of motion correction, in that views beyond 180° are redundant. For example, the 185° view corresponds to the original 5° view. A comparison routine could then be invoked within the computer, with any differences between redundant views assumed to be due to patient motion and averaged (or feathered) out. In typical gantry geometries for dual-slice units, the beam inclination and overlap problems are relatively small, but the resulting artifacts may still be significant. Fortunately, petrous bone imaging is affected only slightly, since petrous bones are usually at the 90° position and not near the center of the picture.

To illustrate the consequences of having nonuniform slice thickness and resulting nonuniform response sensitivity, refer to Figure 1-28. Imagine a dense, high-contrast point placed at different levels along a line perpendicular to the slice plane at the center of the slice (along line AA' in Figure 1-28). Ideally, the response of the CT unit should be rectangular (dashed curve), in that the test point will be detected with equal response as long as it is within the slice thickness (points 1 to 2) and will not be detected at all if it falls outside the slice. In practice, the situation does not follow the ideal; rather a loss of response occurs inside the slice width borders and some response occurs beyond the borders of the slice due to the effects discussed above and to focal-spot penumbra and collimation effects discussed earlier. The final response is as shown in Figure 1-28 (solid line). If a similar test had been conducted along a line closer to the periphery, such as BB', a broader response would have occurred (alternating dash-circle curve). These curves are termed *sensitivity profiles*. By convention the slice thickness is defined as the full width at half maximum of the sensitivity profile through the center of the slice.

A number of methods to measure the slice thickness have been proposed, including use of small beads on a 45° ramp (Goodenough 1975), inclined

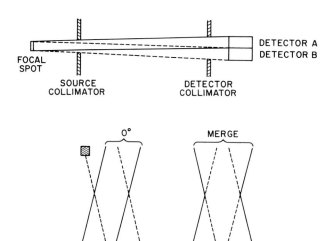

Figure 1-29 *Top:* Asymmetric sensitivity profiles result from dual-slice units due to the partial overlapping and inclination (beams are not perpendicular to axis of the head) which are inherent for extended focal-spot and detector sizes. *Bottom:* Because of beam inclination relative to the axis of the head, there is a possibility of clipping a high-density object (shaded) on the 180° view and missing it on the 0° view, resulting in image streaks. If the unit rotates a full 360° or even just a few degrees beyond 180°, the data merge and the inconsistency and thus the streaking will be minimized.

cylinders (Sorenson 1979) or wires, or an aluminum ramp (AAPM, Report Number I; Brooks 1977). All these methods are based on the fact that projection of the inclined objects will demonstrate different lengths, as seen in Figure 1-28 (bottom). Here, with knowledge of the angle of inclination, one can calculate the slice thickness directly from simple trigonometric considerations. Phantoms can be made up with such inclines at various positions in the field to test for variations in slice thickness. Sensitivity profiles can be approximated by plotting out the CT numbers along the inclination.

SLICE LOCATION AND TABLE INCREMENTATION CT scanners normally have a number of light alignment devices to locate and align the patient. In addition, provision is usually made for automatic incrementation of the table to move the patient into position for consecutive scans. The most recent CT scanners, in fact, provide for both automatic incrementation of the table and inclination of the gantry. These features are indeed convenient and time-saving and offer potentially more accuracy than manual incrementation. Their benefit, however, is clearly compromised if they themselves lack accuracy. The accuracy of all alignments and incrementation features should be verified at regular intervals.

MECHANICAL VIBRATION Inherent to the CT scan process is mechanical motion. Such motion may and usually does create some degree of vibration, which in turn may induce image-degrading effects. The best example of this is the problem of microphonics for third-generation xenon ionization chamber systems. The term *microphonics* refers to the vibrations induced in relatively thin ionization chamber walls by the various gantry motions. These vibrations induce fluctuations in output signals, which result in additive CT image noise. To minimize microphonics, thicker chamber walls with smaller overall area must be used. However, this then affects image quality since ideally walls should be as thin as possible and placed as close to each other as possible. Because of the relatively inefficient quantum absorption of the gas, long chamber walls are required to maintain low patient dosage. This in turn may make the chamber susceptible to further vibration.

CT Imaging Performance

In addition to the problem of artifact sensitivity, as discussed previously, there are three basic descriptors of CT imaging performance: spatial (or high-contrast) resolution, image noise, and tissue (or low-contrast) resolution.

Spatial Resolution

Spatial resolution is the ability of a CT scanner to record fine, high-contrast detail. Various measures of spatial resolution are available (see Table 1-8). What they all have in common is essentially 100 percent contrast and noise-free conditions. These measures do not necessarily predict the actual performance of a CT unit when imaging tissues having similar attenuation coefficients. The resolution-bar pattern is probably the most familiar test object used in general radiology. It can be configured for CT scanning (Goodenough 1977; Maue-Dickson 1979), for instance, with a series of Plexiglas strips (or similar material) in a water bath in such a manner that equal widths of Plexiglas alternate with equal spaces of water. These Plexiglas widths form a *line pair* with the adjoining water space, and each line pair is made progressively narrower—that is, a greater number of line pairs per millimeter, or higher line-pair frequency, is formed. The resolving power of the system is that line-pair frequency which is just barely visible on the image.

Table 1-8 Spatial Resolution Measures (100 Percent Contrast and Noise-Free Conditions)

Measure	Mathematical equivalent
Resolution bar and pin pattern	Zero cutoff of MTF
Sunburst pattern	Zero cutoff of MTF
Point-spread function (PSF)	Basic response function
Line-spread function (LSF)	Integral of PSF along line
Edge-response function (ERF)	Integral of LSF along line (slope of ERF = LSF)
Modulation transfer function (MTF)	Fourier transform of LSF

A variation of the basic resolution bar pattern is the sunburst phantom (Goodenough 1977), in which alternate radial strips and spaces are arranged in a tapered manner around a circle like wheel spokes to provide for continuously varying frequencies. Resolution is given by the distinctly visible tapered pattern closest to the center. This approach was actually used to approximate the modulation-transfer function of a CT system (MacIntyre 1976), which is still another measure of resolution. Instead of repetitive bar patterns, a series of varying-diameter Plexiglas, high-contrast pins in a water bath can be used to assess spatial resolution. Alternatively, one can have holes of varying diameters in Plexiglas. Figure 1-30 shows results for two popular phantoms incorporating various spatial-resolution patterns.

A number of other spatial-resolution descriptors are shown in Table 1-8. Though each is distinct, they are all interrelated. The *point-spread function* (PSF) is the most fundamental measure and is defined as the response of a system to a point object. The PSF can be measured by scanning a high-contrast wire pin which is perpendicular to the long axis of the slice. The *line-spread function* (LSF) is the response of the system to a line object lying within or along the long axis of the slice plane. Mathematically, the LSF can be obtained from the PSF by integrating the PSF along a line. The *edge-response function* (ERF) in turn is merely the mathematical integration of the LSF along a plane. Experimentally, the ERF may be obtained directly by scanning an edge object.

Next to the resolution-bar and pin patterns, the *modulation-transfer function* (Villafana 1978a) approach is probably the most commonly cited descriptor of spatial resolution. The MTF is defined as the response of the system to a sinusoidally varying object. Because of the difficulty of constructing objects with sinusoidally varying CT numbers, usually the PSF (Weaver 1975; Goodenough 1977), LSF (Bishop 1977; Judy 1976), or ERF (Judy 1976) are measured and then mathematically converted to the MTF. For instance, the LSF may be subjected to a Fourier transform operation and converted to an MTF. For the interested reader, Jones (1954) has reviewed in depth the various mathematical relationships between these various measures.

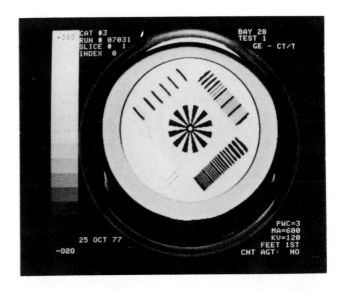

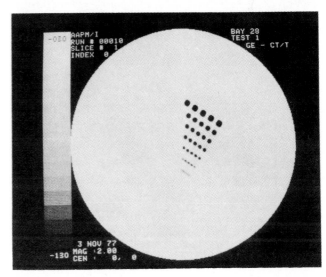

Figure 1-30 Examples of spatial resolution test-scan results for two popular phantom configurations. *Top:* Starburst and bar pattern scans. Four different bar patterns of differing subject contrast can be displayed on the Catphan phantom (Alderson Research Laboratories; Goodenough 1977). *Bottom:* Phantom made up of Plexiglas with different-diameter holes in each row (AAPM phantom; AAPM Report Number 1). Both these phantoms have a variety of test objects in addition to those shown here for evaluating the full range of CT system performance as well as for ongoing quality control tests.

To illustrate the use of MTFs, Figure 1-31 shows for comparison purposes the MTF for GE CT/T 7800 and 8800 systems. The 8800 system has a detector aperture nearly one-half the size of the 7800. As a result, the MTF of the 8800 system is correspondingly better (about twice as good). This can be seen from the fact that the MTF response of the 8800 system drops at higher frequencies than the drop for the 7800 system.

The ideal MTF would correspond to a unit (MTF = 1) response regardless of frequency. Such comparisons can be of great value in assessing performance. Comparisons can also be made between different manufacturers' models and even between subcomponents of a given model CT. This latter application has been admirably demonstrated by Barnes (1979), as shown in Figure 1-32, where it is seen that for the particular CT unit under study, the algorithm (or filter function) represents the limiting system component, since its MTF drops to zero the

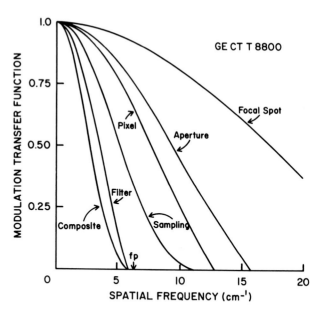

Figure 1-32 Comparison of individual-component MTFs for a given CT system. System shown is the GE CT/T8800 for a 24-cm-diameter patient circle, 0.78-mm pixel size. (Adapted from Barnes et al. 1979.) Here the sampling and the algorithm filter function would be the limiting component, while the focal spot would be the least limiting component. Also shown is the composite or total MTF curve, which is the product of all the component curves. Note that the composite is poorer than any individual component.

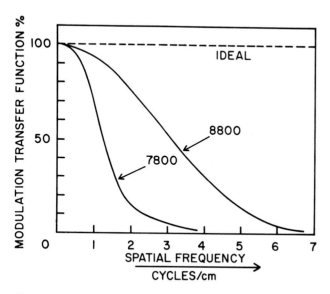

Figure 1-31 The modulation-transfer functions (MTF) for the GE CT/T 7800 and 8800 systems. The GE 8800 system has a detector aperture size nearly half as large as the 7800 and the detectors are correspondingly more closely spaced. The improvement in the MTF is significant (nearly two times). The ideal curve represents the situation in which the system response is unity regardless of how high the frequency is. (Adapted from GE brochure.)

most quickly, and the focal spot is the component least limiting CT performance. The overall total or composite curve is obtained from the product of the MTFs of all the system components at each frequency; that is, in the general case:

$$\text{MTF}_{\text{TOT}} = \text{MTF}_1 \times \text{MTF}_2 \times \text{MTF}_3 \times \ldots \quad (6)$$

Note that the composite MTF is in general lower than, and at most equal to, the lowest MTF response component in the system. Attempts to improve the spatial resolution of this system should be directed to improving the lowest response link in the system. In the specific case shown in Figure 1-32, the sampling MTF would be the next most advantageous component to improve.

As previously seen, insufficient sampling leads to aliasing and artifactual streak formation. Even if algorithms are available to remove such artifacts, a generalized loss of spatial resolution will still be present as predicted by the sampling MTF in Figure 1-32. The pixel MTF refers to the fact that choice of pixel size will affect the resolution of the final image. For instance, a smaller patient or reconstruction circle results in smaller effective pixel size and higher resolution. Finally, the aperture (or collimator) MTF in Figure 1-32 refers to the physical opening at the detector.

It should be noted that some systems having relatively large detectors provide for an absorbing pin which can be placed in front of the detector to reduce its effective size and thus improve its MTF or resolution response. Here again, component MTF curves can predict the possible success of such a maneuver. For instance, in the case of the GE CT/T, such an absorbing pin would be essentially futile, since the aperture MTF is not limiting. This is true for all third-generation xenon ionization chamber systems, since such systems can be configured with small detector face area.

Finally, we again caution that MTF data do not of themselves predict actual clinical performance, since they are defined for 100 percent contrast and for essentially noise-free conditions. Consequently they should be used for comparative purposes only and for imaging high-contrast structures.

Noise

In detecting low-contrast tissue structures (tissues of similar CT numbers), noise plays a dominant role; it is, in general, the limiting factor in CT scanning, since in many applications diagnosis hinges on the visualization of tissue structures having very similar CT numbers. For instance, gray- and white-matter tissues are separated by only 5 to 10 CT numbers. Noise can be defined as the standard deviation in CT numbers in a scanned, uniform water bath. All CT scanners provide for a region-of-interest selector where one can read out automatically the standard deviation of the CT numbers falling within the selected area (usually about 25 pixels in size). To make

the noise measure independent of the particular CT unit and contrast scale (CS) (see Equation 5), the following expression is used:

$$\text{Noise} = \frac{\text{CS} \times \sigma_w}{\mu_w} \times 100 \qquad (7)$$

where μ_w = the linear attenuation coefficient of water (0.195 cm^{-1} for 70 keV) and σ_w is the observed standard deviation for a uniform water-bath region.

It is crucial to note that image noise is directly related to the number of photons received and processed at the detectors. Consequently, to decrease CT noise one must increase the number of photons passing through the patient and available at the detectors. This, of course, increases the patient dose. The statistical variation in the photon number in a uniform beam incident on the detectors is given by the standard deviation of the photon number as follows:

$$\sigma_N = \sqrt{N} \qquad (8)$$

σ_N above, as the fluctuation in the photon number N (which is related to patient dose), must be distinguished from σ_w as specified for the standard deviation in CT numbers of the final reconstructed uniform water field, the difference between these two being the contribution of algorithm noise (Joseph 1978*a*).

From Equation (8) emerges an underlying and crucial conclusion, namely, that *CT imaging performance depends on patient radiation dose*. This is true because the number of photons at the detector is directly related to the number of photons passing through the patient, which in turn determines patient dose. Because of the dependence of image quality on patient dose, one must specify the patent dose associated with any image performance specification. Stated another way, an image may be of very high quality but may have been obtained at the cost of an unacceptably high radiation dose to the patient. Haaga et al. (1981) have recently illustrated how photon levels of different milliamperage affect actual visualization.

Brooks and DiChiro (1976c) have shown that the statistical noise σ_N, pixel size w (representing the limiting resolution measure), slice thickness h, dose D, and the fractional attenuation of the patient B are related as follows:

$$\sigma_N = \left(\frac{KB}{w^3hD}\right)^{1/2} \tag{9}$$

where K is a proportionality constant for any given unit. Equation (9) reveals that in general, as slice thickness decreases, the noise value increases. This is evident, since less thickness h implies a narrower beam and consequently the delivery of fewer photons to the detector. A similar statement is true for the patient-dose factor D, in that a lower dose to the patient (for instance, less tube milliamperage or scan time) results in fewer photons at the detector. Both these factors vary as the square root, which means that halving either one results in a $\sqrt{2}$ times greater noise level. The noise dependence on pixel size, on the other hand, is as the third power. Thus halving the pixel size (which may result in doubling the resolution) results in an eightfold increase in dose to maintain the same level of noise! Not only does CT image performance depend on noise, but attempts at increasing performance by reducing noise may indeed result in a very considerable dose increase to the patient.

If noise is, in fact, limiting CT performance, and not spatial resolution, one may opt, for instance, to increase pixel size. Such a move would reduce noise and might improve visualization of large but low-contrast structures; but care must be taken, since a net reduction of spatial resolution would also result. As discussed above in Equation (9), noise dependence varies with slice thickness to the 1/2 power. Thus increases in slice thickness also reduce noise, but not nearly to the same degree as increases in pixel width, which vary to the 3/2 power. The rationale for the noise dependence on pixel width and slice thickness is simply that reduction in these sizes causes a reduction in the number of photons available to make up the image for each pixel. A reduced number of photons, in turn, creates greater statistical variation, and image noise is increased.

An interesting approach to reducing final noise without increase in dose to the patient is by mathematical smoothing. Algorithms can be configured to include various smoothing routines (referred to as *kernels* or algorithm filters). Such smoothing, however, usually results in blurring and thus a loss of spatial resolution. However, if accomplishment of a particular task is indeed limited by the presence of noise, smoothing may in fact yield significant results, as reported by Joseph (1978a). This area, however, still needs considerable clinical investigation.

Finally, it should be stated that other descriptors of noise even more complete and general are available. For instance, noise power spectra can be constructed (Riederer 1978). These describe noise as a function of spatial frequency; hence they are similar to and can be combined with the MTF descriptor. For further details, the reader is referred to the literature (Barnes 1979; Riederer 1978; Rossman 1972).

Tissue Resolution

Tissue, or low-contrast, resolution may be defined as the smallest object or pin size detectable under low-contrast conditions. Low contrast is considered to exist when scanning CT number differences of less than 0.5 percent or 5 CT numbers. (For a -1000 to $+1000$ CT system, each CT number represents 0.1 percent difference.) Phantoms used are similar to the bar and pin object types already discussed. Recent CT units have a tissue resolution of 4 to 5 mm, compared to a spatial high-contrast resolution of 0.5 mm or less. Tissue resolution is also called *low-contrast detectivity* or *low-contrast sensitivity*.

The tissue-resolution measure is more accurate in predicting clinically expected performance, since low-contrast conditions are more clinically relevant. Also, since low-contrast conditions are specified, the influence of noise is incorporated. Because of crucial interplay among noise, performance, and patient dose, tissue-resolution specifications must be accompanied by statements of pixel size, patient dose, phantom diameter, kilovoltage or filter, and other reconstruction details (McCullough 1980).

Recently another approach describing system resolution has been introduced which uses so-called contrast-detail curves (Cohen 1979a, 1979b). In this approach both the low-contrast and the high-contrast resolution response of a system is specified. Figure 1-33 shows a contrast-detail curve for two levels of radiation dose and two different CT sys-

tems. In general, spatial resolution is relatively good for both units at high contrast and is independent of dose (noise). Note that in both cases spatial resolution still does not get better than a certain minimum detectable size (called the *resolution limit* and occurring at 100 percent contrast). As contrast decreases, resolution falls. At low-contrast levels, curves tend to flatten out (this is referred to as the *noise limit*). Note from Figure 1-33 that if noise levels are reduced (dose increased), detectable size decreases at low-contrast levels but not at high-contrast levels.

Finally, mention should be made of still another approach to quantitating the performance of CT equipment. This consists in using receiver- (or reader) operator-characteristic (ROC) curves. Here, an attempt is made to compare the number of false positive and false negative detection rates as a function of reader bias and decision criteria. The interested reader is referred elsewhere for further details (Weaver 1975; Goodenough 1974a, 1974b; Rossman 1972).

Pixel Sizes, Zoom, and CT Performance

Various aspects of pixels have been previously discussed. Since much discussion concerning CT units centers around statements of pixel sizes, we now summarize some pertinent facts. (1) Pixels are the basic building blocks of the CT image. They represent an element or area of the view over which the reconstruction process has calculated a CT number. (2) Pixels represent a weighted nonlinear average CT number of the various tissues which fall within a given volume element (voxel) within the patient (volume-averaging or partial volume effect) and as a result may be artifactual, especially in regions of the patient where tissue type and structure are rapidly changing. (3) The original EMI Mark I pixel sizes were relatively large, in that they represented a 3 × 3 × 13 mm volume (80 × 80 array). Currently pixel sizes can be configured to less than 1 mm on a side. (4) Changing pixel sizes can indeed improve CT images, in that the partial volume effect is reduced and consequently both spatial and low-contrast tissue resolution can improve. Improvement, however, is dependent on whether there is a corre-

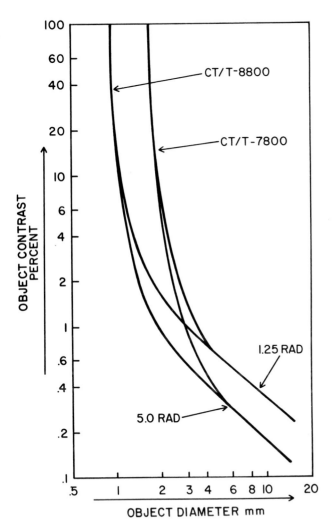

Figure 1-33 Detail-contrast curves. Plot of object diameter visible on both the GE 7800 and the GE 8800 versus object contrast for two different dose levels. At high contrast the smallest possible object diameter is visible (the resolution limit), independent of dose or noise. At low contrast, noise becomes a significant factor and results are highly dependent on dose. (Adapted from GE brochure.)

sponding increase in photon levels to overcome the greater noise levels inherent with smaller pixels (that is, smaller pixel sizes imply a greater number of pixels and thus fewer photons per pixel) and whether the imaging limitation was in fact the pixel size. It is clear that other components such as motion, focal-spot size, or detector-aperture size may be limitations, in which case pixel-size reduction may only result in either image degradation due to noise or an increase in patient dose if photon levels are increased to overcome the higher noise levels for smaller pixel sizes.

Other features which affect pixel size and imaging performance are magnification and zoom. There are a variety of ways in which magnification and zoom can be accomplished. There is as yet no accepted terminology describing these, and the author proposes the terms geometric zoom, interpolated zoom, and reconstructed zoom.

GEOMETRIC ZOOM   Geometric zoom refers to image enlargement accomplished by varying geometric factors such as sampling distances, number of detectors used for the reconstruction process, or mechanical configuration of the gantry. For instance, in first- and second-generation CT systems, a particular detector scans across the total patient cross section. The resulting number of pixels may be the number of intervals over which summing and digitization take place. If a smaller reconstruction area is chosen and if the number of pixels is the same, the patient volume size corresponding to each pixel decreases, allowing for an increase in system performance. For instance, if a particular system is configured for displaying 256×256 pixels for a reconstruction circle of 400 mm, each pixel represents $400/256 = 1.56$ mm. If the reconstruction circle is reduced to 200 mm, each pixel represents $200/256 = 0.78$ mm. To exploit this, CT units have selectable lengths or reconstruction circles over which data can be collected, selection being based on the size of the patient. One must be careful to distinguish between the gantry opening (or patient window), which is the physical opening within which the patient is placed, and the reconstruction circle, which is that region within the gantry opening over which the data are collected and processed, as discussed above. For the best images, the CT operator should select the smallest possible reconstruction circle. Actually, in some applications where resolution is critical, a reconstruction circle even smaller than the patient size is selected and centered around a particular region of interest, as in scanning the cervical spine, for instance.

Sometimes this latter approach is also referred to as *region-of-interest* (ROI) scanning (still a form of geometric zoom). In ROI scanning, caution must be observed in interpreting the resulting CT numbers, since inaccuracies may be introduced by the contribution of patient volumes outside the region of interest. As already stated, the pixel size for small reconstruction circles represents a smaller volume in the patient. As a consequence of this, the actual size of the patient image on the display screen is enlarged. Furthermore, this represents a true zoom, in that enlargement of the image is accomplished with each pixel still representing actual patient data.

In third- and fourth-generation systems, the detectors see the full patient contour, and the millimeters of patient per pixel, and thus data sampling distances, are fixed; thus the use of small detectors is especially necessary. These units, however, still have a selectable reconstruction circle and different possible degrees of final display magnification, in that the smaller regions scanned can still be imaged over the full display with the total pixels available. Image quality is again usually improved, but such improvement will depend on the relative role of the sampling and pixel size MTFs.

One interesting variation of geometric zoom is referred to as *geometrical enlargement*. This configuration provides for variable magnification within the gantry. For example, the detector array, along with the x-ray source, can be moved closer to or farther away from the patient in such a manner that the full array of detectors is always used. When the x-ray source is closer to the patient (and detectors far), a smaller patient diameter is viewed. For larger patient diameter, the source is placed farther away. In either case all the detectors are utilized. With this arrangement, the sampling distances and therefore the image quality can always be optimized.

INTERPOLATED ZOOM   This is quite different from geometric zoom. Interpolated zoom enlarges the image of a relatively small region of interest within an already processed image and, under computer control, expands it to fill the entire display by averaging the CT numbers in each particular pixel over the neighboring pixels. Therefore, while the final pixels represent a smaller patient volume, they do not represent unique and true patient data but arithmetic averages (or interpolations) over adjacent pixels. Note that this type of zoom corresponds to the straight magnification modes made available in the early first- and second-generation units. It is always performed on a finished image without a reconstruction routine. As the ROI decreases the image appears larger but spatial resolution is progressively degraded.

RECONSTRUCTED ZOOM   This type of zoom depends on original data being available to allow reconstruction over a smaller area. Typically, reconstructed zoom can be performed with optimal results when scan sampling disances are smaller than the pixel display sizes. For example, if a third-generation scanner with 576 detectors is used but final reconstruction results are condensed and displayed on a 256 × 256 pixel array, then, if original data are still available, a reconstructed zoom of over two times (576/256 = 2.25) can be invoked on the original image. This is a true zoom in that original patient data are reconstructed and displayed.

In summary, then, it can be stated that pixel size is indeed an important parameter determining CT imaging performance. A statement of array size by itself is not, however, sufficient. Rather, it is important to state what size (or volume) the pixel actually represents in the patient. There are various ways to enlarge or magnify the image which correspond to decreasing the volume each pixel represents. Such zooming in may or may not lead to an increase in perceived image quality.

Patient Radiation Dose

We have already discussed the fact that CT scanning is noise-limited in that image quality increases as the number of x-ray photons utilized increases. A greater number of photons, however, results in greater patient dose. Fortunately, radiation dosimetry, in general, is an established technology. Even though there are some unique aspects to the dose problem in CT scanning, such as highly collimated scanning fields, these can be taken into account.

The radiological units of roentgens and rads are familiar to all. The *roentgen* is a measure of the ionization occurring in air. The International Commission on Radiological Units (ICRU) has recently recommended dropping this unit, and the clinician will be seeing less and less of it. The *rad* is a measure of the absorbed energy per unit mass, or absorbed dose (1 rad = 2.58×10^{-4} joules per kilogram). Given the roentgen exposure, the rad dose may be obtained by multiplication by a suitable factor (0.91 for diagnostic x-ray energies and soft tissue). The ICRU has also recommended the use of the unit *gray* for absorbed dose (1 gray = 1 joule per kilogram) as a replacement for the rad. Presently most dose information is available in rads, but this is expected to shift toward the gray in the future (1 gray = 100 rads).

Table 1-9 summarizes the various factors affecting patient dose. The factors most familiar to the clinician are patient thickness, beam filtration, and the radiographic factors of kilovoltage and milliamperage. To these must be added a number of factors unique to CT scanning such as beam collimation, slice-width effects, and image quality desired.

Table 1-9   Factors Affecting Patient Dose

Patient thickness
Generator and tube factors:
   Kilovoltage and filtration
   Tube current (milliamperage) and scan on time
   Focal-spot size (penumbral spread)
Gantry factors:
   Beam collimation
   Slice width and overlap
   Scan orientation
Image quality desired

PATIENT THICKNESS   It stands to reason that as patient thickness increases, so does the attenuation of the x-ray beam and the amount of radiation which must pass thorugh the patient to provide the required number of photons at the detector level. As a consequence, more total energy is absorbed in the patient. The fact that larger patients have their entry skin surface closer to the x-ray source also results in greater patient skin dose.

KILOVOLTAGE   Kilovoltage affects the dose in two possible ways. If kilovoltage is increased because more photons are needed in the image field, then patient dose is also increased (this is the usual case for CT). Dose is decreased on increasing kilovoltage only if this allows a greater proportional decrease in the milliamperage. This relative decrease comes about because the number of photons arriving at the detector is greater, owing to the higher penetrating ability of the higher-kilovoltage beam.

FILTRATION   Added beam filtration always leads to lower patient doses. The reason for this is the same as in clinical radiography: filtration removes the softer, low-energy photons which are readily absorbed in the patient and have little probability of penetrating through to the detectors. Selection of filters on CT scanners, however, is not to provide for dose saving but rather to harden the beam to avoid beam-hardening effects within the patient. Typically, such added filtration is selected for scanning large body parts as compared to scanning heads. (The filtration referred to here should not be confused with software filters incorporated in an algorithm, which are part of the mathematical reconstruction process.)

TUBE CURRENT AND SCAN ON TIME   Tube current represents the flow of electrons across the x-ray tube, and it controls the final quantity of x-rays emitted. By convention it is measured in milliamperes. Scan "on time" refers to the period of time milliamperes are actually flowing and x-rays are actually on or not shuttered. Pulsing units are configured to fire, or turn on for x-ray pulses or various intervals of time (pulse length). These pulses are repeated at various angles as the x-ray tube rotates around the patient. It is the product of the tube current and the "on time" (the milliamperage product) which is the important dose-determining factor. First- and second-generation units, as well as some fourth-generation units, typically do not pulse, and the x-ray beam is on during the entire scan. Many CT units offer a fast scan at low image quality and a slower scan at higher image quality (if patient motion is not limiting). Typically, the faster scans are accomplished by pulsing at fewer intervals around the patient or an overall reduction in scan times. Since the milliamperes product will be lower for such fast scans, the dose also will be lower.

BEAM COLLIMATION   Typically, CT scanning involves the use of highly collimated beams. First-generation systems used pencil beams approximately 3 mm wide by 30 mm long. Second-generation systems utilized multiple pencils, each having approximately the same dimensions as the first-generation pencil beams. Fan beams, as used in third- and fourth-generation systems, are opened up along the horizontal direction. As far as dose is concerned, the important idea is that the x-ray beam should be collimated down to approximately the height dimensions of the detectors. Figure 1-34 shows examples of a poorly collimated beam and a well-collimated beam. Note that for poor collimation the region which extends beyond the dimensions of the detector unnecessarily adds to the patient dose and forms a region of overlapping dose when the adjacent slice is scanned. To study this in more detail, dose profiles are usually obtained across the patient in a direction perpendicular to the slice plane (along z axis). These can be obtained by the use of thermoluminescent dosimeters (TLD),* for instance, placed on tissue-equivalent phantoms or on patients

---

* TLD detectors usually consist of a small lithium fluoride chip (typically about 1.0 mm $\times$ 3 mm $\times$ 3 mm), which has the advantage of being small and tissue-equivalent; however, it is low-energy-dependent and must be calibrated very carefully. The TLD detector is based on the principle that electrons liberated by the incident radiation are trapped at certain impurity centers, or electron traps, within the crystal. When the crystal is heated, the electron traps are emptied and light is emitted as the electrons fall back to the ground state. This emitted light is proportional to the original incident radiation.

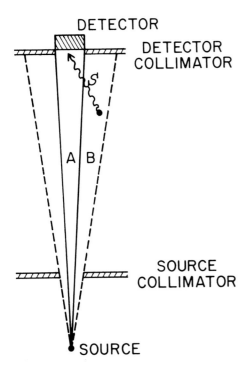

Figure 1-34 **A.** Well-collimated beam confined to the dimensions of the detector. **B.** Poorly collimated beam. Radiation passing through the patient is not utilized at the detector. Additionally, scatter (*S*) may degrade image quality.

directly. Alternatively, ionization chambers on phantoms can also be used.

One of the prime means of evaluating the dose characteristics of a CT scanner is to compare the dose profiles with the sensitivity profiles. It will be recalled that the sensitivity profile is the response of the CT system along the perpendicular (*z* direction) to the scan plane. The dose profile is the radiation distribution along the same direction. Ideally, the dose profile should be identical to the sensitivity profile for a particular set of scan parameters when both are compared at the patient level. Thus the ratio of the two should be 1.0, or 100 percent. This ratio is referred to as *dose utilization*. The practitioner is cautioned that a particular CT unit may have a high dose utilization yet also result in a relatively high dose to the patient, since dose utilization indicates how efficiently the radiation was detected

but does not yield the magnitude of the actual dose received.

SLICE WIDTH AND OVERLAP As slice width decreases, the penumbral region of the field becomes relatively more important, because the tails of the dose profiles then represent a proportionately larger fraction of the dose distribution, and overlapping on multiple scans becomes correspondingly more serious. Additionally, some degree of slice overlap may be incorporated into the scan sequence. Thus a 1.3-mm slice width being scanned may be incremented, for instance, by a 1.2-mm distance. This results in a 1-mm scan overlap, which drives the patient dose even higher. Figure 1-35 shows how total dose distribution for a series of consecutive scans can be obtained by summation of a single-scan dose profile incremented by some known amount; it also shows the case in which peaks may appear in dose distribution, depending on the extent of the tails in the dose profile and the degree of overlap incorporated in the scan sequence.

SCAN ORIENTATION A number of factors associated with scan orientation should be noted. For instance, in a 180° head scanner the x-ray tube should rotate over the posterior of the patient, sparing the eye lens a considerable dose (Villafana 1978*c*; Batter 1977) (a factor of about 10!). Third- and fourth-generation scanners typically rotate 360° around the patient periphery. Some units incorporate an overscan feature

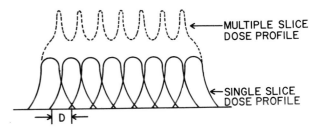

Figure 1-35 Determination of dose distribution over an extended body part when multiple scans are obtained. Appropriate summation of the dose profiles is accomplished by superimposing the dose profiles with incrementation distance *D*. Because of the tailing off of the dose profiles and the degree of overlap in incrementation, dose peaks may appear in the distribution.

for patient-motion and streak correction. In this case, more than 360° is scanned and the dose is greater in the region of overscan. Such a case requires particular attention to avoid having the scan both begin and end over a critical organ such as the eye lens.

Expressing Dose

There are a number of ways to express patient dose. For instance, average or maximum skin dose, or dose at the middepth of the patient, or even the dose at some critical organ such as the eye lens or gonads has been used (Villafana 1978c; Isherwood 1978; Shrivastava 1977; Gyldensted 1977; McCullough 1974; Perry 1973). Other measures include total integrated energy absorbed in the body (integral dose). Since image quality depends on dose and dose in turn depends on many factors (see Table 1-9), care must be exercised in interpreting dose data. For example, the average dose for a 180° scanner would be relatively low in that only half the patient is irradiated directly, but the dose may be averaged over the indirectly irradiated region. Moreover, depending on the extent of the dose profile tails, very high dose regions may exist which may be masked by the average. The simplest adequately descriptive measures of patient dose are the single-scan dose profile and the multiple-scan dose factor (typical values = 1.2 to 2.0). These should be known to the user for the various operating modes of the equipment used. Along with the dose profiles, a plot of dose distribution along the total body part, similar to that in Figure 1-35, should be available.

The most complete description of the patient dose is that using isodose curves (Perry 1973; Agarwal 1979; Jucius 1977; Wall 1979). Figure 1-36 shows such curves. From these the relative dose at any point or level can readily be picked out, since each isodose curve represents the points having the same dose within the patient, and the points falling between the curves can easily be interpolated. If isodoses are stated in terms of percent of peak dose, the peak dose must be explicitly stated.

A way of expressing CT dose which has been recently proposed is the "computed tomography dose index" (CTDI). The CTDI is obtained at a particular

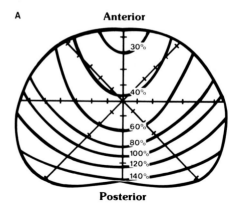

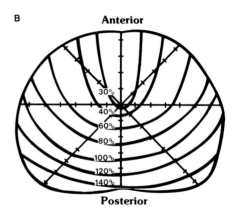

Figure 1-36 Isodose curves in a Rando phantom for a Delta 50FS2 20-second scanner, 140 kVp, 35 mA, 42-cm scan circle, 13-mm slice thickness. **A.** Distribution for a multiple-scan examination average in which 100% = 1.1 R. **B.** Distribution for a single-scan peak exposure at 100% = 1.1 R. (*From Jucius 1977.*)

measurement site by integrating the single-slice dose profile and dividing by the nominal slice thickness (Shope 1981). The volume of the CTDI turns out to be equal to the average dose at the measurement site which would result from scanning a series of contiguous slices as in a typical procedure. The CTDI is usually measured with a special long ionization chamber.

GONAD DOSE   When the head or upper torso is scanned, the gonads receive a relatively low dose (typically 10 mrad or less). The gonads are exposed to both scattered radiation produced within the patient and leakage radiation from the x-ray tube. Scatter in general must pass through and be extensively attenuated by whatever tissue thickness exists between the region scanned and the position of the gonads. Gonad dose increases as the distance to the irradiated region decreases. Tube-leakage levels are limited by law to a maximum of 100 mR/h at 1 meter. As with any diagnostic x-ray tube, most CT tubes have leakage rates well within this maximum because of the lead lining usually placed inside the tube housing. Even for slower scanners requiring 10 to 15 minutes total examination scan time, this would amount to 10 to 15 mR even under maximum leakage levels. In addition to internally scattered and leakage radiation, there is the possibility of radiation scattering from various portions of the gantry components, which also can contribute to patient dose. Each unit should be evaluated as to gonad doses as well as radiation dosages to persons remaining in the scan room to hold or calm patients.

In summary, then, it is recognized that CT scanning-image quality is noise-limited. Noise in turn is dependent on the number of photons utilized to make up the image. Therefore patient dose, noise, and image quality are all intimately related. When evaluating the performance of a CT scanner, the dose must be explicitly stated for the conditions under which the image was obtained.

SECTION B: MAGNETIC RESONANCE IMAGING

Magnetic resonance imaging (MRI) is based on totally different physical principles as compared with computerized tomography (CT). MRI, however, does share in common the fact that radiant energy is beamed into the patient and in turn is detected as it emerges from the patient. In MRI this radiant energy is in the form of radio-frequency waves rather than x-rays as is the case for CT. Like CT, the radiant energy detected correlates with various parameters characteristic of tissue properties. What is important, however, is the fact that magnetic resonance allows us to image much smaller contrast differences between tissues. Just as CT represented a significant increase in tissue contrast sensitivity as compared with classical tomography, so does MRI represent an even greater contrast sensitivity step over CT. To understand why this is so we will look at the magnetic resonance process and the instrumentation necessary for its implementation in this section. The MR process can be broken up into four distinct phases: a preparatory alignment phase, excitation, signal detection, and image generation. Let us look at each of these in turn.

PREPARATORY ALIGNMENT PHASE

All matter, of course, is composed of molecules and atoms. Atoms, in turn, contain nuclei that have different numbers of protons and neutrons. What may not be known is the fact that nuclei have an inherent spin that is due to the spins associated with the individual component protons and neutrons. If charged particles spin or move in any way, a magnetic field is generated around them. Thus, the nucleus in fact has a magnetic field or magnetic moment associated with it due to the fundamental spin properties of its component nucleons. Even the neutrons, which are uncharged, contribute to the spin properties of the nucleus since they in turn are made up of charged particles. The magnitude of the magnetic field associated with any particular nucleus depends on the degree to which the magnetic fields of the individual nucleons add to or cancel each other. In general, nuclei with an even number of protons and an even number of neutrons (even-even nuclei) have zero spin magnetic moment. Examples of these are ^{12}C, ^{16}O, ^{32}S, and ^{40}Ca. Odd-atomic-numbered nuclei with an odd number of neutrons have much stronger magnetic fields associated with them. These "odd-odd" nuclei are most amenable for imaging. Examples of these include ^{1}H, ^{13}C, ^{19}F, and ^{31}P. The odd-even nuclei tend to have intermediate-strength magnetic fields.

Table 1-10

Nucleus	Spin quantum number	Natural abundance, %	Gyromagnetic ratio ($\times 10^{-7}$ MHz/T)	Relative sensitivity for equal number of nuclei at constant field (relative to ^{1}H), %
^{1}H	½	100	42.56	100
^{13}C	½	1.1	10.7	0.25
^{14}N	1	99.6	3.1	0.20
^{15}N	½	0.36	4.3	0.10
^{19}F	½	100	40.1	0.94
^{31}P	½	100	17.2	0.41

Adapted from House 1983.

The magnetic resonance process will depend critically on the net magnetic moment of the nucleus. Of the biologically important nuclei it is the hydrogen nucleus which provides the greatest overall sensitivity to the MR process (see Table 1-10). This is because of both its high magnetic moment and its great abundance in the body in the form of water and other biologically important molecules. Though much interest and research is certainly going on in sodium imaging as well as imaging of other biologically important nuclei, all practical clinical MR imaging is presently done with hydrogen nuclei. We can understand why MRI is so much more sensitive than CT scanning when we realize that the differences in water content (and thus hydrogen content) of biological tissues are greater than the corresponding differences in x-ray attenuation upon which CT depends.

We have established that a magnetic field may exist around any given nucleus. The particular configuration of this magnetic field is always of the dipole type; that is, there are distinct north and south poles. The alignment of the north and south poles defines what is referred to as a magnetic vector. Thus, if a nucleus has a magnetic vector, that vector will always have some magnitude and will be aligned in some particular direction in space. In the case of a spinning nucleus, the vector is aligned perpendicular to the plane of spin as seen in Figure 1-37A. In an extended medium all the various nuclei, because of random interactions with neighboring nuclei and

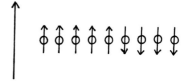

A
MAGNETIC FIELD OF A NUCLEUS

B
RANDOM ORIENTATION OF NUCLEI

C
EXTERNAL MAGNETIC FIELD PRESENT

Figure 1-37   A. Individual nucleus possessing spin manifests a magnetic field directed perpendicular to the plane of spin. This defines a magnetic dipole with north and south poles, and we say the nucleus has a magnetic moment or vector.   **B.** In a medium, individual nuclei with their individual magnetic vectors align randomly. There is no net external magnetic field since they will all cancel each other out.   **C.** When an external magnetic field (B_0) is present, the nuclei of hydrogen, for instance, line up either in the same direction as B_0 (parallel) or in the opposite directon of B_0 (antiparallel). There is only a slight excess aligned in the parallel direction.

with thermal environments, have their magnetic vectors aligned at random in all directions throughout the medium. These vectors will add to or cancel each other (see Figure 1-37B). As a result the overall medium does not have an external magnetic field because each nucleus cancels each other within that medium for the randomly oriented nuclei. Such is the case for biological tissues, which do not normally have externally detectable magnetic fields. Yet the potential for magnetic effects is there since tissues in fact contain nuclei that have magnetic vectors which if properly manipulated can be made to be externally detected.

If the medium is placed in a strong external magnetic field (usually referred to as the B_0 field) the magnetic vectors of the individual nuclei will tend to align with this external magnetic field. Hydrogen, for instance, has two possible alignments, one for the magnetic vector to line up in the same direction as the external magnetic field (referred to as a parallel alignment) and the other for the magnetic vector to align in the direction opposite to the magnetic field (antiparallel alignment) as seen in Figure 1-37C. The parallel direction is a lower-energy state, and as a result a slight excess number of protons are aligned in this direction as compared with the antiparallel direction. Since these two vectors are in opposite directions, they tend to cancel out. Because of the slight excess in the parallel directions, however, some net magnetization will remain in the parallel direction. The magnitude of this net magnetization varies with the strength of the B_0 field, but in general it is due to only about one to three excess parallel aligned protons for every million protons in the medium. Only these relatively few protons enter into the MR process.

One additional very important phenomenon occurs when the nuclear magnetic vectors are under the influence of an external magnetic field: the magnetic vectors will not line up exactly but rather will precess around the direction of the magnetic field. That is, the vector will circle around the B_0 direction as seen in Figure 1-38A. This precession occurs with a particular frequency. Equation (10) shows the relationship between the frequency of precession and the applied external magnetic field.

$$F = KB_0 \qquad (10)$$

In Equation (10), B_0 is the magnitude of the external magnetic field and K is a constant for each different nucleus called the gyromagnetic constant. For hydrogen the gyromagnetic constant equals 42.56 megahertz (MHz) per tesla. Equation (10), also referred to as the Larmor equation, is a fundamental relationship governing the MR process. The tesla is a unit of magnetic field strength and is numerically equal to 10,000 gauss. The gauss is also a measure of magnetic field strength. To give a sense of magnitude for this unit, the natural magnetic field around the earth is approximately ¼ gauss.

Table 1-10 shows the constant K as well as other physical data for various isotopes of interest in medical practice.

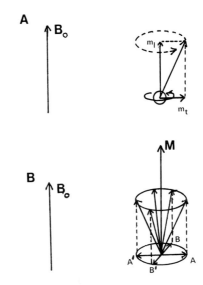

Figure 1-38 **A.** Individual nuclear magnetic vector precessing around the B_0 field. There will be only a couple of protons out of every million whose magnetic field will remain uncancelled and precessing parallel to the external field. Each of these nuclei will have a transverse (m_t) and a longitudinal (m_l) component to the precessing magnetic vector at any instant. **B.** When the ensemble of all nuclei in a particular region of space is considered, each is in a random position in its precessional cycle. As a result all of the transverse components will cancel out (A cancels with A', B with B', etc.). There will, however, be a net longitudinal component since vectors all add up in this direction. This resulting longitudinal component is called the bulk magnetization vector (M).

Figure 1-38*B* shows that the magnetic vectors for the ensemble of all participating nuclei at any one region in space precessing around the static external magnetic field essentially form a cone of vectors. These randomly rotate around the external field. If we look at the projections of each of these vectors onto the transverse plane (the horizontal plane), we see that each vector precesses in a random orientation relative to every other vector, and since there are no preferred directions in space, there are just as many vectors in one direction as in any other direction. In this case, then, all these vectors cancel out in the transverse plane. (In Figure 1-38*B*, *A* cancels with *A'*, *B* with *B'*, etc.) As a result, for any point in the medium, no net magnetic vector exists in the transverse plane. However, when one looks at the projections of the vectors on the longitudinal (up and down or vertical) axis, one sees that each vector in fact adds to every other vector along this longitudinal axis and that a large net longitudinal

vector results composed of the sum of all the various precessing vectors. This net magnetization, also called the bulk magnetization vector (*M*), is seen to lie entirely in the longitudinal direction. At this point we say that the system is in dynamic equilibrium and is relaxed.

We will discuss at length the detection of signals in another section, but suffice it to say here that a signal will be generated whenever there is a net transverse component. In the equilibrium condition just described there is no net transverse component to the bulk magnetization and no net signal is detected. However, any displacement away from equilibrium will shift some magnetization away from the longitudinal direction onto the transverse plane and then a signal will be generated. All these steps are summarized in Table 1-11.

The next step in the MR process is to excite the nuclei, purposely cause a displacement away from the longitudinal alignment, and thus increase transverse magnetization.

Table 1-11   Summary of the MR Preparatory Phase

1. Each nucleus in the medium possesses a magnetic moment due to the inherent spin of its nucleus.

2. The medium possesses no overall externally detectable magnetization since all the individual nuclei are aligned randomly and cancel each other's magnetic fields.

3. When placed in a strong external magnetic field, the nuclear magnetic moments align themselves in either the parallel or the antiparallel directions and in addition precess around the external field direction with frequency given by the Larmor equation ($F = KB_0$).

4. A slight excess population of nuclear magnetic vectors aligned in parallel direction do not cancel out with antiparallel vectors. This yields a net magnetization in the parallel direction (in the direction of the magnetic field).

5. The magnetic vectors precessing in the parallel direction will have their transverse plane projections all cancel out at each point in space because of their random motions. The vectors, however, add up in the longitudinal direction, giving the medium a bulk magnetization along the applied external magnetic field direction. This is the equilibrium or relaxed state.

6. No signal will be detected when the system is in the equilibrium state since no transverse magnetic component exists. However, a signal will be produced when the system is disturbed away from the equilibrium state.

THE EXCITATION PROCESS

We have already seen that under equilibrium conditions no net signal is detected since the net bulk magnetization vector (from now on we will call it the magnetization vector) is entirely along the longitudinal direction. A signal will be detected only if there is some net magnetization along the transverse axis. In the MR process, the intent is to purposely excite nuclei away from the longitudinal alignment into the transverse plane and thus create a signal. As the nuclei relax (return to equilibrium) this signal decays at a time rate characteristic of the particular chemical and tissue milieu of the hydrogen nuclei and will convey information as to the tissue properties at each point in the medium.

What form of energy can be utilized to excite these hydrogen nuclei and their magnetic vectors as they precess around the direction of the external field? Radio-frequency electromagnetic waves are capable of doing just that. The reason for this can be understood by going back to Equation (10), the Larmor relationship. The precessional frequency in megahertz specified there is the key to exciting the nucleus. That is, if one comes in with magnetic energy varying at exactly the Larmor frequency, a resonance absorption effect occurs wherein energy is transferred to the nucleus and the nucleus becomes excited. The frequency expressed in the Larmor relationship in fact falls in the radio-frequency (RF) range for nuclei of clinical interest. To further understand this resonance effect we remember that electromagnetic radiation does in fact have electric and magnetic properties. The magnetic component of these waves having magnitude which we call B_1 is of interest here. Additionally, we know that this magnetic component varies sinusoidally. If the frequency of the RF sinusoidally varying B_1 field exactly matches the Larmor frequency, resonance absorption of RF energy occurs. The net effect is that the bulk magnetization vector is tipped in space away from the longitudinal alignment and into the transverse plane. Additionally, where before all the individual vectors were randomly precessing around the B_0 direction, they now become coherently bundled together so that not only are they tipped toward the transverse plane but they are all spinning in phase relative to each other (phase coherence). This means that they no longer cancel out in the transverse plane. Rather, there is now a very large net transverse plane magnetization. Depending on how long the exciting RF energy is on, the tip angle will increase. Thus, one can tip the vector to any angle such as 90°, 180°, or 270°, as seen in Figure 1-39A. The actual manner in which the magnetization vector is displaced is also seen in this figure. Essentially what occurs is that the RF wave provides a torque on the bulk vector such that the angle with respect to the longitudinal axis increases, resulting in a spiraling precessional motion of the vector away from the original longitudinal alignment. This motion traces out the surface of a sphere as the vector is rotated from equilibrium (0°) to the desired tip angle. As the magnetization vector spirals down, the longitudinal magnetization is reduced. For instance, as seen in Figure 1-39A, at equilibrium (position 1) full magnetization (vector height A) exists.

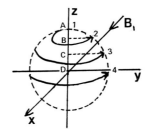

A RF EXCITATION: STATIONARY FRAME

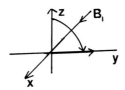

B RF EXCITATION: MOVING FRAME

C LONGITUDINAL AND TRANSVERSE MAGNETIZATION

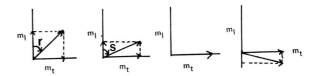

Figure 1-39 **A.** When a radio-frequency wave of appropriate frequency is incident on the nuclei at equilibrium, the magnetic field component B_1 of that RF wave provides a torque such that the magnetization vector precesses in spiral fashion away from the original longitudinal alignment. Longitudinal magnetization goes from maximum (position 1, tip angle 0°) to zero (position 4, tip angle 90°). At intermediate positions (2 and 3) longitudinal magnetization is of intermediate value. Corresponding to each position, the transverse magnetization builds up from zero at position 1 to maximum at position 4. **B.** It is common to use the moving frame representation of excitation whereby the original magnetization vector is tipped directly from the original longitudinal alignment to any tip angle. Here we have a tip angle of 90°. **C.** During excitation over any angle (r or s, for instance) m_l steadily decreases while m_t steadily increases. At 90°, m_l is zero and m_t is maximum. Beyond 90°, m_l assumes negative values while m_t begins to decrease.

At position 2 and 3 there is only a partial longitudinal magnetization projection (vector heights B and C). Notice that we now also have some signal-producing transverse magnetization present (vector lengths B_2 and C_3). At position 4 (90° tip angle) there is zero longitudinal and maximum transverse magnetization (vector length D_4). For simplicity's sake, it is common to depict this spiraling precessional motion as viewed from a moving frame of reference, that is, as if one were riding on the vector. In such a frame of reference the magnetic vector is represented as directly rotating from the longitudinal Z axis to the transverse axis as seen in Figure 1-39B.

What is important to realize here is that RF energy can in fact excite the nuclei of interest and that such excitation results in the perturbation of the equilibrium longitudinal alignment to create a transverse component. This transverse component can generate a detectable electrical signal. It should also be noted that the RF energy incident on the tissues is of such low energy and frequency that it does not disturb the electrostatic bonds of the constituent atoms and molecules within the tissues so that there are no other effects perturbing the MR process.

When the RF field is turned off, the hydrogen protons will be at some given state of excitation manifested by the magnetic vector at some angle relative to the longitudinal axis and generating some signal from the transverse magnetization induced. Individual nuclei will gradually recover back to the longitudinal alignment by losing excitational energy to the overall thermal environment. We call such interactions spin lattice interactions. Nuclei can also exchange energy between themselves and the immediately neighboring nuclei. These interactions cause a dephasing of the individual spinning vectors; that is, nuclear spins which were originally in

phase immediately after excitation interact with each other and rapidly lose their phase coherence. These we call spin-spin interactions. The time constant associated with recovery of the longitudinal magnetization (spin-lattice interactions) is given by T_1, and the time constant associated with loss of phase coherence (spin-spin interactions) is given by T_2. Both of these processes lead to the loss of transverse magnetization and a consequent loss in the detected signal.

SIGNAL DETECTION AND SIGNAL DECAY PROCESSES

We have already seen that RF energy can excite the nuclear spin system, causing the magnetization vector to reorient in space and thus create some transverse magnetization and consequently a detectable signal. But just how is this signal detected? Figure 1-39C shows the magnetization vector M at some intermediate tip angle Q. Note that the vector has projections in both the longitudinal (m_l) and transverse axis (m_t). At a greater tip angle r, m_t is larger and m_l smaller. At the 90° angle m_t is at a maximum while m_l is zero. If M is tipped beyond 90° then m_t decreases while m_l now starts assuming negative values. One can determine the relative amount of transverse magnetization by providing a coil of wire nearby. As the magnetization vector precesses, it induces an electrical signal in the wire coil. This is merely the phenomenon of electromagnetic induction that governs, for instance, the operation of electrical transformers and other devices familiar in x-ray instrumentation. The magnitude of the induced signal is dependent on the angle that exists at a particular moment between the vector and the wires in the coil. A maximum signal will be induced when the vector is cutting across the coil at 90° which corresponds to the situation when transverse magnetization is maximum. As the magnetization angle decreases, the transverse component (m_t) decreases and consequently the signal decreases. It is crucial to emphasize that *the signal detected in MR always*

Table 1-12   Summary of the MR Excitation Phase

1. Magnetic component (B_1) of an RF wave with frequency exactly matching the Larmor precessional frequency provides a torque on the longitudinal magnetization vector.

2. Magnetization vector begins to precess in a spiraling motion away from the longitudinal alignment. As a result the longitudinal magnetization is reduced and the transverse magnetization increases.

3. Nuclei will return to the relaxed original state (longitudinal alignment) with relaxation times (T_1 and T_2) characteristic of particular tissue milieu nuclei sit in.

4. Transverse magnetization component provides a detectable signal allowing the determination of spin relaxation rates as system returns to equilibrium state.

depends entirely on the amount of transverse magnetization present. This therefore forms the basis for signal detection and provides the means of determining m_t and m_l, as will be seen shortly. As the nuclei return to the ground state by losing energy to the thermal lattice environment (via spin-lattice interactions), the magnetic vector gradually returns to the original longitudinal alignment. But as this occurs, the projection on the transverse axis would be expected to gradually diminish and the signal detected would likewise also gradually diminish. The actual manner in which the signal is expected to diminish is exponential.

We define T_1 relaxation in terms of the longitudinal magnetization recovery; specifically T_1 is defined for 63.2 percent recovery as seen in Figure 1-40A. Figure 1-40A also shows different T_1 recovery times expected for a solid as, for instance, when compared with a liquid. In a solid, molecules are closer and are more directly coupled to each other; as a result their energy loss due to spin-lattice interactions is more rapid, and T_1 will be correspondingly shorter. Different biological tissues will also exhibit different T_1's.

In addition to spin-lattice interactions, the nuclei immediately start undergoing spin-spin interactions. These involve individual spins interacting with other spins in their immediate local neighborhood. In this process, energy is transferred back and forth between nuclei, speeding up some and slowing down others. As a result, the initial phase coherence (e.g., vectors precessing in phase) which existed during excitation is degraded. This dephasing drives the MR signal to zero since the individual vectors revert to their random dephased orientations with subsequent cancellation of each other and as a result the transverse magnetization goes to zero independent of longitudinal recovery. The rate at which the vectors dephase and thus the rate at which the signal decays is given by a second time constant, the T_2 relaxation time. Figure 1-40B shows the signal diminishing to zero as dephasing progresses. T_2 is defined in a manner similar to but not exactly like that of T_1. T_2 represents the time necessary for signal to be reduced down to 36.8 percent of its original value. The choice of 36.8 percent signal remaining

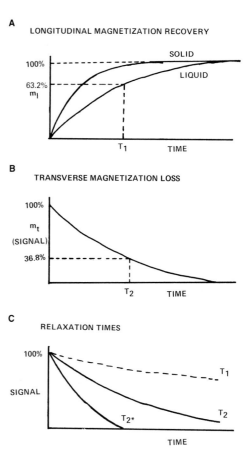

Figure 1-40 **A.** After a 90° RF excitation pulse the longitudinal magnetization begins to recover. T_1 represents the time constant of this recovery and is defined for 63.2 percent recovery. Also shown is the expected elongation in T_1 for a liquid as compared with a solid. **B.** Loss of transverse magnetization (the signal) is principally due to dephasing and is usually very rapid compared with recovery of the longitudinal magnetization. T_2 is the time necessary for signal to decay to 36.8 percent of its original value. **C.** T_2^* decay rate is due to local nonhomogeneities of the magnet. It is the dominant dephasing mechanism and drives the detected signal to zero very quickly. True T_2 signal is shown for the case where T_2^* is absent. T_1 (dashed curve) is relatively long and its signal would normally not be seen.

is not entirely arbitrary—36.8 percent is merely the reciprocal of the exponential number (2.718). This particular factor (and its complement, 63.2) is chosen since it simplifies the mathematical equations related to exponential phenomenon. In general, T_2 values are roughly one-tenth the values of T_1 for biological tissues, T_1 being in hundreds of milliseconds and T_2 in tens of milliseconds.

One more level of complication beyond the two relaxation mechanisms given by T_1 and T_2 must be described. An additional mechanism that contributes to spin-spin interactions is due to the fact that the external magnetic field is not totally uniform. It does have local nonhomogeneities. In general, these local nonhomogeneities serve to enhance spin-spin interactions and speed up the dephasing process and consequently the signal decay. Thus in a simple MR experiment what one would principally measure after excitation is usually the loss of signal due to dephasing as a result of the local magnetic field nonhomogeneities. This dephasing is so rapid that it masks all the T_2 and T_1 signal information. This relaxation time is referred to as T_2^*, and as mentioned previously, it is related to the quality of the magnets and its homogeneity. There is no relationship between it and the tissue properties we desire to study. In a clinically useful MR procedure, one must eliminate the influence of T_2^* and thus get at the more interesting T_1 and T_2 rates.

We now can illustrate the simplest of MR experiments referred to as the free induction decay (FID)

process (Figure 1-41A). The FID is described as follows: a 90° RF pulse is given. This tips the magnetization entirely onto the transverse plane with a correspondingly large signal detected. Notice that the magnitude of this signal is dependent on the number of nuclei (spin density) participating in this process and would be characteristic of the tissue properties at a given point. After cessation of the excitation pulse, all the individual nuclei are in phase with each other. But these rapidly lose their phase coherence owing to spin-spin interactions induced by local magnetic field nonhomogeneities as well as to a lesser extent the true T_2 interactions, and m_t rapidly goes to zero. Figure 1-40C shows the resulting loss of signal that occurs. The T_2^* relaxation dominates the signal in that it quickly drives it to zero. If T_2^* were absent, the signal would follow the T_2 curve. However, T_2 in turn masks the relatively long T_1 relaxation signal. How to unravel T_1 from T_2 from T_2^* is the subject of the next section. Notice in Figure 1-41A that longitudinal magnetization continues to grow and eventually reaches maximum value. If the original tip angle was 180° instead of 90°, an inversion occurs and longitudinal magnetization is maximum in the negative direction (Fig.

A

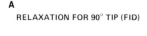

RELAXATION FOR 90° TIP (FID)

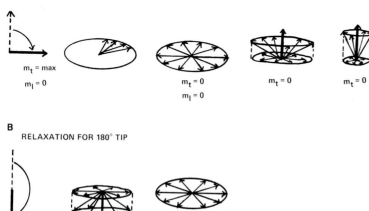

m_t = max
m_l = 0

m_t = 0
m_l = 0

m_t = 0

m_t = 0

m_t= 0
m_l = max

B

RELAXATION FOR 180° TIP

m_t = 0
m_l = max

m_t = 0
m_l = 0

Figure 1-41 Dephasing of vectors. **A.** After a 90° tip angle (FID), the vector rapidly dephases until $m_t = 0$ and $m_l = 0$. No signal is possible after this; however, longitudinal magnetization continues to recover until equilibrium is attained ($m_t = 0$, m_l = max). **B.** If a 180° tip angle is used, the longitudinal magnetization is maximum but negative. No signal is possible since $m_t = 0$. As time goes on, the vectors dephase and m_l assumes smaller negative values. Since vectors are dephased no signal is possible. When vectors arrive at the transverse plane, $m_t = 0$, $m_l = 0$. Progress after this is the same as for the FID response.

1-41*B*). After the cessation of the pulse, as was true of the FID, dephasing proceeds and m_t goes to zero. However, m_l steadily diminishes to zero and then continues growing (recovering) until it becomes a maximum in the positive direction.

Saturation Recovery

To determine T_1 various pulse sequences have been designed. One of these is the saturation recovery pulse sequence.

The saturation recovery pulse sequence is merely a repeated FID sequence, e.g., a series of 90° RF pulses is given as is shown in Figure 1-42*A*. Also shown is the signal which is generated after each pulse. Remember that after each 90° pulse, all of the magnetic vectors are in phase and immediately start to dephase as well as spiraling back to the longitudinal position. (We will indicate the ensemble of dephased vectors as dashed and the in-phase signal-producing vectors as solid throughout this chapter.) Since the 90° pulses are repeated, the second 90°, for instance, will catch the vectors at some intermediate position before they have completely recovered to their longitudinal alignment and will project them 90° into the next quadrant as seen in Figure 1-42*B*. Here there is a net vector projection onto the transverse axis and a signal results. The magnitude of this signal depends on the degree of T_1 relaxation which has occurred at each point. Therefore, we have a way of distinguishing between different T_1's and the different tissue they represent. For instance, if the longitudinal magnetization has recovered to position 1 and the second 90° pulse is given, then these dephased vectors are rephased and are projected 90° into the next quadrant and yields a signal corresponding to the transverse magnetization signal S_1. If T_1 is short, vectors have recovered to position *2* and will project to a larger signal S_2 after the 90° pulse. If a period of time greater than the T_1 values of the tissues in question T_1 elapses before the 90° pulse is repeated, the spin system recovers closer to the full longitudinal magnetization value and subsequent pulses will not distinguish between the different T_1 values as well (point 3 in Figure 1-42*C*).

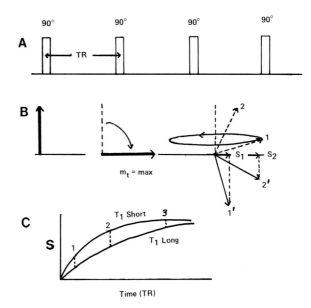

Figure 1-42   A. Saturation recovery. Saturation recovery pulse sequence consisting of a series of 90° pulses separated by some repetition time (TR). A signal whose magnitude correlates with spin density and whose fall-off is governed mainly by T_2^* is detectable after each pulse.   **B.** T_1 can be determined from the saturation recovery sequence by repeating the sequence such that only partial longitudinal recovery has occurred for subsequent pulses. For instance, dephased vectors (dashed) at position 1 yield no signal; however when they are projected 90° to position 1′ they once again are coherent (all add up) and they yield a signal (S_1). A shorter T_1 tissue would have recovered to position 2 and be projected 90° such that signal S_2 is higher.   **C.** Plot of signal magnitude as a function of TR. Contrast is given by the relative T_1 differences between the differing tissues. At short TR (point 1) and long TR (point 3) relatively little contrast results. Higher contrast is found at intermediate TR values (point 2).

If repetition times are short relative to T_1, longitudinal magnetization has only slightly recovered and subsequent 90° pulses will yield both relatively low signals and little signal differences and consequently little contrast. Obviously we must configure an optimal TR timing to achieve both large signal strengths and greater T_1 contrast differences. Sometimes we refer to the above pulse sequence as "partial saturation," partial in the sense that usually TR is sufficiently short that the system recovers only partially before the next pulse is applied. Equation (11) shows the magnitude of the signal as a function of the various timing parameters:

$$S_{ps} = N\,[1 - \exp\,(-TR/T_1)] \qquad (11)$$

where N = a constant dependent on the number of protons present (spin density) and exp represents the exponential function which all MR signal decay processes follow. From Equation (11) it is seen that the signal depends on the ratio TR/T_1 or the fraction that TR represents relative to T_1. It is this fraction which determines the degree of longitudinal recovery occurring between the different tissues (or T_1 weighting) and thus the contrast between them.

The saturation recovery sequence is also applicable in determining proton-weighted images. In Equation (11), if TR is sufficiently long to allow full recovery; then the exponential term goes to zero and the signal is related only to proton density. Since TR intervals are relatively short, there is a high duty cycle for data sampling. However, the saturation recovery sequence is quite sensitive to irregularities in the tip angle accuracy and consistency, as well as having a relatively low contrast scale available as compared, for instance, with inversion recovery. As a result, the latter is usually invoked to obtain T_1-weighted images.

Inversion Recovery

Inversion recovery is a two-pulse sequence used to produce T_1-weighted images. Specifically a 180° pulse is given which inverts the magnetization vector into the 180° antiparallel direction. Immediately after the cessation of the pulse, even though all the vectors are in phase, there is no signal since there is no net transverse magnetization. As time proceeds and vectors recover to longitudinal position, dephasing occurs which prevents a signal from developing. After some appropriate interval of time, called the inversion time TI, the different vectors have recovered to varying decrees according to their T_1 values and a 90° pulse is given. This pulse has the effect of placing the magnetization vector into the next quadrant and of rephasing the spins and thus providing a measurable signal. This signal will depend on T_1 as seen in Figure 1-43.

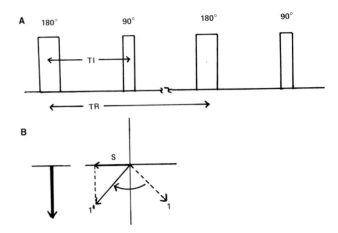

Figure 1-43   A. Inversion recovery pulse sequence consisting of a 180° pulse followed by a 90° pulse after inversion time interval TI. The 90° pulse rephases the spins and allows for a signal readout which depends on the amount of relaxation or recovery which has occurred.

B.   After inversion if dephased vector has progressed to position 1 then after 90° tip it will be at position 1′ and in phase, yielding some signal S.

What occurs is that during the interval TI the magnetization vector reverts to its original longitudinal alignment, at any given time it has recovered some fractional amount, as at position 1 in Figure 1-43B. When the 90° pulse is given, the spins are rephased and shifted 90° to position 1′. At that instant, they have a projection along the transverse axis which constitutes the signal S. The signals generated are dependent on the inversion time TI and magnitude of the TI of the tissues, as can be seen in Figure 1-44A. Correspondingly the image contrast between long and short TI tissues is determined by differences in transverse magnetization for any particular TI. For instance, it can be seen in Figure 1-44 that if the magnetization vector is at position 1, a 90° pulse will drive the magnetization such that a signal S_1 on the negative side results. If the magnetization vector is at position 2 when the 90° pulse is given, no signal is generated since the vector would be projected totally onto the negative longitudinal axis (position 2′) where no transverse magnetization exists. If it is at position 3 a positive signal S_3 results. If we plot the values of the signal as a function of T_1, curves similar to Figure 1-44B (solid curve) result. It is, however, usual to work with the absolute vaues of the signal (dashed portion) at all times to avoid phase effects. Figure 1-44C illustrates how image contrast is generated between two tissues having different T_1 times and plotting absolute values of the signal with varying TI. Image contrast generated at any TI is just the difference in the magnitude of signals produced by the different T_1 tissues. One notes that contrast is relatively low at both short TI (point 1) and long TI (point 4). This is true since at short TI little time has been given to allow a separation in magnetization vectors; at longer TI almost full longitudinal recovery of the different TI tissues has occurred and therefore there is very little difference between them.

One interesting aspect of MR imaging is the fact that relative contrast can be inverted; that is, under one set of timing conditions a particular tissue may appear light and under other timing conditions that tissue may appear dark. This can be seen in Figure 1-44C, where short T_1 (white matter) and long T_1 (gray matter) are plotted. At short TI (region 1 to 2), gray matter, for instance, may have a higher signal and thus appear lighter than the shorter T_1 white matter. At longer T_1 (regions 4 to 6) the shorter T_1 white matter will have a greater signal and thus will appear lighter than the gray matter. Notice also that at point 3, both tissues yield the same signal and therefore there will be no contrast and one could not distinguish between them.

Spin Echo Pulse Sequence

To obtain a T_2-weighted image we must remove the influence of the T_2^* relaxation time. This is done in a unique way as seen in Figure 1-45. One first gives a 90° pulse, which will align the bulk magnetization vector in the transverse plane. Of course, immediately thereafter, dephasing begins to occur. This dephasing, as explained previously, is due to both true T_2 spin-spin interactions, as well as spin-spin interactions due to the local nonhomogeneities of the external magnetic field. As discussed previously, with time the faster precessing vectors separate away from the slower precessing vectors, causing the transverse magnetization and consequently the signal to go to zero. At an appropriate time interval (TE/2), we add an additional 180° pulse. This 180° pulse is designed to drive the vectors around to the opposite side of the transverse plane such that the precessing vectors are now moving toward the original starting

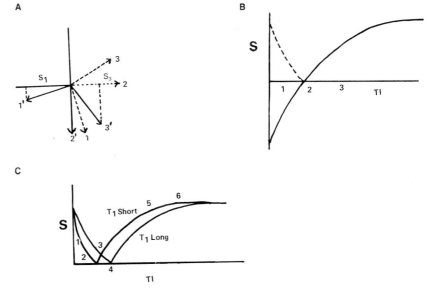

Figure 1-44 In inversion recovery, the magnitude of the signal detected depends on the time interval TI as well as the magnitude of T_1 for the tissues. **A.** Here we see a signal S_1 resulting from a TI such that the dephased vector is arrested at position 1 and which after a 90° pulse is projected to position 1'. Position 2 when projected 90° gives zero signal at 2' (no transverse magnetization) and signal S_3 is gotten when vector 3 is projected 90° to 3'. **B.** Plot of signals resulting as function of TI. Solid curve shows both negative (region 1) and positive signals (regions 2 and 3). In practice only the absolute values are plotted for region 1 (dashed curve). **C.** Contrast between different tissues having different T_1 values as a function of TI. For instance, at long TI (position 6) there is less contrast than at shorter TI (position 1). Notice the inversion of contrast that occurs between positions 4 and 6 where the shorter T_1 tissues appear brighter in the image (because of large signal) as compared with regions 1 to 3 where longer T_1 tissue appears brighter.

point and consequently the vectors are rephasing. That is, the faster ones are catching up to the slower ones. It can be seen that both the slow and the fast will arrive back at the starting line at the same time and be back in phase at time TE. As soon as the vectors begin rephasing, a signal is detectable (the echo signal). This echo signal increases and finally reaches a maximum when the vectors are totally in phase at time interval TE as seen in Figure 1-45*A* and *B*. In actuality, this rephasing occurs only for

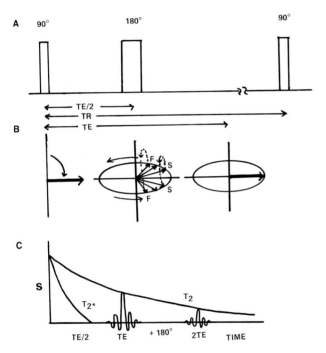

Figure 1-45 The spin-echo pulse sequence.   **A.** After the magnetization vector is tipped 90° into the transverse plane, the individual faster (F) and slower (S) vectors start separating out via spin-spin interactions. This process is dominated by interactions due to local magnet nonhomogeneities (T_2^*). After a time interval TE/2 vectors are flipped 180° onto the opposite side of the transverse plane and rephasing begins till vectors are again in phase coherence at starting point (at time TE). Only the T_2^* interactions are reversible and rephaseable since they are fixed in space. Thus at interval TE the signal obtained is due to the remaining true T_2 interactions.   **B.** Graph of signals decaying from T_2^* and T_2 if T_2^* is absent. As the effects of T_2^* are removed, echo signal increases to the signal value expected if only true T_2 dephasing had been occurring for the period of time TE. Multiple 180° rephasing pulses may be given to collect additional echoes for purposes of signal averaging. These occur, for instance, at 2TE, 3TE, etc., until the T_2 signal is irretrievably dephased away and lost.

dephasing due to the local magnet nonhomogeneities. This is true since these nonhomogeneities are fixed in space and the dephasing they cause is reversible. On the other hand, dephasing due to true T_2 is random and irreversible and will not be affected by rephasing. The signal, in fact, builds up to that corresponding to whatever T_2 dephasing would have been expected if T_2^* had not been present, as seen in Figure 1-45*B*. Notice also that during the echo time interval, the magnetization has had a chance to recover somewhat back to the longitudinal plane; thus the signal may also be influenced by T_1 and be slightly less than its possible maximum value. Also of interest is that if TE is lengthened, more time is given for vectors to dephase and thus the final image is more T_2-weighted.

If TE is very short, very little dephasing occurs and the sequence in fact approximates the partial saturation sequence yielding T_1 information. This can also be appreciated from the spin-echo signal strength equation as follows:

$$S = N \exp\left(-TE/T_2\right)\left[1 - \exp\left(-TR/T_1\right)\right] \quad (12)$$

Here $\exp\left(-TE/T_2\right)$ goes to unity as TE goes to zero (exp of $0 = 1$) and the partial saturation equation (11) depending only on TR and T_1 results. It can also be seen that signal intensity increases as TE or T_1 decreases and TR or T_2 increases (Table 1-13). As is true for the inversion recovery sequence, contrast reversal is also found in the spin-echo sequence. Sometimes to improve signal to noise ratio, multiple echo sampling is done; that is, the spin system is continually rephased, producing succes-

Table 1-13   Signal Strength Increase as Function of Time Parameters

Parameter	Saturation recovery	Inversion recovery	Spin echo
T		Increases	Decrease
TR	Increases	Decreases	Increase
T_1	Decreases	Increases	Decrease
T_2			Increase

T is the interpulse delay time, e.g., TI for inversion recovery and TE for the spin-echo pulse sequence.

sive echoes. Each succeeding echo is of lower magnitude and is located at 2TE, 3TE, etc., as is seen in Figure 1-45C.

It should finally be noted that in clinical practice because of mathematically favorable processing of the echo envelope signal, both saturation recovery and inversion recovery are in fact implemented with a final 180° rephasing pulse. TEs used, however, are so short that final images are essentially T_2-independent.

Before we leave spin-echo imaging, it is interesting to consider an analogy from a foot race that explains the separation of T_2 from T_2^* and features of the spin-echo sequence discussed above. Imagine a foot race with runners lined up at the starting line. Unfortunately, along with the proper runners (analogous to T_2) there are some unwanted runners (analogous to T_2^*). Some of these unwanted runners are very fast and will easily win the race and mask the performance of the proper runners. To eliminate these unwanted runners, we issue them orders that at the signal (corresponding to time TE/2), they are to turn around and run back to the starting line. As soon as the race begins, sure enough, the field is filled with slow and fast runners. At the appropriate time, the unwanted runners turn around and run back toward the starting line. They run at exactly the same velocity that they came out with (the magnetic field nonhomogeneity at a point in space is unchanging). As the faster unwanted runners race off the field and the "faster" ones catch up with the slower unwanted runners back at the starting line, the performance of the appropriate runners which are still racing out on the field becomes more and more apparent (the signal detected is dependent on time T_2 only). At time TE, all the unwanted runners are at the starting line and the field is clear of them. Notice that if TE is very short in this analogy, the appropriate runners have not had enough chance to separate out clearly as to which are faster and which are slower. Thus as we lengthen TE, differences beween runners (tissue T_2) become more pronounced, as we have seen previously.

Up to this point, we have established that given appropriate pulse sequences and timing parameters MR signals weighted for T_1, T_2, or spin density can

Table 1-14 Summary of MR Signal Detection

1. Signal detected always corresponds to the magnitude of the in-phase transverse magnetization.
2. In the original unexcited state, all the magnetization is longitudinal, none transverse, and no signal is available.
3. When the RF wave excites the nuclear spin system, the magnetization vector is tipped away from the longitudinal alignment and a transverse component is formed with a resulting MR signal.
4. Detected signal rapidly goes to zero as magnetization vector is dephased by T_2 and by T_2^* spin-spin interactions. To determine T_2 the effects of T_2^* local magnet nonhomogeneities must be removed.
5. Special pulse sequences are designed to obtain images weighted for proton density, T_1, and T_2 of the biological tissues.

be generated and detected (Table 1-14). MR experiments in this area go back a number of years. What is new for medical imaging is the ability to create image from these parameters; this will now be discussed.

IMAGE GENERATION

To generate an image from the MR signals, one must be able to spatially localize the origin of those signals. To do this, as first suggested by Laturbur (Laturbur 1973), a gradient magnetic field is superimposed upon the external magnetic field. The gradient field is just a linear variation of magnetic intensity across the magnetic field. This means that every point along a given direction experiences a different magnetic field. This, however, would then correspond to a different Lamor frequency [Equation (10)]. Thus, in the presence of the gradient each point in the image precesses at its own particular frequency which then corresponds to a particular spatial position. When the signals along a gradient are detected, they represent the grand sum of all the frequencies present. A means must be had to analyze the various frequencies detected and to determine the amplitude of the signal originating from each particular point along that gradient direction. The mathematical method which is used to accomplish this is called the Fourier transformation. The Fourier transformation has the unique property that it can transform frequency data into spatial position data and as such plays a key role in MRI. In an earlier reconstruction approach one gradient is provided to define a slice, and a second gradient is rotated at 1° intervals to obtain 180 projections around the patient. Data collected are then subjected to conventional back-projection algorithms as in the computerized tomography approach (Laturbur 1973). An approach that is less susceptible to motion artifacts and magnetic field nonhomogeneities as well as having more favorable signal to noise characteristics (Crookes 1983) is referred to as the two-dimensional Fourier transform (2DFT) approach since the Fourier transform has to be done in two directions (Kumar 1975).

To accomplish MR imaging via the 2DFT three gradients must be activated: the slice selection, phase encoding, and readout gradients. These are now discussed.

Slice Selection Gradient

This gradient sets the variation of frequency across the magnetic field (call it the Z direction) such that a slice may be defined. When the slice selection gradient (G_z) is activated, only spins in a particular slice, corresponding to the specific range of RF frequencies used, are excited. Subsequent MR signals must come from this slice. The slice selection gradient can be oriented to yield transverse, coronal, or sagittal views. By increasing the range of frequencies (bandwidth), one in effect increases the slice thickness, as can be seen in Figure 1-46. Notice in this figure that slice thickness can also be varied by increasing the magnitude (or slope) of the gradient. This approach has the effect of encompassing a greater range of frequencies and thus increasing the slice thickness. In practice, the magnitude of the gradients is a small fraction of the overall magnetic field strength.

Phase Encoding Gradient

Having excited the spins in the Z plane, one must proceed to selectively excite spins to define the x-y coordinates. It has been found that rather than varying frequency in all three axes, a phase variation in one of the directions is more advantageous (Edelstein 1980; Kumar 1975). This direction is called the Y direction. In effect, after the spins are excited within a slice, the phase gradient (G_y) alters the phase slightly along each Y column direction. When the phase gradient is turned off, each reverts to precessing at its original frequency. The net effect is that each position within a given Y direction has a slightly different phase angle. That is, each one is slightly ahead of the preceding one. The phase gradient must be repeated for each X position in the matrix array, e.g., 256 times for a 256 × 256 matrix.

Readout Gradient

Finally after the application of the Z and simultaneously with the Y gradients, we apply a final X

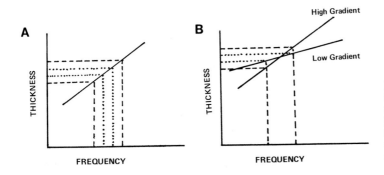

Figure 1-46 Slice thickness dependence on the range of frequencies present and on strength (or slope) of the gradient.   **A.** When a wider range of RF frequencies (dashes) is used, a thicker slice results.   **B.** When a gradient of greater magnitude is used (steeper gradient slope) the thickness which will encompass the fixed frequency range is greater (dashes).

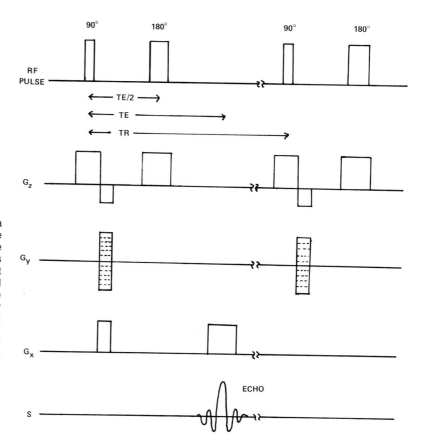

Figure 1-47 Depiction of events occurring in a two-dimensional FT spin-echo pulse sequence. The initial 90° pulse is given in the presence of a slice selection gradient G_z. (Only those spins within this particular slice will be flipped 90°.) The G_z gradient is followed by the phase encoding gradient G_y and a frequency encoded gradient G_x. G_x defines the spatial position of each row in terms of frequency and G_y defines the position along each column in terms of phase. These are followed by a reapplication of G_z when the 180° pulse is given. (This will flip 180° those spins within the slice which had been defined originally by G_z.) Finally G_x is applied as a readout gradient and the spin-echo signal is collected. The whole sequence is repeated for a different value of the phase encoding gradient G_y (dashed lines) for the number of times equal to the matrix size (e.g., 256 times for a 256 × 256 matrix).

axis frequency gradient for reading out the signal. G_x must be applied for each value of G_y. This process essentially goes through the selected slice, interrogating each point defined by the X-Y gradient combination until MR signals from the entire slice are accumulated. Figure 1-47 illustrates the process of gradient application in the specific case of a spin-echo pulse sequence.

It is also interesting to note that the only noise heard by the patient during an MRI scan is from the electric current flowing through the gradient coils, where it experiences a force in the presence of the external magnetic field. As a result the gradient coils "click" back and forth as they are turned on and off. The magnitude of this noise is proportional to the square of the external field strength.

The possibilities of three-dimensional FT techniques are currently much discussed. In this ap-

proach, rather than a narrow (slice selective) bandwidth range of frequencies, a broad (nonselective) band of frequencies is beamed into the patient. This broad frequency range essentially excites the entire volume. Then two variable-phase encoding gradients are applied simultaneously. The data are collected after the readout gradient. Three Fourier transformations must be performed, first along the readout gradient and then along the other two directions. One can reformat these data to yield any combination of planes including oblique ones. Optimal resolution is achieved in 3DFT reformatted images if all the gradient slopes are the same yielding isotropic resolution voxel elements. Anisotropic imaging results if resolution elements are not the same (the voxel shape is not a cube).

There is a distinct signal to noise ratio advantage from the three-dimensional approach in that signals are collected from a larger volume. On the other hand, the penalty paid is increased scan times, especially for isotropic imaging. Compromises can be made to speed up the three-dimensional aproach such as anisotropic imaging, less than 90° flip angles, and shorter TR times. The former affects resolution and the latter two affect signal strength and contrast.

MULTIPLANAR AND MULTIECHO IMAGING ACQUISITION

In general, T_1 relaxation time is relatively long (in hundreds of milliseconds) and limits how short a TR can be used. Additionally the required interpulse delay times (TI or TE) can add up to be considerable when repeating sequences for each point. To efficiently use the inherent TR and delay times, a multiplanar approach can be used. Here one can utilize the TR interval to excite other planes. The result is the acquisition of a multiple number of planar images at the end of the pulse sequence. To illustrate the timing considerations in MR let us look at acquisition times.

Equation (13) can be used to calculate the image acquisition time for a single slice.

$$\text{Time} = (\text{matrix size}) \times (\text{number of acquisitions}) \times (\text{TR}) \quad (13)$$

Notice that this includes not only matrix size and TR but also the number of times the sequence is repeated (number of data acquisitions) for purposes of signal averaging to gain an improvement in the signal to noise ratio. For a simple example, consider a matrix size of 256 × 256, and the number of acquisitions = 2, and TR = 1000 millisec (1 second). Then acquisition time is 512 seconds ($\times 256 \times 2 \times 1$) or 8.53 minutes. For a 10-slice procedure we would, for instance, need 10 × 8.53 or 85.3 minutes. This would be an inordinately long time, and the multiplanar approach becomes very attractive in that rather than repeat this time for each individual slice, multiple slices are acquired utilizing the waiting times between pulses.

The thickness of each slice produced is not rectangular but rather trails off in a gaussian manner (similar to CT slices). One must then be careful of how each plane is excited. The planes are usually acquired in interleaved fashion to avoid crosstalk effects between planes. With interleaving one essentially allows a little more time for recovery before giving the readout pulse.

The multiplanar technique allows not only for the acquisition of multiple planes but for different pulse timing sequences. One can thus, in a particular sequence, obtain two separate and different TE-weighted images. This then can provide additional clinical information to differentiate between different disease states.

OTHER IMAGING FEATURES

Like CT scanning, MR allows for a number of additional imaging features. Examples now follow:

1. Projected scanning. A projected scan is merely a quick scan similar to a "Scoutview" or "Topogram." That is, it is a two-dimensional image wherein all structures are superimposed one on the other. To accomplish this, a broadband RF (non-slice-selective) input is used.
2. True zoom imaging. One can produce a true zoom image by supplying the full gradient not over the entire patient but rather over a limited region of the patient. This has the effect of increasing the gradient over the region of interest. Furthermore, one then applies the full number of available pixels to the desired region. The result is that image is magnified and spatial resolution improves (since each pixel now corresponds to a smaller region of space). In the zoom approach, one must limit the excitation pulses to the specific region of interest to avoid artifacts.
3. Image manipulation. Like CT scanning a number of gray scale and image quality manipulations can be performed. Examples are window width and window level selection. Also available are the usual range of different filtering kernels for such operations as image smoothing and edge

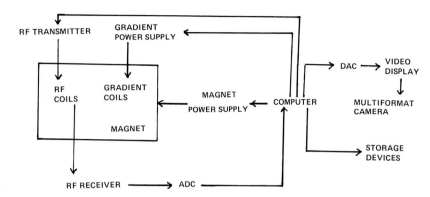

Figure 1-48 Block diagram of MRI imager.

enhancement. Essentially all software functions available to CT can be made available for MRI (distance and angle calculations, histogram analysis, etc.).

INSTRUMENTATION

Figure 1-48 shows a block diagram of a typical MRI system. The major components consist of a large magnet providing the strong magnetic field, the radio-frequency generator and coil, a set of gradient coils with its power supply, and finally the computer, which serves as the control center along with

its peripherals. As in CT, you also have facility for storage and multiformat filming. Given these features, excitational RF energy is generated and made incident on the patient, the signal is detected, and the MR image is finally generated. Let us look closely at some of these instrument components.

Magnets

Magnets are of three general types as currently configured for magnetic resonance imaging. These are permanent, resistive, and superconducting magnets. They are quite distinct in their features (Table 1-15) and result in significant differences in possible

Table 1-15   Major Advantages and Disadvantages of Various Magnet Types

Type	Advantages	Disadvantages
Permanent	Low fringe field	Limited field strength
	Relatively inexpensive upkeep	Relatively heavy
	No cryogens	Temperature-sensitive
	Transverse field (enhanced S/N RF coils)	
Resistive	Good field uniformity	Limited field strength
	Relatively inexpensive	Fringe field problem (for longitudinal fields)
	No cryogens	Field not as stable
	Transverse field possible	Electrical costs higher
Superconducting	Very high fields possible	Expensive to buy and maintain
	High field uniformity	Expensive site preparation
	Very stable field	Cryogens needed
		Quenchable
		Fringe field problem

field strengths, stability, and uniformity as well as expense in their purchase and operation. In all cases, however, a relatively strong, uniform, and temporally stable magnetic field must be produced. To help establish magnetic field uniformity and to counteract the presence of magnetic field warping structures in the environment, small coils (called shim coils) are usually incorporated into the magnet.

The direction of the magnetic field can be aligned either across the bore (transverse) as in the permanent and some resistive magnet types or parallel to the bore (longitudinal), e.g., from head to foot on the patient as in superconducting magnets and certain designs of resistive magnets. These magnet types are now discussed.

Permanent Magnets

Permanent magnets usually consist of two opposing north and south poles within which the patient may be placed. This configuration is as seen in Figure 1-49. The magnetic field in such a configuration is confined between the two poles. These north and south poles are connected via the body of the magnet, creating a return path for the magnetic field lines. Because the magnetic field is directed and confined between the poles, the permanent magnet configuration will result in only minimal magnetic field levels outside and around the magnet. These stray magnetic fields are referred to as fringe fields. The lack of fringe fields greatly facilitates the operation of the MR scanner and the expenses related to its installation. This is true since fringe fields not only affect nearby instrumentation but can also pose a hazard, for instance, to persons wearing cardiac pacemakers. In addition, the interaction of the fringe fields with stationary ferrous structures (structural girders, ducts, etc.) and moving metallic structures (vehicular traffic, elevators, etc.) warps the magnetic field within the magnet gantry with resulting detrimental effects on MR image quality. The continuing upkeep costs for permanent magnets, however, are expected to be relatively low since no field driving electrical power is necessary nor are cryogen replacement costs necessary as is true for superconducting systems.

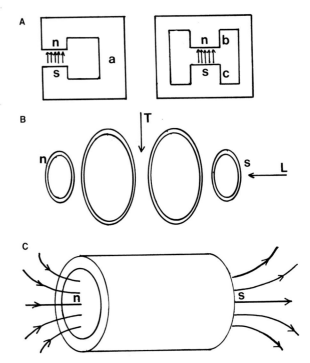

Figure 1-49   A. Permanent magnet of either the C (*left*) or H (*right*) type of pole configurations. These confine the magnetic field between the pole faces. The return path for the magnetic flux is through the body of the magnet, and very little fringe magnetic field is produced. To obtain an iron-core resistive magnet a coil of wire is placed either at **a** or at **b** and **c** for nonpermanent magnet poles. **B.** Resistive magnets are configured with air core Helmholtz coils (two central coils) or a four-coil arrangement as seen above. These coils are arranged around the gantry, and flowing current through these coils generates the desired magnetic field. If the patient is placed along T, a transverse field results. If the patient is placed along L, a longitudinal field results.   **C.** Fringe fields produced by air core resistive and superconducting systems. There is no internal magnetic field line return path. Such a path must be established outside the gantry. Superconducting magnets have coil configured solenoidally around gantry. Magnetic field is maintained without need for continuing electrical current or power. Patient is placed within bore of magnet and magnetic field is longitudinal (along long axis of patient). In both superconducting and air core resistive magnets, significant fringe fields are produced.

One possible disadvantage of the permanent magnet approach is that of relatively large weights (up to and beyond 100,000 pounds). One saving grace, however, concerning weight is that these magnets can usually be shipped and installed in smaller pieces. Another factor is temperature sensitivity; the magnet must be kept under controlled temperature conditions.

Permanent magnets can be made from ceramic materials or from rare earth materials. The latter, however, tend to be more costly and weigh more. Alnico magnets are not used because of possible gradual loss of their field strength. Possible configurations are either the C or H types as per Figure 1-49*A*. Using permanent magnets one need not worry over magnetic field quenching. The quenching phenomenon is characteristically possible for superconducting systems whereby the superconducting state suddenly ceases and there is a sudden reduction and collapse of the magnetic field. Quenching may result in damage to the magnet as well as significant amounts of down time.

One additional very important feature of permanent magnets is the fact that since the magnetic field is confined within and is directed between the pole faces, simple cylindrical RF coils can be designed that provide greater inherent signal to noise characteristics (two to three times better) and correspondingly better image quality.

Resistive Magnets

A resistive magnet is configured with a series of wire coils. These coils are referred to as Helmholtz coils. They are arranged as seen in Figure 1-49*B*. What occurs is that as an electric current flows through the coils, a magnetic field is produced whose direction is perpendicular to the plane of the coils. For optimal field uniformity, the coils should be arranged such that their diameters fall on the surfaces of a sphere. At least four coils in air (air core) are used as a sufficient approximation to produce a homogeneous field. These four coils consist of two large-diameter coils and two of smaller diameter. For clinical scanning, the complete spherical coil arrangement cannot be utilized as there must be at least an opening for the patient. We refer to these type of magnets as resistive since copper from which the coil wires are made provides for a small but yet not insignificant amount of electrical resistance and therefore power consumption. The magnitude of the magnetic field is proportional to the magnitude of the current. The electrical power consumption, however, varies as the square of the current. Thus

to double the magnetic field strength would require quadrupling the electrical power needed to drive the magnets. In addition, considerable heat is produced. The wire coils may in fact be made of hollow copper tubing that allows cooling water to run through to carry off the heat generated. Because of the electrical and heat production problems, resistive magnets are typically limited to field strengths of only up to 0.15 to 0.20 tesla.

Resistive magnets can be configured such that the magnetic field can be either longitudinal (along the length of the patient) or transverse (perpendicular to the patient). The transverse arrangement is obtained by placing the patient at the center of the coils perpendicular to the field lines. To obtain the longitudinal arrangement, the patient is placed down through the bore of the coils parallel to the field lines.

One can also use iron-core resistive magnets. This is accomplished by placing solenoidal coils at region *a* for a C arrangement and at regions *b* and *c* for an H arrangement as seen in Figure 1-49*A*. These iron-core resistive magnets have the advantage of providing a return path for the magnetic field lines and thus having minimal fringe fields beyond the gantry. One important concern with air-core magnets is that fringe fields are produced. There is no internal path for magnetic field lines, and such a path is established outside the gantry.

To date, many consider that resistive magnet technology merely provides a lower-cost, lower-performance alternative to the superconducting systems.

Superconducting Magnets

Superconducting magnet systems operate at very low temperature (near absoute zero). At these temperatures, some metals lose all electrical resistance and flow without additional energy being expended. Under these conditions, very large currents can flow and therefore very large magnetic fields can be produced. Typical units can operate between 0.5 and 2.0 tesla, but there are prototype imaging units operating up to 4.0 tesla. The fringe field problem is present in superconductive systems and is even more critical as these systems operate at much higher magnetic field levels. Unlike air-core Helmholtz coil pair resistive systems, the main field coils are configured in the much simpler solenoidal fashion. This is necessary because of the considerable forces which individual coils would experience. This could result in warping of the coils and the magnetic field. In any case, because of the high currents possible with superconducting systems, the efficiency of Helmholtz coil pairs is not needed. Additionally, for human lengths and for large bores, the solenoidal configuration is quite sufficient. (Crooks 1984; Kaufman 1981) Superconducting systems must be provided with a cryogenic environment to maintain the low temperatures necessary. The coils are thus immersed in liquid helium, surrounded by a vacuum and then a bath of liquid nitrogen. Nitrogen serves to absorb the heat from the environment and to maintain the low temperatures necessary. If there is a loss of helium or loss of the vacuum, the system rises in temperature and the superconducting state is eventually lost, with a resultant collapse of the magnetic field. This is referred to as a "quench" and large electric currents can flow through the conductor which would then revert to operating in the resistive mode. Meltdown of the conductor is then very possible and must be prevented. The material used for the superconductor is NbTi embedded in a copper matrix. In the superconductor state, the copper serves as a heat conductor. When superconductivity is lost, the excess currents flow through the copper and damage to NbTi is avoided.

In addition to high field strengths, another advantage of superconducting systems is the high stability and very high uniformity of the field.

Among the disadvantages is the relatively high cost of purchase and the continuing high cost of operating the system due to cryogen replacement expenses. Because of the large fringe fields produced, siting is also a problem, though this has been minimized recently by using magnetic field containment systems around the magnet gantry or around the room. These field containment systems consist of steel structures that soak up the magnetic fields and greatly reduce the fringe field beyond the containment area.

In addition to the three basic types described above, at least one hybrid system is available commercially (Fonar Corp., Melville, New York). Information on details of this system is proprietary, but presumably it consists of combining technologies from both permanent and resistive magnet systems. It is not clear, however, whether in fact this system is just an iron-core resistive magnet or some other configuration. Other hybrid approaches include (Crooks 1984) using resistive magnets cooled by liquid nitrogen rather than water. This reduces electrical power expended but requires cryogenic technology. Also, one can put iron around resistive or superconductivity magnets that provide a return path for the magnetic field lines and thus reduce fringe field problems.

Gradient Coils

As previously discussed, three gradients in each of three directions must be available to perform MR imaging. These gradients are produced with special additional coils which produce a linearly rising magnetic field superimposed upon the uniform main magnetic field. The magnitude of this gradient field is relatively low and is usually between 0.6 and 1 gauss/cm. A linear gradient can be sufficiently approximated in the magnetic field direction with a Maxwell coil pair. This coil pair is similar to a Helmholtz coil arrangement except that the electric current is flowing in opposite directions. The other two gradients are produced using two Golay coils (Golay 1971). Golay coils consist of opposing coil loops with parallel sides wrapped around the gantry. These coils are displaced one from another by 90° to provide gradients for the two remaining directions.

Since the gradients define spatial position it is important that they be very linear and uniform to within a few percent (Pykett 1983). Their strength must be such that they ride above any nonhomogeneities in the main field magnets. Gradients, along with the bandwidth of the RF pulse, define the slice thickness (see Fig. 1-46) and consequently affect spatial resolution as well as the contrast sensitivity of the system.

Radio-Frequency Coil System

We have seen that to excite the nuclear spin system RF waves must be generated and beamed into the patient. The RF coils used to accomplish this are the so-called head and body coils within which the patient is placed. These coils typically serve as both the transmitter and the receiver of the MRI signal. The design of the coil is of either the saddle shape or solenoidal type. The choice depends on whether the main magnetic field is transverse (perpendicular to the long axis of the patient) or longitudinal (along the long axis of the patient). In the transverse case, we use solenoidal coils. These are simple circularly wound wire loops. If the magnetic field is longitudinal, we must use saddle-shaped coils which are somewhat more complexly configured. The solenoidal RF coils in general provide a signal to noise ratio (SNR) approximately two times that of the saddle-shaped coil of comparable size (Hoult 1976). This enhanced signal to noise ratio can allow for a reduction in imaging time (a factor of 4), or it can allow for an increase in the spatial resolution for the same scan time.

RF field nonuniformities lead to image intensity variations and consequently can also produce errors in the quantitation of T_1 or T_2 values as a function of field position. In all cases, the best RF field uniformity is expected at the center of the coil.

Surface coils have recently gained popularity as a means of significantly increasing the SNR and consequently enhancing spatial resolution and contrast sensitivity. Essentially, a surface coil is merely a coil loop of wire which is placed directly onto the anatomical area to be imaged, and usually serves as the RF receiver coil. The increased SNR of such a surface coil is due to both its small size and its proximity to the region of interest, which allows for enhanced signal reception. One probably minor drawback, however, with surface coils is the possible limited depth response, and the variability in gray scale shading.

Table 1-16   Summary of Coils in MRI

Main field	Configuration
Resistive coils	
Air core	Either 1 coil pair (2 coils) (Helmholtz pair) or 2 pairs (4 coils) whose diameters describe surface of a sphere. Resulting field is either longitudinal or transverse
Iron core	Coil windings are directly around poles of the electromagnet (either C or H configuration). Resulting field is always transverse
Superconducting coils	Windings are solenoidal (around gantry). Conductors are of NbTi filaments in a copper matrix. Resulting fields are always longitudinal
RF coils	
For transverse fields	Solenoidal configuration. Approximately 2 times the SNR advantage over comparable size saddle-shaped coils
For longitudinal fields	Saddle-shaped coils
Surface coil	Circular loop coils placed directly over the anatomical region of interest. Serves as the RF signal receiver
Gradient coils	
Maxwell pair	Pair of coils with current flowing in opposite directions. Used for the slice-selection gradient in the direction of the main field axis
Golay coils	Opposing parallel side coils, curved over the cylindrical surface of the gantry bore. There are 2 sets arranged at a 90° rotation to each other in order to define the two x and y gradient axes
Shim coils	Additional small coils incorporated within gantry to make magnetic field more uniform

Bibliography

AAPM: *Phantoms for Performance Evaluation and Quality Assurance of CT Scanners*, Report Number 1. New York, AAPM, 1978.

AGARWAL SK, FRIESEN EJ, BHADURI D, COURLAS G: Dose distribution from a delta 25 head scanner. *Med Phys* **6**:302–304, 1979.

ALFIDI RJ, MACINTYRE WJ, HOAGAN JR: The effects of biological motion on CT resolution. *Am J Roentgenol* **127**:11–15, 1976.

AMBROSE J: Computerized transverse axial scanning (tomography): Part 2. Clinical application. *Br J Radiol* **46**:1023–1047, 1973.

BAILY NA, KELLER RA, JAKOWATZ CV, KAK AC: The capability of fluoroscopic systems for the production of computerized axial tomograms. *Invest Radiol* **11**:434–439, 1976.

BARNES G, YESTER MV, KING MA: Optimizing computed tomography (CT) scanner geometry. *Proc Soc Photo-opt Eng* **173**:(Med VII) 225–237, 1979.

BASSANO DA, CHAMBERLAIN CC, MOSLEY JM, KIEFFER SA: Physical performance and dosimetric characteristics of the delta 50 whole body/brain scanner. *Radiology* **123**:455–462, 1977.

BATTER S: A philosophy of dose specification for computed tomography. *Med Mundi* **22**:3, 11–12, 1977.

BISHOP CJ, EHRHARDT JC: Modulation transfer function of the EMI head scanner. *Med Phys* **4**:163–167, 1977.

BOYD DP, HERMANNEFELDT WB, QUINN JR, SPARKS RA: "Xray transmission scanning system and method and electron beam Xray scan tube. U.S. Patent 435202-1, September 28, 1982.

BROOKS RA, DICHIRO G: Beam hardening in x-ray reconstructive tomography. *Phys Med Biol* **21**:390–398, 1976a.

BROOKS RA, DICHIRO G: Principles of computer assisted tomography (CAT) in radiographic and radioisotopic imaging. *Phys Med Biol* **21**:689–732, 1976b.

BROOKS RA, DICHIRO G: Slice geometry in computer assisted tomography. *J Comput Assist Tomogr* **1**:191–199, 1977.

BROOKS RA, DICHIRO G: Statistical limitations in x-ray reconstructive tomography. *Med Phys* **3**:237–240, 1976c.

BROOKS RA, DICHIRO G: Theory of image reconstruction in computed tomography. *Radiology* **117**:561–572, 1975.

BROOKS RA, GLOVER AJ, TOLBERT RL, EISNER FA, DIBIANCA FA: Aliasing, a source of streaks in computed tomograms. *J Comput Assist Tomogr* **3**:511–518, 1979.

BRUNDAGE BH, CHOMKE E: Clinical applications of cardiac CT imaging. *Modern Concepts of Cardiovascular Disease* **8**:39–43, August 1985.

CARSON PL, OUGHTON TV, HENDEE WR, AHIYA AS: Imaging soft tissue through bone with ultrasound transmission tomography by reconstruction. *Med Phys* **4**:302–309, 1977.

CHECKLEY DR, ZHU XP, ANTOUN N, CHEN SZ, ISHERWOOD I: An investigation into the problems of attenuation and area measurements made from CT images of pulmonary modules. *J Comput Assist Tomogr* **8**:237–243, 1984.

COHEN G, DIBIANCA FA: The use of contrast-detail-dose evaluation of image quality in a computed tomographic scanner. *J Comput Assist Tomogr* **3**:189–195, 1979a.

COHEN G: Contrast-detail dose analysis of six different computed tomographic scanners. *J Comput Assist Tomogr* **3**:197–203, 1979b.

CORMACK AM, KOEHLER AM: Quantitative proton tomography: Preliminary experiments. *Phys Med Biol* **21**:560–569, 1976.

CRAWFORD CR, KAK AC: Aliasing artefacts in computerized tomography. *App Opt* **18**:3704–3711, 1979.

CROOKS LE, ORTENDAHL D, KAUFMAN L: Clinical efficiency of nuclear magnetic resonance imaging. *Radiology* **146**:123, 1983.

CROOKS LE, KAUFMAN L: Imaging methodology, in James TJ, Margulis AR, eds, in *Bio Medical Magnetic Resonance*, Radiology Research and Education Foundation, 1984.

DICHIRO G, BROOKS RA, DUBAL L, CHEN E: The apical artifact: Elevated attenuation values toward the apex of the skull. *J Comput Assist Tomogr* **2**:65–70, 1978.

DUERINCKX AJ, MACOVSKI A: Polychromatic streak artefacts in computed tomography images. *J Comput Assist Tomogr* **2**:481–487, 1978.

EDELSTEIN WA, HUTCHISON JMS, JOHNSON G, REDPATH T: Spin ways NMR imaging and applications to human whole body imaging. *Phys Med Biol* **25**:751–756, 1980.

Emission computed tomography I. *Semin Nucl Med* vol 10, 1980.

Emission computed tomography II. *Semin Nucl Med* vol 11, 1981.

EXNER GU, ELSASSER U, RUEGSEGGER P, ANLIKER M: Bone densimetry using computer tomography: Parts 1 and 2. *Br J Radiol* **52**:14–28, 1979.

GADO M, PHELPS M: Peripheral zone of increased density in computed tomography. *Radiology* **117**:71–74, 1975.

GENANT HK, ETTINGER B, CANN CE, REISERU; GORDON GS, KOLB FO. Osteoporosis: Assessment by quantitative computed tomography. *Orthop Clin North Am* **16**(3):557–568, 1985.

GLOVER GN, PELC NJ: Nonlinear partial volume artefacts in x-ray computed tomography: *Med Phys* **7**:238–248, 1980.

GOLAY MJE: U/S. Patents Nos. 3569523, 3622869, 1971.

GOODENOUGH DJ, ROSSMAN K, LUSTED LB: Radiographic applications of receiver operating characteristic curves. *Radiology* **110**:89–95, 1974*a*.

GOODENOUGH DJ, ROSSMAN K, LUSTED LB: Factors affecting the detectability of a simulated radiographic signal. *Invest Radiol* **8**:339–344, 1974*b*.

GOODENOUGH DJ, WEAVER KE, DAVIS DO: Potential artefacts associated with the scanning pattern of the EMI scanner. *Radiology* **117**:615–619, 1975.

GOODENOUGH DJ, WEAVER KE, DAVIS DO: Development of a phantom for evaluation and assurance of image quality in CT scanning. *Opt Eng* **16**:52–65, 1977.

GORDON R, HERMAN GT: Three dimensional reconstructions from projections: A review of algorithms. *Int Rev Cytol* **38**:111–151, 1974.

GORDON R, HERMAN GT, JOHNSON SA: Image reconstruction from projections. *Sci Am* pp 56–68, October 1975.

GLYDENSTED C: Gonadal thermoluminescence dosimetry in cranial computed tomography with the EMI scanner. *Neuroradiology* **14**:111–112, 1977.

HAAGA J, MIRALDI F, MACINTYRE W, LIPUMA JP, BRYAN PS, WIESEN E: The effect of mAs variation upon computed tomography image quality as evaluated by invivo and invitro studies. *Radiology* **138**:449–454, 1981.

HERMON G: Demonstration of beam hardening correction in computerized tomography of the head. *J Comput Assist Tomogr* **3**:373–378, 1978.

HINSHAW WS, ANDREW ER, BOTTOMLEY PE, HOLLAND FW, MORRE WS, WORTHINGTON BS: An invivo study of the forearm and hand by thin section NMR imaging. *Br J Radiol* **52**B:6–43, 1979.

HOLLAND GN, HAWKES RC, MOORE WS: Nuclear magnetic resonance (NMR) tomography of the brain: Coronal and sagittal sections. *J Comput Assist Tomogr* **4**:429–433, 1980.

HOULT DI, RICARDS RE: The signal to noise ratio to the nuclear magnetic resonance experiment. *J Mag Res* **24**:71–85, 1976.

HOUNSFIELD N: A Method of and Apparatus for Examination of a Body Part by Radiation such as X-ray or Gamma Radiation. British Patent 1283915, 1972.

HOUNSFIELD N: Some practical problems in computerized tomography scanning, in Ter-Pogossian MM et al (eds.): *Reconstruction Tomography in Diagnostic Radiology and Nuclear Medicine.* University Park Publ., 1977.

HOUSE WV: Theoretical basis for NMR imaging, Chapter 5 in Partain CL, James AE, Rollo FD, Price RR, *Nuclear Magnetic Resonance (NMR) Imaging,* W.B. Saunders Co., 1983.

ISHERWOOD I, PULLON BR, RITCHINGS RT: Radiation dose in neuroradiological procedures. *Neuroradiology* **16**:477–481, 1978.

JONES RC: On the point and line spread functions of photographic images. *J Opt Soc Am* **44**:468, 1954.

JOSEPH PM: Artefacts in computed tomography, in *Radiology of the Skull and Brain: Technical Aspects of Computed Tomography.* vol 5. St. Louis, Mosby, 1981.

JOSEPH PM: Image noise and smoothing in computed tomography (CT) scanners. *Opt Eng* **17**:396–399, 1978a.

JOSEPH PM, SPITAL RD: A method for correcting bone induced artefacts in computed tomography scanners. *J Comput Assist Tomogr* **2**:100–108, 1978b.

JUCIUS RA, KAMBIC GX: Radiation dosimetry in computed tomography. *Proc Soc Photo-Opt Instrument Eng* **127**(Med IV):286–295, 1977.

JUDY PF: The line spread function and modulation transfer function of a computed tomographic scanner. *Med Phys* **3**:233, 1976.

KAK AC: Computerized tomography with x-ray emission and ultrasound sources. *Proc IEEE* **67**:1245–1272, 1979.

KAK AC, JAKOWATZ CV, BAILY NA, KELLER RA: Computerized tomography using video recorded fluoroscopic images. *IEEE Trans BioMed Eng BME* **24**:157–169, 1977.

KAUFMAN SL, CROOKS LE: Hardware for NMR imaging, in Kaufman L, Crook LE, Margulis AR, *Nuclear Magnetic Resource Imaging in Medicine,* IgakuShoin, Publ., 1981.

KIJEWSKI PK, BJARNGARD B: Correction for beam hardening in computed tomography. *Med Phys* **5**:209–214, 1978.

KOEPPE RA, BRIGGER RM, SCHLAPPER GA, LARSEN GN, JOST RJ: Neutron computed tomography. *J Comput Assist Tomogr* **5**:79–88, 1981.

KUMAR A, WELTI D, ERNST RR: NMR Fourier zeugmatography. *J Magn Res* **18**:69–83, 1975.

LATCHAW RE, PAYNE JT, GOLD LHA: Effective atomic number and electron density as measured with a computed tomography scanner: Computation and correlation with brain tumor histology. *J Comput Assist Tomogr* **2**:199–208, 1978.

LATURBUR PC: Image formation by induced local interactions: example employing nuclear magnetic resonance. *Nature* **242**:190–191, 1973.

LEVI C, GRAY JE, MCCULLOUGH EC, HATTERY RR: The unreliability of CT numbers as absolute values. *Am J Radiol* **139**:443–447, September 1982.

LIM ST, SAGE DJ: Detection of subarachnoid blood clot and other flat thin structures by computed tomography. *Radiology* **123**:79–84, 1977.

LIPTON MJ, HIGGINS CB, BOYD DP: Computed tomography of heart: Evaluation of anatomy and function. *J Am Coll Cardiology* **5**:55S–69S, 1985.

LIPTON MJ, BRUNDAGE BH, HIGGINS CH, BOYD DP: Clinical applications of dynamic computed tomography. *Progress in Cardiovascular Diseases* **28**:349–366, 1986.

LITTLETON JT, DURIZCH ML, CROSBY EH, GEORY JC: Tomography: Physical principles and clinical applications, in Robbins LL (ed): *Golden's Diagnostic Radiology*, Sec. 17. Baltimore, Williams & Wilkins, 1976.

MACINTYRE WJ, ALFIDE RJ, HAAGA J, CHERNAK E, MEANY TF: Comparative modulation transfer functions of the EMI and delta scanners. *Radiology* **120**:189–191, 1976.

MAINI R, ISKANDER MF, DURNEY CH: On electro-magnetic imaging using linear reconstruction techniques. *Proc IEEE* **68**:1550–1552, 1980.

MAUE-DICKSON W, TREFLER M, DICKSON DR: Comparison of dosimetry and image quality in computed and conventional tomography. *Radiology* **131**:509–514, 1979.

MCCULLOUGH EC: Factors affecting the use of quantitative information from a CT scanner. *Radiology* **124**:99–107, 1977.

MCCULLOUGH EC: Photon attenuation in computed tomography. *Med Phys* **2**:307–320, 1975.

MCCULLOUGH EC: Specifying and evaluating the performance of computed tomography (CT) scanners. *Med Phys* **7**:291–296, 1980.

MCCULLOUGH EC et al: On evaluation of the quantitative and radiation features of a scanning x-ray transverse axial tomograph: The EMI scanner. *Radiology* **111**:709–715, 1974.

MCCULLOUGH EC, PAYNE JT, BAKER HL, HATTERY RR, SHEEDY PF, STEPHENS DH, GEDGAUDUS E: Performance evolution and quality assurance of computed tomography scanners with illustrations from the EMI, beta and delta scanners. *Radiology* **120**:173–188, 1976.

MCDAVID WD, WAGGENER RG, PAYNE WH, DENNIS MJ: Correction for spectral artefacts in cross sectional reconstruction from x-rays. *Med Phys* **4**:54–57, 1977*a*.

MCDAVID WD, WAGGENER RG, DENNIS MJ, SANK VS, PAYNE WH: Estimation of chemical composition and density from computed tomography carried out at a number of energies. *Invest Radiol* **12**:189–194, 1977*b*.

MEREDITH WJ, MASSEY JB: The effect of x-ray absorption on the radiographic image, in *Fundamental Physics of Radiology*, 2d ed, chap 19. Baltimore, Williams & Wilkins, 1972.

MICHAEL AS, MAFEE MF, VALVASSORI GE, TAN WS: Dynamic computed tomography of the head and neck: differential diagnostic value. *Radiology* **154**:413–419, 1985.

MOORE WS, HOLLAND GN, KNEEL L: The NMR CAT scanner—A new look at the brain. *CT: J Comput Tomogr* **4**:1–7, 1980.

NALCIOGLU O, LOU RY: Post reconstruction method of beam hardening in computerized tomography. *Phys Med Biol* **24**:330–340, 1979.

NEWTON TH, POTTS DG: *Radiology of the Skull and Brain*, Vol 5: *Technical Aspects of Computed Tomography*. St. Louis, Mosby, 1981.

PARTAIN CL, JAMES AE, WATSON JT, PRICE RR, COULAM CM, ROLLO FD: Nuclear magnetic resonance and computed tomography. *Radiology* **136**:767–770, 1980.

PERRY BJ, BRIDGES C: Computerized transverse and axial scanning (tomography): Part III. Radiation dose considerations. *Br J Radiol* **46**:1048–1051, 1973.

PETERS JM, LEWITT RM: Computed tomography with fan beam geometry. *J Comput Assist Tomogr* **1**:429–436, 1977.

PHELPS ME, GADO MH, HOFFMAN EJ: Correlation of effective atomic number and electron density with attenuation co-efficients. *Radiology* **117**:585–588, 1975*a*.

PHELPS ME, HOFFMAN EJ, TER-POGOSSIAN MM: Attenuation coefficients of various body tissues, fluids and lesions at photon energies 18 to 136 Kev. *Radiology* **117**:573–583, 1975*b*.

PICKETT IL: Instrumentation for nuclear magnetic resonance imaging. *Seminars in Nuclear Medicine* **13**:319–328, October 1983.

RAO PS, GREGG EC: Attenuation of monoenergic gamma rays in tissues. *Am J Roentgenol* **123**:631–637, 1975.

RAO PS, SANTOSH K, GREGG EC: Computed tomography with microwaves. *Radiology* **135**:769–770, 1980.

REVAK CS: Mineral content of cortical bone measured by computed tomography. *J Comput Assist Tomogr* **4**:342–350, 1980.

RIEDERER SJ, PELC NJ, CHESTER DA: The noise power spectrum in computed x-ray tomography. *Phys Med Biol* **23**:446–454, 1978.

ROSSMAN K: Image quality and patient exposure. *Curr Probl Radiol* **22**:2–34, 1972.

RUEGSEGGER P, HANGARTNER TH, KELLER HU, HINDERLING TH: Standardization of computed tomography images by means of a material-selective beam hardening correction. *J Comput Assist Tomogr* **2**:184–188, 1978.

RUTHERFORD RA, PULLAN BR, ISHERWOOD I: Measurement of effective atomic number and electron density using an EMI scanner. *Neuroradiology* **11**:15–21, 1976.

SALVOLINI U, CABANIS EA, RODOLLEE A, MENICHELLI F, POSQUINI FU, IBA-ZIZEN MT: Computed tomography of the optic nerve: I. Normal results. *J Comput Assist Tomogr* **2**:141–149, 1978.

SCHULZ RA, OLSON EC, HON KS: A comparison of the number of rays versus the number of views in reconstruction tomography. *Proc SPIE* **127**:25–27, 1977.

SCHWENKER RP: Film selection considerations for computed tomography and ultrasound video photography. *Proc Soc Photo-Opt Instrum Eng* **173** (Med VII): 75–80, 1979

SHEPP LA, STEIN JA: Simulated reconstruction artifacts in computerized x-ray tomography, in Ter-Pogossian M, Phelps M, Brownell GL, Cox JR, Davis DO, Evans RG (eds): *Reconstruction Tomography in Diagnostic Radiology and Nuclear Medicine*, University Park Press, 1977.

SHOPE, T, GAGNE, R, JOHNSON G: A method for describing the doses delivered by transmission x-ray computed tomography. *Med Phys* **8**:488–495, 1981.

SHRIVASTAVA PN, LYNN SL, TING JY: Exposures to patient and personnel in computed axial tomography. *Radiology* **125**:411–415, 1977.

SIEGELMAN SS, ZERHOUNI EA, LEO FP, KHOURI NF, STITIK FP: CT of the solitary pulmonary nodule. *Am J Radiol* **135**:1–13, 1980.

SOM PM, LANZIERI CF, SACHER M, LAWSON W, BILLER HF: Extracranial tumor vascularity: determination by dynamic CT scanning. *Radiology* **154**:401–405, 1985.

SORENSON JA: Technique for evaluating radiation beam and image slice parameters of CT scanners. *Med Phys* **6**:68–69, 1979.

STOCKHAM CD: A simulated study of aliasing in computed tomography. *Radiology* **132**:721–726, 1979.

TER-POGOSSIAN MM: Computerized cranial tomography seminars in roentgenology. **12**:13–25, 1977.

TER-POGOSSIAN MM, PHELPS ME, HOFFMAN EJ, EICHLING JO: The extraction of the yet unused wealth of information in diagnostic radiology. *Radiology* **113**:515–520, 1974.

VILLAFANA T: Advantage of limitations and significance of the modulation transfer function in radiologic practice. *Curr Probl Diagn Radiol* **7**:10, 1978a.

VILLAFANA T, LEE SH, LAPAYOWKER MS: A device to indicate anatomical level in computed tomography. *J Comput Assist Tomogr* **2**:368–371, 1978b.

VILLAFANA T, SCOURAS J, KIRKLAND L, MCELROY N, PARAS P: Health physics aspects of the EMI computerized tomography brain scanner. *Health Phys J* **34**:71–82, 1978c.

WALL BF, GREEN DAC: Radiation dose to patients from EMI brain and body scanners. *Br J Radiol* **52**:189–196, 1979.

WEAVER KE, GOODENOUGH DJ, DAVIS DO: Physical measurements of the EMI computerized axial tomographic imaging system. *Proc Soc Photo-Opt Instrum Eng* **70**:299–309, 1975.

WEHRLI FW, MACTOLL JR, NEWTON TH: Parameter determining the appearance on NMR images. Advanced imaging technique, vol. 2 in Newton TH, Potts DG, eds., *Modern Neuroradiology*, Clavadel Press, 1983.

WEISSBERGER MA, ZOMENHOF RG, ARANON S, NEER RM: Computed tomography scanning for the measurement of bone mineral in the human spine. *J Comput Assist Tomogr* **2**:253–262, 1978.

ZATZ LM: The effect of the kVp level on EMI values. *Radiology* **119**:683–688, 1976.

ZERHOUNI EA, SPIVEY JF, MORGAN RH, LEO FP, STITIK FP, SIEGELMAN SS: Factors influencing quantitative CT measurements of solitary pulmonary nodules. *J Comput Assist Tomogr* **6**:1075–1087, 1982.

2

NORMAL CRANIAL CT ANATOMY

Mokhtar H. Gado

Krishna C.V.G. Rao

The human brain consists of well-known anatomical components. Some parts of these components have been shown to be concerned with certain functions. A complete cranial CT examination consists of a series of several slices obtained in a sequence (Fig. 2-1), usually from the base to the vertex of the cranial vault, in the axial mode. The ultimate goal of this chapter is to pinpoint those slices that depict a given anatomical structure or several structures that deal with a given function. To achieve this goal, the discussion of CT cranial anatomy is presented in three sections.

The first section deals with description of the different components of the brain with reference to the configuration, surfaces, and borders of the brain that one has to be familiar with before addressing

the CT image, with no reference to the detailed internal structure that is not visualized on the CT image.

The second section describes the appearance of the CT images of the cranium taken at different axial levels. The discussion emphasizes the features of each slice that enable one to identify the slice and therefore determine its correct position in the complete stack of cranial CT slices. These distinctive features of a given slice are largely anatomical. Familiarity with the morphologic features of the brain in the first section is therefore essential to the text of the second section.

In the third section the different components of the brain are discussed individually in the context of a CT examination. Each individual structure, such as a lobe of a cerebral hemisphere, is approached

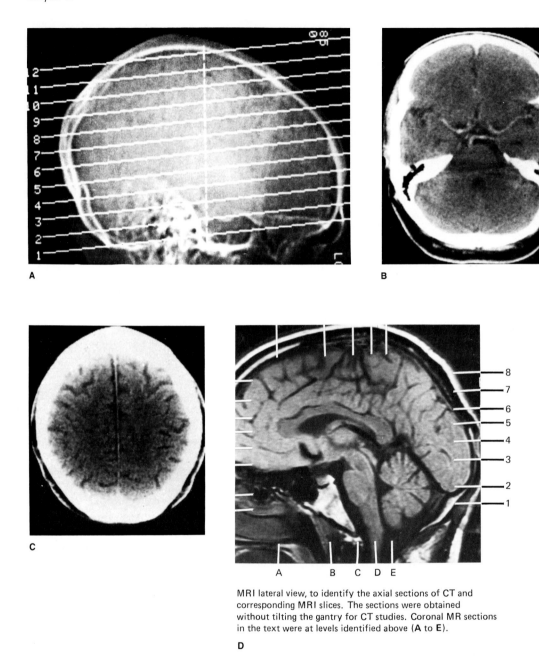

A

B

C

A   B   C D E

MRI lateral view, to identify the axial sections of CT and
corresponding MRI slices. The sections were obtained
without tilting the gantry for CT studies. Coronal MR sections
in the text were at levels identified above (**A** to **E**).

D

Figure 2-1   A. Lateral skull x-ray with the sections superimposed over the calvarium, to denote the location of the sections when viewing
the study. Note the angling of the gantry in relation to orbitomeatal plane.   **B.** Lower section through the posterior fossa. Because of
angulation of the gantry, the fourth ventricle appears in the same plane as the frontal lobes. The linear lucency overlying the brainstem is
a common artifact due to the dense petrous bones.   **C.** At the vertex level, owing to the angulation of the gantry the rolandic fissure
appears more anterior than in a similar section when the gantry of the scanner or the patient's head is not angulated.   **D.** Sagittal MRI to
demarcate the levels of the axial and coronal MR and associated CT sections.

with particular emphasis on which slices may depict that particular structure. The boundaries of the structure within each of the different slices are determined whenever possible. In the same fashion, localization of a particular functional part of that structure in one or more slices is addressed. Familiarity with the terminology and text of the first and second sections is thus necessary for the discussion of the third section.

COMPONENTS OF THE BRAIN

The brain consists of three major components, each of which is composed of several parts:

Forebrain (prosencephalon):
   Telencephalon
   Diencephalon
Midbrain (mesencephalon)
Hindbrain:
   Pons and medulla
   Cerebellum

The ventricular system consists of an interconnected series of cavities lying within the three major components just mentioned. In the forebrain it includes the lateral ventricles within the telencephalon and the third ventricle surrounded by the structures of the diencephalon. In the midbrain it consists of the aqueduct of Sylvius. In the hindbrain it is the fourth ventricle.

The Forebrain or Prosencephalon

The forebrain consists of two components: the diencephalon (the "between brain") and the telencephalon (the endbrain).

The Telencephalon

The telencephalon consists of the two cerebral hemispheres that occupy most of the cranial cavity (Fig. 2-2). In the midline the interhemispheric fissure separates these two hemispheres on both sides. Anteriorly, the interhemispheric fissure extends down to the floor of the cranial fossa. In its middle part the interhemispheric fissure stops at the corpus callosum, which connects the two cerebral hemispheres. Posteriorly, the interhemispheric fissure stops at the upper surface of the cerebellum, which is wedged in pyramidlike fashion between the two occipital lobes (Fig. 2-4*E*,*F*).

The falx cerebri is a midline sheet of dura that lies in the interhemispheric fissure (Fig. 2-3). In the anterior part of the fissure the falx is attached to the anterior part of the bony floor of the cranial cavity. In its middle part the falx has a free edge which hangs over the corpus callosum. In its posterior part the falx cerebri is attached to the tentorium cerebelli, which is a dural partition overlying the superior surface of the cerebellum and separates it from the inferior surfaces of the cerebral hemispheres. The straight sinus lies at the meeting of the falx and the two leaflets of the tentorium cerebelli (Fig. 2-3). The superior sagittal sinus lies at the root of the falx along the inner table of the cranial vault in the midline. At its posterior end, therefore, the superior sagittal sinus meets the posterior end of the straight sinus at the torcular Herophili. From the torcular, on each side of the midline a transverse sinus extends against the inner table of the occipital bone at the line of attachment of the tentorium to this bone.

Each cerebral hemisphere consists of an outer gray substance: the cerebral cortex, an underlying white substance: the centrum semiovale, and a small group of internally located masses of central gray substance: the basal ganglia (Figs. 2-4*B*,*C*, 2-13, 2-14, 2-15).

The *cerebral cortex* covers the surface of the cerebral hemisphere. There are three surfaces for each hemisphere, separated by three borders. The superior border separates the medial and lateral surfaces. The inferolateral border separates the lateral and inferior surfaces, and the inferomedial border separates the medial and inferior surfaces (Fig. 2-4*A*). The medial surface is straight and situated in the midline separated from the opposite side by the falx cerebri. The lateral surface is convex and lies against the inner table of the cranial vault. The inferior surface is irregular. The anterior part of the inferior surface is flat and lies against the floor of the anterior cranial fossa, which separates it from the orbits and nasal cavities (Figs. 2-2A, 2-4A). Posterior to this part, the inferior surface dips downward to occupy the hollow of the middle cranial fossa and thus lies against the inner table of the greater wings of the sphenoid bone and the anterior surfaces of the petrous bones. Farther posterior, this

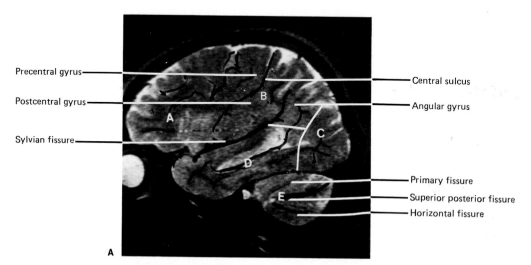

Precentral gyrus — Central sulcus
Postcentral gyrus — Angular gyrus
Sylvian fissure — Primary fissure
Superior posterior fissure
Horizontal fissure

A

MRI lateral view to identify the surface landmarks of the cerebrum and cerebellum. The curved vertical line separates the occipital lobe from the parietal and temporal lobes. It is an arbitrary landmark. A. Frontal lobe; B. parietal lobe; C. occipital lobe; D. temporal lobe; E. cerebellar hemisphere.

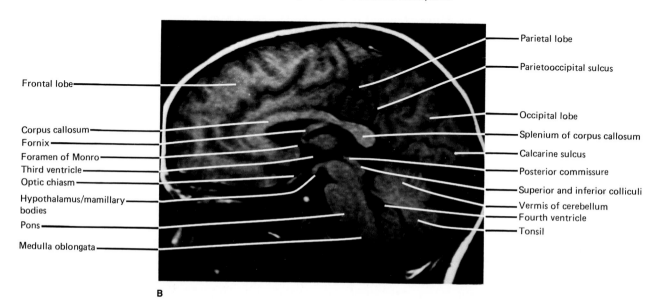

Frontal lobe — Parietal lobe
Parietooccipital sulcus
Corpus callosum — Occipital lobe
Fornix — Splenium of corpus callosum
Foramen of Monro — Calcarine sulcus
Third ventricle — Posterior commissure
Optic chiasm — Superior and inferior colliculi
Hypothalamus/mamillary bodies — Vermis of cerebellum
Pons — Fourth ventricle
Tonsil
Medulla oblongata —

B

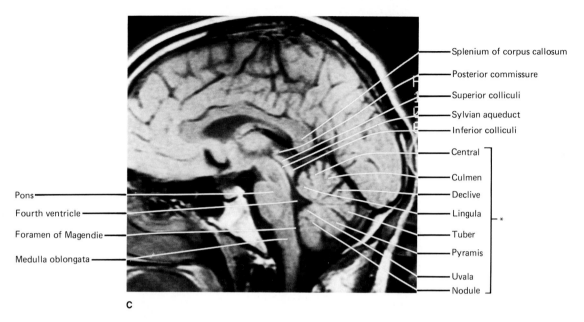

Pons

Fourth ventricle

Foramen of Magendie

Medulla oblongata

Splenium of corpus callosum

Posterior commissure

Superior colliculi

Sylvian aqueduct

Inferior colliculi

Central

Culmen

Declive

Lingula

Tuber

Pyramis

Uvala

Nodule

C

Figure 2-2   (**A**) Lateral and (**B**) medial view of the right hemisphere of the brain section to identify the surface anatomy.   **C.** Detailed view of the medial surface of posterior fossa. (*Various components of the cerebellum in the midline.)

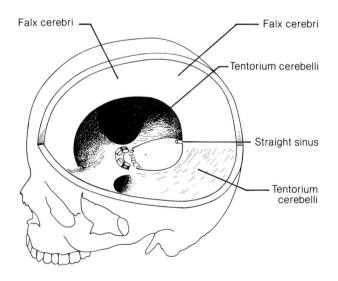

Falx cerebri

Falx cerebri

Tentorium cerebelli

Straight sinus

Tentorium cerebelli

Figure 2-3   Superior lateral view of the cranium. The left half of the vault as well as the soft tissues within the cranium have been removed with the exception of the falx cerebri and tentorium cerebelli.

surface is slanted to fit the slope of the tentorium cerebelli (Figs. 2-2*B*, 2-4*E*,*F*).

The three surfaces of the cerebral hemisphere contain numerous sulci that separate the cerebral gyri. Four of these sulci or fissures are worthy of description, since they are helpful in dividing each cerebral hemisphere into its constituent lobes. The *lateral sulcus (sylvian fissure)* is identified on the lateral surface. It separates the greater part of the temporal lobe below from the frontal lobe and the anterior part of the parietal lobe above (Fig. 2-2*A*). The *central sulcus (rolandic fissure)* begins on the medial surface of the hemisphere at about the middle of the superior border (Figs. 2-4*B*,*D*, 2-5*A*,*B*,*C*). It runs on the lateral surface of the hemisphere downward and forward and stops short of the lateral sulcus. The *parietooccipital sulcus* lies on the medial surface of the cerebral hemisphere (Figs. 2-2*B*, 2-5*C*). It starts at the superior margin at a point about 5 cm from the occipital pole and extends downward and for-

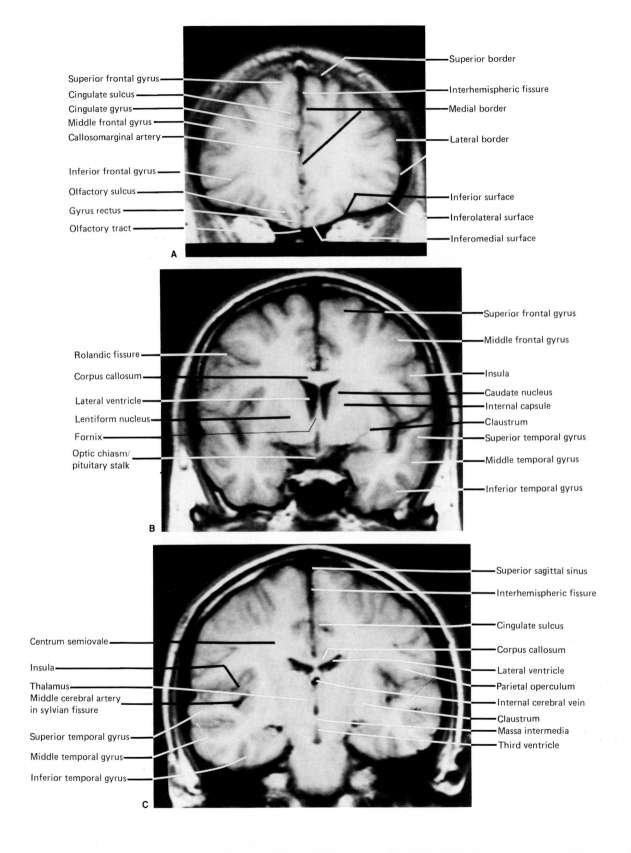

A

Superior frontal gyrus
Cingulate sulcus
Cingulate gyrus
Middle frontal gyrus
Callosomarginal artery

Inferior frontal gyrus
Olfactory sulcus
Gyrus rectus
Olfactory tract

Superior border
Interhemispheric fissure
Medial border
Lateral border

Inferior surface
Inferolateral surface
Inferomedial surface

B

Rolandic fissure
Corpus callosum
Lateral ventricle
Lentiform nucleus
Fornix
Optic chiasm/
pituitary stalk

Superior frontal gyrus
Middle frontal gyrus
Insula
Caudate nucleus
Internal capsule
Claustrum
Superior temporal gyrus
Middle temporal gyrus
Inferior temporal gyrus

C

Centrum semiovale
Insula
Thalamus
Middle cerebral artery
in sylvian fissure
Superior temporal gyrus
Middle temporal gyrus
Inferior temporal gyrus

Superior sagittal sinus
Interhemispheric fissure
Cingulate sulcus
Corpus callosum
Lateral ventricle
Parietal operculum
Internal cerebral vein
Claustrum
Massa intermedia
Third ventricle

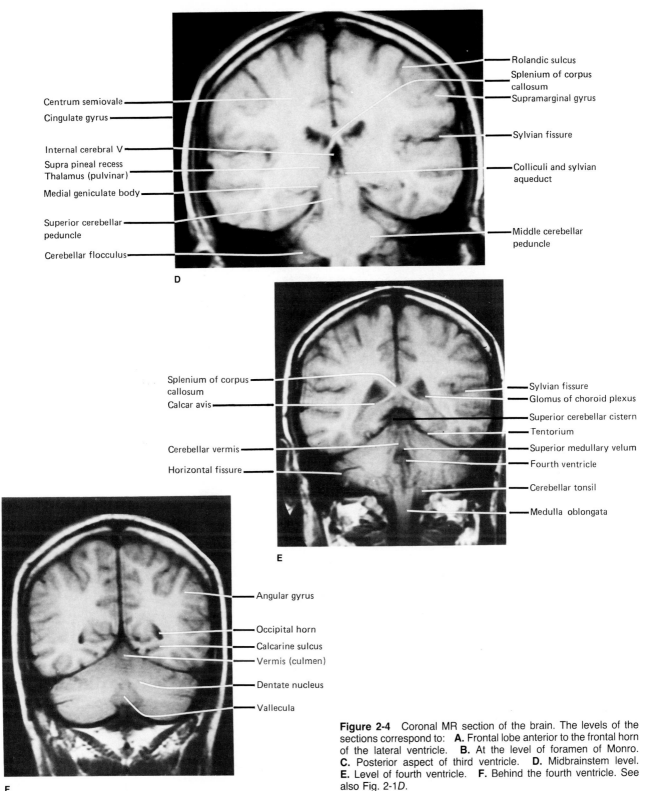

D

Centrum semiovale

Cingulate gyrus

Internal cerebral V

Supra pineal recess
Thalamus (pulvinar)

Medial geniculate body

Superior cerebellar
peduncle

Cerebellar flocculus

Rolandic sulcus

Splenium of corpus
callosum

Supramarginal gyrus

Sylvian fissure

Colliculi and sylvian
aqueduct

Middle cerebellar
peduncle

Splenium of corpus
callosum

Calcar avis

Cerebellar vermis

Horizontal fissure

Sylvian fissure

Glomus of choroid plexus

Superior cerebellar cistern

Tentorium

Superior medullary velum

Fourth ventricle

Cerebellar tonsil

Medulla oblongata

E

Angular gyrus

Occipital horn

Calcarine sulcus

Vermis (culmen)

Dentate nucleus

Vallecula

F

Figure 2-4 Coronal MR section of the brain. The levels of the sections correspond to: **A.** Frontal lobe anterior to the frontal horn of the lateral ventricle. **B.** At the level of the foramen of Monro. **C.** Posterior aspect of third ventricle. **D.** Midbrainstem level. **E.** Level of fourth ventricle. **F.** Behind the fourth ventricle. See also Fig. 2-1*D*.

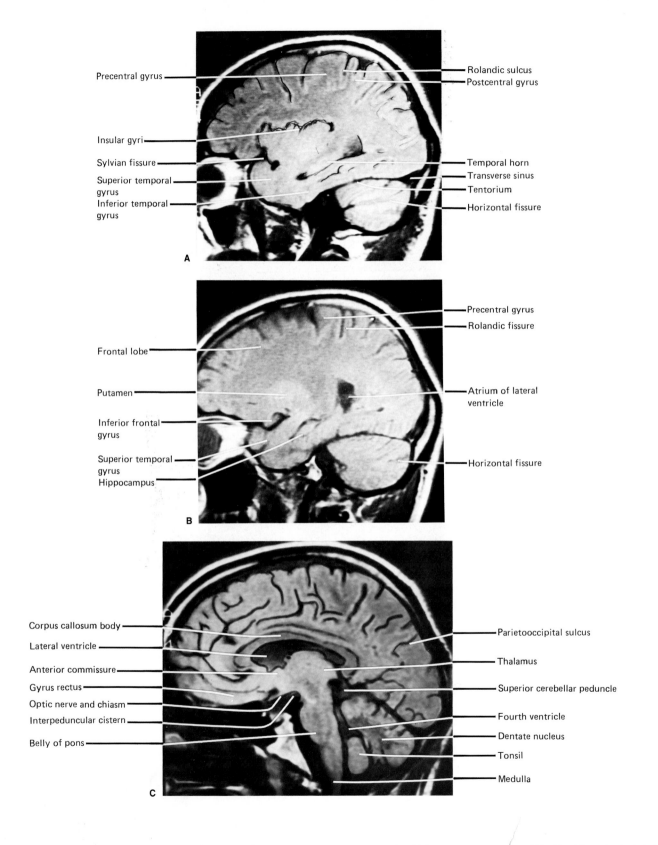

A

Precentral gyrus

Insular gyri

Sylvian fissure

Superior temporal gyrus

Inferior temporal gyrus

Rolandic sulcus

Postcentral gyrus

Temporal horn

Transverse sinus

Tentorium

Horizontal fissure

B

Frontal lobe

Putamen

Inferior frontal gyrus

Superior temporal gyrus

Hippocampus

Precentral gyrus

Rolandic fissure

Atrium of lateral ventricle

Horizontal fissure

C

Corpus callosum body

Lateral ventricle

Anterior commissure

Gyrus rectus

Optic nerve and chiasm

Interpeduncular cistern

Belly of pons

Parietooccipital sulcus

Thalamus

Superior cerebellar peduncle

Fourth ventricle

Dentate nucleus

Tonsil

Medulla

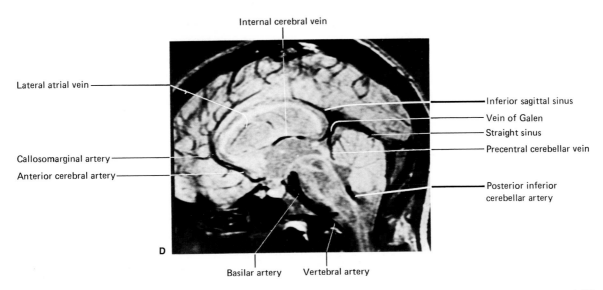

Figure 2-5   Sagittal MR section to identify the components of the brain parenchyma.   **(A)** Extreme lateral, **(B)** atrial level, and **(C)** more medial.   **(D)** Demonstrates the vascular anatomy on T$_2$ weighted image. (*Courtesy of Dr. Zimmerman, Hospital of University of Pennsylvania.*)

ward, where it meets the *calcarine sulcus* near the splenium of the corpus callosum. The calcarine sulcus extends from this point backward on the medial surface of the occipital lobe and ends at the occipital pole (Fig. 2-2*B*).

Each cerebral hemisphere is divided into five lobes. The boundaries separating these lobes are in part formed by the sulci mentioned above and in part by imaginary lines, as will be described. The *frontal lobe* is the anterior part of the hemisphere. On the lateral surface (Fig. 2-2*A*) it is limited posteriorly by the central sulcus (rolandic fissure) and inferiorly by the lateral sulcus (sylvian fissure). On the medial surface (Fig. 2-2*B*) it is limited posteriorly by a line drawn downward and anteriorly from the end of the central sulcus to the corpus callosum. The *occipital lobe* is the small posterior part of the cerebral hemisphere. On the medial surface it is limited anteriorly by the parietooccipital sulcus (Fig. 2-2*B*). Its anterior border on the lateral surface (Fig. 2-2*A*) is an imaginary line extending from the upper end of the parietooccipital sulcus at the superior border of the hemisphere to the preoccipital notch on the inferolateral border.

The *parietal lobe* lies between the frontal lobe anteriorly and the occipital lobe posteriorly. The inferior border of the parietal lobe on the lateral surface (Fig. 2-2*A*) is formed by the posterior part of the lateral sulcus and an arbitrary line extending from the lateral sulcus toward the other arbitrary line which forms the anterior border of the occpital lobe described above. It will be seen, therefore, that the separation between the parietal, temporal, and occipital lobes on the lateral surface is formed by arbitrary lines and thus they are rather ill-defined. The area could be referred to as a zone and may be termed the *parietotemporooccipital junction*. On the medial surface (Fig. 2-2*B*), the posterior border of the parietal lobe is formed by the parietooccipital sulcus which separates it from the occipital lobe. The *insula (central lobe)* is hidden in the depth of the lateral sulcus and can be seen only if the lips of the sulcus are bent back or cut away. These lips are parts of the frontal, parietal, and temporal lobes. They are called the frontal, parietal, and temporal opercula, respectively. These regions can be best appreciated in the coronal and sagittal sections on MRI studies and by CT (Figs. 2-4*C*, 2-5*A*–*C*).

The *centrum semiovale* constitutes the white matter of the internal portion of the cerebral hemisphere. The *corpus callosum* is a great band of central white matter that connects the two cerebral hemispheres (Fig. 2-2B). Its anterior end is bent downward and is called the *genu*. The main part of the corpus callosum is called the *body*. Its posterior end, which has a thick, rounded free edge and is called the *splenium*, overhangs the pineal body and the colliculi (see below under Midbrain).

The *basal ganglia* represent the central gray matter of the telencephalon (Figs. 2-13, 2-14). The *caudate nucleus* has an enlarged anterior end, the head, that indents the lateral wall of the anterior horn of the lateral ventricle. It has a narrow posterior portion, the tail, which follows the superolateral border of the thalamus. The *lentiform nucleus* has a wedge-shaped configuration in the axial section (Figs. 2-13, 2-14, 2-4B). The *internal capsule* is a thick band of white matter situated between the thalamus (see below) and the caudate and lentiform nuclei. The part of the internal capsule that lies between the caudate and lentiform nuclei is called the anterior limb. The part between the thalamus and lentiform nucleus is called the posterior limb. Both limbs meet in a right angle at the genu (Fig. 2-14).

The Diencephalon

The diencephalon consists of several structures that lie around the third ventricle. It connects the midbrain on one side to the cerebral hemispheres on the other side. Its structures include the thalami, the geniculate bodies, the epithalamus, the subthalamus, and the hypothalamus.

1. The *thalami* are two large ovoid masses, small in size anteriorly and more voluminous posteriorly. Each thalamus is 4 cm long. Its medial surface forms the lateral wall of the third ventricle. It is covered with ependyma and is separated from the opposite thalamus by the third ventricle itself (Fig. 2-4C,D). Its superior surface forms part of the floor of the lateral ventricle on each side. The medial part of the superior surface which does not form part of the floor of the lateral ventricle is covered with the fold of pia called tela choroidea, which forms the velum

interpositum in the roof of the third ventricle (Fig. 2-14). The fornix lies on top of the superior surface of the thalamus, separating the lateral part from the medial part (Fig. 2-2B). The anterior end of the thalamus is small and forms the posterior boundary of the foramen of Monro, while the column of the fornix that overlies the thalamus forms at this point the anterior border of the foramen of Monro (Fig. 2-2B). Each foramen of Monro forms a communication between the lateral ventricle of that side and the third ventricle. The voluminous posterior end of the thalamus is the pulvinar. It extends farther posteriorly beyond the posterior end of the third ventricle (Fig. 2-4D), so each pulvinar overlies a superior colliculus. In the space between the two pulvinars the pineal rests in the midline just above the two superior colliculi (Figs. 2-2B, 2-6, 2-8). Unlike the superior and medial surfaces of the thalamus, which form part of the walls of the lateral and third ventricles, the inferior and lateral surfaces lie against other parts of the brain tissue. The inferior surface is continuous with the upper end of the tegmentum of the midbrain (see below). The lateral surface lies against the white matter that constitutes the posterior limb of the internal capsule (Fig. 2-14). The medial surfaces of the thalami are separated by the cavity of the third ventricle, but they are connected by the massa intermedia (Fig. 2-4C).

2. The *geniculate bodies* (Figs. 2-4D, 2-6, 2-13) are a medial and a lateral one on each side. All four structures constitute the metathalamus. The geniculate bodies serve as relay stations. The lateral geniculate body is connected by the superior brachium to the superior colliculus and serves as part of the visual pathways that end in the visual cortex of the occipital lobe. The medial geniculate body is connected by the inferior brachium to the inferior colliculus and serves as part of the auditory pathways that end in the auditory cortex of the superior temporal gyrus.

3. The *habenula*, the *pineal body*, and the *posterior commissure* constitute the epithalamus (Figs. 2-4D, 2-2D, 2-8). The stalk which attaches the pineal gland consists of a superior and an inferior lamina. The superior lamina is formed by the habenula. The inferior lamina is formed by the posterior commis-

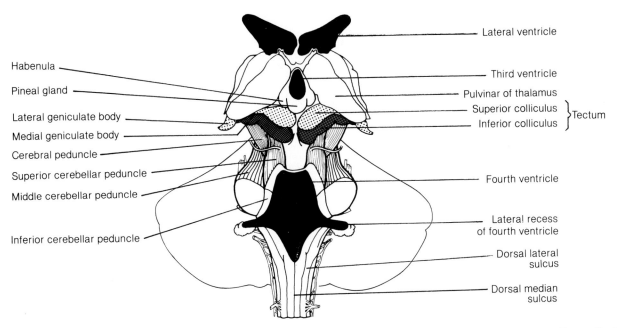

Figure 2-6   Dorsal view of the diencephalon and brainstem. (*Modified from Nieuwenhuys, Vougd, Van Huijzen: The Human Central Nervous System. Berlin, Heidelberg, New York, Springer-Verlag, 1979.*)

sure. Between these two laminae is the pineal recess of the third ventricle.

4. The *subthalamus* is the transition zone between the thalamus and the tegmentum of the midbrain, upon which it lies and with which it is continuous.

5. The *hypothalamus* forms the wall of the anterior end of the third ventricle. It consists of several small parts: the mamillary bodies, the tuber cinereum, the infundibulum, the hypophysis, and the optic chiasm (Figs. 2-2*B*, 2-2*C*, 2-4*B*, 2-7).

The Midbrain or Mesencephalon

The midbrain (mesencephalon) is a short segment of the brainstem. It connects the pons and the cerebellum on the one hand with the forebrain on the other hand. The brainstem thus consists of the midbrain, the pons, and the medulla. The latter two are part of the hindbrain.

The midbrain consists of a smaller dorsal portion called the *tectum* (Fig. 2-6) and a larger anterior portion formed by the *cerebral peduncles* (Fig. 2-7). Between the tectum and the cerebral peduncles, the central gray substance of the midbrain surrounds the aqueduct which connects the fourth and third ventricles. The cerebral peduncles are viewed on the ventral surface of the brain as two prominent ridges (Fig. 2-7), diverging as they approach the cerebral hemispheres. Thus a triangular area, the interpeduncular fossa, separates the two cerebral peduncles. The triangular configuration of this fossa is seen in the ventral view as well as the axial view of the midbrain. The floor of the interpeduncular fossa is the posterior perforated substance.

The tectum of the midbrain consists of four rounded prominences, the *corpora quadrigemina* or *colliculi* (Fig. 2-2*B*). The superior colliculi are continuous on both sides with the superior brachia; each connects one superior colliculus to the ipsilateral lateral geniculate body where the ipsilateral optic tract

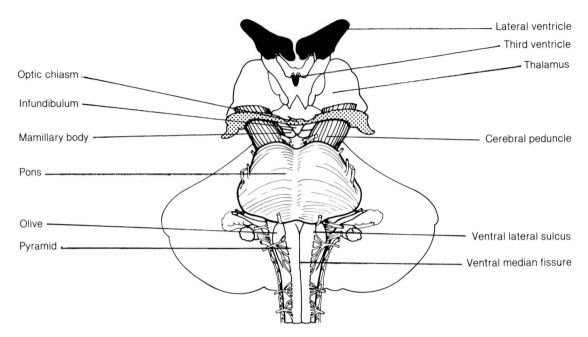

Figure 2-7   Ventral view of the diencephalon and brainstem. (*Modified from Nieuwenhuys, Vougd, Van Huijzen: The Human Central Nervous System. Berlin, Heidelberg, New York, Springer-Verlag, 1979.*)

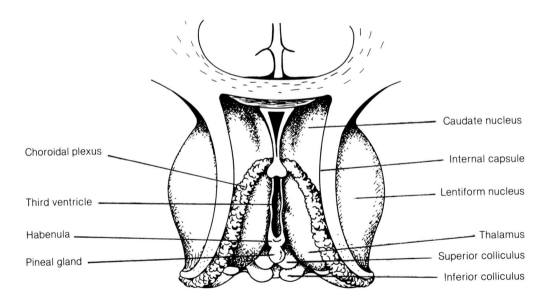

Figure 2-8   Superior view of the diencephalon. (*Modified from Carpenter MB: Human Neuroanatomy, 7th ed. Baltimore, Williams and Wilkins, 1976.*)

ends. Thus the fibers of the superior brachium connect the superior colliculus and the visual cortex. Likewise, the inferior brachia extend from the inferior colliculi to the medial geniculate bodies, connecting the inferior colliculus and auditory cortex.

Each cerebral peduncle consists of a ventral part, the crus (or basis pedunculi), and a dorsal part, the tegmentum of the midbrain. The superior cerebellar peduncle (brachium conjunctivum) penetrates deeply into the tegmentum of the inferior part of the midbrain from the dorsal aspect on each side of the midline (Fig. 2-6).

The Hindbrain

The hindbrain consists of two parts. The anterior part is the *medulla oblongata* inferiorly and the *pons* superiorly. The posterior part is the *cerebellum*. Between the anterior and posterior parts of the hindbrain is the fourth ventricle. This communicates with the third ventricle through the aqueduct of Sylvius and the extraaxial CSF space, the subarachnoid cistern, via its midline foramen of Magendie and the two lateral recesses, the foramina of Luschka.

The Medulla Oblongata

The medulla oblongata is continuous inferiorly with the spinal cord and superiorly with the pons (Figs. 2-2B, 2-4E). It measures 3 cm in length. Its cross-sectional dimensions are 2 cm from side to side and 1.25 cm anterioposteriorly. There are two midline grooves, a ventral and a dorsal. Anteriorly, the ventral median fissure starts below at the pyramidal decussation and ends superiorly at the inferior border of the pons (Fig. 2-7). The dorsal median sulcus is present only on the dorsal aspect of the inferior half of the medulla and stops at the superior half, where the dorsal surface of the medulla forms the floor of the fourth ventricle (Fig. 2-2B). These two midline grooves thus bisect the medulla. Each half furthermore shows two longitudinal grooves, the

ventral lateral sulcus and the dorsal lateral sulcus (Figs. 2-6, 2-7).

The two lateral sulci enable several structures to be identified on the surface of each lateral half of the medulla. Anteriorly, the *pyramid* lies between the ventral median fissure and the ventral lateral sulcus (Fig. 2-7). The *olive* lies between the two lateral sulci (Fig. 2-7). Behind the dorsal lateral sulcus and lying between it and the dorsal median fissure are the cuneate and gracile tubercles (Fig. 2-6). As previously mentioned, the dorsal median sulcus is present only over the dorsal aspect of the lower half of the medulla, so these tubercles are present only on that portion of the medulla.

The upper half of the dorsal surface of the medulla shows two diverging prominences forming the lateral boundaries of the floor of the fourth ventricle (Fig. 2-6). These prominences contain the *inferior cerebellar peduncles* (restiform bodies), which connect the spinal cord and medulla with the cerebellum.

The Pons

The pons connects the medulla below with the midbrain above. It forms a massive protuberance, with well-defined borders, on the ventral surface of the brainstem (Fig. 2-7). This protuberance is separated from the medulla oblongata by the inferior pontine sulcus and from the cerebral peduncles of the midbrain by the superior pontine sulcus (Fig. 2-7). The ventral prominence consists of transverse strands across the midline. At each side these strands form the middle cerebellar peduncle. There is a shallow midline depression on the ventral surface of the pons, the basilar sulcus. The basilar artery lies in this depression.

In addition to the massive ventral component of the pons, which is also called the *basis pontis*, there is a smaller dorsal component, the tegmentum of the pons. The dorsal surface of the tegmentum forms the upper half of the floor of the fourth ventricle (Figs. 2-4E, 2-6), so the floor of the fourth ventricle is formed in part by the dorsal aspect of the medulla and in part by the dorsal aspect of the pons. These two components form the rhomboid fossa.

The Cerebellum

The cerebellum occupies the greater part of the posterior cranial fossa. It is located on the dorsal aspect of the pons and medulla, separated from these two structures by the cavity of the fourth ventricle (Figs. 2-2*B*, 2-5*A,B*, 2-4*E,F*).

The upper surface of the cerebellum lies under the tentorium cerebelli, which separates it from the occipital lobes. As a result of the upward slope of the leaflets of the tentorium toward the midline, the high point of the cerebellum is in the midline anteriorly. The posterior surface of the cerebellum lies against the inner table of the occipital bone. The cerebellum is attached to the brainstem by three cerebellar peduncles. The superior peduncle (brachium conjunctivum) connects it with the midbrain, the middle peduncle (brachium pontis) connects it with the pons, and the inferior peduncle (restiform body) connects it with the medulla. The cerebellum consists of a narrow medial portion, the vermis, and two hemispheres which extend laterally and posteriorly (Fig. 2-9).

The superior part of the vermis begins at the anterior medullary velum, which forms the superior part of the roof of the fourth ventricle. The farthest anterior part of the superior vermis is the lingula, which can be visualized from the ventral aspect of the cerebellum after removal of the brainstem (Fig. 2-9*C*). The part of the superior vermis behind the lingula is the central lobule, and farther posterior is the culmen. When viewed from the superior aspect (Fig. 2-9*A*), the cerebellum has a midline shallow concavity anteriorly (the anterior cerebellar fissure) and a narrow deep groove posteriorly (the posterior cerebellar fissure); the anterior part of the culmen appears at the bottom of the shallow anterior cerebellar fissure (Fig. 2-9*A*), and the folium lies at the bottom of the narrow and deep posterior cerebellar fissure (Fig. 2-9*A*). Between the culmen and the folium is the declive. When viewed from the dorsal aspect, the culmen, declive, and folium of the superior vermis appear in continuity with the tuber, pyramid, and uvula of the inferior vermis (Fig. 2-9*B*). The farthest forward structure of the inferior vermis is the nodulus; this cannot be visualized from

the dorsal aspect of the cerebellum but only from the ventral aspect after removal of the brainstem (Fig. 2-9*C*). In the ventral aspect of the cerebellum (Fig. 2-9*C*), the lingula and central lobule of the cerebellum lie above the cavity of the fourth ventricle, while the nodulus and uvula lie below the fourth ventricle. On both sides of the fourth ventricle and inferolateral to the cut edges of the middle cerebellar peduncles, the flocculus is seen on each side in relation to the lateral recess of the fourth ventricle (Figs. 2-9*C*, 2-4*D–F*).

The cerebellar tonsils are the most anterior inferior structures of the cerebellar hemispheres (Fig. 2-9*B*). The rest of the cerebellar hemispheres on the inferior aspect consist of the biventral lobules (Fig. 2-9*C*), followed posteriorly by the inferior semilunar lobules. The horizontal fissure separating the inferior semilunar lobule from the superior semilunar lobule is best visualized on the dorsal view of the cerebellum (Fig. 2-9*B*). The superior surface of the cerebellar hemisphere is formed at its posterior end by the superior semilunar lobule (Fig. 2-9*A*). In front of the superior semilunar lobule and separated from it by the superior posterior fissure is the lobule simplex, which in turn is separated from the quadrangular lobule by the primary fissure (Fig. 2-9*A*).

CT AND MR IMAGE CORRELATION

A complete set of CT slices consists of sections from the base of the cranium to the vertex. Although CT studies are still performed at a plane 20 degrees above the orbitomeatal line, with the improvement in CT technology and availability of MRI it is not unusual to obtain CT axial sections without angling the gantry or the patient's head. It makes comparison with MR studies optimal. Also if reformatted CT images are desired it is easier to obtain them when the axial slices have not been performed with the 15- to 20-degree angulation.

In the following text the distinctive features of CT and corresponding MR slices are described. Wherever appropriate, coronal and sagittal MR slices

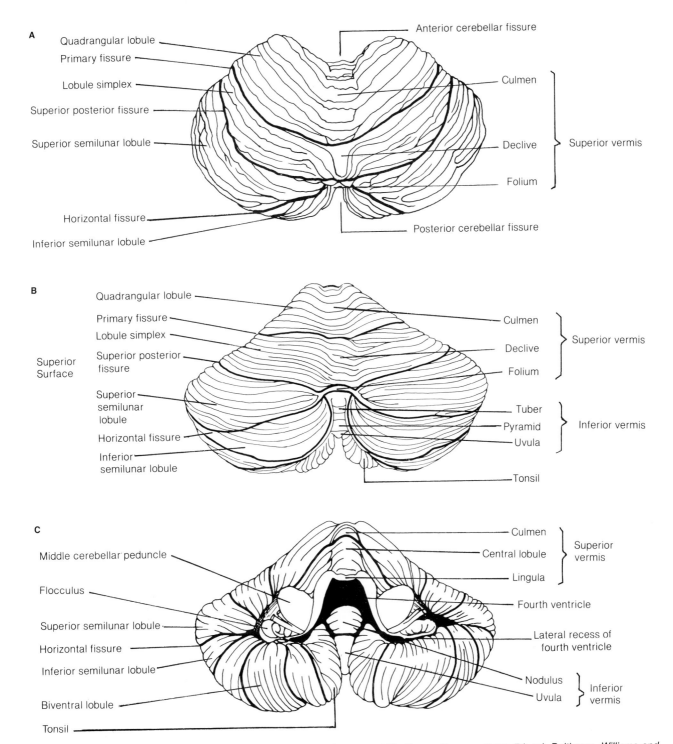

Figure 2-9 The cerebellum. **A.** Superior view. (*Modified from Carpenter MB: Human Neuroanatomy, 7th ed. Baltimore, Williams and Wilkins, 1976.*) **B.** Dorsal view. (*Modified from Nieuwenhuys, Vougd, Van Huijzen: The Human Central Nervous System. Berlin, Heidelberg, New York, Springer-Verlag 1979.*) **C.** Ventral view. (*Modified from Nieuwenhuys, Vougd, Van Huijzen: The Human Central Nervous System. Berlin, Heidelberg, New York, Springer-Verlag 1979.*)

(Figs. 2-2, 2-4, 2-5) provide a three-dimensional perspective of the normal anatomy. For purposes of identifying the vascular territory of each section, correlate with the vascular topography demarcated on the cerebral surfaces (Fig. 2-19C,D).

For descriptive purposes the CT and MR slices are divided into infraventricular, ventricular, and supraventricular sections (Fig. 2-1D).

The infraventricular or infratentorial series is the lowest subset (Figs. 2-10 to 2-12). In these sections the petrous bone and the occipital bones delineate the walls of the posterior fossa while the temporal fossa is delineated by the petrous segment of the temporal bones posteriorly, the squamous temporal bones laterally, and anteriorly by the wings of the sphenoid bones, which separate the intracranial contents from the intraorbital compartment. In the lowermost section from this region (Fig. 2-10), the cerebellar hemispheres are separated from the brainstem anteriorly by the inferior aspect of the fourth ventricle. On CT the fourth ventricle appears slitlike (Fig. 2-10A); however, on the MRI slice at a similar level the anteroposterior concave appearance is due to the projection of nodules of the vermis. On CT it may appear as a hyperdense structure and should not be confused as hemorrhage or tumor nodule. In front of the brainstem is the prepontine cistern which extends laterally and continues as the cerebellopontine angle cistern. Coursing

through the cisternal space into the internal auditory meatus are the seventh and eighth cranial nerves. On CT sections it is difficult to appreciate these nerves or for that matter the gray and white matter of the cerebellum. In addition it is not unusual to observe a lucent band overlying the brainstem. An artifact caused by beam hardening due to the thick petrous bone, this is termed the Hounsfield effect. On MR sections at a similar level, all of the above structures can be well visualized, since owing to an absence of signal intensity from the petrous bone the brainstem and the cisterns can be visualized without artifacts. In addition occasionally the seventh and eighth cranial nerves (Fig. 2-10) as well as, on sagittal and coronal MR images, the foramina of Luschka and Magendie can also be visualized (Fig. 2-2B).

In the next higher slice (Fig. 2-11) above the previous level, the bony landmarks still are the same, except anteriorly in the midline the superior part is formed by the clivus and the posterior wall of the sella forms part of the anterior osseous boundary for the posterior fossa structures. The fourth ventricle has an oblong shape. The fourth ventricle separates the belly of the pons from the cerebellar hemispheres. On either side are the middle cerebellar peduncles. Projecting from the inner table of the occipital bone is the inion where the torcula or confluence of the venous sinuses is attached. In front of the pons is the prepontine cistern wherein on a

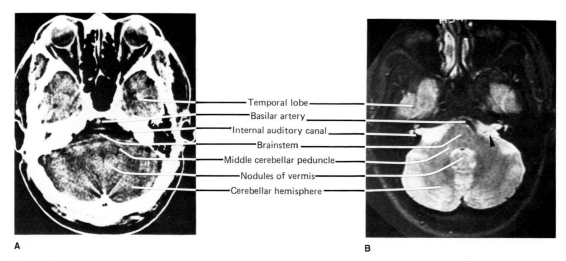

Temporal lobe
Basilar artery
Internal auditory canal
Brainstem
Middle cerebellar peduncle
Nodules of vermis
Cerebellar hemisphere

A

B

Figure 2-10 (**A**) CT and (**B**) MR anatomy of the brain in the lowermost level of the infraventricular series.

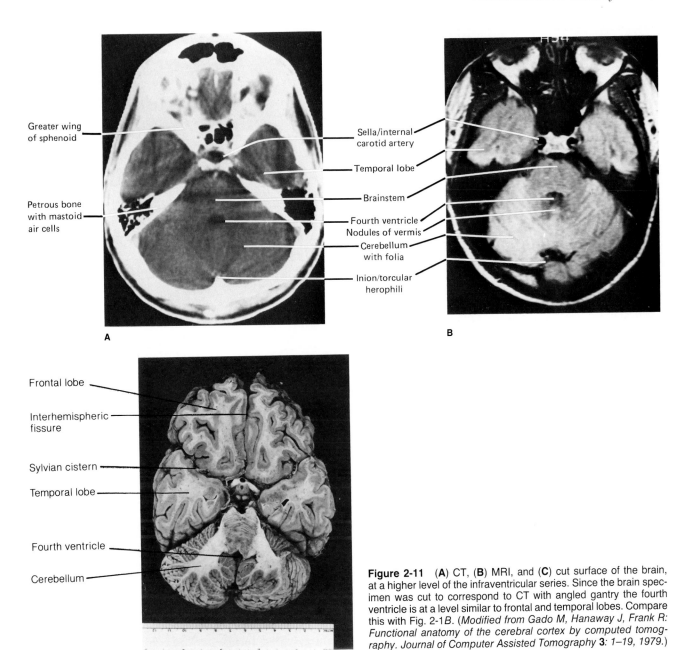

Greater wing of sphenoid

Petrous bone with mastoid air cells

A

Sella/internal carotid artery

Temporal lobe

Brainstem

Fourth ventricle

Nodules of vermis

Cerebellum with folia

Inion/torcular herophili

B

Frontal lobe

Interhemispheric fissure

Sylvian cistern

Temporal lobe

Fourth ventricle

Cerebellum

C

Figure 2-11 (**A**) CT, (**B**) MRI, and (**C**) cut surface of the brain, at a higher level of the infraventricular series. Since the brain specimen was cut to correspond to CT with angled gantry the fourth ventricle is at a level similar to frontal and temporal lobes. Compare this with Fig. 2-1*B*. (*Modified from Gado M, Hanaway J, Frank R: Functional anatomy of the cerebral cortex by computed tomography. Journal of Computer Assisted Tomography 3: 1–19, 1979.*)

contrast-enhanced CT the basilar artery can be visualized. MR through the same region in addition to visualization of the above structures can also show the dentate nucleus, the gray, white matter of the cerebellar hemisphere, and the cerebellar folia. An-

teriorly in the temporal fossa the temporal lobe and occasionally the tips of the temporal horn can also be seen.

The next cephalad section (Fig. 2-12) of the infraventricular series lies just above the level of the

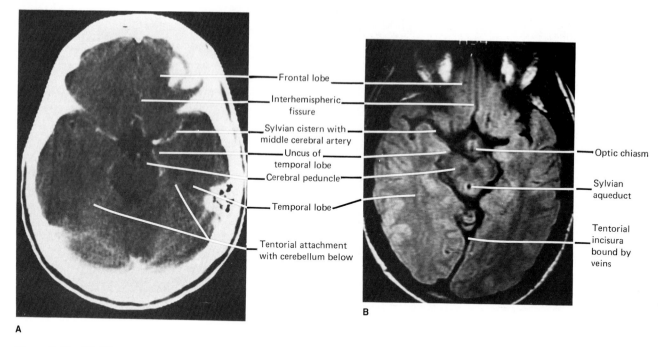

Figure 2-12   (**A**) CT and (**B**) MR anatomy at the brainstem level.

petrous bone and therefore is bounded by the occipital, temporal, and frontal bones. The superior vermis is located in the midline, bounded on either side in an anteromedial and posterolateral direction by the tentorium. The free margin of the tentorium and thus the anterior border of the tentorial hiatus is demarcated by the ambient cistern which communicates anteriorly with the interpeduncular and suprasellar cisterns by means of the circummesencephalic cistern. Anterolaterally on either side are the temporal lobes. Anteriorly in front of the suprasellar cistern are the frontal lobes separated by the interhemispheric fissure. The posterior border of the frontal lobes is demarcated by the suprasellar cistern medially and the sylvian cisterns anterolaterally. The suprasellar cistern has a hexagon or pentagonal shape. The lateral wall of the cistern is formed by the medial margin of the temporal lobe consisting of the uncus. The posterior margin of the cistern is formed by the two cerebral peduncles. The two temporal lobes are demarcated from the peduncles by continuation of the intrapeduncular cistern laterally

forming the circummesencephalic cistern. On the contrast-enhanced CT vascular structures which may be identified include the circummesencephalic vein and/or the posterior cerebral arteries. Occasionally in the midline along the posterior margin of the brainstem one can identify the slitlike aqueduct of Sylvius. Posterolaterally there is a sharp demarcation extending from the lateral margin of the ambient cistern to the inner table of the calvarium separating the temporal lobes on each side from the superior portion of the cerebellar hemisphere. The sharp lucent area demarcates the lateral portion of the superior cerebellar cistern, and adjacent linear hyperdensity represents the attachment of the dural lining which forms the tentorium. Because of the medial convergence of the tentorium one will notice that on higher sections the cerebellar tissue is more in midline and laterally the parenchymal tissue represents the posterior temporal lobe and the occipital lobe. The attachment of the tentorium and the hiatus is best visualized on a contrast-enhanced CT and MRI (Fig. 2-4 *D,E,F*) in the axial and coronal planes.

On contrast-enhanced CT the tentorium appears as a relatively hyperdense structure due to the venous plexus within the dural sinuses.

Low Ventricular Series

The next subset in a cephalad sequence are the low ventricular series (Figs. 2-13, 2-14). These slices lie above the level of the petrous bones and therefore are bounded peripherally by the occipital, temporal, parietal, and frontal bones. They include parts of the frontal horns, trigones, and temporal horn as well as posterior horns of the lateral ventricles. In addition, depending on the angling of the gantry, these slices may include the superior vermis of the cerebellum and the brainstem together with the thalamus and the basal ganglia. In the section through the lower level of the subset (Fig. 2-13) the CSF cisternal space has a consistent pattern and includes sequentially from front to back the intrahemispheric fissure, the inferior part of the frontal horns, the third ventricle, the quadrigeminal cistern, and occasionally the superior cerebellar cistern. Laterally, on both sides, separating the temporal lobes from midline structures, are the sylvian fissures. The inferior parts of the frontal horns appear as oblique curved slits that converge on the midline. The interhemispheric fissure and the third ventricle lie in a line with each other. The quadrigeminal cistern lies more or less in a transverse position; it is curved with concavity anterior, and it caps the posterior aspect of the tectal plate of the midbrain. For purposes of description, this slice can be divided into an anterior, a middle, and a posterior third. Thus, the anterior third is bounded anteriorly by the frontal bones and is demarcated by the bony projections (pterion) which also is helpful since it demarcates the posterior limit of the frontal lobe from the temporal lobe which is separated by the sylvian fissure on both sides laterally. Toward the midline, along the lateral aspect of the frontal horns, are two slightly hyperdense structures, the caudate nucleus (Figs. 2-13A, 2-4B). Anteriorly, the two frontal lobes are separated by the interhemispheric fissure. On the MR slice at a similar level, one can identify in the

posterior aspect of the interhemispheric fissure the anterior cerebral artery as it lies in front of the genu of the corpus callosum. In the middle third of the slice, the surface of the insula appears buried underneath the surface of the cerebral hemisphere (Figs. 2-13A,C, 2-5C). The CSF space on the surface of the insula is the circular sulcus. The brain parenchyma separating the circular sulcus and the insula from the surface of the hemisphere is formed by the opercula, while deep to the insula the lentiform and caudate nuclei are visualized by the slightly higher density compared with the surrounding white matter (Figs. 2-13A,B,C and 2-4B). Owing to absence of angling the gantry, the posterior inferior aspect of the thalamus is also noted in the slice located just anterior to the tectal plates. The posterior third of this section comprises the temporal lobe and the inferior aspect of the occipital pole. In the midline, behind the quadrigeminal cistern, is the superior aspect of the vermis representing the midportion of the cerebellar hemisphere projecting through the tentorial hiatus. Behind the vermis is the top portion of the superior cerebellar cistern. The demarcation between the cerebellar tissue and the temporooccipital poles can be better identified on a CT performed following intravenous contrast injection. The same, however, can be well visualized on coronal CT as well as MR sections (Fig. 2-4D,E,F).

The next higher slice of the low ventricular subset has distinctive features shown in Fig. 2-14A and the corresponding MR section in Fig. 2-14B. The CSF structures in the central part of this slice differ in appearance from those of the lower slice just described. The frontal horns each appear as a triangular CSF space with a concave lateral border. The medial limb of the triangle is straight and lies against the opposite frontal horn separated by the thin septum pellucidum. The third ventricle lies in the midline, starting at the posterior end of the frontal horns. The foramen of Monro connecting the frontal horns to the third ventricle may occasionally be visualized in this section (Fig. 2-14A,B). The quadrigeminal cistern in this slice has a rhomboid configuration with four extensions; the anterior extension is in the velum interpositum of the roof of the third ventricle, the posterior extension forms or joins the superior cerebellar cistern, and the two lateral extensions form the retrothalamic cisterns. On contrast-enhanced CT within the cistern can be visualized the posterior end of the internal cerebral vein and/or the vein of Galen. If the pineal gland is calcified, that also can be identified. The trigones of the lateral ventricles are situated away from the midline, one on each

side in the depth of a cerebral hemisphere. For purposes of description, the slice is again divided into an anterior, middle, and posterior third. The middle third of the slice contains, in addition to the caudate and lentiform nuclei, the two thalami, one on each side of the third ventricle. On each side, the internal capsule appears as an L-shaped band of lower den-

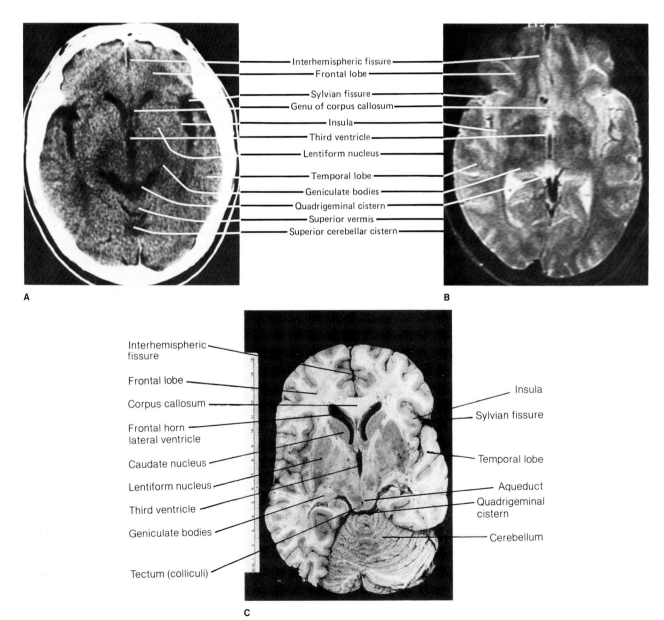

A

Interhemispheric fissure
Frontal lobe
Sylvian fissure
Genu of corpus callosum
Insula
Third ventricle
Lentiform nucleus
Temporal lobe
Geniculate bodies
Quadrigeminal cistern
Superior vermis
Superior cerebellar cistern

B

Interhemispheric fissure
Frontal lobe
Corpus callosum
Frontal horn lateral ventricle
Caudate nucleus
Lentiform nucleus
Third ventricle
Geniculate bodies
Tectum (colliculi)

Insula
Sylvian fissure
Temporal lobe
Aqueduct
Quadrigeminal cistern
Cerebellum

C

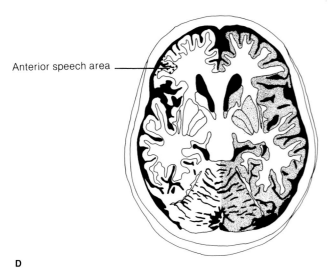

Anterior speech area

D

Figure 2-13 (**A**) CT, (**B**) MRI, (**C**) cut surface of the brain at the low ventricular level and (**D**) corresponding line diagram, showing the speech area. Discrepancy between the anatomical specimen and CT, MRI section is due to the absence of angling the gantry on CT and MRI. (*Modified from Gado M, Hanaway J, Frank R: Functional anatomy of the cerebral cortex by computed tomography. Journal of Computer Assisted Tomography* **3**: *1–19, 1979.*)

sity separating the caudate nucleus, lentiform nucleus, and thalamus (Figs. 2-14*A,B,* 2-4*B*). The insula is visualized lateral to the lentiform nucleus. The circular sulcus appears on the surface of the insula. The sylvian fissure is shown as a deep fissure that extends from the surface of the hemisphere to the posterior end of the insula (Fig. 2-14*A,B,C*). The posterior third of the slice is occupied by the temporal and occipital poles. On an enhanced CT, the two occipital poles are separated by the straight sinus running in the junction of the falx and the tentorial dura. The anterior third of the slice is occupied by the frontal lobes, separated in the midline by the interhemispheric fissure (Figs. 2-14*A,* 2-4).

High Ventricular Series

The next subset of slices is the high ventricular series (Figs. 2-15 and 2-16). The main distinctive feature of these slices is the presence of the bodies of the lat-

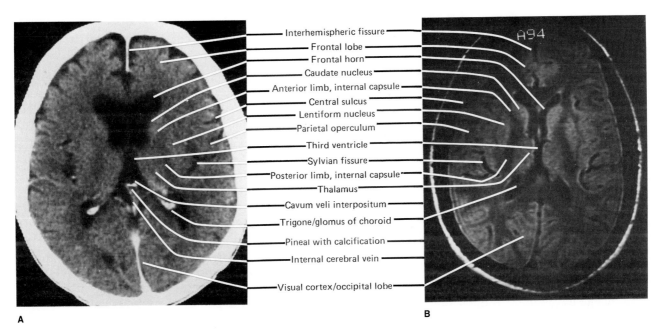

Interhemispheric fissure
Frontal lobe
Frontal horn
Caudate nucleus
Anterior limb, internal capsule
Central sulcus
Lentiform nucleus
Parietal operculum
Third ventricle
Sylvian fissure
Posterior limb, internal capsule
Thalamus
Cavum veli interpositum
Trigone/glomus of choroid
Pineal with calcification
Internal cerebral vein
Visual cortex/occipital lobe

A   **B**

Figure 2-14 (**A**) CT, (**B**) MRI, at the low ventricular level through the thalamus. (*Continued on p. 92*)

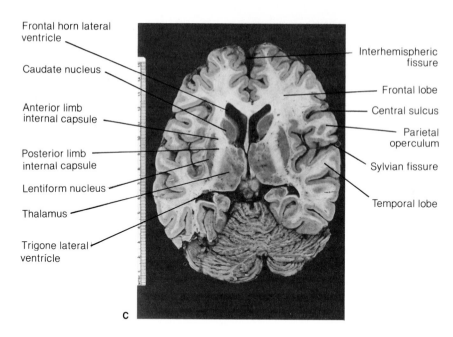

Frontal horn lateral ventricle

Caudate nucleus

Anterior limb internal capsule

Posterior limb internal capsule

Lentiform nucleus

Thalamus

Trigone lateral ventricle

Interhemispheric fissure

Frontal lobe

Central sulcus

Parietal operculum

Sylvian fissure

Temporal lobe

C

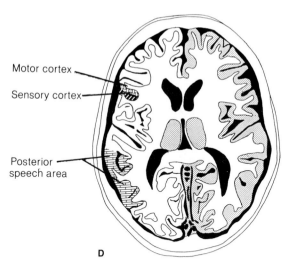

Motor cortex

Sensory cortex

Posterior speech area

D

Figure 2-14 (*cont.*)   (**C**) Brain specimen. (**D**) Line drawing to demonstrate anatomy of brain at the low ventricular level through the thalamus. The line diagram shows the location of the motor and sensory areas as well as the posterior speech area. (*Modified from Gado M., Hanaway J, Frank R: Functional anatomy of the cerebral cortex by computed tomography. Journal of Computer Assisted Tomography* **3**: *1–19, 1979.*)

eral ventricles. The lower and the higher slices in this subset are distinguishable by certain anatomic features. In the lower slice of this subset (Fig. 2-15*A*,*B*) the bodies of the lateral ventricles lie close to midline separated only by the septum pellucidum. In the posterior part, the lateral ventricles diverge away from the midline into the depth of each

cerebral hemisphere, where the body of the ventricle joins the trigone (Fig. 2-14*A*). The basal ganglia is not visualized, except occasionally the superior border of the caudate nucleus, which may appear as a narrow band of density at the lateral border of the body of the lateral ventricle (Fig. 2-15*A*,*B*). The rest of the brain parenchyma in this slice consists of

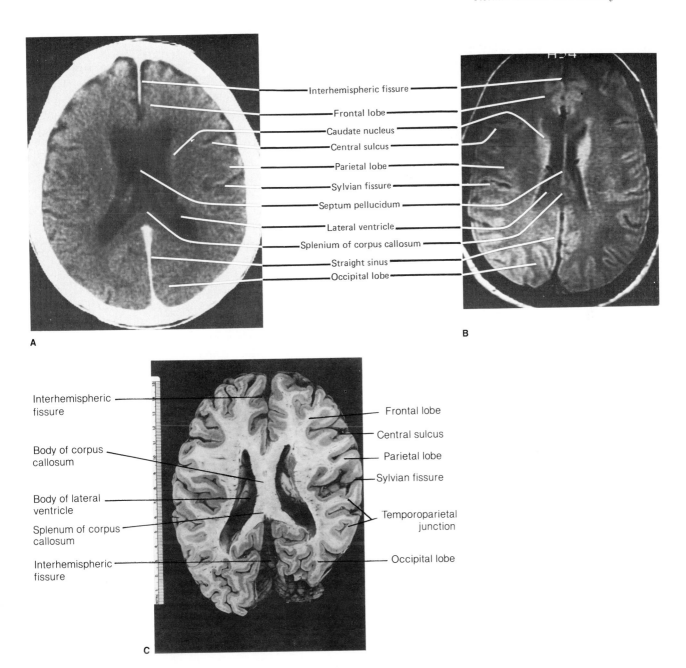

Interhemispheric fissure
Frontal lobe
Caudate nucleus
Central sulcus
Parietal lobe
Sylvian fissure
Septum pellucidum
Lateral ventricle
Splenium of corpus callosum
Straight sinus
Occipital lobe

A

B

Interhemispheric fissure
Body of corpus callosum
Body of lateral ventricle
Splenum of corpus callosum
Interhemispheric fissure

Frontal lobe
Central sulcus
Parietal lobe
Sylvian fissure
Temporoparietal junction
Occipital lobe

C

Figure 2-15 (**A**) CT, (**B**) MRI, (**C**) brain specimen, and (**D**) corresponding line diagram at the high ventricular level through the body of the lateral ventricles (see text). The discrepancy between the CT, MRI sections and the brain specimen is due to lack of tilting of head in the former. The location of the motor, sensory, and speech area is identified in the line diagram. (*Modified from Gado M, Hanaway J, Frank R: Functional anatomy of the cerebral cortex by computed tomography. Journal of Computer Assisted Tomography* **3**: *1–19, 1979.*)

(*Continued on p. 94*)

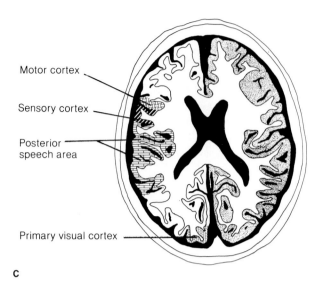

Motor cortex

Sensory cortex

Posterior
speech area

Primary visual cortex

C

Figure 2-15 (*Cont.*)

the white matter of the centrum semiovale and over-lying cerebral cortex. At the convexity, the sylvian fissure appears in the middle of this slice in the same place as the trigone of the lateral ventricle (Fig.

2-14*A*,*B*). In the anterior half of the convexity, the central sulcus lies in the same plane as the anterior end of the body of the lateral ventricle. In the mid-line, the parietooccipital sulcus is seen in the posterior third of the slice separating the parietal lobe and the occipital lobe (Fig. 2-14*A*,*B*). On intravenous enhanced CT at the same level and on MRI, one can identify the lateral atrial vein most often situated in the anterior and mid third junction of the body of the lateral ventricle as well as the anterior cerebral artery as it courses forward over the corpus callosum. In the midline, the parietooccipital sulcus is seen in the posterior third of the slice separating the parietal lobe from the occipital lobe (Fig. 2-15*A*,*B*). The next higher slice in this subset is distinct from the lower slice by the obvious separation between the bodies of the lateral ventricles (Fig. 2-16*A*,*B*). The gap between the two lateral ventricles is occupied by the corpus callosum and cingulate gyrus. The most remarkable sulcus in the midline is the parietooccipital sulcus in the posterior third of the slice (Fig. 2-16*A*,*B*). At the convexity, the central sulcus can occasionally be visualized. The central sul-

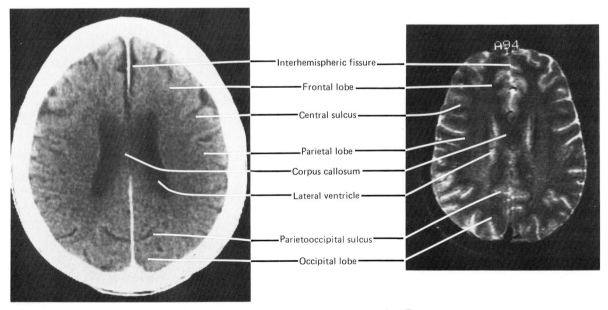

Interhemispheric fissure

Frontal lobe

Central sulcus

Parietal lobe

Corpus callosum

Lateral ventricle

Parietooccipital sulcus

Occipital lobe

A

B

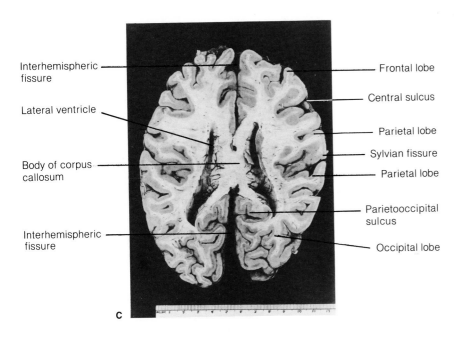

Interhemispheric fissure

Lateral ventricle

Body of corpus callosum

Interhemispheric fissure

Frontal lobe

Central sulcus

Parietal lobe

Sylvian fissure

Parietal lobe

Parietooccipital sulcus

Occipital lobe

C

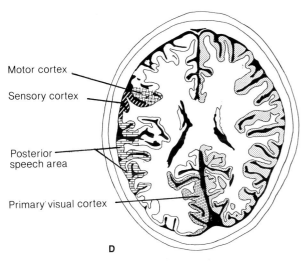

Motor cortex

Sensory cortex

Posterior speech area

Primary visual cortex

D

Figure 2-16 (**A**) CT, (**B**) MRI, (**C**) brain specimen, and (**D**) corresponding line diagram at the high ventricular level through the roof of the lateral ventricle (see text). Discrepancy in CT, MRI sections and brain specimen is due to the lack of tilting of gantry in the former.

cus when visualized lies at a level opposite the anterior third of the body of the lateral ventricle.

Supraventricular Series

The last subset is the supraventricular component (Fig. 2-17). Slices at yet higher levels in this series show decrease in size toward the vertex. Also the higher the slice, the more conspicuous the sulci appear, and they extend farther toward the central part of each hemisphere. The feature common to all slices in this subset is the absence of any central CSF space other than the straight midline intrahemispheric fissure. On each side, the cerebral hemisphere consists of the centrum semiovale and the overlying cerebral cortex (Fig. 2-17A,B). The only recognizable feature in the midline is the intrahemispheric fissure (Fig. 2-17A,B). Over the convexity, the central sulcus is not distinguishable from the other sulci. Its location is approximately at the junction between the ante-

rior one-fourth and the posterior three-fourths of the convexity. Several features not identifiable on the axial CT or even coronal CTs can be well visualized on MR images performed in the sagittal and coronal planes (Figs. 2-3, 2-4, 2-5).

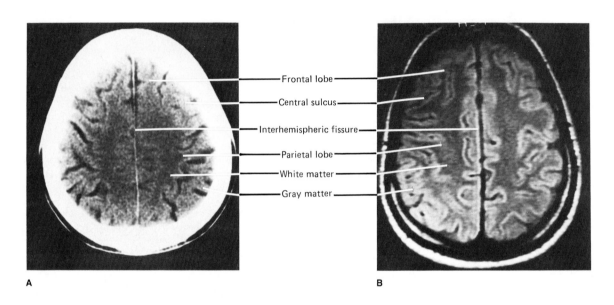

A   B

Frontal lobe

Central sulcus

Interhemispheric fissure

Parietal lobe

White matter

Gray matter

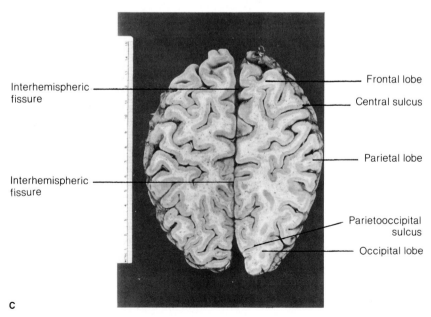

C

Interhemispheric fissure

Interhemispheric fissure

Frontal lobe

Central sulcus

Parietal lobe

Parietooccipital sulcus

Occipital lobe

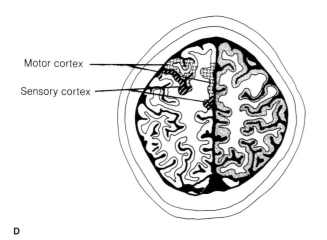

Motor cortex

Sensory cortex

D

Figure 2-17 (**A**) CT, (**B**) MRI, (**C**) brain specimen, and (**D**) line diagram at the supraventricular level (see text). Discrepancy between (**A**) (**B**), and (**C**) (**D**) is related to lack of angling in the former. (*Modified from Gado M, Hanaway J, Frank R: Functional anatomy of the cerebral cortex by computed tomography. Journal of Computer Assisted Tomography **3**: 1–19, 1979.*)

CT AND MRI CORRELATION WITH FUNCTIONAL ANATOMY

In this section, the CT and MRI anatomy of the different lobes of the cerebral hemisphere is described,

each lobe being dealt with separately. The question of which sections contain each lobe is addressed, and within each slice borders of the lobe are defined. Since the architectonic mapping of the cerebral cortex by Brodmann in 1909, several functional areas of the cerebral cortex have been described (Figs. 2-18*A,B*, 2-19*A,B*). In this section the anatomy of the motor, sensory, speech, and visual cortical areas is described. In addition, utilizing the vascular topography which has been demonstrated by CT sectional anatomy (Hayman 1981; Berman 1980, 1984), the CT and MRI sections can be helpful to correlate with the vascular and functional anatomy within that slice (Fig. 2-19*A–D*).

Frontal Lobe

Identification of the Borders of the Frontal Lobe

In the infraventricular subset of slices, the frontal lobes occupy approximately the anterior third of the section (Fig. 2-12*A,B,C*). Two borders of the frontal lobe can be identified. The lateral border lies against the inner table of the cranium. Anteriorly, it starts at the interhemispheric fissure, where it joins the medial border. Posteriorly, the lateral border of the

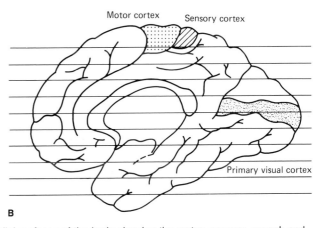

A

B

Figure 2-18 Diagramatic representation of the (**A**) lateral and (**B**) medial surfaces of the brain showing the motor, sensory, speech and primary visual areas of the cerebral cortex. The levels of the CT and MRI sections are represented by the straight lines across the diagram. (*Modified from Gado M, Hanaway J, Frank R: Functional anatomy of the cerebral cortex by computed tomography. Journal of Computer Assisted Tomography **3**: 1–19, 1979*).

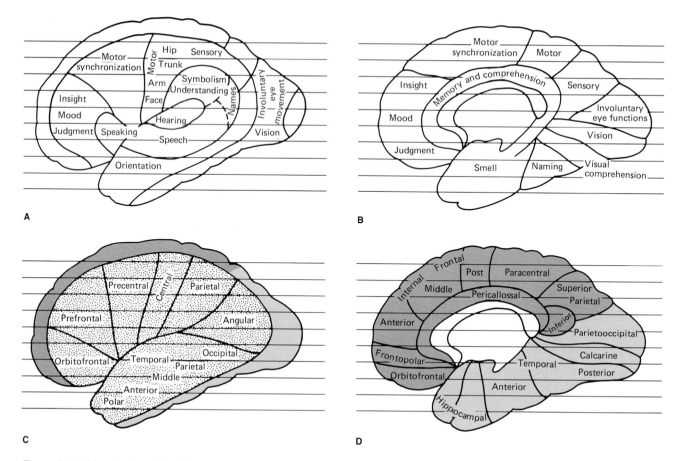

Figure 2-19 Line drawing of the (**A**) lateral and (**B**) medial surface of the brain showing functional localization of the brain. Corresponding (**C**) lateral and (**D**) medial surface demarcation of the vascular territories to match the functional areas and corresponding vascular component. (*Light gray:* anterior cerebral artery. *Stippled:* middle cerebral artery. *Dark gray:* posterior cerebral artery.) (*Modified from Berman et al., Hayman et al.: Correlation of CT cerebral vascular territories with function by computed tomography. 1. Anterior cerebral artery. AJNR **1:** 259–263, 1980. 2. Posterior cerebral artery. AJNR **2:** 219–225, 1981. 3. Middle cerebral artery. AJNR **5:** 161–166, 1984.*)

frontal lobe joins the sylvian cistern which extends across the slice toward the suprasellar cistern in the midline (Fig. 2-12*A*,*B*). The medial border of the frontal lobe extends in the midline from the inner table of the frontal lobe to the suprasellar cistern.

In the low ventricular subset of slices (Figs. 2-13*A*,*B*, 2-14*A*,*B*), the medial borders of the frontal lobe are clearly marked by the interhemispheric fissure which separates them. The intrahemispheric fissure occupies only the anterior fourth of the midline in these slices. The posterior limit of the interhemispheric fissure varies from one slice to the other.

In the lower slice of this subset the intrahemispheric fissure and the third ventricle appear almost continuous, being separated only by a thin layer of gray matter, the lamina terminalis. In the higher slice, however, the posterior limit of the interhemispheric fissure is at the corpus callosum which separates it from the septum pellucidum (Fig. 2-14*A*). The lateral border of the frontal lobe lies against the inner table of the skull. In the lower slice of this subset (Fig. 2-13*A*,*B*), the lateral border of the frontal lobe starts anteriorly in the midline at the interhemispheric fissure and extends posteriorly to the sylvian fissure. The sylvian fissure is therefore a definable landmark for the posterior limit of the frontal lobe in this slice (Fig. 2-13A,B). On the other hand, in the higher slice of the subset, the lateral border of the frontal lobe does not extend to the sylvian fissure (Fig. 2-14A,B) but is separated from it by the part of the parietal lobe that contributes to the formation of the operculum, separating the surface of the insula from the inner table of the skull. The central sulcus, which marks the separation of the frontal lobe from the parietal lobe within the operculum, may not be visible. Its location is approximately in the same transverse plane that passes through the anterior end of the septum pellucidum and can be seen in a coronal section through the same level (Figs. 2-2A, 2-4B). The sylvian fissure, on the other hand, is clearly recognizable by its extreme depth. At its deepest point, the sylvian fissure marks the posterior limit of the insula (Fig. 2-14A,B). In the high ventricular subset of slices (Figs. 2-15, 2-16), the medial border of the frontal lobe is marked by the interhemispheric fissure extending in the midline between the inner table of the frontal bone and the corpus callosum, which lies between the anterior ends of the two lateral ventricles (Fig. 2-15A,B). The lateral border of the frontal lobe lies against the inner table of the skull, starting anteriorly at the interhemispheric fissure and ending posteriorly at the central sulcus, which separates the frontal lobe from the parietal lobe. The central sulcus is not as easily recognizable as the sylvian fissure. Its location is approximately in the same transverse plane that passes through the anterior ends of the lateral ventricles or slightly posterior to it (Figs. 2-15A,B, 2-16A,B). In the supraventricular set of slices (Fig. 2-17A,B), the interhemispheric fissure extends through the entire length of midline and the lateral ventricles are absent. We therefore have no anatomical landmark to determine the posterior limits of the frontal lobe at the medial or lateral borders. One may arbitrarily take the frontal lobes to be occupying the anterior one-fourth of the cerebral hemisphere in each slice of this subset (Fig. 2-17A,B). However, the borders of the frontal lobe can be defined utilizing the sagittal MR sections (Figs. 2-2A,B, 2-5A,B).

Functional Localization in the Frontal Lobe

The anterior cortical speech area (Broca's speech area) is located in the dominant hemisphere. It occupies the posterior end of the inferior frontal gyrus on the lateral surface of the frontal lobe (Fig. 2-18A). It is thus located in the upper slice of the infraventricular subset and the next slice of the low ventricular subset (Figs. 2-13, 2-14). The posterior part of the lateral border of the frontal lobe in both slices forms the anterior cortical speech area. The motor cortical area occupies the precentral gyrus. It starts inferiorly just behind the speech area (Figs. 2-18A, 2-19A) and extends superiorly to the superior margin of the cerebral hemispheres, with an extension for a short distance downward from the medial surface forming part of the paracentral lobule (Fig. 2-18B). The motor and premotor cortex thus is represented in slices of the low ventricular, high ventricular, and supraventricular subsets.

Temporal Lobe

Identification of the Borders of the Temporal Lobe

In the infraventricular slices, the temporal lobe is limited anteriorly by the sylvian cistern or sphenoid ridge (Figs. 2-10A,B, 2-11A,B). The lateral border of the temporal lobe lies against the inner table of the cranium posteriorly and medially; the temporal lobe lies against the anterior surface of the petrous bone and the lateral border of the clivus, dorsum sella, and suprasellar cistern (Fig. 2-11A,B). In the slices of this subset, the temporal lobe occupies a small area in the middle third of the slice on both sides of the clivus. In the highest of this subset and in the low ventricular subset, the lateral border of the temporal lobe is limited anteriorly by the sylvian fissure (Figs. 2-12A,B, 2-13A,B). Posteriorly, it blends imperceptibly into the occipital lobe. There is no demarcating anatomical structure that separates the lateral border of the temporal lobe from the occipital lobe (Fig. 2-13A,B). Also, medially the temporal lobe is continuous with the region of the basal ganglia and thalamus (Figs. 2-13*A*,*B*, 2-14*A*,*B*).

In the slices of the high ventricular subset, the temporoparietal junction is seen at the lateral border of the cerebral hemisphere behind the sylvian fissure in the lower of the subset slices (Fig. 2-15*A* and *B*).

Functional Localization
in the Temporal Lobe

The acoustic cortical area is located in the superior temporal gyrus. It is located in the lateral border of the temporal lobe where the borders close in to form the posterior limit of the sylvian fissure. The sizes of the low ventricular subset contain that portion of the superior temporal gyrus.

The posterior speech area is located in the dominant hemisphere. It occupies an extensive area of the posterior parts of the superior and middle temporal gyri and extends into the inferior part of the parietal lobe (Fig. 2-18*A*), being located at the lateral border of the cerebral hemisphere in the slices of the high ventricular subset (Figs. 2-14, 2-15, 2-16). In these slices, the posterior speech area extends in front of and behind the sylvian fissure. In addition, part of the posterior speech area is also located in the high slice of the low ventricular subset (Fig. 2-14), in which, however, it is located only behind the sylvian fissure.

Parietal Lobe

Since presently the CT is done without angling the gantry, the parietal lobe is situated in line with the superior part of the temporal lobe. However, if there is tilting of the gantry by 20 degrees of the orbital meatal plane, the anterior inferior part of the parietal lobe will appear in the low ventricular slices anterior to and in line with the superior posterior part of the temporal lobe separated from it by the sylvian fissure. This part of the parietal lobe is referred to as the parietal operculum, to distinguish it from the rest of the parietal lobe, which appears in slices of higher levels as one continuous structure

extending from the central sulcus anteriorly to the parietooccipital junction posteriorly (Fig. 2-16).

Identification of the Borders
of the Parietal Lobe

In the slices of the low ventricular subset, only the parietal operculum is visualized. Its lateral border lies against the inner table of the cranium. Its posterior border is clearly defined by the deep sylvian fissure, which separates the posterior border of that portion of the parietal lobe from the temporal lobe. The slices of the low ventricular subset thus do not include any part of the parietal lobe behind the sylvian fissure. This is in contrast to the slices of the high ventricular subset as discussed below.

In the slices of the high ventricular subset, the sylvian fissure is recognized. The central sulcus lies approximately at the same transverse line that passes through the anterior ends of the lateral ventricles (Figs. 2-15*A*,*B*, 2-16*A*,*B*) so the lateral border of the parietal lobe lies between these two sulcal landmarks easily recognized. In the lower section (Fig. 2-15*A*,*B*), the lateral border of the cerebral hemisphere behind the sylvian fissure belongs to the temporoparietal junction. The lateral border of the temporoparietal junction becomes continuous posteriorly with the lateral border of the occipital lobe. There is no recognizable structure separating the two. In the upper slice of the high ventricular series (Fig. 2-16*A*,*B*), however, the parietal lobe forms the lateral border of the cerebral hemisphere from the central sulcus anteriorly to the parietooccipital junction posteriorly. Again, the parietooccipital junction is not defined by an anatomical structure. A clue to the approximate location of the parietooccipital junction may be obtained from the conspicuous parietooccipital sulcus on the medial surface of the cerebral hemisphere (Figs. 2-16*A*,*B*, 2-4). In the supraventricular section (Fig. 2-17), the interhemispheric fissure extends the entire length of the midline. Both the medial and the lateral borders of the parietal lobe are therefore identified in the slices of this subset, the lobe occupying the middle half of the slice, with the frontal lobe occupying the anterior one-fourth and the occipital lobe the posterior one-fourth (Fig. 2-17*A,B*). The parietooccipital junction is recognized on the medial border of the hemisphere by the parietooccipital sulcus (Figs. 2-17*A,B*, 2-4). In the higher supraventricular slices, the extent of the occipital lobe gradually diminishes; the topmost one or two slices of this subset may contain no part of it. In these extremely high levels, the slice consists solely of frontal and parietal lobes. The size of the portions occupied by the frontal and parietal lobes, respectively, would depend upon the orientation of the slice and the slope of the vertex.

Functional Localization in the Parietal Lobe

The sensory cortex occupies the postcentral gyrus of the parietal lobe. On the lateral surface of the parietal lobe, the cortical area starts inferiorly in the parietal operculum (Fig. 2-18*A*) and extends superiorly to the superior border of the cerebral hemisphere, with an extension of the medial surface forming part of the paracentral lobule (Fig. 2-18*B*). The sensory cortex is thus represented in the sections of the low ventricular (Figs. 2-13*C*, 2-14*C*), high ventricular (Figs. 2-15*C*, 2-16*C*), and supraventricular (Fig. 2-17*C*) subsets. Since the localization of the central sulcus may be difficult, the anterior end of the septum pellucidum may be used as a guide to its location in the low ventricular series and the anterior ends of the lateral ventricles in the high ventricular series; in the supraventricular series, it lies at the junction of the anterior one-fourth and the rest of the slice. The sensory cortex lies in the posterior side of the central sulcus. In the top slices, the sensory cortex is seen in both the lateral and medial borders of the parietal lobe (Figs. 2-17*C* and 2-4). The posterior speech area is a large area (Fig. 2-18*A*) curving around the posterior extremity of the sylvian fissure in the dominant hemisphere, occupying the inferior part of the parietal lobe and extending into a more extensive area of the adjoining parts of the superior and middle temporal gyri (Fig. 2-18*A*). In the slices of the high ventricular subset (Figs. 2-14, 2-15*C*), the posterior speech area is lo-

cated in the lateral border of the dominant hemisphere extending in front of as well as behind the sylvian fissure. In addition, part of it is also located in the higher slice of the low ventricular subset (Fig. 2-13*C*), in which it is located only behind the sylvian fissure.

The Occipital Lobe

Identification of the Borders of the Occipital Lobe

The occipital lobe can be visualized in the low ventricular series (Fig. 2-13) and extending into the high ventricular series where it is demarcated posteriorly from the parietal lobe by the parietooccipital sulcus (Fig. 2-16*A,B*). In the low ventricular subset the anterior limit of the occipital lobe at the medial border is demarcated by the parietooccipital sulcus. At the occipital pole, the medial border of the occipital lobe is continuous with the lateral border, which lies against the inner table of the skull. The anterior limit of the occipital lobe at the lateral border is not defined by any anatomical structure.

In the slices of the high ventricular subset (Figs. 2-15, 2-16), the configuration is the same as just described. Extremely deep convolutions of visual cortex around the calcarine sulcus may be recognized in slices of this subset. However, these are better visualized on both axial as well as sagittal MR sections since the parietooccipital sulcus as well as the calcarine sulcus can be clearly identified (Figs. 2-2*B*, 2-4). The calcarine sulcus is situated within the substance of the occipital lobe and encroached upon the white matter in the deep part of the occipital lobe.

In the supraventricular subset, it is difficult to identify the calcarine fissure. It is the cuneus of the occipital lobe that is represented in the slices of this subset. In the higher slices of the supraventricular subset, the distinction between the parietooccipital sulcus and the posterior end of the cerebral hemisphere diminishes. This results in the decrease of the length of the position of the medial border of the hemisphere that belongs to the occipital lobe. In the top one or two slices of the supraventricular subset, the parietooccipital sulcus, enhanced occipital lobe, may not be recognizable at all. For this reason, if it is necessary to identify lesions and/or anatomical description of this area, MR is more useful, particularly in the sagittal plane.

Functional Localization in the Occipital Lobe

The primary visual area, referred to as the striate cortex, occupies the upper and lower lips and the depth of the calcarine sulcus (Fig. 2-18*B*). It thus lies largely on the medial surface of the occipital lobe, extending posteriorly into the occipital pole and limited laterally by the lunate sulcus (Fig. 2-18*A*). The primary visual area receives fibers of the optic radiation from the lateral geniculate body. The geniculate radition spreads out through the white matter of the occipital lobe, terminating in the occipital cortex.

CT Anatomy of the Basal Ganglia

The basal ganglia are parts of the telencephalon. They represent the central gray matter of the telencephalon. They include the caudate nucleus, the lentiform nucleus, the claustrum, and the amygdala. The caudate nucleus consists of an enlarged anterior portion, or head, and a narrow posterior portion, or tail. The head occupies most of the lateral wall of the anterior horn of the lateral ventricle. The tail curves along the lateral aspect of the thalamus. At its terminal portion, the tail forms the amygdala.

The basal ganglia are not visualized in the intraventricular subset of slices. It is the low ventricular subset that includes these deep gray-matter structures (Figs. 2-13, 2-14). In addition, only the superior surface of the body of the caudate nucleus is visualized in the lower slice of the high ventricular subset (Fig. 2-15).

The internal capsule is a thick band of white matter situated between the thalamus, which is part of the diencephalon, and the caudate and lentiform nuclei, which are parts of the telencephalon (Fig. 2-14). As previously stated, both the telencephalon and the diencephalon are parts of the forebrain (prosencephalon). The internal capsule is thus visualized only in the slices of the low ventricular subset (Figs. 2-13, 2-14). The anterior limb of the internal capsule lies between the caudate nucleus and the lentiform nucleus. The posterior limb lies between the thalamus and the lentiform nucleus. The posterior limb contains the motor fibers from the cerebral cortex to the spinal motor nuclei and the sensory fibers from the thalamus to the sensory cortex, as well as fibers of the auditory and optic radiations from the geniculate bodies to the temporal and occipital cortices. The superior inferior extent of the structures comprising the basal ganglia is best visualized in coronal MR and occasionally in CT (Fig. 2-4*B,C,D*).

The claustrum appears in the axial section as a thin band of deep gray matter that lies between the lentiform nucleus medially and the cortex of the insula laterally (Figs. 2-14, 2-4*C*). The white matter between the claustrum and the lentiform nucleus is the external capsule, while that between the claustrum and the insular cortex is the extreme capsule.

Bibliography

BERMAN SA, HAYMAN LA, HINCK VC: Correlation of CT cerebral vascular territories with function. 3. Middle cerebral artery. *AJNR* **5**(2):161–166, 1984.

BERMAN SA, HAYMAN LA, HINCK VC: Correlation of cerebral vascular territories with cerebral function by computed tomography. 1. Anterior cerebral artery. *AJNR* **1**:259–263, 1980.

CARPENTER MB: *Human Neuroanatomy*, 7th ed. Baltimore, Williams and Wilkins, 1976.

GADO M, HANAWAY J, FRANK R: Functional anatomy of the cerebral cortex by computed tomography. *J Comput Assist Tomogr* **3:**1–19, 1979.

GOSS CM (ed): *Gray's Anatomy* 29th Am. Ed. Philadelphia, Lea & Febiger, 1973.

HANAWAY J, SCOTT W, STROTHER C: *Atlas of the Human Brain and the Orbit for Computed Tomography.* St. Louis, Warren Green Inc., 1977.

HAYMAN LA, BERMAN SA, HINCK VC: Correlation of CT cerebral vascular territories with function: II, posterior cerebral artery. *AJNR* **2:**219–225, 1981.

MATSUI, T, HIRANO A: *An Atlas of the Human Brain for Computerized Tomography.* Tokyo, New York, Igaki-Shon, 1978.

NIEUWENHUYS, VOUGD, VAN HUIJZEN: *The Human Central Nervous System.* Berlin, Heidelberg, New York, Springer-Verlag, 1979.

WILLIAMS, WARWICK: *Functional Neuroanatomy of Man.* Philadelphia and Toronto, Saunders, 1975.

3

THE ORBIT

Scott W. Atlas

Robert A. Zimmerman

Larissa T. Bilaniuk

INTRODUCTION AND TECHNIQUE

The application of computed tomography (CT) to the evaluation of orbital disease constitutes a major advance (Forbes 1980; Trokel 1979; Forbes 1982; Jacobs 1980). Computed tomography provides information regarding the presence, location, and extent of intraorbital lesions, as well as the involvement of the orbit by lesions arising in the adjacent bone and paranasal sinuses (Mancuso 1978; Weber 1978; Som 1985). The introduction of high-resolution scanners with thin sections, short scan times, and magnification and reformation capabilities has extended the scope and increased the accuracy of the CT evaluation of orbital lesions.

TECHNIQUE

The examination of the orbit by CT should be tailored to the clinical problem at hand but should also be anatomically complete. Contiguous thin sections, no larger than 5 mm in thickness, are obtained routinely in at least two planes: (1) transverse, (2) coronal and/or sagittal (Baleriaux-Waha 1977; Hoyt 1979; Osborn 1980; Tadmor 1978; Unsold 1980a; Wing 1979). The entire orbit is encompassed, as well as the adjacent portions of the brain and of sinus, facial, and pharyngeal soft tissues. The authors' experience indicates that examination is necessary in the transverse plane usually at an angulation of $-10°$ to the orbitomeatal base line (Fig. 3-1) and that the initial

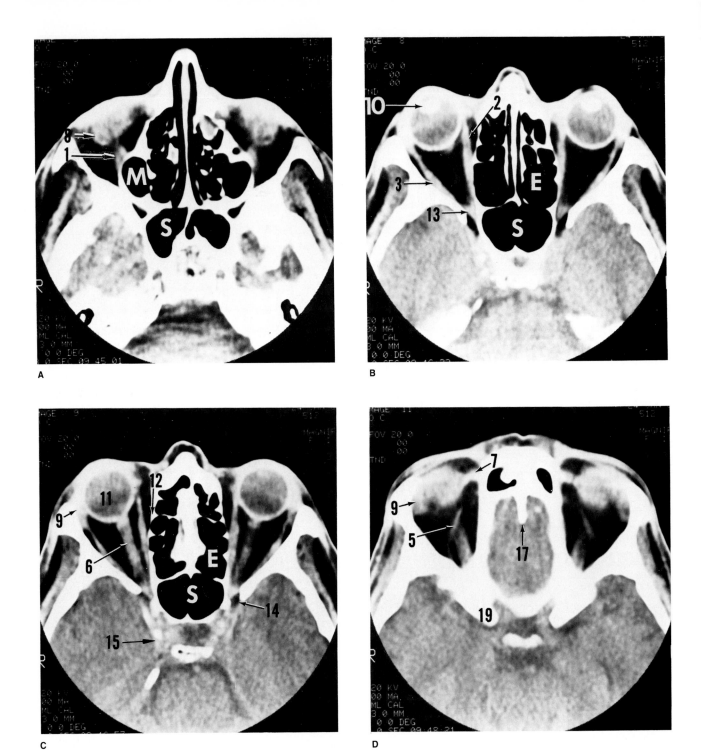

Figure 3-1 (**A–D**) Normal orbit, axial plane, inferior to superior. 1 = inferior rectus, 2 = medial rectus, 3 = lateral rectus, 4 = superior rectus, 5 = superior ophthalmic vein, 6 = optic nerve, 7 = superior oblique, 8 = inferior oblique, 9 = lacrimal gland, 10 = lens, 11 = vitreous, 12 = lamina papyracea, 13 = optic canal, 14 = superior orbital fissure, 15 = cavernous sinus, 16 = floor of orbit, 17 = crista galli, 18 = cribriform plate, 19 = anterior clinoid, 20 = planum sphenoidale, 21 = inferior orbital fissure. M = maxillary sinus, E = ethmoid sinus, S = sphenoid sinus.

examination should be made both before and after the injection of an adequate amount of iodinated contrast material. Coronal sections are made in addition to the transverse section (Fig. 3-2). Where 1.5- or 2-mm sections are possible, sagittal reformation, and even satisfactory coronal reformation from the transverse sections can be made, provided the patient has not moved during the examination. Oblique reformation, so that the plane of the optic nerve (Unsold 1980a) or of the superior ophthalmic vein can be followed, may be of value in specific cases.

Because of its sinuous course in two places, the appearance and course of the optic nerve depend on the thickness and plane of the CT section as well as on the direction of gaze (Unsold 1980b). Unsold recommends a negative angulation of $-20°$ to the orbitomeatal base line with the eye in upgaze position in order to stretch the nerves and have their course parallel to the plane of section.

The adequacy of the CT examination of the orbit can be assured only if the study is carefully monitored and if images that are marred by motion or artifacts are repeated. Following completion of the examination, the study must be carefully reviewed. Such a review is best done on a diagnostic display console, so that the sections may be examined for the osseous and soft-tissue structures at a variety of window widths with different window levels. For permanent film record, two setings are recommended at approximately 30/300 and 350–700/ 1000–2000 with image magnifications.

NORMAL ANATOMY OF THE ORBIT

Orbital Walls

The orbit is a pyramidal bony compartment that houses the eyeball and its functional components (extraocular muscles, blood vessels, nerves, lacrimal gland, and fat) (Tadmor 1978). The orbital walls separate the intraorbital components from surrounding brain and facial structures (Hesselink 1978).

The *roof* of the orbit (Fig. 3-2) is formed for the most part by the orbital plate of the frontal bone and separates the orbit from the anterior cranial fossa. The lacrimal gland (Figs. 3-1, 3-2) forms a fossa, the lacrimal fossa, in the superolateral aspect of the orbit. Overall, the bone that forms the roof of the orbit is relatively thin. To a variable extent, the frontal sinus and sometimes the ethmoid sinuses extend into the roof of the orbit. The posterior component of the roof of the orbit that is formed by the lesser wing of the sphenoid may also contain air cells derived from either the posterior ethmoidal cells or the sphenoid sinus.

The *floor* of the orbit (Fig. 3-2) is composed primarily of the orbital plate of the maxilla. It has a triangular shape, with contributions from portions of the zygoma and the palatine bone. The infraorbital nerve courses along the orbital surface of the floor of the orbit. The orbital floor is thin, except at its most anterior margin, where the orbital rim is formed, which is a thicker osseous structure in continuity below with the anterior wall of the maxillary sinus. The floor of the orbit separates the intraorbital structures from the maxillary sinus (Fig. 3-2) which lies beneath.

The *lateral wall* of the orbit is formed by the zygoma (Figs. 3-1, 3-2) anteriorly and the greater wing of the sphenoid posteriorly (Figs. 3-1, 3-2). The lateral orbital wall is the thickest and strongest of the orbital walls. Lateral to this structure lies the temporal fossa, which contains the temporal muscle.

The *medial wall* (Figs. 3-1, 3-2) is the thinnest component of the orbital walls. It serves to separate the orbital contents from the ethmoid and sphenoid air cells. Contributions to the structure of the medial wall are made by the maxilla, lacrimal bone, ethmoid bone, and body of the sphenoid. The largest component is that contributed by the ethmoidal orbital plate (lamina papyracea).

Orbital Fissures and Canals

At the apex of the pyramidal structure of the orbit lie three openings that communicate with adjacent extraorbital areas.

The *optic canal* (Figs. 3-1, 3-2) is formed by the sphenoid bone and serves to conduct the optic nerve and ophthalmic artery between the orbit and the

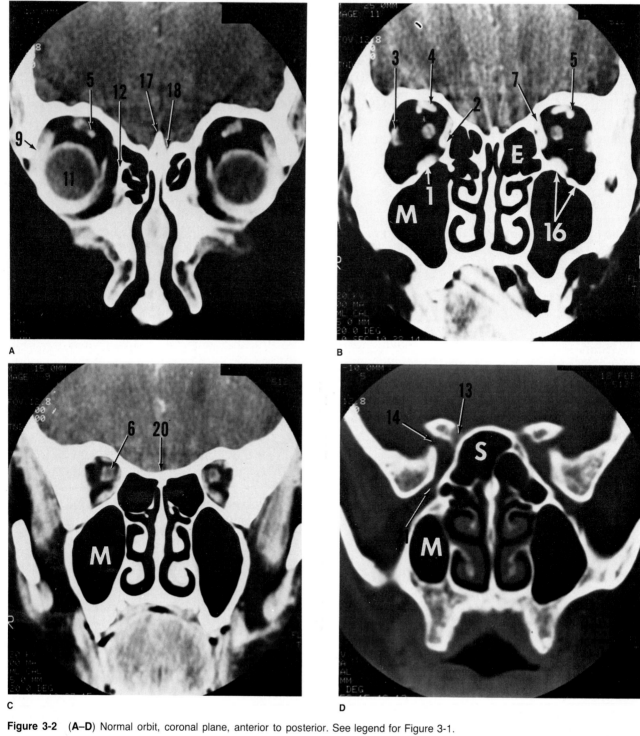

Figure 3-2 (**A–D**) Normal orbit, coronal plane, anterior to posterior. See legend for Figure 3-1.

middle cranial fossa. The optic nerve is surrounded by a small subarachnoid space which contains cerebrospinal fluid (CSF) and is surrounded by the arachnoid. The ophthalmic artery lies beneath the optic nerve. The roof of the optic canal measures 10 to 12 mm in length and is formed by the lesser wing of the sphenoid. The medial wall of the optic canal is formed by the body of the sphenoid bone, while its inferior and lateral walls are formed by the roots of the lesser wing of the sphenoid (optic strut), which also serves to separate the optic canal from the superior orbital fissure.

The *superior orbital fissure* (Fig. 3-2) is a space between the greater and lesser wings of the sphenoid. It is separated medially from the optic canal by the optic strut. Transmitted through the superior orbital fissure between the middle cranial fossa and orbit are the superior ophthalmic vein, the third, fourth, and sixth cranial nerves, and the first division of the fifth cranial nerve.

The *inferior orbital fissure* (Fig. 3-2) permits communication between the orbit and the pterygopalatine and infratemporal fossae. Through it runs the infraorbital nerve and the communication between the inferior ophthalmic vein and the pterygoid venous plexus. The maxilla, palatine bone, and greater wing of the sphenoid bone contribute to its margins.

Periosteum

Periosteum lines the bones of the orbit and is in communication with the periosteum covering the intracranial compartment, through the various fissures. The septum orbitale (Fig. 3-1) is a periosteal reflection from the anterior orbital margin which is continuous with the tarsal plates. It serves to separate the orbit into pre- and postseptal components. The intraorbital fat is limited anteriorly by the orbital septum. The eyelids lie anterior to the orbital septum.

Orbital Soft Tissue

The wall of the *globe* consists of three layers. The innermost, the retina, contains the nerve elements that allow visual perception. The middle layer consists of the choroid, ciliary body, and iris (uveal tract), a set of structures of vascular and nutritive function. The outermost layer is a fibrous protective coating that constitutes the sclera and, anteriorly, the transparent cornea. The lens (Fig. 3-1) is a transparent crystalline body approximately 1 cm in diameter that serves to transmit light and lies between the iris and the vitreous humor (Fig. 3-1). Between the cornea and the lens is a space containing aqueous humor that is divided by the iris into an anterior chamber and a posterior chamber.

The *optic nerve* (Figs. 3-1, 3-2), the second cranial nerve, extends from the papilla on the posterior surface of the globe to the optic chiasm. Its length is between 35 and 50 mm, with its intraorbital component 20 to 30 mm, the intracanalicular portion 4 to 9 mm, and the intracranial portion 3 to 6 mm. The diameter of the optic nerve is approximately 3 to 4 mm. Running beneath the optic nerve as it enters the optic canal from the intracranial compartment is the ophthalmic artery, which remains beneath the optic nerve in its intracanalicular segment and in its initial intraorbital segment. Surrounding the optic nerve throughout its intraorbital course is the central orbital fat.

Six *extraocular muscles* (Figs. 3-1, 3-2) insert on the sclera. These are the medial and lateral recti, the superior and inferior recti, and the superior and inferior oblique muscles. The superior rectus is the longest, 40 mm, with the medial, lateral, and inferior recti being of progressively shorter length. The medial rectus has the largest diameter of the ocular muscles. The superior oblique muscle is the thinnest muscle and lies in the superomedial aspect of the orbit. The levator palpebrae superioris muscle lies just under the roof of the orbit as a thin flat structure, above the superior rectus. It attaches to the skin of the upper eyelid. Below the superior rectus muscle lies the superior ophthalmic vein, and below it, the optic nerve. The lateral rectus lies adjacent to the periosteum of the lateral orbital wall, and only anteriorly does a slight amount of fat intervene between the periosteum and the muscle. The medial rectus is separated from the lamina papyracea by some peripheral orbital fat. The posterior portion of the inferior rectus muscle lies in contact with the floor of the orbit, but its anterior portion is separated from the roof of the maxillary sinus by peripheral orbital fat.

Orbital fat (Figs. 3-1, 3-2) fills the space that is not occupied by nerve, muscle, or vessels. It extends from the orbital septum anteriorly and from the optic nerve to the orbital wall. It is divided by the intermuscular membrane into a central portion and a more peripheral (extramuscular) portion. The peripheral fat lies between the periosteum of the orbital walls and the rectus muscles.

The *superior ophthalmic vein* (Figs. 3-1, 3-2) forms at the root of the nose, at the juncture of the frontal and angular veins, and enters the orbit, passing around the trochlea for the superior oblique muscle. After coursing posterosuperiorly for a very short segment, it passes posterolaterally into the muscle cone and comes to lie adjacent to the inferior surface of the superior rectus muscle. It then turns medially to course between the superior rectus and lateral rectus muscles and at the orbital apex enters the superior orbital fissure. After it passes through the superior orbital fissure it joins the cavernous sinus. The diameter of the superior ophthalmic vein varies in size from 2 to 3.5 mm, and can change with head position. Asymmetry may be present in a normal patient.

A small space filled with cerebrospinal fluid surrounds the optic nerve. The space lies within the nerve sheath and extends from the optic canal forward to the papilla. The size of the space varies, and its degree of communication with the chiasmatic cistern may also vary (Haughton 1980). Entrance of both Pantopaque (Tabaddor 1973) and air (Tenner 1968) has been reported at the time of myelography and pneumoencephalography. The radiographic visualization of the space has not been a regular phenomenon and has not been without risk of optic nerve injury (Tabaddor 1973). Water-soluble intrathecal contrast medium opacifies the *intracranial subarachnoid space*, putting into relief structures which lie within, such as the optic chiasm. Opacification of the *perioptic subarachnoid space* has been recognized on CT following the intrathecal injection of metrizamide (Fox 1979; Manelfe 1978).

Intravenous enhanced high-resolution CT, along with surface coil magnetic resonance (MR), have obviated the need for metrizamide instillation for evaluation of possible optic nerve pathology. (See Chapter 8, Figure 8-26.)

ORBITAL INFLAMMATION

Bacterial Infection

Bacterial infection of the orbit is most often due to sinus infection, foreign body, skin infection, or bacteremia (Krohel 1982). The orbital septum, the reflected periosteum from the anterior bony margin of the orbit, functions as a barrier that prevents preseptal cellulitis from extending back into the orbital soft tissues (Fig. 3-3) (Kaplan 1976). The postseptal portion of the orbit may become involved by bacterial infection transmitted through the orbital sep-

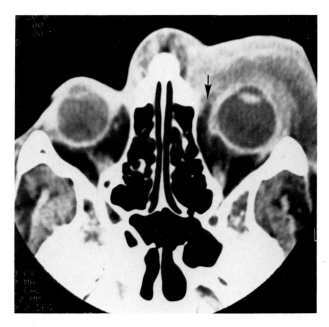

Figure 3-3 Preseptal cellulitis. Enhancing mass anterior to orbital septum (arrow) with normal retrobulbar fat.

tum. The infection may extend into the orbit proper along venous pathways or through the orbital wall and then through the periosteum.

The chief clinical manifestation of orbital infection is swelling and redness of the eyelids. This may be either edematous swelling or actual cellulitis. In either situation, adequate physical examination of the eye is often difficult or impossible, and the extent of the infection cannot be delineated or its source determined clinically.

The absence of valves in the facial veins (including the orbit and paranasal sinuses) leads to the free transmission of elevated pressure between sinus and orbit. In the child and adolescent, orbital infection is most often a concomitant of sinusitis. Increased pressure in the sinus cavity is transmitted to the orbit and causes preseptal edema. Septic thrombophlebitis leads to cellulitis and possibly to orbital cellulitis. Direct extension of infection through congenital osseous dehiscences or involvement of the thin bony walls of the orbit by osteomyelitis can lead to subperiosteal abscess formation (Fig. 3-4). The orbital periosteum is loosely attached except at the suture line, so that subperiosteal collections are eas-

ily formed. In the young child with ethmoid sinusitis, the subperiosteal collection is along the medial orbital wall and produces lateral proptosis of the globe. In the adolescent with frontal sinusitis, the subperiosteal collection is in the superior aspect of the orbit and produces anterior and downward displacement of the globe.

While skull radiographs and pluridirectional tomography of the paranasal sinuses can demonstrate free introrbital air, osteitis of the sinus wall, and mucosal thickening or sinus opacification, CT is capable of showing not only the bony changes and sinus opacification but the orbital soft tissue changes as well. Zimmerman (1980*a*) reported a series of 18 patients with orbital infection with or without cerebral complications studied by CT. All cases of acute periorbital cellulitis showed septal swelling, and the majority showed proptosis, scleral thickening, subperiosteal abscesses, and occasionally infection of the peripheral surgical space. Frontal lobe cerebritis and epidural inflammation are also well shown by CT. Soft tissue scarring of the retrobulbar space can be seen 2 years after bacterial orbital cellulitis. In patients with trauma or foreign body, CT not only

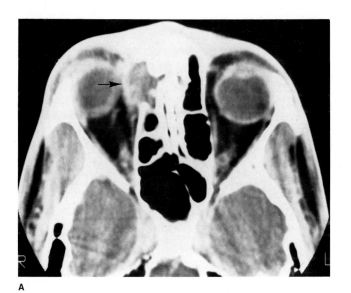

A

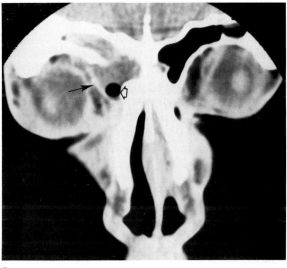

B

Figure 3-4 **(A, B)** Subperiosteal abscess. Soft-tissue density extending from right frontoethmoid sinus into orbit. Note focal defect in nonexpanded sinus wall, enhancing periosteal lining (arrow) and air within abscess (open arrow).

localized the radiodense foreign body but also demonstrated intraorbital, subperiosteal, and intracranial abscesses (Zimmerman 1980*a*).

Infection within the orbit proper can be classified as (1) intraconic, within the muscle cone (central surgical space); (2) extraconic, extrinsic to the intermuscular fibrous septum (within the peripheral surgical space); or (3) subperiosteal, between the orbital wall and its periosteal covering. Most cases of postseptal cellulitis are limited to the extraconal space (Towbin 1986). Infection of the central surgical space obliterates the soft-tissue planes that exist normally between the optic nerve, orbital fat, and rectus muscles. Infection in the peripheral surgical space obliterates the plane between the rectus muscles, peripheral fat, and wall of the orbit. Infection in the subperiosteal space is demonstrated by displacement of the contrast-enhanced periosteal membrane away from the orbital wall (Fig. 3-4).

The rapid increase in the use of CT in evaluation of patients with orbital infection at the authors' institution reflects its clinical value in such cases. Treatment of orbital infection, whether medical or surgical, must be timely, specific, and sufficient. It is imperative that the disease process be recognized quickly and treated aggressively and that operative drainage be carried out whenever indicated. Subperiosteal abscesses need to be drained, and often also the offending infected sinuses. The danger of cavernous sinus thrombosis is real, and it carries with it, even in the antibiotic era, a significant morbidity and mortality. The consequences of inadequate treatment remain potentially catastrophic, because blindness and death may result. The consequences of cerebritis and cerebral abscess formation, even when the condition is adequately treated, may appear as seizures, motor weakness, and psychological aberrations.

Foreign Bodies

Localization of an intraorbital foreign body by routine radiographic means may be difficult. In order to facilitate surgical planning for removal, it is necessary to localize the foreign body accurately. With radiodense foreign bodies this is easier, as they are well shown on routine x-rays, tomography, and CT (Figs. 3-5, 3-6). However, CT is clearly superior to conventional radiography in demonstrating precise anatomic localization of foreign bodies within the globe and sequelae thereof (i.e., ruptured globe, retinal detachment, lens disruption, or vitreal hemorrhage) in patients who may be difficult to thoroughly examine clinically (Sevel 1983). In addition, often unsuspected fragments, retrobulbar or intracranial in location, are detected by CT. Prognostic information may also be obtained by CT in penetrating injuries of the globe (Sternberg 1984; Brown 1985; Weisman 1983). Double penetration of the globe and optic nerve injury by foreign bodies are relevant to surgical planning and prognosis.

With the nonopaque foreign body (Fig. 3-7), such as a wood splinter, CT may show only the granulomatous reaction (Macrae 1979) or focal air density. In the patient who presents wth proptosis or with evidence of granulomatous reaction in the vicinity

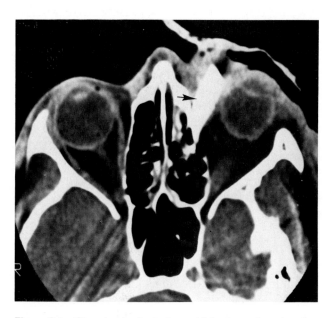

Figure 3-5 Glass foreign body. Large high-attenuation glass foreign body (arrows) just medial to left globe, leaving globe intact.

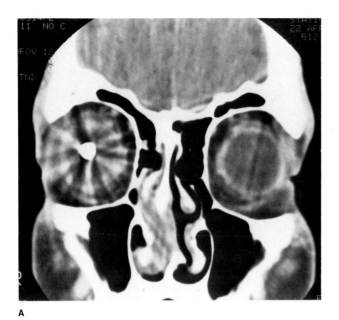

A

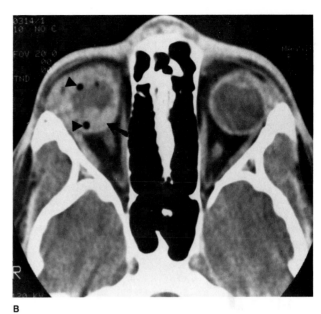

B

Figure 3-6 **(A, B)** Intraocular foreign body. Metallic foreign body on coronal image **(A)** in vitreous, with secondary intraocular hemorrhage and air. Note subretinal hemorrhage (arrow) and air (arrowheads) on axial view **(B)**.

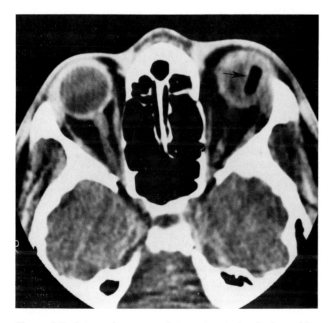

Figure 3-7 Intraocular sponge. Intraocular air density (arrow) indicates retained surgical sponge in left globe.

of the orbit, consideration should be given to a forgotten minor trauma produced by an intraorbital foreign body. In such a case, CT is capable of revealing metallic fragments and other radiodense foreign bodies such as pencil lead or glass (Fig. 3-5).

Pseudotumor

Between the ages of 10 and 40, the most common cause of an intraorbital mass is the orbital pseudotumor (Bernardino 1977). The classic clinical triad includes proptosis, pain, and impaired ocular motility. To a variable degree there may also be diplopia, decreased vision, papillitis, and retinal striae. The symptomatology and clinical signs simulate an intraorbital tumor. Orbital pseudotumor is one of the most common causes of unilateral exophthalmos (Bernardino 1977), but bilaterality is common (Rothfus 1984; Dresner 1984).

The cause of orbital pseudotumor is not known, but experimental work has implicated an autoimmune response of the retrobulbar tissues to antigens (Wilner 1978). Pathologically, two categories of disease exist: (1) an acute form, in which the reaction is that of a vasculitis with vessel wall necrosis and fibrinoid changes, and (2) a chronic inflammatory process, with diffuse infiltration of the affected tissues with lymphocytes, plasma cells, macrophages, and occasionally eosinophils (Jones 1979). The changes of orbital pseudotumor may be found in association with certain clinical conditions, including Wegener's midline granuloma (Vermess 1978), fibrosing mediastinitis, thyroiditis, and cholangitis (Bernardino 1978).

The classic CT finding originally described is that of contrast-enhancing uveal-scleral thickening (Bernardino 1977). The scleral-uveal thickening may obliterate both the sharply demarcated insertion of the optic nerve at the papilla and the insertion of the tendons of the rectus muscles onto the sclera (Figs. 3-8, 3-9). Intraorbitally the involved tissue is usually isodense to slightly hyperdense compared with muscle prior to the injection of contrast. On contrast-enhanced CT (CECT), there is enhancement of the involved tissue. The disease process may present as uveal-scleral thickening, as an isolated discrete mass without uveal-scleral thickening (Fig. 3-10), as an obliteration of all retrobulbar soft-tissue planes, as a thickening of the rectus muscle(s) (Fig. 3-11), or as a lacrimal mass (Fig. 3-12) (Nugent 1981). Occasionally, perioptic enhancement mimicking optic nerve sheath meningioma may be the sole CT manifestation of pseudotumor (Fig. 3-13). Single-muscle involvement in the form of a myositis is thought to be a variant in the manifestations of orbital pseudotumor. One or multiple muscles may be involved. Although classically described as having muscle insertion involvement, pseudotumor may involve any part of the muscle and often spares insertions. Therefore, if the muscle insertion is involved, pseudotumor is more likely than thyroid ophthalmopathy, but a normal muscle insertion with enlargement of the muscle belly has no differential

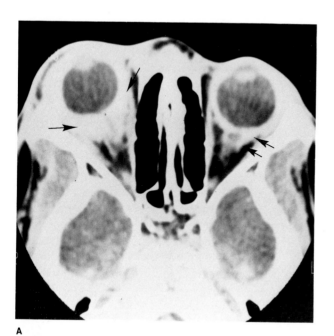

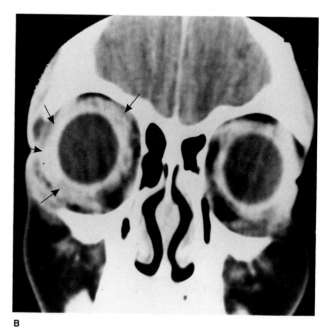

A

B

Figure 3-8 (**A, B**) Bilateral pseudotumor. Axial (**A**) and coronal (**B**) images demonstrate marked bilateral irregular enhancement (worse on the right) involving uveal-scleral regions (arrows) and extending posteriorly along optic nerve sheath.

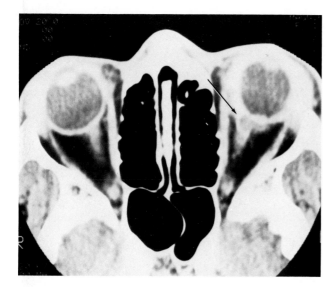

Figure 3-9 Pseudotumor. Enhancing, thickened uveal-scleral region along insertion of optic nerve on left (arrow).

ment may be seen in connection with other causes of intraorbital inflammation (Fig. 3-15) (trauma, surgery, and bacterial infection), as well as in connection with infiltrating neoplasm (i.e., lymphoma or metastases).

Orbital pseudotumor usually shows a dramatic clinical response to steroids, with evidence of improvement on CT (Fig. 3-14). In fact, the diagnosis is clinched on the basis of response to steroids. Biopsy is rarely indicated, being reserved for the infrequent lesions that are steroid unresponsive, which therefore require radiation therapy (Sergott 1981; Leone 1985). Pseudotumor may occasionally be difficult to differentiate both clinically and on CT from Graves' disease. Orbital pseudotumor may be mimicked clinically by other infiltrative disease processes, including lymphoma and metastatic carcinoma (breast), as well as retrobulbar hemorrhage.

utility (Dresner 1984). Lateral rectus muscle enlargement with extension into an enlarged lacrimal gland (Fig. 3-14) is a relatively common manifestation of this disease. Uveal-scleral thickening with enhance-

Thyroid Exophthalmos

The exophthalmos of Graves' disease is of unknown etiology. Inflammatory infiltration and proliferation

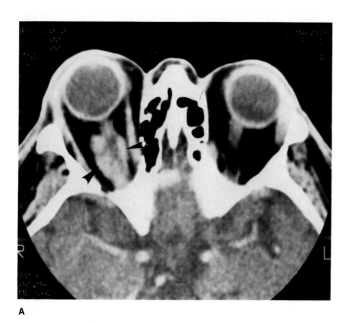

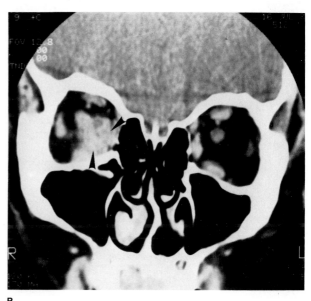

A   B

Figure 3-10 (**A, B**) Pseudotumor. Enhancing irregular intraconal mass (arrowheads) surrounding right optic nerve.

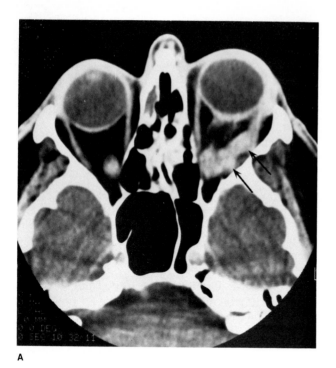

A

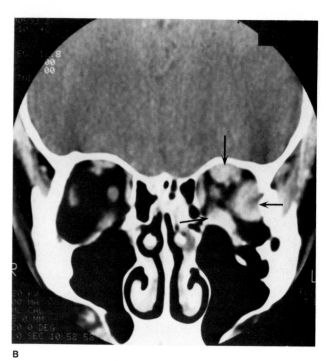

B

Figure 3-11 (**A, B**) Pseudotumor. Involvement of left superior, lateral, and inferior rectus muscles (arrows) demonstrated on axial (**A**) and coronal (**B**) images. Note sparing of left medial rectus, in contrast to thyroid myositis.

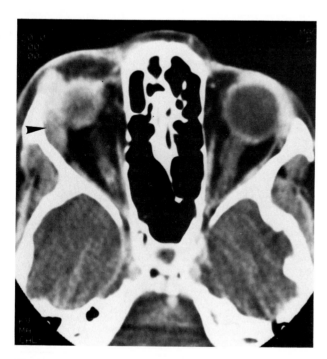

Figure 3-12 Pseudotumor. Mass in right lacrimal fossa (arrowhead) as sole manifestation of pseudotumor.

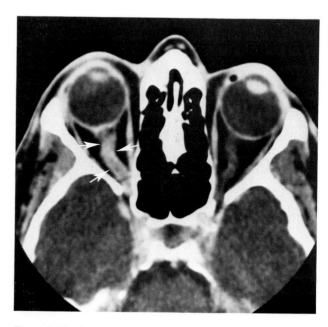

Figure 3-13 Pseudotumor. Enhancing thickening along periphery of right optic nerve/sheath complex ("tram-track" sign), mimicking optic nerve meningioma (arrows).

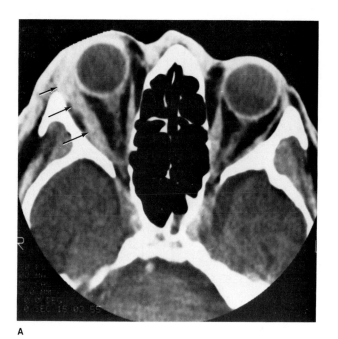
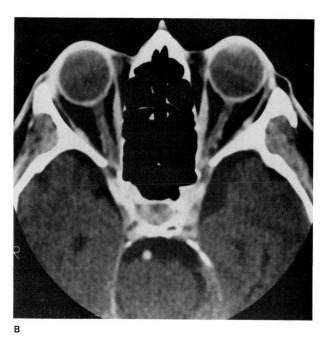

A

B

Figure 3-14   Pseudotumor.   **A**. Enlarged right lateral rectus with involvement of insertion and lacrimal gland (arrows), on presentation. **B**. After steroid therapy, total resolution.

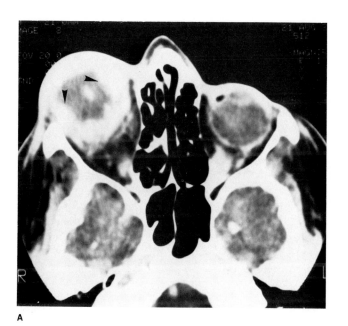
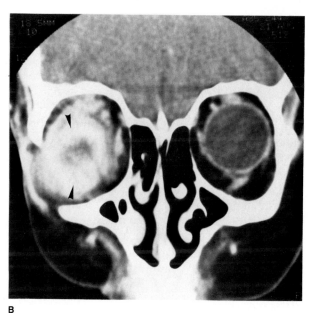

A

B

Figure 3-15   (**A, B**) Endophthalmitis-periophthalmitis. Note markedly thickened, enhancing ill-defined sclera with streaky densities in retrobulbar fat. Lobulated thickened soft tissue within peripheral vitreous (arrowheads) indicates endophthalmitis.

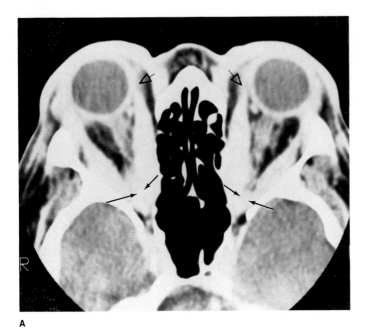

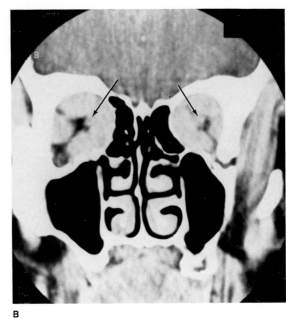

A

B

Figure 3-16   (A, B) Thyroid ophthalmopathy. Bilateral, marked enlargement of all extraocular muscles with typical tapering at insertions (open arrowheads). Streaky increased densities in fat can be seen in severe thyroid ophthalmopathy, as well as pseudotumor. Note compression of optic nerves at orbital apex on axial (**A**) and coronal (**B**) images (arrows).

of connective tissue occurs in the soft tissues of the orbit, especially the extraocular muscles (Alper 1977).

The histopathologic picture of the muscles in Graves' disease is similar to that found in orbital pseudotumor (Jones 1979). It is possible that auto-immune responses may be the cause of both the thyroid exophthalmos of Graves' disease and the changes associated with orbital pseudotumor. Most easily recognized is the massive swelling of the extraocular muscles (Fig. 3-16), which may be enlarged volumetrically up to eight times normal size. Interstitial inflammatory edema and lymphocytic infiltration of the muscles account for their enlargement. When the condition occurs in association with thyrotoxicosis, orbital fat content may be increased (Fig. 3-17) (Peyster 1986). However, increased orbital fat may also be seen in Cushing's disease (or syndrome) and in obesity (Cohen 1981; Carlson 1982). The increase in volume of the orbital tissues produces proptosis. Ulceration of the cornea, occlusion of the central retinal vein or artery, and compressive

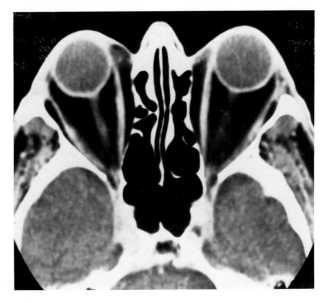

Figure 3-17 Thyroid ophthalmopathy. Note bilateral proptosis with marked increase in orbital fat, bowing orbital septum and separating medial rectus from medially bowed lamina papyracea.

optic neuropathy may be seen as a result. Muscle dysfunction occurs, and ocular motility is impaired. Pain is usually not a feature of thyroid ophthalmopathy.

The exact incidence of thyroid exophthalmos is not known. It occurs in both hyperthyroid and euthyroid patients. Its presentation is usually bilateral; it is unilateral in 5 to 10 percent of cases (Rothfus 1984; Peyster 1986). The classic, mild form is characterized clinically by a prominent stare, mild proptosis, eyelid retraction, and lid lag (Alper 1977). This is most frequently found associated with thyrotoxicosis in young females, and it is bilateral. Most often the patient is asymptomatic (Alper 1977). Typically, the more severe clinical form occurs in the middle-aged patient and is associated with gradual onset of severe proptosis and varying degrees of ophthalmoplegia. Thyrotoxicosis is usually present. Overall, women predominate in the incidence of both thyroid disease (4:1) and Graves' exophthalmos (Alper 1977).

Soon after the introduction of CT, its efficacy in the study of Graves' disease was recognized (Brismar 1976; Enzmann 1976b). Graves' disease accounts for more cases of unilateral and bilateral exophthalmos in the adult than any other single disease entity (Enzmann 1976b; Jacobs 1980). While CT is not always necessary for the diagnosis of Graves' disease, it has been useful in indicating the degree of muscle involvement and its bilaterality and has proved useful when there is ophthalmopathy without clinical or laboratory evidence or history of thyroid disease (Enzmann 1979). Additionally, CT is useful for evaluating results of orbital decompressive surgery. In the transverse section, the inferior and superior recti are cut tangentially (Fig. 3-1). These muscles are better evaluated either in the coronal projection (Fig. 3-2) or on reformed sagittal CT sections. In the direct sagittal CT section, the inferior and superior recti are visualized in their entire length, so that minimal changes of Graves' disease can be recognized (Wing 1979).

Enzmann (1979) reported the CT findings in 107 hyperthyroid and 9 euthyroid patients with thyroid exophthalmopathy. The CT revealed bilateral involvement in 85 percent (Figs. 3-16, 3-18), unilateral

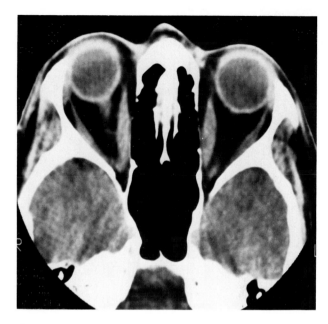

Figure 3-18 Thyroid ophthalmopathy. Medial rectus muscles are enlarged and taper anteriorly at insertions.

involvement in 5 percent (Fig. 3-19), and no abnormality in 10 percent. Seventy percent of Enzmann's cases with bilateral involvement had symmetrical muscle disease, whereas 30 percent had asymmetrical muscle involvement. Most commonly, all four of the above-mentioned recti were involved (Fig. 3-16). The inferior and medial recti were involved in approximately three-fourths of the cases and had the most severe degree of enlargement, whereas the superior and lateral recti were involved in approximately half the cases and had a lesser degree of enlargement. Indeed, any or all extraocular muscles may be involved in nearly any combination. However, if isolated lateral rectus enlargement exists, another etiology is suggested. Enzmann (1979) found a rough linear parallel between the clinical assessment of the degree of ophthalmopathy and the severity of the muscle enlargement. However, no correlation was found between the degree of muscle enlargement and the degree of abnormal thyroid function. Enzmann points out, further, that in 6 of 12 patients who had given a clinical impression of unilateral disease, CT revealed the presence of

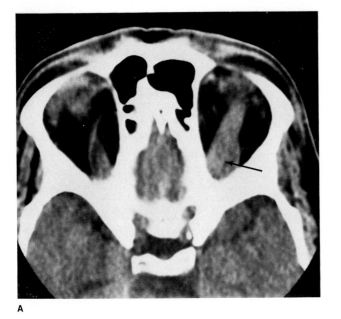

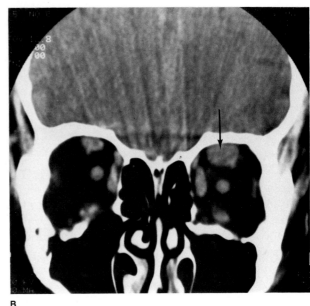

A   B

Figure 3-19 Thyroid ophthalmopathy. Isolated enlargement of left superior rectus muscle (arrow), on axial (**A**) and coronal (**B**) images.

Table 3-1   Etiologies of Extraocular Muscle Enlargement

Thyroid ophthalmopathy
Myositis
   Pseudotumor
   Bacterial (sinus extension)
Carotid-cavernous fistula
   Traumatic
   Dural AVM
Lymphangioma
Hemorrhage (spontaneous)
Malignant neoplasm
   Metastases (especially breast)
   Lymphoma
   Leukemia
   Rhabdomyosarcoma
Trauma (edema, hemorrhage)
Acromegaly
Orbital apex mass

bilateral disease. Table 3-1 lists the causes of extraocular muscle enlargement.

ORBITAL TRAUMA

A blow to the face or head may result in injury to the osseous orbit and the orbital soft tissues. Overlying soft-tissue hematoma may preclude adequate physical examination of the orbit. In such circumstances, CT is a useful adjunct in demonstrating the presence or absence of underlying osseous and soft-tissue injury (Figs. 3-20, 3-21). Fractures of the orbit are classifiable as external (e.g., the tripod fracture of the zygoma and anterior orbital rim) (Fig. 3-22) or internal (blowout fracture into the maxillary or ethmoid sinuses) (Figs. 3-21, 3-23, 3-24). In fractures of the orbital floor, trapping of the inferior rectus and inferior oblique muscles along with ad-

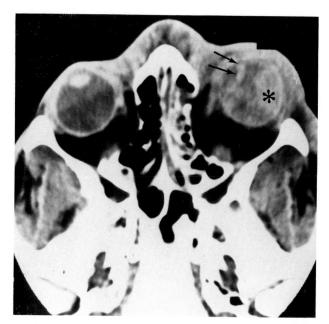

Figure 3-20 Blunt trauma. Left globe is filled with hemorrhage (asterisk). Lens is disrupted (arrows). Note medial wall blowout fracture has opacified left ethmoid sinus.

jacent fat and connective tissue, as the fragment projects into the roof of the maxillary sinus, leads to vertical muscle imbalance. CT is able to demonstrate herniation of the soft-tissue contents into the roof of the maxillary sinus (Grove 1978; Hammerschlag 1982). Grove (1978) found that coronal CT was better than pluridirectional tomography in depicting the bony fragments in such blowout fractures. CT also may detect unsuspected fracture of the orbital apex (Unger 1984).

In addition to damage to the bony orbit, trauma of sufficient force and direction can also lead to damage to the globe and optic nerve. Rupture of the globe is most often associated with blows to the lateral aspect of the orbit that strike the globe just anterior to the lateral wall. CT demonstrates the deformity of the eyeball and the presence of intraocular hemorrhage (Figs. 3-20, 3-21, 3-25). Direct damage to the optic nerve and bleeding within the subarachnoid, subdural, or intradural space can lead to loss of vision, due either to the primary optic nerve injury or to secondary optic nerve injury by

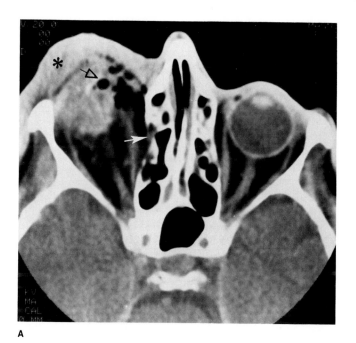

A

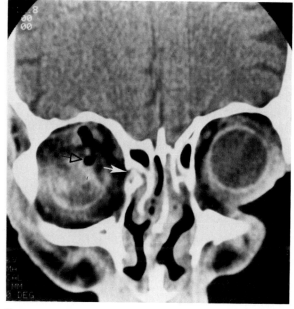

B

Figure 3-21 (A, B) Medial wall fracture with ruptured globe. Axial (A) and coronal (B) images demonstrate right medial wall blowout fracture (arrow) and orbital emphysema. Signs of ruptured globe include distortion of normal shape with intravitreal hemorrhage and intraocular air (open arrow). Lens cannot be identified. Note extensive preseptal hemorrhage (asterisk).

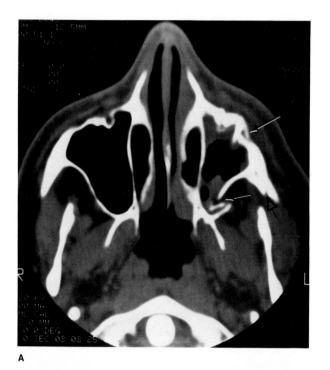

A

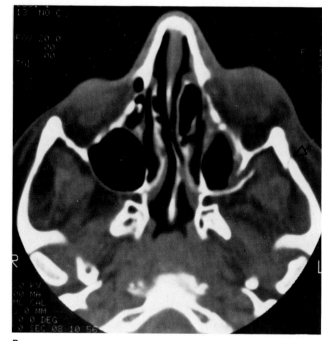

B

C

Figure 3-22   (**A–C**) Tripod fracture. Axial images demonstrate fractures involving anterior and lateral walls of the right maxillary sinus (arrows) and widening of the frontozygomatic suture (open arrow). Note intact pterygoids.

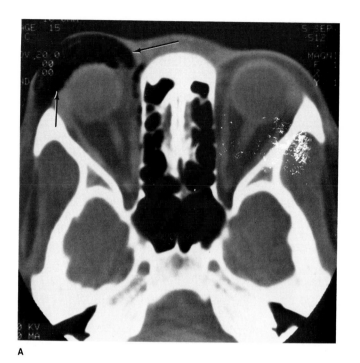
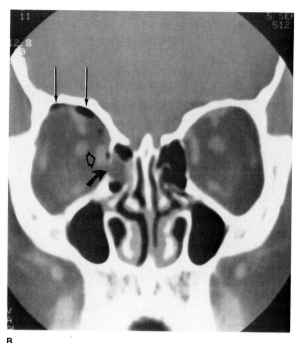

Figure 3-23 (**A, B**) Medial wall fracture. Medial orbital wall fracture (curved arrow) is best demonstrated in coronal view (**B**), with soft tissue and fat herniating into right ethmoid. Medial rectus is in its normal position (open arrow). Extensive orbital emphysema is also present (straight arrows).

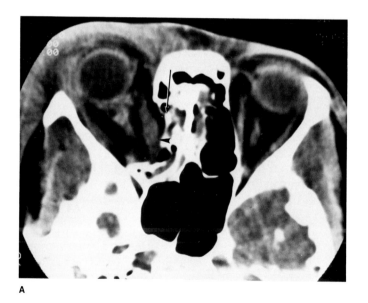
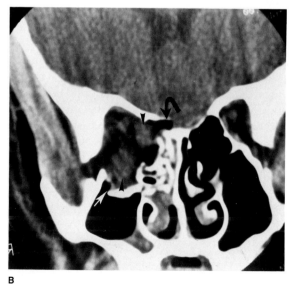

Figure 3-24 (**A, B**) Double blowout fractures. Medial wall fracture (arrow) and floor fracture (white arrow) from blunt trauma. Medial and inferior recti are engorged, but not entrapped (arrowheads). Note air going into intracranial cavity (curved arrow).

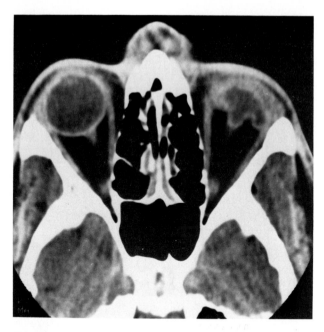

Figure 3-25 Perforated globe. Left globe is markedly decreased in size and has abnormal configuration after perforating injury, indicating rupture.

vascular compression or injury. Fractures in the vicinity of the optic foramen, especially those associated with local subperiosteal hemorrhage, may compress the optic nerve focally. This is an indication for emergency decompression. Intradural hemorrhage in the optic nerve sheath occurs most frequently at the apex of the orbit, where the tendinous attachments insert onto the optic nerve sheath. Intraneural optic nerve hemorrhage also occurs at the apex of the orbit. Subarachnoid and subdural hemorrhage are more frequent just posterior to the papilla, where they are associated with subhyloid retinal hemorrhages (Lindberg 1973).

VASCULAR LESIONS

Orbital Hemangioma

Cavernous hemangiomas have an equal sex distribution and occur most frequently from the second to the fifth decade of life. They are characterized by a slowly progressive course. The symptoms consist of proptosis and difficulty with extraocular motility. Hemangioma is one of the most common benign intraorbital lesions (Forbes 1982), and is most often located within the muscle cone (Fig. 3-26), although extraconal hemangiomas are not uncommon (Fig. 3-27). In the pediatric age group, orbital hemangiomas are classified as capillary, rather than cavernous, on pathologic examination. The CT appearance of these lesions is identical.

Cavernous hemangiomas consist of large, dilated, endothelium-lined vascular channels. They are encompassed by a fibrous pseudocapsule. The arterial blood supply is not prominent, and the blood flow is relatively stagnant. Thrombosis, phlebolith formation with calcification (Fig. 3-26), fibrosis, and chronic inflammation are not infrequent. Spontaneous hemorrhage is not a feature of this lesion.

CT demonstrates the cavernous hemangioma as a homogeneously dense mass usually within the muscle cone with smooth margins and uniform contrast enhancement (Figs. 3-26, 3-27) (Davis 1980). These lesions often do *not* deform the globe when abuttng it, distinguishing hemangioma from many retrobulbar metastases (Fig. 3-28). Lymphoma is similarly a soft mass which often does not deform the globe. Expansion of the adjacent orbital wall is common but bone destruction does not occur, and if present, suggests a more aggressive lesion. The detection on CT of a calcified phlebolith is an infrequent but highly suggestive characteristic of this lesion. In Davis' series, 83 percent of the cavernous hemangiomas were intraconic, with 67 percent being lateral to the optic nerve; 22 percent of his cases extended to the orbital apex. On CT it is possible to demarcate the cavernous hemangioma from the adjacent optic nerve and muscles. This is important in planning for operative removal. Because the cavernous hemangioma is encapsulated, it is easily peeled off from the extraocular muscles and optic nerves. The tumors show no tendency to recur or to undergo malignant transformation (Jones 1979). It is important to differentiate hemangioma from lymphangioma of the orbit, a lesion that is not easily removed surgically, frequently recurs, and is more often

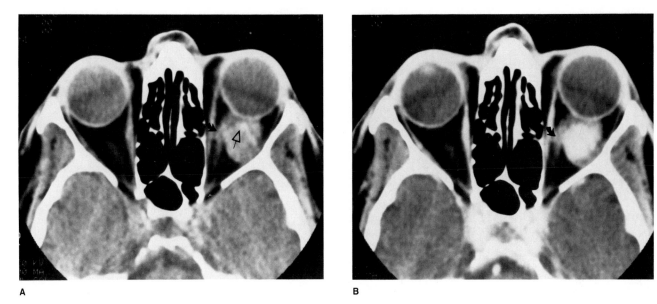

Figure 3-26 (**A, B**) Intraconal hemangioma. NCCT (**A**) demonstrates well-circumscribed intraconal mass deviating right optic nerve (curved arrow) medially. Note artifacts emanating from calcified phlebolith (open arrow) within mass. Note absence of deformity of posterior globe. Mass enhances homogeneously on CECT (**B**).

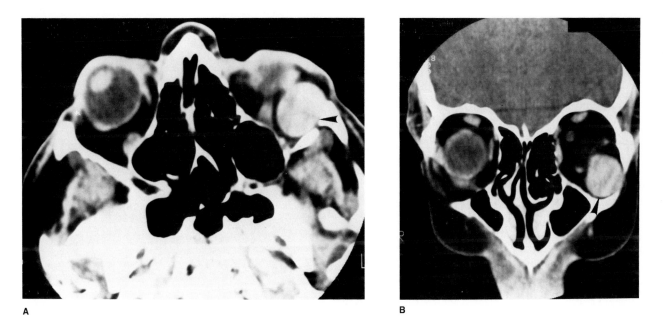

Figure 3-27 (**A, B**) Extraconal hemangioma. Well-circumscribed, homogeneously enhancing mass (arrowhead) in inferolateral aspect of left orbit is outside of muscle cone on axial (**A**) and coronal (**B**) images.

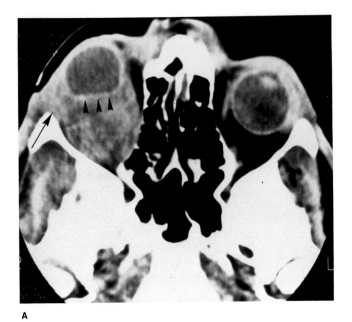

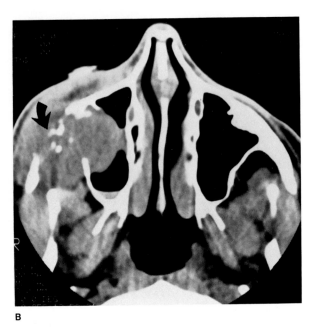

A

B

Figure 3-28 **(A, B)** Metastatic melanoma. **A**. Slightly nonhomogeneous mass fills right orbit, infiltrates lacrimal gland (arrow), and deforms posterior aspect of globe (arrowheads). **B**. Mass destroys right malar eminence (curved arrow) and erodes into maxillary sinus.

extraconic, ill-defined, and less homogeneous in its enhancement.

Lymphangioma

Lymphangiomas are less frequent than cavernous hemangiomas. They are most often extraconic in location and present at a younger age (mean age 22) than the cavernous hemangioma (mean age 45). Lymphangiomas have a slow, progressive growth without evidence of regression. They are characterized by thin vascular spaces filled with clear fluid and by lymphoid follicles. Unlike hemangiomas, which have a propensity to thrombosis, lymphangiomas are likely to hemorrhage (Fig. 3-29), producing acute symptoms such as pain or rapidly progressive proptosis. They tend to infiltrate along planes without a capsule and for that reason do not lend themselves to surgical extirpation.

On CT, lymphangiomas have the same density

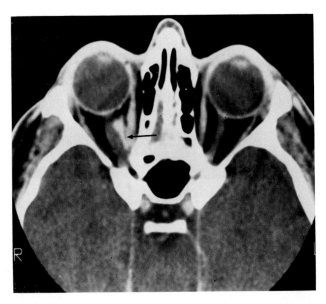

Figure 3-29 Lymphangioma. High-attenuation region of acute hemorrhage (arrow) in ill-defined intraconal mass along right optic nerve.

before injection of contrast material as do hemangiomas; that is, they appear hyperdense within the orbit. Contrast enhancement is mottled and less marked than with hemangiomas. Davis (1980) described lymphangiomas as nonhomogeneous masses with irregular margins due to their infiltrative nature, most often extraconic (Davis 1980). Bone expansion may be present. Differentiation of lymphangiomas from cavernous hemangiomas is important. The hemangioma may be safely excised because of its encapsulation, whereas the lymphangioma is usually not completely removable because it lacks a capsule.

Varix

Vascular malformations of the venous system are infrequent orbital lesions which include orbital varices, varicoceles, and venous angiomas. They are characterized by the production of intermittent exophthalmos, most often associated with activities that produce an increase in venous pressure (coughing, straining, the Valsalva maneuver). The lack of valves within the jugular vein allows back pressure to be transmitted to the orbital veins and the venous malformation. The distension of the vascular spaces within the venous malformation produces the exophthalmos. Recurrent episodes of extreme proptosis have been reported to lead to blindness in as many as 15 percent of patients with orbital varix. Other causes of intermittent exophthalmos are bleeding into lymphangiomas, sinus infection with edema of the orbital soft tissue, and allergic edema. Venous variceal formations associated with arteriovenous fistulas, carotid-cavernous in nature, are usually pulsatile and do not regress.

Routine skull radiographs are usually normal, although phleboliths may be present within the varix. Orbital venography has been the most useful diagnostic modality in the past, prior to the advent of high-resolution CT. Rosenblum and Zilkha (1978) reported a case of sudden visual loss secondary to an orbital varix in which the orbital venogram was negative but the lesion was demonstrated by CT.

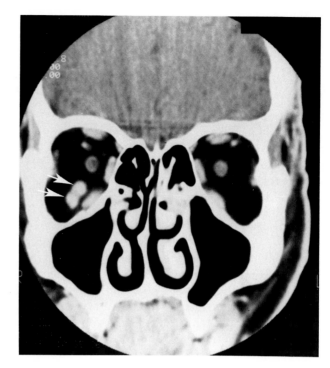

Figure 3-30 Varix, inferior ophthalmic vein. Enhanced coronal CT demonstrates "double-barrel" enlarged inferior ophthalmic vein (arrows) consistent with tortuous venous varix.

CT clearly demonstrates the location of the soft-tissue mass of the varix (Fig. 3-30) and characterizes it by showing enlargement of the varix with the Valsalva maneuver and diminution in its size with a Muller maneuver. Alternatively, varix can be documented by appearance and disappearance on CT with change in head position.

Carotid-Cavernous Fistula

A communication between the internal carotid artery (or branches of the external carotid artery) and the cavernous sinus leads to the development of a fistula in which the veins are under arterial pressure. Valveless venous intercommunication between the cavernous sinus and the superior ophthalmic vein leads to a transmission of arterial pressure into the veins of the orbit. Proptosis, motility disturbances, pulsating exophthalmos (with a bruit), and suffusion of the globe, sclera, and conjunctiva are the hallmarks of the carotid-cavernous fistula. The etiology is most often traumatic (Fig. 3-31), but fistulas may occur spontaneously, either secondary to atherosclerotic disease or from communications between dural branches of the external carotid artery and the basilar venous plexus (dural arteriovenous malformations) (Fig. 3-32). The exophthalmos and ocular symptoms that accompany the fistula are usually ipsilateral to the site of the fistula but are contralateral in 10 percent, and may be bilateral, as intercavernous sinus connections exist.

While carotid arteriography remains the definitive method of demonstrating the site of the fistula and its pattern of venous drainage (Zimmerman 1977), CT is contributory in the initial diagnosis of cases that are not clinically obvious. Enlargement of the superior ophthalmic vein, engorgement of the rectus muscles, proptosis, and distension of the involved cavernous sinus can be demonstrated on CT (Figs. 3-31, 3-32). While traumatic fistulas require surgical or neurointerventional treatment, dural fistulas may thrombose spontaneously. The differential diagnosis of an enlarged superior ophthalmic vein is shown in Table 3-2.

OCULAR TUMORS

Ocular Melanoma

Both benign and malignant melanomas arise intraocularly and have been classified according to their site of origin (uveal or retinal). Extraocular extension through the vortex veins occurs in approximately 13 percent of ocular melanomas (Starr 1962). Local recurrence of the melanoma following exenteration is extremely high if extraocular extension has already occurred. The diagnosis of melanoma as a primary tumor in the orbit requires the exclusion of a primary intraocular focus as well as the exclusion of an extracranial primary site (Jones 1979).

Malignant melanoma of the uveal tract (i.e., iris, choroid, ciliary body) is the most common intraocular malignancy in adults (Shields 1977), predominantly occurring in whites and rare in blacks (Shields 1977; Yanoff 1975). Primary malignant melanoma of the choroid is nearly always unilateral. Melanomas usually occur in older patients and are uncommon in the pediatric population. The clinical presentation varies from visual field defects or decreased visual acuity to pain or inflammation.

On CT, melanoma usually presents as a focal mass of slight hyperdensity which extends into the vitreous (Fig. 3-33). These tumors may show slight enhancement (Mafee 1985; Peyster 1985). The shape of the mass varies from polypoid (Fig. 3-33) to flat or crescentic (Figs. 3-34 to 3-36); associated retinal detachment is common and often requires intravenous contrast for CT differentiation (Figs. 3-35, 3-36). Rarely, choroidal melanoma can manifest as predominantly inflammatory (i.e., endophthalmitis, episcleritis, or iridocyclitis). Calcification in uveal melanomas has not been seen on CT (Table 3-3). The usefulness of CT is mainly in detecting episcleral extent, tumor recurrence, and as an aid to differential diagnosis (Figs. 3-37, 3-38), as many benign and malignant lesions can simulate melanoma funduscopically (Table 3-4).

Choroidal Hemangioma

Hemangiomas of the choroid are benign lesions, usually detected in patients 10 to 20 years of age. Fifty percent of patients have Sturge-Weber (Reese 1976). Histologically, these lesions are cavernous, and up to 90 percent have associated retinal detachments microscopically. CT demonstrates focal areas of intense contrast enhancement in the choroid (Fig. 3-38); indeed, the lesion may not be detected on an NCCT. These lesions can spontaneously hemorrhage.

Retinoblastoma

Retinoblastoma, the most common intraocular malignancy of childhood, has an incidence of between

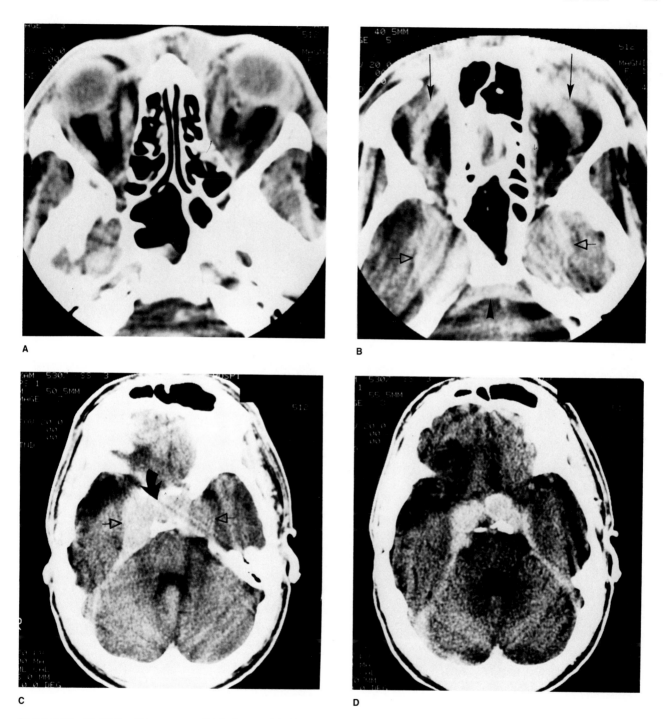

Figure 3-31 **(A–D)** Carotid-cavernous fistula (traumatic). Note bilateral proptosis and engorgement of all muscles with markedly enlarged superior ophthalmic veins bilaterally (arrows). The cavernous sinuses are bulging (open arrows) and there appears to be an intra- and suprasellar mass (curved arrows). The basilar venous plexus is also engorged (arrowhead).

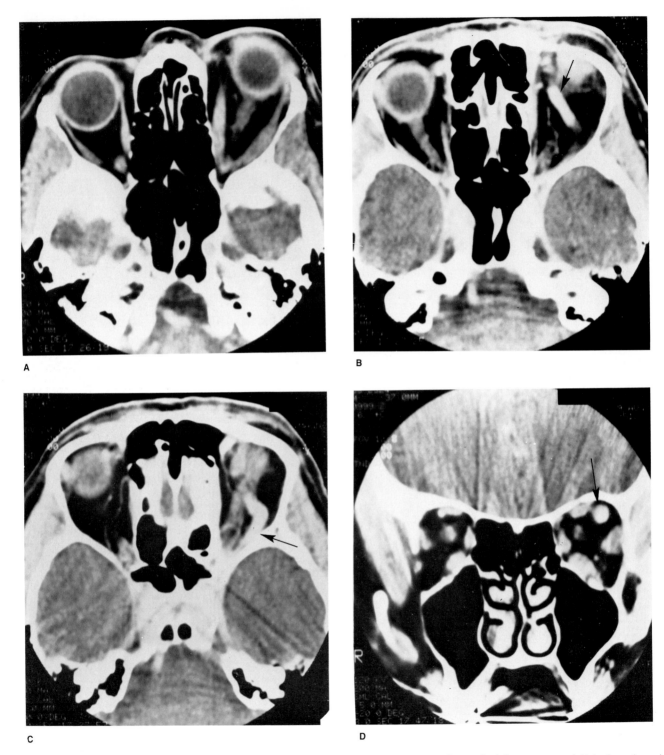

Figure 3-32 **(A–D)** Dural cavernous fistula. The left globe is proptotic, and extraocular muscles on the left are engorged. Note the enlarged left superior ophthalmic vein (arrow).

Table 3-2 Etiologies of Enlarged Superior Ophthalmic Vein

Carotid-cavernous fistula
  Traumatic
  Dural fistula (AVM)
Varix
Orbital apex mass (compressing vein)
Thyroid ophthalmopathy
Pseudotumor
Normal variant

1 in 15,000 and 1 in 30,000 (Zimmerman 1978). It accounts for 1 percent of early childhood deaths and 5 percent of childhood blindness (Zimmerman 1979). While the tumor is of congenital origin, it is not necessarily recognized at birth. The average age at time of diagnosis is 18 months (Reese 1976). In 25 to 33 percent of patients with retinoblastoma, the disease is bilateral and represents an autosomal dominant form of genetic transmission that has a variable penetrance (Zimmerman 1979); 50 percent of the offspring of the affected parent are at risk, and thus in the bilateral cases there is a frequent familial history. Conversely, 60 percent of familial cases are bilateral. The typical presentation of leukokoria, strabismus, glaucoma, or vision loss occurs in 90 percent of cases, while the remaining 10 percent mimic a variety of illnesses, including orbital cellulitis, ophthalmitis, conjunctivitis, and systemic illness (Appelboom 1985).

Retinoblastoma arises in the nuclear layer of the retina as a primary malignant neuroectodermal neoplasm composed of small round or ovoid cells (Russell 1977). It is characterized by multicentric origin, rapid growth, and ability to invade the adjacent tissues. As the tumor outgrows its blood supply, cell necrosis occurs and DNA is released that has a propensity to form a calcified complex. It is this calcified complex that enables the tumor to be identified with confidence radiologically (Brant-Zawadzki 1979; Klintworth 1978; Zimmerman 1979). X-ray studies of enucleated eyes have shown a characteristic pattern of calcification, consisting of closely packed dis-

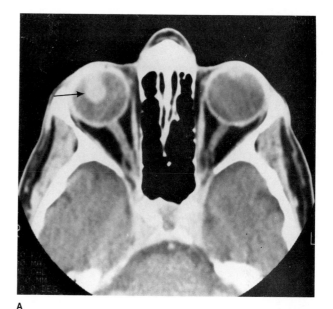

A

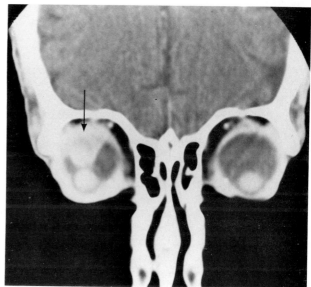

B

Figure 3-33 (**A, B**) Melanoma. Large enhancing polypoid mass (arrow) projects from superior choroid of right globe. Its site of attachment is best appreciated on coronal view (**B**).

crete radiodensities (Klintworth 1978) 1 mm in diameter.

Intraocular spread of retinoblastoma occurs when the malignant cells disseminate throughout the eye

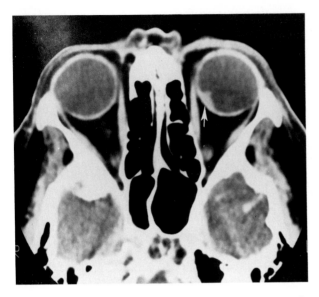

Figure 3-34   Melanoma. Small crescentic enhancing mass (arrow) with nodular irregularity in posteronasal choroid.

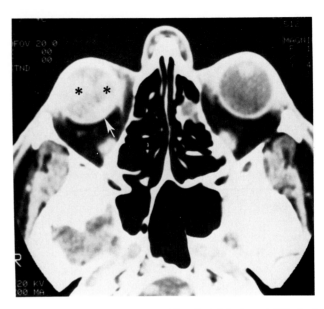

Figure 3-36   Ocular melanoma with retinal detachment. "Kissing" retinal detachments (asterisks) meet in midline. Note enhancing melanoma posteriorly (arrow), revealing etiology of extensive detachment.

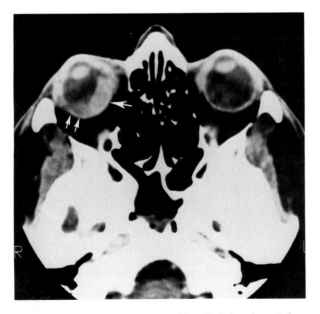

Figure 3-35   Ocular melanoma with retinal detachment. Large plaquelike melanoma enhances (single arrow) and is therefore distinguishable from associated nonenhancing retinal detachment (double arrow).

Table 3-3   Ocular Calcification

Optic nerve drusen
Phthisis bulbi
Neoplasm
  Retinoblastoma
  Choroidal osteoma
  Astrocytic hamartoma
    Tuberous sclerosis
    Neurofibromatosis
    Isolated abnormality
Infection (congenital)
  Toxoplasmosis
  Cytomegalic virus
  Herpes
  Rubella
Metabolic
  Hyperparathyroidism
  Hypervitaminosis D
  Milk-alkali syndrome

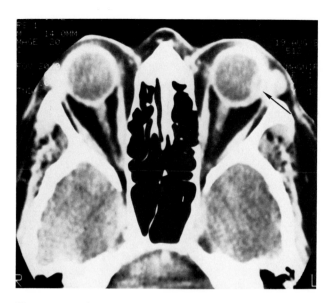

Table 3-4   Differential Diagnosis of Choroidal Melanoma

Malignant melanoma (melanotic or amelanotic)
Benign melanoma
Optic nerve melanocytoma
Choroidal hemangioma
Hemorrhage
Astrocytic hamartoma
Detached choroid
Choroidal metastasis (especially breast)
Inflammation (granuloma, endophthalmitis)
Retinal astrocytoma
Retinal cyst
Sarcoidosis
Arterial macroaneurysm (Brown 1985)

Figure 3-37   Choroidal metastases. Enhancing choroidal mass temporal aspect of left globe (arrow) proven to be breast carcinoma metastases.

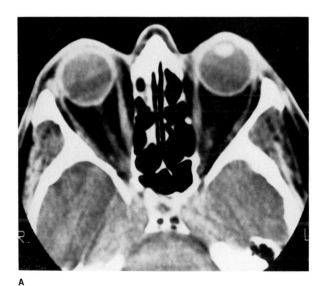

A

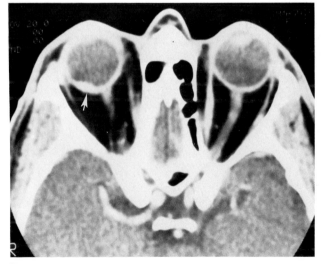

B

Figure 3-38   (**A, B**) Choroidal hemangioma. Precontrast scan (**A**) is normal. After intravenous contrast, markedly enhancing mass posterotemporally (arrow), a typical appearance of this entity.

and implant at other sites (choroid, retina, posterior surface of the cornea) (Reese 1976). Extension of the tumor along perineural and perivascular spaces results in intraorbital and optic nerve spread of the tumor. Extension of the tumor into the subarachnoid space surrounding the optic nerve allows its dissemination by the cerebrospinal fluid throughout the nervous system. Involvement of the intraorbital vascular system by tumor permits systemic extracranial spread to distant sites such as long bones, lymphatics, and viscera (Jones 1979).

The development of more sensitive diagnostic techniques, including CT, has led in recent years to better detection and earlier treatment. This has led to an increase in survival of patients with retinoblastoma. However, spread beyond the globe carries a poor prognosis.

CT recognition of retinoblastomas is dependent upon the identification of a soft-tissue mass involving the retina with calcification (Figs. 3-39 to 3-42). The presence of calcification helps to differentiate the tumor from other causes of retinal thickening, such as astrocytic hamartoma (Fig. 3-43) or retinal detachment. CT is particularly valuable in demonstrating the extension of the tumor to other sites

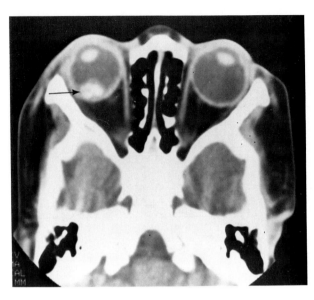

Figure 3-40   Unilateral retinoblastoma. Typical nodular calcification in right retinal mass (arrow).

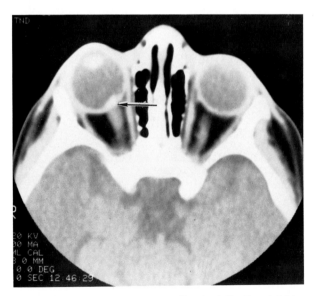

Figure 3-39   Small retinoblastoma. Focal calcification at right optic nerve head (arrow) in young child suggests retinoblastoma.

within the globe (or multifocal origins) and bilaterality of the tumor (Fig. 3-41). Rarely, retinoblastoma can involve the entire globe, diffusely infiltrating the vitreous and aqueous humor (Fig. 3-44). In these cases, calcification may be difficult to detect. In addition, the globe may be buphthalmic (Fig. 3-44).

Associated retinal detachment (Fig. 3-42) can be distinguished from the true tumor mass with intravenous contrast, as most retinoblastomas with noncalcified portions enhance. Thickening of the optic nerve shadow may indicate extension of the tumor into the perineural subarachnoid space, a poor prognostic sign. The presence of tumor within the intracranial subarachnoid space can be demonstrated with contrast enhancement. In addition, intracerebral metastases and the rare "trilateral" retinoblastoma (bilateral retinoblastoma with associated pineal tumor) can also be detected by CT (Johnson 1985).

Concomitant with an improvement in the survival of patients with congenital bilateral retinoblastomas, there has been an appreciation that these patients have a predisposition to the development of radiation-induced neoplasm (Soloway 1966). This

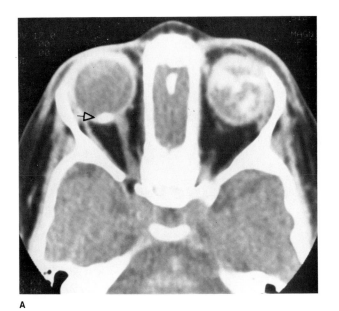

A

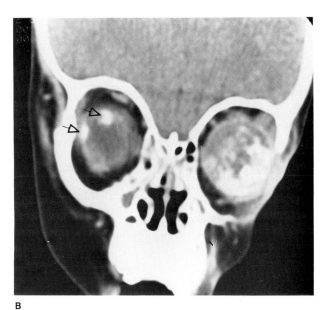

B

Figure 3-41 Bilateral retinoblastoma. Large mass occupying most of left globe with irregular margin and nodular calcifications. Multiple calcifications in right globe (open arrows) denote multifocal, bilateral retinoblastoma.

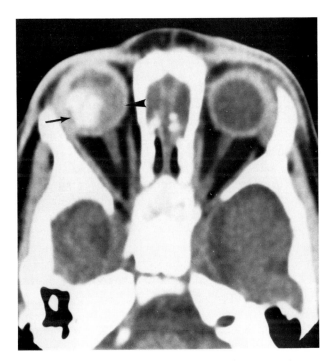

Figure 3-42 Unilateral retinoblastoma with retinal detachment. Densely calcified mass (arrow) with associated massive retinal detachment (arrowhead).

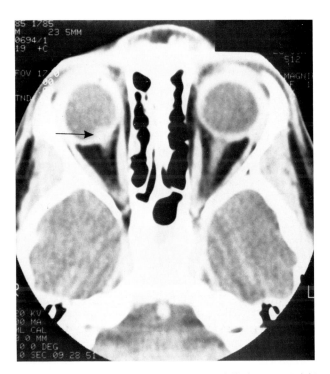

Figure 3-43 Astrocytic hamartoma. Noncalcified mass at right optic nerve head (arrow) in a patient without tuberous sclerosis.

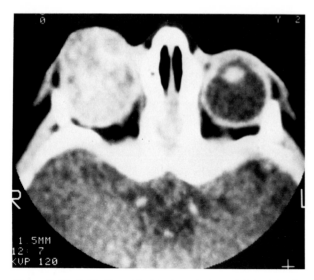

Figure 3-44 Infiltrative retinoblastoma. Enlarged right globe filled by diffuse, heterogeneous mass in buphthalmic globe.

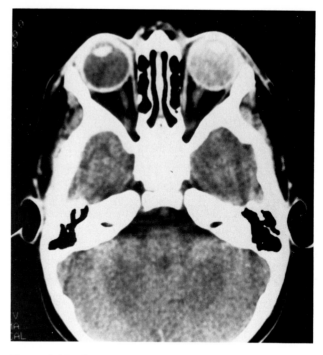

Figure 3-45 Coat's disease. Uniformly hyperdense left globe, presenting as leukokoria. Absence of calcifications helps distinguish this condition from retinoblastoma.

occurs in about one-fifth of survivors with bilateral retinoblastomas who have been irradiated. The site of secondary tumor is usually within the field of radiation. These tumors are most commonly manifested within 10 years of radiation therapy. The majority of them are of mesenchymal origin, in the form of sarcomas. However, carcinomas have also been reported (Zimmerman 1979). In addition, second malignancies in nonirradiated patients apparently occur more frequently than in the general population (Abramson 1984).

OTHER CAUSES OF LEUKOKORIA

Coat's Disease

This benign entity consists of unilateral retinal telangiectasia with associated massive subretinal exudative fluid accumulation causing retinal detachment. Males (80 percent) of ages 6 to 8 years are typically affected (Reese 1976). CT demonstrates relatively homogeneous hyperdensity involving the entire vitreous cavity (Fig. 3-45), secondary to lipoproteinaceous exudate underlying a (usually) total retinal detachment (Sherman 1983). Calcification is nearly always absent, although tiny foci of calcified cholesterol plaques may rarely be seen on funduscopy. Features distinguishing this entity from retinoblastoma include an older age at presentation, exclusively unilateral occurrence, lack of calcification or enhancement, and of course, absence of extraocular spread (Haik 1985). CT can therefore obviate the need for globe exenteration in these patients and instead lead to appropriate laser therapy. Coat's disease is the primary differential diagnosis to distinguish from retinoblastoma.

PHPV

Persistent hyperplastic primary vitreous (PHPV) is an abnormal congenital persistence of embryonic

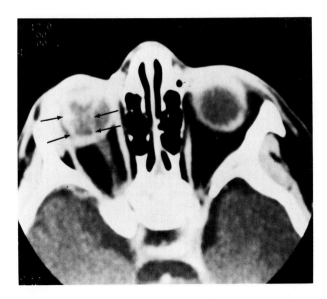

Figure 3-46 PHPV. Irregular linear densities (arrows) extend posteriorly from malformed lens to region of optic disc.

hyaloid vasculature. CT demonstrates a linear density extending anteriorly through the vitreous to the lens (Fig. 3-46), which represents the remnant of the hyaloid stalk, and regions of increased attenuation consistent with retrolental membranes. Hyaloid remnants often cannot be differentiated from retinal detachment. PHPV is unilateral and noncalcified. Enhancement is variable. The globe is frequently microphthalmic (Haik 1985). Lens abnormalities, including cataract and abnormally shaped lenses, can also be seen.

Retinopathy of Prematurity

Retinopathy of prematurity, or retrolental fibroplasia, is usually seen in premature infants receiving high oxygen concentrations. Recent literature suggests that high oxygen concentration in inspired air is not a requisite for the development of this entity (Patz 1985). Bilateral retinal detachments with variable enhancement and occasional calcification may be seen. Microphthalmia has also been described (Haik 1985).

Ocular Toxicariasis

Toxocara canis infestation can also present with leukokoria and retinal detachment secondary to endophthalmitis. "Pseudomicrophthalmia" (Haik 1985) from focally thickened sclera with enhancement is common. CT may also demonstrate a nonenhancing, hyperdense mass occupying most of the vitreous cavity (Edwards 1985).

GLOBE SHAPE ABNORMALITIES

Coloboma

Colobomas are congenital defects in the retina, choroid, iris, optic nerve, and/or lens which result from deficient closure of the fetal optic fissure, along the inferonasal aspect of the globe and optic nerve (Simmons 1983). The posterior globe and optic nerve are most commonly affected. They are transmitted as an autosomal dominant trait with variable penetrance, occurring bilaterally in 60 percent of cases. Visual field defects and decreased visual acuity are present. CT demonstrates defects in the posterior globe extending into the optic nerve (Fig. 3-47). Microphthalmia and retinal cysts may accompany optic nerve colobomas. CT is useful for identifying retinal cysts posterior to the globe, as well as revealing any CNS abnormality which can be associated with these lesions, such as encephalocele or callosal agenesis (Corbett 1980).

Staphyloma

Staphylomas are acquired defects in the wall of the globe resulting in protrusion of either cornea or sclera. These defects are lined with iris or choroid tissue. In severe myopia, accompanying staphylomas typically are seen as focal bulges in the posterior surface of the globe, on the temporal side of the optic disc (Anderson 1983). Anterior staphylomas can be seen in inflammatory entities, such as rheumatoid arthritis.

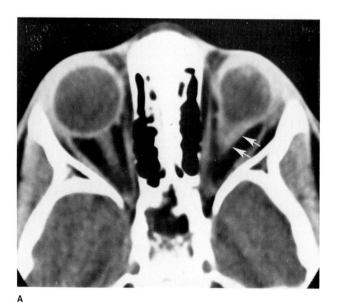
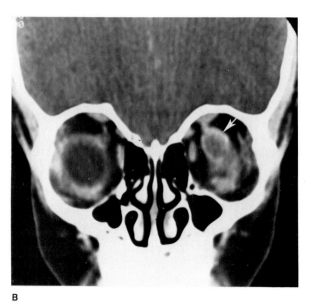

A

B

Figure 3-47   (A, B) Microphthalmos with coloboma. Conical defect in posterior globe extending into optic nerve (arrows) seen on axial (**A**) and coronal (**B**) views in microphthalmic globe.

Axial Myopia

Axial myopia is characterized by anteroposterior elongation of the globe (Fig. 3-48). Anterior protrusion may be noted and result in proptosis (Brodey 1983). It is distinguished from staphyloma by the absence of focal bulge in an elongated globe. Retinal detachment and staphyloma may accompany the myopic globe.

Buphthalmos

Buphthalmos, or congenital glaucoma, is usually detected because of clouding or enlargement of the cornea, or because the child acts insensitive to light (Gittinger 1984). It is unilateral in approximately 25 percent of cases, and is caused by maldevelopment of aqueous humor outflow channels in the anterior chamber angle. Glaucoma in a child results in an enlarged globe (Fig. 3-49). Macrophthalmos may be unrelated to intraocular pressure, however, and can

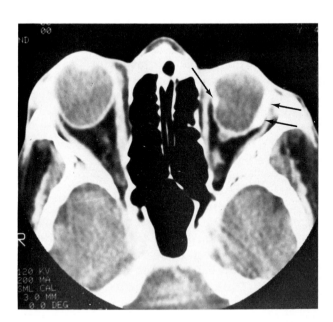

Figure 3-48   Myopia, status postscleral banding. Both globes have myopic configuration. High-density structures at periphery of left globe (arrows) with waistlike deformity represent scleral band placed for prior retinal detachment.

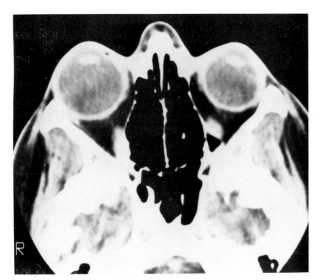

Figure 3-49 Buphthalmos. Note macrophthalmic right globe in patient with glaucoma.

be seen as an isolated entity, secondary to massive intraocular tumor, or in association with neurofibromatosis.

GLOBE CALCIFICATIONS

The etiology of calcification in the globe is varied (Hedges 1982; Turner 1983), and differential diagnosis is highly dependent on the age of the patient (Table 3-3). In an infant or young child, any focal calcification in the globe must be considered retinoblastoma until proven otherwise. The contralateral eye must be examined thoroughly for calcification, as up to one-third of retinoblastomas are bialteral (Fig. 3-41). Calcification is seen in up to 95 percent of cases (Bullock 1977). Other etiologies of globe calcification in a child include astrocytic hamartoma, a nodular mass frequently associated with tuberous sclerosis (Fig. 3-43). Choroidal osteoma is a rare tumor seen usually in young women as a focal area of calcification near the optic disc (Hedges 1982).

In adults, the most common cause of focal calcification in the globe is optic nerve drusen. These lesions are commonly bilateral (Fig. 3-50), and represent benign accumulations of hyalinelike material beneath the surface of the optic disc (Hedges 1982;

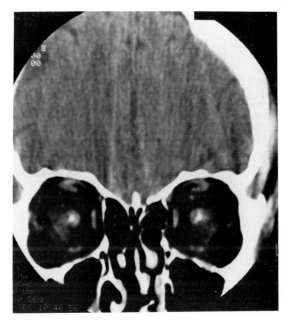

A   B

Figure 3-50 (**A, B**) Bilateral optic nerve drusen. Axial (**A**) and coronal (**B**) images demonstrate round, focal calcification at optic discs, diagnostic of optic nerve drusen.

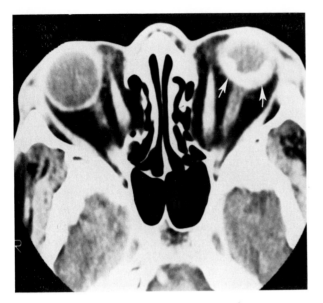

Figure 3-51   Phthisis bulbi. Small left globe with extensive choroidal calcification (arrows) in patient many years after trauma to globe.

(Savage 1985). Interestingly, visual field defects typically occur in areas not corresponding to the funduscopic location of the drusen (Savage 1985). The etiology of optic nerve drusen is not clearly established but is considered to represent a developmental anomaly or degenerative process (Ramirez 1983). There is a familial tendency for the development of these lesions.

Phthisis bulbi is an end-stage calcified, shrunken globe which is blind. Extensive calcification is seen on CT in a small, irregularly shaped globe (Fig. 3-51). Etiologies include trauma, recurrent retinal hemorrhage, prior surgery, chronic ocular inflammation (Fig. 3-52), and radiation.

Ramirez 1983). Funduscopically, drusen can masquerade as papilledema. Although frequently asymptomatic, optic nerve drusen can be associated with visual field defects in up to 80 percent of cases

RETINAL DETACHMENT

When the retinal pigment epithelial layer is separated from the sensory retina by fluid, a retinal detachment is present (Fig. 3-53). A choroidal detachment can mimic a retinal detachment radiographically and often occurs after intraocular surgery. These can be quite extensive and meet in the midline to result

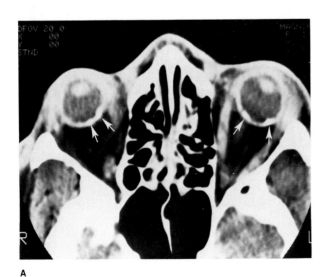

A

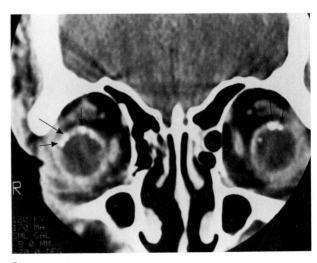

B

Figure 3-52   (**A, B**) Congenital toxoplasmosis. Multiple associated foci of calcification bilaterally (arrows), consistent with chorioretinitis.

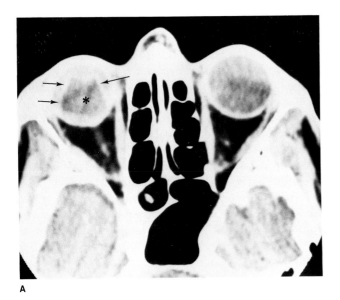

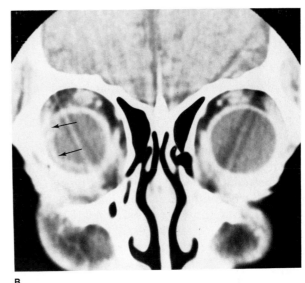

A   B

Figure 3-53 **(A, B)** Serous retinal detachment. Thin line of high density (arrows) representing detached retinal membrane separates vitreous from subretinal fluid (asterisk).

in "kissing detachments." Retinal detachments can be classified as rhegmatogenous or nonrhegmatogenous, depending upon whether a rhegma, or hole, exists in the sensory retina. Most detachments are rhegmatogenous; retinal holes are secondary to retinal degeneration or vitreous traction from liquefaction of the vitreous. Spontaneous detachments occur in under 10 per 100,000 per year (Gittinger 1984). Predisposing factors include high myopia, surgical aphakia (lens absence), and a history of detachment in the contralateral eye. There may be no acute symptoms, but gradual vision loss may be noted.

Treatment of retinal detachment can be divided into two major techniques: scleral buckle (Fig. 3-48) and pars plana vitrectomy. In some cases, temporary tamponade is obtained with intraocular silicone oil (Fig. 3-54) (Gonvers 1985).

Nonrhegmatogenous detachments are caused by subretinal fluid accumulation from abnormal vessels, most often in neoplastic tissues (i.e., choroidal melanoma, metastases, choroidal hemangioma, retinoblastoma, etc). Nonneoplastic causes include Coat's disease and inflammation.

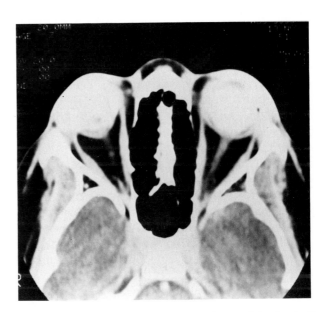

Figure 3-54 Silicone oil for retinal detachment. Intravitreal silicone appears as markedly high attenuation in this patient with recurrent retinal detachment.

ORBITAL TUMORS

Optic Glioma

Optic gliomas are uncommon tumors of the orbit (1 in 100,000 eye complaints; Jones 1979). The peak age for presentation is between 2 and 6 years, with 75 percent presenting by age 10, and 90 percent by age 20. In approximately 12 to 38 percent, there is an association with neurofibromatosis. The symptoms of the intraorbital optic glioma include progressive, nonpulsatile exophthalmos, limitation of eye movement, optic atrophy, and papilledema. The proptosis precedes a decrease in vision and the onset of strabismus. Histologically, these lesions are low-grade astrocytomas.

CT has replaced other radiographic modalities in the diagnostic evaluation of optic gliomas (Byrd 1978; Peyster 1983; Rothfus 1984), because CT is able to demonstrate the posterior extent of the optic glioma. A significant number of optic gliomas are part of a more extensive disease process, one that involves the visual pathway, including not only the optic nerve but the optic chiasm, optic tract, lateral geniculate body, and optic radiation (Fig. 3-55). It has been the authors' experience that unsuspected involvement of the optic tracts and geniculates has been present in one-fourth of patients (Bilaniuk 1981). Preliminary experience by the authors suggests that MR may detect extensive visual pathway involvement in a significantly higher percentage of these patients.

Optic gliomas appear most often as irregular nodular enlargements of the optic nerve, or occasionally as fusiform enlargements, most of which show contrast enhancement (Figs. 3-55, 3-56). Bilateral involvement, which in some cases is clinically unsuspected (Fig. 3-55), may be diagnostic of neurofibromatosis. Management of these lesions remains controversial. Table 3-5 lists the causes of enlarged optic nerve/sheath complex (Fig. 3-57).

Meningioma

Meningiomas may originate within the orbit, most often from the optic nerve sheath (Figs. 3-58, 3-59) and less frequently from the periosteum of the orbital wall or arachnoidal nests randomly located within the orbit (Fig. 3-60, 3-61). Meningiomas also secondarily involve the orbit by extension from a primary intracranial meningioma. Primary intraorbital meningiomas (5 percent of primary orbital tumors) are less frequent than those which secondarily involve the orbit. If one considers only primary tumors of the optic nerve, optic nerve meningiomas account for one-third (Reese 1976). Bilateral lesions are often associated with neurofibromatosis.

Meningiomas that arise along the course of the optic nerve may do so intraorbitally (sheath meningioma), within the optic canal (intracanalicular meningioma), or at the intracranial opening to the optic canal (foraminal meningioma). Most commonly they occur in females (up to 80 percent) in the third, fourth, and fifth decades of life. The predominant feature of optic nerve sheath meningioma is early visual loss, with proptosis occurring later (Wright 1979). Papilledema and optic atrophy are common accompaniments.

High-resolution CT accurately delineates the size of the optic nerve shadow and its components: subarachnoid space, surrounding arachnoid, and optic nerve. Significant enlargement, whether of the nerve, subarachnoid space, or arachnoidal membrane, is easily visualized. The problem is in differentiating the perioptic meningioma from other lesions that occur at the same anatomical site. To a large extent optic nerve gliomas occur in children, whereas perioptic meningioma occurs in adults. The bilateral enlargement of the optic nerve shadow due to distension of the subarachnoid space by CSF (papilledema) can usually be differentiated from other causes of optic nerve shadow enlargement (optic glioma, perioptic meningioma). Tumor enlargement is more nodular and irregular or fusiform (Bilaniuk 1981) than the smooth, parallel, symmetric enlargement that is seen in distension of the subarachnoid space (Cabanis 1978). The perineural location of the perioptic meningioma may actually be shown on CT as a mass surrounding a relatively less dense center (compressed optic nerve). Contrast enhancement of the optic nerve sheath meningioma is usually present and marked, resulting in the "tram-track" appear-

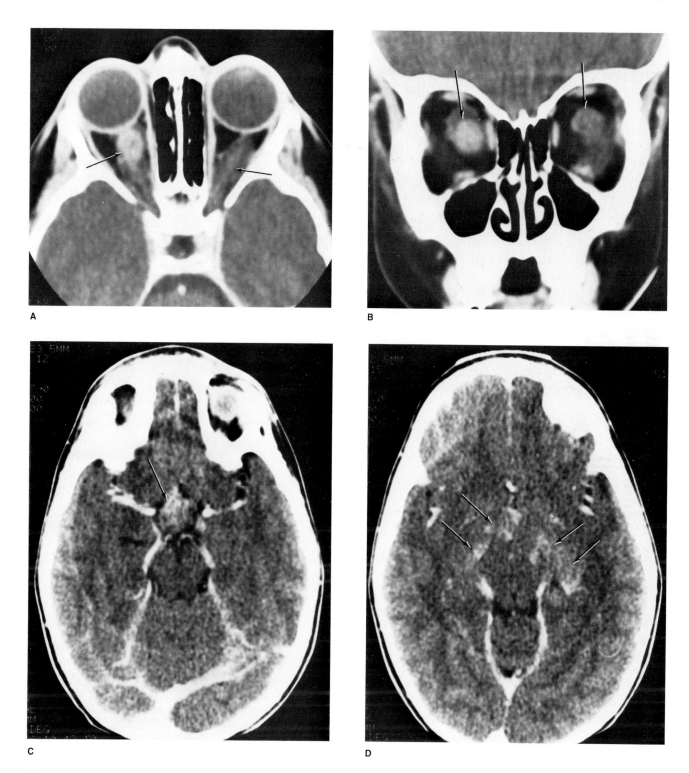

Figure 3-55 (**A–D**) Visual pathway glioma. Extensive optic pathway glioma involves optic nerves, chiasm, and optic tracts bilaterally (arrows).

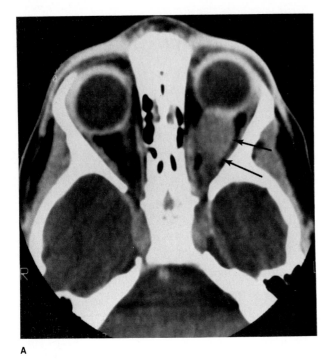
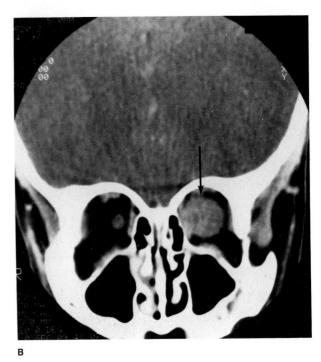

A   **B**

Figure 3-56 (**A, B**) Optic glioma. Massive lobulated enlargement of left optic nerve (arrow) in axial (**A**) and coronal (**B**) planes. Note slight flattening of globe.

Table 3-5 Etiologies of Enlarged Optic Nerve/Sheath Complex

Neoplasm
  Optic nerve glioma
  Meningioma
  Hemangioblastoma (especially in von Hippel–Lindau)
  Neuroma
  Leukemia
  Lymphoma
  Metastases
Other
  Orbital pseudotumor
  Optic neuritis
  Distended subarachnoid space
  Sarcoidosis
  Perioptic hematoma
  Thyroid ophthalmopathy
  Tuberculosis
  Toxoplasmosis

Modified from Peyster 1983.

ance seen on axial and coronal views (Figs. 3-58, 3-59). This finding distinguishes meningioma from optic nerve glioma (or any other true nerve mass), but is not specific (Table 3-6). Calcification helps confirm the diagnosis. Optic canal widening, hyperostosis, and intracranial extent are well seen on CT.

Rhabdomyosarcoma

Orbital rhabdomyosarcoma is the most common primary malignant orbital tumor of childhood. It is rarely seen in the adult. The tumor is composed of striated muscle cells and is thought to arise from undifferentiated mesenchymal elements that possess the ability to differentiate into striated muscle. In the orbit, rhabdomyosarcomas appear to arise from the orbital soft tissues and not from the extraocular muscles. The most common clinical presentation is that of rapidly progressive exophthalmos over days to weeks, often mimicking orbital cellulitis. The su-

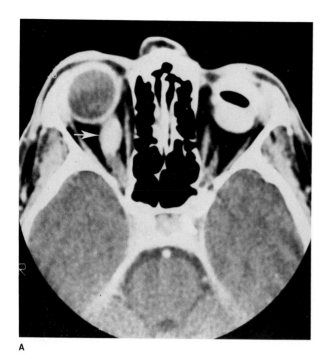

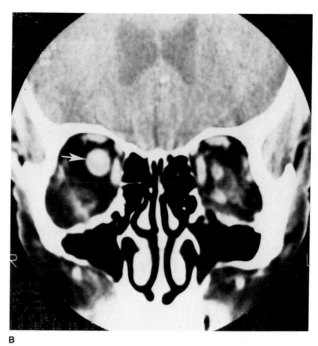

A

B

Figure 3-57 (**A, B**) Hemangioblastoma, optic nerve, von Hippel–Landau. In this patient, status/post left enucleation and prosthesis placement after multiple hemorrhages from retinal angiomas, axial (**A**), and coronal (**B**) images show markedly enhancing mass enlarging right optic nerve (arrow).

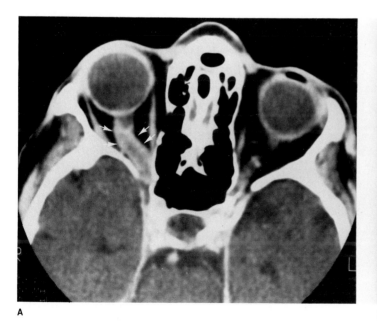

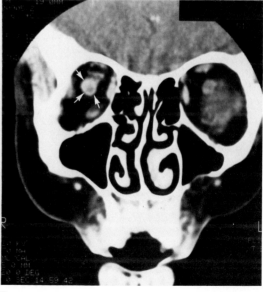

A

B

Figure 3-58 (**A, B**) Optic nerve meningioma. Axial (**A**) and coronal (**B**) images demonstrate "tram-track" enhancement along right optic nerve periphery (arrows).

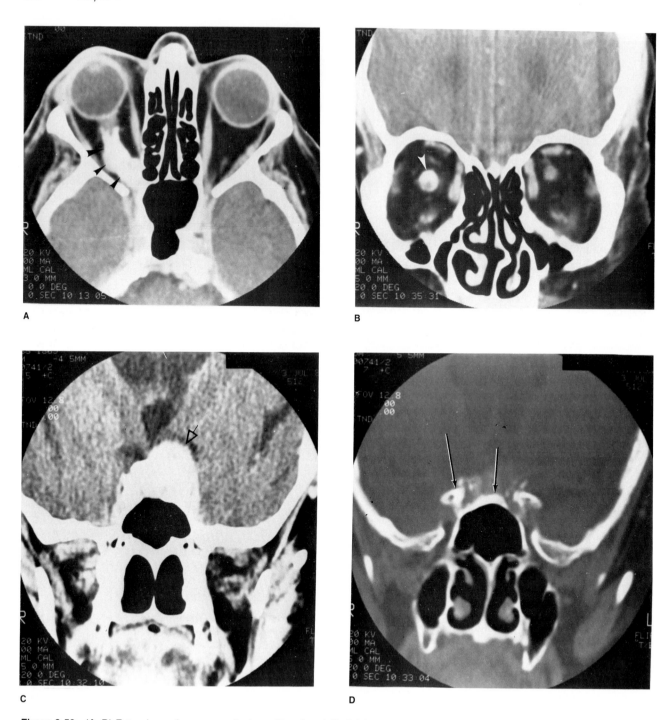

Figure 3-59 (**A–D**) Extensive optic nerve meningioma. Heavily calcified right perioptic meningioma (arrowheads, **A, B**) extends posteriorly into sellar region (open arrow, **C**). Note ''blistering'' of sellar floor and right optic strut (arrows, **D**).

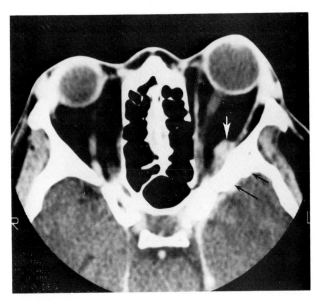

Figure 3-60 Orbital meningioma. Enhancing extraconal mass (white arrow) along posterolateral aspect left orbit. Note adjacent bony thickening of left sphenoid wing (black arrows).

peromedial aspect of the orbit is the most common site. In the authors' experience, rhabdomyosarcomas arising in the adjacent paranasal sinuses and extending into the orbit through the thin bony walls, thereby presenting with orbital symptoms, have been almost as frequent.

CT is an ideal method of evaluating the location and extent of the sarcoma; differentiation between primary orbital rhabdomyosarcoma and that arising from paranasal sinuses is usually possible (Zimmerman 1978). In one series of craniofacial sarcomas (Zimmerman 1978) there were six orbital rhabdomyosarcomas and none of these had CT evidence of bone destruction at the time of presentation; the tumors were all confined to the orbital soft tissues. In four paranasal sinus rhabdomyosarcomas which presented with orbital symptoms, the CT scan showed a more extensive process within the paranasal sinus, with destruction of the sinus wall and intraorbital extension (Bilaniuk 1980). CT is of further use in that it demonstrates intracranial epidural and subarachnoid extension of the tumor, which may be subclinical at the time of presentation (Zimmerman 1978). Intracranial spread into the subarach-

noid or epidural space is a poor prognostic sign, associated with an almost 100 percent recurrence rate.

On CT, rhabdomyosarcoma appears as an enhancing isodense to slightly hyperdense mass which may infiltrate the retrobulbar fat and muscle planes and often involves the posterior aspect of the globe (Fig. 3-62). The contrast enhancement of the tumor is often uniform.

The local response to chemotherapy and radiotherapy is often dramatic, with almost complete disappearance of the tumor in 6 weeks (Jereb 1985).

Lacrimal Gland Tumors

The lacrimal fossa is located extraconically in the superolateral aspect of the orbit. The lacrimal gland, the size and shape of an almond, lies within the lacrimal fossa, adjacent to the tendons of the lateral and superior rectus muscles. Histologically the lacrimal gland tissue is similar to that of the salivary gland, and pathologically it is affected by similar disease processes. Of the masses that arise within the lacrimal gland, 50 percent are tumors of epithelial origin. Approximately half of these are benign mixed tumors, while the other half comprise a variety of carcinomas. The remaining 50 percent of the masses arising in the lacrimal gland are either tumors of lymphomatous origin or are inflammatory masses.

The correct surgical management of the benign mixed lacrimal gland tumor is excision of the whole gland. This avoids the risk of seeding the tumor cells into the adjacent tissues and minimizes the possibility of recurrence (Wright 1979). Other lesions arising in the lacrimal fossa, such as inflammatory pseudotumor, epidermoid, and dermoid cysts, are only biopsied for tissue diagnosis. Thus it is important to know the extent of the disease process and whether the tumor is infiltrative or merely displaces adjacent soft tissues.

Benign mixed lacrimal gland tumors characteristically present in an age range that extends from the late twenties to the early sixties. They present as slowly progressive, painless swellings beneath

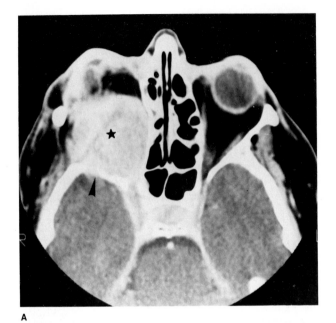

A

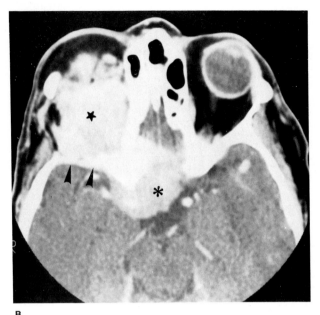

B

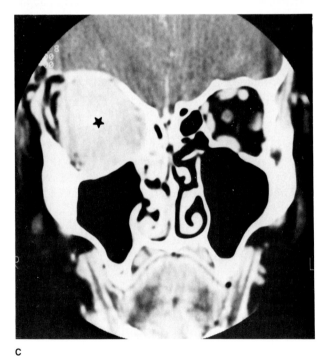

C

Figure 3-61 **(A–C)** Orbital meningioma. Homogeneously enhancing mass (star) filling right orbit and extending into suprasellar cistern (asterisk) impinging upon right uncus. Destruction of right sphenoid wing (arrowheads).

Table 3-6   Etiologies of the "Tram-Track" Sign

Optic nerve meningioma
Orbital pseudotumor
Perioptic neuritis
Sarcoidosis
Leukemia
Lymphoma
Perioptic hemorrhage
Metastases
Normal variant

the upper eyelid, with duration of symptoms usually over 12 months (Wright 1979). Carcinomas of the lacrimal gland characteristically have a rapidly worsening clinical course that usually lasts less than 9 months (Wright 1979). Adenoid cystic carcinoma is the most common malignant epithelial cell tumor of the lacrimal gland, comprising 29 percent of all epithelial neoplasms of the gland (Lee 1985). These tumors present in adults, with a mean age of 45 years, with no sex predilection. Approximately 50 percent of patients survive 2½ years after diagnosis (Lee 1985).

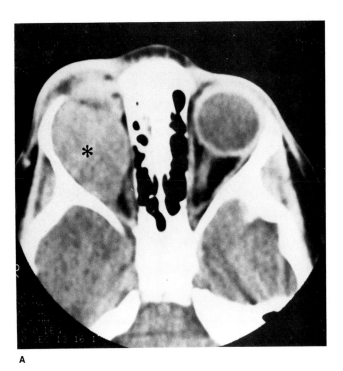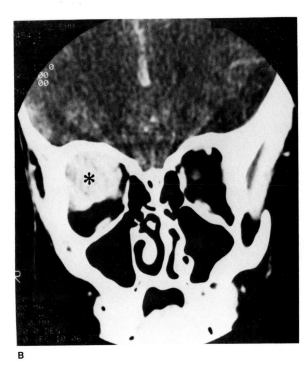

A **B**

Figure 3-62 (**A, B**) Rhabdomyosarcoma. Large homogeneous mass (asterisk) in superolateral aspect of right orbit is well circumscribed on precontrast axial image (**A**). Coronal postcontrast scan (**B**) shows marked enhancement in this mass, presenting as rapidly progressive proptosis.

Both benign and malignant tumors of the lacrimal gland expand and go on to produce unilateral exophthalmos. Because of their location in the superolateral aspect of the orbit, the globe is displaced inferiorly and medially (Fig. 3-63). The mass tends to enlarge posteriorly, so that the muscle cone and optic nerve are displaced along with the globe. The largest lesions extend to the orbital apex. The benign mixed adenomas do not invade the bone nor do they invade the muscle cone. They are usually well-defined masses of the same density as brain tissue that erode and expand the adjacent lacrimal fossa. Contrast enhancement in the benign mixed adenomas is variable, with only half enhancing (Forbes 1980). Hesselink et al. (1979*b*) have reported three cases of mucoepidermoid carcinoma of the lacrimal gland that were of hyperdensity and contrast-enhanced. Malignant neoplasms of the lacrimal gland have a tendency to invade the muscle cone and to destroy adjacent margins of the orbital wall. They may also produce sclerosis of the adjacent bone and may contain calcifications. In general, however, although CT can show precise location and extent of lacrimal masses, specific etiologies are not differentiated in the majority of cases (Balchunas 1983) (Figs. 3-12, 3-63, 3-64). Preliminary data suggest that MR may aid in differentiating neoplastic from inflammatory etiologies (Atlas 1986).

Lymphoma

The incidence of orbital involvement by lymphoma is approximately 1 percent (Jones 1979). The lacrimal gland is the most frequent site of lymphomatous disease within the orbit. Lymphomas presenting in the lacrimal gland either may be due to systemic disease or may indicate the primary site. Bilateral involvement of the lacrimal glands in patients with

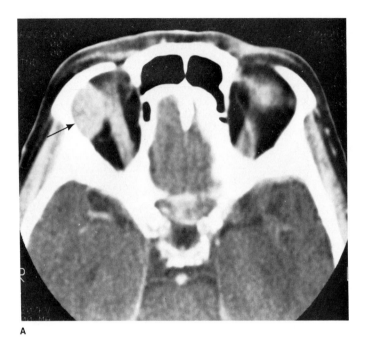

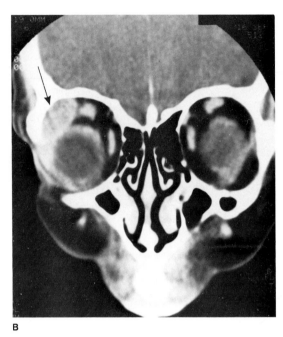

A

B

Figure 3-63 (**A, B**) Lymphoma. Enhanced axial (**A**) and coronal (**B**) images show well-circumscribed right lacrimal mass with peripheral rim enhancement (arrows).

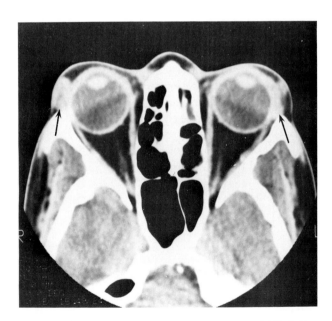

Figure 3-64 Sarcoid. Bilaterally prominent lacrimal glands (arrows) in patient with sarcoid.

systemic lymphoma is not unusual. Undifferentiated lymphomas produce symptoms with a duration of weeks to months, while the more differentiated ones often are associated with symptoms of longer duration. The patient with involvement of the lacrimal region presents with lid swelling and a palpable mass. Response to radiation therapy and chemotherapy may be in the form of a dramatic reduction in tumor size.

Lymphoma may also present as an infiltrative process in the retroconic space that obliterates the normal soft-tissue planes. Thus, it may mimic orbital pseudotumor and may be difficult to differentiate from it histologically, clinically, and by CT. On CT, lacrimal gland lymphoma appears as a mass in the lacrimal fossa of increased density that shows contrast enhancement and displaces the globe medially and forward (Fig. 3-63). Not infrequently there is extension of the lacrimal lymphomatous process into the eyelid and into the fossa temporalis.

Orbital Metastases from Distant Sites

In a large series of orbital neoplasms, metastases from distant primary sites were relatively rare (5 percent, Albert 1967). This may be a misleadingly low figure, because the orbital structures are rarely examined in patients who die with disseminated metastases. The patterns of orbital metastases differ in children and in adults. The tumors that metastasize most frequently to the orbit in the child are those which arise from embryonal tumors, neuroblastoma (Fig. 3-65), and Ewing's sarcoma (Jones 1979). Leukemia may also involve the orbit. In the child, the orbit is more frequently involved and the globe less often. In the adult, metastases are most often from carcinomas of breast and lung, and are more frequently linked to the globe (Hesselink 1980). In the adult, 70 percent of metastases are ocular (Fig. 3-37), whereas only 30 percent are orbital (Jones 1979). In 50 percent of these orbital metastases, the primary is unknown. In such a situation the site of the unknown primary is more likely to be the lung than the breast.

Symptoms of orbital metastatic disease include an abrupt onset of proptosis, external ophthalmoplegia, and orbital pain early in the course of the disease (Jones 1979).

Metastases to the orbit most often have indistinct boundaries and are diffusely infiltrating (Figs. 3-28, 3-66 to 3-68). A minority of metastatic lesions are discrete and well circumscribed. Metastatic retrobulbar carcinoma from breast carcinoma has been relatively frequent in the authors' experience. This most often appears on CT as a diffusely infiltrative, contrast-enhancing mass lesion without clear-cut margins. At times, metastases may have a CT appearance similar to that seen with extensive orbital pseudotumor. MR may aid in differentiating these entities (Atlas 1986). When the metastasis is from a scirrhous carcinoma, the fibrous response produces enophthalmos (Fig. 3-66).

In children, orbital metastases most often involve the walls of the orbit. The tumors extend subperiosteally into the orbital space. Neuroblastoma frequently presents with simultaneous metastases to both orbits but often also as unilateral metastatic disease (Fig. 3-65). The bone is infiltrated, and the orbital periosteum is displaced (Zimmerman 1980*b*).

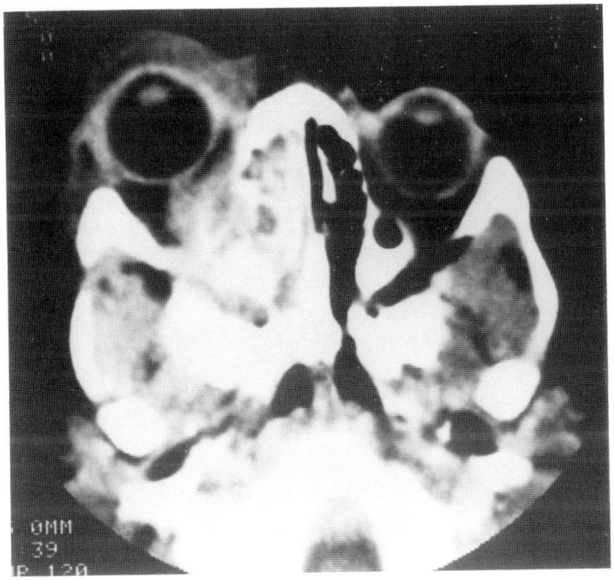

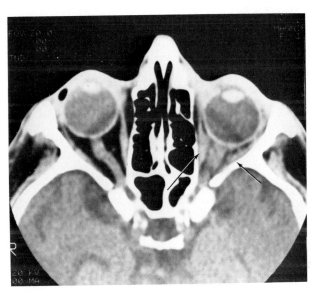

Figure 3-65 Neuroblastoma metastases. Destructive mass involving right medial orbit and ethmoid sinus causes proptosis.

Figure 3-66 Metastatic breast carcinoma. Extraconal masses in left orbit (arrows) with secondary enophthalmos, typical of scirrhous breast carcinoma metastasis.

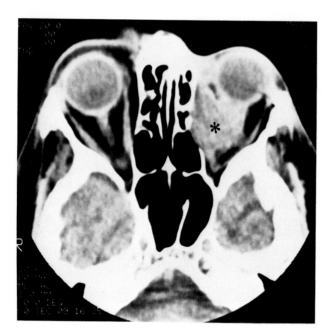

Skull radiographs may show mixed lytic and hyperostotic bone changes, spiculated periosteal bone reaction, and obliteration of adjacent paranasal sinuses. In addition to revealing similar bone changes, CT demonstrates the subperiosteal portion of the tumor, which shows contrast enhancement (Zimmerman 1980*b*). The orbital tumor in neuroblastoma may be dense on NCCT, owing to hemorrhage within the tumor.

Distant metastases to the orbital bones and paranasal sinuses also occur in adults and may resemble pediatric neuroblastoma. Metastatic prostate carcinoma is typified by its sclerotic bone reaction and subperiosteal extension, often presenting with large intraorbital soft-tissue masses (Fig. 3-68).

Orbital Wall and Paranasal Sinus Tumors
Benign Tumors

Fibrous Dysplasia

Fibrous dysplasia is probably a developmental mesodermal disorder that presents in either a mono-

Figure 3-67 Metastatic melanoma. Irregular, ill-defined mass (asterisk) in left retrobulbar space from primary cutaneous malignant melanoma.

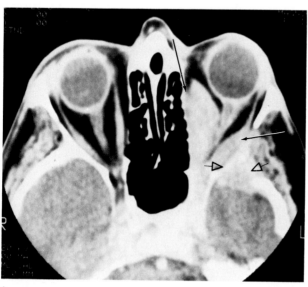

A

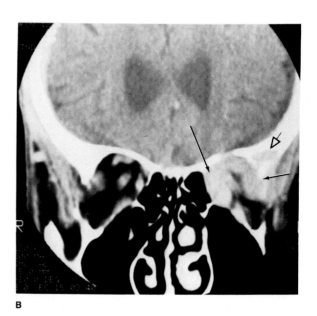

B

Figure 3-68 (A, B) Metastatic prostate carcinoma. Axial (A) and coronal (B) images demonstrate enhancing mass in the medial, superior, and lateral aspects of the left orbit (arrows) with destruction of the sphenoid wing (open arrow). Note extra axial mass anterior to left temporal lobe, a common site for metastasis.

stotic or a polyostotic form. In its polyostotic form there may be an associated skin pigmentation abnormality and an endocrine disorder (Albright's syndrome). There is no sex predilection. The disease is most often encountered in children and young adolescents. The monostotic facial form presents clinically with headaches, facial asymmetry, and painless swelling of the cheek and periorbital region. When the craniofacial bones are involved it is not unusual to find encroachment upon the paranasal sinuses, orbit, and foramina that transmit nerves. This encroachment can produce visual loss, proptosis, diplopia, and epiphora (tearing) (Liakos 1979). Depending upon the location of the fibrous dysplasia, the symptoms affecting the orbit will differ. Fibrous dysplasia involving the cranial base may produce an extraocular palsy and fifth nerve neuralgia, whereas fibrous dysplasia involving the optic canal will produce visual loss and optic atrophy. Proptosis and bony prominence are common when there is involvement of the frontal bones (Moore 1985).

CT, like skull radiography, reveals obliteration of the medullary canal by expansile homogeneous matrix denser than that of the normal bone but occasionally containing focal sclerotic and lytic areas. CT is excellent in defining the constrictive effect of the osseofibrous lesion upon the orbit, the optic canal, and the adjacent paranasal sinuses. Treatment of fibrous dysplasia is surgical, with unroofing of the optic canal or cosmetic remodeling of the orbit in order to provide adequate room for the intraorbital contents. Radiation therapy is not advised, because osteogenic sarcoma may develop as a result (Jones 1979).

Ossifying Fibroma

Ossifying fibromas are controversial lesions, often linked to fibrous dysplasia. They are benign tumors which grow without regard to skeletal maturity and may occur in the mandible, maxilla, and paranasal sinuses, especially in the frontal and ethmoid sinuses (Margo 1985). They are found most often after 10 years of age with no sex predilection. When they arise in the paranasal sinuses adjacent to the orbit, they most often present as exophthalmos. Histologically they are highly cellular, with a fibrous stroma, and osteoid, having a calcific matrix. Ossifying fibromas are more apt to show aggressive growth than fibrous dysplasia.

The radiologic picture of an ossifying fibroma reflects the variable composition of the lesion (fibrous tissue, osteoid, and calcific matrix). Conventional roentgenography shows opacification and expansion of the involved paranasal sinus. The lesion is relatively lucent when compared to a typical case of fibrous dysplasia. CT demonstrates the expansion of the paranasal sinus, the homogeneous matrix which shows contrast enhancement, and the admixture of bone spicules within it.

Osteoma

The incidence of osteomas on routine skull radiographs is on the order of 0.3 percent. They are found rising most often within the paranasal sinuses (Arger 1977) but on rare occasions may arise from the wall of the orbit. The most frequent location is within the frontal sinuses (40 to 80 percent), with the incidence decreasing in the ethmoid, maxillary, and sphenoid sinuses (2 percent). They are usually found after age 20 and more often in males than in females. The lesion consists mainly of thick lamellar bone (Margo 1985).

The osteoma expands within and conforms to the shape of the sinus. As the osteoma grows, it may produce obstruction of the ostia, which leads to infection or possibly the development of a mucocele. Pneumoencephalus has been reported as a complication of ethmoidal and frontal osteomas that have eroded through the floor of the anterior cranial fossa.

Visual symptoms are due to encroachment on the orbit or compression of the optic nerve. Frontal osteomas may produce both facial asymmetry and downward displacement of the globe. Ethmoidal osteomas can produce lateral displacement of the globe. Sphenoidal osteomas may encroach upon the optic canal and orbital apex (Jones 1979).

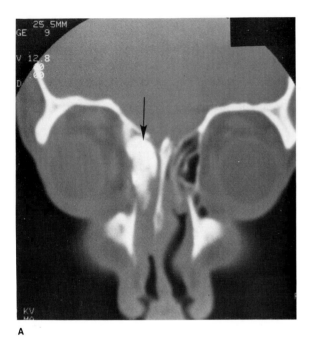
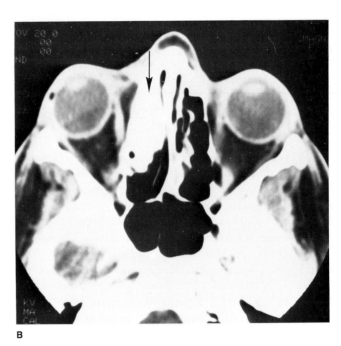

A

B

Figure 3-69 (**A, B**) Osteoma. Bone density within right ethmoid sinus involving medial wall or right orbit (arrows).

CT reveals the osteoma to be smoothly demarcated, frequently lobulated, homogeneously hyperdense (Fig. 3-69), and most often lying within the expanded paranasal sinuses. Encroachment on the orbit is graphically demonstrated in the coronal and transverse CT sections.

Inclusion Cyst

Sequestration of ectoderm in the wall of the orbit during embryogenesis leads to the formation of dermoid cysts. These consist of an epidermal lining which contains dermal appendages and ectodermal material (sebaceous glands, hair follicles, and occasional sweat glands) sequestered during embryogenesis. The desquamated contents consist of laminated keratin and cholesterol crystals. Epidermoid cysts are less common than dermoid cysts; they consist of a true epidermis and contain only desquamated keratin. Epithelial cysts also arise in the orbit and in the lacrimal gland as intrinsic lesions due to dilatation of the lacrimal ducts.

Dermoid cysts occur most often in the first decade of life, when they present with physical signs of proptosis or progressive swelling of the upper eyelid. A smooth mass may be palpable in the upper outer quadrant of the orbit.

Dermoid cysts are most often attached to the osseous structures surrounding the orbit. Most frequently they arise in the superolateral portion, in the vicinity of the lacrimal fossa. Extension through the bone, against the dura mater of the anterior cranial fossa, is not uncommon, nor is extension into the orbit with displacement of the orbital periosteum.

On CT, dermoid cysts have well-defined margins and appear cystic, with the density of their center ranging from that of CSF to that of fat (Figs. 3-70, 3-71) (Hesselink 1979*b*). On CECT the wall is noted to enhance, whereas the central portion remains the same in density. CT is of value in that it identifies a relatively characteristic benign lesion and shows both its intraorbital and its intracranial extent. Surgical treatment is indicated for cosmetic purposes; total removal without dissemination of the

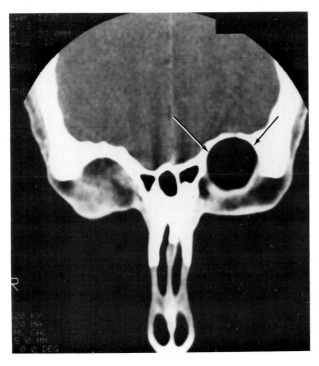

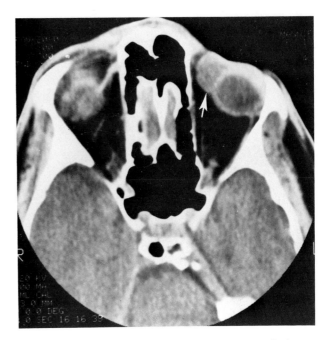

Figure 3-71 Dermoid. Soft-tissue density, well-circumscribed mass (arrow) medial to left globe.

Figure 3-70 Dermoid. Extraconal mass of fat attenuation (arrows) with thinning of adjacent left orbital roof.

contents is necessary. The contents, if ruptured, may incite a granulomatous inflammatory reaction. Recurrences are unusual.

Mucocele

A mucocele consists of a sac lined by respiratory epithelium, often containing a thin serous fluid but at times showing evidence of hemorrhage or previous infection. There is a history of sinusitis in approximately half the patients with mucocele, a history of trauma in about one-quarter, and a history of allergy in one-eighth. The cause of the mucocele is blockage of the ostium of the involved sinus. The ostium obstruction may be due to inflammation, fibrosis, trauma, prior surgery, anatomic abnormality, or osteoma. The developing mucocele produces an expansion of the sinus, with thinning and remodeling of the sinus wall. The expanded sinus may

protrude upon the orbital contents or encroach on the optic canal or cavernous sinus. Mucoceles are uncommon before age 13, as the paranasal sinuses are in the process of developing during childhood. Those which occur in the younger child usually do so as a result of problems in sinus drainage (cystic fibrosis). The most frequent location for mucoceles is the frontal sinus (60 percent); 30 percent occur in the ethmoid sinus. The sphenoid and maxillary sinuses are involved considerably less frequently (Som 1985). The type of symptoms depends on the location of the mucocele. Mucoceles that arise in the frontal and ethmoidal sinuses classically present as palpable masses in the superomedial aspect of the orbit. They produce proptosis and limitation of eye movement (resulting in diplopia). The swelling is usually painless but may be crepitant to palpation.

Skull radiography, pluridirectional tomography, and CT all show the involved sinus to be opacified and expanded and the sinus wall thinned. CT, because of its ability to show both bone and soft tissue, is an ideal method of evaluating the extent of the

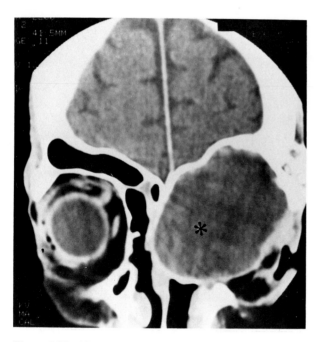

Figure 3-72 Mucocele. Markedly expanded left frontal and ethmoid sinuses secondary to huge mucocele (asterisk).

mucocele. Lateral extension of the frontoethmoidal mucocele produces erosion of the lamina papyracea (Fig. 3-72) and lateral displacement of the medial rectus (Hesselink 1979*a*). There is preservation of the fat plane between the mucocele and the medial rectus muscle (Som 1980). Proptosis is often evident on CT. Less commonly, there may be medial extension of the ethmoidal mucocele, so that the medial wall of the ethmoid sinus is eroded, with the mucocele projecting into the nasal cavity and against the perpendicular plate of the ethmoid. Superior extension of frontal and ethmoidal mucoceles can occur through the roof of the ethmoid or the cribriform plate. The use of the term *frontoethmoidal* mucocele points to the high incidence of contiguous sinus involvement (Figs. 3-72, 3-73). The expanded sinus is most often isodense and rarely calcified. Contrast enhancement is infrequent, unless the mucocele is infected (mucopyocele) (Som 1985) (Fig. 3-73).

Mucoceles that arise in the sphenoid sinus can produce extraocular muscle palsies by involvement of the cavernous sinus and can damage the optic

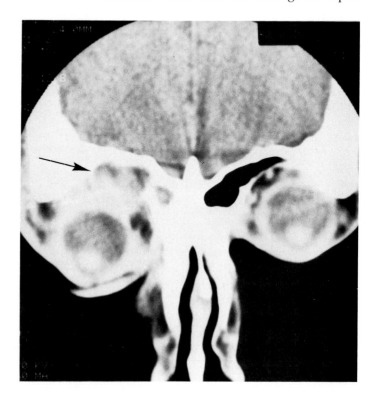

Figure 3-73 Mucopyelocele. Enhancing, opacified right frontal sinus (arrow) which is slightly expanded.

nerve and chiasm by direct compression. They may also interfere with pituitary function and mimic a primary intrasellar tumor (Chap. 13). CT shows expansion and opacification of the sphenoid sinus and may show a soft-tissue mass that extends out of the sphenoid sinus superiorly intracranially, inferiorly into the nasopharynx, or laterally into the cavernous sinus. Destruction of the sellar floor, erosion of the optic canals, widening of the superior orbital fissure, and elevation of the anterior clinoid processes are other manifestations of sphenoidal mucoceles. The clinical picture depends on the direction of expansion: there may be ophthalmoplegia and proptosis (anterolateral expansion into the orbit and cavernous sinus); chiasmal compression and pituitary dysfunction (with superior intracranial extension); airway obstruction (with expansion into the nasopharynx); and multiple cranial nerve (third, fifth, sixth) deficits (with posterolateral extension against the petrous apex) (Osborn 1979).

Malignant Tumors

Sinus Carcinoma

The thin osseous walls separating the orbit from the adjacent four paranasal sinuses offer little resistance to the direct spread of tumor. It has been estimated that in anywhere from 40 to 65 percent of paranasal sinus carcinomas the orbit is at risk. Preoperative management of these tumors necessitates an accurate evaluation of the extent of the malignancy and the presence or absence of orbital involvement. To this extent, CT has added a new dimension to the preoperative evaluation and treatment planning of sinus carcinomas. With CT it is possible to identify osseous involvement of the orbital wall and extension of the tumor extraconically, as well as intraconal extension (Mancuso 1978) (Fig. 3-74). Any degree of orbital extension is particularly devastating, because it necessitates either orbital exenteration or orbital reconstruction (Jones 1979). This same information is also valuable in postoperative radiotherapy planning. Evaluation of the sinus and orbit should include both transverse sections as well as

coronal sections. Sagittal sections, direct or reformatted, are also extremely valuable. Three-dimensional reconstruction may also be useful.

Malignant tumors of the paranasal sinuses are relatively rare, constituting between 0.26 and 0.31 percent of cancers. The most frequent site of involvement is the maxillary sinus, with the ethmoid sinus being the next most frequent and the frontal or sphenoid sinus relatively uncommon. The most common forms of paranasal sinus malignancy are squamous cell carcinomas and undifferentiated carcinomas. Less frequent is lymphoma, and relatively uncommon are melanoma, plasmocytoma, and various sarcomas. Squamous cell carcinoma represents over 50 percent of the lesions in the series reported by Weber et al. (1978), constituting over half of those that arose in the maxillary antrum.

Not infrequently, the clinical diagnosis is delayed (over 50 percent of cases) and the tumor is advanced at the time of diagnosis. Frequently more than one of the paranasal sinuses is involved. Early symptoms are often trivial, so the delay between onset of symptoms and histologic diagnosis may be as long as a year. Presenting symptoms depend on the site of origin and the degree of extension of the tumor at the time of diagnosis. The most frequent locations of carcinomas of the maxillary sinus have been described by Baclesse (1952): (1) tumors arising within the inferior portion of the maxillary sinus— these do not involve the orbit; (2) tumors arising in the roof of the antrum—these not infrequently extend posteriorly and laterally to the infratemporal fossa and superiorly into the ethmoid sinuses and orbit; (3) a generalized growth arising from the mucosal surfaces of the antrum and tending not to involve the osseous wall but filling the sinus; (4) medial wall neoplasms which often extend from the maxillary sinuses into the nasal fossa; (5) those which arise in the superior-medial angle at the ethmoidomaxillary septum—these classically have extensive involvement of the medial orbit.

Swelling of the face is the most common symptom with maxillary sinus carcinoma (40 percent). Involvement of the nasal cavity causing pain, unilateral obstruction, and nasal discharge is present in another 35 percent. The orbit is involved at the time

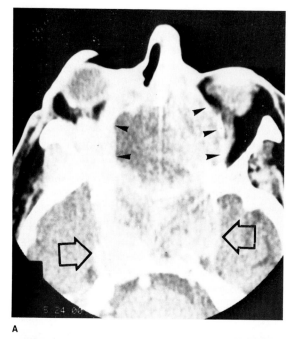

A

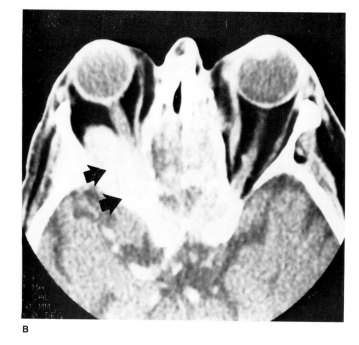

B

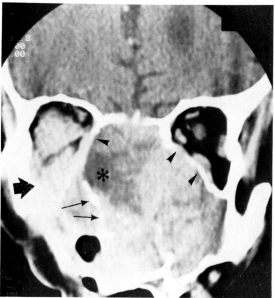

C

Figure 3-74 (**A–C**) Adenocystic carcinoma. Axial images (**A, B**) demonstrate large mass replacing midline sinuses, extending into right orbital apex (large arrows), bowing medial orbital walls laterally (arrowheads), and invading cavernous sinuses (open arrows). Coronal image (**C**) defines extent of mass; destroyed bone fragments (small arrows) present within mass adjacent to necrotic area (asterisk).

of presentation in only 10 percent. Ethmoidal carcinomas have a higher incidence of nasal involvement (55 percent) and a much higher incidence of orbital involvement (35 percent) at the time of initial presentation. Orbital signs are proptosis, diplopia, visual loss, paresthesias, and involvement of such structures as the infraorbital nerve.

The hallmarks of sinus carcinoma, detected by routine radiography, pluridirectional tomography, and CT, are the presence of a sinus soft-tissue mass in association with extensive bone destruction (Fig. 3-74). Bone remodeling, as opposed to overt bone destruction, may be seen in malignant as well as benign lesions. Some of these malignancies (adenoid cystic carcinoma) have worse five-year survival percentage than squamous cell carcinoma, which is more destructive radiographically (Som 1985). Extension of the mass outside the sinus cavity into the face, other paranasal sinuses, adjacent orbit, or intracranial contents is most typical of a carcinoma, but on rare occasions it can be seen with *Aspergillus* infection or Wegener's granulomatosis (Vermess 1978) (Fig. 3-75). It should be noted that opacification of adjacent paranasal sinuses does not necessarily indicate tumor involvement but may merely represent fluid retained within the sinus secondary to ostium obstruction. Intravenous contrast enhancement may aid in this distinction.

Chondrosarcoma

Of the chondrosarcomas occurring in the skeleton, approximately 9.4 percent occur in the bones of the face and cranium. Chondrosarcomas arise from cartilaginous rests in the walls of the orbit and paranasal sinuses. The bones of the base of the skull are preformed in cartilage, and rests from this formation give rise to the tumors. Thus the ethmoid region, maxilla, cribriform plate, and sphenoid bone are frequently involved. It is also possible for chondrosarcomas as well as other cartilaginous tumors to arise within the orbit from the cartilage of the trochlea (Jones 1979).

Chondrosarcomas of the craniofacial bones frequently are slowly progressive and form an expansile mass, most often in the maxilloethmoid region. One-third of patients are less than 20 years of age. Unlike osteogenic sarcomas of the facial bones, chondrosarcomas are not known to be painful during their initial growth. In contrast to the chondrosarcoma, osteogenic sarcomas involving the orbit are rare. They occur predominantly in the older patient (that is, between 20 and 50 years of age), are painful, have a rapid onset of symptoms (less than 3 months), and are much more likely to occur in the mandible or alveolar ridge of the antrum than in the orbital region.

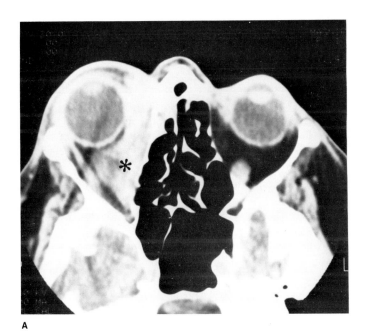
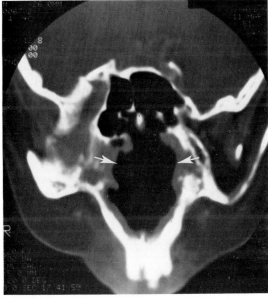

A

B

Figure 3-75 (**A, B**) Wegener's granulomatosis. (**A**) Enhancing intra- and extraconal mass extends along medial aspect right orbit (asterisk). (**B**) Destroyed nasal septa typical of necrotizing aggressive process (arrows).

On CT, chondrosarcoma is a densely calcified mass, often showing a whorled pattern (with central hypodensity) and capped by a soft-tissue mass that is not calcified. Both calcified and noncalcified tumor components show contrast enhancement. Adjacent normal bone is destroyed and the local soft-tissue planes are obliterated as a result of invasion.

Bibliography

ABRAMSON DH, ELLSWORTH R, KITCHIN S: Second non-ocular tumors in retinoblastoma survivor. *Ophthalmol* **91**:1351–1355, 1984.

ALBERT DM, RUBENSTEIN RA, SCHEIE HG: Tumor metastases to the eye: I. Incidence in 213 adult patients with generalized malignancy. *Am J Ophthalmol* **63**:723–726, 1967.

ALPER MG: Endocrine orbital disease, in Arger PH, ed.: *Orbit Roentgenology,* New York, Wiley, 1977.

ANDERSON RL, EPSTEIN GA, DAUER EA: Computed tomographic diagnosis of posterior ocular staphyloma. *AJNR* **4**:90–91, 1983.

APPELBOOM T, DURSO F: Retinoblastoma presenting as a total hyphema. *Ann Ophthalmol* **17**:508–510, 1985.

ARGER PH: Tumor and tumor-like conditions, in Arger PH, ed.: *Orbit Roentgenology,* New York, Wiley, 1977.

ATLAS SW, GROSSMAN RI, SAVINO PJ, et al: High field surface coil MR of orbital pseudotumor. *AJNR* 1986 (in press).

BACLESSE F: Les cancers du sinus maxillaire de l'ethmoide et des fosses nasales. *Ann Otolaryngol* **69**:465, 1952.

BACON KT, DUCHESNAU PM, WEINSTEIN MA: Demonstration of the superior ophthalmic vein by high resolution computed tomography. *Radiol* **124**:129–131, 1977.

BALCHUNAS WR, QUENCER RM, BYRNE SF: Lacrimal gland and fossa masses: Evaluation by computed tomography and A-mode echography. *Radiol* **149**:751–758, 1983.

BALERIAUX-WAHA D, MORTELMANS LL, DUPONT MG, TERWINGHE G, JEANMART L: The use of coronal scans for computed tomography of the orbits. *Neuroradiol* **14**:89–96, 1977.

BERNARDINO ME, ZIMMERMAN RD, CITRIN CM, DAVIS DO: Scleral thickening: A sign of orbital pseudotumor. *Am J Roentgenol* **129**:703–706, 1977.

BERNARDINO ME, DANZIGER J, YOUNG SE, WALLACE S: Computed tomography in ocular neoplastic disease. *Am J Roentgenol* **131**:111–113, 1978.

BILANIUK LT, ZIMMERMAN RA: Computer-assisted tomography: Sinus lesions with orbital involvement. *Head Neck Surg* **2**:293–301, 1980.

BILANIUK LT, ZIMMERMAN RA, SCHUT L, BRUCE D: Computed tomography in the diagnosis and post-treatment evaluation of the visual pathway gliomas. Presented at XVth International Congress of Radiology, Brussels, Belgium, 1981.

BRANT-ZAWADZKI M, ENZMANN DR: Orbital computed tomography: Calcific densities of the posterior globe. *J Comp Assist Tomogr* **3**:503–505, 1979.

BRISMAR J, DAVIS KR, DALLOW RL, BRISMAR G: Unilateral endocrine exophthalmos. Diagnostic problems in association with computed tomography. *Neuroradiol* **12**:24, 1976.

BRODEY PA, RANDEL S, LANE B, FISCH AE: Computed tomography of axial myopia. *JCAT* **7**:484–485, 1983.

BROWN GC, TASMAN WS, BENSON WE: BB-gun injuries to the eye. *Ophthal Surg* **16**:505–508, 1985.

BROWN GC, WEINSTOCK F: Arterial macroaneurysm on the optic disk presenting as a mass lesion. *Ann Ophthalmol* **17**:519–520, 1985.

BULLOCK JD, CAMPBELL RJ, WALKER RR: Calcification in retinoblastoma. *Invest Ophthalmol Vis Sci* **16**:252–255, 1977.

BYRD SE, HARDWOOD-NASH DC, FITZ CR, BARRY JF, ROGOVITZ DM: Computed tomography of intraorbital optic nerve gliomas in children. *Radiol* 129:73–78, 1978.

CABANIS EA, et al.: Computed tomography of the optic nerve: II. Size and shape modifications in papilledema. *J Comput Assist Tomogr* **2**:150–155, 1978.

CARLSON RE, SCHERIBEL KW, HERING PJ, WOLIN L: Exophthalmos, global luxation, rapid weight gain: Differential diagnosis. *Ann Ophthalmol* **14**:724–729, 1982.

COHEN BA, SOM PM, HAFFNER PH, FRIEDMAN AH: Steroid exophthalmos. *J Comput Assist Tomogr* **5**:907–908, 1981.

CORBETT J, SAVINO PJ, SCHATZ NJ, ORR LS: Cavitary developmental defects of the optic disc. *Arch Neurol* **37**:210–213, 1980.

DANZIGER A, PRICE HI: CT findings in retinoblastoma. *Am J Roentgenol Radium Ther Nucl Med* **133**:783–785, 1979.

DAVIS KR, HESSELINK JR, DALLOW RL, GROVE AS JR: CT and ultrasound in the diagnosis of cavernous hemangioma and lymphangioma of the orbit. *CT: J Comput Tomogr* **4**:98–104, 1980.

DRESNER SC, ROTHFUS WE, SLAMOVITZ TL, KENNERDELL JS, CURTIN HD: Computed tomography of orbital myositis. *AJR* **143**:671–674, 1984.

EDWARDS MG, PORDELL GR: Ocular toxocariasis studied by CT scanning. *Radiol* **157**:685–686, 1985.

ENZMANN D et al.: Computed tomography in Graves' ophthalmopathy. *Radiol* **118**:615–620, 1976a.

ENZMANN D, DONALDSON SS, MARSHALL WH, KRISS JP: Computed tomography in orbital pseudotumor (idiopathic orbital inflammation). *Radiol* 120:597–601, 1976b.

ENZMANN DR, DONALDSON SS, KRISS JP: Appearance of Graves' disease on orbital computed tomography. *J Comput Assist Tomogr* **3**:815–819, 1979.

FORBES G: Computed tomography of the orbit. *RCNA* **20**:37–49, 1982.

FORBES GS, SHEEDY PF, WALLER RR: Orbital tumors evaluated by computed tomography. *Radiol* **136**:101–111, 1980.

FOX AJ, DEBRUN G, VINUELA F, ASSIS L, COATES R: Itrathecal metrizamide enhancement of the optic nerve sheath. *J Comput Assist Tomogr* **3**:653–656, 1979.

GITTINGER JW: *Opthalmology: A Clinical Introduction.* Boston, Little, Brown and Co., 1984.

GONVERS M: Temporary silicone oil tamponade in the management of retinal detachment with proliferative vitreoretinopathy. *Am J Ophthalmol* **100**:239–245, 1985.

GROVE AS JR, TADMOR R, NEW PFJ, MOMOSE KJ: Orbital fracture evaluation by coronal computed tomography. *Am J Ophthalmol* **85**:679–685, 1978.

HAIK BG, SAINT LOUIS L, SMITH ME, ABRAMSON DH, ELLSWORTH RM: Computed tomography of the nonrhegmatogenous retinal detachment in the pediatric patient. *Ophthalmol* **92**:1133–1142, 1985.

HAMMERSCHLAG SB, HUGHES S, O'REILLY GV, NAHEEDY MH, RUMBAUGH CL: Blow-out fractures of the orbit: A comparison of computed tomography and conventional radiography with anatomical correlation. *Radiol* **143**:487–492, 1982.

HAUGHTON VM, DAVIS JP, HARRIS GJ, HO KC: Metrizamide optic nerve sheath opacification. *Invest Radiol* **15**:343–345, 1980.

HEDGES TR, POZZI-MUCELLI R, CHAR DH, NEWTON TH: Computed tomographic demonstration of ocular calcification: Correlations with clinical and pathologic findings. *Neuroradiol* **23**:15–21, 1982.

HESSELINK JR, DAVIS KR, WEBER AL, DAVIS JM, TAVERAS JM: Radiological evaluation of orbital metastases with emphasis on computed tomography. *Radiol* **137**:363–366, 1980.

HESSELINK JR, et al.: Computed tomography of the paranasal sinus and face. I. Normal anatomy. *J Comput Asisst Tomogr* **2**:559–567, 1978.

HESSELINK JR, WEBER AL, NEW PFJ, DAVIS KR, ROBERSON GH, TAVERAS JM: Evaluation of mucoceles of the paranasal sinuses with CT. *Radiol* **133**:397–400, 1979*a*.

HESSELINK JR, DAVIS KR, DALLOW RL, ROBERSON GH, TAVERAS JM: Computed tomography of masses in the lacrimal gland region. *Radiol* **131**:143–147, 1979*b*.

HOYT WF: Coronal sections in the diagnosis of orbital disease, in Thompson HS, ed, *Topics in Neuro-ophthalmology*. Baltimore, London, Williams & Wilkins, 1979, pp. 369–371.

JACOBS L, WEISBERG LA, KINKEL WR: *Computerized Tomography of the Orbit and Sella Turcica*, New York, Raven Press, 1980.

JEREB B, HAIK BG, ONG R, GHAVIMI F: Parameningeal rhabdomyosarcoma (including the orbit): Results of orbital irradiation. *Int J Radiat Oncol Biol Phys* **11**:2057–2065, 1985.

JOHNSON DL, CHANDRA R, FISHER WS, HAMMOCK MK, MCKEOWN CA: Trilateral retinoblastoma: Ocular and pineal retinoblastomas. *J Neurosurg* **63**:367–370, 1985.

JONES IS, JAKOBIEC FA: *Diseases of the Orbit*. Hagerstown, Md., Harper & Row, 1979.

KAPLAN RJ: Neurological complications of infections of the head and neck. *Otolaryngol Clin North Am* **9**:729–749, 1976.

KLINTWORTH GK: Radiographic abnormalities in eyes with retinoblastoma and other disorders. *Br J Ophthalmol* **62**:365–372, 1978.

KROHEL GB, KRAUSS HR, WINNICK J: Orbital abscess: Presentation, diagnosis, therapy and sequelae. *Ophthalmol* **85**:492–498, 1982.

LEE DA, CAMPBELL RJ, WALLER RR, ILSTRUP OM: A clinicopathologic study of primary adenoid cystic carcinoma of the lacrimal gland. *Opohthalmol* **92**:128–134, 1985.

LEONE CR, LLOYD WC: Treatment protocol for orbital inflammatory disease. *Ophthalmol* **92**:1325–1331, 1985.

LIAKOS GM, WALKER CB, CARRUTH JAS: Ocular complications in craniofacial fibrous dysplasia. *Br J Ophthalmol* **63**:611–616, 1979.

LINDBERG R, WALSH FB, SACHS JG: *Neuropathology of Vision: An Atlas*. Philadelphia, Lea & Febiger, 1973.

MACRAE JA: Diagnosis and management of a wooden orbital foreign body: Case report. *Br J Ophthalmol* **63**:848–851, 1979.

MAFEE MF, PEYMAN GA, MCKUSICK MA: Malignant uveal melanoma and similar lesions studied by comuted tomography. *Radiol* **156**:403–408, 1985.

MANCUSO AA, HANAFEE WN, WARD P: Extensions of paranasal sinus tumors and inflammatory disease as evaluated by CT and pluridirectional tomography. *Neuroradiol* **16**:449–453, 1978.

MANELFE C, PASQUINI U, BONK WO: Metrizamide demonstration of the subarachnoid space surrounding the optic nerves. *J Comput Assist Tomogr* **2**:545–548, 1978.

MARGO CE, RAGSDALE BD, PERMAN KI, ZIMMERMAN LE, SWEET DE: Psammomatoid (juvenile) ossifying fibroma of the orbit. *Ophthalmol* **92**:150–159, 1985.

MOORE AT, BUNCIC JR, MUNRO IR: Fibrous dysplasia of the orbit in childhood: Clinical features and management. *Ophthalmol* **92**:12–20, 1985.

NUGENT RA, ROOTMAN J, ROBERTSON WD, LAPOINTE JS, HARRISON PB: Acute orbital pseudotumors: Classification and CT features. *AJR* **137**:957–962, 1981.

OSBORN AG, JOHNSON L, ROBERTS TS: Sphenoidal mucoceles with intracranial extension. *J Comput Assist Tomogr* **3**:335–338, 1979.

OSBORN AG, ANDERSON RE, WING SD: Sagittal CT scans in the evaluation of deep facial and naso-pharyngeal lesions. *CT: J Comput Tomogr* **4**:19–24, 1980.

PATZ A: Observations on the retinopathy of prematurity. *Am J Ophthalmol* **100**:164–168, 1985.

PEYSTER RG, AUGSBERGER JJ, SHIELDS JA, SATCHELL TV, MARKOE AM, CLARKE K, HASKIN ME: Choroidal melanoma: Comparison of CT, fundoscopy and US. *Radiol* **156**:675–680, 1985.

PEYSTER RG, HOOVER ED, HERSHEY BL, HASKIN ME: High-resolution CT of lesions of the optic nerve. *AJNR* **4**:169–174, 1983.

PEYSTER RG, GINSBURG F, SILBER J, ADLER L: Exophthalmos caused by excessive fat: CT volumetric analysis and differential diagnosis. *AJNR* **7**:35–40, 1986.

RAMIREZ H, BLATT ES, HIBRI NS: Computed tomographic identification of calcified optic nerve dru-sen. *Radiol* **148**:137–139, 1983.

REESE AB: *Tumors of the Eye.* New York, Harper & Row, 1976.

ROSENBLUM P, ZILKHA A: Sudden visual loss secondary to an orbital varix. *Surv Ophthalmol* **23**:49–56, 1978.

ROTHFUS WE, CURTIN HD, SLAMOVITZ TL, KENNERDELL JS: Optic nerve/sheath enlargement. *Radiol* **150**:409–415, 1984.

ROTHFUS WE, CURTIN HD: Extraocular muscle enlargement: A CT review. *Radiol* **151**:677–681, 1984.

RUSSELL DS, RUBENSTEIN LJ: *Pathology of Tumours of the Nervous System.* Baltimore, Williams & Wilkins, 1977.

SALVOLINI U, CABANIS EA, RODALLEC A, MENICHELLI F, PASQUINI U, IBA-ZIZEN MT: Computed tomogra-phy of the optic nerve. I. Normal results. *J Comput Assist Tomogr* **2**:141–149, 1978.

SAVAGE GL, CENTARO A, ENOCH JM, NEWMAN NM: Drusen of the optic nerve head: An important model. *Ophthalmol* **92**:793–799, 1985.

SERGOTT RC, GLASER JS, CHARYULU K: Radiotherapy for idiopathic inflammatory pseudotumor: Indi-cations and results. *Arch Ophthalmol* **99**:853–856, 1981.

SEVEL D, KRAUSZ H, PONDER T, CENTENO R: Value of computed tomography for the diagnosis of a ruptured eye. *J Comput Assist Tomogr* **7**:870–875, 1983.

SHERMAN JL, MCLEAN IW, BRAILLIER DR: Coat's disease: CT—pathologic correlation in two cases. *Radiol* **146**:77–78, 1983.

SHIELDS JA: Current approaches to the diagnosis and management of choroidal melanomas. *Surv Ophthalmol* **21**:443–463, 1977.

SIMMONS JD, LAMASTERS D, CHAR D: Computed tomography of ocular colobomas. *AJR* **141**:1223–1226, 1983.

SOLOWAY HB: Radiation-induced neoplasms following curative therapy for retinoblastoma. *Cancer* **12**:1984–1988, 1966.

SOM PM, SHUGAR JMA: The CT classification of ethmoid mucoceles. *J Comput Assist Tomogr* **4**:199–203, 1980.

SOM PM: CT of the paranasal sinuses. *Neuroradiol* **27**:189–201, 1985.

STARR H, ZIMMERMAN L: Extrascleral extension and orbital recurrence of malignant melanomas of the choroid and ciliary body. *Int Ophthalmol Clin* **2**:369, 1962.

STERNBERG P, DE JUAN E, MICHELS RG, AUER C: Multivariate analysis of prognostic factors in penetrat-ing ocular injuries. *Am J Ophthalmol* **98**:467–472, 1984.

TABADDOR K: Unusual complications of iophendylate injection myelography. *Arch Neurol* **29**:435–436, 1973.

TADMOR R, NEW PFJ: Computed tomography of the orbit with special emphasis of coronal sections: 1. Normal anatomy. *J Comput Assist Tomogr* **2**:24–34, 1978.

TENNER NS, TROKEL SL: Demonstration of the intraorbital portion of the optic nerves by pneumoencephalography. *Arch Ophthalmol* **79**:572–573, 1968.

TOWBIN R, HAN BK, KAUFMAN RA, BURKE M: Post-septal cellulitis: CT in diagnosis and management. *Radiol* **158**:735–737, 1986.

TROKEL SL, HILAL SK: CT scanning in orbital diagnosis, in Thompson HS, ed., *Topics in Neuro-ophthalmology.* Baltimore, Williams & Wilkins, 1979, pp. 336–346.

TURNER RM, GUTMAN I, HILAL SK, BEHRENS M, ODEL J: CT of drusen bodies and other calcific lesions of the optic nerve: Case report and differential diagnosis. *AJNR* **4**:175–178, 1983.

UNGER J: Orbital apex fractures: The contribution of computed tomography. *Radiol* **150**:713–717, 1984.

UNSOLD R, NEWTON TH, HOYT WF: Technical note—CT examination of the optic nerve. *J Comput Assist Tomogr* **4**:560–563, 1980a.

UNSOLD R, DEGROOT J, NEWTON TH: Images of the optic nerve: Anatomic CT correlation. *Am J Roentgenol* **135**:767–773, 1980b.

VERMESS M, HAYNES BF, FANCI AS, WOLFF SM: Computed assisted tomography of orbital lesions in Wegener's granulomatosis. *J Comput Assist Tomogr* **2**:45:48, 1978.

WEBER AL, TADMOR R, DAVIS R, ROBERSON G: Malignant tumors of the sinuses. *Neuroradiol* **16**:443–448, 1978.

WEISMAN RA, SAVINO PJ, SCHUT L, SCHATZ NJ: Computed tomography in penetrating wounds of the orbit with retained foreign bodies. *Arch Otolaryngol* **109**:265–268, 1983.

WILNER HI, COHN EM, KLING G, JAMPEL RS: Computer assisted tomography in experimentally induced orbital pseudotumor. *J Comput Assist Tomogr* **2**:431–455, 1978.

WING SD, HUNSAKER JN, ANDERSON RE, VANDYCK HJL, OSBORN AG: Direct sagittal computed tomography in Graves' ophthalmopathy. *J Comput Assist Tomogr* **3**:820–824, 1979.

WRIGHT JE: Primary optic nerve meningiomas: Clinical presentation and management. *Trans Am Acad Ophthalmol Otolaryngol* **83**:617–624, 1977.

WRIGHT JE, STEWART WB, KROHEL GB: Clinical presentation and management of lacrimal gland tumors. *Br J Ophthalmol* **63**:600–606, 1979.

YANOFF M, FINE BS: *Ocular Pathology. A Text and Atlas.* Harper & Row, Hagerstown, Md., 1975.

ZIMMERMAN RA, BILANIUK LT, LITTMAN P: Computed tomography of pediatric craniofacial sarcoma. *CT:J Comput Tomogr* **2**:113–121, 1978.

ZIMMERMAN RA, BILANIUK LT: Computed tomography in the evauation of patients with bilateral retinoblastomas. *CT: J Comput Tomogr* **3**:251–257, 1979.

ZIMMERMAN RA, BILANIUK LT: CT of orbital infection and its cerebral complications. *Am J Roentgenol Radium Ther Nucl Med* **134**:45–50, 1980a.

ZIMMERMAN RA, BILANIUK LT: Computed tomography of primary and secondary craniocerebral neuroblastoma. *Am J Neuroradiol* **1**:431–434, 1980b.

ZIMMERMAN RA, VIGNAUD J: Ophthalmic arteriography, in Arger PH, ed., *Orbit Roentgenology,* New York, Wiley, 1977.

4

CRANIOCEREBRAL ANOMALIES

Krishna C.V.G. Rao

Derek C. Harwood-Nash

Congenital craniocerebral anomalies of the brain and its coverings are the result of deviation in form and structure during intrauterine development of the nervous system. The combination of genetic and intrauterine environmental factors is the cause of craniocerebral anomalies in nearly 40 percent of intracranial malformations. Of these, chromosomal deviations account for 10 percent, inheritance (either recessive or dominant) for 20 percent, and intrauterine environmental factors such as hypoxia, maternal disease, and infection for 10 percent of the anomalies (Ebaugh 1963). In the remaining 60 percent no single pathogenetic factor has been implicated.

In many of these anomalies a logical cause cannot be deduced, since dysgenesis can occur during the gestational period (initial 3 weeks of intrauterine life), during intrauterine maturation, or during subsequent development. Inflammatory reaction within the fetal brain is uncommon before the sixth month of intrauterine life. Thus most anomalies in which infection is a factor affect the developing fetus during the maturation period, except in unusual situations.

Craniocerebral anomalies have been classified either according to the phases of development (Yakovlev 1959; Adams 1968) or according to anatomical (organogenetic) or cellular (histogenetic) alterations (DeMeyer 1971). Because of the variety of causative factors involved, the etiology in many of the malformations is not clearly established. The classification adopted here (Table 4-1) is the one proposed by DeMeyer.

Prior to the availability of CT, diagnosis of many

Table 4-1   Classification of Cerebral Malformations*

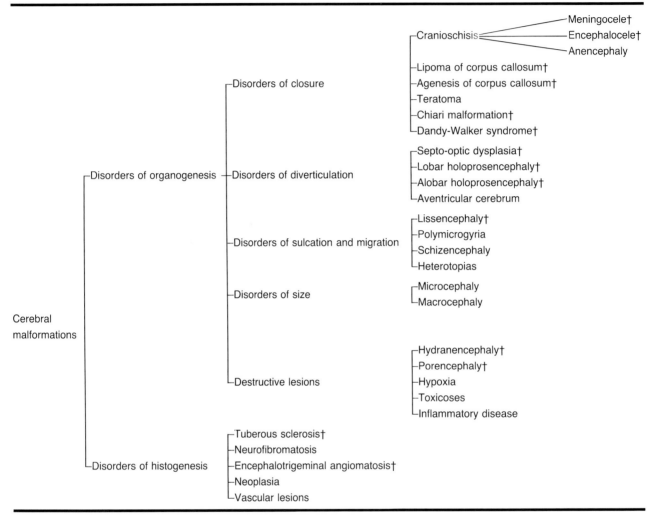

* Modified from DeMeyer 1971.
† Dealt with in this chapter.

of these anomalies was possible only at autopsy or by invasive neurodiagnostic studies such as angiography and air studies. In some cases diagnostic studies were not possible because of a variety of factors, such as unavailability of sophisticated units except in certain institutions, the maturity and size of the infant, or lack of experience in dealing with pediatric-age patients. Computed tomography has provided a noninvasive method of evaluating in vivo the complex structural changes associated with congenital craniocerebral anomalies. A majority of malformations, because of the presence of associated neurological or craniofacial anomaly, are studied in the neonatal period or infancy. A few craniocerebral anomalies, however, may be seen at later ages. Some of the craniocerebral anomalies are detected incidentally by CT. In these patients an understanding of the underlying developmental anomalies may prevent confusion and the need for further diagnostic studies. In pediatric patients, CT studies may be performed for a variety of reasons such as to exclude an associated intracranial malformation when there is a visible structural defect such as midline craniofacial anomaly; the presence of neurological findings although no structural abnormality can be detected clinically, as in septo-optic dysplasia; or the presence of an enlarging head or abnormal skull x-rays, with or without evidence of increased intracranial pressure.

In most of the congenital malformations, a precise diagnosis of the anomaly can be made by CT, in both the axial and coronal planes. With the refinements in ultrasonography and availability of appropriate transducers, many of the anomalies can be detected by sonography either in utero or in the neonatal period without exposure to ionizing radiation (Rumack 1984). Till quite recently CT following intrathecal or intraventricular water-soluble contrast (Fitz 1978a) (CT cisternography) was necessary to provide detailed morphological visualization of the subarachnoid space and its alterations resulting from or due to the malformation. MRI in many instances is replacing the need for such studies. MR, with its capacity to generate images in a three-dimensional plane, provides a precise morphological demonstration of the various anomalies. CSF spaces can be analyzed without recourse to CT cisternography. With the above additional armamentarium in imaging presently available, the need for cisternography and even vascular studies is gradually diminishing. Angiography may be indicated if the above studies demonstrate the need to identify the vascular topography.

DISORDERS OF ORGANOGENESIS

Chiari Malformations

The hindbrain dysgenesis known as Chiari malformation was first described by Cleland in 1883. Chiari in 1891 described three types of cerebellar malformation and added a fourth type in 1896. The type I malformation consists of tonsillar invagination through the foramen magnum into the spinal canal, with variable degree of displacement of the cerebellum and a normal position of the fourth ventricle. Symptoms are related to the lower cranial and spinal nerves. Symptomatic patients are commonly older children and adults. Although they do not have myelomeningocele, syringohydromyelia is an associated finding.

Chiari II malformation (Arnold-Chiari malformation) is commonly seen in neonates and infants. Along with a more severe hindbrain dysgenesis, myelomeningocele and a variety of cerebral malformations are common findings. Chiari's type III and later type IV malformations are variations in the degree of hindbrain dysgenesis. In type III there is a high cervical or occipital encephalocele, and in type IV there is extreme cerebellar hypoplasia without associated downward displacement. In clinical practice the two most common anomalies associated with Chiari's name are the Chiari I malformation in adults and the type II malformation in the pediatric age group.

Chiari I Malformation

In the adult, or Chiari type I, malformation the essential pathology is herniation of the inferior cerebellum and tonsils through the foramen magnum, with peglike projections from tonsils and adhesions. There is often associated syringomyelia or hydromyelia. Cranial and skeletal anomalies are uncommon. Very few reports dealing with the CT appearance of Chiari I malformation have appeared in the literature (Forbes 1978; Weisberg 1981), probably because of the difficulty in identifying the cervical spinal cord and cerebellar tonsils, as well as the unreliability in detecting a dilated cord with enlarged central canal or cystic spaces within the cord without utilizing intrathecal contrast. With the availability of water-soluble contrast agent and high-resolution scanners, CT is the primary mode for screening and demonstrating the findings of Chiari I malformation. However, MRI is rapidly replacing CT as an imaging modality in the craniocervical region. The

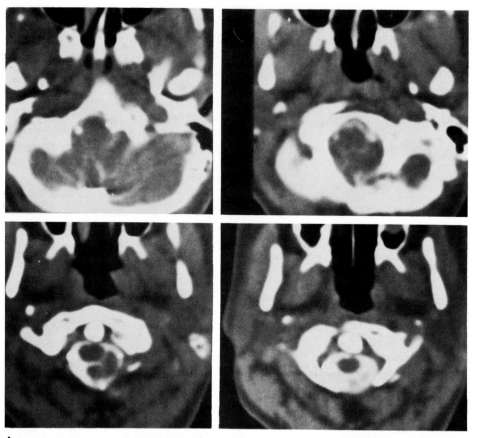

A

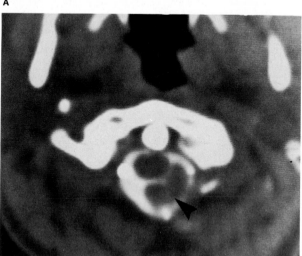

B

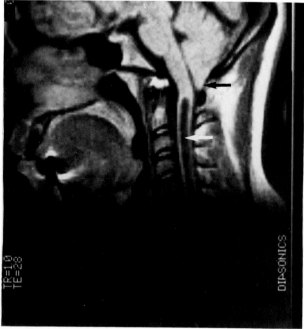

C

Figure 4-1 Chiari type I malformation: CT following intrathecal metrizamide. **A.** Four CT sections demonstrating herniation of the cerebellar tonsil. **B.** Close-up showing the cervicomedullary portion of cord and the tonsil (arrow). **C.** Chiari type I malformation. Sagittal MRI demonstrates the peglike (black arrow) tonsils which protrude below the foramen magnum. The foramen is small. Associated syringohydromyelia involving the cervical segment of cord (white arrow). Signal intensity is similar to CSF (TR—1.0 sec, TE—28 msec). (*Courtesy of Dr. William Bradley, Pasadena, California.*)

two components for a diagnosis of Chiari I malformation are (1) cerebellar tonsillar herniation and (2) syringomyelia. For CT evaluation CT of the head and spine was performed before and after intrathecal metrizamide. The syrinx or the cavitation in the cord is visualized better on the delayed CT of the spine performed 6 to 8 hours after the intrathecal contrast.

CT through the posterior fossa and craniocervical junction usually demonstrates normal or small posterior fossa. In the majority of cases there is basilar impression and/or assimilation of first cervical vertebrae with the basiocciput. This results in a relatively small foramen magnum. The fourth ventricle is in normal position. The ventricles may not be dilated. None of the changes seen in Chiari II malformation are present intracranially. CT myelography with water-soluble myelographic agents demonstrates the cervicomedullary portion of the cord as a sagittally flat, narrow structure. The tonsils are situated posteriorly and separated from the cord by the contrast agent (Fig. 4-1). In the presence of an associated syringomyelia or hydromyelia there is an associated widening of the cord, either localized to the cervical region or extending to the midthoracic region. The CT appearance of syringohydromyelia has been extensively documented (Bonate 1980; DiChiro 1975; Vignaud 1979; Resjo 1979; Aubin 1983). Delayed CT is helpful in demonstrating the intrathecal contrast which on initial study is within the subarachnoid space later concentrating within the central cavity of the cord (Fig. 4-2), further confirming the diagnosis of syringohydromyelia. MRI, however, is a more ideal method of imaging patients suspected of this anomaly (DeLaPaz 1983; Yeats 1983; Lee 1985; Spinos 1985). It replaces the need for CT

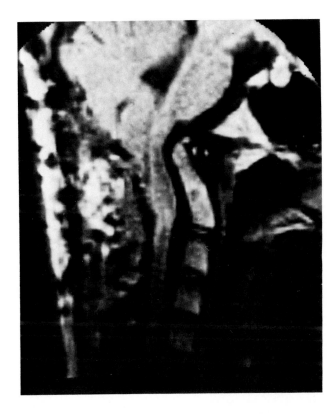

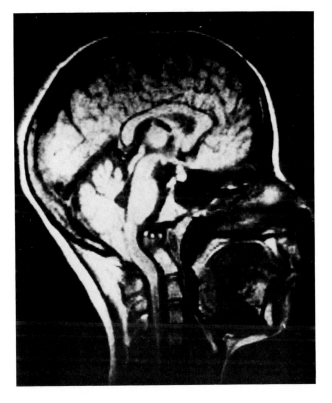

Figure 4-2 Chiari type I malformation. **A.** Sagittal MRI demonstrates downward herniation of the cerebellum and tonsils, associated with cavitation involving the medulla and upper cervical cord. There is associated basilar invagination with occipitalization of C-I.

and multiple imaging following intrathecal contrast. Moreover MRI provides a nondistorted image of the extent of the syringohydromyelia and the extent of associated tonsillar invagination into the cervical spinal canal. Sagittal MR images are the most informative (Fig. 4-2). Even very early syrinxes which were difficult to demonstrate on CT can be clearly defined.

Chiari II Malformation

The hallmark of the Chiari II malformation is dysgenesis of the hindbrain, resulting in a caudally displaced, elongated fourth ventricle and associated caudal herniation of the medulla and vermis. A host of concurrent anomalies involve the neural axis. They include myelomeningocele, mesencephalic beaking, enlarged massa intermedia, accessory anterior commissure, beaking of the frontal horn, absence of the corpus callosum, gyral malformation, and hypoplasia or partial absence of the falx and/or the tentorium. The bony vault is also involved, resulting in the presence of lückenschädel (craniolacunia, lacunar skull), scalloping of the petrous bone as well as the clivus, and enlargement of the foramen magnum.

Not all these findings are necessary for the diagnosis of the Chiari II malformation, and indeed many of them may not be detected on computed tomog-

raphy except in older children. The computed tomography findings in this anomaly have been reviewed in detail by Naidich (1980*a, b, c*).

LÜCKENSCHÄDEL   Lückenschädel is present in a majority of children with meningocele or encephalocele. The condition is due to dysplasia of the membrane bones. The lacunae disappear after 6 months of age. They do not signify increased intracranial pressure secondary to hydrocephalus. They can be seen in a majority of infants below 6 months by computed tomography. Although obvious in routine CT settings, they are especially easy to identify in wide window settings (Fig. 4-3). They appear as pits which involve predominantly the inner aspects of the calvarium, most prominent in the vertex and upper half of the calvarium involving the parieto-occipital region.

CLIVUS AND PETROUS SCALLOPING   Because of the small posterior fossa, as the cerebellum and midbrain develop there is pressure erosion of the clivus and posterior medial aspect of the petrous part of the temporal bone (Kruyffe 1966). Since the changes start in infancy, there is molding of the bones forming the boundaries of the posterior fossa. On computed tomography the characteristic changes involve the petrous pyramids, sparing the jugular

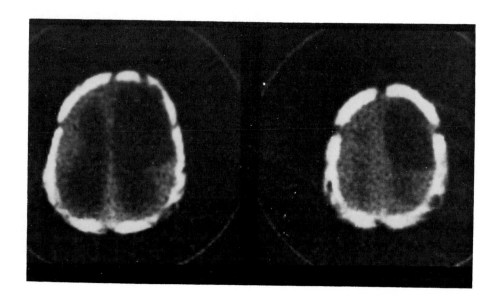

Figure 4-3   Chiari II malformation: craniolacunia appearing on CT as pits involving the inner table of the skull. (See also Fig. 6-8.)

tubercles and the petrous ridges. There is resultant shortening of the internal auditory canals, which also appear to be directed posteromedially (Fig. 4-4). These findings are better visualized in older children and may not be significant in infants. The changes in the clivus cannot be appreciated in routine axial sections unless sagittal reconstruction images can be obtained; they are more commonly seen in infants than in neonates. These findings can be better appreciated on sagittal views of the MRI (Fig. 4-4*B–D*).

ENLARGED FORAMEN MAGNUM The enlarged foramen magnum in the Chiari II malformation is more commonly seen in older children. The enlargement occurs in the sagittal direction (Fig. 4-5). Evaluation

of an enlarged foramen magnum by CT may be difficult in the axial plane unless the CT section is done parallel to the foramen magnum. Enlargement can occasionally be appreciated if sagittal and coronal reconstructions are available.

DURAL ANOMALIES

Hypoplasia or Fenestration of Flax Cerebri Pathological specimens demonstrate varying degrees of hypoplasia as well as fenestration of the falx separating the two cerebral hemispheres (Peach 1965) (Fig. 4-6). This finding has been demonstrated on contrast-enhanced CT (CECT) (Naidich 1980*a*). Fenestration can also be demonstrated by CT in the coronal plane. The indirect sign of fenestration of the

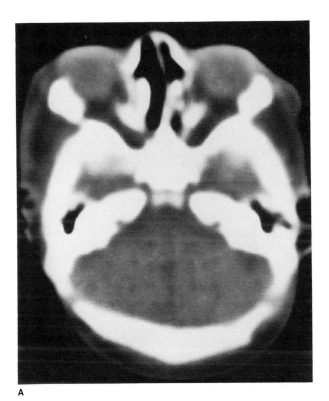

A

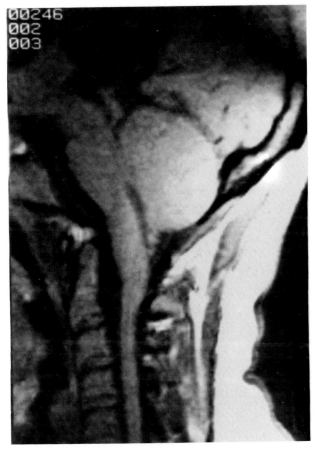

B

Figure 4-4 **A.** Chiari II malformation: mild petrous scalloping with the internal auditory canal directed posteromedially. (See also Fig. 6-9.) **B.** Sagittal MRI of the craniovertebral region demonstrates small posterior fossa; low torcula (1); narrow deformed fourth ventricle (2); scalloping of the clivus (3); syrinx involving the cord (4).
(Continued on p. 172)

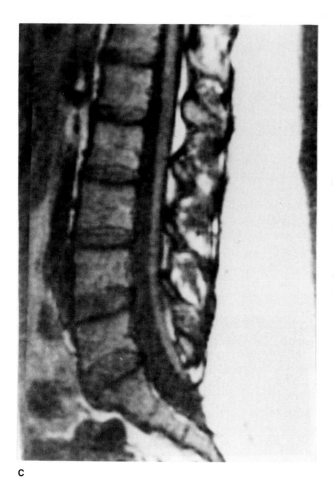

C

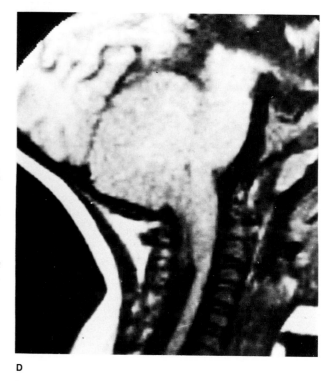

D

Figure 4-4 (*cont.*)   **C.** Same patient, midsagittal MRI demonstrates tethered cord with its distal end at the level of S-1 (arrow). **D.** Another patient with similar findings.

falx, which can be appreciated on CT in coronal plane, is the close apposition, with interdigitation between the two cerebral hemispheres. In the axial sections the interhemispheric fissure may be narrow in the hydrocephalic infant, although more commonly it is wide following treatment of hydrocephalus. The enhanced falx may not be visualized throughout its length or in segments.

Hypoplasia of the Tentorium   On CECT, the normal tentorial hiatus has a V-shaped configuration in nearly 90 percent of normal CT images (Naidich 1977*b*), being wider in the lower sections and becoming narrower until the straight sinus is seen. In Chiari II malformation, hypoplasia of the tentorium

and resultant upward direction as well as foreshortening of the straight sinus has a characteristic CT appearance. The free margin of the tentorium, instead of having the normal V configuration, has a U configuration, with the limbs of the U bowed laterally, creating a wide space between the two edges of the tentorium (Fig. 4-7).

HINDBRAIN AND MIDBRAIN ANOMALIES   Along with the bony and dural components which form part of the spectrum of Chiari II malformation, the essential feature of this malformation is the pathological downward displacement of the fourth ventricle. This results in an elongated, sagitally flattened fourth ventricle, extending into the cervical canal to a var-

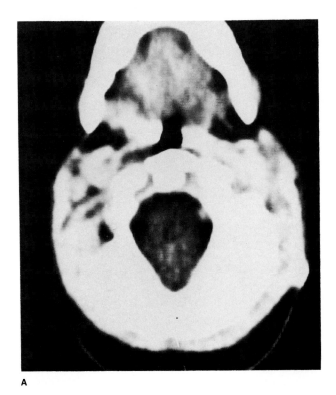

A

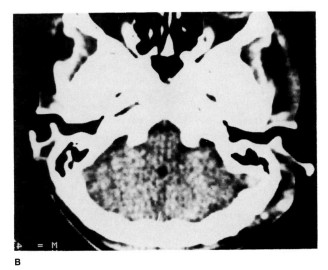

B

Figure 4-5 Chiari II malformation. **A.** Sagittally enlarged foramen magnum. **B.** Slitlike fourth ventricle at a slightly higher level.

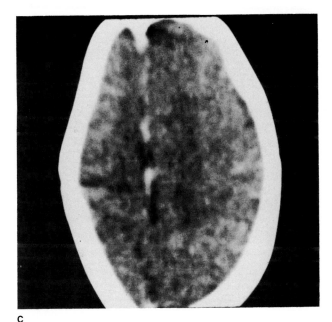

C

Figure 4-6 Chiari II malformation: interdigitation of the gyri with fenestration in the falx.

iable extent. Because of the downward displacement of the medulla and occasionally the pons, the cranial nerves pursue a longer intracranial course (Naidich 1983). This, however, cannot be appreciated on CT or present MRI. Because of these changes, nonvisualization of the fourth ventricle by CT is fairly common. In the series reported by Naidich (1980c), the fourth ventricle was not visualized in 70 percent of cases, was sagitally flattened but identifiable in 15 percent, and in 5 percent was dilated but low in position. The most common feature suggestive of the Chiari II malformation is failure to demonstrate a normal fourth ventricle at or above the level of the petrous pyramids (Zimmerman RD 1979). In infants, even on high-resolution CT the posterior fossa appears full, because of a shallow posterior fossa in which the cerebellum is pushed anteriorly to wrap the surface of the brainstem laterally and anterolaterally fills the cerebellopontine angle cistern. In 70 percent of cases, the medulla buckles backward and on itself, creating a cervicomedullary kink, behind

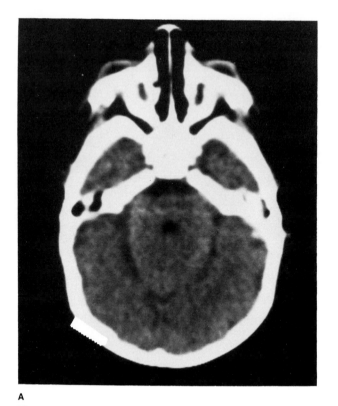

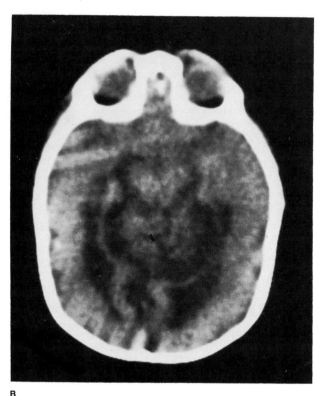

A   B

Figure 4-7   Chiari II malformation.   **A.** CECT demonstrates wide tentorial hiatus.   **B.** Compressed cerebellar tissue with prominent pericerebellar cistern at a higher level.

and below the upper cervical cord (Naidich 1983; Emery 1973). This kink is variable and depends on the thickness and variable length of the dentate ligament (Emery 1973). This finding may occasionally be seen on sagittal MRI. This finding is more commonly seen in children than in infants (Fig. 4-8). The slitlike fourth ventricle, when visualized, has an appearance of being displaced forward, with a voluminous cerebellar hemisphere. The midline cerebellum in infants with the Chiari II malformation has been found to be denser than the normal cerebellar vermis (Harwood-Nash 1977). The exact cause for the relatively increased density is not known, although this may be a manifestation of a tight posterior fossa.

Because of the low position as well as hypoplasia of the tentorium, the cerebellum projects upward through the wide incisura (Fig. 4-9). Wide or prominent cisternal space called the *pericerebellar cistern* (Naidich 1980*b*) is commonly seen and is presumed to be due to the large CSF pool created by the shallow posterior fossa. This is more commonly seen following shunting procedures. The portion of the cerebellum visualized through the incisura has an appearance of prominent sulci, suggestive of an atrophic process but more probably created from invagination of the cerebellum by the midbrain. The third ventricle may show some dilatation. This, however, is less common than dilatation of the lateral ventricles. The massa intermedia is larger and closer to the foramen of Monro (Fig. 4-10). In the majority of cases axial CT demonstrates relatively small third ventricles, with parallel or biconcave side walls, the concavity being maximum at the insertion of the massa intermedia. This has been reported in nearly 80 percent of cases (Naidich 1980*c*). Similarly,

Figure 4-8 Metrizamide CT cisternogram. **A.** CT section shows enlarged foramen magnum. The cervicomedullary portion of the cord is flattened, with the two tonsils (arrows) situated posteriorly. **B.** Section at higher level demonstrating the narrow cisternal space filled with metrizamide. The cerebellar hemisphere wraps the medulla. (See also Fig. 4-4*B–D* for MRI comparison.)

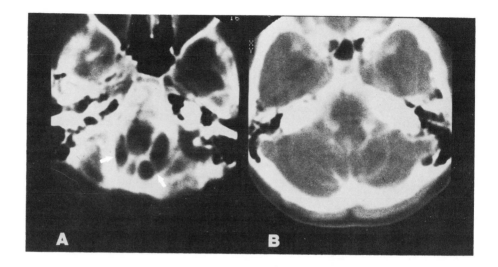

the tectum has a pointed appearance and is best visualized in a section through the superior colliculi (Fig. 4-11). This finding is often seen in the older child and following shunting.

FOREBRAIN ANOMALIES Dilatation of the lateral ventricles is common in the majority of patients. The degree of dilatation is variable and depends to some degree on the time interval between the closure of the myelomeningocele and detection of the cranial enlargement both clinically and by CT. Dilatation is usually bilateral and symmetrical, involving predominantly the atria and occipital horns, the cortical mantle being thinnest in the region of the occipital

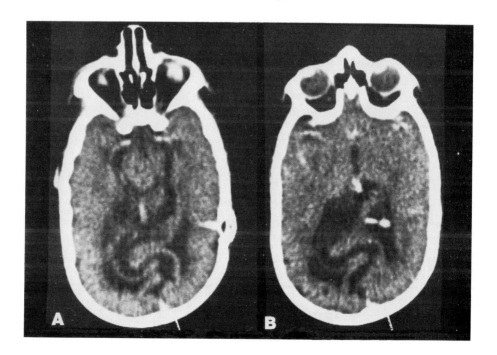

Figure 4-9 **A.** CECT through midbrain, Chiari II malformation. The cerebellum projects through the wide tentorial incisura. Prominent pericerebellar cistern and deep indentations in the cerebellum are due to infolding of the cerebellum. **B.** At a slightly higher level.

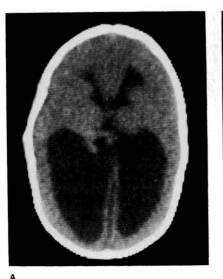

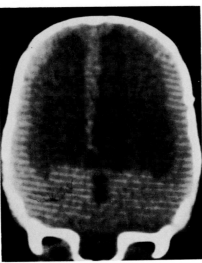

Fiugure 4-10   Massa intermedia in Chiari II malformation.   **A.** Axial.   **B.** Coronal noncontrast CT. The massa intermedia bulges into the third ventricle and is situated higher and farther anterior than normal.

A

B

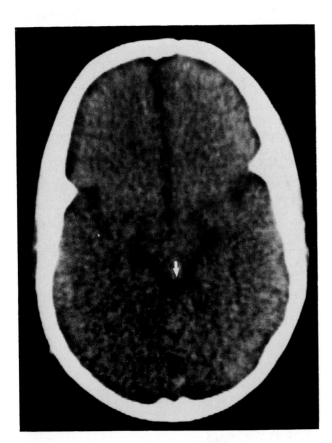

Figure 4-11   Chiari II malformation: pointed tectum (arrow) in a section through level of superior colliculi.

lobes and vertex. Flattening of the superolateral angle of the frontal horns in spite of significant ventricular dilatation is a common finding (Naidich 1980c). This is better appreciated in direct coronal CT. Although asymmetry of the lateral ventricles has been reported in 42 percent of cases (Naidich 1980c), this has not been the authors' experience in nonshunted infants. In the presence of massive enlargement of the ventricles atrial diverticulation can also be seen (Fig. 4-12C–F). Similar changes have been reported in severe hydrocephalus from any cause in children (Naidich 1982). Air studies in infants with Chiari II malformation demonstrate a characteristic pointed inferior angle of the frontal horns (Gooding 1967). A similar appearance can be seen on direct coronal CT in sections through the frontal horns (Fig. 4-12). This appearance is due to a prominent caudate nucleus and absence of the forceps major. The septum pellucidum may occasionally be absent. In CT sections above the level of the ventricles the interhemispheric fissure appears narrow, although in some patients before shunting and occasionally afterward this space may be wide (Fig. 4-13). Contrast-enhanced CT in both the axial and the coronal plane demonstrates not only the fenestration and hypoplasia of the falx but also the interdigitation of the gyri between the two cerebral hemispheres (Fig. 4-6). In the majority of cases the various

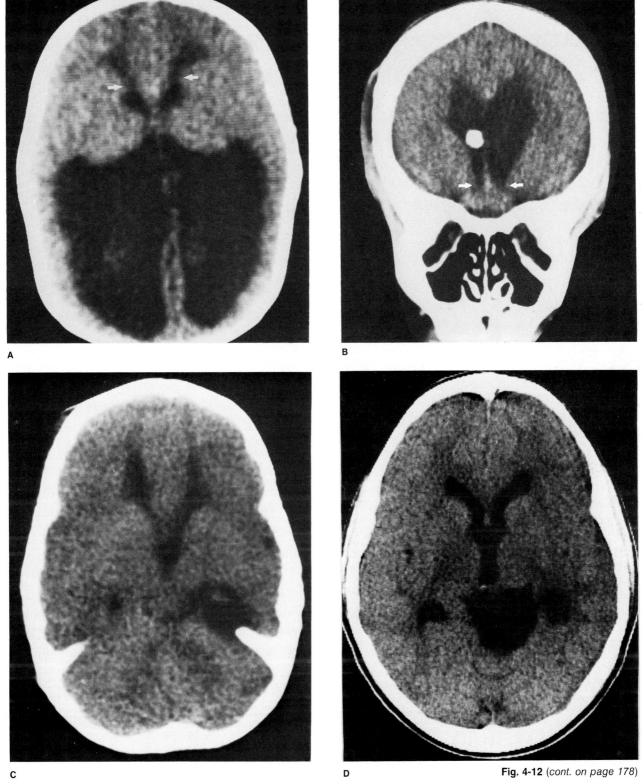

A

B

C

D **Fig. 4-12** *(cont. on page 178)*

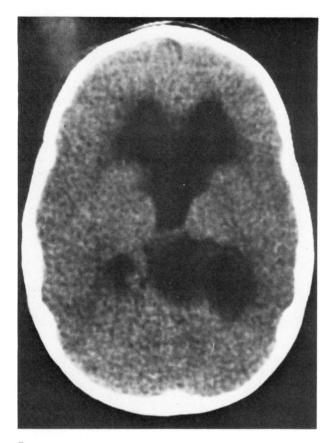

E

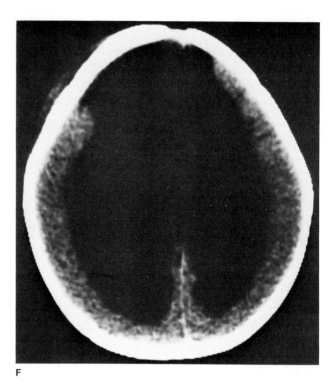

F

Figure 4-12   Chiari II malformation: axial image **(A)** shows prominence of the caudate nuclei (arrows). Coronal image **(B)** demonstrates the beaked appearance of the frontal horns along their inferior aspect (arrows). (See also Fig. 6-12.)   **C–F**. Chiari type II malformation. Apart from the above findings, there is severe hydrocephalus and a lateral atrial cyst (arrow).

components of the anomaly described can be diagnosed; however, if surgical intervention other than shunting is being planned, further neurodiagnostic studies such as MR imaging provide a precise understanding of the anatomical changes in the posterior fossa and the craniovertebral junction. The majority of children with Chiari malformation may also later demonstrate syringohydromyelia.

Dandy-Walker Syndrome

Hydrocephalus associated with a posterior fossa cyst and atresia of the foramina of Magendie and of Luschka was first described by Dandy and Blackfan in 1914 and subsequently by Taggart and Walker

(1942). They also described midline cerebellar hypoplasia, thus the eponym Dandy-Walker cyst. Although the anomaly is well recognized, the pathogenesis is not clearly defined. The posterior fossa cyst which replaces the fourth ventricle may not in all cases be secondary to atresia of the outlet foramina, since patency of the foramina has been shown in some cases (Hart 1972; Gardner 1975). Hydrocephalus, which was part of the original description, may not be present in all cases. Absence of hydrocephalus, however, is more commonly seen in the so-called Dandy-Walker variant. A variety of congenital anomalies may coexist with the posterior fossa cyst. Dysgenesis of the corpus callosum is the most frequently noted coexisting anomaly. That the anomaly is more complex than the simple atresia of the outlet foramina is well recongized (Benda 1954;

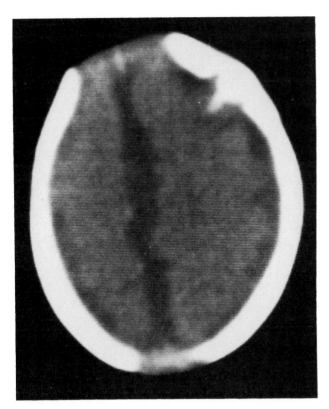

Figure 4-13 Chiari II malformation: wide interhemispheric fissure in a shunted child, also showing the gyral pattern. (Compare with Figs. 4-6 and 6-11.)

Brodal 1959; Gibson 1955; Gardner 1960). Current views indicate the importance of dysgenesis of the cerebellar roof rather than the foraminal atresia. Because of the complexity of the anomalies associated with the posterior fossa cyst, the condition is more commonly recognized as Dandy-Walker syndrome.

In its most common form the fourth ventricle is replaced by a symmetrically enlarged midline cyst with hypoplasia of the inferior vermis. The superior vermis is stretched and displaced upward. The aqueduct is foreshortened. The bony calvarium of the posterior fossa is enlarged. The torcular and the transverse sinus are above the lambdoid suture. This results in inversion of the torcular-lambdoid relationship, not seen with posterior fossa intra- or extraaxial cysts (Harwood-Nash 1976) or giant cisterna magna. The tentorium is elevated. The CT appear-

ance of a Dandy-Walker cyst is a large, low-density cystic mass occupying most of the posterior fossa (Fig. 4-14). The pons and medulla are seen anteriorly, with a thin rim of cerebellar tissue anterolaterally. The cerebellopontine angle cisterns and, in appropriate thin sections, the lateral recess of the fourth ventricle as well as the vallecula cannot be identified. The third and lateral ventricles are usually enlarged, perhaps because of atresia of the outlet foramina of the fourth ventricle, although often there is kinking of the aqueduct which may result in multiple levels of obstruction. This may be of clinical importance, since isolated shutting off of one compartment (lateral ventricle or cystic fourth ventricle) may result in herniation in the opposite direction of the other compartment (Carmel 1977). The relative obstruction of the aqueduct can be easily resolved by CT study with use of a small amount of dilute nonionic intrathecal contrast introduced into the ventricles, or more appropriately with MRI. The tentorium can be demarcated on noncontrast CT (NCCT) because of the massive cystic dilatation of the posterior fossa midline cyst and resultant thinning of the cerebellar mantle and its compression against the elevated, stretched tentorium. The tentorial margins are elongated and stretched outward (Fig. 4-15). The malpositioned tentorium is seen as diverging bands, usually at a level higher than expected. The tentorial margins have an inverted V configuration. This finding is highly suggestive of Dandy-Walker syndrome and may be seen even in the absence of dilated third and lateral ventricles (Naidich 1977*a,b*). Similar changes may, however, be seen occasionally with larger retrocerebellar arachnoid cysts as well as ependymal cyst.

Dandy-Walker variant is a milder form of the syndrome, in which a diverticular outpouching of varying size and shape extends from the inferior medullary velum, the upper part of the fourth ventricle having a normal shape although being somewhat dilated. The cerebellar hypoplasia is also milder. The incomplete development of the vermis and the nodules results in a wide vallecula. The CT findings in Dandy-Walker variant may often be confusing. The characteristic findings described above in Dandy-Walker cyst may not be present (Lipton 1978). Un-

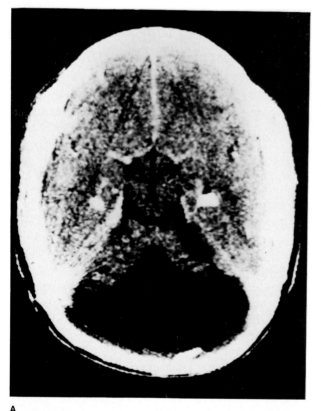

A

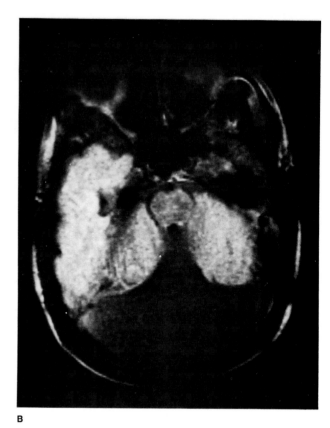

B

C

Figure 4-14   Dandy-Walker cyst.   **A**. CT axial study. A large cystic CSF containing space replaces the fourth ventricle. No cerebellar tissue is seen posteriorly.   **B**. Axial and (**C**) sagittal MRI demonstrates the cyst and its relationship to other posterior fossa structures. Note absence of hydrocephalus.

Figure 4-15 Noncommunicating Dandy-Walker cyst. **A.** Axial and reformed sagittal and coronal CT demonstrates the metrizamide within the lateral and third ventricles. **B.** Coronal with reformed axial and sagittal CT following instillation of metrizamide within the dilated cystic fourth ventricle. (*Continued on p. 182*)

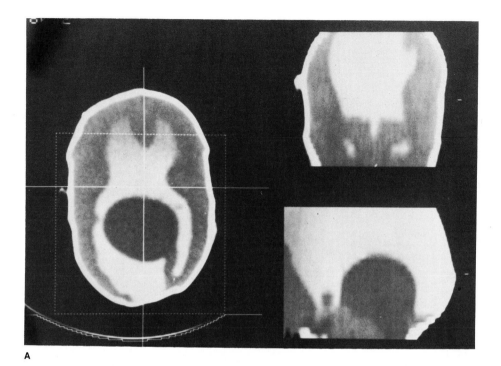

A

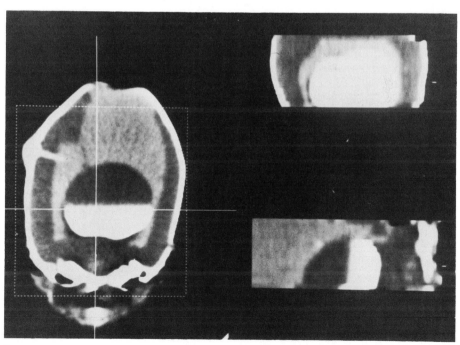

B

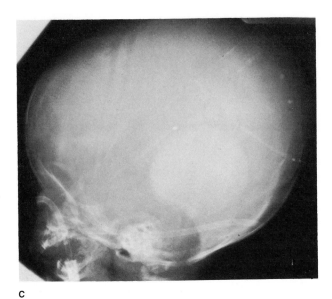

c

Figure 4-15 (*cont.*)   **C.** Lateral skull x-ray showing the metrizamide within the posterior fossa cyst.

like Dandy-Walker cyst, which is commonly seen in neonates and infants, the Dandy-Walker variant may not be recognized until later in life. The typical calvarial changes described above may also not be present. CT findings include (Fig. 4-16) a wide vallecula with a cystic space separating the two cerebellar hemispheres. Either because of the extension of the outpouching or the plane of the CT section, the fourth ventricle may be seen separate from the cyst. The fourth ventricle appears in normal position in its upper half but is moderately dilated. The lateral and third ventricles may or may not be dilated.

Dandy-Walker cyst and its variant form may be difficult to differentiate from other midline posterior fossa cystic lesions such as retrocerebellar arachnoid cyst, ependymal cyst, giant or "mega" cisterna magna, trapped fourth ventricle, and, rarely, cystic midline neoplasms.

Giant (mega) cisterna magna is occasionally seen in children and adults, its incidence by CT being 0.4 percent (Adams 1978). Megacisterna magna can extend upward, communicating with the superior cerebellar cistern (Fig. 4-17). It is considered to be a benign developmental anomaly, often identified as an incidental finding (Adams 1968; Harwood-Nash

1977). The adjacent cerebellar hemispheres may show atrophy, although the vallecula is not wide as in Dandy-Walker variant. In megacisterna magna the fourth ventricle is in normal position (Fig. 4-18). The prepontine- and cerebellopontine-angle cisterns are well visualized and occasionally may be prominent. Aqueduct stenosis with resulting hydrocephalus may be associated with megacisterna magna (Fig. 4-19) and mistaken for a Dandy-Walker variant. In occasional cases diagnosis can be established by ventriculography. Enlargement of the third and lateral ventricles secondary to a megacisterna magna, although rare, has been reported (Archer 1978).

Retrocerebellar arachnoid cyst may occasionally be difficult to differentiate from the Dandy-Walker syndrome by CT. The extraaxial cyst may invaginate between the two cerebellar hemispheres, resulting in nonvisualization of the fourth ventricle. Even when a slitlike fourth ventricle is seen (Fig. 4-20), differentiation from Dandy-Walker variant may be difficult. Metrizamide CT cisternography following intrathecal metrizamide (Drayer 1977) will help in the diagnosis of the noncommunicating arachnoid cyst. Occasionally, a few of the arachnoid cysts communicate with the fourth ventricle or the adjacent subarachnoid space, in which metrizamide CT cisternography may be confusing. Further evaluation by pneumoencephalography or angiography may become necessary in symptomatic patients. Delayed CT 6 to 8 hours later may demonstrate metrizamide within the cyst. This probably either represents intermittent communication of the cyst or is due to membrane transportation. The belated appearance of metrizamide in the cyst allows differentiation from an epidermoid tumor (Drayer 1977), which can also occur in the midline posterior fossa as a low-density lesion.

Ependymal cysts which are noncommunicating, CSF-containing cavities usually occur in the midline and may be located behind the fourth ventricle.

Blake (1900) indicated that evagination of the roof of the fourth ventricle into an ependyma-lined diverticulum occurs between the eighth and sixteenth week of gestation (Brocklehurst 1969). The so-called Blake's pouch may result in formation of the intraaxial supracollicular cyst. Although in Blake's

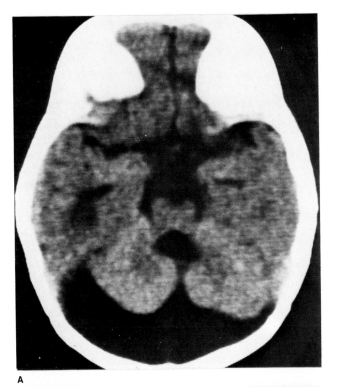

A

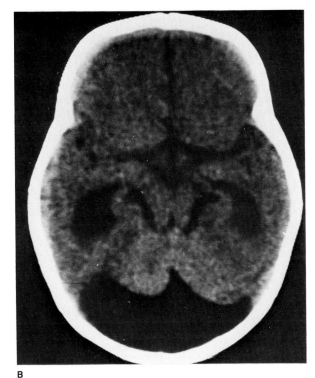

B

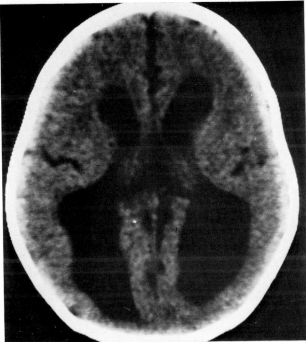

C

Figure 4-16   Dandy-Walker variant.   **A–C**. Axial CT sections demonstrate the dilated fourth ventricle with its posterior extension through the widened vallecula. There is dilatation of both lateral and third ventricle. Splaying of the medial walls of the lateral ventricle (**C**) is due to dysgenesis of the corpus callosum. (*Continued on p. 184*)

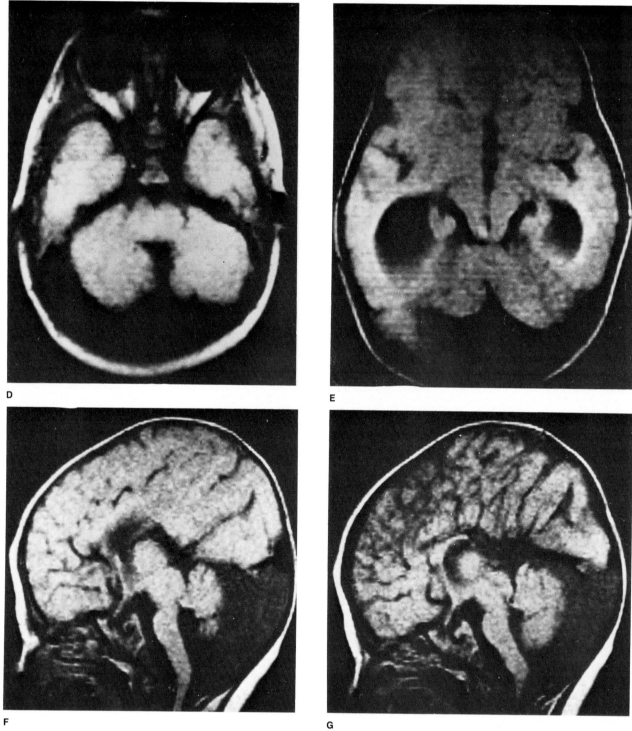

Figure 4-16 (*cont.*) **D, E.** MRI same patient. Similar findings on axial images. **F, G.** Sagittal MRI: Radiating sulci from roof of third ventricle characteristic of dysgenesis of corpus callosum in (**G**). The communication between the cyst and the fourth ventricle is precisely demonstrated.

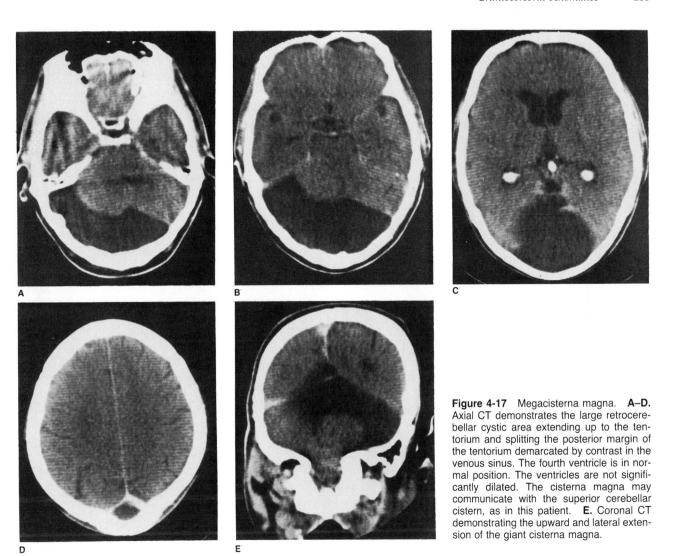

Figure 4-17 Megacisterna magna. **A–D.** Axial CT demonstrates the large retrocerebellar cystic area extending up to the tentorium and splitting the posterior margin of the tentorium demarcated by contrast in the venous sinus. The fourth ventricle is in normal position. The ventricles are not significantly dilated. The cisterna magna may communicate with the superior cerebellar cistern, as in this patient. **E.** Coronal CT demonstrating the upward and lateral extension of the giant cisterna magna.

original description the pouch was lined by cuboidal epithelium, case reports in the literature have used this eponym to designate cysts separate from the fourth ventricle, with different cell types forming the wall (Alvord 1962). It is conceivable that the ependyma-lined cyst located within the cerebellum but close to the normal fourth ventricle may represent a form of Blake's cyst. The extraaxial arachnoid cyst may represent a variation with a similar origin where the orifice of the cyst remains small or separated from the roof of the fourth ventricle. Since

some of these cysts are recognized in adult life, their relation to past intracerebellar infarction or hematoma may not be recognized if definite clinical history is not available.

Both axial and coronal CT (Fig. 4-21) will demonstrate the cyst separate from the fourth ventricle. Metrizamide CT cisternography will help differentiate the ependymal cyst from Dandy-Walker variant or retrocerebellar arachnoid cyst. Ependymal cyst may represent a form of Dandy-Walker variant; where it is due to coarctation, the cyst wall, al-

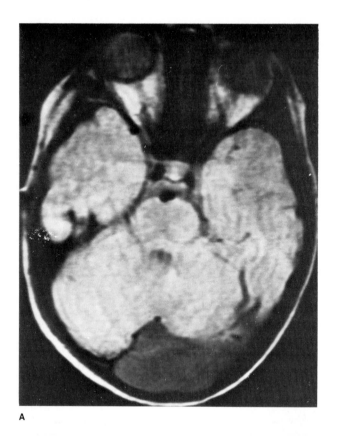

A

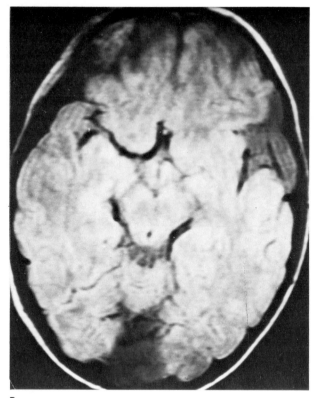

B

C

Figure 4-18 Megacisterna magna.   **A.** Axial MRI demonstrates a large CSF containing space posterior to the cerebellar hemisphere. Note the lateral deviation of the torcula and straight sinus. **B.** Higher section shows upward extension of the cisterna magna. There is also encephalomalacia of the temporal tip on right side. **C.** Sagittal MRI. Upward extension of cisterna magna through the tentorium. Note normal size of fourth and lateral ventricles.

Figure 4-19 Giant cisterna magna in association with aqueduct stenosis. Axial CT **(A–D)** demonstrates a large retrocerebellar midline hypodense area. The prepontine cistern is well visualized. The fourth ventricle is not enlarged. Dilatation of the third and lateral ventricles is due to associated aqueduct stenosis.

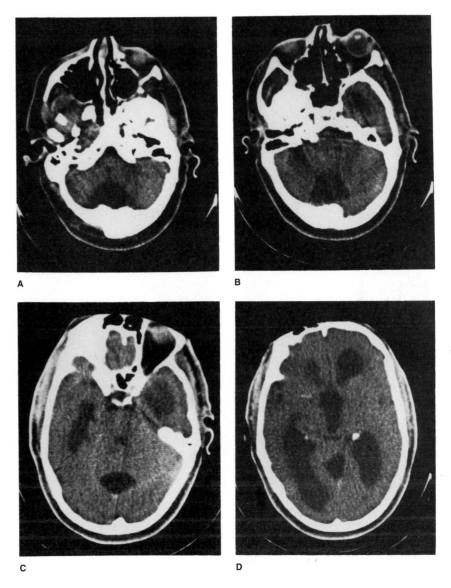

though glia- and ependyma-lined, is separated from the fourth ventricle. Controversy exists as to whether this is a form of arachnoid cyst (Harwood-Nash 1976) or a separate entity (Friede 1973; Bouch 1973). A trapped fourth ventricle (Zimmerman 1978; Scotti 1980) or a dilated fourth ventricle secondary to communicating hydrocephalus (Fig. 4-22) can be easily differentiated from the Dandy-Walker syndrome,

since although the fourth ventricle may be markedly dilated, it still retains its shape.

CECT usually does not provide additional information in any of the above entities. The choice of additional studies following conventional NCCT or CECT depends on the clinical history and age of the patient as well as the resultant hydrocephalus.

The most common midline neoplasms which may

occasionally be confused with relatively benign cystic conditions are cystic hemangioblastoma (Fig. 4-23) and cystic astrocytoma. They can be differentiated from the above entities following CECT.

Hydranencephaly

Virtual absence of the cerebral hemispheres except for basal parts of the occipital and sometimes the temporal poles is defined as hydranencephaly, the most severe form of porencephaly implying a destructive or encephaloclastic process (Probst 1979).

They usually do not demonstrate an enlarging head circumference. The walls of the fluid-filled sac consist of pia-arachnoid with an inner lining of glial tissue. These infants have normal falx cerebri, basal ganglia, and infratentorial structures. The exact causative factor or factors are not known. CT demonstrates a fluid-filled cranium with visible falx cerebri and tentorium (Fig. 4-24). CECT accentuates the basal ganglia, the falx, and the tentorium. When these findings are present in a microcephalic infant, hydranencephaly can be easily diagnosed. More commonly, though, infants with hydranencephaly show increase in head circumference. In these chil-

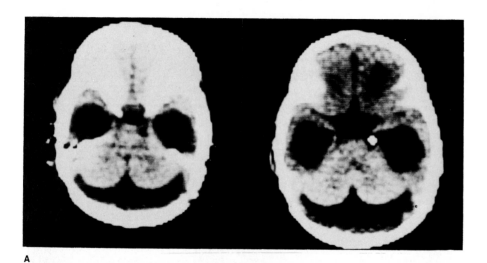

A

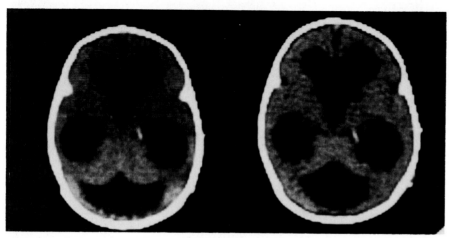

B

Figure 4-20 Retrocerebellar extraaxial cyst. **A.** The fourth ventricle is sagittally compressed by a large low-density retrocerebellar cyst. **B.** Enlarged third and lateral ventricles. (*Continued on p. 189*)

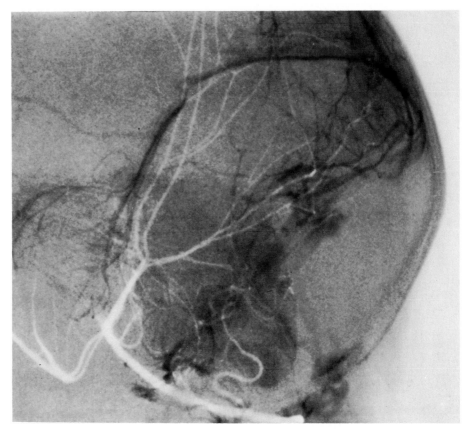

Figure 4-20 (*cont.*) **C.** Angiogram, lateral view: arterial and venous phases are superimposed to demonstrate the retrocerebellar avascular mass. This angiographic finding is typical of retrocerebellar extraaxial cyst.

C

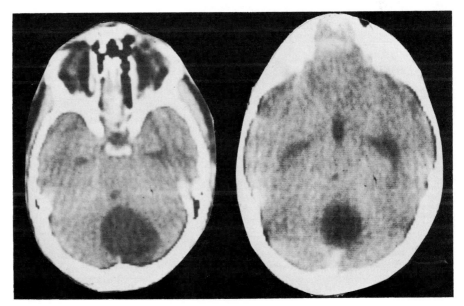

Figure 4-21 Noncommunicating ependymal cysts. **A.** Axial CECT. (*Continued on p. 190*)

A

Figure 4-21 (*cont.*)   **B.** Coronal CECT. Neoplasm is excluded by absence of enhancement. The fourth ventricle is compressed in the sagittal plane.

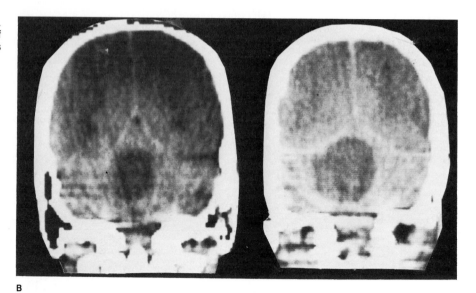

B

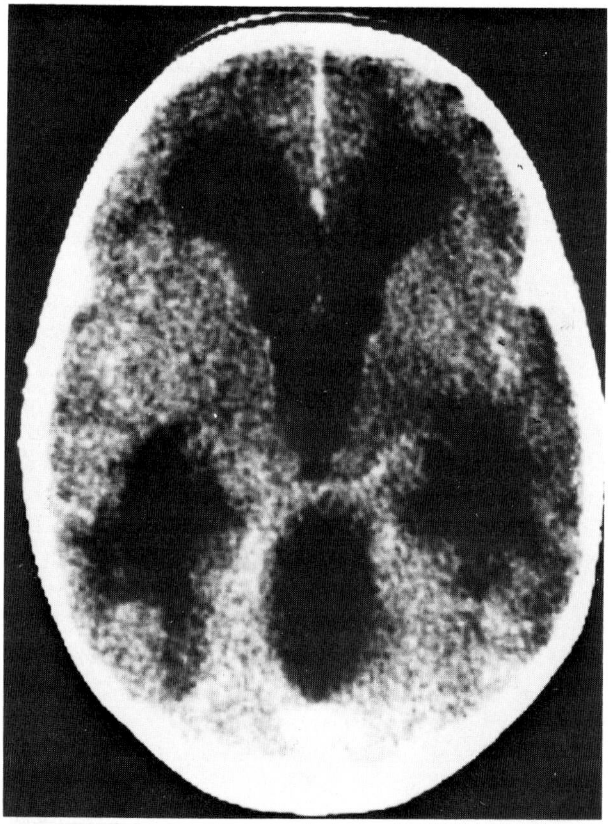

Figure 4-22   Dilated fourth ventricle secondary to a communicating hydrocephalus.

dren, the condition cannot be differentiated from severe forms of hydrocephalus (Dublin 1980). On rare occasions, CECT may show contrast within vascular structures in the sylvian fissures. Vascular studies are usually helpful in the differentiation.

Even in severe hydrocephalus, a normal but stretched complement of middle and anterior cerebral branches can be visualized on angiography; these are usually absent in hydranencephaly (Fig. 4-25). MRI in combination with sonography may replace the need for angiography in many cases.

Porencephaly

Porencephaly denotes a cavitation, most often seen on CT as a focal area of low density following infarction and as a result of gliosis. Porencephaly can be due to a variety of etiological factors (Ramsey 1977), either developmental or acquired. In adults it is almost always acquired (from trauma, hemorrhage, infection, surgery, or a vascular process). The variety seen in neonates and children is probably part of a devlopmental anomaly, although infection is an added factor, as shown in a few recent reports (DuBois 1979). The proencephalic cavity is often lined with ependymal cells, and the cavitation may be isolated, although more commonly it communicates

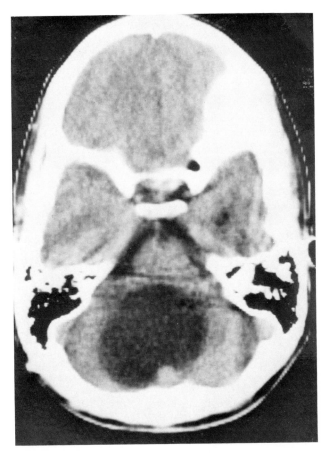

Figure 4-23 Cystic hemangioblastoma. NCCT demonstrates a large cystic lesion similar to a dilated fourth ventricle. Soft-tissue nodular density along the posterior wall represents the tumor nodule.

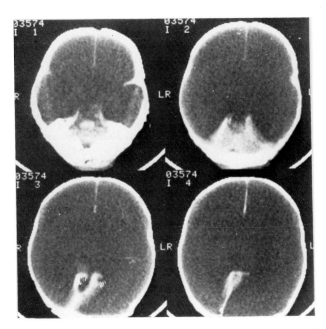

Figure 4-24 CT in hydranencephaly. There is no evidence of cortical mantle. The falx cerebri, the tentorium, and the midbrain structures appear prominent.

with either the ventricles or the subarachnoid space. Thus in children and neonates porencephalic cavities may be due to vascular insult (*encephaloclastic*) or may be developmental (*schizencephalic*). The two variants cannot be differentiated on the basis of CT. It has been presumed that when CT demonstrates bilateral deep fissures extending through the gray matter into the ventricular system it most likely represents schizencephaly (Raybaud 1983). Because of the variations in pattern of the malformation it is difficult to classify the lesion utilizing CT, whether it is of developmental origin or is the result of vas-

cular and/or infectious cause. CT is useful in demonstrating whether the lesion is focal or multiple (*multiple encephalomalacia*), involving one or both cerebral hemispheres (Fig. 4-26). Similar encephaloclastic changes may also involve the cerebellum. In both these conditions, unlike hydranencephaly, identifiable brain parenchyma and the ventricles can be seen. Communication of the cystic cavities with the ventricular system can also be defined by CT following intraventricular or intrathecal metrizamide, depending on the clinical setting. Most often the developmental variety will show thickening of the calvarium on the side of the cyst. This is secondary to brain atrophy, giving the appearance of Dyke-Davidoff syndrome (Fig. 4-27). The contents of the cystic cavity, whether or not communicating with the ventricles or subarachnoid space, have a density similar to the CSF within the ventricles. Absence of a vascular capsule on CECT excludes the possibility of a necrotic tumor or abscess in isolated porencephalic cavities.

Holoprosencephaly

Holoprosencephaly is the result of failure of normal development of the forebrain (prosencephalon). Failure of the forebrain to divide during the period of differentiation (from three brain vesicles to five) between the fifth and sixth week of embryogenesis results in this complex facial and craniocerebral anomaly (Harwood-Nash 1976). Depending on the severity of the forebrain anomaly, holoprosence-

phaly has been classified as alobar, semilobar, and lobar. In the alobar and semilobar variety, midline facial anomalies are common. In all three types the septum pellucidum and the olfactory bulb are absent. In all forms of holoprosencephaly the sylvian fissures are poorly developed and the temporal horns may not be clearly defined. Although diagnosis can be confirmed by ventriculography (Harwood-Nash 1976), characteristic CT findings have been described (Byrd 1977; Hayashi 1979; Derkhshan 1980).

Figure 4-25   A. Hydranencephaly.   **B.** Massive hydrocephalus. The CT in these two entities appears similar. (*Continued on p. 193.*)

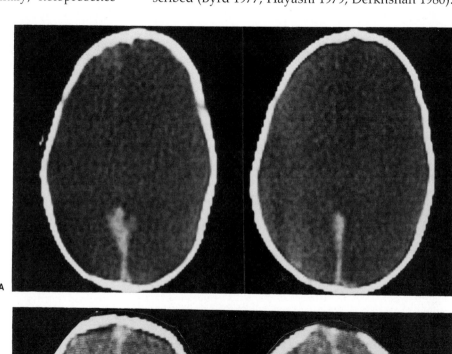

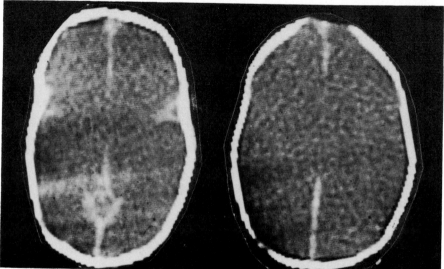

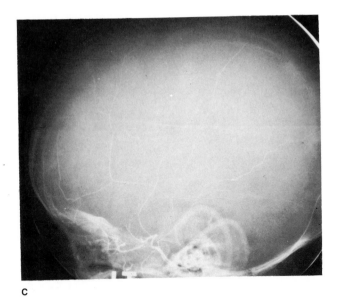

C

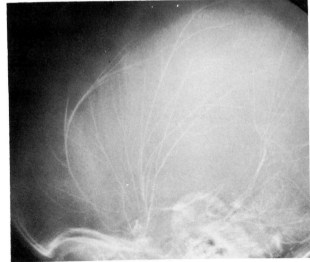

D

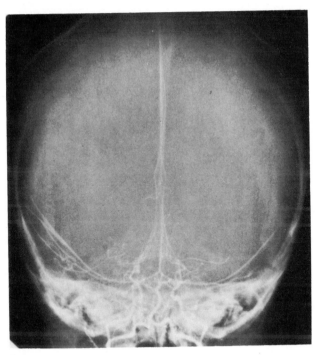

E

Figure 4-25 (*cont*.) **C.** Angiogram in hydranencephaly: absence of middle and anterior cerebral arteries. **D** and **E.** Angiogram in hydrocephalus. Both the anterior and middle cerebral arteries are present, although they are stretched from massive ventricular dilatation. (*Continued on p. 194*)

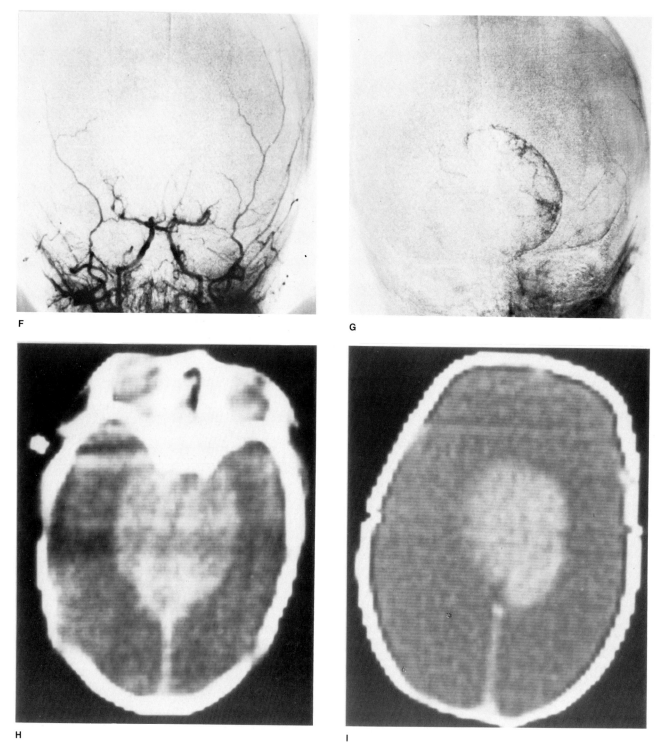

Figure 4-25 (*cont*.)   **F, G.** Axial CT demonstrates a hyperdense midbrain and thalami surrounded by CSF.   **H, I.** Vascular study demonstrates lack of cortical vessels in another case of hydranencephaly.

Figure 4-26 Encephalomalacia. Contrast-enhanced **(A)** axial and **(B)** coronal CT demonstrate ventricular dilatation with large CSF-containing spaces communicating with the dilated ventricles. The subarachnoid space is prominent, indicating an atrophic process. (*Continued on p. 196*)

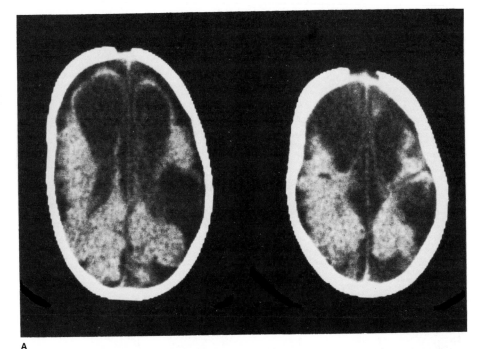

A

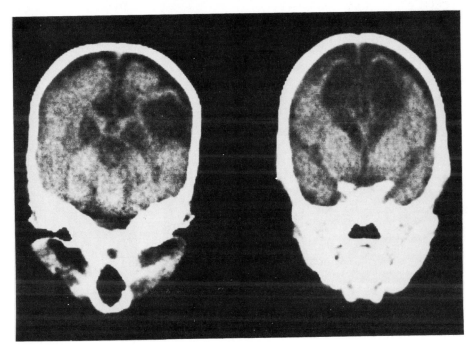

B

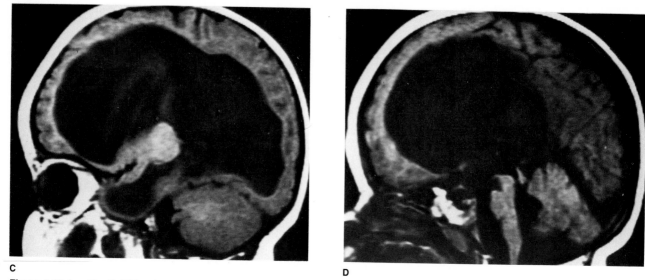

C   D

Figure 4-26 (*cont.*)   **C.** Midsagittal MRI demonstrates markedly enlarged lateral ventricle.   **D.** Slightly lateral sagittal image demonstrates loss of brain parenchyma, a characteristic finding in diffuse encephalomalacia.

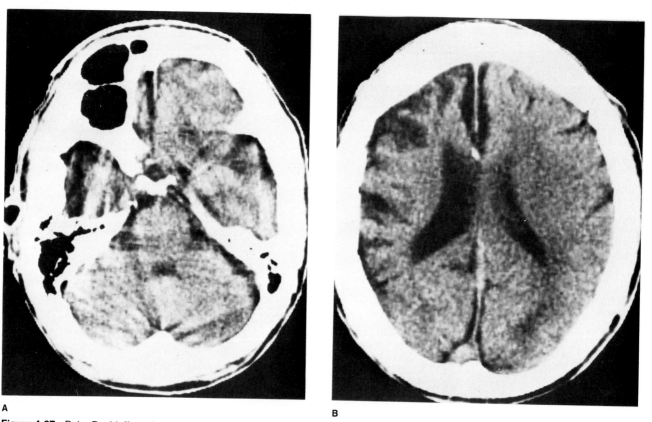

A   B

Figure 4-27   Dyke-Davidoff syndrome. Axial NCCT.   **A.** There is compensatory hyperaeration of the air sinuses associated with thickening of the adjacent calvarium on the left side.   **B.** At a higher level there is diffuse atrophy of the left cerebral hemisphere, evidenced by enlarged subarachnoid cistern and ventricle.

Alobar Prosencephaly

This is the extreme form of holoprosencephaly, resulting in a single ventricle with thin cortical tissue. Some amount of cerebral tissue can be identified. On CT, alobar holoprosencephaly is seen as a large, low-density area with a thin rim of brain tissue in either the frontal or the occipital region (Fig. 4-28). The thalami are fused. The third ventricle, which cannot be identified, becomes part of the single lateral ventricle. The septum pellucidum and the interhemispheric fissure which separate the two lateral ventricles, as well as the two cerebral hemispheres, are not seen. On coronal CT, there is a single ventricle bounded by a thin rim of cortical mantle, with absence of the midline structures as well as the flax cerebri. Holoprosencephaly can be diagnosed by CT when associated facial anomalies such as cleft lip and palate, microophthalmia, anophthalmia, micrognathia, or trigonocephaly are present. Skull x-rays demonstrate absence of the nasal septum, cleft palate, and trigonocephaly. Infants with alobar holoprosencephaly do not usually survive.

Semilobar Holoprosencephaly

CT in infants with semilobar holoprosencephaly differs from the alobar variety in that, although there is a single lateral ventricle, more cerebral tissue is present. An attempt at formation of the frontal and occipital horns is seen (Fig. 4-29). As in the alobar form, midline structures such as the falx cerebri, corpus callosum, and septum pellucidum are not visualized. Although the interhemispheric fissure is not seen on CT, autopsy specimens may show a midline ridging. The facial anomalies are less severe, infants presenting most commonly with cleft palate and cleft lip.

Lobar Holoprosencephaly

In this, the mildest form of holoprosencephaly, CT demonstrates (Fig. 4-30) well-formed lateral ventricles and cerebral hemisphere. The ventricles appear dilated. There is a distinct third ventricle. The roof of the frontal horn appears flat or squared off, in both axial and coronal CT. The septum pellucidum may or may not be present. The falx cerebri, as well

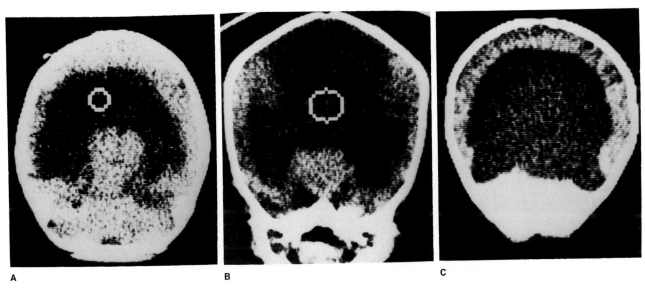

A   **B**   **C**

Figure 4-28 Alobar holoprosencephaly: **(A)** axial and **(B** and **C)** coronal CT. A single midline ventricle is noted. Absence of the interhemispheric fissure and falx in the midline is indicative of the alobar form of holoprosencephaly.

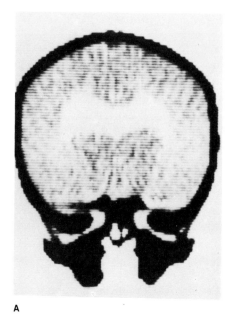

A

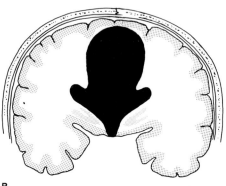

B

Figure 4-29 Semilobar holoprosencephaly. **A.** Coronal CT demonstrates absence of the falx cerebri and septum pellucidum. The thalami are in close apposition, a clue to diagnosis. **B.** Line drawing in semilobar and lobar holoprosencephaly.

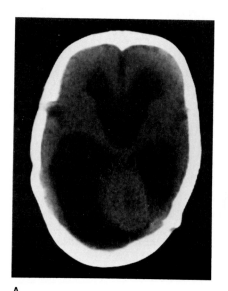

A

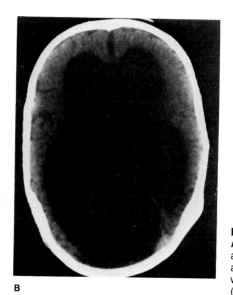

B

Figure 4-30 Lobar holoprosencephaly. **A–D.** Axial CT demonstrates presence of a third ventricle and well-defined frontal and occipital horns. The falx may not always be in the midline, as in this case. (*Continued on p. 199*)

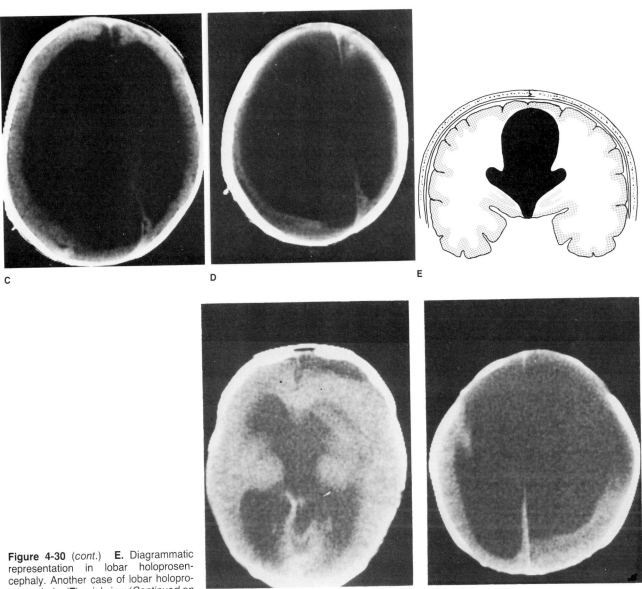

Figure 4-30 (*cont.*)   **E.** Diagrammatic representation in lobar holoprosencephaly. Another case of lobar holoprosencephaly. (**F**) axial view (*Continued on p. 200*)

(*Continued on p. 200*)

as the corpus callosum, may not be present. The sylvian fissures are absent. In the presence of facial anomalies, it is usually possible to differentiate lobar from the semilobar form of holoprosencephaly. When facial anomalies are not seen, differentiation of alobar or semilobar forms of holoprosencephaly from severe forms of hydrocephalus or hydranencephaly

may become difficult. However, in both hydranencephaly and severe hydrocephalus the falx cerebri is present (Hayashi 1979); this is not seen in holoprosencephaly.

Lobar holoprosencephaly can be differentiated from simple absence of the septum pellucidum as well as septo-optic dysplasia by the absence of the

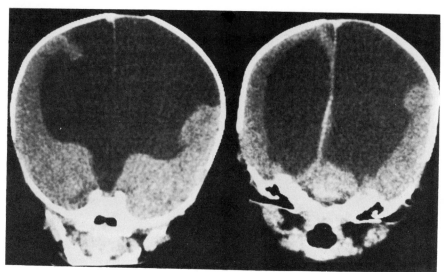

Figure 4-30 (*cont.*)   (**G**) Coronal views. Note prominent thalamus which is separated because of enlarged third and lateral ventricle.

G

falx cerebri in lobar holoprosencephaly and its presence in the latter two conditions. The CT findings of septo-optic dysplasia are detailed separately in the next section. Lobar and semilobar holoprosencephaly should also occasionally have to be differentiated from dysgenesis of the corpus callosum (Fig. 4-31), dysgenesis with associated interhemispheric

arachnoid cyst, absent septum pellucidum. In the majority of cases coronal CT and occasionally vascular studies may be indicated.

Occasionally bilateral subdural hygromas may be confused with alobar or semilobar holoprosencephaly (Byrd 1977). Clinical findings usually help in the differentiation. In most of the conditions which

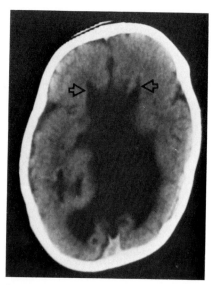

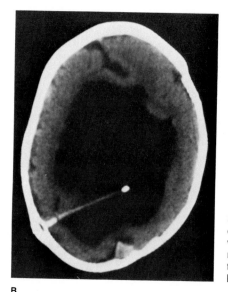

Figure 4-31   Dysgenesis of the corpus callosum.   **A, B.** Axial NCCT. There is wide separation of the frontal horns (arrowheads) associated with a midline cystic sac which could be mistaken for lobar holoprosencephaly.

A

B

need to be differentiated from the various forms of holoprosencephaly, the presence of coexisting facial anomalies helps in the CT diagnosis. When no facial anomalies are found, angiography is the next most useful diagnostic modality. In all forms of holoprosencephaly, unlike hydranencephaly, the middle and anterior cerebral arteries are present. In bilateral subdural hygromas, the cerebral vascular architecture is normal but compressed, whereas in holoprosencephaly the vascular architecture has a characteristic appearance (Harwood-Nash 1976).

Septo-Optic Dysplasia

Septo-optic dysplasia is a rare congenital anomaly first described by deMorsier (1956). The anomaly involves anterior midline structures of the brain and consists in absence of the septum pellucidum, primitive optic ventricle, and hypoplasia of the optic nerves, chiasma, and infundibulum, resulting in a prominent chiasmatic recess. On physical examination there is hypoplasia of one or both optic discs and blindness with wandering nystagmus. Hypothalamic-hypopituitary disorders are frequently associated with septo-optic dysplasia, the most com-

mon being diabetes insipidus. The malformation probably occurs about the fourth to sixth week of gestation. Many of the features seen in septo-optic dysplasia appear to be a minor form of lobar holoprosencephaly (Harwood-Nash 1976). Neuroradiological diagnosis has been based on pneumoencephalographic and plain film findings and associated clinical presentation (Harwood-Nash 1976). Very few CT descriptions in septo-optic dysplasia have been reported recently (Manelfe 1979*a*; Byrd 1977; Bush 1978; O'Dwyer 1980). CT demonstrates some or all of the following features (Fig. 4-32). There is absence of the septum pellucidum. The ventricles are enlarged, especially the lateral ventricles. The temporal horns are normal and may not be visualized. The anteromedial aspect of the frontal horns is flat or squared off in both axial and coronal CT. These findings are similar to those seen in lobar holoprosencephaly. With high-resolution CT the atrophic optic nerve can be demonstrated in both axial and coronal CT. The suprasellar and chiasmatic cisterns are prominent. On coronal CT, beaking of the floor of the lateral ventricles similar to the appearance seen in Chiari II malformation and lobar holoprosencephaly has been noted (Manelfe 1979*a*). When septo-optic dysplasia is associated with diabetes in-

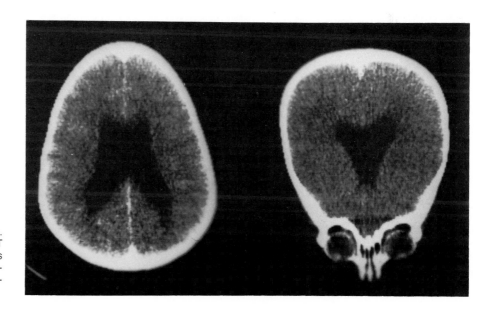

Figure 4-32 Septo-optic dysplasia. Axial (*left*) and coronal (*right*). CT demonstrates mildly dilated ventricles with absent septum pellucidum. Normally the suprasellar cistern is prominent.

sipidus, enlargement of the pituitary stalk and infundibulum can occur (Manelfe 1979*b*). This is best seen after contrast enhancement.

Diagnosis of septo-optic dysplasia may thus be confirmed by CT examination in the presence of appropriate clinical findings, without the need for invasive studies.

Cavum Septi Pellucidi and Cavum Vergae

The two leaves of the septum pellucidum which separate the lateral ventricle usually fuse in the neonatal period, around the second month. In the majority of neonates and occasionally in older children as well as adults, nonfusion of the two leaves results in a potential space, the cavum septi pellucidi, or cavity of the septum pellucidum. Its posterior extension results in the cavum Vergae. Most often they communicate with the ventricular system through the interventricular foramina. Cavum septi pellucidi and cavum Vergae are thus developmental anomalies without any clinical significance, common in children and found in 12 to 15 percent of adults (Shaw 1969; Nakano 1981). Their appearance has been well documented by CT and other diagnostic studies (Berkowitz 1939; Dandy 1931; Dyke 1936; Lowman 1948; Harwood-Nash 1977; Byrd 1978*a*). Cavum septi pellucidi is seen on CT (Fig. 4-33) as a CSF-containing space separated by thin septi from the frontal horns of the two lateral ventricles. Even though the septi are thin, they are well visualized because of the density of the CSF. The walls are parallel, extending posteriorly up to the foramen of Monro. Unlike the situation in dysgenesis of the corpus callosum, the lateral walls are not formed by the callosal bundles.

Cavum Veli Interpositi

Cavum veli interpositi, or interventricular cistern, is dilatation of the normal cistern of the velum interpositum (cistern of the tranverse sinus) (Williams

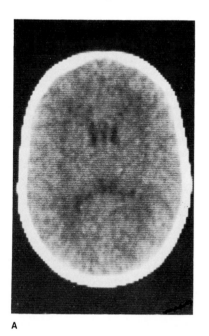
A

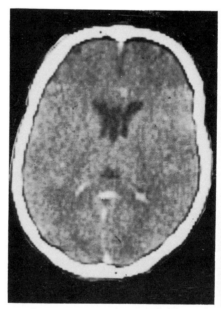
B

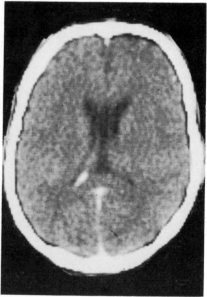

Figure 4-33 Cava septi pellucidi et Vergae. **A.** The two frontal horns are separated by a linear CSF-containing cavum septi pellucidi. This is a common finding in infants. **B.** Axial CT in an adult with cava septi pellucidi et Vergae. The CSF-containing midline space extends posteriorly beyond the foramen of Monro.

1975). It is situated over the roof of the third ventricle and communicates with the quadrigeminal cistern. It is frequently seen in infants and children (Byrd 1978a; Harwood-Nash 1977) and has been observed more commonly than cavum septi pellucidi or cavum Vergae (Strother 1978). It has been well documented both by pneumoencephalography (Picard 1976; Harwood-Nash 1976; Amundsen 1978) and by CT (Harwood-Nash 1977; Byrd 1978a). Cavum veli interpositi on CT (Fig. 4-34) usually has a triangular appearance and is situated between the bodies of the lateral ventricles, with its base directed posteriorly. Occasionally it may have a "mitre hat" appearance due to confluence of the adjacent quadrigeminal cistern.

Cyst of the Cavum Septi Pellucidi

Sometimes the cavum septi pellucidi, instead of having a CSF density with parallel walls, may appear distended, with its lateral walls outwardly convex. Cystic dilatation of the septum pellucidum is presumed to be secondary to occlusion at the foramen of Monro. Most often this may be an incidental finding, although occasionally the condition may be symptomatic. The symptoms usually are similar to those of the patient presenting with intermittent obstruction of the foramen of Monro, as can occur with colloid cyst of the third ventricle. There are no criteria which allow a distinction by CT between a dilated cavum septi pellucidi and a cyst of the septum pellucidum (Shaw 1969) or between a symptomatic and a nonsymptomatic cyst. Cystic dilatation of the cavity of the septum pellucidum commonly involves the cavum Vergae. Pathological or symptomatic cyst of the cavity of the septum pellucidum results in dilatation of the lateral ventricles, due to intermittent or complete obstruction of the interventricular foramina, and may require surgical intervention for relief of symptoms (Heiskanen 1973; Berkowitz 1939). On CECT the wall of the bulging cyst is well demarcated by the enhanced choroid plexus (Fig.

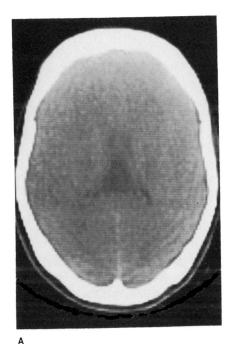
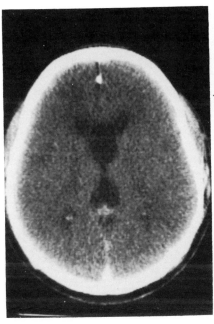
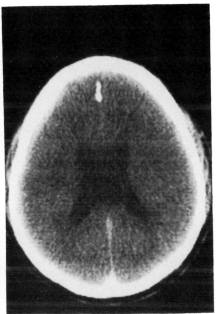

A B

Figure 4-34 A. Cavum veli interpositi. A triangular CSF-containing region is noted in the midline above the third ventricle and between the two lateral ventricles. This is compared with **(B)** cavum septi pellucidi et Vergae.

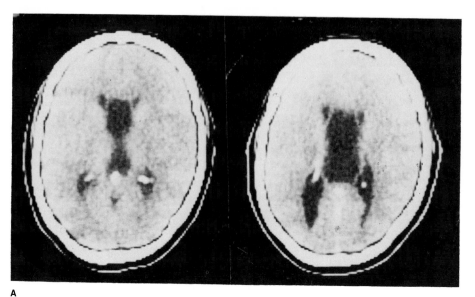

Figure 4-35 Cyst of cavum septi pellucidi. Occasionally, due to non-communication, cavum septi pellucidi may become cystic. **A.** Contrast-enhanced CT in axial plane demonstrates the septum pellucidum cyst demarcated by the choroid plexus and the wall of the septum. **B.** Antero-posterior blow-up view during pneumopolytomography: the walls of the cyst (arrow) encroaching on the lateral ventricle demarcate the cyst of the septum pellucidum.

A

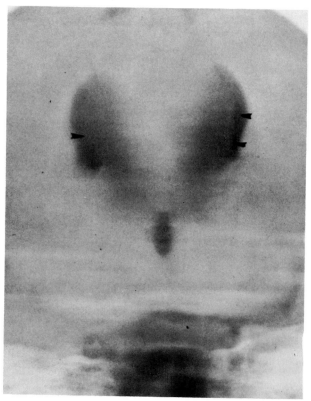

B

4-35) (Cowley 1979). Coronal CT is useful in demonstrating the cyst associated with enlargement of the lateral ventricles and a normal third ventricle. In symptomatic patients the CT findings can be confirmed either by CT metrizamide ventriculography or by penumoencephalography, thus differentiating the cyst from atresia or inflammatory obstruction of the interventricular foramina.

Cyst of the cavum septi pellucidi may be mistaken for dysgenesis of the corpus callosum or arachnoid cyst. In dysgenesis of the corpus callosum, the interposed third ventricle is separated from the lateral ventricles by the longitudinal columns of the corpus callosum as well as the infolded cerebral tissue. This results in wide separation of the frontal horns and body of the two lateral ventricles, both on axial and on coronal CT. Interhemispheric arachnoid cyst, when small and close to the corpus callosum, may be mistaken for a cyst of the septum pellucidum. The two conditions can be differentiated by coronal CT. Interhemispheric cysts are rare and are commonly associated with partial or complete absence of the corpus callosum (Solt 1980).

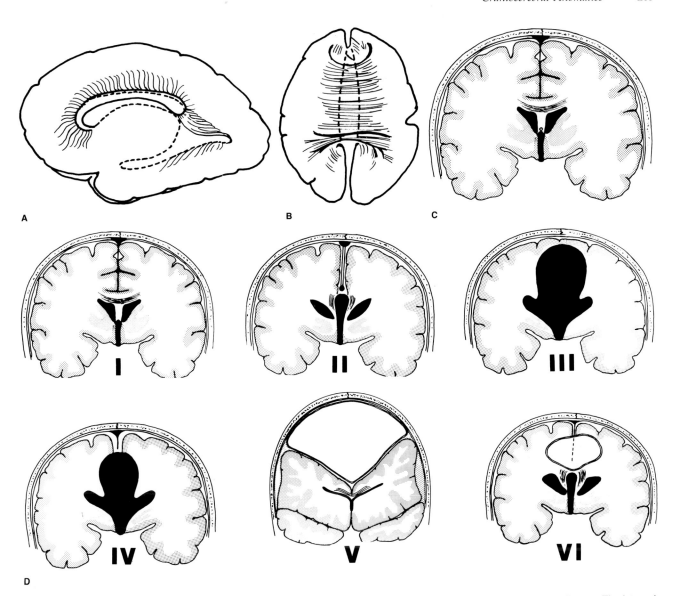

Figure 4-36 **(A)** Sagittal, **(B)** axial, and **(C)** coronal diagrams demonstrating the normal appearance of the corpus callosum. The internal cerebral vein lies over the roof of the third ventricle, separated from the corpus callosum by the medial walls of the lateral ventricles and the septum pellucidum. **D.** Diagrams demonstrating anomalies associated with the corpus callosum: (I) normal appearance, (II) dysgenesis of corpus callosum, (III) alobar holoprosencephaly, (IV) lobar holoprosencephaly, (V) intradural cyst, and (VI) dysgenesis of corpus callosum with interhemispheric arachnoid cyst.

Dysgenesis of Corpus Callosum

The corpus callosum is the transverse commissure connecting the two cerebral hemispheres. The corpus callosum begins to form around the twelfth week of gestation and is fully developed by 18 to 20 weeks. The fibers develop in a medial and longitudinal direction from front to back. The normal anatomy of the corpus callosum is better defined by axial and coronal CT (Fig. 4-36) than by other diagnostic stud-

Table 4-2   Anomalies Associated with Dysgenesis of Corpus Callosum

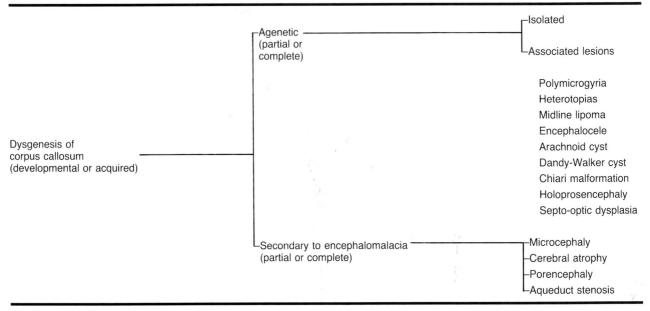

		Isolated
Agenetic (partial or complete)		Associated lesions

Polymicrogyria
Heterotopias
Midline lipoma
Encephalocele
Arachnoid cyst
Dandy-Walker cyst
Chiari malformation
Holoprosencephaly
Septo-optic dysplasia

Dysgenesis of corpus callosum (developmental or acquired)

Secondary to encephalomalacia (partial or complete)
Microcephaly
Cerebral atrophy
Porencephaly
Aqueduct stenosis

Modified from Byrd et al: *J Can Assoc Radiol* **20:** 108–112, 1978.

ies (Wing 1977). Absence of the corpus callosum may be complete or partial and may be developmental or acquired. A variety of causes such as genetic, metabolic, and mechanical factors involving the commissural plate early in development have been implicated to explain the defect. Dysgenesis of the corpus callosum may occur as an isolated lesion or as part of another craniocerebral anomaly, such as the Dandy-Walker cyst. Byrd (1978a) has classified the spectrum of anomalies and variations associated with this dysgenesis (Table 4-2) and the association with other malformations.

CT and MRI findings are characteristic and well defined in both axial and coronal sections (Fig. 4-37) (Byrd 1978a; Lynn 1980). CT in the axial plane normally demonstrates wide separation of the frontal horns. The frontal horns also appear narrow, unless there is dilatation secondary to hydrocephalus or associated with other anomalies. The bodies of the lateral ventricles and frontal horns have sharply angled lateral beaks. This is better defined in the coronal sections. Because of the long callosal bundles running longitudinally, the medial walls of the

bodies of the lateral ventricles are concave (Fig. 4-38). The occipital horns may show relative dilatation when compared to the width of the bodies of the lateral ventricles. The most important CT finding is interposition of the third ventricle between the bodies of the lateral ventricles. The third ventricle usually appears wider than normal. The height of the interposed third ventricle may vary, sometimes extending upward between the interhemispheric fissure to the vertex.

Differentiation from cavum septi pellucidi and cyst of the cavum septi pellucidi and cavum Vergae is possible in most instances when both axial and coronal CT are performed; a distinct separation of the third ventricle from the cavity or cyst of the septum pellucidi and cavum Vergae can be demonstrated. With a cavity or cyst of the septum pellucidum and cavum Vergae the corpus callosum is normally situated both in axial and in coronal CT, unlike dysgenesis of the corpus callosum, in which the frontal horn and bodies of the lateral ventricles are separated by the callosal bundles. Rarely, dysgenesis of the corpus callosum may be associated

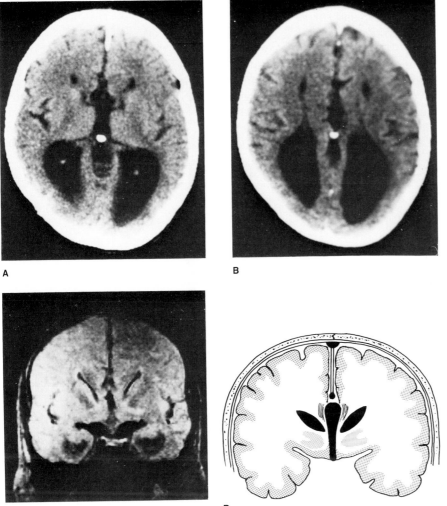

A

B

C

D

Figure 4-37 Dysgenesis of corpus callosum: **A.** Axial NCCT demonstrates wide displacement of the frontal horns (arrowheads) with midline dilated third ventricle. **B.** At a higher level there is wide separation of the medial wall of the ventricles with convex borders. The dilated third ventricle is seen between the callosal fibers in the midline. **C.** Coronal MRI demonstrates the relationship of the third ventricle, corpus callosum, and the lateral ventricle precisely. **D.** Diagrammatic representation.

with an interhemispheric cyst (Solt 1980) (Fig. 4-39) and may be mistaken for semilobar holoprosencephaly. However, three features help distinguish the two entities (Kendall 1983): (1) In holoprosencephaly the lamina terminalis appears thickened whereas in dysgenesis it is completely absent. (2) In holoprosencephaly the thalamus is fused, but it is widely separated in dysgenesis. (3) In holoprosencephaly the fornices cannot be identified. MRI demonstrates all these features; in addition appropriate sections in the midsagittal plane also demonstrate

the characteristic pattern of the sulci on the medial surface of the hemisphere, radiating from the elevated roof of the third ventricle, and failure of the parieto-occipital and calcarine fissure to converge (Fig. 4-40). Direct coronal CT is helpful in demonstrating the cyst separate from the roof of the third ventricle. In rare situations there may be difficulty in demonstrating the cyst wall separate from the roof of the third ventricle; metrizamide CT cisternogram then becomes useful. Computed tomography in both axial and direct coronal plane is also helpful in distinguishing porencephalic cavities, when they are close to or communicating with the ventricular system and associated with dysgenesis of the corpus callosum. Very rarely, a large cyst of the dura (Fig. 4-41) or an intraventricular arachnoid cyst may mimic dysgenesis of the corpus callosum. Diagnosis can often be made following metrizamide CT cisternography but rarely may require angiography. MRI will replace the need for these studies in the future.

Lipoma of Corpus Callosum

The corpus callosum is the most common site of this fatty tumor of maldevelopmental origin. It is caused by incorporation of the mesodermal adipose tissue into the neural tube during its closure, between the third and fifth weeks of fetal gestation. Intracranial lipomas, although more common in the anterior

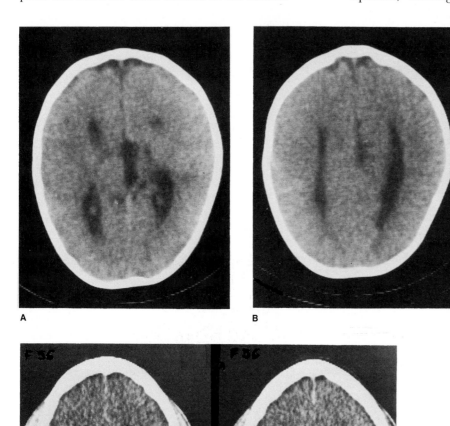

A

B

C

Figure 4-38 Dysgenesis of corpus callosum. **A** and **B.** CT in axial plane. The bodies of the lateral ventricles are widely separated by the longitudinal rearrangement of the corpus callosum fibers, resulting in the characteristic concave configuration of the bodies of the lateral ventricles. **C.** Contrast-enhanced axial CT in another case of dysgenesis of corpus callosum demonstrating separation of the internal cerebral veins by the upward displacement of the third ventricle and the characteristic dilated occipital horns.

portion of the corpus callosum, may also be seen in other areas, most commonly close to the midline cisterns. The location of the tumor relative to the midsagittal plane is probably related to the stage of fetal development (Zimmerman RA 1979). Intracranial lipomas have been reported in the suprasellar region, the quadrigeminal cisterns, and the crural cisterns as well as the cerebellopontine-angle cistern (Fukui 1977) (Fig. 4-42).

Lipoma of the corpus callosum is occasionally associated with dysgenesis of the corpus callosum, another midline dysraphic condition. Calcification of the fatty tumor is infrequent and probably depends of the size of the tumor. It is seen most often

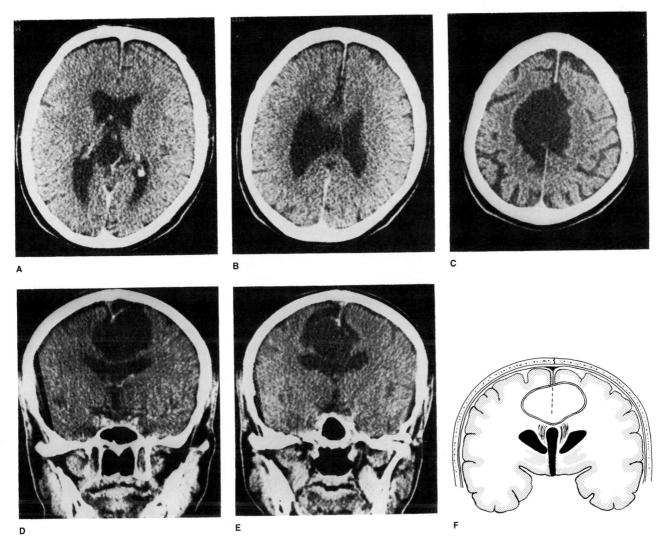

Figure 4-39 Partial dysgenesis of corpus callosum associated with interhemispheric arachnoid cyst. **A, B,** and **C.** Axial CT demonstrating dysgenesis of the corpus callosum with a midline hypodense area. **D.** Coronal CT demonstrating the cyst separated from the roof of the lateral ventricles in its anterior position. **E.** Posteriorly the cyst is contiguous with the lateral ventricles. This is due to partial dysgenesis, which primarily involves the posterior component of the corpus callosum. **F.** Diagrammatic representation. (*Courtesy of Dr. TerBrugge; previously published in Journal of Neurosurgery, vol. 52, 1980.*)

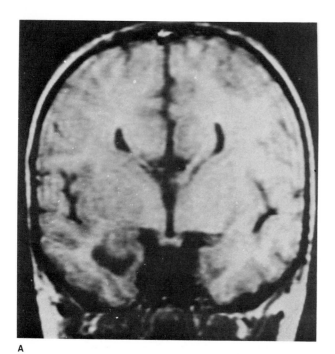

A

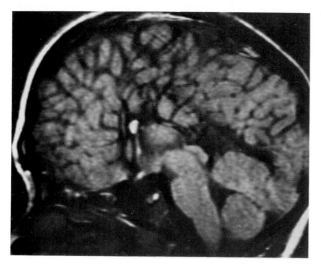

B

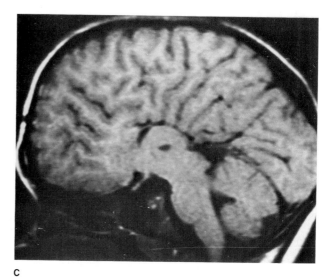

C

Figure 4-40 Dysgenesis of corpus callosum. **A.** Coronal MRI demonstrates upward migration of the third ventricle. **B.** Midsagittal and (**C**) off center MRI. The sulci radiate from the roof of the third ventricle characteristic of this anomaly. Other findings are nonconvergence of the parietooccipital sulci, laterally displaced fornix (**B**), and elevated internal cerebral vein.

in large tumors located in the corpus callosum but not at other sites (Zimmerman RA 1979; Faerber 1979; Fukui 1977). When calcification occurs, it is curvilinear and mural in location, although atypical calcification can rarely be encountered (Fig. 4-43). CT diagnosis is characteristic because of the low attenuation values indicative of fat within the tumor. In large lipomas involving the corpus callosum, the anterior cerebral artery is incorporated within the fatty tumor and on angiography is dilated, having the appearance of an elongated fusiform aneurysm. This can be demonstrated within the fatty tumor on CECT (Zimmerman RA 1979). The tumor does not show any change in density on CECT. As with dysgenesis

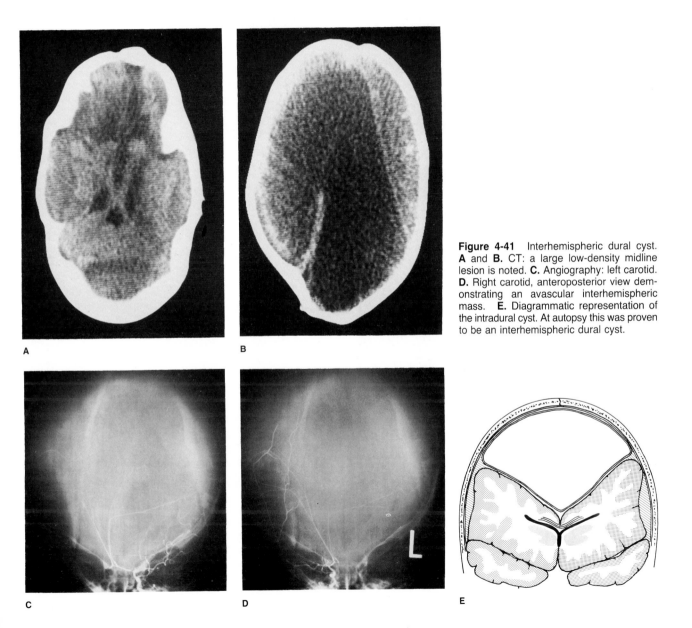

Figure 4-41 Interhemispheric dural cyst. **A** and **B.** CT: a large low-density midline lesion is noted. **C.** Angiography: left carotid. **D.** Right carotid, anteroposterior view demonstrating an avascular interhemispheric mass. **E.** Diagrammatic representation of the intradural cyst. At autopsy this was proven to be an interhemispheric dural cyst.

A

B

C

D

E

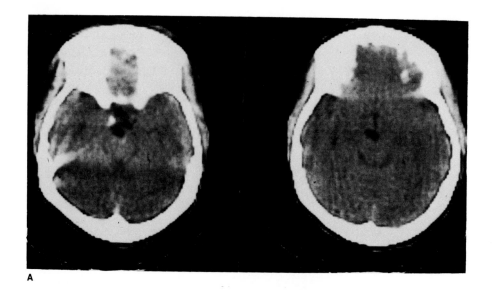

A

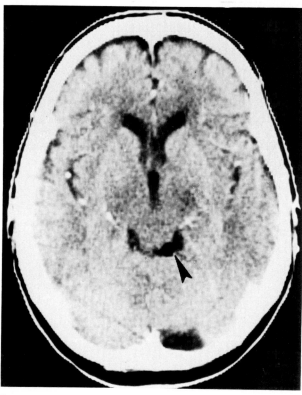

B

Figure 4-42   Intracranial lipoma.   **A.** Nonsymptomatic lipoma in another patient located in the prepontine cistern.   **B.** Another incidental lipoma (arrowhead) in the ambient cistern.

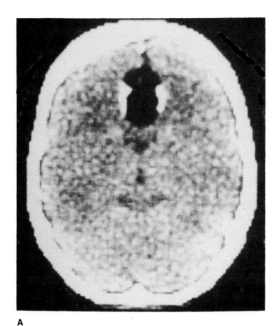

A

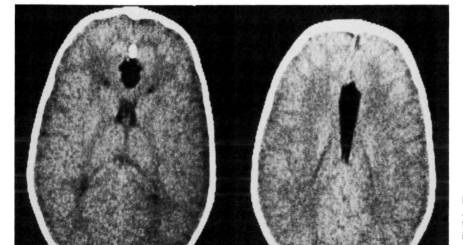

B   C

Figure 4-43   Lipoma of corpus callosum. **A.** The fatty tumor is located anteriorly in the genu of the corpus callosum, with typical calcification in the periphery of the tumor. **B.** Another patient with lipoma of the corpus callosum with minimal calcification. **C.** A third patient with lipoma involving the whole extent of the corpus callosum.

of the corpus callosum, in which the third ventricle is interposed between the frontal horns and bodies of the lateral ventricles, lipoma of the corpus callosum is seen as a low-density mass between the two lateral ventricles, with the third ventricle situated below the tumor. This can be characteristically seen in coronal CT (Fig. 4-44). Detection of dysgenesis of the corpus calosum or lipoma of the corpus callosum by CT may be incidental to evaluation of a nonrelated neurological deficit. A history of seizures is the most frequent clinical presentation in patients with dysgenesis of the corpus callosum or lipoma (Gastaut 1980).

Differentiation of dysgenesis of the corpus callosum from noncalcified lipoma of the corpus callosum is usually easy because of the characteristic difference in the CT numbers of fat and CSF, as well as the appearance in axial and coronal CT. Rarely, because of their location, lipomas may result in hydrocephalus, necessitating a shunting procedure (Kazner 1980).

Megalencephaly

Megalencephaly, or enlargement of the head, can by symmetrical, involving both cerebral hemispheres, or, very rarely, unilateral. In symmetrical enlargement of the head, the head circumference is above the ninety-fifth percentile or may show rapid increase in size. A variety of disorders can result in symmetrical enlargement of the head, such as obstructive or communicating hydrocephalus, intracranial neoplasm, tuberous sclerosis, spongy sclerosis (Canavan's disease), Tay-Sachs disease, and Hurler's disease. Excluding the above entities as the causative factor, there remains a rare malformative disorder in which there is symmetrical or unilateral enlargement of the head due to a developmental anomaly. Children with this disorder usually present with seizures, delayed milestones, and mental retardation. The etiology is not known, although the developmental anomaly is presumed to be caused by a defect of cell migration about the third month of gestation (Townsend 1975).

Very few reports have appeared in the CT literature (Fitz 1978b; Michaels 1978). The CT findings in symmetrical enlargement of the head of developmental origin consist in increase in size of the lateral ventricles compared to normal children. The temporal horns are not commonly enlarged. The enlarged lateral ventricles are presumed to be secondary to a cerebral atrophic process. CT diagnosis of megalencephaly is by a process of exclusion of other known pathological processes.

Megalencephaly can, rarely, be unilateral (Fitz 1978b; Townsend 1975); the whole hemisphere or a lobe may be involved. On CT the findings suggest an enlarged hemisphere, occasionally obliterating the ventricles but more commonly associated with dilatation of the ventricles. No change in density is seen following contrast enhancement. Absence of the insula, with a smooth hemispheric surface, is seen at autopsy. This can occasionally be appreciated on high-resolution CT. Even in the presence of these CT findings, the possibility of a neoplasm or nonneoplastic hamartoma such as occurs in tuberous sclerosis cannot be excluded. Angiography and radionuclide brain scan do not provide additional information.

Lissencephaly or Agyria

In lissencephaly there is a lack of gyral formation. The sylvian fissures are wide, with absence of operculation of the insula, resulting in a smooth hemispheric surface lacking primary fissures. The basic mechanism is interruption of neuronal migration from the ventricular matrix to the cortical surface. Since gyral formation occurs between the twenty-sixth and twenty-eighth week of gestation, the anomaly represents cessation of development at that stage.

Children with lissencephaly have microcephaly and micrognathia. They usually present with seizures, psychomotor retardation, decerebrate posture, and failure to thrive. Most children die before 2 years.

Very few cases with well-documented clinical, pathological, and CT findings have been reported (Ohno 1979; Garcia 1978) (Fig. 4-45). CT demonstrates wide sylvian fissures and subarachnoid space. Absence of sulcal patterns over the surface and

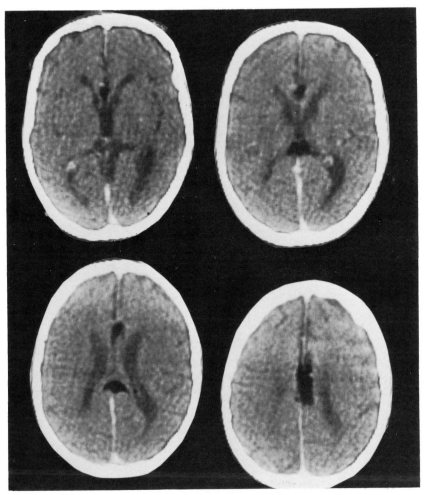

A

Figure 4-44 Noncalcified lipoma of the corpus callosum in **(A)** axial sections and **(B)** coronal sections.

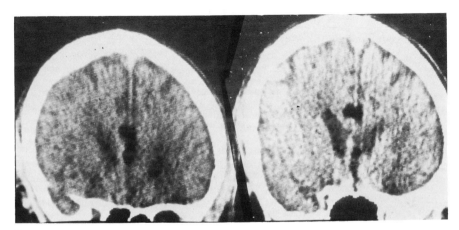

B

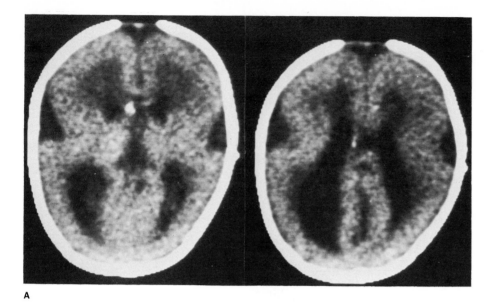

A

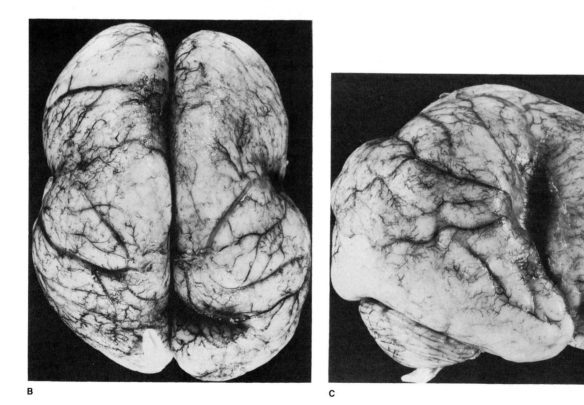

B   C

Figure 4-45   Lissencephaly.   **A.** CT demonstrates absence of gyri, prominent subarachnoid space and sylvian fissures, and moderate ventricular enlargement and punctate calcification of the ependymal lining of ventricle. Autopsy specimen of the same case: **(B)** dorsal and **(C)** lateral views showing the prominent sylvian groove and absence of gyral folds. *(Courtesy of Dr. Powell Williams.)*   **D.** Another case of lissencephaly, with calcification in the region of the caudate nucleus.   **E.** MRI in lissencephaly. Microcephalic head with deformed enlarged ventricles, absence of sulci over convexity. There is an associated Dandy-Walker cyst involving the posterior fossa.

moderate ventricular enlargement are commonly seen. Differentiation from cerebral atrophy is based on the absence of sulci, with dilated ventricles and sylvian fissures. Angiography has been performed in a few cases but does not provide additional information. A combination of CT and clinical findings should suggest the diagnosis.

Schizencephaly

When there is failure of formation of the brain due to segmental failure either in the germinal matrix or during neuronal migration there are resultant clefts in the brain parendyma. These are usually bilateral but need not be symmetrical (Zimmerman 1983).

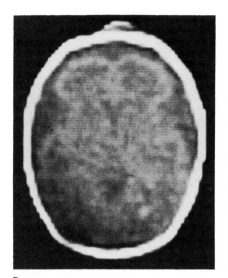
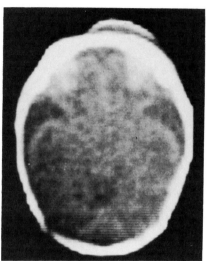

D

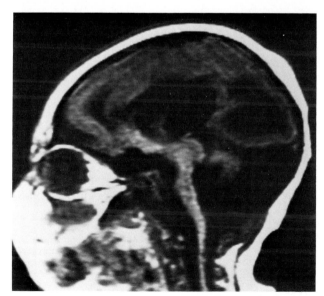

E

Schizencephaly represents thus clefts involving the cerebral hemisphere (Fig. 4-46) which extends through the entire section, communicating with the ventricles medially and laterally with the subarachnoid space. The clefts are lined by pial-ependymal lining. Similar appearance can also be the result of vascular insult, in which case they may be termed porencephalic cavitation. The clefts in schizencephaly tend to involve the pre- and postcentral gyri and extend downward into the insula (Friede 1975). Heterotopic tissue may be present on the walls of the cleft or adjacent ventricles. Polymicrogyria may be seen on the surface of the cortex. Clinically the patient is mentally retarded and prone to seizures. Spastic or hypotonic motor disturbance is not uncommon. The patient may also be mute and blind.

Meningoencephalocele

Herniation of glial tissue as well as meninges through a congenital defect in the skull vault results in meningoencephalocele. The contents of the herniated sac may be meninges containing CSF, when the anomaly is defined as *meningocele;* when the contents include brain tissue, it is called an *encephalocele.* This congenital anomaly probably results from a defect in the overlying mesoderm (Emery 1970). Meningoencephalocele may also be acquired, following trauma or surgery. Meningoencephaloceles are midline anomalies, most often involving the occipital region. Although involvement of the frontoethmoidal region is not uncommon, it is more often seen in Southeast Asia (Suwanwela 1972; Diebler 1983). A variety of classifications have been proposed (Suwanwela 1972; Gisselsson 1947), depending on the site of the cranial defect. Byrd (1978b) has modified the classification and described the common associated congenital anomalies of the brain. The encephalocele may be of varying size; sometimes the whole cerebellum may be present within the herniated sac. A large occipital encephalocele may cause hydrocephalus. Frontal encephaloceles produce facial deformities. Evaluation of these anomalies by CT is useful in determining the precise location, extent, and contents of the sac (Fig. 4-47).

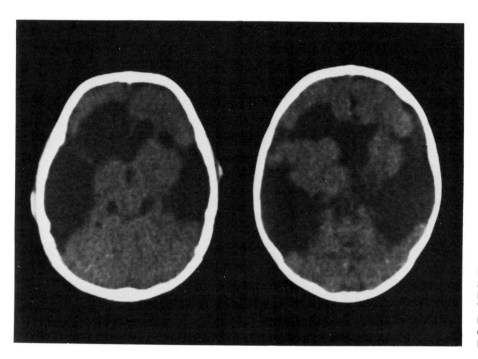

Figure 4-46 Schizencephaly: NCCT axial sections demonstrate large clefts involving both cerebral hemispheres. The CSF containing spaces communicates with both the ventricles medially and the subarachnoid spaces laterally.

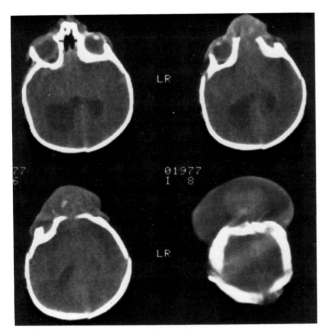

Figure 4-47 Frontal encephalocele: CT demonstrates a soft-tissue mass associated with a bony defect at the nasal bridge.

CT will also define other associated intracranial anomalies such as Dandy-Walker cyst and dysgenesis of the corpus callosum. Encephalocele, although rarely, may also occur at the base of the skull (Manelfe 1978; Byrd 1978b; Sakoda 1979). Diagnosis of the basal encephalocele may be more difficult. It may be mistaken for a polyp or soft-tissue mass in the nasal cavity or the nasopharynx. Occult clinical signs which suggest possible basal encephalocele include broad nasal bridge, hypertelorism, wide bitemporal diameter, and, rarely, intermittent CSF rhinorrhea. CT in the routine axial plane may not show the bony defect if the cranial defect is small. Diagnosis requires high-resolution CT in both axial and coronal planes (Fig. 4-48). CT is better than pluridirectional tomography. Metrizamide CT cisternography provides additional information in demonstrating a small encephalocele as well as encroachment of the subarachnoid space into the sac (Manelfe 1978). Once diagnosis of an encephalocele rather than a meningocele has been confirmed by CT, depending on the size of the cranial defect and

its contents, angiography may be necessary prior to surgery in evaluating the relationship of the intracranial vasculature to the herniated brain tissue.

DISORDERS OF HISTOGENESIS

Under this category are included the developmental anomalies classified as phakomatoses. The ectoderm, mesoderm, and endoderm are all involved to a variable extent in each of these entities. The more common phakomatoses are tuberous sclerosis, Sturge-Weber encephalotrigeminal angiomatosis, von Hipple–Lindau disease, and neurofibromatosis.

Tuberous Sclerosis or Bourneville's Disease

Tuberous sclerosis is a heredofamilial disease with the clinical triad of adenoma sebaceum, seizures, and mental retardation. The condition was first described by von Recklinghausen, and a more detailed description was provided by Bourneville in 1880. The disease is characterized by hamartomas involving virtually all organs, although not commonly in the same patient. Hamartomas in the brain are present in every case of tuberous sclerosis. The disease is autosomal-dominant but may skip generations. Sporadic cases thus are common. Occasionally the disease may not be clinically manifested until later in life. Since mental retardation and seizures are the earliest features, definitive diagnosis is useful for genetic counseling of the patient's family. CT, being noninvasive, provides a useful modality for this evaluation.

Intracranially the most common site of the hamartomas is the cerebrum, although the cerebellum, medulla, and spinal cord may be involved (Critcley 1932). The hamartomas may vary in size and number. The vast majority lie adjacent to the CSF pathway, predominantly along the ventricular surface as subependymal nodules close to the foramen of Monro. Obstructive hydrocephalus may result from the location of the hamartomas and change in size. Ten to fifteen percent of the hamartomas have been reported to undergo malignant changes (Fitz 1974; Kapp 1967). These neoplasms are relatively benign, slow-growing, and histologically classified as giant-cell astrocytomas. Malignant change of the hamartomas is common in the subependymal nodules, most commonly in the nodules closest to the foramen of Monro.

CT Findings

CT findings in tuberous sclerosis are characteristic (Gomez 1975; Lee 1978). On NCCT the subependymal nodules appear as rounded projections of varying size. They are denser than the rest of the brain parenchyma. Calcification is fairly common, even faint calcification being well defined by CT (Fig. 4-49). Noncalcified hamartomas within the parenchyma may be difficult to demonstrate. There is normally no change in density following contrast enhancement. When malignant changes have occurred there is significant enhancement (Fig. 4-50). Any change in density following contrast enhancement should arouse suspicion of malignant changes. A few patients will show mild to moderate enlargement of the ventricles with prominence of the cortical sulci, indicative of cerebral atrophy. Thickening of the diploic spaces may also be noted occasionally. This is usually seen in patients who have had severe mental retardation and seizures for a long time. The thickened calvarium may be the result of tuberous sclerosis or, more likely, the effect of prolonged Dilantin medication (McCrea 1980).

The differentiation of the noncalcified subependymal and cortical hamartomas of tuberous sclerosis from cerebral heterotopias may occasionally be difficult. Heterotopias are projections of normal brain tissue in areas where they should not exist. On CT they are seen as projections along the ventricular surface, more commonly along the medial wall. They usually have a density similar to that of the adjacent brain parenchyma and do not enhance on CECT. Presence of associated intracranial congenital anomalies and absence of associated clinical findings of tuberous sclerosis usually help in the diagnosis.

In children below 2 years, calcific nodules in the periventricular area as well as in the parenchyma due to tuberous sclerosis may be difficult to differentiate from an intrauterine infectious process such

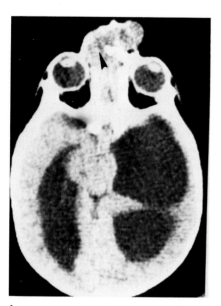

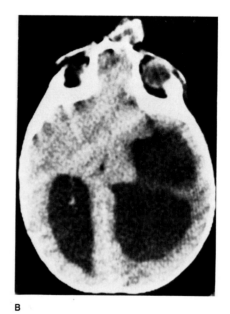

Figure 4-48 Nasoethmoidal encephalocele. NCCT **(A, B)**. A large soft-tissue mass protrudes through the bridge of the nose. This mass is contiguous with the intracranial contents. Bony defect in the nasoethmoid region (arrowhead) can be seen. There are associated encephaloclastic changes involving the brain parenchyma.

A

B

as toxoplasmosis or cytomegalic inclusion disease. Cerebral atrophy and microcephaly are more commonly associated with these two conditions. Differentiation from a vascular malformation with calcification of the vessels may be difficult when only a few calcific areas of parenchymal density are seen on the same side. CECT usually will show enhancement.

Rarely, when there is only a slight nodule in the region of the third ventricle, differentiation from a colloid cyst can be difficult. Most colloid cysts have a higher density than the nodule of tuberous sclerosis. The hamartomas of tuberous sclerosis do not increase in density on CECT unless malignant change has occurred. Similar diagnostic problems may also occur when a single nodule enhances on CECT. Differentiation from other varieties of neoplasm such as an ependymoma or other types of glioma is not possible. In these situations other diagnostic studies, short of surgical proof, do not prove helpful.

Sturge-Weber Syndrome

This syndrome, also known as encephalotrigeminal angiomatosis, was first described in 1879. It consists of port-wine nevus of the face, along the first branch of the trigeminal nerve, mental retardation, seizure disorder, leptomeningeal angiomatosis, glaucoma, hemiatrophy, and hemiparesis. The facial nevus and the leptomeningeal angiomatosis are usually on the same side as the cerebral atrophy. Calcification, which starts beneath the leptomeningeal angiomatosis, is rarely seen on routine skull x-rays below 2 years. The angiomatosis and calcification predominantly involve the temporoparietooccipital region. In older children and adults the cranial and facial manifestations are easily identifiable. Skull x-rays demonstrate the dense calcification, with hemiatrophy. The bony changes consist of elevation of the base of the skull and enlargement and increased aeration of the mastoid air cells. These are secondary to the developmental changes in the brain, with resultant remodeling of the calvarium.

CT (Fig. 4-51) usually shows the calcification involving the periphery of the cerebral hemispheres and having a gyral pattern. The sulci on the affected side are prominent, with mild to moderate enlargement of the ventricle, indicating some amount of cerebral atrophy. This finding is more commonly seen in older children and adults. CT is helpful in detecting the intracranial calcification and atrophic process in children less than 2 years of age (Welsh 1980). In older children and adults, CT helps define

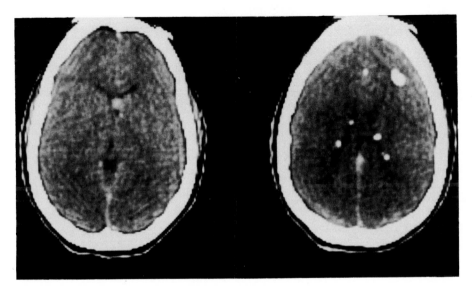

Figure 4-49 Tuberous sclerosis. Calcified hamartomas noted within the parenchyma as well as along the ependymal surface of the ventricles are characteristic.

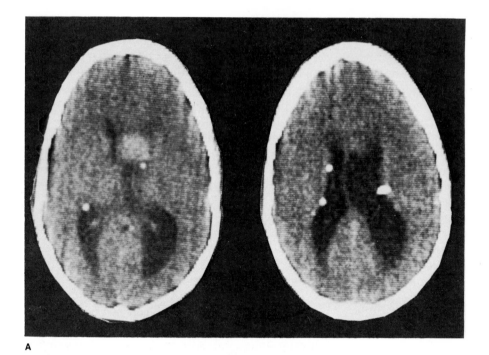

A

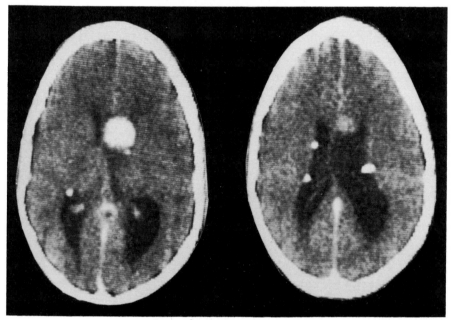

B

Figure 4-50   Malignant transformation in hamartoma of tuberous sclerosis. CT before contrast **(A)** and after contrast **(B)** demonstrates intense enhancement of the large tumor located in the region of the foramen of Monro. This is the typical appearance and location of giant cell astrocytoma.

the extent of the calcification and any associated abnormalities. Calcification has ben reported to involve the cerebral hemisphere not only on the same side as the nevus but also on the opposite side, as well as the cerebellum (Kendall 1978). Very rarely, instead of hemiatrophy, enlargement of the hemicranium on the side of the nevus may occur (Enzmann 1977). Contrast-enhanced CT in most cases will show diffuse superficial enhancement on the side of the nevus, extending beyond the calcification. This is similar to the sustained stain seen on angiography (Poser 1957). There is an apparent shift of the falx toward the site of the lesion which reflects calvarium remodeling. The superior sagittal sinus may not be well defined in vertex sections. Nonvisualization of the cortical veins on the affected side, associated with resultant tortuous collateral deep venous channels, has been shown by angiography (Bentson 1971). On CECT these tortuous collateral deep veins are seen as linear densities (Kendall 1978; Enzmann 1977).

Most often Sturge-Weber disease can be diagnosed on the basis of the clinical findings, the skull films, and CT. There are rare instances in which the clinical features of Sturge-Weber syndrome may be present although the CT findings are not characteristic. In the absence of typical gyral calcification on CT, the venous angiomatosis and associated sinovenous thrombosis of Sturge-Weber syndrome (Fig. 4-52) cannot be differentiated from arteriovenous malformation or the CT features of sinovenous thrombosis (Buonanno 1978). Angiography and the clinical features are usually helpful (Wagner 1981).

Neurofibromatosis

Von Recklinghausen syndrome, or neurofibromatosis, may have a localized or systemic manifestation. CNS manifestation occurs in the form of cranial nerve tumors such as schwanomas, optic

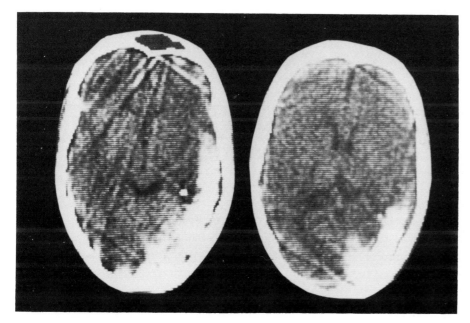

Figure 4-51 Typical calcification in Sturge-Weber syndrome.

chiasmatic gliomas, brainstem gliomas, and a high incidence of meningiomas. Bone dysplasia is also a not uncommon manifestation. It may present as dysplasia involving the greater and lesser wing of the sphenoid resulting in herniation of intracranial contents into the orbit, presenting as pulsating exophthalmos. There may be associated plexiform neurofibroma (Fig. 4-53). Petrous bone dysplasia results in widening of the internal auditory canal mimicking bilateral schwanomas.

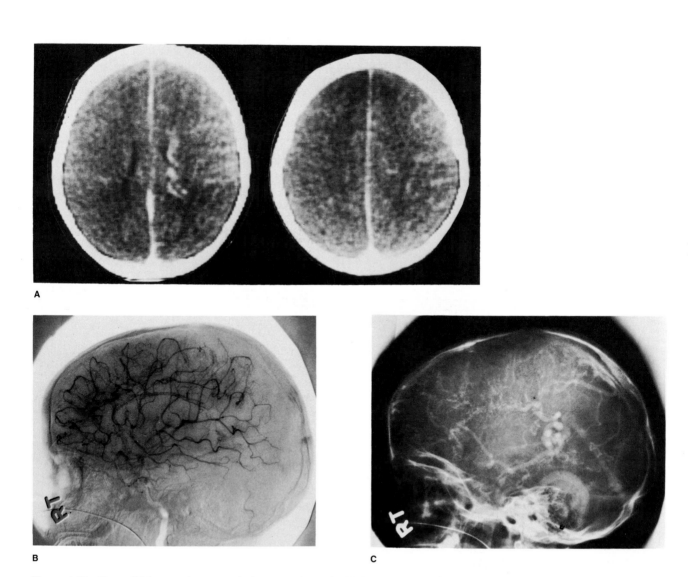

Figure 4-52   Sturge-Weber syndrome, atypical presentation.   **A.** CECT with enhancing gyral and subependymal vessels. Note slight thinning of the calvarium.   **B.** Lateral view of angiograms: note faint vascular stain in arterial phase.   **C.** Thrombosed superior sagittal sinus and prominent deep medullary veins.

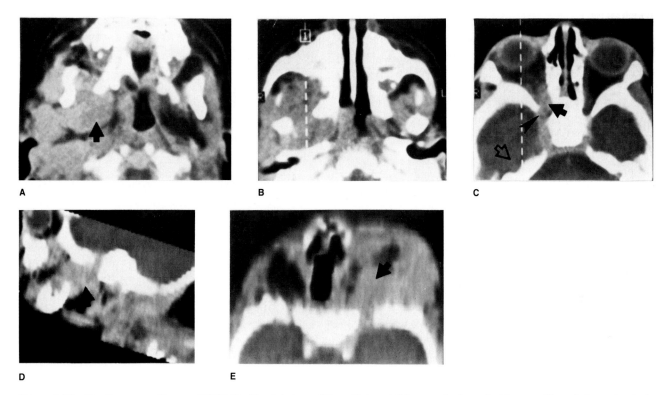

Figure 4-53 Plexiform neurofibroma: NCCT **(A–C)** axial views, **(D)** sagittal, and **(E)** coronal reformatted images. There is bone dysplasia involving the greater wing of the sphenoid (arrowhead) and the floor of the temporal fossa. The slightly hyperdense mass arising in the Meckles cave and in the temporal fossa (arrow) extends through the bone defect and foramen ovale into the orbit and pterygomaxillary fossa (black arrow).

Bibliography

ADAMS RD, SIDMAN RL: *Introduction to Neuropathology.* New York, McGraw-Hill, 1968.

ADAMS RD, GREENBURG JO: The mega cisterna magna. *J Neurosurg* **48:**190–192, 1978.

ALTMAN NR, ALTMAN DH, SHELDON JJ, LEBORGNE J: Holoprosencephaly classified by computed tomography. *AJNR* **5:**433–437, 1984.

ALVORD EC JR, MARCUSE PM: Intracranial cerebellar meningoencephalocele (posterior fossa cyst) causing hydrocephalus by compression at the incisura tentorii. *J Neuropathol Exp Neurol* **2:**50–69, 1962.

AMUNDSEN P, NEWTON TH: Subarachnoid cisterns, in Newton TH, Potts DG (eds): *Radiology of the Skull and Brain: Ventricles and Cisterns.* St. Louis, Mosby, vol 4, 1978.

ARCHER, CR, DARWISH H, SMITH K: Enlarged cisterna magna and posterior fossa cysts simulating Dandy-Walker syndrome in computed tomography. *Radiology* **127**:681–686, 1978.

ARMSTRONG EA, HARWOOD-NASH DCF, HOFFMAN H et al: Benign suprasellar cysts, the CT approach. *AJNR* **4**:163–166, 1983.

BENDA CE: The Dandy-Walker syndrome or so-called atresia of the foramen of Magendie. *J Neuropath Exp Neurol* **13**:12–29, 1954.

BENTSON JR, WILSON GH, NEWTON TH: Cerebral venous drainage patterns of Sturge-Weber syndrome. *Radiology* **101**:111–118, 1971.

BERKOWITZ NJ: Non-communicating cyst of the septum pellucidum with recovery following ventriculography. *Minn Med* **22**:402–405, 1939.

BLAKE JA: The roof and lateral recess of the fourth ventricle, considered morphologically and embryologically. *J Comp Neurol* **10**:79–108, 1900.

BONAFE A, ETHIER R, MELANCON D, BELANGER G, PETERS T: High resolution computed tomography in cervical syringomyelia. *J Comput Assist Tomogr* **4**(1):42–47, 1980.

BOUCH DC, MITCHELL I, MALONEY AFS: Ependymal lined paraventricular cerebral cyst: A report of 3 cases. *J Neurol Neurosurg Psychiatry* **36**:611–617, 1973.

BROCKLEHURST G: The development of the human cerebrospinal fluid pathway with particular reference to the roof of the fourth ventricle. *J Anat* **105**:467–479, 1969.

BRODAL A, HAUGLIE-HANSEN E: Congenital hydrocephalus with defective development of the cerebellar vermis (Dandy-Walker syndrome): Clinical and anatomical findings in two cases with particular reference to the so-called atresia of the foramina of Magendie and Luschka. *J Neurol Neurosurg Psychiatry* **22**:99–108, 1959.

BROOKS BL, EL GAMMAL T: Metrizamide CT ventriculography in the evaluation of a pseudoballooned fourth ventricle. *AJNR* **5**:825–827, 1984.

BUONANNO FS, MOODY DM, BALL MR, LASTER DW: Computed cranial tomographic findings in cerebral sino-venous occlusion. *J Comput Assist Tomogr* **2**:281–290, 1978.

BUSH JA, BAJANDA FJ: Septo-optic dysplasia (deMorsier's). *Am J Ophthalmol* **86**:202–205, 1978.

BYRD SE, HARWOOD-NASH DC, FITZ CR, ROGOVITZ DM: Computed tomography evaluation of holoprosencephaly in infants and children. *J Comput Assist Tomogr* **1**:456–463, 1977.

BYRD SE, HARWOOD-NASH DC, FITZ CR: Absence of corpus callosum: Computed tomographic evaluation in infants and children. *J Can Assoc Radiol* **20**:108–112, 1978*a*.

BYRD SE, HARWOOD-NASH DC, FITZ CR, ROGOVITZ DM: Computed tomography in the evaluation of encephaloceles in infants and children. *J Comput Assist Tomogr* **2**:81–87, 1978*b*.

CARMEL PW, ANTUNES JL, HILAL SK, GOLD AP: Dandy-Walker syndrome: Clinico-pathological features and re-evaluation of modes of treatment. *Surg Neurol* **8**:132–138, 1977.

COULAM CM, BROWN LR, REESE DF: Sturge-Weber syndrome. *Semin Roentgenol* **11**(1):56–60, January 1976.

COWLEY AR, MOODY DM, ALEXANDER E, BALL MR, LASTER DW: Distinctive C.T. appearance of cyst of the cavum septi pellucidi. *Am J Roentgenol* **133**:548–550, 1979.

CRITCLEY N, EARL CJ: Tuberous sclerosis and allied conditions. *Brain* **55**:311–346, 1932.

DANDY WE, BLACKFAN KD: Interval hydrocephalus: An experimental, clinical and pathological study. *Am J Dis Child* **8**:406–482, 1914.

DANDY WE: Congenital cerebral cysts of the cavum septi pellucidi (fifth ventricle) and the cavum Vergae (sixth ventricle). *Arch Neurol Psychiatry* **25**:44–66, 1931.

DEMEYER W: Classification of cerebral malformations. *Birth Defects* **7**:78–93, 1971.

DEMORSIER G: Etudes sur les dysraphies cranioencéphaliques: III. Agénésie du spetum lucidum avec malformations du tractus optique: La Dysplasie septo-optique. *Schweiz Arch Neurol Neurochir Psychiatr* **77**:267–292, 1956.

DERKHSHAN I, SABOUR-DEYLAMI M, LOTTI J: Holoprosencephaly: Computed tomographic and pneumographic findings with anatomical correlation. *Arch Neurol* **37**:55–57, 1980.

DICHIRO G, AXELBAUM SP, SCHELLINGER D, TWIGGS HL, LEDLEY RS: Computerized axial tomography in syringomyelia. *N Engl J M* **292**:13–16, 1975.

DIEBLER C, DULAC O: Cephaloceles, clinical and neuroradiological appearance, asociated cerebral malformations. *Radiology* **151**:825, 1984.

DOBYNS WB, MCCLUGGAGE CW: Computed tomographic appearance of lissencephaly syndromes, *AJNR* **6**:545, 1985.

DRAYER BP, ROSENBAUM AE, MAROON JC, BANK WO, WOODFORD JE: Posterior fossa extra-axial cyst: Diagnosis by metrizamide C.T. cisternography. *Am J Roentgenol* **128**:431–436, 1977.

DUBLIN AB, FRENCH BN: Diagnostic image evaluation of hydranencephaly and pictorially similar entities with emphasis on computed tomography. *Radiology* **137**:81, 1980.

DUBOIS P, HEINZ ER, WESSEL HB, ZAIAS BW: Multiple cystic encephalomalacia of infancy: Computed tomographic findings in two cases with associated intracerebral calcification. *J Comput Assist Tomogr* **3**:97–102, 1979.

DYKE CG, DAVIDOFF LM: The pneumonencephalographic diagnosis of tumors of the corpus callosum. *Bull Neurol Inst NY* **4**:602–623, 1936.

EBAUGH FG, HOLT AW: Congenital malformations of the nervous system. *Am J Med Sci* **246**:106–113, 1963.

EMERY JL, KALHAN SC: The pathology of exencephalus. *Develop Med Child Neurol* **12**(suppl. 22): 51–64, 1970.

EMERY JL, MACKENZIE N: Medullo-cervical dislocation or deformity (Chiari II deformity) related to neurospinal dysraphism (meningomyelocele). *Brain* **96**:155–162, 1973.

ENZMANN DR, HAYWARD RW, NORMAN D, DUNN RP: Cranial C.T. scan appearances of Sturge-Weber disease: Unusual presentation. *Radiology* **122**:721–724, 1977.

FAERBER EN, WOLPERT SM: The value of computed tomography in the diagnosis of intracranial lipoma. *J Comput Tomogr* **2**:297–299, 1979.

FITZ CR, HARWOOD-NASH DC, THOMPSON JR: Neuroradiology of tuberous sclerosis in children. *Radiology* **110**:635–642, 1974.

FITZ CR: Metrizamide ventriculography and computed tomography in infants and children. *Neuroradiology* **16**:6–9, 1978a.

FITZ CR, HARWOOD-NASH DC, BOLDT DW: The radiographic features of unilateral megalencephaly. *Neuroradiology* **15**:145–148, 1978b.

FITZ CR, HARWOOD-NASH DC: Computed tomography in hydrocephalus. *Comput Tomogr* **2**:91–108, June 1978c.

FITZ CR: Holoprosencephaly and related entities. *Neuroradiology* **25**:225–238, 1983.

FORBES W, ISHERWOOD I: Computed tomography in syringomyelia and the associated Arnold-Chiari Type I malformation. *Neuroradiology* **15**:73–78, 1978.

FRIEDE RL, YASARGIL MG: Supratentorial intracerebral (ependymal) cysts: Review, case reports, and the fine structure. *J Neurol Neurosurg Psychiatry* **36**:611–617, 1973.

FRIEDE RL: *Developmental Neuropathology.* New York, Springer Verlag, 1975.

FUKUI M, TANAKA A, KITMURAK K, OKUDERA T: Lipoma of the cerebellopontine angle: Case report. *J Neurosurg* **46**:544–547, 1977.

GARCIA CA, DUNN D, TREVOR R: The lissencephaly (agyria) syndrome in siblings: Computerized tomographic and neuropathological findings. *Arch Neurol* **35**:608–611, 1978.

GARDNER WJ, MCCORMACK LJ, DOHN DF: Embryonal atresia of the fourth ventricle, the cause of arachnoid cyst of the cerebellopontine angle. *J Neurosurg* **17**:226–237, 1960.

GARDNER E, O'RAHILLY R, PROLO D: The Dandy-Walker and Arnold-Chiari malformation. *Arch Neurol* **32**:393–407, 1975.

GASTAUT H, REGIS JL, GASTAUT E, YERMENOS E, LOW MD: Lipomas of the corpus callosum and epilepsy. *Neurology* **30**:132–138, 1980.

GIBSON JB: Congenital hydrocephalus due to atresia of the foramen of Magendie. *J Neuropathol Exp Neurol* **14**:244–262, 1955.

GISSELSSON L: Intranasal forms of encephalomeningocele. *Acta Otolaryngol (Stockh)* **35**:519–531, 1947.

GOMEZ MR, MELLINGEN JF, REESE DF: The use of computerized transaxial tomography in the diagnosis of tuberous sclerosis. *Mayo Clin Proc* **50**:553–556, 1975.

GOODING CA, CARTER A, HOARE RD: New ventriculographic aspects of the Arnold-Chiari malformation. *Radiology* **89**:626–632, October 1967.

HART MN, MALAMUD N, ELLIS WG: The Dandy-Walker syndrome: A clinicopathological study based on 28 cases. *Neurology* **22**:771–780, 1972.

HARWOOD-NASH DC, FITZ CR: *Neuroradiology in Infants and Children*. St. Louis, Mosby, 1976.

HARWOOD-NASH DC: Congenital cranio-cerebral abnormalities and computed tomography. *Semin Roentgenol* **12**(1):39–51, 1977.

HAYASHI T, YOSHIDA M, KURAMOTO S, TAKYA S, HASHIMOTO T: Radiological features of holoprosencephaly. *Surg Neurol* **12**:261–265, 1979.

HEISKANEN O: Cyst of the septum pellucidum causing increased intracranial pressure and hydrocephalus. *J Neurosurg* **28**:771–773, 1973.

KAPP JP, PAULSON GW, ODOM GL: Brain tumors with tuberous sclerosis. *J Neurosurg* **26**:191–202, 1967.

KAZNER E, STOCHDORP O, WENDE S, GRUMME T: Intracranial lipoma: Diagnostic and therapeutic considerations. *J Neurosurg* **52**:243–245, 1980.

KENDALL BE, KINGSLEY D: The value of computed axial tomography (CAT) in cranio-cerebral malformations. *Br J Radiol* **51**:171–190, March 1978.

KENDALL BE: Dysgenesis of the corpus callosum. *Neuroradiology* **25**:225–238, 1983.

KRUYFFE E, JEFF SR: Skull abnormalities associated with the Arnold-Chiari malformation. *Acta Radiol [Diagn] (Stockh)* **5**:9–24, 1966.

LARSEN PD, OSBORN AG: Computed tomographic evaluation of corpus callosum agenesis and associated malformations. *Radiology* **148**: 883, 1983.

LEE BCP, GAWLER J: Tuberous sclerosis: Comparison of computed tomography and conventional neuroradiology. *Radiology* **127**:403–407, 1978.

LEE BCP, ZIMMERMAN RD, MANNING JJ, DECK MDI: MR imaging of syringeomyelia and hydromyelia. *AJNR* **6**:221–228, 1985.

LIPTON HL, PREZIOSI TJ, MOSES H: Adult onset of the Dandy-Walker syndrome. *Arch Neurol* **35**:672–674, 1978.

LOWMAN RM, SHAPIRO R, COLLINS LC: The significance of the widened septum pellucidum. *Am J Roentgenol* **59**:177–196, 1948.

LYNN RB, BUCHANAN DC, FENICHEL GM, FREEMON FR: Agenesis of the corpus callosum. *Arch Neurol* **37**:444–478, 1980.

MANELFE C, ROCHICCIOLE P: C.T. of septo-optic dysplasia. *Am J Roentgenol* **133**:1157–1160, 1979a.

MANELFE C, LOUVET JP: Computed tomography in diabetes insipidus. *J Comput Assist Tomogr* **3**:309–316, 1979*b*.

MANELFE C, STARLING-JARDIM D, TOUIBI S, BONAFE A, DAVID J: Transsphenoidal encephalocele associated with agenesis of the corpus callosum: Value of metrizamide computed cisternography. *J Comput Assist Tomogr* **2**:356–361, 1978.

MCCREA ES, RAO KCVG, DIACONIS JN: Roentgenographic changes during long-term diphenylhydantoin therapy. *South Med J* **73**(3):310–311, 1980.

MEDELEY BE, MCLEOD RA, WAYNE HO: Tuberous sclerosis. *Semin Roentgenol* **11**(1):33–54, January 1976.

MILLER EM, NEWTON TH: Extraaxial posterior fossa lesions simulating intraaxial lesions on computed tomography. *Radiology* **127**:675, 1978.

MICHAELS LG, BENTSON JR: Computed assisted tomography and pneumoencephalography in nonhydrocephalic, nontumorous head enlargement. *J Comput Assist Tomogr* **2**:439–447, 1978.

NAIDICH TP: Primary tumors and other masses of the cerebellum and fourth ventricle: Differential diagnosis by computed tomography. *Neuroradiology* **14**:153–174, 1977*a*.

NAIDICH TP, LEEDS NE, KRICHETT II, PUDLOWSKI RM, NAIDICH JB, ZIMMERMAN RD: The tentorium in axial section: I. Normal C.T. appearance and non-neoplastic pathology. *Radiology* **123**:631–638, 1977*b*.

NAIDICH TP, PUDLOWSKI MR, NAIDICH JB, GORNISH M, RODRIGUEZ FJ: Computed tomographic signs of the Chiari II malformation: I. Skull and dural portions. *Radiology* **134**:64–71, 1980*a*.

NAIDICH TP, PUDLOWSKI MR, NAIDICH JB: Computed tomographic signs of the Chiari II malformation: II. Midbrain and cerebellum. *Radiology* **134**:391–398, 1980*b*.

NAIDICH TP, PUDLOWSKI MR, NAIDICH JB: Computed tomographic signs of the Chiari II malformation: III. Ventricles and cisterns. *Radiology* **134**:657–663, 1980*c*.

NAIDICH TP, MCLONE DG, HAHN YS, HANAWAY J: Atrial diverticulation in severe hydrocephalus. *AJNR* **3**:257–266, 1982.

NAKANO S, HOJO H, KATAOKA K, YAMASAKI S: Age-related incidence of cavum septi pellucidi and cavum Vergae on CT scans of pediatric patients. *J Comput Assist Tomogr* **5**:348–349, 1981.

O'DWYER JA, NEWTON TH, HOYT WF: Radiologic features of septooptic dysplasia. *Am J Neuroradiol* **1**:433–448, 1980.

OHNO K, ENOMOTO T, IMAMOTO J, TAKESHILA K, ARIMA M: Lissenecephaly (agyria) on computed tomography. *J Comput Asst Tomogr* **3**(1):92–95, 1979.

OKAMOTO S, HANDA H, YAMASHITA J et al: Computed tomography in intra- and suprasellar epithelial cysts (symptomatic Rathke cleft cysts). *AJNR* **6**:515, 1985.

OSBORN AG, WILLIAMS RG, WING SD: Low-attenuation lesions in the midline posterior fossa: Differential diagnosis. *Comput Tomogr* **2**(4):319–329, 1978.

PEACH B: Arnold-Chiari malformation: Anatomic features of 20 cases. *Arch Neurol* **12**:613–621, 1965.

PICARD L, LEYMARIE F, ROLAND J, SIGIEL M, MASSON JP, ANDRE JM, REARD M: Cavum veli interpositi: Roentogen anatomy-pathology and physiology. *Neuroradiology* **10**:215–220, 1976.

POSER CM, TAVERAS JM: Cerebral angiography in encephalotrigeminal angiomatosis. *Radiology* **68**:327–336, 1957.

RAMSEY RG, HUCKMAN MS: Computed tomography of porencephaly and other cerebrospinal fluid-containing lesions. *Radiology* **123**:73–77, 1977.

RAO KCVG, GUNADI IK, DIACONIS IN: Congenital interhemispheric dural cyst: A case report. In press.

RAO KCVG, KNIPP H, WAGNER E: Computed tomographic findings in cerebral sinus and venous thrombosis. *Radiology* **140**:391–398, 1981.

RAYBAUD C: Destructive lesions of the brain. *Neuroradiology* **25**:265–291, 1983.

REED D, ROBERTSON WD, ROOTMAN J, DOUGLAS G: Plexiform neurofibromatosis of the orbit: CT evaluation. *AJNR* **7**:259–263, 1986.

RESJO IM, HARWOOD-NASH DC, FITZ CR, CHUANG S: Computed tomographic metrizamide myelography in syringohydromyelia. *Radiology* **131**:405–407, 1979.

SAKODA K, ISHIKAWA S, VOZUMI T, HIRAKAWA K, OKAZAKI H, HARADA Y: Sphenoethmoidal meningoencephalocele associated with agenesis of the corpus callosum and median cleft lip and palate: Case report. *J Neurosurg* **51**:397–401, 1979.

SCOTTI G, MUSGRAVE MA, FITZ CR, HARWOOD-NASH DC: The isolated fourth ventricle in children: CT and clinical review of 16 cases. *Am J Neuroradiol* **1**:419–424, 1980.

SHAW CM, ALVORD EC: Cava septi pellucidum et verge: Their normal and pathological studies. *Brain* **92**:213–224, 1969.

SOLT LC, DECIC JHN, BAIM RG, TERBRUGGE K: Interhemispheric cyst of neuroepithelial origin in association with partial agenesis of the corpus callosum: Case report. *J Neurol* **52**:399–403, 1980.

SPINOS E, LASTER DW, MOODY DM, BALL MR et al: MR evaluation of Chiari I malformation at 0.15T. *AJNR* **6**:203–208, 1985.

STROTHER CM, HARWOOD-NASH DC: Congenital malformations in radiology of the skull and brain, in Newton TH, Potts DG (eds): *Radiology of the Skull and Brain: Ventricles and Cisterns*. St. Louis, Mosby, 1978, vol 4, pp 3712–3748.

SUWANWELA C, SUWANWELA N: A morphological classification of sincipital encephalomeningocele. *J Neurosurg* **36**:201–211, 1972.

TAGGART JK, WALKER AE: Congenital atresia of the foramens of Luschka and Magendie. *Arch Neurol Psychiatr* **48**:583–594, 1942.

TOWNSEND JJ, NIELSON SL, MALAMUD N: Unilateral megalencephaly: Hamartoma or neoplasm. *Neurology* **25**:448–453, 1975.

VIGNAUD J, AUBRIN ML, JARDIN C: Computed tomography in 25 cases of syringomyelia. Presented at the American Society of Neuroradiology meeting, Toronto, 1979.

WAGNER E, RAO KCVG, KNIPP H: Sturge-Weber syndromes. CT angiographic correlation. *CT: J Comput Tomogr* **5**:324–327, 1981.

WEISBERG L, STRABERG D, MERIWETHER RD, ROBERTSON H, GOODMAN G: Computed tomography findings in the Arnold Chiari type I malformation. *Comput Tomogr* **5**:1–11, 1981.

WELSH K, NAHEEDY MH, ABROMS IF, STRAND RD: Computed tomography of Sturge-Weber syndrome in infants. *J Comput Assist Tomogr* **4**:33–36, 1980.

WILLIAMS PL, WARWICK R: *Functional Neuroanatomy of Man*. Philadelphia, Saunders, 1975.

WING SD, OSBORN AG: Normal and pathological anatomy of the corpus callosum by computed tomography. *Comput Tomogr* **1**:183–192, 1977.

YAKOVLEV PI: Pathoarchitectonic studies of cerebral malformation. *J Neuropathol Exp Neurol* **18**:22–55, 1959.

ZETTNER A, NETSKY MG: Lipoma of the corpus callosum. *J Neuropathol Exp Neurol* **19**:305–319, 1960.

ZIMMERMAN RA, BILANIUK LA, GALLO E: Computed tomography of the trapped fourth ventricle. *Am J Roentgenol* **130**:503–506, 1978.

ZIMMERMAN RA, BILANIUK LT, DOLINSKAS C: Cranial computed tomography of epidermoid and congenital fatty tumors of maldevelopmental origin. *Comput Tomogr* **3**(1):40–47, 1979.

ZIMMERMAN RD, et al: Cranial C.T. findings in patients with meningomyelocele. *Am J Roentgenol* **132**:623–629, April 1979.

ZIMMERMAN RA, BILANIUK LT, GROSSMAN RL: Computed tomography in migratory disorders of human brain development. *Neuroradiology* **25**:257–263, 1983.

5

HYDROCEPHALUS AND ATROPHY

Karel G. TerBrugge

Krishna C.V.G. Rao

Seungho Howard Lee

Hydrocephalus (nonatrophic ventricular enlargement) is defined as ventricular enlargement secondary to an increase in the intracranial content of cerebrospinal fluid, associated with an elevation in intracranial CSF pressure which may be intermittent or present at some times. Hydrocephalus is a dynamic process in which there is an active and progressive increase in the volume of the ventricles because of relative obstruction of the passage of CSF between its place of origin and the site of absorption.

The term *hydrocephalus ex vacuo* has been used in the past where increased intracranial CSF spaces are associated with enlarged ventricles secondary to a destructive process involving brain parenchyma. In this chapter the term *atrophy*, which is synonymous with hydrocephalus ex vacuo, is used.

Nonatrophic ventricular enlargement (hydrocephalus) in the adult population may be caused by increased CSF production or decreased CSF absorption. Increased production of CSF, such as occurs in patients with choroid plexus papillomas, is an extremely rare cause for ventricular enlargement in the adult population. Nonatrophic distention of the cerebral ventricles in adults is most commonly the result of obstruction somewhere along the pathway of the CSF circulation. If the obstruction is within the ventricular system, which may be as far distal as the outlet foramina of the fourth ventricle, then it is defined as *noncommunicating* (obstructive) hydrocephalus. In *communicating* hydrocephalus, the obstruction in the CSF pathway can be due to causes between the outlet foramina of the fourth ventricle, or involving the various compartments of the subarachnoid spaces, or secondary to the pathological processes involving the arachnoid villi and the venous sinuses.

If the condition develops acutely, it is usually accompanied by headaches, vomiting, papilledema, and obtundation; but if the mode of onset is slower, these symptoms may be absent. Depending on the location and etiology of the obstructing lesion, localizing neurological symptoms and signs may be present.

COMPUTED TOMOGRAPHY IN HYDROCEPHALUS AND ATROPHY

Computed tomography has proved a reliable method in evaluating the ventricular system and intracranial cerebrospinal fluid (CSF) spaces. A variety of characteristic CT findings have been described which help in distinguishing nonatrophic ventricular enlargement (hydrocephalus either communicating or noncommunicating) from ventricular enlargement due to atrophy. Presence of sulcal prominence, as well as the cisternal spaces, provides features which are useful in distinguishing the CT findings as being due to an atrophic process rather than secondary to hydrocephalus. A variety of measurements have been described utilizing pneumoencephalography in determining the normal range of measurements of the ventricular and CSF spaces. Unlike pneumoencephalography, CT provides a reliable noninvasive method to evaluate the size of the ventricles and the sulcal prominence (Epstein 1977).

Linear measurements of the ventricular system utilizing either the axial sections or direct coronal sections in the different age groups have been established (Barron 1976; Gyldensted 1975; Gyldensted 1977; Hahn 1976; Haug 1977; Huckman 1975; Meese 1980; Pedersen 1979; Wolpert 1977). Another method has been to calculate the area using planimetry, comparing ventricles to brain volume from single sections (Synek 1976; Gomori 1984). Synek et al. (1976) felt the reliability of measurements of the ventricular system by CT to be similar to that obtained by pneumoencephalography. However, the measurements can be in error because of a variety of factors such as the partial-volume averaging and the spatial resolution of the scanner. The measurements are less precise when the ventricles are not enlarged (Wolpert 1977) or when they are rapidly enlarging (Penn 1978). Penn et al. (1978) suggested that even though there was a discrepancy of 16 percent, a more reliable analysis could be done on the basis of estimating the volume of the ventricles. The ventricular system increases only slightly in size from the second to the sixth decade. A significant increase in the size of the ventricular system is apparent after the sixth decade, together with a progressive increase in width of the cerebral sulci, as part of the normal aging process (Zatz 1982). In most cases, experience will suffice to judge the size of the ventricular system and sulci, but in borderline cases one still has to rely on certain measurments which have been established. Utilizing the EMI scanner, the combined width of the anterior horns of the lateral ventricles normally does not exceed 45 mm on the transaxial CT scan. The normal intercaudate distance measures about 15 mm, with an upper limit of 25 mm. The normal width of the third ventricle is 4 mm, with an upper limit of 6 mm. The normal width of the fourth ventricle is about 9 mm. Since actual measurements utilizing different scanners may differ, it is better to use an index system. This also may be more reliable, since slight change in angulation of the patient's head may result in different values in each study. The frontal-horn ratio which divides the maximum width of the anterior horns by the transverse inner diameter of the skull at that level is normally not more than 35 percent. In cases of atrophic ventricular enlargement, the ratio is above 40 percent, with an upper limit of 50 percent. In obstructive hydrocephalus the frontal-horn ratio is more than 45 percent in the majority of cases and frequently exceeds 55 percent.

Several morphological features may help to distinguish ventricular enlargement in noncommunicating (obstructive) hydrocephalus from that in atrophy (Fig. 5-1). Distention of the ventricular system in obstructive hydrocephalus is symmetrical and characterized by concentric expansion. The ventric-

Ventricular size index

$$\text{V.S.I.} = \frac{\text{Bifrontal diameter}}{\text{Frontal horn diameter}}$$

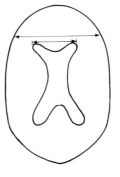

Normal	30%
Mild enlargement	30-39%
Moderate enlargement	40-46%
Severe enlargement	47%

	Atrophy		Obstructive hydrocephalus		Remarks
Angle of frontal horn		Obtuse		Acute	
Frontal horn ratio		Small		Wide	FHR: Measured at the widest part of the frontal horn perpendicular to the long axis of the frontal horn.
Temporal horn ratio		Not visible or small		Wide	Width of temporal horn measured at the genu.
Sulci and cistern		Wide		Obliterated	

Figure 5-1 Differentiating features between atrophic and obstructive ventricular enlargement. (*Adapted from Heinz et al., J Comput Assist Tomogr 4:320–325, 1980.*)

ular walls bulge as if they were expanded by multiple vectors of force radiating from a central axis (Heinz 1970). This causes a change in the appearance of, in particular, the anterior horns of the lateral ventricles, which become balloon-shaped (Fig. 5-2), as opposed to cerebral atrophy, which enlarges the ventricles without significantly changing their shape (Fig. 5-3). In cerebral atrophy, all parts of the ventricle may be affected equally, while in obstructive hydrocephalus, the larger parts of the ventricular system become distended first (anterior horns), to be followed by distention of the smaller parts (temporal horn, fourth and third ventricles). Enlargement of the temporal horns as a sign of obstructive hydrocephalus was noted by Sjaastad in 1969. LeMay et al. (1970) further defined this sign for CT and suggested that obstructive hydrocephalus is probable when the temporal horns are enlarged and the sylvian and interhemispheric fissures are normal in appearance or not visible (Fig. 5-4). A

discrepancy between the ventricular enlargement and the degree of cortical cerebral atrophy is suggestive of obstructive hydrocephalus.

Periventricular decreased density has been noted as an important but sometimes transient feature of obstructive hydrocephalus (Di Chiro 1979; Hopkins 1977; Hiratsuka 1979; Mori 1980). It is most often present in acute noncommunicating hydrocephalus but has been recognized in as high as 40 percent of cases with communicating hydrocephalus (Mori 1980). The periventricular hypodensity starts and is best recognized along the dorsolateral and dorsomedial angles of the anterior horns of the lateral ventricles (Fig. 5-5). Di Chiro et al. in 1979 attempted to characterize the periventricular hypodensity phenomenon in a variety of pathological conditions. When density measurements were done from the anterior horn toward the cortex in acute hydrocephalus, most often a linear pattern was noted; that is, the ventricular wall was not evident and the

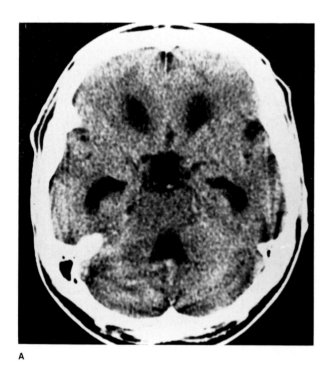

A

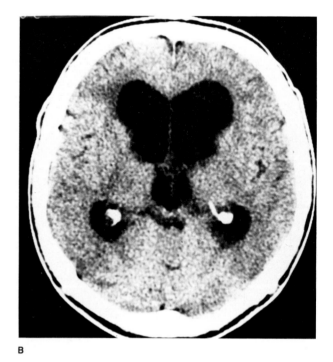

B

Figure 5-2 **A** and **B.** Primary communicating hydrocephalus in a 58-year-old male who presented with a 5-month history of dementia, ataxia, and urinary incontinence. Note generalized ventricular enlargement and ballooning of the anterior horns in the presence of normal cortical sulci.

Figure 5-3 Cerebral atrophy, with dilatation of the lateral ventricle and the cisterns. The cortical sulci over the convexity are also dilated. The fourth ventricle is normal size. Even though the ventricles are enlarged, they retain their shape.

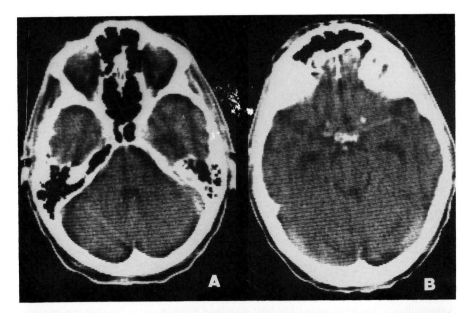

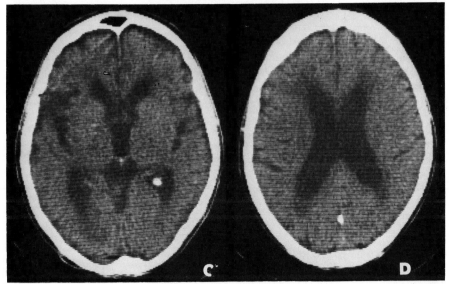

density increased linearly toward the cortex. When the hydrocephalus had been present for some time, a double-slope pattern was evident; that is, a moderately steep increase in density at the ventricular wall was present, followed by a slower increase in density in the parenchyma. The steeper initial slope presumably reflected partial restoration of the damaged wall. The periventricular hypodensity patterns

in the leukoencephalopathies were different because of nonuniform involvement of the white matter, although sometimes overlap occurred when secondary hydrocephalus was present (Di Chiro 1979). Periventricular hypodensity is sometimes noted in elderly patients with cerebral atrophy (Mori 1980) and might be associated with hypertension under these circumstances (Hatazawa 1984). But it differs

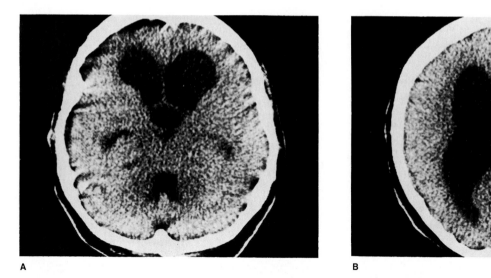

A   **B**

Figure 5-4 **A** and **B.** Communicating hydrocephalus secondary to previous subarachnoid hemorrhage. Note characteristic generalized ventricular enlargement with absent sulci in this 53-year-old female who underwent aneurysm surgery 8 months prior to the CT scan. Gait disturbance and dementia disappeared after ventricular shunting.

from the appearance in noncommunicating hydrocephalus in that the ventricular wall is usually preserved on the CT scan (Fig. 5-6).

The etiology of the periventricular hypodensity in obstructive hydrocephalus is still under investi-

gation. It can be inferred, however, that if the drainage of the CSF from the ventricular system is inhibited, as in noncommunicating hydrocephalus, there will be progressive ventricular enlargement with ependymal changes due to the pressure and rupture

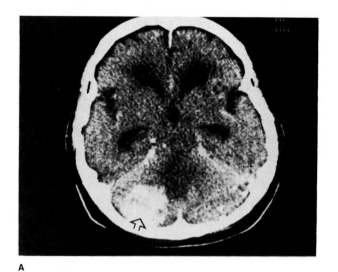
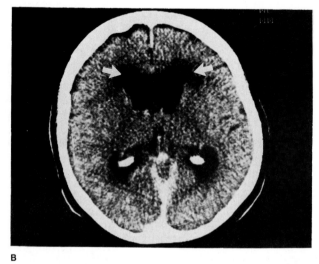

A   **B**

Figure 5-5 Noncommunicating (obstructive) hydrocephalus caused by metastasis of lung carcinoma to the right cerebellar hemisphere (open arrow), with obliteration of the fourth ventricle. Note the symmetrical enlargement of the third ventricle and both lateral ventricles, as well as the periventricular hypodensity adjacent to the anterior horn (white arrow), in this 68-year-old male.

of cell junctions, in particular at the dorsolateral angles of the anterior horn (James 1980). Water and salts pass freely across the ependyma into the periventricular tissue, causing decreased density on the CT scan. In communicating hydrocephalus, a steady state may be obtained when proteins pass through the damaged ependyma into the subependymal tissue, leading to a fall in effective intraventricular colloid osmotic pressure, and the ventricular protein concentration will reach a normal level characterized by an increased amount of CSF (Jensen 1979). In time, repair mechanisms take effect, with a glial and ependymal scar covering the previously exposed brain parenchyma in an incomplete manner

(James 1980). This possibility explains why in most cases of long-standing communicating hydrocephalus the periventricular hypodensity is no longer present.

Noncommunicating Hydrocephalus

In noncommunicating hydrocephalus there is symmetrical distention of the ventricular system proximal to the obstruction and a ventricular system of normal or less than normal size distal to the obstruction. The possible site of the obstruction should be examined in detail with thin sections and if necessary overlapping cuts, using the transaxial and possibly the coronal mode as necessary to establish the pathogenesis of the obstruction. In noncommunicating hydrocephalus, depending on the nature and location of the obstructing process, the ventricular dilatation may be focal or generalized (Table 5-1). It may be caused by a congenital narrowing of the lumen (web formation, aqueduct stenosis) (Fig. 5-7) or the lumen may be obliterated by the presence of mass effect. The mass lesion may be located within the lumen of the ventricle (colloid cyst, meningioma) (Fig. 5-8), the wall of the ventricular system (ependymal cyst, ependymoma) (Fig. 5-9), or the adjacent brain tissue (primary and secondary brain tumors).

The effectiveness of CT for reliably demonstrating such lesions has been established, and CT is without doubt the method of choice in the investigation of patients with noncommunicating (obstructive) hydrocephalus. The role of ventriculography and pneumoencephalography after an intraventricular drain has been installed is extremely limited to the demonstration of intraventricular webs, aqueduct stenosis, and fourth-ventricle outlet obstruction, if one wants to pursue the probable cause of the hydrocephalus demonstrated on CT (Fig. 5-10). Similar information can also be obtained by CT examination following intrathecal instillation of water-soluble contrast medium or magnetic resonance imaging (Fig. 5-7). The treatment of these conditions, however, would still be ventricular shunting, and most institutions would probably omit ventriculography and pneumoencephalography and perform a

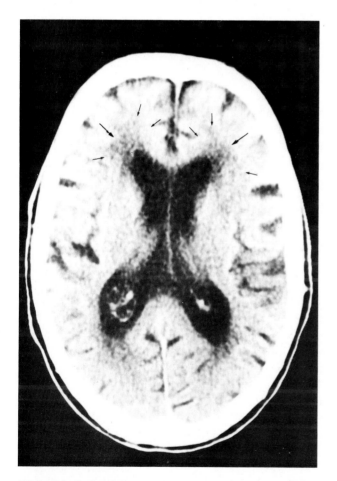

Figure 5-6 Perientricular hypodensity and atrophy: The ventricles are dilated and sulci are prominent. Hypodensities are noted around the ventricles, especially the frontal horns (arrows).

Table 5-1   Hydrocephalus: Classification and Causative Factors

Overproduction	*Noncommunicating*	*Communicating*
Choroid plexus papilloma	1. Postinflammatory 2. Congenital anomalies 3. Posthemorrhagic 4. Tumors	Infection Neoplastic Subarachnoid hemorrhage Congenital anomalies Dural venous thrombosis Normal-pressure hydrocephalus

	Anterior third ventricle		*Posterior third ventricle*
	Intraaxial	*Extraaxial*	
	Trauma	Pituitary adenoma	Pinealoma
	Colloid cyst	Craniopharyngioma	Teratoma
	Arachnoid cyst	Giant aneurysm	Collicular/paracollicular cysts
	Hypothalamic glioma	Arachnoid cyst	Galenic venous aneurysm
	Ependymoma	Ectopic teratoma	
		Dermoid	

shunting procedure, to be followed by a repeat CT scan to examine the ventricular size and the possible development of complications such as extacerebral fluid collections.

Communicating Hydrocephalus

In communicatng hydrocephalus, the ventricular enlargement is due to obstruction in the normal CSF pathway distal to the fourth ventricle. The obstruction usually involves the subarachnoid space between the basal cisterns and cisterns over the convexity of the brain, and may involve the Pacchionian granulations of the venous sinuses as well. The entity of symptomatic hydrocephalus in adults with normal CSF pressure was first described by Hakim in 1964 and subsequently by Adams et al. in 1965. The patients presented with symptoms of ataxia, dementia, and urinary incontinence. At pneumoencephalography a communicating type of hydrocephalus was demonstrated, and dramatic relief of symptoms occurred after ventricular shunting had been carried out. Subsequently, two types of communicating hydrocephalus were identified. In the primary, or idiopathic, form, no cause for the hydrocephalus is apparent (Fig. 5-2). In the second-

ary form, a previous history of trauma (Fig. 5-11), subarachnoid hemorrhage (Fig. 5-4), meningitis (Fig. 5-12), or meningeal carcinomatosis is supposedly responsible for the defect in absorption of CSF and subsequent development of communicating hydrocephalus.

Unfortunately, not all patients with the clinical triad suggestive of so-called *normal pressure hydrocephalus* (NPH) have responded favorably to shunting. Pneumoencephalography (LeMay 1970; Benson 1970), radionuclide cisternography (Tator 1968; Benson 1970; Heinz 1970; McCullough 1970), metrizamide cisternography (Hindmarsh 1975; Enzmann 1979), and cerebral blood flow studies (Greitz 1969a; Greitz 1969b) have all been used to identify those patients who would benefit from ventricular shunting. The predictive value of these tests has been disappointing (Black 1980; Coblentz 1973; Jacobs 1976b; Salmon 1972; Shenkin 1973; Stein 1974; Wolinsky 1973). Encouraging treatment results have been reported in patients with a positive lumbar CSF infusion test (Katzman 1970; Coblentz 1973; Nelson 1971; TerBrugge 1980; Wolinsky 1973). This test examines the compliance (CSF volume change per unit change of CSF pressure) of the cerebral and spinal compartments, which is in part governed by the collapsibility of the cerebral venous vascular system

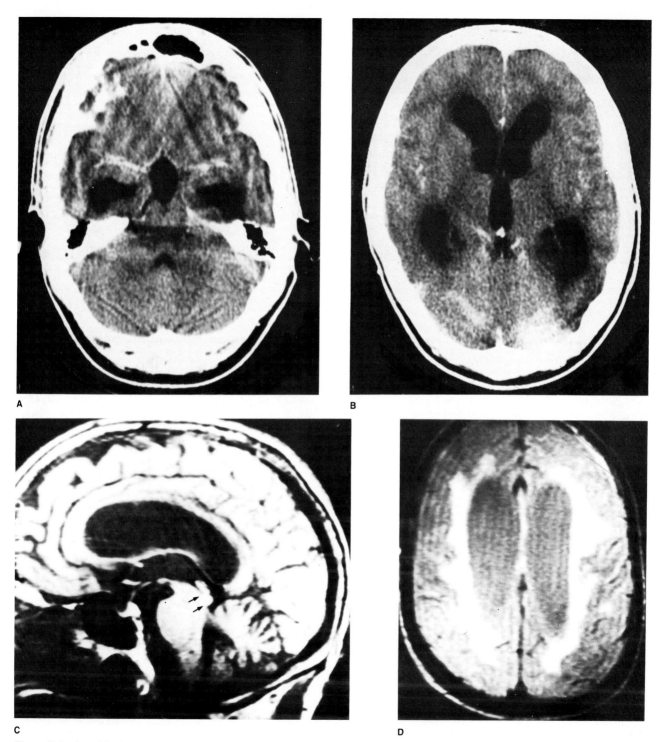

A

B

C

D

Figure 5-7 **A** and **B.** Aqueduct stenosis in 15-year-old male with recent onset of headaches and vomiting. Note normal-size fourth ventricle and enlarged third and both lateral ventricles. **C** and **D.** Obstructive hydrocephalus due to aqueductal stenosis—adult-type: MRI in sagittal T$_1$-WI (**A**) demonstrates occlusion of the aqueduct (arrows) with normal fourth ventricle. Axial T$_1$/T$_2$-WI shows periventricular hyperintense signals representing transventricular CSF absorption. Marked ventricular dilatation is apparent on both images. (*Courtesy of Dr. Robert Fisher, Plainfield, N.J.*)

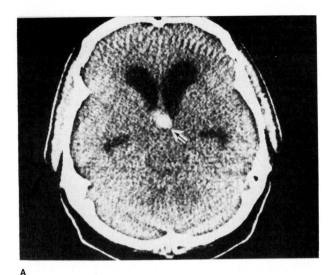

A

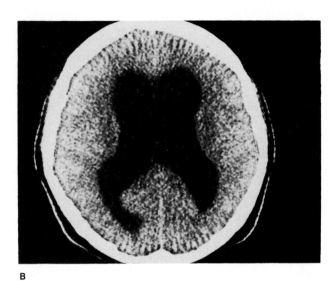

B

Figure 5-8 Noncommunicating hydrocephalus caused by a colloid cyst (arrow) within the third ventricle. Note the symmetrical distention of both lateral ventricles in this 29-year-old female, who presented with a 5-month history of increasing headaches. The third and fourth ventricles were less than normal in size.

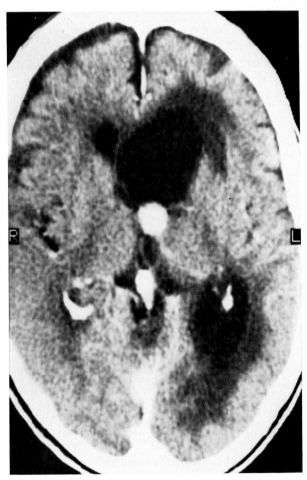

A

B

Figure 5-9 Unilateral intraventricular hydrocephalus due to (**A**) basilar artery aneurysm and (**B**) an ependymoma compressing and obstructing ipsilateral foramen of Monro. Obstructive hydrocephalus may also occur because of a mass at a distant focus associated with edema and herniation.

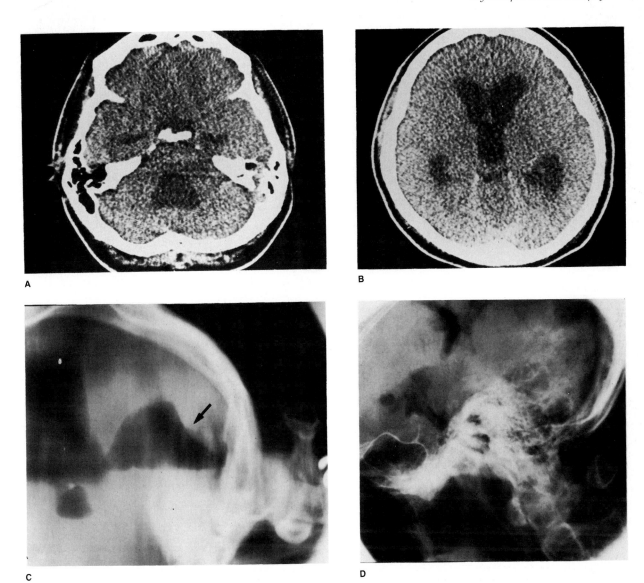

A

B

C

D

Figure 5-10 **A** and **B.** Noncommunicating hydrocephalus caused by outlet obstruction of the fourth ventricle in a 38-year-old male who presented with positional vertigo. Note the generalized symmetrical enlargement of the entire ventricular system. Air ventriculogram in **C** showed no exit of air from the enlarged fourth ventricle (arrow). **D.** Subsequent pneumoencephalogram revealed air within the basal cisterns, but no entry into the ventricluar system.

(Marmarou 1975). It has also become apparent that the intracranial pressure in patients with occult hydrocephalus is not necessarily low or normal at all times; high-pressure waves have been demonstrated during prolonged intracranial-pressure monitoring (Gunasekera 1977; Symon 1977; Ter-Brugge 1980).

Generalized ventricular enlargement on CT with normal or absent sulci has proved to be a useful sign indicative of communicating hydrocephalus (Gunasekera 1977; Black 1980). Gado et al. (1976) proposed a scoring system in which lateral ventricular enlargement was scored as mild (+1), moderate (+2), or severe (+3); the third ventricle as normal

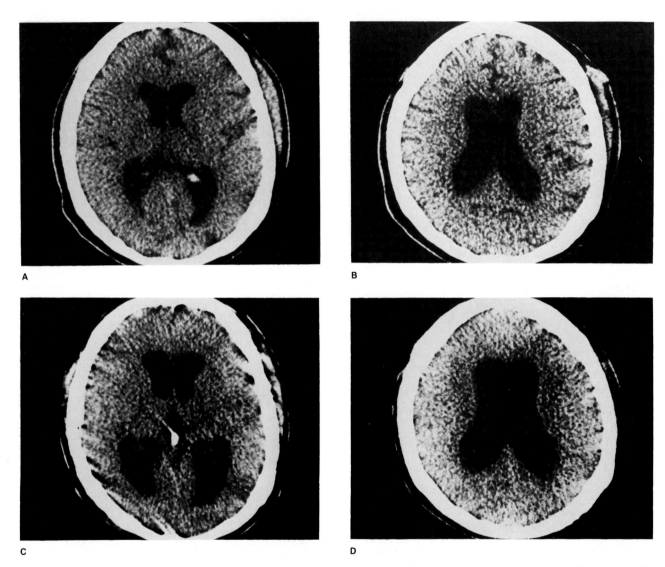

A

B

C

D

Figure 5-11 Communicating hydrocephalus secondary to trauma. CT at the time of the head injury (**A** and **B**) showed moderate diffuse cortical atrophy in this 40-year-old male. CT scan done 4 days later (**C** and **D**) shows progressive generalized ventricular enlargement and absent sulci. The clinical condition improved after ventricular shunting.

(0) or enlarged (+ 2); and the sulci as normal (0) or enlarged (− 2). Communicating hydrocephalus was suggested if the algebraic sum of the score was 3 or more. TerBrugge et al. (1980) showed that in a group of patients with clinical evidence of NPH who responded favorably to shunting, only 56 percent had CT evidence of communicating hydrocephalus, while 24 percent showed evidence of atrophy and 20 per-

cent had a normal CT scan. The findings were identical for the primary and secondary types of communicating hydrocephalus.

Computed tomography, because of its proven ability in evaluating the size of the ventricular system and the cortical sulci, should be the first investigative procedure when clinically the diagnosis of NPH is suspected. While generalized ventricular en-

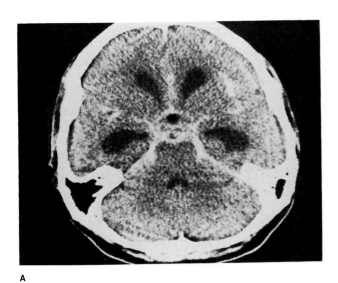

A

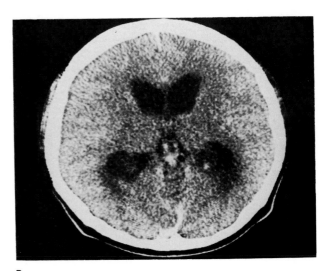

B

Figure 5-12 Obstructive hydrocephalus in a 49-year-old female with previous history of tuberculous meningitis. Note symmetrical enlargement of the lateral ventricles and, in particular, the temporal horns. The fourth ventricle is relatively normal in size. Obliteration of the basal cisterns is due to previous inflammatory disease. The obstruction of CSF is probably at the level of the midbrain.

largement and normal or absent sulci represent excellent CT evidence of communicating hydrocephalus, the diagnosis should not be rejected when the CT is normal or reveals evidence of cerebral atrophy. In such cases further investigations, such as the lumbar CSF infusion test, intraventricular pressure monitoring, and possibly radionuclide or contrast cisternography, should be carried out to assess whether the patient may benefit from CSF shunting. The change in ventricular size following a shunting procedure is best appreciated by CT. Clinical improvement, however, does not necessarily correspond to a diminished ventricular size, and therefore additional tests may be needed to assess whether a ventricular shunt is functioning properly (Schutz 1983). Further investigation utilizing MRI is in progress (see Chapter 17).

ATROPHY OF THE BRAIN

Brain atrophy is defined as loss of substance within the brain, which may involve the white matter, the gray matter, or both. Depending on the etiology (Table 5-2), brain atrophy can be focal or diffuse (generalized).

Focal Brain Atrophy

Focal brain atrophy presents on CT as a region of hypodensity within the brain parenchyma or as focal dilatation of a part of the ventricle or subarachnoid space. Most often there is a combination of components. Occasionally the pathogenesis of the atrophy is suggested by the location of the focal atrophic process, but more often a clinical history is necessary for correlation with the CT findings.

Posttraumatic Atrophy

The atrophic process is usually seen 3 to 6 months following the trauma (Kishore 1980; see Chap. 11). Focal atrophy is common when a hemorrhagic contusion is present in the acute phase. Surgical evacuation of a large hematoma or spontaneous resolution of an intracerebral hematoma may result in focal atrophy. Although hemorrhagic contusions or

Table 5-2   Brain Atrophy

Focal	*Diffuse*
Posttrauma	Alzheimer's disease
Postinfarction	Pick's disease
Postinflammatory	Multifocal infarct
Postvascular anomalies	Huntington's disease
Cerebellar	Parkinson's disease
	Wilson's disease
	Cerebral anoxia
	Binswanger's disease
	Jakob-Creutzfeldt disease
	Neoplasia and metabolic disorder
	Drug related atrophy
	Demyelinating disease
	Chronic schizophrenia

hematoma may involve any portion of the brain, they are often located peripherally, predominantly involving the frontal lobe and the anterior temporal lobes (Fig. 5-13). When hemorrhagic contusion or hematoma involves the parenchyma close to the ventricular margins or subarachnoid space, they appear as porencephaly. Posttraumatic atrophy may occasionally be diffuse.

Postinflammatory Atrophy

Postinflammatory atrophy secondary to brain abscess is most often due to necrosis of the brain, although surgical drainage may also, indirectly, be a factor, resulting in focal atrophy even when resolution of the abscess has been achieved with medical treatment. Diffuse cerebral atrophy may occasionally be seen in patients surviving low-grade infection, as in Reye's syndrome.

Postinfarction Atrophy

Cerebral infarction can be ischemic or hemorrhagic. Usually there is an antecedent history of frequent transient ischemic attacks and of hypertension. Since infarcts, both ischemic and hemorrhagic, involve major arterial branches, the atrophic process tends to be confined to their distribution. Postischemic infarcts tend to be evident on CT as early as 3 to 6 months after the episode (Fig. 5-14). It is not surprising to find a discrepancy between the neurologic deficit and the volume of focal atrophic process demonstrated by CT. CT may show mild ventricular dilatation with prominence of the cortical sulci without a focal low density in the parenchyma, although the patient may have a profound neurological deficit.

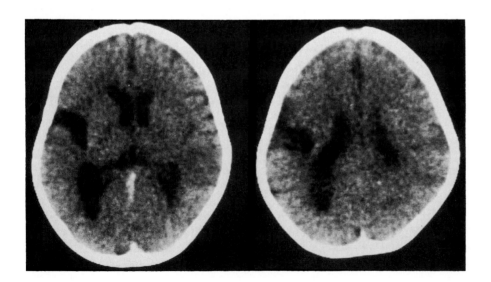

Figure 5-13 Focal atrophy following trauma: CT in a young man who had a head trauma 4 months earlier and who presented with seizures. There is focal atrophy involving the right temporal lobe. The right lateral ventricle is larger than the left.

Figure 5-14 Focal atrophy following cerebral infarction: CT 3 months after stroke in a 58-year-old female. There is mild prominence of the cortical sulci. The ventricles are slightly enlarged. Focal low density in the right occipital pole is noted, indicating parenchymal loss rather than mass. The clinical history was consistent with cerebral infarction.

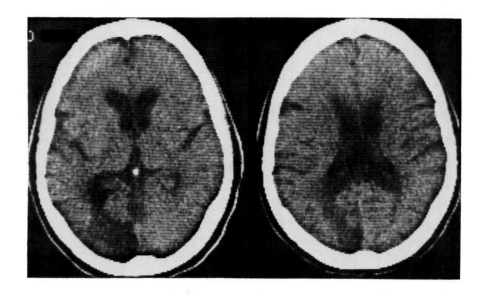

An increased incidence of cerebral atrophy has been noted in patients with migraine headaches of more than five years' duration (du Boulay 1983). Whether these changes are related to infarction or to the treatment with various medications (propranolol, ergotamine) remains to be clarified.

Cerebral Hemiatrophy

Cerebral hemiatrophy (Davidoff-Dyke syndrome) usually manifests itself during adolescence. The hemiatrophy is secondary to neonatal or intrauterine vascular occlusion, resulting in massive infarction. Rarely, the vascular occlusion may occur in childhood. CT demonstrates atrophy involving almost the entire hemisphere, with the ventricles shifted toward the side of the atrophy (Fig. 5-15). The sulci on the involved side are widened and occasionally may not be visible. Thickening of the calvarium on the involved side is common. CT will also occasionally show elevation of the roof of the orbit on the involved side, associated with prominent mastoid and adjacent paranasal sinuses. Focal cerebral atrophy associated with calcification of the cortical surface is seen in Sturge-Weber syndrome, in which a capillary angioma of the cortical surface is associated with a cutaneous facial nevus on the ipsi-

lateral side (see Chap. 13). The cause of the atrophy is the angioma combined with the associated cortical venous thrombosis.

Atrophy Associated with Vascular Anomalies

Arteriovenous malformation may occasionally be associated with focal atrophic changes, usually located distal to the vascular malformation (see Chap. 13). On CT this is most often seen as prominence of the cortical sulci in a focal area adjacent to the vascular malformation, predominantly over the cortical surface. Ventricular dilatation on the same side as the vascular malformation may be seen when the vascular anomaly is located deep within the parenchyma. The atrophy is most often due to ischemia of the adjacent parenchyma, probably resulting from a "steal" or from repeated small hemorrhages within the vascular malformation, or a combination of these factors.

Diffuse Atrophy

Diffuse cerebral atrophy may involve primarily the gray matter or the white matter, but most often it is mixed. Diffuse atrophy has also been classified as

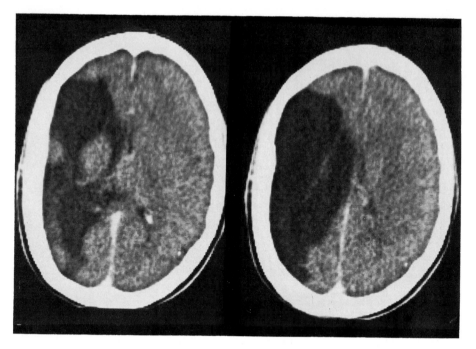

Figure 5-15 Cerebral hemiatrophy: enhanced CT in a young male with uncontrolled seizures. There is extensive loss of parenchyma involving the right cerebral hemisphere. The volume loss is partly compensated by an apparent shift of the opposing cerebral hemisphere. There is also compensating thickening of the calvarium on the affected side. These changes indicate a process that occurred during the neonatal period.

either central atrophy, in which the ventricular enlargement is more prominent than widening of the sulci (Fig. 5-3), or cortical atrophy, in which the sulci are wide relative to the enlarged ventricles (Fig. 5-16).

Diffuse cerebral atrophy can be due to a variety of entities (Table 5-2). The atrophic process, although diffuse, may involve the ventricle, sulci, or both (Fig. 5-17).

Numerous studies have been conducted eval-

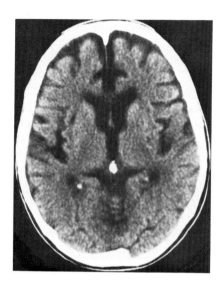

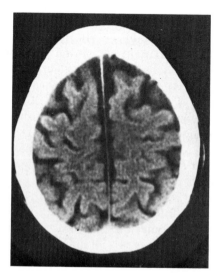

Figure 5-16 Cortical atrophy. CT in a 63-year-old male. The cortical sulci over the convexities are prominent while the ventricles are the upper limit of normal in size. Note several small lacunar infarcts.

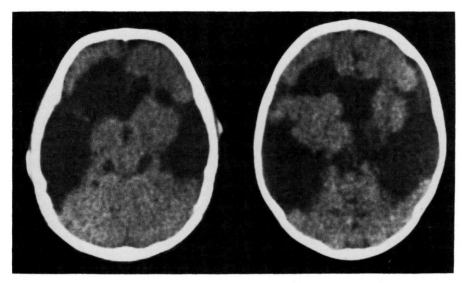

Figure 5-17 Diffuse cerebral atrophy. A 2-year-old child with large CSF spaces involving the temporal poles as well as the frontal pole on the right side. The CSF space between the ventricles and subarachnoid space are communicating. The lateral ventricle is dilated. The third ventricle is normal. This is another form of diffuse cerebral atrophy and does not require ventricular subarachnoid shunting.

uating the role of CT in predicting the degree of intellectual impairment in persons demonstrating evidence of cerebral atrophy (Huckman 1975; Fox 1975; Gado 1976; Roberts 1976; deLeon 1979; Jacoby 1980*a*, *b*; Gado 1983*a*), as well as CT correlation with aging (Barron 1976; Brinkman 1981; Hughes 1981; Jacoby 1980*a*; Yamaru 1980; Gado 1983*b*; Laffey 1984; Takeda 1984). All previous studies have shown that an increase in the size of ventricles and cerebral sulci occurs with aging and results from loss of brain substance. The decrease in brain substance involves both gray and white matter. Neuropathological studies indicate that the decrease in brain volume is due to progressive neuronal loss (Brody 1955) as well as decrease in Betz cells (Scheibel 1975). Decrease in brain volume and weight, however, may be more significant in patients with dementia (Tomlinson 1970). In the earliest CT study dealing with the subject Huckman et al. (1975) felt that there was a correlation between the severity of atrophy detected by CT and the dementia, though they were cautious in their analysis of the inconsistency between the CT pattern and the clinical rating of dementia. Hughes et al. (1981) have utilized linear measurements on CT in patients over 60 years old in defining the demented group as distinguished from the normal control group. They found that linear indices

(measurements of ventricular space and sulcal width at appropriate levels) which have been utilized by other authors were not, in their own evaluation, useful in separating the two groups. More recently, Gado (1981, 1983*a*, *b*) has shown that although linear indices may not be useful, volumetric indices derived from CT can be utilized in identifying dementia. In evaluating patients over 60, while the CT may show ventricular and sulcal prominence indicative of cerebral atrophic process, volumetric analysis from CT will show greater loss of brain substance in demented patients than in a control group of the same age, sex, and socioeconomic status.

Other methods of quantifying dementia by means of CT incude measuring the mean Hounsfield number in the centrum semiovale. In patients over 60 years old Naeser et al. (1980) found a mean CT number below 40 HU for patients with dementia while normal individuals had a mean CT number above 41. George et al. (1980) noted a loss in discriminability of gray and white matter by CT in patients demonstrating cognitive impairment, and did not find this to be age-related.

CT is useful in demonstrating treatable causes of dementia, and thus is a useful screening test (Huckman 1975; Jacobson 1979; Hughes 1981). With the limitations discussed above borne in mind, CT features found in some of the causes of diffuse cerebral atrophy are described below.

Alzheimer's Disease

Alzheimer's disease, or presenile dementia, is a diffuse form of cerebral atrophy, although there is predominant involvement of the gray matter. Senile dementia is considered to be a progression of the presenile stage. The latter is one of the most common forms of dementia encountered in clinical practice. Neuropathological studies demonstrate atrophy of the brain secondary to neuronal loss, vascular degeneration, neurofibrillary tangles, and plaques within the perikaryon of the cerebral cortex. The CT findings are nonspecific. The most common CT findings are symmetrically enlarged ventricles with prominence of the cortical sulci (Gado 1983a) (Fig. 5-18), which, as shown earlier, are not characteristic of Alzheimer's disease and may not be confirmed on pathological studies. Occasionally the cortical sulci may appear more prominent, and in other instances the ventricles are significantly increased in size. It is not usual to have a normal CT in a demented patient with abnormal psychometric test and cognitive functions. In a few cases, further studies such as radioisotope cisternography may be indicated to evaluate for normal-pressure hydrocephalus—a treatable cause of dementia.

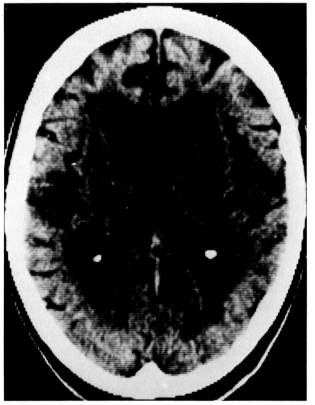

A

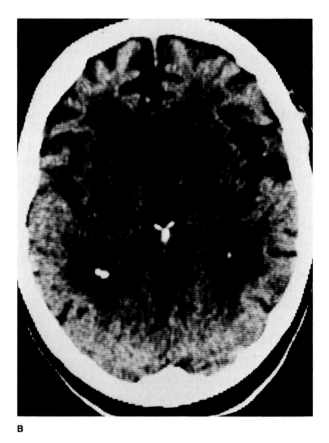

B

Figure 5-18 Alzheimer's disease: The ventricles are symmetrically dilated and the cortical sulci are prominent; a diffuse, nonspecific form of central and cortical atrophy.

Pick's Disease

Clinically, differentiation of Pick's lobar atrophy from the diffuse atrophy of Alzheimer's disease may be difficult. In both, the clinical progression is gradual and downhill. Pick's disease is more commonly seen in females. The disease is occasionally familial and may be inherited. The atrophic process, although diffuse, predominantly involves the temporal and frontal lobes. CT findings include dilatation of frontal and temporal horns (McGeachi 1979). The cisterns and sylvian fissure also appear prominent. Significant cortical atrophy over the convexity may be absent.

Huntington's Disease

Huntington's disease is characterized by choreiform movement and dementia. It is autosomal dominant, predominantly involving males and manifesting itself in the fourth and fifth decade. The disease starts with choreiform movement of the extremities, followed by dementia and personality changes. The hallmark in neuropathologic studies is atrophy of the caudate nucleus and putamen. In later stages diffuse atrophy of frontal and temporal regions occurs. CT in this disease is characterized by atrophy of the caudate nucleus, resulting in increased bicaudate diameter of the ventricles (Fig. 5-19). This may or may not be associated with enlargement of the ventricles and cortical sulci. Presence of this CT picture confirms the clinical diagnosis, although in the authors' series, four of nine patients did not show CT evidence of caudate nucleus atrophy.

Recently, Simmons et al. (1986) demonstrated that MRI is superior to CT in the detection of atrophy of the caudate nucleus and corpus striatum in all four patients with Huntington's disease (see Chap. 17 also).

Parkinson's Disease

Brain atrophy in Parkinson's disease predominantly involves the subcortical regions, primarily resulting in degeneration of the cells and fibers of the corpus striatum, the globus pallidus, and the substantia ni-

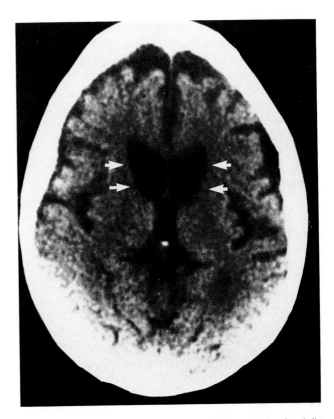

Figure 5-19 Huntington's disease. NCCT demonstrates focal dilation of the frontal horns, especially the lateral walls (arrows), secondary to atrophy of the caudate nucleus. This is characteristic of Huntington's disease.

gra. Postencephalitic Parkinson's disease is presently uncommon. Most cases present in the sixth and seventh decades. CT in Parkinson's disease is associated with enlarged ventricles and calcification of the basal ganglia. Isolated calcification of the basal ganglia per se is not an indication of Parkinson's disease, since it can be seen in the normal population; and CT findings of enlarged ventricles and prominent cortical sulci associated with aging are difficult to differentiate from those caused by the disease process. No significant correlation between the severity of the tremor and akinesia and the severity of the cerebral atrophy as shown by CT has been documented. Numerous studies, however, have shown that the atrophic process on CT is more marked in patients with Parkinson's disease than in persons in the same age group without the disease (Schneider 1979; Becker 1979; Johnstone 1976; Weinberger 1979; Adam 1983). A higher degree of cognitive impairment, not age-related, has been associated with severity of the atrophic process as detected by CT (Johnstone 1976). Other studies have shown that patients with Parkinson's disease demonstrating basal ganglia calcification respond poorly to L-dopa therapy.

Wilson's Disease

Wilson's disease is due to impairment in copper metabolism. Pathologic changes in the brain consist of loss of neurons and fibrillary gliosis involving the basal ganglia and cerebral cortex. Because of deficiency of ceruloplasmin there are deposits of copper both in the liver and within the basal ganglia in the brain. The authors failed to detect any abnormal CT findings in two cases of proven Wilson's disease. Ropper (1978), Harik (1981), and Kvicala (1983) have described hypodense regions within the basal ganglia, occasionally involving the cerebellar nuclei and adjacent white matter. There was, however, no correlation between the severity of dementia and the degree of atrophic process on CT in a majority of their cases.

Cerebral Anoxia

Anoxia results in neuronal loss associated with gliosis and edema. The end result in persons surviving anoxia is diffuse cortical atrophy disproportionate to the dilatation of the lateral ventricles. Correlation between CT and autopsy in premature and full-term neonates that suffered from perinatal asphyxia showed generalized ventricular enlargement and prominent CSF spaces to be a frequent occurrence (Flodmark 1980). In children and adults who survive the acute episode, the CT shows diffuse cortical and ventricular enlargement. Changes similar to those seen in neonates are also seen in adults exposed to carbon monoxide poisoning. In the acute stage the CT may appear normal, or there may be an increase in hypodensity of the white matter. Some have described symmetrical necrosis involving the globus

pallidus, usually in those surviving beyond 48 hours (Sawa 1981; Kono 1983). Late changes include enlargement of the ventricles and cortical sulci (see Chap. 14).

Binswanger's Disease

Binswanger's disease (Binswanger 1894) is progressive dementia associated with periods of remission and exacerbation. The disease is usually manifested in the fifth or sixth decade of life, usually in the form of intellectual impairment and alteration of personality progressing to dementia. The gradual but progressive course of the disease is presumed to be due to arteriosclerotic involvement of the small vessels in the subcortical region, with sharply demarcated areas of necrosis and demyelination involving the white matter. The CT findings described in Binswanger's disease (Rueck 1980; Zeumer 1980; Rosenberg 1979; Agnoli 1984) consist of hypodense lesions in the periventricular white matter, lacunar infarcts in the basal ganglia, and dilatation of the ventricles. Similar CT findings are also seen in dementia secondary to multifocal infarcts. The diagnosis of Binswanger's disease is based on the clinical progression of the dementia and findings on CT (see Chap. 14).

Jakob-Creutzfeldt Syndrome

Jakob-Creutzfeldt disease is characterized by rapidly progressive dementia. Other neurological findings include altered perception, myoclonus, increased response to startle stimulus, and cerebellar dysfunction. Although initially believed to be caused by a slow virus (Gajdusek 1977), it is now thought to be related to a transmissible protein substance (prion). Neuropathological studies demonstrate enlarged ventricles, with atrophy predominantly involving the gray matter, but white matter lesions have also been described (Macchi 1984). Spongiform changes of the cerebral cortex predominantly involve the temporal and occipital lobes. In the few cases in which CT findings have been reported (Rao 1977), the pattern is that of diffuse cerebral atrophy (Fig. 5-20). Although this finding is not character-

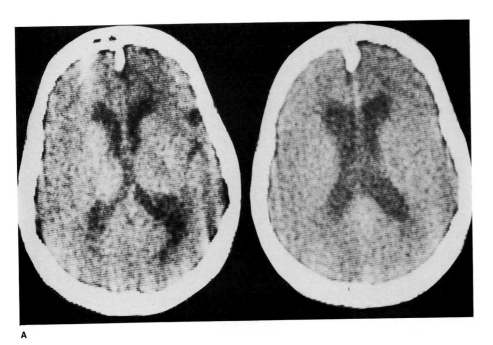

A

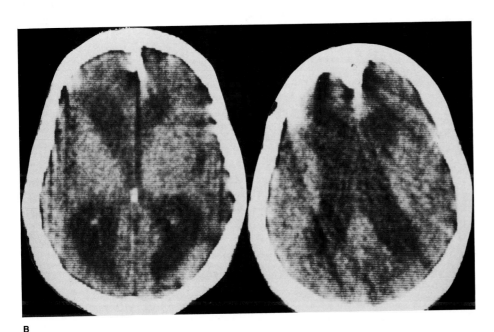

B

Figure 5-20   Jakob-Creutzfeldt disease. The rapid change in ventricular size is a characteristic feature in this disease.   **A.** Initial CT.   **B.** CT a few weeks later, demonstrating rapid progression of atrophic process. (*Continued on page 252*)

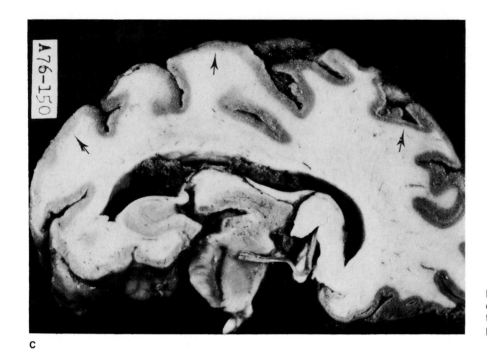

Figure 5.20 (*cont.*)   **C.** Significant loss of gray matter (arrows) characteristic of this disease at autopsy in the same patient.

C

istic, diagnosis is based on rapid clinical deterioration and progression of the atrophic process on sequential CT (Chap. 15).

Neoplasia and Metabolic Disorder

Huckman (1975) reported on patients with neoplasia without metastatic brain disease, enlarged ventricles, and cortical sulci, indicative of atrophy, matched with a control group of similar age and sex. The atrophic appearance is believed to be related to nutrition; similar findings have been reported in patients with anorexia nervosa (Enzmann 1977; Kohlmeyer 1983). The atrophy is reversible following restoration of proper nutrition. Prominence of the cortical sulci with apparent ventricular enlargement is also seen in patients with acquired immunodeficiency syndrome (AIDS) (Bursztyn 1984) and in patients with chronic renal failure who are on hemodialysis (Kretzschmar 1983; Savazzi, 1986). Similar

CT findings are noted in patients with hepatic encephalopathy: they are most likely nonspecific and may even be attributed to alcohol intake and nutritional status.

Reyes et al. (1985) reported intracranial calcifications in three adult patients with raised serum lead levels and known exposure to lead for 30 or more years working in a lead smelting plant. Puntiform, curvilinear, specklike, and diffuse calcifications are noted in the subcortical, basal ganglioma, and cerebellum.

Drug-Related Atrophy

Atrophic changes have been reported on CT studies with a variety of drugs such as steroids, Dilantin, methotrexate, amphetamines, and cannabis (including marijuana) and in alcoholics.

Persons on steroids for a prolonged period demonstrate enlarged ventricles with prominence of the cortical sulci. In addition, an increase in hypodensity of the white matter has been reported (Bentson 1978). Return to normal ventricles and sulci has been documented when the steroid medication is stopped (Heinz 1977; Bentson 1978; Okuno 1980).

Increase in periventricular hypodensity and focal ventricular enlargement may also be seen in patients on methotrexate. But with methotrexate, focal enhancement of the white matter occurs in periventricular regions. The enhancement is presumed to be due to focal areas of drug-induced vasculitis.

A few reports have dealt with the CT findings in patients who are on amphetamines, cannabis, and marijuana (Rambaugh 1980; Co 1977; Kuehnle 1977). Patients on amphetamines were reported to have changes indicative of cerebral atrophy. However, in these cases, since there was an associated history of head trauma and use of alcohol, amphetamine may not have been the cause of atrophy. Animal studies do, however, suggest that chronic use of intravenous amphetamines can produce cerebral atrophy (Rambaugh 1980).

Prolonged use of Dilantin has been shown to result in atrophy predominantly involving the cerebellar hemisphere. This finding has been shown both by pneumoencephalography and by CT studies (Ghatak 1976; McCrea 1980; Baier 1984; Lindvall 1984) (Fig. 5-21). Dilantin in toxic doses, however, does not result in cerebral atrophy.

Numerous studies document the effect of chronic alcoholism by CT studies. Chronic alcoholism results in enlargement of the ventricles and sulci when compared to controls of similar sex and age. It is possible that in a few patients the cerebral atrophic process may be due also to hepatic encephalopathy, since studies have shown liver damage in a majority of patients who are chronic alcohol abusers. Chronic alcohol abusers show not only cerebral but also cerebellar atrophy (Fox 1976). It has also been shown that the degree of cerebral atrophy correlates with impairment of the nondominant hemisphere functions but not of the intelligence quotient (Cala 1978). There have been a few studies in which, following abstinence from alcohol, there was a reversal of the atrophic process as documented by CT (Carlen 1978;

Artmann 1981). The reversal involved the cortical sulci more than the ventricles. In one series, the reversal in CT appearance occurred and corresponded to the clinical improvement between 9 and 20 months following abstinence (Artmann 1981).

Cerebellar Atrophy

Isolated atrophy of the cerebellum is seen in a variety of degenerative disorders (Abe 1983; Andreula 1984), as well as being secondary to the toxic effect or prolonged use of drugs such as alcohol and diphenylhydantoin. In chronic alcoholism, cerebellar degeneration primarily involves the vermis and, to a lesser extent, the cerebellum (Allen 1979). Prolonged use of diphenylhydantoin in toxic doses has been shown to produce degeneration of the Purkinje cells of the cerebellum in animals. Similar findings can also be seen with CT (Fig. 5-22). In *olivopontocerebellar degeneration*, one form of spinocerebellar degeneration, atrophic changes involve the inferior olive, pons, and cerebellum (Fig. 5-22) (Savoiardo 1983).

The CT changes are similar in all the above-described clinical processes. Atrophy of one component may be more significant than the other. CT diagnosis of cerebellar atrophy is based on demonstrating two or more of the following features (Allen 1979):

1. Enlargement of the cerebellar sulci by more than 1 mm
2. Enlargement of the cerebellopontine cisterns by more than 1.5 mm, the measurement being taken at the superior lateral margin of the cerebellar hemisphere and adjacent petrous bone
3. Enlargement of the fourth ventricle by more than 4 mm
4. Enlargement of the superior cerebellar cistern

Isolated enlargement of the fourth ventricle and presence of a giant cisterna magna, as proposed by Baker et al. (1976), do not signify cerebellar atrophy.

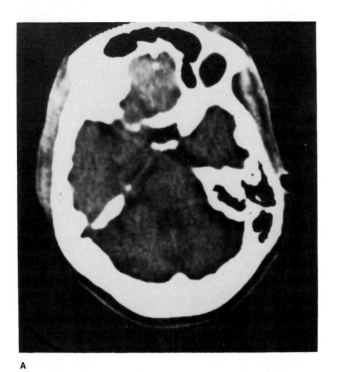

A

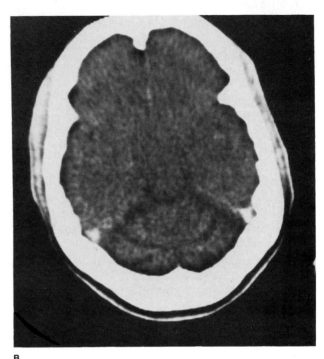

B

C

Figure 5-21 Drug-related cerebellar atrophy: CT in a patient on prolonged diphenylhydantoin medication. The folia of the vermis and to a lesser extent the cerebellar folia are prominent. The fourth ventricle and the cerebellopontine cisterns are mildly dilated. Prolonged use of diphenylhydantoin results in cerebellar atrophy predominantly involving the vermis. Similar changes can also be seen with chronic ethanol use.

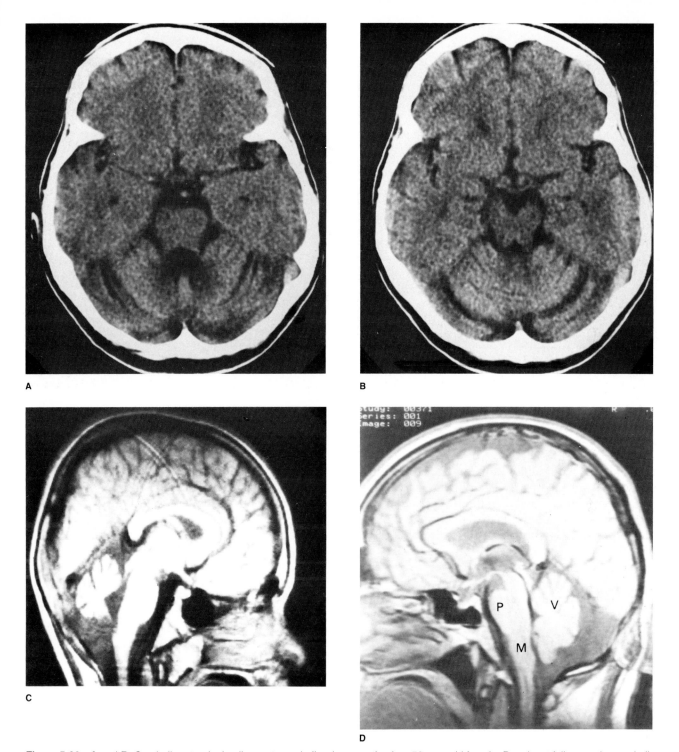

Figure 5-22 **A** and **B.** Cerebellar atrophy in olivopontocerebellar degeneration in a 58-year-old female. Prominent folia over the cerebellar hemispheres are noted as well as generous CSF spaces at the prepontine, interpeduncular, and ambient cistern levels. **C** and **D.** MRI (sagittal T$_1$-WI) shows atrophic cerebellum and vermis (V) and small anterior pons (P) and medulla oblongata (M). Large vermian cistern and cisterna magna and frontal lobe atrophy are also present on two different patients.

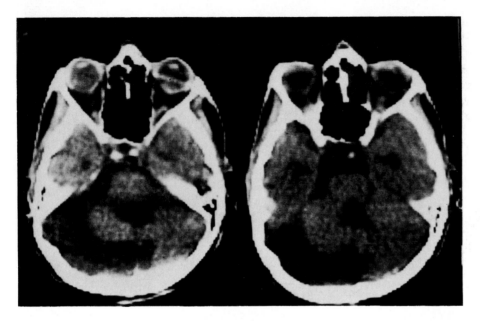

Figure 5-23 Cerebellar atrophy secondary to vascular occlusion. There is focal loss of cerebellar parenchyma on the right side with resulting widening of the cerebellopontine cistern. The fourth ventricle is dilated. Absence of deformity and contralateral displacement of the dilated fourth ventricle excludes the possibility of a cerebellopontine angle mass.

Focal cerebellar atrophy is most often secondary to a vascular process or trauma (Fig. 5-23).

Schizophrenia

In chronic schizophrenics, enlargment of the third and fourth ventricles and bilateral widening of the sylvian fissures are noted without sulcal dilation, similar to NPH (Pandurangi 1984). Lateral ventricular enlargement (Johnstone 1976; Andreasen 1982), third ventricular enlargement (Dewan 1983*a*), and evidence of cerebellar atrophy (Dewan 1983*b*) are also presented. Density increase in both periventricular nuclei and cerebellum (Dewan 1983*a,b*) is of uncertain significance. The exact neuropathologic correlation and clinical implication of these CT findings are not clear at this time.

Magnetic Resonance Imaging

Magnetic resonance imaging allows for excellent visualization of the brain and CSF spaces. Whether signal characterization will be able to determine etiological factors in certain atrophic brain conditions and CSF circulation disturbances is presently under investigation (see Chapter 17). CT, at present, is valuable in recognizing not only space-occupying treatable lesions, but also in diagnosing numerous primary degenerative diseases (LeMay, 1986).

Bibliography

ABE S, MIYASAKA K, TASHIRO K, TAKEI H, ISU T, TSURU M: Evaluation of the brainstem with high-resolution CT in cerebellar atrophic processes. *AJNR* **4**(3):446–449, May–June 1983.

ADAM P, FABRE N, GUELL A, BESSOLES G, ROULLEAU J, BES A: Cortical atrophy in Parkinson's disease: correlation between clinical and CT findings with special emphasis on prefrontal atrophy. *AJNR* **4**(3):442–445, May–June 1983.

ADAM RD, FISHER CM, HAKIM S, OJEMANN RG, SWEET WH: Symptomatic occult hydrocephalus with "normal" cerebrospinal fluid pressure. *N Engl J Med* **273**:117–126, 1965.

AGNOLI A, RUGGIERI S, DENARO A, MARTUCCI N, TANFANI G, STOCCHI F: White matter disease (Binswanger's encephalopathy) in chronic cerebrovascular disorders. *Monogr Neural Sci* **11**:144–149, 1984.

ALLEN JH, MARTIN JT, MCLAIN LW: Computed tomography in cerebellar atrophic processes. *Radiology* **130**:379–382, 1979.

ANDREASEN NC, SMITH MR, JACOBY CG et al: Ventricular enlargement in schizophrenia; definition and prevalence. *Am J Psych* **139**:292–296, 1982.

ANDREULA CF, CAMICIA M, LORUSSO A, D'APRILE P, FEDERICO F, BRINDICCI D, CARELLA A: Clinical and CT parameters in degenerative cerebellar atrophy in aged patients. *Neuroradiology* **26**(1):29–30, 1984.

ARTMANN H, GAIL MV, HACKER H, HERRHICH J: Reversible enlargement of cerebral spinal fluid spaces in chronic alcoholics. *Am J Neuroradiol* **2**:23–27, 1981.

BAIER WK, BECK U, DOOSE H, KLINGE H, HIRSCH W: Cerebellar atrophy following diphenylhydantoin intoxication. *Neuropediatrics* **15**(2):76–81, May 1984.

BAKER HL, HOUSER OW: Computed tomography in the diagnosis of posterior fossa lesions. *Radiol Clin N Am* **14**:129–147, 1976.

BANNA M: The ventriculo-cephalic ratio on CT. *J Can Assoc Radiol* 1977.

BARRON SA, JACOBS L, KINKEL WR: Changes in size of normal lateral ventricles during aging determined by computerized tomography. *Neurology* **26**:1011–1013, 1976.

BECKER H, SCHNEIDER E, HACKER H, FISCHER PA: Cerebral atrophy in Parkinson's disease—represented by CT. *Arch Psychiat Nervenkr* **227**:81–88, 1979.

BENSON DF, LEMAY M, PATTEN DH, RUBENS AB: Diagnosis of normal pressure hydrocephalus. *N Engl J Med* **283**:610–615, 1970.

BENTSON J, REZA M, WINTER J, WILSON G: Steroids and apparent cerebral atrophy on computed tomography scans. *J Comput Assist Tomogr* **2**:16–23, 1978.

BINSWANGER O: Die Abgrenzung der allgemeinen progressive Paralyse. *Berl Klin Wochenschr* **31**:1103–1105, 1137–1139, 1180–1186, 1894.

BLACK PM: Idiopathic normal-pressure hydrocephalus. *J Neurosurg* **52**:371–377, 1980.

BRINKMAN SD, SARWAR M, LEVINE HS, MORRIS HS: Quantitative index of computed tomography in dementia and normal aging. *Radiology* **138**:89, 1981.

BRODY H: Organization of the human cerebral cortex: III. A study of aging in the human cerebral cortex. *J Comp Neurol* **102**:511–556, 1955.

BURSZTYN EM, LEE BC, BAUMAN J: CT of acquired immunodeficiency syndrome. *AJNR* **5**(6):711–714, November–December 1984.

CALA LA, JONES B, MASTAGLIA FL, WILEY B: Brain atrophy and intellectual impairment in heavy drinkers—a clinical, psychometric and computerized tomography study. *Aust NZ J Med* **8**:147–153, 1978.

CALA LA, MASTAGLIA FL: Computerized axial tomography in the detection of brain damage. *Med J Aust* **2**:616–620, 1980.

CARLEN PL, WORTZMAN G, HOLGATE RC, WILKINSON DA, RANKIN JG: Reversible cerebral atrophy in recently abstinent chronic alcoholics measured by computed tomography scans. *Science* **200**:1076–1078, 1978.

CO BT, GOODWIN DW, GADO M, MIKHAEL M, HILL SY: Absence of cerebral atrophy in chronic cannabis users—evaluation by computerized transaxial tomography. *JAMA* **237**:1229–1230, 1977.

COBLENTZ JM, MATTIS S, ZINGESSER LH, KASOFF SS, WISNIEWSKI HM, KATZMAN R: Presenile dementia. *Arch Neurol* **29**:299–308, 1973.

DELEON MJ et al: Correlations between computerized tomographic changes and behavioural deficits in senile dementia. *Lancet* **2**:859–860, 1979.

DEWAN MJ, PANDURANGI AK, LEE SH et al: Central brain morphology in chronic schizophrenic patients: a controlled CT study. *Biol Psych* **18**:1133–1140, 1983a.

DEWAN MJ, PANDURANGI AK, LEE SH et al: Cerebellar morphology in chronic schizophrenic patients: a controlled CT study. *Psych Research* **10**:97–103, 1983b.

DI CHIRO G, REAMES PM, MATHEWS WB: RISA vetriculography and RISA cisternography. *Neurology* **14**:185–191, 1964.

DI CHIRO G, ARIMITSU T, BROOKS RA, MORGENTHALER DG, JOHNSTON GS, JONES AE, KELLER MR: Computed tomography profiles of periventricular hypodensity in hydrocephalus and leukoencephalopathy. *Radiology* **130**:661–666, 1979.

DU BOULAY GH, RUIZ JS, ROSE FC, STEVENS JM, ZILKHA KJ: CT changes associated with migraine. *AJNR* **4**(3):472–473, May–June 1983.

ENZMANN DR, LANE B: Cranial computed tomography findings in anorexia nervosa. *J Comput Assist Tomogr* **1**:410–414, 1977.

ENZMANN DR, NORMAN D, PRICE DC, NEWTON TH: Metrizamide and radionuclide cisternography in communicating hydrocephalus. *Radiology* **130**:681–686, 1979.

EPSTEIN F, NAIDICH T, KRICHEFF I, CHASE N, LIN J, RANSOHOFF J: Role of computerized axial tomography in diagnosis, treatment and follow-up of hydrocephalus. *Child Brain* **3**:91–100, 1977.

FLODMARK O, BECKER L, HARWOOD NASH D, FITZHARDINGE P, FITZ C, CHUANG S: Correlation between CT and autopsy in premature and fullterm neonates that have suffered perinatal asphyxia. *Radiology* **137**:93–103, 1980.

FOX JK, KASZNIAK AW, HUCKMAN M: Computerized tomographic scanning not very helpful in dementia—nor in craniopharyngioma. *N Engl J Med* **300**:437, 1979.

FOX JK, RAMSEY RG, HUCKMAN MS, PROSKE AE: Cerebral ventricular enlargement: Chronic alcoholics examined by computed tomography. *JAMA* **236**:365–368, 1976.

FOX JH, TOPEL JL, HUCKMAN MS: Use of computerized tomography in senile dementia. *J Neurol Neurosurg Psychiatry* **8**:948–953, 1975.

GADO MH, COLEMAN RE, LEE KS, MIKHAEL MA, ALDERSON PO, ARCHER CR: Correlation between computerized transaxial tomography and radionuclide cisternography in dementia. *Neurology* **26**:555–560, 1976.

GADO MH, HUGHES CP, DANZIGER W, CHI D, JOST G, BERG L: Volumetric measurements of the cerebrospinal fluid spaces in subjects with dementia and controls. Presented in the Neuroradiology Section of the 67th Annual Meeting of the Radiological Society of North America, December 1981.

GADO M, PATEL J, HUGHES CP, DANZIGER W, BERG L: Brain atrophy in dementia judged by CT scan ranking. *AJNR* **4**(3):499–500, May–June 1983a.

GADO M, HUGHES CP, DANZIGER W, CHI D: Aging, dementia, and brain atrophy: a longitudinal computed tomographic study. *AJNR* **4**(3):699–702, May 1983b.

GAJDUSEK DC, GIBBS CJ, ASHER DM, BROWN P, DIWAN A, HOFFMAN P, NEMO G, ROBWER R, WHITE L: Precautions in medical care of, and in handling materials from, patients with transmissible virus dementia (Jakob-Creutzfeldt disease). *N Engl J Med* **297**:1253–1258, 1977.

GEORGE AE, DELEON MJ, FERNS SH, KRICHEFF II: Parenchymal CT correlates of senile dementia (Alzheimer's disease)—loss of grey-white matter discriminability. *Am J Neuroradiol* **2**:205–213, 1981.

GHATAK NR, SANTOSO RA, MCKINNEY WM: Cerebellar degeneration following long-term phenytoin therapy. *Neurology* **26**:818–820, 1976.

GLUCK E, RADU EW, MUNDT C, GERHARDT P: A computed tomogaphic protective study of chronic schizophrenics. *Neuroradiology* **20**:167–169, 1980.

GOMORI JM, STEINER I, MELAMED E, COOPER G: The assessment of changes in brain volume using combined linear measurements. A CT-scan study. *Neuroradiology* **26**(1):21–24, 1984.

GREITZ TVB: Cerebral blood flow in occult hydrocephalus studied with angiography and the xenon 133 clearance method. *Acta Radiol* **8**:376–384, 1969a.

GREITZ TVB, GREPE AOL, KALMER SF, LOPEZ J: Pre- and postoperative evauation of cerebral blood flow in low-pressure hydrocephalus. *J Neurosurg* **31**:644–651, 1969b.

GUNASEKERA L, RICHARDSON AE: Computerized axial tomography in idiopathic hydrocephalus. *Brain* **100**:749–754, 1977.

GYLDENSTED C, KOSTELJANETZ M: Measurements of the normal hemispheric sulci and computer tomography. *Neuroradiology* **10**:147–149, 1975.

GYLDESTED C, KOSTELJANETZ M: Measurements of the normal ventricular system with computer tomography of the brain. *Neuroradiology* **10**:205–213, 1976.

GLYDENSTED C: Measurements of the normal ventricular system and hemispheric sulci of 100 adults with computed tomography. *Neuroradiology* **14**:183–192, 1977.

HACKER H, ARTMANN H: The calcification of CSF spaces in CT. *Neuroradiology* **16**:190–192, 1978.

HAHN FJY, KEAN RIM: Frontal ventricular dimensions on normal computed tomography. *Am J Roentogenol Radium Ther Nucl Med* **126**:593–596, 1976.

HAKIM S: Some observations on C.S.F. pressure: Hydrocephalic syndrome in adults with "normal" CSF pressure. Thesis No. 957, Javeriana University, School of Medicine, Bogota, Colombia, 1964.

HARIK SI, POST MJD: Computed tomography in Wilson's disease. *Neurology* **31**:107–110, 1981.

HATAZAWA J, YAMAGUCHI T, ITO M, YAMAURA H, MATSUZAWA T: Association of hypertension with increased atrophy of brain matter in the elderly. *J Am Geriat Soc* **32**(5):370–374, May 1984.

HAUG G: Age and sex dependence of the size of normal ventricles on computed tomography. *Neuroradiology* **14**:201–204, 1977.

HEINZ E, DAVIS DO, KARP HR: Abnormal isotope cisternography in symptomatic occult hydrocephalus. *Radiology* **95**:109–120, 1970.

HEINZ E, MARTINEX J, HAWNGGELI A: Reversibility of cerebral atrophy in anorexia nervosa and Cushing's syndrome. *J Comput Assist Tomogr* **1**:415–418, 1977.

HINDMARSH T, GREITZ T: Computer cisternography in the diagnosis of communicating hydrocephalus. *Acta Radiol* **346**:91–97, 1975.

HIRATSUKA H, FUJIWARA K, OKASA K, TAKASATA Y, TSUYUMU M, INABA Y: Modification of periventricular hypodensity in hydrocephalus and ventricular reflux in metrizamide CT cisternography. *J Comput Assist Tomogr* **3**:204–208, 1979.

HOPKINS LN, BAKAY L, KINKEL WR, GRAND W: Demonstration of transventricular CSF absorption by computerized tomography. *Acta Neurochir (Wien)* **39**:151–157, 1977.

HUCKMAN MS, FOX J, TOPEL J: The validity of criteria for evaluation of cerebral atrophy by computed tomography. *Radiology* **116**:85–92, 1975.

HUGHES CP, GADO M: Computed tomography and aging of the brain. *Radiology* **139**:391–396, 1981.

JACOBS L, KINKEL WR: Computerized axial transverse tomography in normal pressure hydrocephalus. *Neurology* **26**:501–507, 1976a.

JACOBS L, CONTI D, KINKEL WR, MANNING EL: Normal pressure hydrocephalus. *JAMA* **235**:510–512, 1976*b*.

JACOBSON PL, FARMER TW: The "hypernormal" CT scan in dementia: Bilateral isodense subdural hematoma. *Neurology* **29**:1522–1524, 1979.

JACOBY RJ, LEVY R, DAWSON JM: Computed tomography in the elderly: 1. The normal population. *Br J Psychiatry* **136**:249–255, 1980*a*.

JACOBY RJ, LEVY R: Computed tomography in the elderly: 2. Senile dementia: Diagnosis and functional impairment. *Br J Psychiatry* **136**:256–269, 1980*b*.

JACOBY RJ, LEVY R: CT scanning and the investigation of dementia: A review. *J Roy Soc Med* **73**:366–369, 1980*c*.

JAMES AE, FLOR WJ, NOVAK GR, RIBAS JL, PARKER JL, SICKEL WL: The ultrastructural basis of periventricular edema: Preliminary studies. *Radiology* **135**:757–760, 1980.

JENSEN F: Acquired hydrocephalus: III. A pathophysiological study correlated with neuropathological findings and clinical manifestations. *Acta Neurochir (Wien)* **47**:91–104, 1979.

JOHNSTONE EC, CROW TJ, FRITH CD, HUSBAND J: Cerebral ventricular size and cognitive impairment in chronic schizophrenia. *Lancet* **30**:924–926, 1976.

JOHNSTONE EC, CROW TJ, FRITH CD et al: Cerebral ventricular size and cognitive impairment in chronic schizophrenia. *Lancet* **2**:924–926, 1976.

KATZMAN R, HUSSEY F: A simple constant-infusion manometric test for measurement of CSF absorption. *Neurology* **20**:534–544, 1970.

KISHORE PRS, LIPPER MH, DASILVA AAD, GUDEMAN SK, ABBAS SA: Delayed sequelae of head injury. *Comput Tomogr* **4**:287–295, 1980.

KOHLMEYER K, LEHMKUHL G, POUTSKA F: Computed tomography of anorexia nervosa. *AJNR* **4**(3):437–438, May–June 1983.

KONO E, KONO R, SHIDA K: Computerized tomographies of 34 patients at the chronic stage of acute carbon monoxide poisoning. *Arch Psychiatr Nervenkr* **233**(4):271–278, 1983.

KRETZSCHMAR K, NIX W, ZSCHIEDRICH H, PHILIPP T: Morphologic cerebral changes in patients undergoing dialysis for renal failure. *AJNR* **4**(3):439–441, May–June 1983.

KUEHNLE J, MENDELSON J, DAVIS K, NEW P: Computed tomographic examination of heavy marijuana smokers. *JAMA* **237**:1231–1232, 1977.

KVICALA V, VYMAZAL J, NEVSIMALOVA S: Computed tomography of Wilson's disease. *AJNR* **4**(3):429–430, May–June 1983.

LAFFEY PA, PEYSTER RG, NATHAN R, HASKIN ME, MCGINLEY JA: Computed tomography and aging: results in a normal elderly population. *Neuroradiology* **26**(4):273–278, 1984.

LEMAY M, NEW PFJ: Radiological diagnosis of occult normal pressure hydrocephalus. *Radiology* **96**:347–358, 1970.

LEMAY M CT changes in dementing diseases: A review. *Neuroradiology* **7**:841–853, 1986

LEMAY M, HOCHBERG FH: Ventricular differences between hydrostatic hydrocephalus and hydrocephalus ex vacuo by computed tomography. *Neuroradiology* **17**:191–195, 1979.

LINDVALL O, NILSSON B: Cerebellar atrophy following phenytoin intoxication. *Ann Neurol* **16**(2):258–260, August 1984.

MACCHI G, ABBAMONDI AL, DI TRAPANI G, SBRICCOLI A: On the white matter lesions of the Creutzfeldt-Jakob disease. *Can J Neurol Sci* **63**(2):197–206, February 1984.

MARMAROU A, SHULMAN K, LAMORGESE J: Compartmental analysis of compliance and outflow resistance of the cerebrospinal fluid system. *J Neurosurg* **43**:523–534, 1975.

MCCREA ES, RAO KCUG, DIACONIS JN: Roentgenographic changes during long-term diphenylhydantoin therapy. *South Med J* **73**(3):310–311, 1980.

MCCULLOUGH DC, HARBERT JC, DICHIRO G, OMMAYA SK: Prognostic criteria for cerebrospinal fluid shunting from isotope cisternography in communicating hydrocephalus. *Neurology* **20**:594–598, 1970.

MCGEACHI RE, FLEMING JO, SHARER LR, HYMAN RA: Diagnosis of Pick's disease by computed tomography. *J Comput Assist Tomogr* **3**:113–115, 1979.

MEESE W, KLUGE W, GRUMME T, HOPFENMULLER W: CT evauation of the CSF space of healthy persons. *Neuroradiology* **19**:131–136, 1980.

MORI K, HANDA T, MURATA T, NAKANO Y: Periventricular lucency in computed tomography of hydrocephalus and cerebral atrophy. *J Comput Assist Tomogr* **4**:204–209, 1980.

NAESER MA, GEBHARDT C, LEVINE HC: Decreased computerized tomography numbers in patients with presenile dementia. *Arch Neurol* **37**:401–418, 1980.

NARDIZZI LR: Computerized tomographic correlate of carbon monoxide poisoning. *Arch Neurol* **36**:38–39, 1979.

NELSON JR, GOODMAN SJ: An evaluation of the cerebrospinal fluid test for hydrocephalus. *Neurology* **21**:1037–1053, 1971.

OKUNO T, MASATOSHI I, KONISHI Y, MIEKO Y, NAKANO Y: Cerebral atrophy following ACTH therapy. *J Comput Assist Tomogr* **4**:20–23, 1980.

PANDURANGI AK, DEWAN MJ, LEE SH et al: The ventricular system in chronic schizophrenic patients: a controlled CT study. *Brit J Psych* **144**:172–176, 1984.

PEDERSEN HM, GYLDENSTED M, GYLDENSTED C: Measurement of the normal ventricular system and supratentorial subarachnoid space in children with computed tomography. *Neuroradiology* **17**:231–237, 1979.

PENN WD, BELANGER MG, YASNOFF WA: Ventricular volume in mass computed from CT scans. *Ann Neurol* **3**:216–223, 1978.

RAMBAUGH CL et al: Cerebral CT findings in drug abuse: Clinical and experimental observations. *J Comput Assist Tomogr* **4**:330–334, 1980.

RAMSEY RG, HUCKMAN MS: Computed tomography of porencephaly and other cerebrospinal fluid–containing lesions. *Radiology* **123**:73–77, 1977.

RAO KCVG, BRENNAN TG, GARCIA JH: Computed tomography in the diagnosis of Creutzfeldt-Jakob disease. *J Comput Assist Tomogr* **1**:211–215, 1977.

REYES PF, GONZALEZ CF, ZALEWSKA MK, BESARAB A: Intracranial calcifications in adults with chronic lead poisoning. *AJNR* **6**:905–908, 1985.

ROBERTS MA, CAIRD FL: Computerized tomography and intellectual impairment in the elderly. *J Neurol Neurosurg Psychiatry* **39**:986–989, 1976.

ROPPER AH, HATTEN HP, DAVIS KR: Computed tomography of Wilson's disease: Report of two cases. *Ann Neurol* **5**:102–103, 1979.

ROSENBERG GA, KORNFELD M, STOVRING J, BICKNELL JM: Subcortical arteriosclerotic encephalopathy (Binswanger) and computerized tomography. *Neurology* **29**:1102–1106, 1979.

RUDICK RA, JOYUT RT: Normal pressure hydrocephalus: A treatable dementia. *Tex Med* **76**:46–49, 1980.

RUECK JD, CREVITS L, COSTER WD, SIEBEN G, ECKEN H: Pathogenesis of Binswanger chronic progressive subcortical encephalopathy. *Neurology* **30**:920–928, 1980.

SALMON JH: Adult hydrocephalus: Evaluation of shunt therapy in 80 patients. *J Neurosurg* **37**:423–428, 1972.

SAVAZZI FGM: Cerebral CT in uremic and hemodyalized patients. *J Comput Assist Tomogr* **10:** 567–570, 1986.

SAVOIARDO M, BRACCHI M, PASSERINI A, VISCIANI A, DI DONATO S, COCCHINI F: Computed tomography of olivopontocerebellar degeneration. *AJNR* 4(3):509–512, May–June 1983.

SAWA G, WATSON C, TERBRUGGE K, CHIU M: Delayed encephalopathy following carbon monoxide intoxication. *Can J Neurological Sci* **8:**77–79, 1981.

SCHEIBEL ME et al: Progressive dendritic changes in aging human cortex. *Exp Neurol* **47:**392–403, 1975.

SCHNEIDER E, BECKER H, FISHER PA, GRAU H, JACOBY P, BRINKMAN R: The course of brain atrophy in Parkinson's disease. *Arch Psychiatr Nervenkr* **227:**89–95, 1979.

SCHUTZ H, TERBRUGGE K, CHIU M, MONGUL A, TAYLOR F: Determination of C.S.F. shunt patency with a lumbar infusion test. *Neurosurgery* **58:**553–556, 1983.

SHENKIN HA, GREENBERG J, BOUZARTH WF, GUTTERMAN P, MORALES JO: Ventricular shunting for relief of senile symptoms. *JAMA* **225:**1486–1489, 1973.

SIMMONS JT, PASTAKIA B, CHASE TN, SCHULTZ CW: MRI in Huntington disease. *AJNR* **7:**25–28, 1986.

SJAASTAD O, SKALPE IO, ENGESET A: The width of the temporal horn in the differential diagnosis between pressure hydrocephalus and hydrocephalus ex vacuo. *Neurology* **19:**1087–1093, 1969.

STEIN SC, LANGFITT TW: Normal pressure hydrocephalus: Predicting the results of cerebrospinal fluid shunting. *J Neurosurg* **41:**463–470, 1974.

SYMON L, HINZPETER T: Enigma of normal pressure hydrocephalus. *Clin Neurosurg* **24:**285–315, 1977.

SYNEK V, REUBEN JR, GAWLER J, DUBOULAY GH: Comparison of the measurements of the cerebral ventricles obtained by CT scanning and pneumoencephalography. *Neuroradiology* **17:**149–151, 1976.

TAKEDA S, MATSUZAWA T: Brain atrophy during aging: a quantitative study using computed tomography. *J Am Geriatr Soc* **32**(7):520–524, July 1984.

TATOR CH, FLEMING JFR, SHEPPARD RH, TURNER VM: A radioisotope test for communicating hydrocephalus. *J Neurosurg* **28:**327–340, 1968.

TERBRUGGE KG, SCHUTZ H. CHIU MC, TAYLOR F: CSF dynamics in adults with hydrocephalus. Presented at the 18th annual meeting, American Society of Neuroradiology, March 16–21, 1980, Los Angeles.

TERRENCE CF, DELANEY JF, ALBERTS MC: Computed tomography for Huntington's disease. *Neuroradiology* **13:**173–175, 1977.

TOMLINSON BE, BLESSED G, ROTH M: Observations on the brains of demented old people. *J Neurol Sci* **11:**205–242, 1970.

WEINBERGER DR, TORREY EF, NEOPHYTIDES AN, WYATT RJ: Lateral cerebral ventricular enlargement in chronic schizophenia. *Arch Gen Psychiatry* **36:**735–739, 1979.

WOLINSKY JS, BARNES BD, MARGOLIS MT: Diagnostic tests in normal pressure hydrocephalus. *Neurology* **23:**706–713, 1973.

WOLPERT S: The ventricular size on computed tomography. *J Comput Assist Tomogr* **1:**222–226, 1977.

YAMARU H, ITO M, KUBOTA K, MAFSUZAWA T: Brain atrophy during aging: A quantitative study with computer tomography. *J Gerontol* **35:**492–497, 1980.

ZATZ LM, JERNIGAN TL, AHUMADA AJ JR: Changes on computed cranial tomography with aging: intracranial fluid volume. *Am J Neuroradiol* 3(1):1–12, 1982.

ZEUMER H. SCHONSKY B, STRUM KW: Predominant white matter involvement in subcortical arteriosclerotic encephalopathy (Binswanger disease). *J Comput Assist Tomogr* **4:**14–19, 1980.

ZILKHA A: CT of cerebral hemiatrophy. *Am J Roentgenol Radium Ther Nucl Med* **135:**263–267, 1980.

6

THE VENTRICLES AND SUBARACHNOID SPACES IN CHILDREN

Charles R. Fitz

HYDROCEPHALUS

Ventricular dilatation does not necessarily mean hydrocephalus. Several other causes of ventricular dilatation can be identified by CT. Physiologic dilatation occurs in premature infants (Fig. 6-1), being greatest in those born early in the mother's pregnancy and approaching normal size in those born after approximately 36 weeks of gestation. Mild ventricular enlargement occurs in some megalencephalies such as Soto's syndrome (Fig. 6-2). Congenital malformations may have a developmental or dysplastic ventricular enlargement. Atrophic ventricular enlargement, to be discussed later in this chapter, may be present with or secondary to hydrocephalus.

The definition of hydrocephalus as a dynamic process (Harwood-Nash and Fitz 1976, Chap. 10) due to a blockage of CSF flow somewhere along its pathway or an overproduction of CSF remains valid. Because it is a dynamic process, the static image of a single CT examination may not be sufficient to indicate clearly whether the ventricular enlargement is secondary to hydrocephalus. Experience, however, often offers the physician clues to help decide whether true hydrocephalus is present.

CT Evaluation of Suspected Hydrocephalus

Most hydrocephalus in childhood begins and is diagnosed in early infancy. Most cases are congenital,

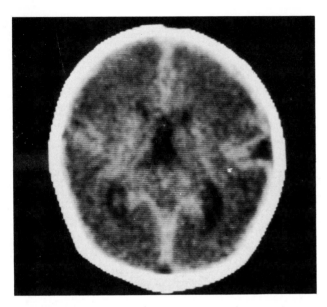

Figure 6-1 CT of premature infant (30-week gestation age) showing physiologic mild dilatation of the lateral ventricles. The sylvian fissures are also wide. CT done without contrast.

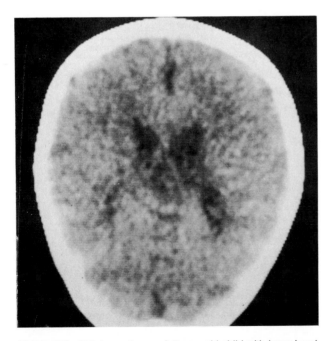

Figure 6-2 Soto's syndrome. A 5-year-old child with large head and mild retardation shows mild ventricular and sulcal enlargement suggestive of Soto's syndrome. There was no evidence of increased intracranial pressure.

though they result from a variety of causes. Given a short history of enlarging head in an infant under 3 months of age, with no obvious preceding event such as infection or hemorrhage, it is the author's routine practice to perform the CT examination without contrast, using 10-mm slices. If the results of the initial examination are unusual or suggestive of a disease process that would become clearer with intravenous contrast injection, this is given and the examination is repeated. Other views, especially coronal or clival perpendicular, may be obtained, as well as thinner, 5-mm slices in areas where greater detail is needed, though this is uncommon.

The radiation dose should be kept as low as possible in the newborn. Most examinations of infants are done at the author's institution at a dose of approximately 13 rad (GE 9800 third-generation scanner) if extra views or contrast enhancement are not required. The dose is even lower for premature infants.

In a child of 6 months or more, intravenous contrast is always part of the examination, since congenital causes for hydrocephalus are less common at that age and tumor in particular must be excluded as a cause of hydrocephalus. Signs of inflammation or trauma, such as subdural membranes, may also be seen.

Intraventricular contrast thus continues to have a limited, though important, role in the diagnosis of hydrocephalus. It is no longer necessary to outline the ventricles with air, but air or metrizamide can give important information as to the sites of obstruction and the location of cysts that are the occasional cause of hydrocephalus (Marc 1980) and can be introduced via the shunt reservoir after treatment of hydrocephalus. An average of 1 to 3 ml of 210 to 220 mg I per ml metrizamide is injected very slowly through the shunt tubing so as to layer on the floor of the frontal horns or directly into the third ventricle, with the patient in a sitting position. The head is flexed slightly forward to hold the metrizamide in the frontal horns if it has not already entered the third ventricle. The head is slowly extended or rotated toward the supine position to allow the contrast to drain into the third ventricle and outline its floor, the aqueduct, and the fourth ventricle if the aqueduct is patent. The initial part of

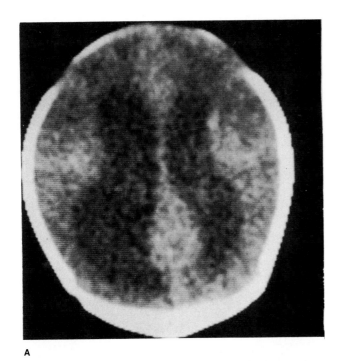

A

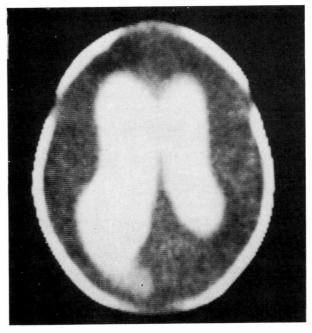

B

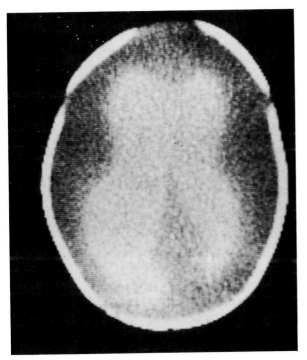

C

Figure 6-3 Transependymal absorption of metrizamide. **A.** CT without contrast in an infant with aqueduct stenosis shows large lateral ventricles. **B.** CT immediately following metrizamide ventriculogram shows the contrast agent within the ventricular system. **C.** Examination 24 hours later using the same window setting shows transmission of ventricular contrast through the entire brain. Further examination showed continued decrease in ventricular density and increase in brain density.

this examination is best done on a conventional pneumoencephalographic unit. If an obstruction is encountered, CT can be done to see if any metrizamide passes the obstruction. If the ventricular system is patent, CT can be used to follow the metrizamide flow into the subarachnoid space and to watch for any block. The examination can in this way substitute for a radionuclide study of the cerebral spinal fluid flow. In an infant with bulging fontanelle, injection of similar amounts of metrizamide following a ventricular tap may provide the diagnosis in occasional cases.

A serendipitous observation in examinations done in this manner has been the transependymal absorption of the metrizamide through the brain parenchyma (Fig. 6-3)(Fitz 1978*b*), confirming the conclusion of others that periventricular hypodensities are due to transependymal passage of CSF (Milhorat 1970; Hiratsuka 1979).

Metrizamide has little or no place in the primary CT investigation of hydrocephalus. In infants in whom a cyst or intraventricular adhesions are suspected, the use of ultrasound is often very helpful. Cyst walls and membranes can often be well seen.

Intraventricular Obstructive Hydrocephalus

This term refers to the obstruction of CSF flow anywhere along the ventricular pathways from the lateral ventricles to the fourth ventricular outlets, commonly called *noncommunicating hydrocephalus*. The cause of congenital intraventricular obstructive hydrocephalus (IVOH), excluding toxic, infectious, and posthemorrhagic causes, is usually aqueduct stenosis, often associated with the Chiari II malformation.

OCCLUSION OF THE FORAMEN OF MONRO IVOH due to occlusion of one or both of the foramina of Monro is uncommon. Intraventricular hemorrhage from trauma or other causes of bleeding, such as arteriovenous malformation or hemophilia, can cause a temporary clot in the foramen with resulting hydrocephalus, but this is usually temporary in children. Infection is also an uncommon cause of obstruction at this site. Congenital atresia is extremely rare (Taboada 1979).

The most common obstructing lesion is tumor of various types. Suprasellar masses, especially craniopharyngiomas, extend upward and sometimes compress the third ventricle and cause a partial obstruction of the foramen of Monro (Fig. 6-4). Intraventricular tumors or cysts and arachnoid cysts of the suprasellar cistern (Fig. 6-5) may also obstruct the foramen of Monro, as can hypothalamic astrocytomas.

In the case of tumors in the midline, the obstruction is usually bilateral but not always equal on both sides. Colloid cyst is one such tumor, although rare in childhood, with the youngest case recorded being 11 years old (Ganti et al. 1981). Unilateral tumors, such as those arising in the hypothalamus, basal

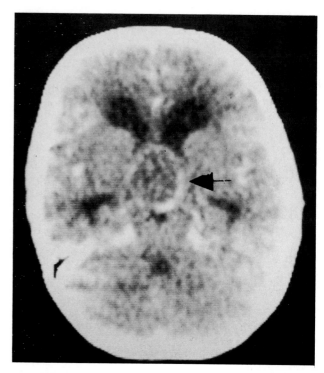

Figure 6-4 Occlusion of the foramen of Monro. CT with intravenous contrast shows ring enhancement of suprasellar craniopharyngioma (arrow) partially blocking the foramen of Monro and causing hydrocephalus.

ganglia, or cerebral parenchyma, may obstruct only one side (Fig. 6-6), but a large tumor can compress both foramina. In the latter case it is common for the ipsilateral ventricle to be compressed by the tumor mass and the opposite ventricle dilated.

AQUEDUCT STENOSIS Congenital aqueduct stenosis, or occlusion without the Chiari malformation, does occur but is uncommon (Table 6-1). A hereditary type has also been reported (Edwards 1961) but is, in the author's experience, extremely rare.

Hydrocephalus, especially that following repair of the meningocele, is invariably associated with the Chiari II malformation. It is by far the most common cause of hydrocephalus and aqueduct stenosis seen in early childhood. Most aqueduct occlusions in association with the Chiari malformation were previously thought, on the basis of air or Pantopaque

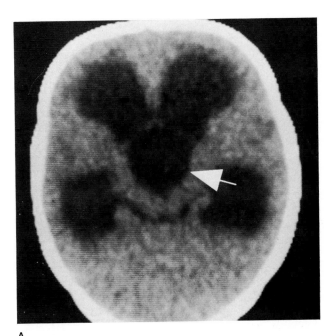

A

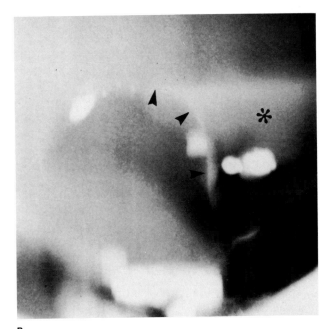

B

Figure 6-5 Occlusion of the foramen of Monro. **A.** Five-month-old with suprasellar cyst obstructing the third ventricle and causing severe hydrocephalus. Even in severe hydrocephalus the third ventricle is usually not this wide. **B.** Metrizamide ventriculogram, lateral view. Metrizamide is visible in the frontal horns (asterisk) and in the anterior third ventricle, which is compressed upward by the large suprasellar cyst (arrows). Denser contrast material is a small amount of Pantopaque also injected.

Figure 6-6 Occlusion of the foramen of Monro. The right lateral ventricle is totally obstructed by a huge thalamic tumor. There is partial obstruction of the left lateral ventricle. A large subacute subdural hematoma is also present on the left side secondary to previous shunting and operative procedures.

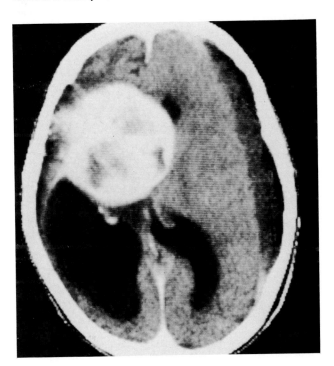

Table 6-1   Lesions Causing Aqueduct Obstruction

Intrinsic
    Infection
    Congenital factors
    Hemorrhage
    Chiari II malformation
Extrinsic
    Neoplasm
    Dilated vein of Galen
    Quadrigeminal cyst
    Brainstem edema

ventriculography, to be total. Metrizamide examination has shown, however, that a majority have some contrast flow through the aqueduct and fourth ventricle, with a significant blockage of CSF flow within the subarachnoid cisterns at the tentorial level (Fig. 6-7)(Fitz 1978*a*). Other specific abnormalities of the Chiari malformation that can be identified on CT are dealt with in greater detail in Chapter 4. The bony abnormalities of the lacunar skull (Fig. 6-8) are seen in the neonatal period, usually up to 3 to 6 weeks. Outer table scalloping is a normal finding having no relation to any congenital anomaly. Scalloping of the posterior wall of the petrous bones (Fig. 6-9) can be seen from birth onward. The steep tentorium and low transverse sinuses are visible with intravenous contrast enhancement in clival perpendicular views (Fig. 6-10).

Features of the brain and ventricular system are also identifiable (Naidich 1980*b*). As the falx is usually deficient, the medial cortices of the cerebral hemisphere are not separated and may show interdigitation (Fig. 6-11). This is better defined in the older child. The lateral ventricles have a peculiar configuration, best seen when they are not grossly

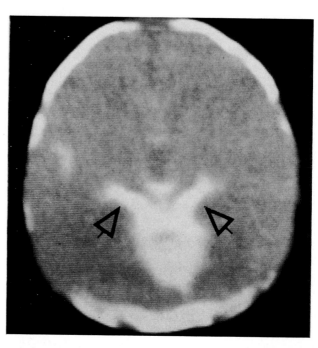

Figure 6-7 Chiari II malformation. CT 2 hours after metrizamide ventriculography shows most of the contrast trapped in the quadrigeminal cistern and against the hiatus (arrows). A small amount of contrast is visible in one sylvian fissure.

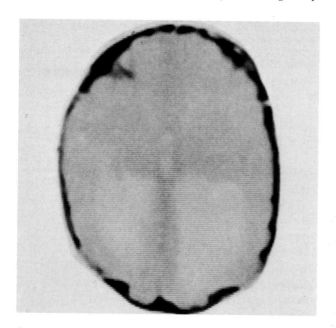

Figure 6-8 Chiari II malformation: lacunar skull. CT with reversed gray scale shows scalloping of the inner table of the skull in 5-day-old infant.

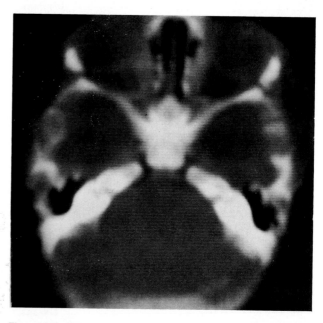

Figure 6-9 Chiari II malformation. Scalloping of the petrous bones due to compression of the hindbrain is visible in a two-week-old infant.

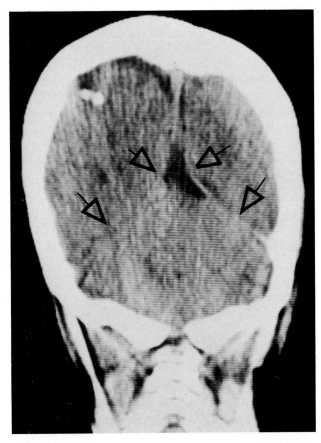

Figure 6-10 Chiari II malformation. Clival perpendicular view with contrast in 2-year-old shows the steepness of the tentorium (arrows).

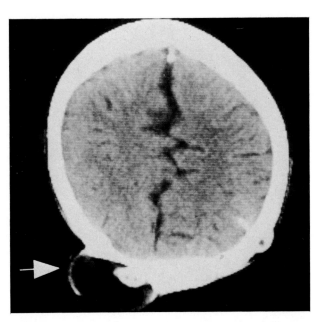

Figure 6-11 Chiari II malformation. Interdigitation of the sutures across the interhemispheric fissure is easily visible in this shunted child. An unusual shunt complication—leakage of CSF along the shunt into the scalp around the reservoir— is also visible (arrow).

enlarged. The occipital horns are relatively larger than the ventricular bodies in many cases, and the bodies of the lateral ventricles are parallel, as seen in dysgenesis of the corpus callosum. The frontal horns also have a peculiar configuration (Fig. 6-12), visible in both standard and coronal views, due to the prominence of the caudate nuclei. Such findings were previously described from air studies (Gooding 1968; Harwood-Nash and Fitz 1976, Chap. 16). The fourth ventricle is usually small and can be missed if the CT sections are 10 mm or thicker. The cerebellar tonsils may be seen below the foramen magnum, especially if they are outlined with metrizamide (Fig. 6-13). The larger-than-normal foramen magnum may also be recognizable. The beaking of the tectum, the inverted V shape of the tentorial

hiatus, and other features (Naidich 1980*a*) are best seen after shunting in older children.

Congenital aqueduct stenosis without the Chiari malformation is most often a structural lesion of unknown cause. Infrequently it can be an inherited autosomal dominant trait. It is not known to be commonly related to any specific insult. In aqueduct stenosis, or in any IVOH for that matter, the ventricles are usually larger than in extraventricular obstructive hydrocephalus (communicating hydrocephalus), indicating that the obstruction is more severe. The lateral and third ventricles are moderately to severely enlarged (Fig. 6-14). The shapes of the ventricles are not specific. However, in neonates and infants with hydrocephalus, the occipital horns appear more dilated than the frontal horns. Subsequently, in the untreated infant, progressive enlargement of all segments of the lateral ventricles takes place. If a Chiari malformation is not present the fourth ventricle is usually normal in size, but on occasion it, too, is mildly enlarged for unknown reasons.

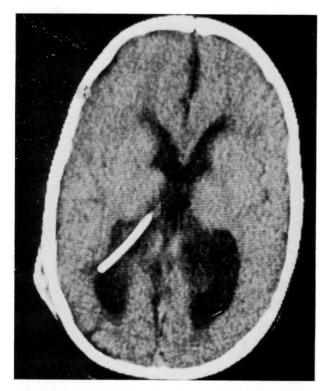

Delayed aqueduct stenosis of childhood is a relatively specific entity. It is usually diagnosed around ages 8 to 11 years. The head is mildly enlarged. The patient may present with signs or symptoms of hydrocephalus of relatively recent onset. On CT, the ventricles resemble those seen in infantile aqueduct stenosis. Usually only moderately large, they can sometimes be quite sizable (Fig. 6-15). The skull usually shows signs of chronic increased intracranial pressure, with sutural splitting and prominent digital markings of the inner table.

CT after intravenous contrast should always be performed to rule out enhancing masses or acute inflammation, though these are uncommonly found in hydrocephalus without specific neurological signs in children. Because CT spatial resolution does not show the aqueduct well, contrast ventriculography with air, metrizamide, or MRI should also be done

Figure 6-12 Arnold-Chiari malformation: frontal horns. Prominent caudate nuclei give the frontal horns their characteristic appearance, as though they are being compressed from their lateral surfaces.

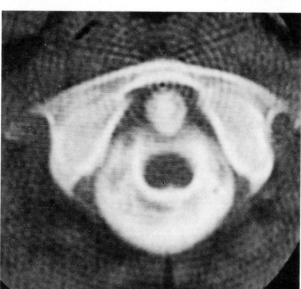

A

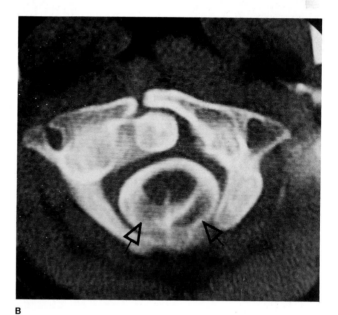

B

Figure 6-13 Chiari II malformation: tonsillar herniation. **A.** CT metrizamide myelogram through C1 shows the cerebellar tonsils as slight posterior bulges not separable from the cervical cord. **B.** A CT metrizamide myelogram of an 11-year-old child. At the

C1–C2 level CT image shows larger tonsils that can be seen separate from the cord (arrows). The right tonsil is more poorly seen because of averaging of the CT numbers between the inferior tip of the tonsil and metrizamide below it. Also note bony anomaly.

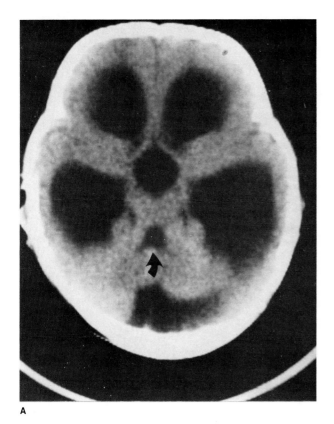

A

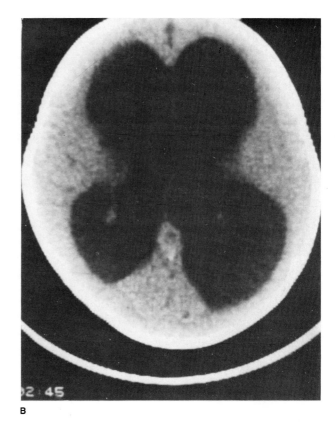

B

Figure 6-14 Congenital aqueduct stenosis. **A.** Inferior CT slice shows marked enlargement of the lateral and third ventricles, with a normal-size fourth ventricle (arrow). **B.** Marked enlargement of the lateral ventricles on a higher cut.

when there is a clinical suspicion of a tumor. The simplest method is the injection of metrizamide via a shunt reservoir into the ventricular system to outline the posterior third ventricle and aqueduct. In the author's experience, the posterior third ventricle and proximal aqueduct commonly have some irregularity suggesting previous inflammation (Fig. 6-16), and care is required to avoid overdiagnosis of tumor in such cases. For this portion of the examination, CT has not been an adequate substitute. MRI in sagittal plane would resolve if a neoplastic process is the cause of the obstruction. In many cases the cause of the stenosis may not be known (Chuang 1981); most probably it is inflammatory and of post-neonatal onset.

Tumors causing aqueduct stenosis are not uncommon, though rare in the first 3 months, when most aqueduct stenosis is found. Any posterior fossa

mass may obstruct the aqueduct, usually by a forward displacement and kinking of the passage. Brainstem gliomas do not usually cause aqueduct stenosis or significant hydrocephalus except when they are exophytic and growing superiorly into the cerebellum. Direct compression by pineal tumors has the same result as posterior fossa masses.

Cysts of the quadrigeminal cistern likewise cause aqueduct obstruction (Fig. 6-17). In the author's experience, nearly all quadrigeminal cysts have occurred in children with the Chiari malformation who have had previous shunts. The tumor or cyst is nearly always clearly visible on CT as the cause of aqueduct stenosis in such cases. If the tumor can be successfully removed, the hydrocephalus will not require shunting in most cases.

Aqueduct stenosis may also be secondary to edema, with uncal herniation or generalized swell-

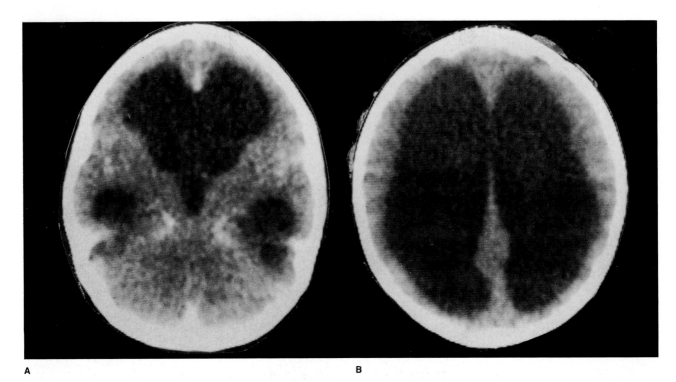

A   B

Figure 6-15   Delayed-onset aqueduct stenosis.   **A** and **B** resemble the findings in Figure 6-14 in this 10-year-old. The **A** view is slightly above the fourth ventricle.

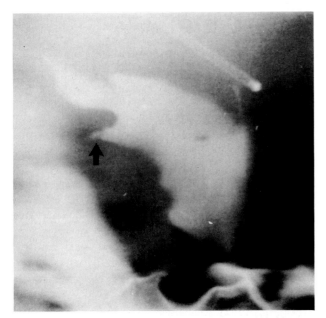

Figure 6-16   Delayed-onset aqueduct stenosis: metrizamide ventriculogram. Lateral view shows some irregularity of the third ventricle–aqueduct junction area (arrow).

ing and downward compression of the midbrain into the posterior fossa. The stenosis is self-limited and temporary if the edema is treatable. In association with vascular malformation, aneurysmal dilatation of the vein of Galen is one of the less common causes of aqueduct obstruction and resulting hydrocephalus.

Acute infection is usually not a cause of aqueduct stenosis, but it may be suspected, inasmuch as the aqueduct is the narrowest and longest intraventricular passage. Neonatal hemorrhage as a cause of aqueduct stenosis is dealt with separately in a later section of this chapter.

OBSTRUCTION OF THE FOURTH VENTRICULAR OUTLETS
Although it is relatively uncommon in childhood, obstruction of the fourth ventricular outlets is second to aqueduct stenosis as a cause of hydrocephalus in infancy. Most often, regardless of age, the fourth ventricle is quite dilated and proportionately slightly larger than the third ventricle (Fig. 6-18) in

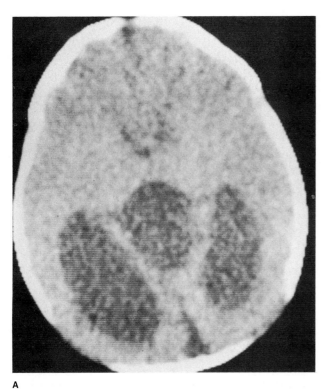

A

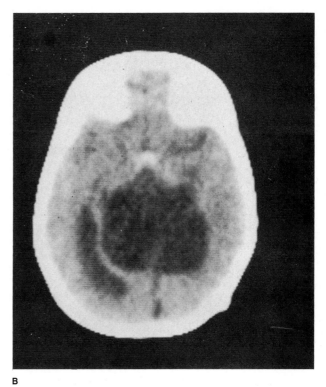

B

Figure 6-17 Aqueduct stenosis: quadrigeminal cyst. **A.** CT slice through level of the quadrigeminal cistern shows CSF space between occipital horns interpreted as a large quadrigeminal cistern in this infant with Chiari malformation. **B.** CT at 1 year shows marked enlargement of the quadrigeminal cyst.

this condition. Occasionally the fourth ventricle can be of normal size in spite of the outlet obstruction (Fig. 6-19). Such discrepancy is not easily explainable by CSF dynamics, as it is most commonly the ventricle closest to the obstruction that is the most dilated.

The specific causes of fourth ventricular outlet obstruction are similar to those of other ventricular narrowings. Ventricular hemorrhage or infection can obstruct the foramina, though proven cases are uncommon. Tumors are usually not located in such a position as to cause this obstruction, though inferior vermis medulloblastomas, brainstem tumors of the inferior medulla, and congenital or malignant extraaxial tumors may rarely do this.

Extraaxial cysts such as arachnoid cysts of the cisterna magna may cause hydrocephalus by occluding the fourth ventricular outlets (Fig. 6-20). The specific diagnosis is of some importance, since per-

manent collapse of the cyst may obviate the need for ventricular shunting. Enlargement of the cisterna magna or a CSF space is obvious in such cases, but the cause may not be. A congenitally large cisterna magna and some Dandy-Walker malformations may also resemble an arachnoid cyst (Fig. 6-21). Unless one sees an obvious mass effect and compression of the cerebellar hemispheres, radionuclide or contrast material such as metrizamide should be injected. If the contrast is injected into the ventricles, CT will usually show contrast within the ventricles with demonstration of the extraaxial arachnoid cyst (Fig. 6-20*B*). If injected by the lumbar subarachnoid space, it will either not enter the posterior fossa or entry will be delayed.

In the Dandy-Walker cyst, a developmental obstruction of the fourth ventricular outlets with absence or hypoplasia of the vermis (Hart 1972), a large fourth ventricle that empties directly into a cystic

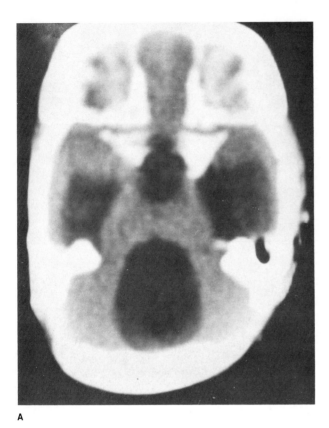

A

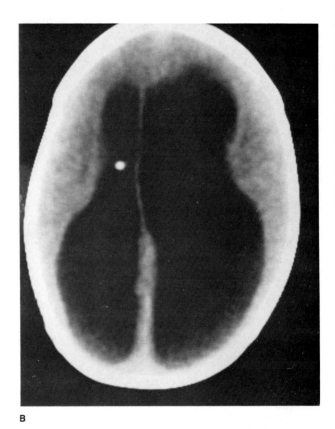

B

Figure 6-18 Obstruction of the fourth ventricular outlet following IVH in an infant. **A.** CT through the posterior fossa shows the markedly enlarged fourth ventricle and associated lateral and third ventricular expansion. **B.** There is marked enlargement of the lateral ventricles, though a recent shunt has caused some decrease in size on the right.

cavity resembling the cisterna magna is common (Fig. 6-22). The vermis is not visible, and the cerebellar hemispheres are hypoplastic. The cyst is nearly always in direct communication with the fourth ventricle.

The Dandy-Walker variant is a less well-defined lesion in which the fourth ventricle has a wide but formed foramen of Magendi. Some inferior vermis may also be visible. The torcular-lambdoid inversion of the classical Dandy-Walker cyst is usually not present. Differentiation from an arachnoid cyst may be quite difficult (Archer 1978) without ventricular instillation of contrast that fills the cyst in the Dandy-Walker variant and the normal fourth ventricle in the extraaxial arachnoid cyst. Even this is not a completely reliable sign, with variations reported. Dandy-Walker cysts are said to have open foramina at times

(Raimondi 1969), and arachnoid cysts may communicate with the ventricular system or subarachnoid space (di Rocco 1981).

Extraventricular Obstructive Hydrocephalus

In extraventricular obstructive hydrocephalus (EVOH), or *communicating hydrocephalus*, the obstruction is distal to the ventricles and may be anywhere along the subarachnoid space. The basal cisterns, the tentorial hiatus, the spaces over the cerebrum and arachnoid granulations, or any combination of these may be sites of obstruction. Identification of the sites is usually not of clinical importance except in certain situations. If a shunt from the lumbar arachnoid space to the peritoneum is planned, one must be sure that the obstruction is at least above the basal cisterns. If IVOH is to be treated by ventriculotomy—most commonly puncture of the third ventricle (Hoffman 1980)—one would like to know that the subarachnoid space is not obstructed.

Children with hydrocephalus, unlike adults, may show dilatation of the subarachnoid space over the hemisphere. Most commonly this occurs in EVOH (Fig. 6-23), and it is, in the author's experience, a reasonably reliable sign that the obstruction is outside the ventricular system.

The lateral ventricles are usually only moderately dilated in EVOH, and the third and fourth ventricles also show mild dilatation. There are, of

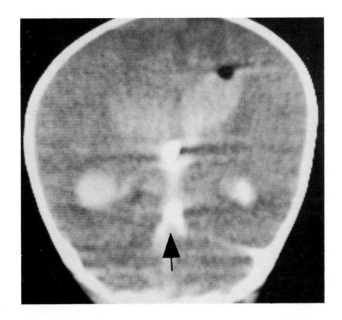

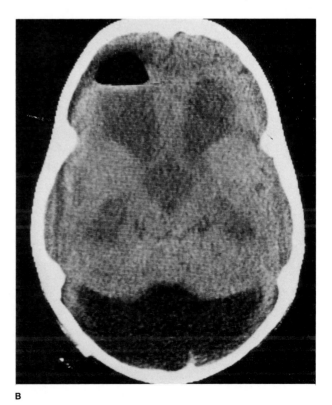

Figure 6-19   Obstruction of the fourth ventricular outlet. CT in clival parallel position following metrizamide ventriculography shows dense collection of metrizamide in obstructed fourth ventricle (arrow). Artifacts due to motion are present.

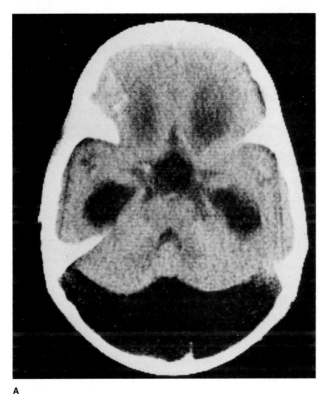

A

Figure 6-20   Posterior fossa arachnoid cyst.   **A.** CT in a 9-year-old shows a large posterior fossa cyst with enlargement of the lateral and third ventricles but a normal-size, possibly compressed,

B

fourth ventricle.   **B.** After metrizamide ventriculography, CT shows metrizamide in the ventricular system but none in the arachnoid cyst. A small amount of air is present in the right frontal horn.

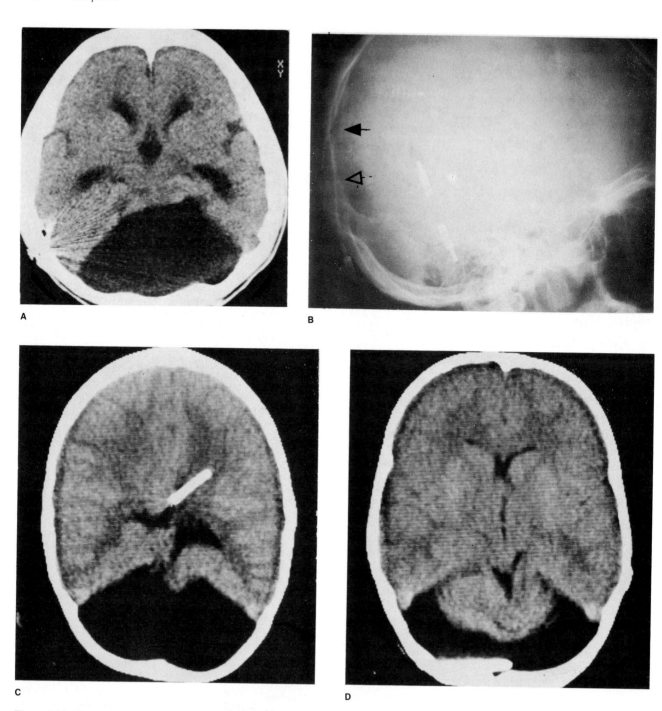

A

B

C

D

Figure 6-21 Posterior fossa cyst. **A.** Twelve-year-old with Dandy-Walker cyst and shunted hydrocephalus. **B.** In spite of extreme cerebellar hypoplasia, the torcular (open arrow) is not higher than lambda (closed arrow). **C.** Posterior fossa arachnoid cysts re-semble **A** at higher level. **D,** at lower levels, shows compressed fourth ventricle and more development of the cerebellum. Both the hydrocephalus and the cyst are shunted (**C** and **D**).

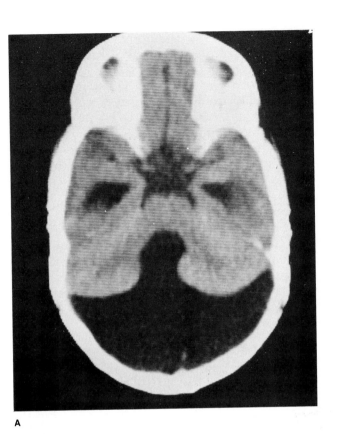

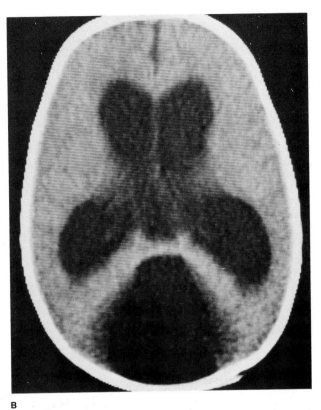

A

B

Figure 6-22 Dandy-Walker cyst. **A.** Enlarged fourth ventricle opening directly into the posterior fossa cyst owing to absence of the vermis. **B.** Higher cut shows hydrocephalus and lack of cerebellar tissue.

course, exceptions to this rule, and considerable dilatation of all ventricles or of only the lateral and third ventricles occasionally occurs (Fig. 6-24). The reasons for these variations are not certain, though one may speculate that the cause of the hydrocephalus may currently or previously have been affecting the outlets of the more dilated ventricles. Generally, this information is not of much clinical significance.

Because the appearance of EVOH is similar no matter what the level of obstruction, this entity is discussed here by cause rather than by site. For the most part the causes are the same as in IVOH, but they are more likely to be documented. This is because EVOH more frequently is diagnosed after the neonatal period and after a clinically evident causal event. Because the ventricles are less enlarged, the head is relatively less enlarged. In an older child the

head also will not expand as rapidly as in an infant. Symptoms may be mild, and the obstruction to CSF flow is usually incomplete.

TUMORS Primary brain tumors do not obstruct the subarachnoid space. The possible exception to this might be a large posterior fossa mass that compresses the cerebellum against the tentorium and causes obstruction at the hiatus at the same time as it occludes the aqueduct.

In children, secondary seeding of the subarachnoid space from almost any malignant disease except leukemia is rare. In leukemia, a blockage of the basal cisterns or subarachnoid space (or both) over the hemispheres may occur. Contrast examination should be carried out to confirm this leukemic spread, though in the author's experience, enhancement of

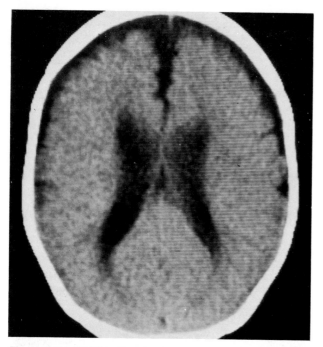

Figure 6-23 EVOH: dilated sulci. Five-month-old with mild to moderate hydrocephalus showing enlargement of the sulci. Compare with normal sulcal prominence in Figure 6-55.

the subarachnoid space is uncommon in spite of the presence of hydrocephalus and of visible leukemic cells in the CSF on microscopy.

Ventricular and sulcal dilatation in leukemia presents a problem to the radiologist. It is a common event, even in leukemic children who do not have symptoms of hydrocephalus (Fig. 6-25). A possible cause other than hydrocephalus in such cases is treatment with methotrexate and/or radiation, producing atrophic enlargement. Treatment with steroids is also known to give the brain an atrophy-like appearance (Okuno 1980).

Primary tumor of the subarachnoid space is a very rare cause of hydrocephalus. The author has seen only one such case, a primary melanosarcoma of the meninges. Here the contrast enhancement of the meninges could not be distinguished from that caused by metastases or inflammation (Flodmark 1979).

INFECTION Acute meningitis can cause permanent or temporary obstruction of the flow of CSF by inflammatory reaction and later adhesions. In the acute stage one will usually see contrast enhancement in

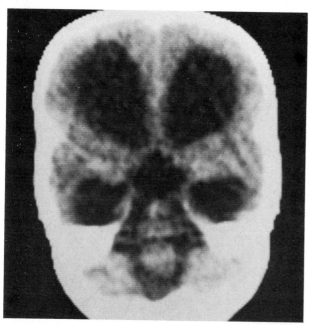

A

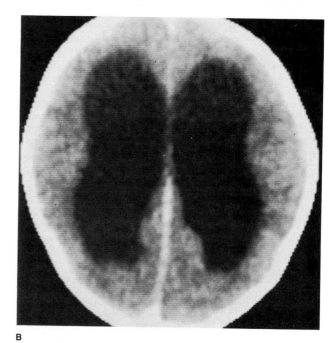

B

Figure 6-24 EVOH. Clival parallel projection in **A** shows large suprasellar cistern and cisterns around the brainstem. This may occur in spite of marked ventricular dilatation, as noted in **B**.

cephalus in infants. Experience has shown that this is not a common sequela, especially in our own series of patients (Flodmark 1980). While intraventricular hemorrhage usually causes temporary dilatation of the ventricles and hydrocephalus, the condition most often resolves. It has also been found that intraventricular hemorrhage is usually accompanied by subarachnoid hemorrhage (Flodmark 1980), and hydrocephalus that occurs after ventricular bleeding can be a combination of partial obstruction in both areas. Subarachnoid hemorrhage as a primary event in neonates usually occurs only in the term infant who has had a traumatic delivery. Here too, hydrocephalus is not necessarily a subsequent condition.

SUBDURAL HEMATOMA Subdural hematoma, especially in the chronic stage, is commonly a cause of EVOH. From about 1 week after the hematoma oc-

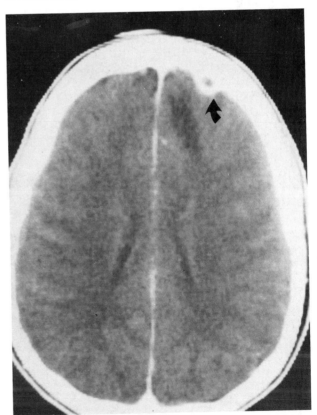

Figure 6-26 Subdural empyema in a 13-year-old. Following intravenous contrast, a small empyema is visible in the left frontal subdural space (arrow). Focal white matter edema is also present although there is no brain abscess.

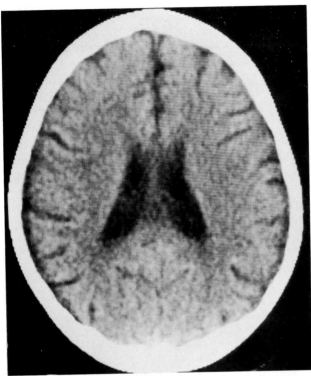

Figure 6-25 Leukemia. CT in 8-year-old child being treated for acute lymphocytic leukemia shows mild enlargement of the sulci and lateral ventricles.

the cisterns or other subarachnoid spaces along with the ventricular enlargement (Chap. 13). After treatment only the history may suggest the cause of hydrocephalus.

Subdural or extradural empyema is also a cause of EVOH. In the acute phase, contrast enhancement is visible (Fig. 6-26). The hydrocephalus is secondary to both the inflammatory reaction and the pressure, which may compress a portion of the subarachnoid space.

Small empyemas along the floor and inferior part of the frontal lobe may be difficult to see without thin axial or coronal sections (Fig. 6-26). As frontal sinusitis is a relatively common cause of this entity, extra views should be considered in such clinical situations.

NEONATAL HEMORRHAGE Before the availability of CT and ultrasound, it was thought that intraventricular hemorrhage was a common cause of hydro-

curs, an inflammatory membrane is often visible on the inner surface of the hematoma after contrast enhancement. This can persist for an indefinite period. Subdural hematoma also causes dilatation of the subarachnoid space over the cortex, presumably because the CSF accumulates in the subarachnoid space near the site of obstruction.

In the author's experience, subdural hematoma fairly quickly reaches the density of the brain in about 4 to 7 days, then appears decreasingly less dense and reaches a chronic appearance that is of approximately CSF density in about 4 weeks. It may be possible to see evidence of recurrent subdural hematoma bleeding by visualization of layers of different density (Fig. 6-27).

The hydrocephalus caused by subdural hematoma is usually mild to moderate, though nonetheless clinically significant.

CONGENITAL FACTORS Communicating hydrocephalus is often seen in children with achondroplasia. The ventricles are dilated moderately in association with prominent subarachnoid spaces, especially over the convexity. Although the exact mechanism is not known, the condition is presumed to be secondary to a relative outlet obstruction from the narrow foramen magnum. More recently it has been postulated that the communicating hydrocephalus is secondary to decreased venous outflow at outlet foramina such as the sigmoid sinus (Yamada 1981). Similar patterns of communicating hydrocephalus have also been reported in craniometaphyseal dysplasia (Fig. 6-28) (Allen 1982). Communicating hydrocephalus possibly due to hypoplasia of the arachnoid granulations has also been reported (Gilles 1971).

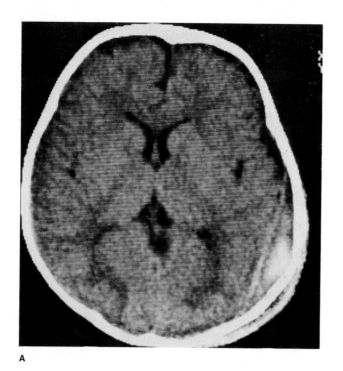

A

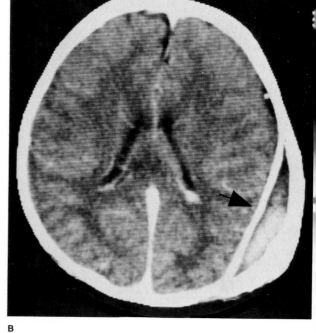

B

Figure 6-27 Subdural hematoma. CT before intravenous contrast **(A)** and after contrast **(B).** Marked enhancement of inner membrane of subacute or chronic subdural hematoma is seen in **B** (arrow). Recurrent nonenhancing bleeding is seen as increased density in both **A** and **B** within the isodense hematoma. No hydrocephalus is present in this 7-year-old.

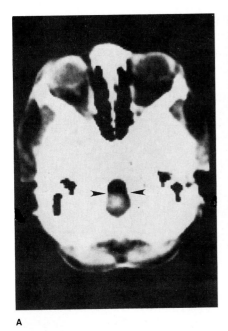
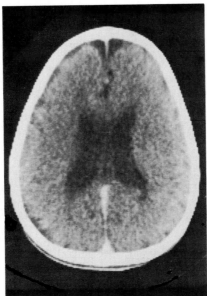
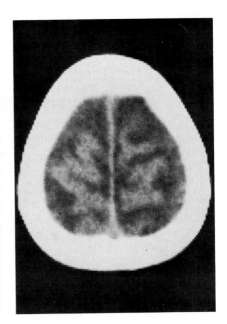

A

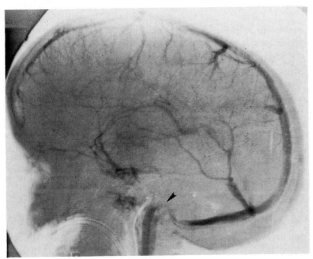

B

Figure 6-28 **A.** Cranial CT. Thickening of skull base; moderately enlarged ventricular size with prominent frontal subarachnoid space; frontal bossing; prominent cortical sulci due to CSF stasis. **B.** Right side: narrowing at the origin of the jugular vein (arrowhead).

Increased Production of CSF

Overproduction of CSF in children is a rare event caused by choroid plexus papilloma or carcinoma. In the adult these are usually in the fourth ventricle; in children, in the lateral ventricle. When these tumors are large, they are fairly easy to diagnose on CT (Fig. 6-29) and can be differentiated from other intraventricular masses by their choroid location and typical choroidal contrast enhancement. With a small tumor, diagnosis by CT may be difficult, because the tumor may not be obviously larger than the prominent choroid plexus on the normal side. This usually occurs in children under the age of 2 years,

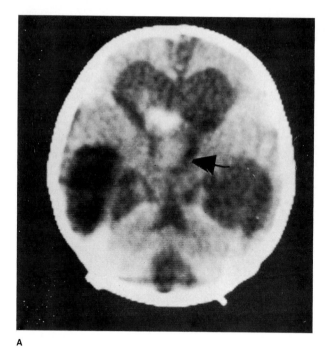

A

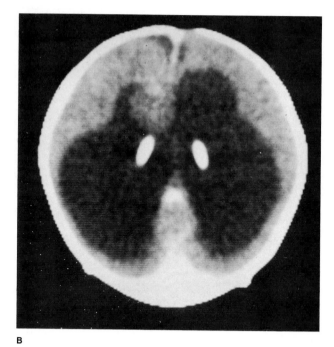

B

Figure 6-29 A large choroid plexus papilloma visible in contrast-enhanced CT in a 3-month-old. Papilloma is unusual in that it extends in **A** from the third ventricle (arrow) into the frontal horn in

both **A** and **B**. Only a portion of the papilloma adjacent to the third ventricle shows enhancement. Note the marked hydrocephalus in spite of the biventricular shunts.

a group that has prominent choroid plexuses even in the normal situation (Fig. 6-30). When the tumors are small, angiography may be needed to visualize an abnormal choroid vasculature. In some cases measurement of CSF output by ventricular cathe-terization may be necessary to be certain of the diagnosis.

Normal-Pressure Hydrocephalus

Normal-pressure hydrocephalus, a condition that occurs in older adults, is not a diagnosis made in children. It may be that children investigated for hydrocephalus who have mild ventricular and sul-cal dilatation on CT but no definite clinical symp-toms of raised intracranial pressure have a condition that is equivalent to the adult normal-pressure

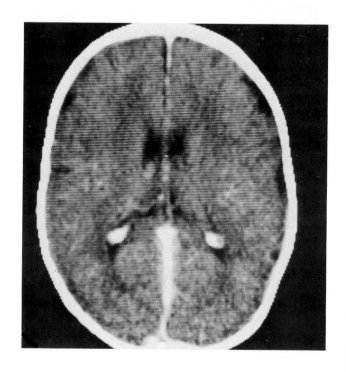

Figure 6-30 CT with intravenous contrast shows prominence of the normal choroid plexus in an 8-month-old child.

hydrocephalus. They do not, however, have the clinical triad of gait ataxia, urinary and fecal incontinence, and dementia.

Arrested Hydrocephalus

It may be said in some seriousness that the only arrested hydrocephalic is one who is under police custody. A better term is *compensated hydrocephalus*, since a person with hydrocephalus, treated or untreated, may have an activation of the disease even though it has been asymptomatic for several years. It must again be emphasized that a single CT examination may be noninformative as to the dynamic state of the patient's hydrocephalus. This is especially true when the first CT examination available to the radiologist is made after treatment or there has been an interval of 2 or more years between examinations. Ventricular size may change considerably over a short period of time—a week to a month (Fig. 6-31).

Treated Hydrocephalus

Normal Posttreatment Status

The ideal situation following shunting is a decrease in intracranial pressure and ventricular size. The amount of change in ventricular size and apparent gain in brain tissue can be significant (Fig. 6-32). On CT it may be unclear whether the ventricular size after treatment is ideal, as patients with small normal or mildly enlarged ventricles may be asymptomatic. Most treated children in either of these states show enlargement of the sulci following shunting (Fig. 6-33). This is probably mostly brain remolding to the smaller ventricular size but may reflect some degree of atrophy. It is especially common when shunting has been done after age 2, when the skull is less compliant.

In a recent study of uncomplicated hydrocephalus, there was surprisingly little difference in IQ levels between most treated hydrocephalic patients

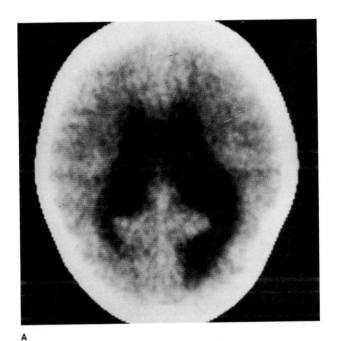

A

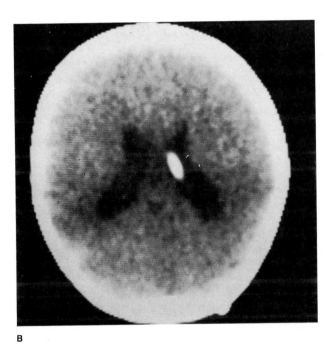

B

Figure 6-31 A. Moderate hydrocephalus before shunting in a 7-year-old. **B.** One week after shunting, the lateral ventricles have shrunk to nearly normal size.

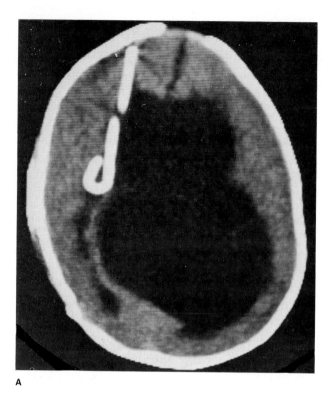

A

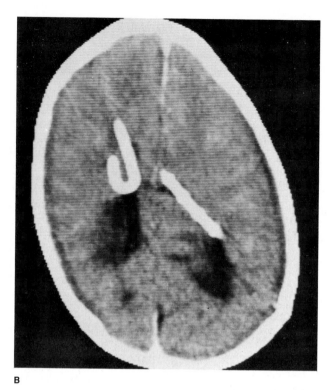

B

Figure 6-32 Ventricular shunting. **A.** Huge encysted lateral ventricle in a 6-month-old with thinning of the cortex on both ipsilateral and contralateral side. The contralateral ventricle is small, with a functioning shunt. **B.** Five months later, after shunting to the en-cysted ventricle, both ventricles are small and there is an apparent thickening of the cortex. Note that some of this increased brain volume is actually due to a narrowing of the calvarium.

and normal children (Dennis 1981) and no relationship between the IQ and the number of shunt revisions, indicating that the complications of shunt blockage may not be as severe as usually thought.

Complications

Blocked shunts are the most common problem in treated hydrocephalus. An abnormal shunt position is easily diagnosed on CT, though the significance is not always known when several shunts are present. Indeed, it is not too uncommon to see an extraventricular shunt tip in a patient who no longer needs a shunt or where there is CSF going along the shunt tract to its tip. With a suspected shunt block, a previous CT is most helpful to confirm the change in ventricular size and thus the obstruction in CSF flow.

Shunt types change from year to year as neurosurgeons continue to look for the ideal shunt that will find its way into the proper position and never block. All intracranial shunts are visible on CT, even if not seen on plain skull x-ray. A short shunt in the subdural space against the inner table can be missed unless the window settings are adjusted to see it.

Shunt disconnection between the reservoir and intracerebral tubing is quite uncommon, because there is no motion between these two parts. It may be missed because of its proximity to the inner table, or it may be overlooked when multiple tubes are present (Fig. 6-34). Plain radiographs are of great help in such cases.

When no previous knowledge of ventricular size is available and the shunt system is connected and in good position, two other clues are sometimes

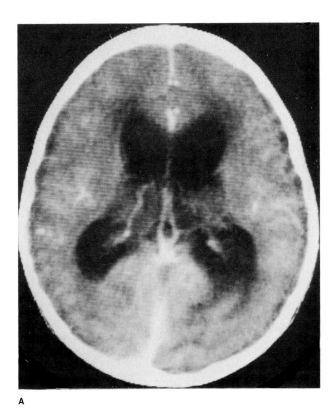

A

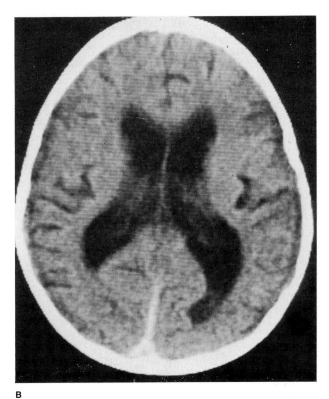

B

Figure 6-33 Ventricular shunting.   **A.** Four-year-old child with hydrocephalus secondary to posterior fossa tumor.   **B.** Two weeks after shunting and tumor removal, there is some decrease in ven-tricular size and visibly dilated sulci. The patient had not received chemotherapy or radiation.

available for the radiologist. One is the periventricular hypodensity of transependymal absorption of CSF. This is usually most visible at the tips of the frontal horns and the lateral atrial regions. It is uncommon following shunt blockage unless there is a rapid and large change in intracranial pressure. The other clue is the plain film finding of split sutures or resplit sutures in the older child. Because a child's skull, even up to age 14 or 15, responds quickly to changes in increased intracranial pressure, x-ray should be done along with CT. Usually a postero-anterior and a lateral film are sufficient to evaluate sutural changes.

Excessive shunt function is a complication at the opposite end of the spectrum. This is nearly always an acute phenomenon following shunting in children or infants for the very large ventricles. It is especially a danger in the child beyond infancy, where the decreased compliance of the calvarium (and perhaps the brain) no longer allows as much physiological "collapse" in response to the decreased ventricular size. In such a case the ventricles quickly get smaller, allowing the brain to "shrink" and enlarging the subdural-subarachnoid space. Stretching of the bridging veins occurs, and subdural hematomas, often of large size and extent, may result (Fig. 6-35). If this occurs, the surgeon is often in the position of trying to balance the two spaces—ventricular and subdural-subarachnoid—and may be forced to allow the ventricles to reexpand in order to prevent recurrence of the subdural hematoma. Shunting of the subdural space itself is sometimes necessary in such cases.

Intracerebral hematomas and subdural hemato-

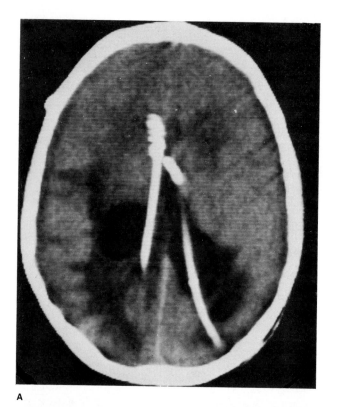

A

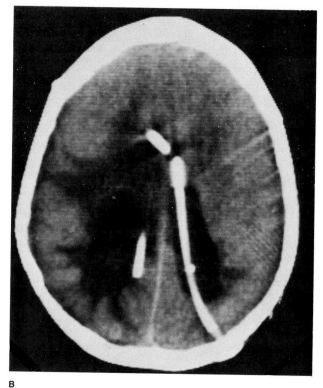

B

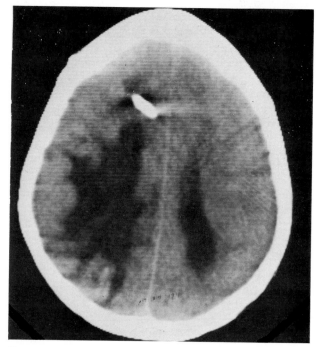

C

Figure 6-34 Ventricular shunting: seven-year-old hydrocephalic child with multiple shunts and clinical signs of a blocked shunt. **A.** Ventricular catheters are noted in both lateral ventricles. **B.** Left-sided catheter can be followed to the calvarium, while right-sided catheter is disconnected and does not reach the inner table. A third Hakim catheter is seen anteriorly in **B** and **C.** This catheter was seen to be connected in higher cuts. Note periventricular edema due to right-sided block and encystment of a portion of the right lateral ventricle.

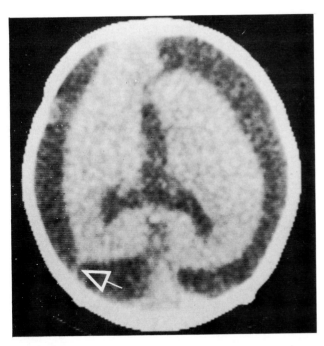

Figure 6-35 Ventricular shunting: same patient as in Figure 6-29. After removal of the choroid plexus papilloma and shunting of the ventricles, the patient developed huge bilateral subdural hematomas. A bridging vein (arrow) is visible posteriorly.

mas from shunt insertion are quite uncommon, and have no features that distinguish them from other hemorrhages in the same regions of other etiology.

ISOLATED FOURTH VENTRICLE   This complication occurs only in shunted hydrocephalus, usually as a result of repeated infection. The fourth ventricle becomes blocked at both the aqueduct and its outlets, causing the ventricle to expand in spite of good shunt function in the lateral ventricles (Fig. 6-36). Often the patients are those with Chiari malformation and previous aqueduct stenosis, but the condition can also occur in EVOH (Scotti 1980).

Treatment is by shunting of the fourth ventricle. It is often difficult to pass a shunt into this dilated ventricle in spite of its size and closeness to the skull vault. This complication has been diagnosed only since CT became available (see Chap. 13).

SLIT-VENTRICLE SYNDROME   Also known as *shunt dependency*, this is said to occur when shunting allows

the ventricles to become very small. Either by adhesions or other mechanisms, the ventricles lose their compliance and ability to reexpand. Neither the clinical symptoms nor the CT appearance are necessarily clear-cut, and small ventricles may reexpand (Fig. 6-37). When the problem is clinically diagnosed and the ventricles are slitlike on CT, one possible treatment is decompression of the temporal lobe by so-called subtemporal craniectomy. This may allow both expansion of the temporal horn and bulging of the brain when shunt blockage occurs (Fig. 6-37) (Holness 1979).

INFECTION   On occasion, especially following shunt revision, the shunt system becomes infected and causes a ventriculitis. This can be diagnosed by contrast enhancement of the ventricular walls (Fig. 6-38). Although usually suspected clinically, it is sometimes masked by the symptoms of shunt obstruction.

MISCELLANEOUS   Migration of shunt tubing outside the cranial vault is not a common occurrence, but radiologists and neurosurgeons are familiar with it. Intracranial migration of shunt tubing is extremely rare but may also occur. The author has experience in one such case, in which the tubing migrated intracranially. In this case there was no reservoir, and neck motion was assumed to have caused the shunt tubing to move continually upward.

In shunting in the older child with very large ventricles, considerable thickening of the skull may be seen, caused by the decrease in brain size and growth of the bone on the inner table to fill the space. Because skull thickness is not accurately demonstrated on CT without using a very wide window (Fig. 6-39), mild thickening is often overlooked unless accompanying skull x-rays are done.

Johnson et al. (1986) recently found that nonvisualization of the quadrigeminal cistern in a child with symptoms of a blocked shunt is an ominous sign, even when the ventricles do not appear to be significantly enlarged. Rapid deterioration and death may occur. The exception to this is the child with a lumboperitoneal shunt. This cistern is usually small and difficult to see in these patients (Fig. 6-37A) (Chuang et al. 1985).

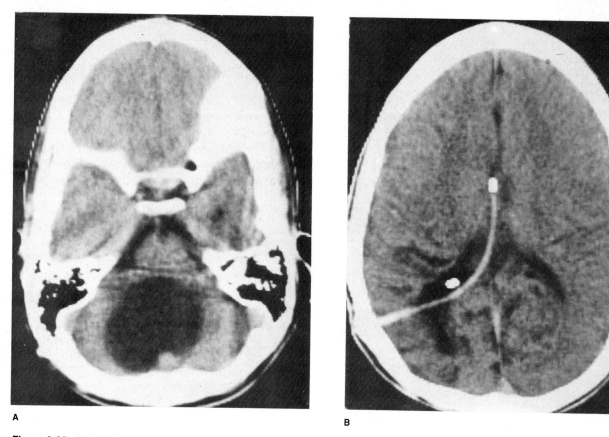

A

B

Figure 6-36 Isolated fourth ventricle in a 9-year-old. **A.** There is marked dilatation of the fourth ventricle. **B.** A higher slice shows small lateral ventricles with two shunts.

ATROPHY

As stated at the beginning of this chapter, ventricular enlargement is not necessarily hydrocephalus. The same condition causing hydrocephalus may cause atrophy. The two abnormalities may also be seen combined in the same patient. This is especially true for ventricular dilatation secondary to hemorrhage or infection. On a single CT examination it may be impossible to state whether the abnormal findings are due to hydrocephalus alone, atrophy alone, or a combination of the two problems. However, focal atrophy or porencephaly may be a result of shunt complications such as bleeding along a shunt insertion tract. Such a damaged area

will allow disproportionate focal ventricular enlargement when shunt blockage occurs.

There are signs to help distinguish atrophy from hydrocephalus. If the subarachnoid space and sulci are relatively larger than the ventricles, it is fairly certain that hydrocephalus is not the primary diagnosis (Fig. 6-40). Local areas of enlargement of the ventricles are a sign of focal atrophy and suggest that atrophy is the predominant condition, especially if combined with the above-mentioned relatively large sulcal dilatation.

Calcifications of the brain secondary to infection, radiation, or other insult are signs of damage. There is usually an accompanying sulcal or ventricular enlargement or both.

Heinz et al. (1980) noted that in atrophy the fron-

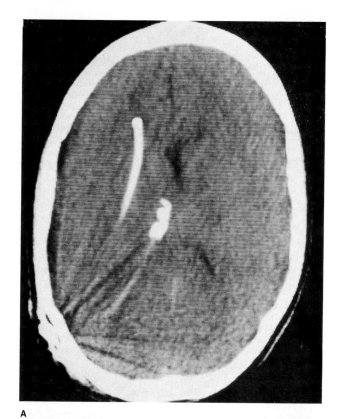

A

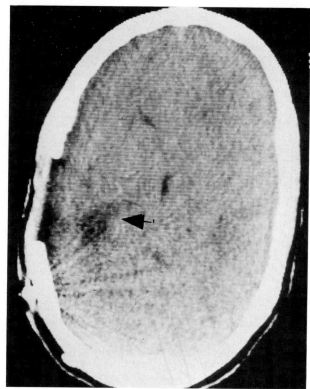

B

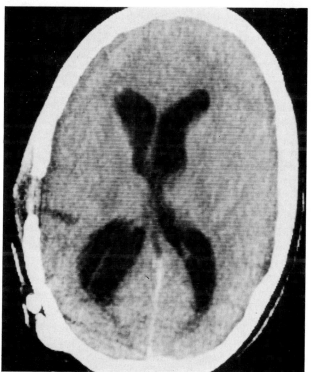

C

Figure 6-37 Slit-ventricle syndrome. **A.** This 9-year-old shunted hydrocephalic child had symptoms of increased intracranial pressure and small ventricles on CT. **B.** Five and a half months later, after temporal decompression, there is some enlargement of the right temporal horn (arrow). **C.** Approximately 1 year later, child again returned with signs of increased intracranial pressure. CT at this time showed that the entire ventricular system had reexpanded.

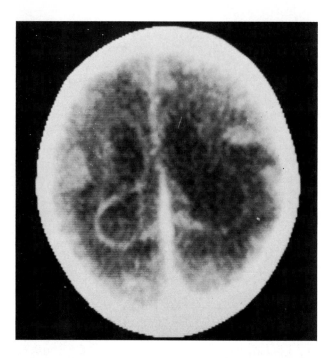

tal horns keep their normal shape but expand, whereas in hydrocephalus the angle formed by the corners of the tips of the frontal horns becomes much more obtuse. The author believes that while this is usually the case, it is not a completely reliable criterion, as atrophic ventricular dilatation may mimic hydrocephalus on occasion (Fig. 6-40). One must make use of the clinical information available: if a child has clinical evidence of brain damage and no evidence of hydrocephalus, the radiological diagnosis should take such information into account even if the ventricular enlargement appears to be hydrocephalic on CT.

Figure 6-38 Ventriculitis. CT following intravenous contrast shows enhancement of the ventricular walls secondary to an infected shunt which had been removed. Hydrocephalus and white-matter edema are present. The picture is the same as that seen in ventriculitis from other causes.

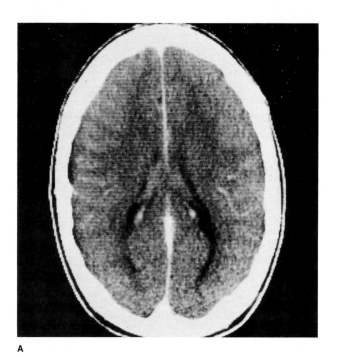

A

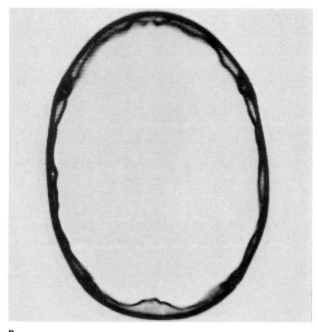

B

Figure 6-39 Skull thickness. **A.** An 11-year-old retarded child with a thickened skull vault that is not especially prominent with the standard window. **B.** Wide windows and reverse gray scale show true skull thickness, which is greater than normal but again not appreciated unless one is used to this window setting.

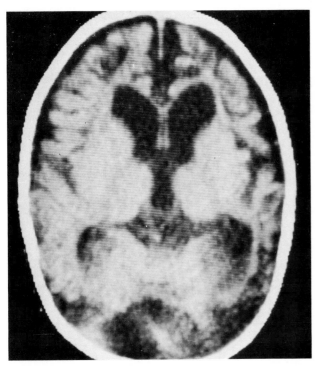

Figure 6-40 Severe atrophy. CT in a 10-month-old with marked atrophy shows both enlargement of the lateral ventricles with rounding of the frontal horns and marked dilatation of the sulci disproportionate to what would be seen in EVOH.

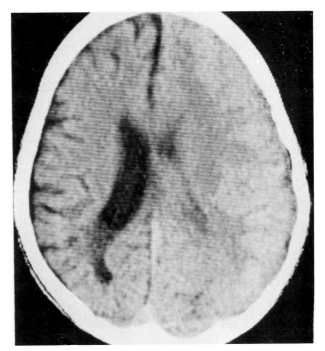

Figure 6-41 Hemiatrophy. A 6-year-old with hemiatrophy shows mild dilatation of the lateral ventricle and sulci on the affected side. The affected hemisphere is smaller.

Hemiatrophy

This can occasionally be difficult to tell from a mass effect on CT, though differentiation is much less of a problem with better scanners. In hemiatrophy, the atrophic side usually has the larger ventricle, the midline shift, if present, is to the atrophic side, and the sulci on that side are equal to or larger than those on the contralateral side (Fig. 6-41), although infrequently the larger ventricle is seen on the more normal side (Fig. 6-42). With hemiatrophy, it is difficult to tell how much damage is also present on the opposite side or how much any ventricular and sulcal dilatation is simply a reaction to occupy the atrophic space.

Focal Atrophy

This is usually easy to diagnose on CT. It can be seen as local ventricular enlargement or local sulcal enlargement or a combination of the two (Fig. 6-43). The term *infarction* usually refers to atrophy resulting from a vascular accident, but probably most atrophy is the result of a partial or complete loss of blood supply to the area involved. Exceptions are direct toxic insults, infection, and perhaps edema.

Central Atrophy

This term usually refers to a condition in which a child shows mild ventricular enlargement with no sulcal enlargement and has clinical signs of delayed development or brain injury or similar evidence not compatible with hydrocephalus.

Cortical Atrophy

This term refers to enlargement of the sulci without enlargement of the ventricles, with a clinical condition similar to that described in the above para-

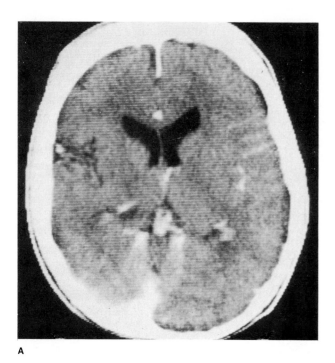

A

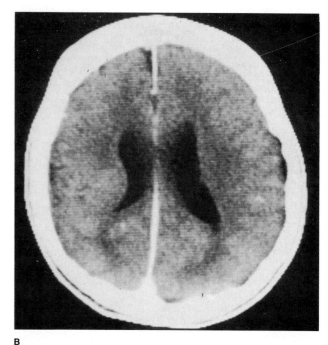

B

Figure 6-42 Hemiatrophy. A 5-year-old with hemiatrophy shows slight enlargement of the sulci on the right side in both **A** and **B.** The left frontal horn is slightly larger in **A.** The left lateral ventricle is slightly larger in **B,** in spite of the fact that the right hemisphere is visibly smaller, with a shift of the straight sinus **(A)** and falx **(B)** from the atrophy.

graph. In the author's experience, these two radiological diagnoses, though affecting very different areas of the brain, do not have significant differences in clinical symptoms or history.

Microcephaly

Microcephaly is often due to brain damage, yet it is surprising that there is often no enlargement of the ventricles or sulci on CT. The reason for this is not known, though one may speculate that the damage occurred very early in utero and retarded the overall growth rate of the brain. An interesting finding in microcephaly is the frequent visualization of normal brain markings of the inner skull table despite obvious lack of brain growth (Fig. 6-44). Some microcephalic children, however, show obvious ventricular and sulcal enlargement, and at least some of these enlargements are secondary to severe postnatal damage such as neonatal meningitis.

Total Brain Infarction

A very small number of infants undergo what can probably be best described as total brain infarction. This is an unusual postnatal or perinatal event, usually secondary to a severe insult, most often infection but occasionally birth anoxia or intracranial hemorrhage. In such cases one initially sees ventricular and sulcal enlargement due to hydrocephalus from the active process such as encephalitis or infarctions. Following this there is a decrease in the density of the brain to that of the enlarged ventricles, or nearly so. If this is due to anoxia, there is initial severe edema and small ventricles (Fig. 6-45*A*), followed by marked ventriculomegaly and continued low brain density with sparing of the basal ganglia and cerebellum (Fig. 6-45*B*). It may become nearly impossible to distinguish brain from ventricle on CT. In most cases the subarachnoid space is not visibly large, but occasionally the brain may shrink consid-

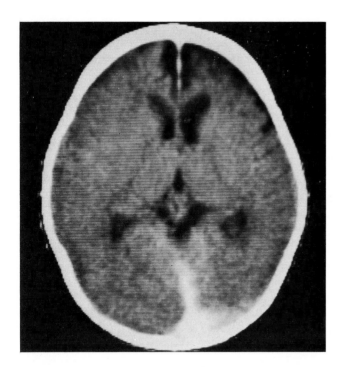

erably, leaving only a thin rim around the enlarged ventricles and a huge subarachnoid space.

Porencephaly

Porencephaly is a condition defined in different ways in different specialties and by medical dictionaries (Anderson 1977; Dorland's 1974; Blakiston's Gould 1979; Stedman's 1976). To the neuroradiologist it is a fluid-filled cavity (presumably CSF-filled) in the brain secondary to the local infarction. It may be noncommunicating—that is, separate from the ventricle—or communicating—that is, connecting to the ventricles and most often a portion of one of the lateral ventricles. It may be associated with hydro-

---

Figure 6-43 Focal atrophy. CT following intravenous contrast shows focal enlargement of the sulci over much of the left frontal area and the right frontal region at the midline. The atrophy was secondary to birth anoxia.

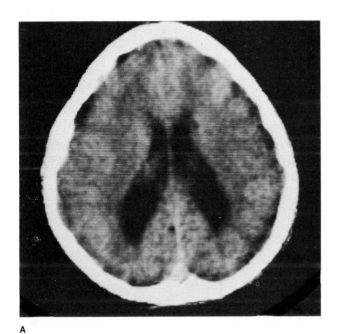

A

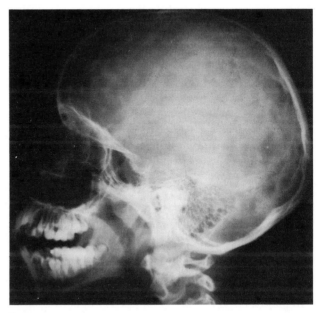

B

Figure 6-44 Microcephaly. **A.** CT in an 11-year-old child with severe microcephaly shows mild dilatation of the lateral ventricles and sulci. **B.** Lateral skull x-ray in the same patient.

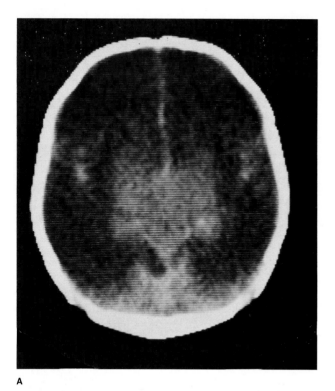

A

B

Figure 6-45 Brain infarction. **A.** CT in a 2-day-old full-term infant who suffered marked birth asphyxia. The brain is of low density except for the central basal ganglia and thalami, the posteriorly located cerebellum, and a small portion of cortex in the area of each sylvian fissure. **B.** Repeat CT at 17 days of age shows mild ventricular enlargement. The apparent increased density of the basal ganglia and thalami is due to the marked decrease in density in the remainder of the brain, which can be seen to be of nearly the same density as the ventricular CSF.

cephalus as discussed earlier. It is thought to be usually due to vascular occlusion and can arise from a variety of insults, varying from neonatal anoxia (Fig. 6-46) to infection to simple vascular occlusion. When the porencephalic defect connecting the ventricles is associated with hydrocephalus and expands from the transmitted increased ventricular pressure, it becomes a porencephalic cyst.

Developmental defects may leave underdeveloped areas of brain. These may form cavities that are usually considered to be porencephaly and are indistinguishable from the type caused by damage of an already developed area.

Puncture porencephaly is an uncommon condition that occurs when hydrocephalus dilates the tract of the ventricular needle (Fig. 6-47); it will usually not occur if shunting is done or other means are taken to control the increased pressure within 1 or 2 days of puncture. Such cysts more commonly occur when repeated ventricular punctures are performed for instillation of antibiotics in ventriculitis when shunting is not feasible because of existing infection.

Hydranencephaly

This may be thought of as a gross polyporencephaly. It is usually believed to be due to a vascular accident early in utero with complete or nearly complete infarction of the territories of the brain supplied by the middle cerebral and anterior cerebral arteries (Crome 1972). Evidence of other malformations of the brain, however, suggests anomalous development (Halsey 1971). Typically, the basal

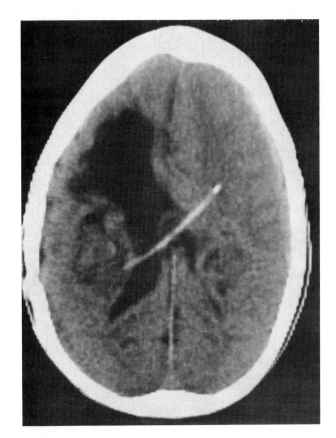

Figure 6-46 Porencephaly. A 7-year-old shunted hydrocephalic child has a porencephaly communicating with the ventricular system. The porencephaly was secondary to neonatal interventricular hemorrhage with extension into the brain parenchyma.

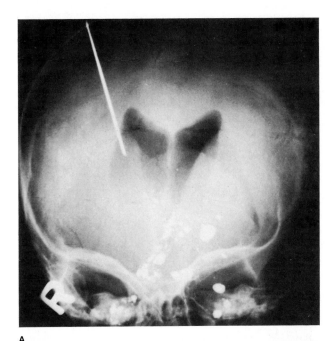

A

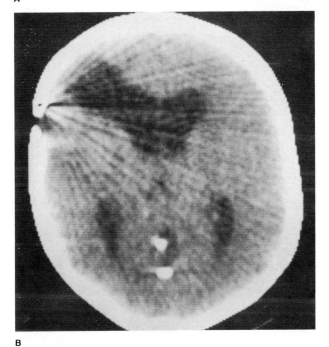

B

Figure 6-47 Puncture porencephaly. **A.** Anteroposterior film during a ventriculogram shows the needle in the right frontal horn in a 1½-year-old child. **B.** CT after shunting and 5-year interval shows a large porencephalic cyst in the frontal horn. (*Fitz CR and Harwood-Nash DC 1978a. Reprinted with permission from the publisher.*)

ganglia are spared and a collapsed strip of occipital lobe is visible against the tentorium (Fig. 6-48). The cranial cavity is mostly filled with CSF, but no ventricles except the fourth ventricle can be identified on CT. Occasionally a partial hydranencephaly can occur, with sparing of portions of the inferior, frontal, and temporal lobes (Fig. 6-49). Patients usually present in infancy, sometimes with a large head but often with a normal head and normal brainstem function but with transillumination over the entire skull.

In extreme hydrocephalus, on rare occasions, the cortex is so thin as not to be clearly visible on CT. In such cases the resemblance to hydranencephaly may be so great that angiography is needed to dis-

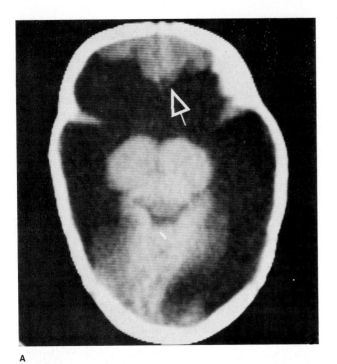

A

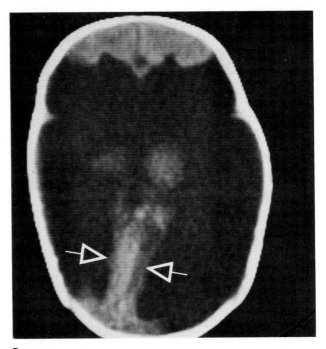

B

Figure 6-48 Hydranencephaly. **A.** CT at level of the tentorium shows small amount of residual frontal lobe anteriorly (arrow), central thalami, and cerebellum and inferior occipital lobes posteriorly.

B. Slightly higher cut shows residual frontal cortex, tops of the thalami, and thin strips of occipital lobe (arrow) on either side of the falx.

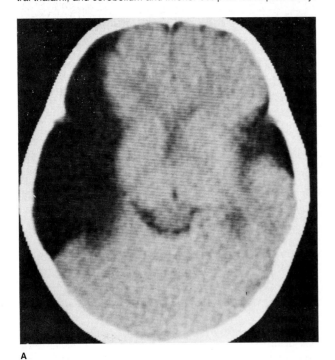

A

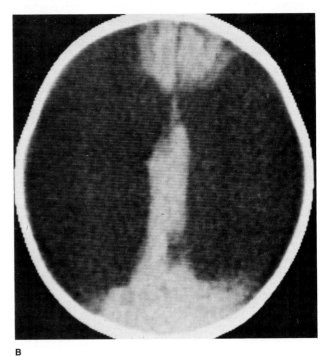

B

Figure 6-49 Partial hydranencephaly. The child presented with an enlarging head at 6 months. **A.** CT shows far better preservation of the brain than in Figure 6-48, although there is consid-

erable damage on the right. **B.** CT through the level of the ventricular bodies shows severe damage but some preservation of brain in the midline to a greater degree than in Figure 6-48.

tinguish the two entities. At angiography, hydrocephalus, no matter how severe, will show cortical arteries and veins over the brain surface beneath the inner table.

MISCELLANEOUS CONDITIONS

Encephalocele

This anomaly, a disorder of the midline closure, is rare, being said to occur in 4 of 10,000 births (Leck 1966). It is most commonly seen in the occipital region. When large, it is easily diagnosed clinically and by CT. The exact contents of the encephalocele may be difficult to determine if brain has herniated into it (Fig. 6-50). Enlargement of the ventricles invariably accompanies large encephaloceles, though this is probably in part developmental rather than hydrocephalic.

Small encephaloceles that present only with a small lump on the scalp can be difficult to diagnose on CT. Since they are only 1 to 3 cm in size outside the cranial vault, the Hounsfield numbers are usually not accurate enough to determine whether they contain CSF. Those in the occipital region will usually show an enlarged interhemispheric space from

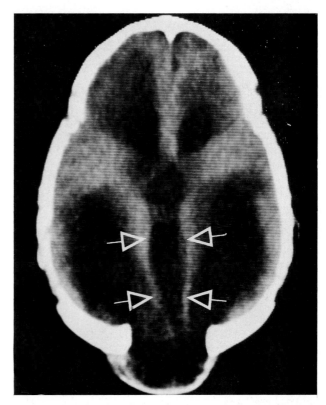

Figure 6-51 Encephalocele. Six-month-old infant with occipital bony defect and moderate encephalocele protruding posteriorly. Tract of encephalocele (arrows) extends to the quadrigeminal cistern.

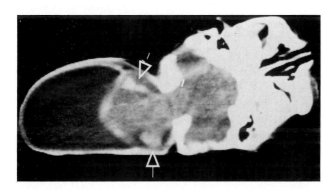

Figure 6-50 Encephalocele. CT shows a large occipital encephalocele containing considerable brain and CSF. In spite of inferior location, there are two enhancing regions suggestive of lateral ventricle choroid plexus (arrows). The infant had to be examined on its side because of the large encephalocele.

vault to quadrigeminal cistern (Fig. 6-51), or occasionally the third or even the lateral ventricle. This is a reliable indication that the mass is an encephalocele.

Arachnoid Cyst

Arachnoid cysts causing hydrocephalus have been discussed in the hydrocephalus section. It is the location of the cyst in or beneath the third ventricle, in the quadrigeminal cistern, and in the cisterna magna region that is the cause of the hydrocephalus rather than any other quality of the cyst itself. Arachnoid cysts are probably congenital lesions that arise in utero. Their exact cause is not known.

The most common location for arachnoid cyst is in the region of the sylvian fissure. A gradual dila-

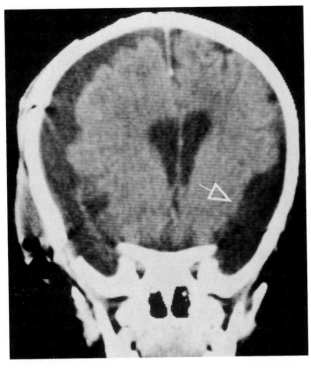

Figure 6-52 Arachnoid cyst. Coronal view in a 14-month-old shows a left-sided unoperated temporal arachnoid cyst (arrow) and a right-sided arachnoid cyst with superimposed large subacute subdural hematoma that has reaccumulated after evacuation. The hematoma causes a shift of the ventricles to the left.

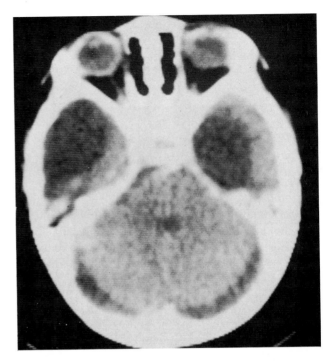

Figure 6-53 Arachnoid cyst. Bilateral temporal arachnoid cysts are seen in this inferior CT slice in a 6-year-old child examined for behavior problems. The cisterna magna is prominent but normal.

tation of the cyst is thought to occur over a period of months or years until it becomes clinically evident by local enlargement of the skull vault, seizures, or bleeding into the subdural space outside the cyst following an injury. CT shows the enlarged sylvian fissure and cystic space (Fig. 6-52). It often goes beneath the temporal lobe to the midline and is occasionally bilateral (Fig. 6-53). The brain adjacent to the cyst, especially the temporal tip, is usually atrophic in appearance on CT (Fig. 6-54) and hypovascular on angiography. Although surgical treatment is usually given to create communication between the cyst and the normal subarachnoid space and to remove any abnormal vasculature of its covering that might reintroduce bleeding, the brain often will not reexpand to fill the space even though it is no longer under pressure, or this may occur only over a period of several years.

Subdural Hygroma

The sulci are normally visible up to 6 months of age and probably up to 1 year (Fig. 6-55). A subarachnoid space showing more sulcal separation or displacement of the cortex farther away from the inner table than seen in Fig. 6-55 is abnormal. It is not uncommon to see on CT large subarachnoid spaces, especially frontally in children examined for possible hydrocephalus, who usually present with increased head size and no other symptoms (Fig. 6-56). If there is no contrast enhancement of membranes to indicate a traumatic or infectious cause, the diagnosis is often perplexing. The ventricles frequently are minimally enlarged (Robertson 1979; Mori 1980). It is the author's belief that these lesions are subdural hygromas which are benign accumulations of CSF of unknown cause.

At the author's hospital, a CSF flow study (cisternogram) is recommended to evaluate the dynamics of CSF absorption. There is frequently a mild abnormality involving fourth ventricle reflux and slight delay of passage of radionuclide over the cerebral hemisphere but no clear-cut evidence of EVOH. These children are usually followed without treatment. Follow-up studies including CT demonstrated either no change or decrease in the size of the wide subarachnoid spaces. A few have undergone tapping of the fluid collection, which reaccumulated fairly quickly. The psychomotor development and neurologic examinations have been normal in the majority of these children.

The collections tend to be located over the frontal lobes. It was our original thought that examination of such children in the prone position might differ-

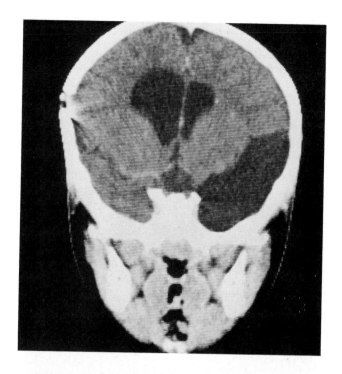

Figure 6-54 Arachnoid cyst. Coronal view of a 3-year-old with a large left temporal arachnoid cyst shows a deepening of the temporal fossa in comparison with the normal side. Temporal lobe is replaced by cyst back to the level of this slice at the sella.

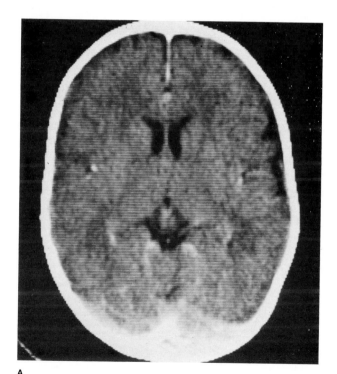

A

Figure 6-55 Normal subarachnoid space. **A.** The frontal sulci and interhemispheric fissure are slightly visible in this 8-month-old.

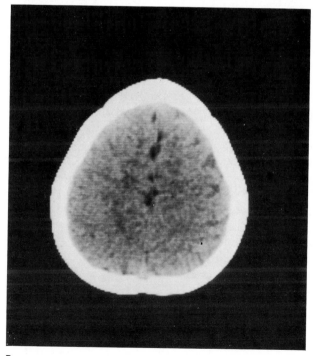

B

B. At the level of the vertex, the sulci are also slightly visible in another child of 8 months.

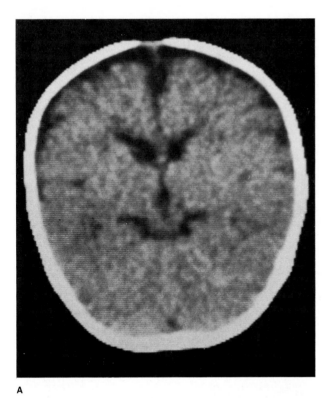

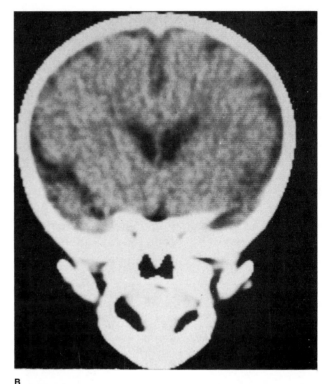

A

B

Figure 6-56 Subdural hygroma. Enlargement of the extracerebral space is seen, especially in the frontal region, in **(A)** the standard semiaxial view and **(B)** the coronal view. No enhancing membrane was visible following intravenous contrast.

entiate a loculated collection from a simple atrophy, because an atrophic brain might change position and sink forward in the prone position. This, however, did not prove to be the case, and such examination could not reliably differentiate the two conditions.

Though the radiologist can easily diagnose the enlarged extracerebral space, it can sometimes be hard to tell whether it is in the subdural or the subarachnoid compartment and whether it is clinically significant.

Bibliography

ALLEN HA, HANEY P, RAO KCVG: Vascular involvement in cranial hyperostosis. *Am J Neuroradiol* **3**:193–195, 1982.

ANDERSON WAD, KISSANE JM: *Pathology,* 7th ed. St. Louis, The C.V. Mosby Company, 1977, chap. 48.

ARCHER C, DARWISH H, SMITH K JR: Enlarged cisternae magnae and posterior cysts simulating Dandy-Walker syndrome on computed tomography. *Radiology* **127**:681–686, 1978.

Blakiston's Gould Medical Dictionary, 4th ed. New York, McGraw-Hill Book Company, 1979.

CHUANG SH, FITZ CR, HARWOOD-NASH DC: The use of metrizamide ventriculography in pediatric hydrocephalus. Presented at the Society of Pediatric Radiology, March, 1981.

CROME L: Hydraencephaly. *Dev Med Child Neurol* **14**:224–234, 1972.

DENNIS M et al: The intelligence of hydrocephalic children. *Arch Neurol* **38**:607–615, 1981.

DI ROCCO C, CALDARELLI M, DI TRAPANI G: Infratentorial arachnoid cysts in children. *Child's Brain* **8**:119–133, 1981.

Dorland's Illustrated Medical Dictionary, 25th ed. Philadelphia, W.B. Saunders Company, 1974.

EDWARDS JH: The syndrome of sex-linked hydrocephalus. *Arch Dis Child* **36**:486–493, 1961.

FITZ CR, HARWOOD-NASH DC: Computed tomography in hydrocephalus. *CT: Comput Tomogr* **2**:91–108, 1978a.

FITZ CR, HARWOOD-NASH DC, CHUANG S, RESJO M: Metrizamide ventriculography and computed tomography in infants and children. *Neuroradiology* **16**:6–9, 1978b.

FLODMARK O et al: Correlation between computed tomography and autopsy in premature and full-term neonates that have suffered perinatal asphyxia. *Radiology* **137**:93–103, 1980.

FLODMARK O, FITZ CR, HARWOOD-NASH DC, CHUANG S: Neuroradiological findings in a child with primary leptomeningeal melanoma. *Neuroradiology* **18**:153–156, 1979.

GANTI SR, ANTUNES JL, LOUIS KM, HILAL SK: Computed tomography in the diagnosis of colloid cysts of the third ventricle. *Radiology* **138**:385–392, 1981.

GILLES FH, DAVIDSON RI: Communicating hydrocephalus associated with deficient dysplastic parasagittal arachnoidal granulations. *J Neurosurg* **35**:421–426, 1971.

GOODING, CA, CARTER A, HOARE RD: New ventriculographic aspects of the Arnold-Chiari malformation. *Radiology* **89**:626–632, 1968.

HALSEY JA, ALLEN N, CHAMBERLIN HR: The morphogenesis of hydraencephaly. *J Neurol Sci* **12**:187–217, 1971.

HART MN, MALAMUD N, ELLIS WG: The Dandy-Walker syndrome: A clinicopathological study based on 28 cases. *Neurology* **22**:771–780, 1972.

HARWOOD-NASH DC, FITZ CR: *Neuroradiology in Infants and Children.* St. Louis, C.V. Mosby Company, 1976.

HEINZ ER, WARD A, DRAYER BP, DUBOIS PJ: Distinction between obstructive and atrophic dilatation of ventricles in children. *J Comput Assist Tomog* **4**:320–325, 1980.

HIRATSUKA H et al: Modification of periventricular hypodensity in hydrocephalus with ventricular reflux in metrizamide CT cisternography. *J Comput Assist Tomog* **2**:204–208, 1979.

HOFFMAN HJ, HARWOOD-NASH DC, GILDAY DL: Percutaneous third ventriculostomy in the management of non-communicating hydrocephalus. *Neurosurgery* **7**:313–321, 1980.

HOLNESS RO, HOFFMAN HJ, HENDRICK EB: Subtemporal decompression for the slit-ventricle syndrome after shunting in hydrocephalic children. *Child's Brain* **5**:137–144, 1979.

JOHNSON DL, FITZ CR, MCCULLOUGH DC, SCHWARZ S: Perimesencephalic cistern obliteration: a CT sign of life-threatening shunt failure. *J Neurosurg* **64**:386–389, 1986.

LECK I: Changes in the incidence of neural tube defects. *Lancet* **2**:791–793, 1966.

MARC JA et al: Positive contrast ventriculography combined with computed tomography: Technique and applications. *J Comput Assist Tomog* **4**:608–613, 1980.

MILHORAT TH, CLARK RG, HAMMOCK MK, MCGRATH PP: Structural, ultrastructural, and permeability changes in ependyma and surrounding brain favoring equilibration in progressive hydrocephalus. *Arch Neurol* **22**:397–407, 1970.

MORI K, HANDA H, ITOH M, OKUNO T: Benign subdural effusions in infants. *J Comput Assist Tomgr* **4**(4):466–471, 1980.

NAIDICH TP, PUDLOWSKI RM, NAIDICH JB: Computed tomography signs of Chiari II malformation: II. Midbrain and cerebellum. *Radiology* **134**:391–398, 1980*a*.

NAIDICH TP, PUDLOWSKI RM, NAIDICH JB: Computed tomography signs of Chiari II malformation: III. Ventricles and cisterns. *Radiology* **134**:657–663, 1980*b*.

OKUNO T, ITO M, YOSHIOKA M, NAKANO Y: Cerebral atrophy following ACTH therapy. *J Comput Assist Tomogr* **4**:20–23, 1980.

RAIMONDI AJ, SAMUELSON G, YARZAGARAY L, NORTON T: Atresia of the foramina of Luschka and Magendie: The Dandy-Walker cyst. *Neurosurgery* **31**:202–216, 1969.

ROBERTSON WC JR, CHUN RWM, ORRISON WW, SACKETT JF: Benign subdural collections of infancy. *J Pediatr* **94**:382–385, 1979.

SCOTTI G, MUSGRAVE MA, FITZ CR, HARWOOD-NASH DC: The isolated fourth ventricle in children. *Am J Neuroradiol* **1**:419–424, 1980.

Stedman's Medical Dictionary, 23d ed. Baltimore, Williams & Wilkins Company, 1976.

TABOADA D, ALONSO A, ALVAREZ JA, PARAMO C, VILA J: Congenital atresia of the foramen of Monro. *Neuroradiology* **17**:161–164, 1979.

YAMADA H, NAKAMURA S, TATIMA M, KAGEYAMA N: Neurological manifestations of pediatric achondroplasia. *J Neurosurg* **54**:49–57, 1981.

7

PRIMARY TUMORS IN ADULTS

Seungho Howard Lee

Krishna C.V.G. Rao

GENERAL CONSIDERATIONS

After Roentgen's discovery of x-rays, the first radiographic means of evaluating intracranial pathology, apart from plain skull roentgenograms, was pneumoencephalography. This consisted in injection of small amounts of air or inert gas into the ventricular and subarachnoid spaces so as to study the effects of intracranial masses on these structures and to localize the masses. The limited information obtained was enough for carrying out appropriate treatment. With the availability of angiography and development of more sophisticated pneumoencephalographic equipment, there was significant improvement in the diagnosis of intracranial disease. By judicious use of these two study tools, a mass could be diagnosed and its vascular anatomy defined in a majority of cases; one provided information dealing with the encroachment of intracranial masses on the CSF compartments, either directly or indirectly, and the other provided the vascular topography. In fact, specificity as defined then related to the ability to specify the nature of an intracranial lesion by utilizing these two techniques.

Craniocerebral radionuclide studies provided an added dimension, since the radionuclide accumulated in tissues, cerebrospinal fluid spaces, or vascular structures altered by various pathological processes. Thus radionuclide studies, although not specific, were more sensitive than pneumoencephalography or angiography. Specificity in the past

303

could not be attributed to any single study but was a function and outcome of the judicious utilization of a combination of studies.

Sensitivity and Specificity of CT

Sensitivity and specificity have a slightly different connotation when applied to CT images. As used in the CT literature, *sensitivity* is defined as the ability to distinguish between two similar objects of a certain size or to differentiate a single object from an adjacent or surrounding region. In CT parlance, it is the ability to detect a single lesion (or more than one lesion) within the brain parenchyma which is slightly more dense or less dense than the surrounding parenchyma. Extending this concept further, it is the ability, as applied to tumors, to discern a small lesion (less than 1 cm) wthin the brain parenchyma. Several factors contribute to the detectability of such a lesion (Table 7-1), most of them by an instrument-related characteristic designated *resolution capacity*. The resolution capacity of the most recent scanners is excellent when viewing a dense object such as a 1-mm pinhead, but it may not be adequate to detect an object with a density slightly greater or less than water.

Table 7-1   Factors Influencing Sensitivity

Instrument-related	
Spatial resolution:	Detector aperture
	Tube focal spot size
	Magnification geometry
	Radiation dose
Contrast resolution:	Spatial sampling frequency
	Slice thickness
	Reconstruction algorithm
	Target reconstruction
Patient-related	Size of body organ
	Size of lesion
	Nature of pathological process
	Patient motion
Observer-related	Visual perception
	Level of expertise

Since the detection of a given lesion also depends on the linear attenuation of the x-ray beam, certain lesions may be better visualized if the study is performed with different energies (kilovoltages). Section thickness also plays an important part in the detectability of a lesion, inasmuch as a larger section thickness (10 mm) may obscure a lesion because of partial volume averaging, while the lesion may be visible when a smaller (2 to 5 mm) section thickness is used. In evaluating sellar and petrous bone, the process of target reconstruction, which involves reconstruction of the detector readings, results in an image with better spatial resolution (Shaffer 1980). These factors are explained in greater detail in Chapter 1. Patient-related factors such as the size of the organ in relation to the size of the lesion can also result in decreased sensitivity, as can the type of lesion. A small or pinhead-size hematoma can be detected by CT, whereas a hematoma having a density similar to the brain parenchyma can easily be missed. Patient motion resulting in artifacts may also be responsible for nonvisualization of a lesion.

Sensitivity has also been used in CT literature to compare CT with other diagnostic modalities, that is, to evaluate the ability of procedures to distinguish between normal and abnormal processes. After the introduction of CT, several investigators compared the sensitivity of CT with cranial radionuclide studies and indicated that the two modalities were equally sensitive in the detection of acute lesions, with almost the same rate of accuracy (Pendergrass 1975; Clifford 1976; Alderson 1976). The sensitivity of CT for the detection of certain lesions can also be increased significantly by utilizing intravenous iodinated contrast. Lesions which are small or isodense may be detected by their vascularity and their disruption of the blood-brain barrier. The amount of iodinated contrast also appears to play a role in increasing the sensitivity of CT. Initially, small volumes of contrast (50 ml of 60 percent iodinated contrast) were felt to be adequate. Davis (1979) and Hayman (1980) have shown that certain lesions, because of either their small size or their ultrastructure, may be seen only if very large amounts of contrast (300 ml of 60 percent iodinated contrast; close to 80 g of iodine) are utilized.

Even without the use of high doses of contrast, the sensitivity of CT in the detection of intracranial neoplasms is uniformly high, varying between 85 and 98 percent in the different series (Ambrose 1975a; Wende 1977; Claveria 1977b; Evens 1977; Baker 1980). With presently available scanners and judicious utilization of iodinated contrast, the detection rate in neoplastic processes may approach 100 percent.

Numerous similar studies have evaluated the specificity of CT. *Specificity* can be defined as the ability to determine the exact nature of the lesion and, if possible, its histological nature. The approaches adopted by various authors have been to correlate the pathology data with the histological variance. A variety of factors influence the attempt to be specific about a given lesion (Table 7-2). Some are related to the CT equipment and the utilization of different software; others depend on the pathological process itself.

The specificity of CT in establishing histologic types and grades of intracranial tumors has not proved nearly as high as its sensitivity in the careful qualitative analysis of CT patterns (Steinhoff 1976; Thomson 1976; Tchang 1977; Butler 1978; Tans 1978; Hilal 1978b; Oi 1979). Qualitative analyses have utilized the structural composition of tumors as seen on CT both before and after contrast enhancement. Circular or irregular homogeneous contrast enhancement was noted in 89 percent of meningiomas, mixed or ring enhancement in 77 percent of glioblastomas, and no enhancement in 100 percent of grade I atrocytomas (Steinhoff 1977). Although these contrast-enhancement CT characteristics are of assistance in histologic diagnosis, others have not been able to duplicate these results (Tans 1978). The specificity is somewhat limited because of significant overlap among different tumors.

Different methods of quantitative analysis have also been attempted. Huckman (1977) utilized quantitative measurement of the mean values of CT numbers to delineate the different varieties of intracranial lesions. Hilal et al. (1978) attempted histological diagnosis by correlation between the initial density on NCCT and the extent of uptake on CECT. Their study revealed an often inverse relationship between the degree of enhancement and the grade

Table 7-2   Factors Influencing Specificity

Instrument-related	Differences in linear attenuation coefficient
	Effective atomic number
	Dual energy
Patient-related	Clinical history (mode of onset, etc.)
	Age and sex
Pathological process	Size and shape of lesion
	Location of lesion
	Extent of mass effect
	Presence or absence of Ca^{++} or hemoglobin
	Nature of enhancement (ring, homogeneous, etc.)
	Time/density curve of CECT

of malignancy: the higher the initial density the less the contrast uptake and usually the lower the grade of malignancy, whereas the lower the density on NCCT the higher the contrast uptake and the grade of malignancy. However, it is doubtful that a consistent linear relationship exists between the initial density of a tumor and the degree of enhancement which is specific for each group of tumors. The use of histograms in the region of interest has been reported to be an additional help in the pathologic definition of tumors when careful analysis of pre- and postcontrast curves is carried out (Dorsch 1978; Vonofakos 1978; Mances 1978; Gardeur 1977).

Contrast-enhancement response as a function of time has been investigated in various types and grades of intracranial tumors as an aid to diagnostic specificity (Steinhoff 1976; Lewander 1978). The time-response curve of enhancement has been divided into an initial and a delayed phase. Rapid early rise of the curve is noted in the initial phase and slow minimal variation in the late phase extending from ½ hour to 3 hours. Although delayed scanning is at least minimally useful in the grading of certain tumors, its practicality in many institutions is limited. CT numbers on the CECT may not be dependable, since multiple variables such as the amount of contrast injected, the mode of injection, and variation in scanner calibration may compound the difficulty in evaluation of the contrast-enhancement pattern. Several authors have shown that when the same lesion is scanned at different voltages before and after contrast enhancement, the effective atomic numbers change. Latchaw (1978*b*, 1980) has shown that the percentage change in the effective atomic number following contrast enhancement can be helpful in differentiating major categories of intracranial neoplasms such as gliomas, meningiomas, and metastases. A potential role of the new-generation scanners with extremely fast scanning time (dynamic CT study) is to help divorce the intravascular and extravascular elements in the early phase of contrast enhancement, although the usefulness of the response curve in various tumors remains to be proved. The rapid-high-dose (80 g of iodine) infusion technique (Hayman 1979, 1980) may be of further help in defining tumor pathology when combined with delayed scans; it needs to be further evaluated.

Histologic diagnosis and grading of a tumor as a means of estimating its biologic behavior have intrinsic problems. The fraction of tissue histologically examined may not be representative of the total tumor; also, mixed grades and types may occur in a tumor. The gross pathology of a tumor observed at operation or autopsy frequently suggests its histology. Correct diagnosis based on gross pathology is possible, especially after consideration of the location of the tumor, which may indicate cells of origin in some cases. A similar dilemma in making a histologic diagnosis on the basis of CT characteristics is to be expected, since CT depicts very closely the gross pathology of a tumor as seen at autopsy or surgery.

Nevertheless, one of the advantages, and a significant contribution, of CT is its ability to distinguish a tumor mass from surrounding edema, which can be accomplished only with some difficulty and limited accuracy by cerebral angiography. Cerebral edema is associated with most, if not all, primary and metastatic tumors and is present in the distribution of the white matter. Malignant intracerebral tumors, specifically glioblastoma and metastatic tumor, usually incite the greatest degree of edema. Slow-growing intracerebral tumors have been considered to incite less edema and extradural tumors

the least edema. But edema is notably absent in intraventricular and some midline tumors, probably because of lack of contact with the white matter. However, the frequency, extent, and degree of edema are not pathognomic and, taken alone, lack specificity.

Technical Considerations

The earlier CT scanners with fixed section thickness and other limitations in flexibility resulted in nonvisualization of neoplasms less than 8 to 10 mm in size, particularly when the tissue density of the lesion did not change significantly on CECT. Some of the larger lesions were also not detected, either because of their location or because of motion artifacts resulting from the long scanning time. With the present generation of scanners, which are not only faster but have more flexible options (slice thickness, scanning time, and high resolution), very small lesions can be easily detected. Most centers have evolved protocols for CT studies, with guidelines for contrast enhancement (Latchaw 1978*a*; Kramer 1975). Most centers perform CT studies in the noncontrast mode (NCCT) followed by the contrast-enhanced mode (CECT), although others (Latchaw 1978*a*; Butler 1978) believe that NCCT does not add further information, and its omission will decrease the radiation dose to the patient. Cost-saving factors such as more patient throughput in a given unit are also a consideration in deciding not to perform the NCCT. Eliminating the NCCT, however, may cause the examiners to miss fresh hemorrhage or calcification in a tumor—findings that may be of immediate clinical importance or may help to characterize the tumor histologically. Occasionally, thinner sections (2 to 5 mm) following a high dose of contrast are necessary to demonstrate smaller lesions, especially when the decision as to treatment modality depends on the CT findings.

CT Contrast Enhancement

When CT first became available, Ambrose (1975*b*) observed that intravenous iodinated contrast enhanced the visualization of brain tumors. Contrast enhancement can be attributed to two mechanisms, (1) extravascular and (2) intravascular accumulation of contrast material (Gado 1975). Contrast enhancement in tumors depends to a significant extent on the contrast agent accumulation in an extravascular compartment due to the leakage of contrast medium across the blood-brain barrier, analogous to that of radionuclide (Gado 1975). The portion contributed by increased intravascular accumulation of contrast agent in tumors may not be as significant as in cerebrovascular anomalies. In the early period of CT utilization, there were significant differences of opinion regarding the necessity of and indications for contrast enhancement (New 1975; Paxton 1974). The total dosage of iodine, its concentration, and the mode of administration (bolus, infusion, or both) were set arbitrarily by different groups. At present the consensus (Norman 1978; Davis 1976) is to use a dose which provides about 40 g of intravenous iodine (150 ml of 60 percent iodinated contrast), given intravenously as a bolus (Deck 1976) in 4 to 5 minutes, or else 300 ml of 30 percent solution as a drip infusion (Kramer 1975; Butler 1978; Huckman 1975) for an adult patient of average weight. Even larger amounts of up to 80 g of iodine have been utilized (Kramer 1975; Davis 1979; Hayman 1979) and have been useful in detecting very small neoplasms. The only contraindication to the use of a large volume

of contrast appears to be poor renal function. Various studies have shown that the incidence of untoward reactions is not dose-related (Hayman 1979). As a guideline, Table 7-3 gives the total amount of iodine at different volumes and concentrations.

The time interval between administration of intravenous iodinated contrast and CT has also been debated. In general, CECT, when performed immediately following injection of contrast, demonstrates enhancement of the lesion unless the patient is on large doses of steroids. Delayed CT studies may occasionally be helpful in demonstrating smaller lesions or for those patients who are on high doses of steroids. Although the exact mechanism is not clearly understood, it is presumed that steroids restore the normal blood-brain barrier and reverse the abnormal capillary permeability associated with metastatic and primary brain tumors. Hayman (1980) has shown that in patients on heavy doses of steroids, the smaller metastases can be demonstrated by CT immediately following large doses of intravenous contrast (80 g of iodine), suggesting that visualization of certain neoplasms, regardless of their size or histology, may be related to the volume of contrast material. The authors believe that both the disruption of the blood-brain barrier and the volume of contrast influence detection of the lesion. CECT may also show varying degrees of enhancement of the cisternal spaces in leptomeningeal carcinoma-

Table 7-3   Iodine Content Based on Volume and Concentrations

Volume (mL)	Concentration (%)	Iodine (mg/mL)	Total amount of iodine (g)
50	50	300	15.0
50	60	282	14.1
		292	14.6
100	60	282	28.2
		292	29.2
100	76	370	37.0
150	60	282	42.3
150	76	370	55.5
200	60	282	56.4
300	30	141	42.3

Prepared by M.G. Lee & S.H. Lee.

tosis (Enzmann 1979). Enhancement of epidural and subdural metastases is common on CECT. Delayed examination is useful in determining whether a lesion is truly cystic or is solid and necrotic (Afra 1980).

Approach to Diagnosis

When an intracranial neoplasm is suspected, certain features are helpful in identifying the mass, its location, and the effect of the mass on the normal intracranial contents.

A neoplasm, whether it is enhancing or nonenhancing, most often will produce a mass effect, which may be focal or hemispheric. There is often distortion or obliteration of the adjacent CSF-containing spaces such as the sulci, subarachnoid cisterns, or ventricles. Enhancement of the neoplasm often helps in defining its precise location and its remote effects

on the adjacent structures. Focal areas of hemorrhage or calcification on NCCT often provide information on the nature of the tumor.

CT also provides evidence of brain herniation within the rigid compartments resulting from the attachment of the dural folds. In herniation across the falx, the characteristic CT findings consist of slight bowing of the falx (since only the inferior margin is free), associated with distortion of the various components of the lateral ventricles (Fig. 7-1). This effect is most often seen when the mass is located below the level of the corpus callosum. In lesions located at a higher level, the only evidence is obliteration of the sulcal pattern.

In masses located in the temporal lobe, there is first medial and then downward herniation of the temporal lobe through the tentorial hiatus (Fig. 7-2). The earliest sign of transtentorial herniation consists of encroachment on the lateral recess of the

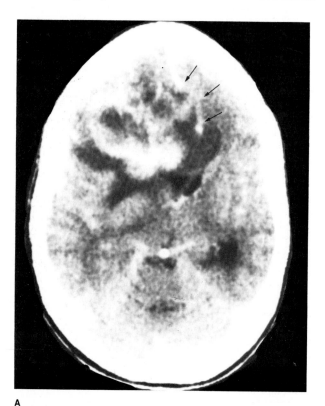
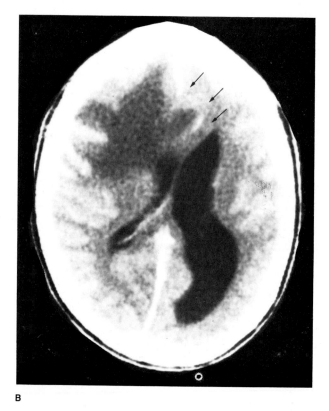

A

B

Figure 7-1 Subfalcine herniation. CECT demonstrating the bowing of the free margin of the falx (arrows) secondary to the large frontal glioblastoma involving the corpus callosum.

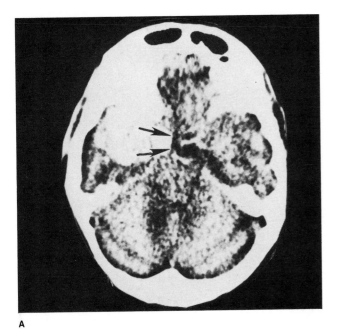

A

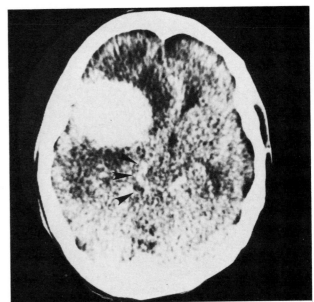

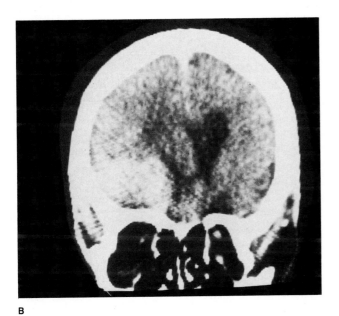

B

Figure 7-2 Uncal herniation. CECT. **A.** Axial section. A large glioblastoma involving the temporal pole has resulted in deformity of the suprasellar cistern (arrows), as well as mild rotation of the brainstem (arrowheads). **B.** Coronal section not only demonstrates the encroachment of the cistern but also the associated subfalcine herniation (arrowheads).

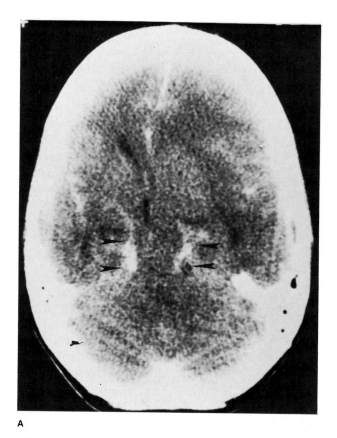

A

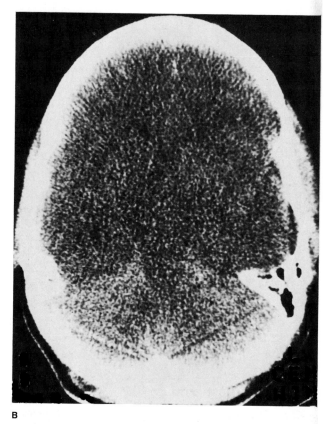

B

Figure 7-3 Transtentorial downward herniation. **A.** Left temporoparietal glioma with transtentorial downward herniation. Compression, displacement, and elongation of the brainstem (arrowheads) are shown on CECT. **B.** Complete obliteration of the quadrigeminal cistern due to diffuse severe cerebral edema in the supratentorial compartment.

suprasellar cistern, resulting in flattening of the normal pentagonal cistern (Osborn 1977; Stovring 1977). With further herniation of the hippocampus and uncus, there is widening of the crural, ambient, and lateral pontine cisterns on the ipsilateral side of the lesion. Because of associated rotation of the brainstem, the opposite cistern is obliterated (Fig. 7-2). Widening of the contralateral temporal horn is a common feature, caused by downward herniation and compression of the mesencephalon with resulting hydrocephalus (Stovring 1977).

If the condition is unrelieved, the uncus and hippocampus are forced through the tentorial hiatus by the combination of the mass and the associated hydrocephalus. This results in nonvisualization of the interpeduncular and parasellar cistern, with anteroposterior elongation of the brainstem (Fig. 7-3). The posterior cerebral artery, which travels in the mesencephalic cistern, if caught between the tentorial margin and the herniating brain tissue, can become occluded, with resultant infarction (see Chapter 14).

In massive transtentorial downward herniation which is rapid, as in diffuse cerebral edema, the CT findings may indicate slitlike ventricles and absence of the gyral pattern, associated with obliteration of the suprasellar cistern anteriorly. The crural and ambient cisterns are obliterated laterally and the superior cerebellar cisterns posteriorly (Fig. 7-3).

Similarly, masses located in the infratentorial

compartment may result in upward herniation of the midline posterior fossa structures through the tentorial incisure. The highly variable size and configuration of the tentorial incisure, as well as the size of the superior cerebellar cisterns, determine the CT appearance.

The earliest sign of upward herniation of the vermis may be compression or asymmetry of the quadrigeminal cistern (Fig. 7-4). In later stages, obliteration of the superior cerebellar cistern and flattening of the quadrigeminal cistern occur. With massive upward herniation, the "toothy smile" configuration of the quadrigeminal cistern changes to a "toothless frown" (Osborn 1978*a*). The resulting flattening of the posterior aspect of the third ven-

tricle, with associated obstructive hydrocephalus, is the end stage of the upward herniation (Fig. 7-4). Associated with the above findings there is usually obliteration of the cerebellopontine angle cistern and the prepontine cistern and anterior displacement of the brainstem. Depending on the pathological process and the location of the mass, there may also be distortion or nonvisualization of the fourth ventricle.

CT, however, is not useful in demonstrating tonsillar herniation, unless intrathecal water-soluble contrast has been injected. In most situations where tonsillar herniation is suspected as a secondary effect rather than as the primary pathological process (e.g., Chiari I malformation), lumbar puncture and thus use of intrathecal contrast are contraindicated.

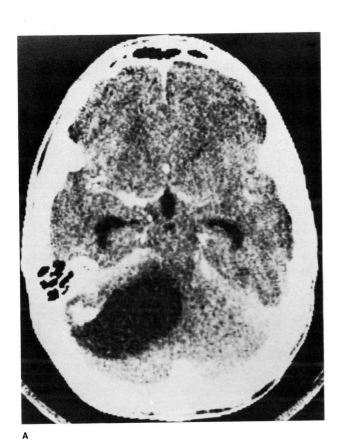
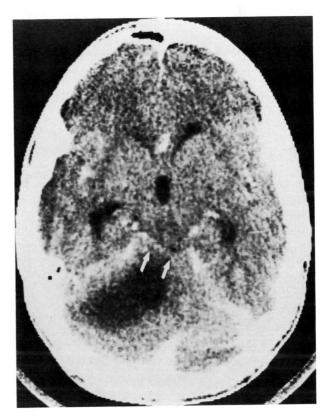

A

Figure 7-4 Transtentorial upward herniation. **A.** A large hemangioblastoma in the right cerebellar hemisphere compresses and obliterates the quadrigeminal cistern (arrows). (*Continued on p. 312.*)

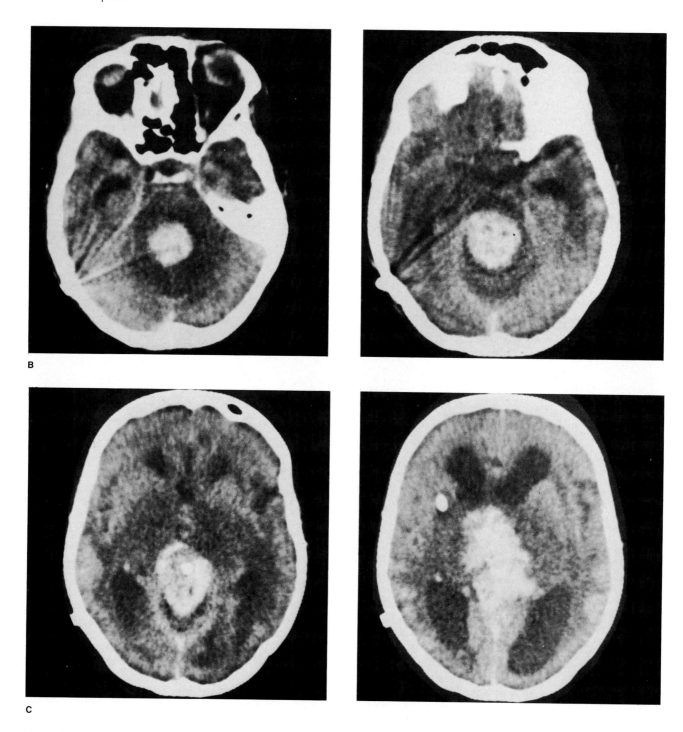

B

C

Figure 7-4 (*cont.*)   **B.** CECT in another patient with ependymoma growing through the tentorial hiatus. The prepontine and superior vermian cisterns are obliterated.   **C.** The tumor is growing through the incisura, with resulting hydrocephalus.

In such a situation, angiography and, if available, MRI due to its noninvasive characteristics, should be the obvious choice of examination.

Other Diagnostic Modalities

The diagnostic accuracy of angiography has proved to be slightly inferior to that of CT, since the latter provides considerably more information. However, cerebral angiography of high quality has a role to play even in this sophisticated era of CT. Preoperative cerebral angiography has certain advantages. These include its ability to delineate (1) exact and accurate arterial anatomy—multiple feeding vessels, tumor infiltration and arterial encasement, aneurysm formation, and stenosis or occlusion; (2) tumor angioarchitecture—vascularity and blush and arteriovenous shunting; and (3) venous anatomy—thrombosis, collateralization, and variations in the vascular filling and draining pattern. Frequently angiography is necessary in order to obtain detailed anatomic information relating the lesion to familiar angiographic landmarks for satisfactory therapeutic planning and also to assess the histologic diagnosis preoperatively. More important, whenever vascular anomalies are a consideration in the differential diagnosis of a tumor, angiography should be performed prior to surgery in order to prevent potential catastrophe. Angiography should be utilized when CT alone may not be sufficient to determine the pathophysiological changes of a suspected tumor.

The detectability of cerebral tumors by radionuclide scan ranges from 84 to 93 percent (Alderson 1977; Buell 1977). Perhaps the major problems with radionuclide scan are its nonspecificity and, to a lesser degree, its lack of sensitivity. Pneumoencephalography and ventriculography utilizing air or water-soluble contrast medium are rarely needed in elucidating detailed relationships with other structures, as in the midline situations of posterior fossa lesions, because, with recent technologic improvements, such as CT reformation in multiple planes, CT images can yield exquisite details with demonstration of precise anatomic relationships.

There is no doubt that MRI has a distinctive advantage in relation to CT in localization and detection of intracranial lesions because of its ability to demonstrate exquisite anatomical details in orthogonal planes without x-ray exposure (see Chap. 17). Although better localization of the lesion may increase the diagnostic capabilities, the specificity based on MR characteristics has become frequently disappointing in our limited experience. Perhaps, complexity of various changing signal intensities depending upon different parameters may be a contributing factor. Definitely, its sensitivity surpasses specificity at present, and we hope both will equilibrate in the near future.

TYPES OF ADULT PRIMARY INTRACRANIAL TUMORS

The major categories of primary intracranial tumor in the adult population are astrocytoma and meningioma. Other histologic varieties of tumor are less common. Diagnosis of the specific histology of a tumor purely on the basis of CT is often difficult. In the authors' experience, certain CT features are helpful in identifying the type of neoplasm (Table 7-4), but variations from the usual pattern are not uncommon.

Congenital Intracranial Tumors

This group of tumors makes up less than 5 percent of all intracranial tumors. Epidermoids are the most common within the group, followed closely by lipomas, dermoids, and teratomas (Russell 1977). Embryologically, these tumors arise from incorporation of one or more of the three germ layers (ectoderm, mesoderm, and endoderm) into the neural tube during its closure. This closure occurs at 3 to 5 weeks' gestation. The stage of fetal development during which the incorporation takes place determines the location of the tumor. If inclusion is early (3 weeks), the lesion is usually midline. Later inclusions place the tumor further from the midline, and

Table 7-4 Features Useful in CT Identification of Various Types of Neoplasm*

Tumor	Initial density	Frequency calcification	Edema	Enhancement pattern	Age/sex group	Location	Other findings
Extraaxial							
Meningioma	↑	20%	+1	+3 H	A/F	Dural attachment	Occasional hemorrhage
Pineoblastoma	↑	Rare	0	+3 M	P/M	Pineal region	Irregular margin and hypodense center
Choroid plexus papilloma	↑	Rare	0	+3 H	P	Ventricular system	Occasional hemorrhage
Choroid plexus carcinoma	↑	Rare	0	+3 H	P	Ventricular system	Irregular margin
Colloid cyst	↑	0	0	0/+1 H	A	Anterior 3d ventricle	
Germinoma	↑/↔	Rare	0	+3 H	A/M	Pineal region	Meningeal and ependymal seeding
Pituitary adenoma	↔/↑	<5%	0	+3 H	A	Sella	Rare hemorrhage or infarction
Neuroma	↔/↑	0	+1	+3 H	A	Cerebellopontine angle	Occasonally cystic
Pineocytoma	↔/↑	Rare	0	+2 H	P	Pineal region	
Craniopharyngioma	↔/↓	30/80%	0	+2 M/R	A/P	Suprasellar	Some cystic
Teratoma	↓	Frequent	+1/0	0	P/A/M	Midline supratentorial	Some cystic, rupture, seeding
Dermoid	↓	Frequent	+1/0	0	P/A/F	Post-fossa base of skull	Some cystic
Epidermoid	↓	Frequent	+1/0	0	P/A	Post-fossa base of skull	Some cystic
Lipoma	↓	Rare	+1/0	0	P/A	Supratentorial midline	
Intraaxial							
Primary lymphoma	↑/↔	0	+2	+2/+3 H	A	Peripheral and deep structures	Irregular margin, multiplicity
Medulloblastoma	↑	10%	+2	+2 H	P	Vermis	Irregular margin
Oligodendroglioma	↑	>90%	+1	+2 M	A	Supratentorial	Irregular margin
Ependymoma	↔/↑	30–40%	+2	+2 H	P	4th ventricle	Irregular margin
Embryonal cell carcinoma	↑/↓	Rare	+1	+3 H	P	Pineal	
Hemangioblastoma	↔	0	+1	+3 H	A	Post-fossa	Cystic, mural nodule
Ganglioglioma	↓/↔	>30%	0	+1 M	P/A	Temporal lobe	Irregular margin, cystic
Neuroblastoma	↔/↓	Common	+2	+2 M	P	Supratentorial	Hemorrhage
Low-grade astrocytoma	↔/↓	<30%	+1	0/+1 M	A	Supratentorial	Indistinct margin
High-grade astrocytoma (glioblastoma)	↔/↓	Rare	+2	+2-3 M/R	A	Supratentorial	Can be cystic, irregular margin
Brainstem glioma	↓/↔	0	0	+1/M	P	Brainstem	Indistinct margin
Cystic astrocytoma	↓	Rare	+1	+1H	P	Post-fossa	Mural tumor nodule

TABLE 7-4 KEY

Key: ↑ = Hyperdensity   H = Homogeneous
     ↔ = Isodensity   M = Mixed
     ↓ = Hypodensity   R = Ring pattern
    +1 = Minimal enhancement   A = Adult: P = Pediatric
    +2 = Moderate enhancement M = Male predominance
    +3 = Intense enhancement   F = Female predominance

*This table was prepared by Russell A. Blinder, M.D., and S. H. Lee, M.D., in 1982 and modified by S. H. Lee, M.D., in 1986.

if extremely late, the lesion becomes intradiploic (Toglia 1965).

Epidermoid

The incidence of this tumor ranges from 0.2 to 1.8 percent of all intracranial neoplasms (Banerjee 1977). The age of occurrence encompasses the years from 25 to 60. Males are affected at a rate of 2 to 1. Ectodermal inclusion of the neural tube gives rise to this lesion, which occurs in the midline or laterally.

Epidermoids may have a multiobulated and grayish white appearance suggesting a pearl. They may be intradural, extradural, or intraventricular but are predominantly intradural and occur most commonly at the cerebellopontine angle. Other sites, in order of frequency, include the parapituitary and midposterior cranial fossa. Intradural lesions rarely

calcify and are difficult to diagnose because of minimal neurological findings and normal skull radiographs. Extradural masses make up 25 percent of all epidermoids and are easier to recognize because of well-marginated radiolucent defects and bone erosion of the base of the skull or diploe. Their edges are sclerotic and may be scalloped (Chambers 1977). This radiographic appearance is not specific and may require differentiation from neuroma, meningioma, aneurysm, chordoma, and metastatic lesion (Tadmor 1977). Some epidermoids are found in the ventricles: the fourth ventricle is the most common location, followed by the temporal horn of the lateral ventricles (Chambers 1977). Epidermoids may also rupture into the ventricular system, exhibiting a fat-CSF fuid level (Laster 1977; Zimmerman 1979*a*).

On CT, epidermoids most frequently show low density similar to that of the CSF (Fig. 7-5). The

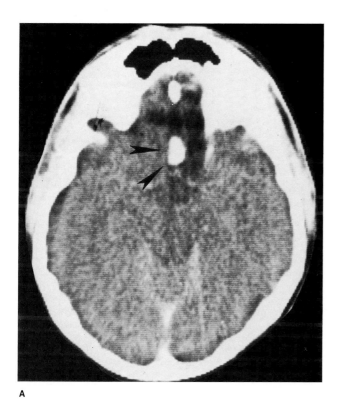

A

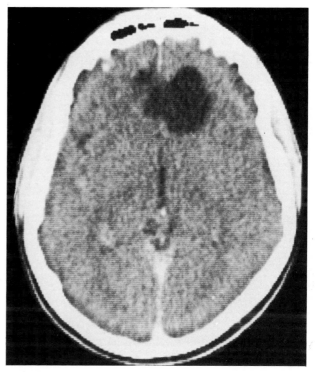

B

Figure 7-5 Epidermoid tumors. **A** and **B**. Multiple areas of hypodensity in the basal frontal area, with the crista galli anteriorly and a calcification posteriorly (arrowheads) within the tumor. Lobulated epidermoid crosses the midline. The absence of contrast enhancement of the wall and the absence of mass effect are noteworthy. (*Continued on p. 316.*)

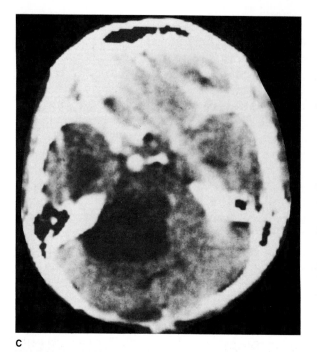

C

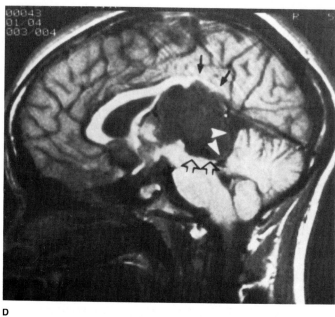

D

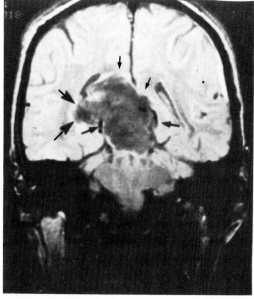

E

Figure 7-5 (*cont.*)   **C.** A large epidermoid tumor in the cerebellopontine angle. Hypodensity and sharp margination of the lesion are noteworthy.   **D** and **E.** Epidermoid tumor of the pineal region. MRI: Sagittal T_1-WI (**D**) shows a large lobulated hypointense mass (arrows) with slight nonhomogeneous signal. Coronal MRI (**E**) shows the boundary of the tumor with clarity. (*Courtesy of Robert A. Zimmerman, University of Pennsylvania, Philadelphia, Pennsylvania.*)

tumor density reflects the composition of the two major contents, keratinized cellular debris and cholesterin (Davis 1976*b;* Zimmerman 1979*a*). Frequently, the density on CT is greater than the negative value of lipids, which is accounted for by the presence of a large amount of nonlipid material (keratin) compared to the chief lipid content, cholesterin. Less often, the cholesterin is present in greater proportion than the keratin, so that the tumor density falls into the minus range (-16 to -80 HU) (Cornell 1977; Laster 1977). Calcification of the epidermoid is generally an inconstant feature of epidermoids. However, occasional increased density ($+80$ to $+120$ HU) and mural calcification (Figs. 7-5*A*, 7-6) are thought to be due to calcification of the keratinized debris, with saponification to calcium salts (Fawcitt 1976; Braun 1977). The absence

of enhancement on CECT is a constant finding. This reflects the structureless, avascular nature of the contents of these tumors and their thin avascular wall (Davis 1976; Chambers 1977). Cerebral arteriogram merely confirms the avascular nature of this tumor. Rare occurrence of contrast enhancement at the periphery of the lesion is considered to be a result of the surrounding vascular connective tissue and dura mater (Tadmor 1977), the presence of gliosis (Mikhael 1978), and cerebral arteries stretched around the mass (Chambers 1977). Nosaka (1979) reported that primary epidermoid carcinoma presents as an isodense or slightly increased density which enhances homogeneously throughout the lesion on CECT.

Absence of hydrocephalus, relative absence of a mass effect, and lack of surrounding edema in spite

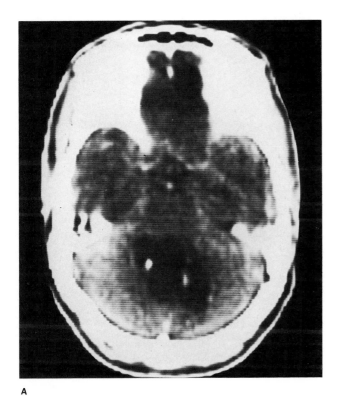

A

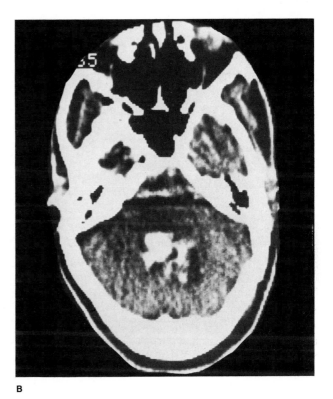

B

Figure 7-6 Intraventricular epidermoid. **A.** The fourth ventricle is enlarged and deformed, with flecks of calcification within and at the periphery of the hypodense lesion. The lateral and third ventricles are normal on a higher level. **B**. CT following intrathecal metrizamide. The metrizamide fills the interstices of the epidermoid within the fourth ventricle.

of the size and site of these lesions are noteworthy and are due to the soft consistency, the slow rate of growth, and the expansion of tumor into the available spaces (Mikhael 1978). Rupture of the capsule further reduces the mass effect. Intraventricular epidermoids may not be readily detected because their density is similar to that of CSF. They may rarely be accompanied by focal dilatation or noncommunicating hydrocephalus. Diagnosis of intraventricular epidermoid can be made following intrathecal contrast. The characteristic CT pattern shows the contrast demonstrating the tumor and occasionally filling its interstices (Fig. 7-6)—a finding diagnostic of intraventricular epidermoid. Rupture of the tumor, with escape of keratin and cholesterin into the ventricular system, allows the less dense cholesterin to float, while the heavier keratin sinks (Laster 1977). As a result, a fat-CSF level is present in the ventricles, which can be clearly detected by CT.

Rupture of the tumor into the subarachnoid space may deposit cholesterin droplets in the adjoining spaces.

Early diagnosis may permit curative surgery. Satisfactory treatment consists of surgical removal of the mass with its capsule. Iatrogenic liberation of its contents into the CSF compartments during surgery can stimulate a chemical or granulomatous meningitis.

Dermoid

Dermoids occur less frequently than epidermoids and account for approximately 1 percent of all intracranial tumors. The age range includes primarily the first three decades, with only a slight female predominance. The inclusion of ectodermal and mesodermal elements at the time of closure of the neural

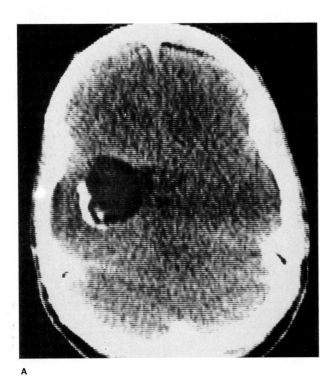

A

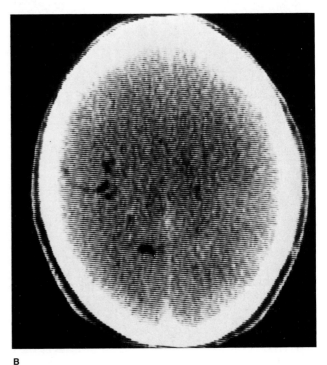

B

Figure 7-7 Dermoid tumor in the temporal lobe.   **A.** Temporal-lobe hypodense mass (− 70 HU) with mural calcification. Soft-tissue mass within the cavity is faintly visible.   **B.** Multiple small fat densities (lipomatosis) are noted in the sylvian cisterns and convexity sulci.

groove leads to the development of sebaceous, apocrine, and adipose tissue within the tumor. These buttery contents fill in between hairs, and toothy calcifications are also found in the dermoid. It is the demonstration of hair, skin, and fat elements that distinguishes dermoids from epidermoids. Calcifications are also more frequent in dermoids. A stratified squamous epithelium lines the inside of the tumor.

Dermoids occur throughout the posterior fossa and at the base of the brain, near the midline. On skull radiographs, dermoids may be seen as radiolucent masses, occasionally with peripheral calcifi-

cations (Gross 1945; Lee 1977). On angiography an avascular mass is usually found. CT demonstrates the low-density masses ranging from −20 to 120 HU (Amendola 1978; Handa 1979) (Fig. 7-7). This fat density actually represents secretions of sebaceous glands and desquamated degenerated epithelium. In vitro the fluid in the cyst has been noted to measure −80 HU (Handa 1979). Incomplete mural calcification may be visible at the periphery of the cavity (Figs. 7-7A, 7-8), and at an appropriate setting of center and window levels, a matted hair ball inside the cavity can also be visualized (Lee 1977) (Fig. 7-8). Contrast enhancement of the capsule is

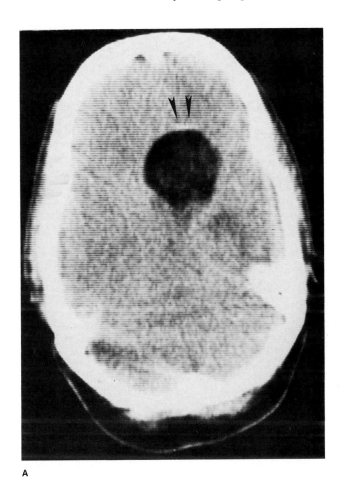

A

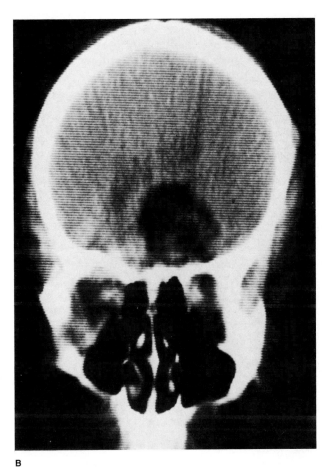

B

Figure 7-8 Dermoid containing a hair ball. **A.** A large, hypodense, round lesion (−80 HU) with minimal mural calcification (arrowheads) and a soft-tissue mass inside which turned out at surgery to be a hair ball. **B.** Coronal view shows a large soft-tissue mass within. (*With permission from Lee, 1977.*)

extremely unusual. The mass effect is usually slight when compared to the size of the lesion.

Spontaneous or iatrogenic rupture of dermoids may result in egress of the contents into the ventricles and subarachnoid spaces, causing a granulomatous meningitis with marked foreign-body giant cell reaction due to irritant cholesterin from keratin breakdown; CT clearly demonstrates an intraventricular fat-fluid level (Zimmerman 1979a) (Fig. 7-9) or freely movable fatty material in the ventricles (Fawcitt 1976; Laster 1977) and in the subarachnoid cisterns (Fig. 7-7) (Laster 1977; Amendola 1978). Hydrocephalus may follow the intraventricular rupture of the cyst (Fig. 7-9), leading to death from severe chemical meningitis. As with epidermoids, surgery should include removal of tumor contents and capsule, since incomplete removal of the capsule may lead to recurrence of the tumor.

Lipoma

Intracranial lipomas are rare tumors, evidently of developmental origin, implicating both the leptomeninges and subjacent neural tissue by inclusion of the mesodermal germ layer early in gestation. About 50 percent of all lipomas are asymptomatic. They are commonly found at or near the midsagittal plane, most frequently in the corpus callosum and occasionally in the cerebellopontine angle and quadrigeminal plate cisterns. Other sites of involvement are the base of the cerebrum, brainstem, roots of the cranial nerves, ventral aspect of the diencephalon, choroid plexus of the lateral ventricles, and dorsal aspect of the midbrain. Some lipomas include elements other than fat, notably calcification, and are associated with dysraphism, such as hypertelorism, myelomeningocele, agenesis of the cerebel-

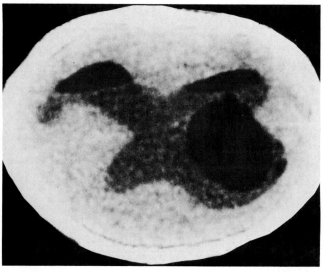

B

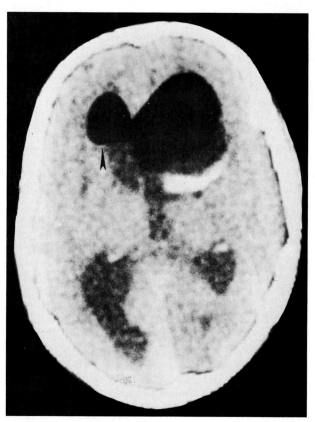

A

Figure 7-9 Frontal dermoid with intraventricular rupture. **A.** Axial CT in supine position demonstrates a large fat-containing mass projecting into the right frontal horn of the lateral ventricle. Calcification is present in the inferior wall of the mass. A fat-CSF level is present in the left frontal horn (arrowhead). **B.** Right lateral decubitus axial CT demonstrates multiple fat-CSF levels in the left lateral ventricle. Hydrocephalus and the right frontal dermoid are well visualized (*Zimmerman, 1979a*). *(Continued on p. 321.)*

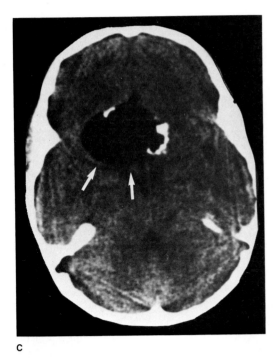

C

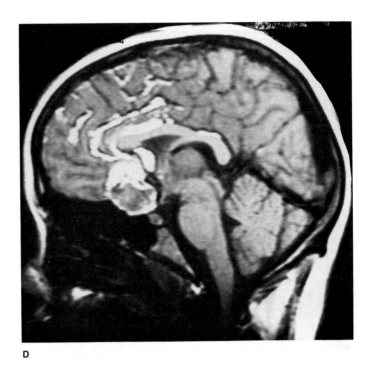

D

Figure 7-9 (*cont.*) **C** and **D.** Rupture of a dermoid into the subarachnoid space. Axial NCCT (**C**) demonstrates a parasellar fatty mass (arrows) with peripheral calcifications. A sagittal MRI, T_1-weighted (**D**) discloses a hyperintense parasellar mass (dermoid) with hyperintense frontal sulci representing fatty tissue in the adjacent and distant sulci. Sulcal widening by fat is a characteristic MR finding of a ruptured intracranial dermoid. (*Courtesy of Dr. Francis J. Hahn, University of Nebraska Medical Center, Omaha, Nebraska.*)

lar vermis, and cranium bifidum (Zettner 1960; Kushnet 1978).

Lipoma of the corpus callosum is associated with agenesis of the corpus callosum in about 50 percent of cases (Zettner 1960). Plain skull radiographs show curvilinear mural calcifications in the genu of the corpus callosum with radiolucency within the lipoma. Symmetrical separation of the anterior portions of the frontal horns and bodies of the lateral ventricles, with elevation of the third ventricle, has been described on ventriculography and pneumoencephalography. Cerebral angiography demonstrates dilated anterior cerebral arteries that are incorporated within the lipoma. All these findings can be clearly depicted on CT (Chapter 4). The diagnosis on CT is made by the characteristic appearance of an area of low density consistent with fat (−100 HU). Except for lipomas involving the corpus

callosum, mural calcification is infrequent. Lipomas in other locations can be easily diagnosed by CT (Figs. 7-7B, 7-10), obviating invasive investigative procedures. Absence of contrast enhancement is characteristic, as with epidermoid. Surgical mortality for lipoma of the corpus callosum is reported to be as high as 65 percent (Patel 1965). Occasionally hydrocephalus is an associated finding, for which surgical relief may be indicated.

Teratoma

The occurrence rate for this tumor is about 0.5 percent but in patients under 15 years of age can be as high as 2 percent. It presents slightly more frequently in males and involves the first two decades of life. Elements of all three germ layers are incorporated early into the neural tube, so that bone,

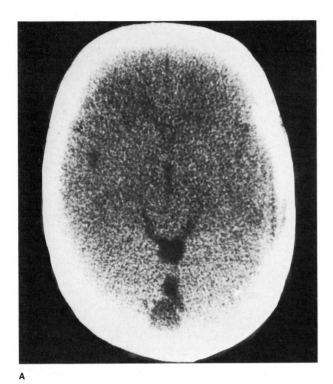

A

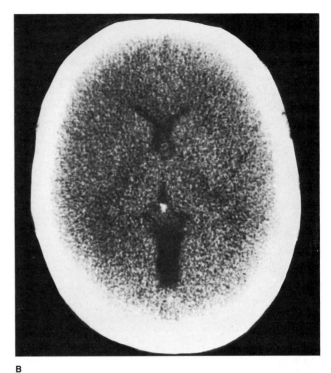

B

Figure 7-10 Lipoma in the quadrigeminal and superior vermian cisterns. **A.** Well-demarcated areas of fat density in the quadrigeminal cistern with no mass effect to the midbrain or cerebellum. **B.** Superior extension into the superior vermian cistern and the vein of Galen cistern is shown. Sharp margination, homogeneous fat density, and conformation to the adjacent structure with no mass effect and no contrast enhancement are characteristic CT findings.

cartilage, teeth, hair, fat, and sebum may all be present at the same time. Calcification generates from the developing dentine and enamel portions of the teeth. The term *teratoid* is employed for forms of teratoma in which derivatives of all three germinal layers are not clearly identified.

The pineal body is chiefly affected (42 percent). Midline locations, such as the pituitary and third ventricle (16 percent), come next, followed by the posterior fossa (11 percent). The remaining 31 percent are widely distributed intracranially (Russell 1977). Clinical presentation depends upon the expanding pressure and infiltration of the surrounding structures, such as the pituitary gland, hypothalamus, optic chiasm and tracts, inferior and superior colliculi, and medial geniculate body. Cerebellar signs, due to downward pressure against the

tentorium, and hydrocephalus, may also be present (Camins 1978).

The pineal region is the most common site for teratomas (45 percent) (Gawler, 1979; McCormack 1978; Zimmerman 1979a, 1980b; Ganti 1986). The tumor consists of fat, soft tissue, hair, as well as tooth elements, characterized on CT as areas of mixed density (Fig. 7-11A). Spontaneous rupture of the tumor into the ventricles results in fat-CSF interfaces, as with epidermoid and dermoid tumors (Goshhajra, 1979). The preponderant location in the pineal region and presence of osseous structures help to make a CT diagnosis.

Germinoma (atypical teratoma) is the most common form of growth at the site of the pineal body. The tumor may present either simultaneously or sequentially in the anterior and posterior third ven-

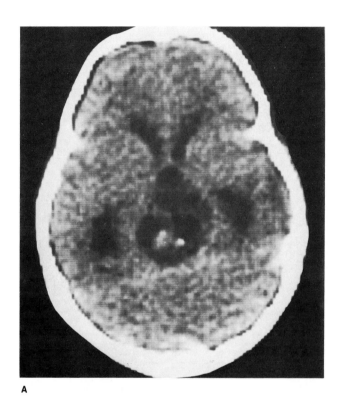

A

B

Figure 7-11 **A.** Teratoma: a large tumor of mixed density in the pineal region. Calcifications and lipid contents are evident. **B.** Germinoma. A large oval, well-marginated, homogeneously enhancing lesion in the region of the anterior third ventricle. The suprasellar cistern and the anterior third ventricle are obscured by the tumor. NCCT (not shown) demonstrated an isodense lesion without calcification and a normal sella turcica. (*Courtesy of Dr. R. A. Zimmerman.*)

tricular region. Frequently the point of origin is difficult to establish. The tumor may grow by direct continuity or by metastasis from the primary site (Camins 1978). NCCT demonstrates a density equal to or slightly higher than the normal brain, whereas CECT exhibits intense homogeneous enhancement (Takeuchi 1978; Neuwelt 1979; Naidich 1976; Zimmerman 1980*b*; Ganti 1986). The tumor is usually rounded, with well-defined margins (Fig. 7-11*B*). Frequently an irregular, indistinct margin suggesting infiltration into the adjacent brain and along the ventricular wall is noted. Complete and rapid disappearance of the tumor following irradiation is usual

in germinomas (Ganti 1986). Although Futrell (1981) found no consistent CT criteria for an accurate histologic diagnosis or for predicting the benign or malignant character of a pineal region tumor, differential diagnosis from other pineal tumors, such as pineoblastoma, pineocytoma, embryonal carcinoma, other glial tumors in the pineal region, and meningioma, may be possible according to Ganti (1986). Tumors arising from the pineal cells (pinealblastoma and pinealcytoma) appear to have a lesser tendency to calcify than do teratomas (Fig. 7-12*A*) (Zimmerman 1980*b*; Ganti, 1986). Perhaps, age and gender may be of help in the differential diagnosis,

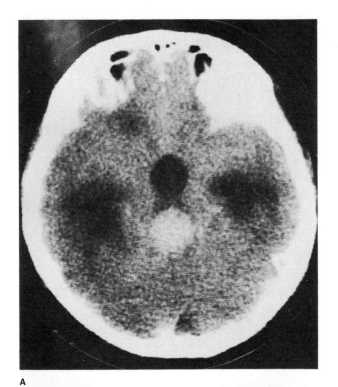

A

Figure 7-12 Pineal tumors. **A.** Pinealcytoma: a round, well-circumscribed lesion at the site of the pineal gland with intense homogeneous contrast enhancement. No calcification is present. Dilated anterior third lateral ventricles (temporal horns) are evident, as well as obliteration of adjacent cisterns. **B–E.** Pineoblastoma: NCCT (**B**) & CECT (**C**) show a slight hyperdense mass exhibiting mild CE. Sagittal and axial MRIs (**D** and **E**) demonstrate a hyperintense mass (arrows) compressing on the 3rd ventricle (3). A solid pineal tumor with no cyst or hemorrhage was found at surgery, which was proven to be a pineablastoma on histologic examination. (*Courtesy of William Cunningham, Somerville, NJ.*)

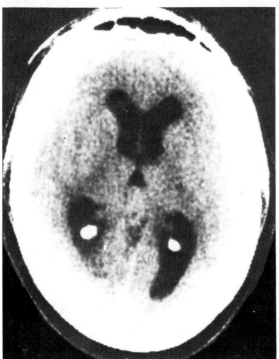

B

C

(*Continued on p. 325.*)

Figure 7-12 (*cont.*)

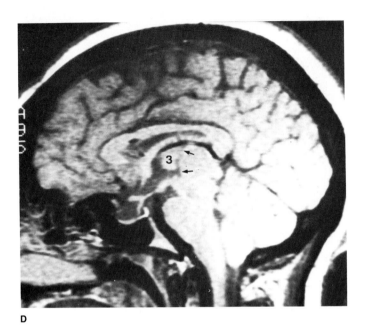

D

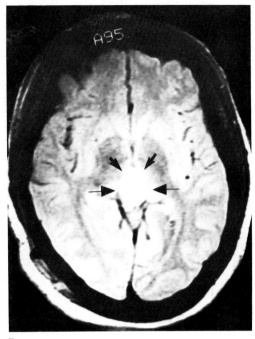

E

since certain pineal tumors, such as teratomas, germinomas, and pineoblastomas, occur either exclusively or predominantly in males.

The role of positive-contrast ventriculography or pneumoencephalography in detecting small lesions in the sella and pineal regions is severely limited and rarely needed with utilization of high-resolution CT scanner with diverse rearrangement ability in different planes. Occasionally, the exact identification of intra- versus extra-axial lesions may still require positive-contrast CT ventriculography or cisternography. However, MRI in orthogonal planes can be a definitive diagnostic study of choice in this situation (Fig. 7-12B).

Gliomas

Gliomas are the most common primary brain tumors. The incidence in larger series varies from 30 to 60 percent of all intracranial neoplasms, but most investigators would accept 45 percent as a representative figure (Russell 1977). Preponderant occurrence in childhood and in males is well known (Bodian 1953; Penman 1954). In dealing with gliomas as

with other tumors, it is highly desirable to know preoperatively the type and grade of tumor so that the appropriate management strategy can be established and an adequate patient treatment plan initiated (Oi 1979).

Astrocytoma

As a group, astrocytomas make up 30 to 35 percent of all gliomas. The low-grade types have been classified by the predominant cell form, but cellular composition and biologic behavior may vary to a considerable degree according to site. Microscopically there are various histologic types such as fibrillary, protoplasmic, gemistocytic, and anaplastic forms. Macroscopically all these types have a firm, gray, granular appearance (Russell 1977).

The majority of low-grade astrocytomas (grades I and II) present on NCCT as irregular, nonhomogeneous low-density lesions (20 HU), less well demarcated than the high-grade tumors (Fig. 7-13). Occasionally, however, low-grade astrocytomas may be relatively well defined, low-density lesions which

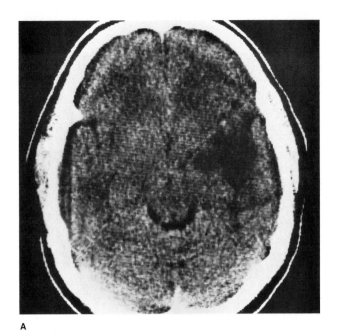

A

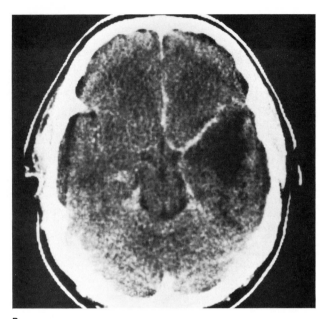

B

Figure 7-13 Low-grade astrocytoma presenting as a cystic lesion. **A.** A poorly marginated mass in the temporal lobe shows nonhomogeneous hypodensity suggestive of a cystic lesion. **B.** CECT shows no apparent contrast enhancement at the periphery of or within the tumor. The central area of hypodensity, at surgery, revealed a solid tumor, not a cyst. Differentiation between the solid and cystic components of a tumor may be difficult on the basis of CT appearance alone.

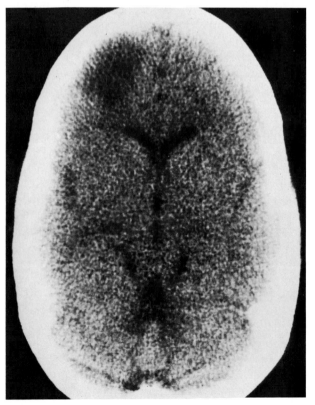

A

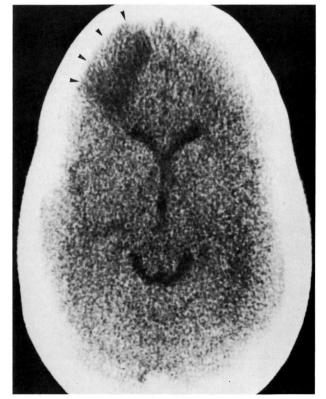

B

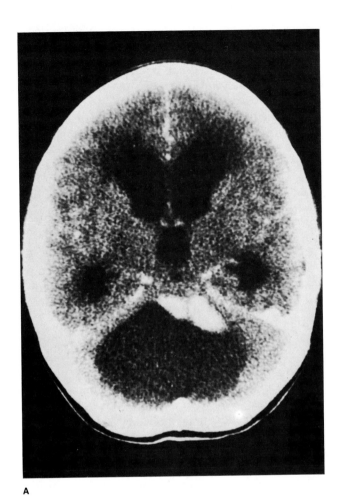

A

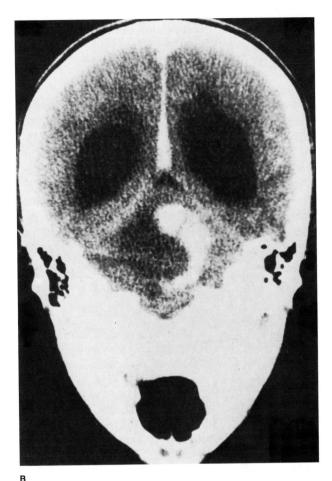

B

Figure 7-15 Cerebellar cystic astrocytoma. Axial **(A)** and coronal **(B)** CECT show a large cerebellar cystic astrocytoma with mural tumor nodules. The remainder of the cyst wall, devoid of tumor tissue, shows no contrast enhancement.

are regular in shape (Fig. 7-14). Calcification is sometimes present, probably in more cases than the reported incidence of 13 percent on plain skull roentgenograms (Gilbertson 1956). Edema around the lesion is slight or absent (Tchang 1977). Some low-grade tumors may contain isodense areas, making it difficult to distinguish the periphery from the surrounding edema or brain. These CT findings are

◀ **Figure 7-14** Low grade astrocytomas (grade II). **A.** NCCT shows a fairly well marginated, hypodense lesion in the right frontal lobe with no mass effect on the frontal horn. **B.** CECT shows minimal contrast enhancement within the lesion (arrowheads). Cerebral angiogram (not shown) demonstrates slight tumor blush. At surgery, a solid low-grade astrocytoma was found.

not unexpected, since gliomas, in general, are not encapsulated and are poorly demarcated from the surrounding parenchyma, particularly in the low-grade gliomas, on histologic examination. The low density on CT usually represents a cystic component (Fig. 7-15), but infrequently, the solid tumor also may present as a low-density lesion, as in microcystic astrocytoma (Fig. 7-13). The distinction between the two may be difficult to make on the basis of CT alone. On CECT, 45 to 50 percent of low-grade astrocytomas enhance, with a wide range of absorption values (Oi 1979). Grade I tumors generally show minimal enhancement (Steinhoff 1978) (Fig. 7-14) or no enhancement at all (Tans 1978) (Fig. 7-13). Steinhoff (1977) reported contrast enhancement in grade II neoplasms in as many as 89 percent of cases and ring enhancement in 26 percent.

High-grade astrocytomas (grades III and IV) on NCCT show nonhomogeneous moderately decreased (Fig. 7-16), mixed, or rarely increased (Fig. 7-17) densities. The low-density area usually measures 16 to 18 HU when cystic and 21 to 24 HU when necrotic. Occasionally, differentiation between cystic and necrotic components may not be possible because of the minimal CT number differences between the two, although morphologically, tumor cysts show a relatively thin enhancing rim and very smooth inner margins (Fig. 7-15), while central tumor necrosis exhibits irregular inner margins and relatively thick walls (Fig. 7-17). It has been reported (Afra 1980) that on delayed CECT, intracystic contrast fluid levels may be demonstrated in cystic centers but not in necrotic centers.

Tans (1978) described three types of CECT appearance of astrocytomas: (1) the annular (ring) type, characterized by an irregular wall of varying thickness with a central area of necrosis; (2) the nodular type, marked by the presence of one or more rounded nodules with fairly sharp margins and of homogeneous contrast enhancement; (3) the mixed type, showing patches of increased density distributed irregularly in a low-density lesion. Most high-grade astrocytomas are of the nodular type, with irregular, indistinct margins (Fig. 7-16). Nodular-appearing tumors usually show the most enhancement and are the most vascular. Although the degree of contrast enhancement correlates well with the amount of vascularity on histologic studies (Tans 1978), there is less correlation on angiograms. In the annular type, a faintly visible ring of isodensity or slightly increased density may surround the tumor, demarcating it from edema (Fig. 7-17). The amount of edema tends to increase with the grade of malignancy, as do ventricular distortion and mass effect. Thomson (1976) suggests that lesions showing patterns of less homogeneity or low density are more likely to be rapidly growing tumors of high malignancy; slow-growing tumors are represented by a higher-density pattern, especially one which is homogeneous.

Tans and Jongh (1978) reported that in 98 percent of astrocytomas the lesions were detected and in 93 percent were recognized as tumors. The specific diagnosis of astrocytoma was correctly made in 68 percent, and the grade of tumor was correct in 78 percent. Only one false negative was seen, and no false positives. According to Kendall (1979), a correct diagnosis was possible in 87.3 percent of 314 supratentorial gliomas, but 1.5 percent were not detected on CT; 6.5 percent were false negatives and 6.5 percent false positives (more significant in patient management). The wrong diagnoses were hemangioma, metastasis, infection, infarction, hemorrhage, and vascular malformation. All these should be considered in the differential diagnosis of gliomas.

Glioblastoma Multiforme

Glioblastoma is rare in persons under the age of 30, and its peak incidence is at about 50 years of age, with males predominanting. It constitutes 50 percent of all gliomas. Average survival after surgery is 12 months (Reeves 1979). The white matter is usually affected, with the common sites being in the frontal lobes. More than one lobe may be involved. If the corpus callosum is implicated, a butterfly pattern in coronal section is seen where the mass links both hemispheres. Next in order of frequency are the temporal lobe and basal ganglia. A well-circumscribed mass may penetrate the cortex and invade the leptomeninges and dura. The tumor very often has a creamy-yellow center of necrosis with a variegated surface and contains small cysts. Rapidly growing glioblastomas may be demarcated from the surrounding brain parenchyma like the high-grade astrocytoma. A clear histologic distinction between glioblastoma and high-grade astrocytoma may not always be possible—a fact that compounds the difficulty of CT differentiation between them. Even in cases with definite histologic diagnosis, CT differentiation can be extremely difficult.

On NCCT, glioblastoma density may present as increased (8.5 to 18 percent), decreased (11.8 to 27 percent), isodense (14.4 to 16.5 percent), or mixed (38.5 to 65.3 percent) (Steinhoff 1977, 1978). Mixed density is the most frequent CT appearance prior to contrast injection (Figs. 7-18, 7-19, 7-21). Calcification is not a common feature in glioblastoma.

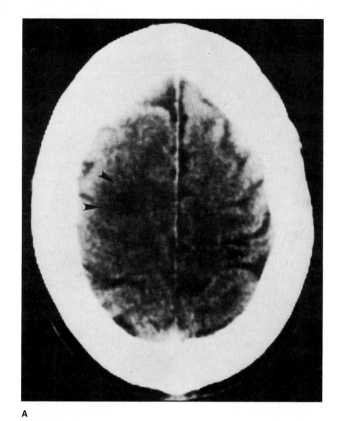

A

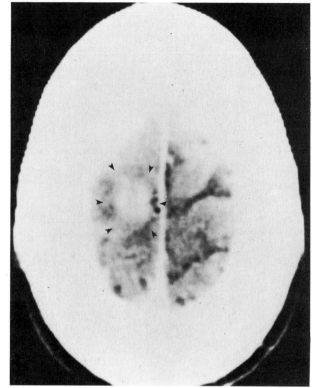

B

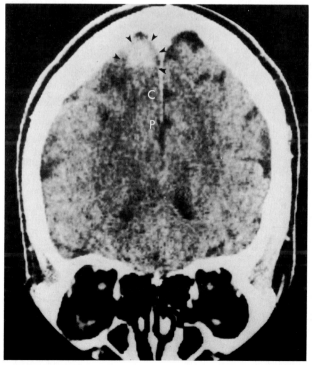

C

Figure 7-16 High-grade astrocytoma: hypodensity with nodular contrast enhancement. **A.** NCCT shows a focal area of hypodensity in the frontoparietal white matter (arrowheads). Effacement of convexity cortical sulci reflects mass effect **B.** CECT displays a nodular enhancement in the superior border of the tumor (arrowheads). **C.** Coronal CECT exhibits nodular contrast enhancement in the cortex, with irregular hypodense areas underneath indicating deep white-matter involvement. Note effacement of ipsilateral pericallosal (*P*) and cingulate (*C*) sulci.

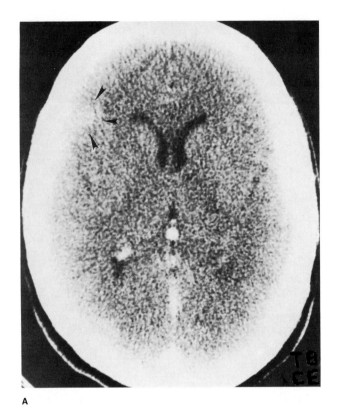

A

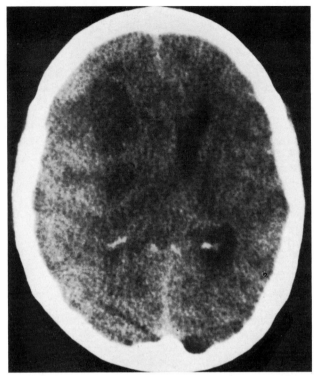

B

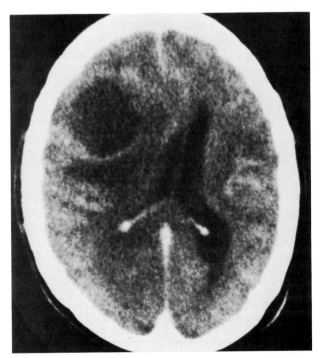

C

Figure 7-17 High-grade (grade IV) astrocytoma with necrosis.
A. CECT shows slightly hyperdense area in the frontal lobe (arrowheads).   **B.** Three months later, NCCT displays a large mixed-density lesion in the frontal lobe. The wall is partly hyperdense and irregular. Marked shift and compression of the ipsilateral ventricle is present.   **C.** CECT demonstrates a ringlike, irregularly enhancing wall of varying thickness at the periphery of the tumor. The central hypodense area represents necrosis. Minimal surrounding edema is present in the white matter.

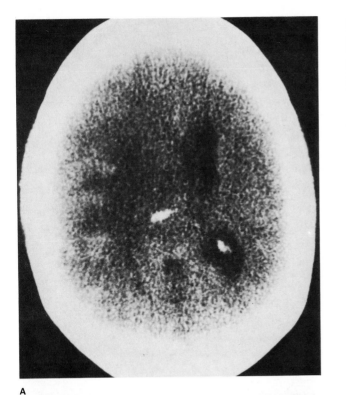

A

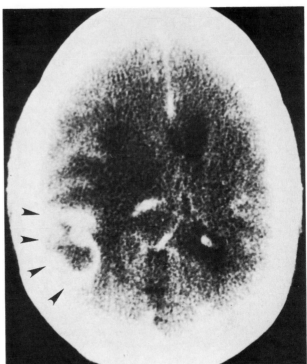

B

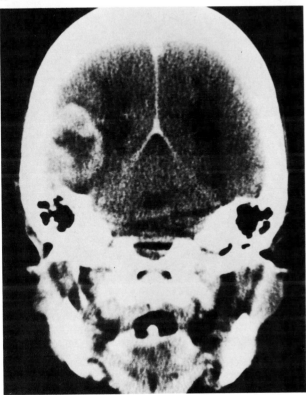

C

Figure 7-18 Glioblastoma multiforme in temporoparietal lobe.
A. On NCCT, a poorly defined area of mixed density in the right temporoparietal lobe. Marked compression and contralateral shift of the right choroid plexus and the lateral ventricles are evident. **B.** CECT shows irregular, thick walls of the tumor (arrowheads). Central tumor necrosis and severe white-matter edema are evident. **C.** Coronal CECT displays the tumor to better advantage.

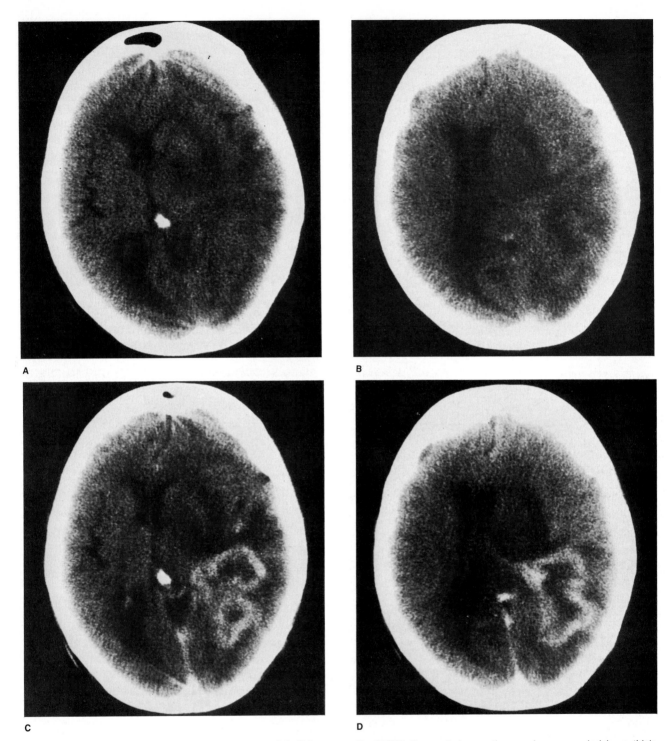

Figure 7-19 Glioblastoma multiforme in the temporooccipital lobe. **A.** and **B.** NCCT demonstrates ventricular compression and shift of the midline structures. A large mixed-density (isodense and hypodense) area is noted in the left temporooccipital lobe **C** and **D.** On CECT, the central necrotic area is surrrounded by a thick, irregular wall of ameboid appearance. Note the involvement of the ventricular wall and extension into the choroid plexus.

On CECT, almost all glioblastomas—91 percent (Tchang 1977) to 100 percent (Steinhoff 1978)—show enhancement, although hypodense glioblastomas without any change after contrast injection have been reported (Tchang 1977; Steinhoff 1977). According to Steinhoff (1978), the annular type with central low density is the most frequent pattern (55 percent) (Figs. 7-18, 7-19). The annular zone of high density represents solid vascularized tumor, while the central zone of low density usually corresponds to tumor necrosis and occasionally intratumoral cyst (Fig. 7-20). The enhanced rim of a glioblastoma is usually thick (more than 5 mm) and irregular, in contrast to the usual thin, homogeneous wall of the abscess cavity. The mixed type of enhancement, the second most frequent manifestation (27 percent), is characterized by variable density zones and heterogeneous enhancement of the glioblastoma (Fig. 7-21). The pathological substrate of this type consists of solid and necrotic parts. The nodular type (18 percent) represents homogeneous solid tumor, which can easily be differentiated from perifocal edema on CECT.

Perifocal edema expands in the subcortical white matter, typically exhibiting a digital configuration (Fig. 7-18). The frequency of this tumor-induced edema is 88 percent in glioblastomas (Steinhoff 1978). Grading the extent of edema was considered to be helpful: grade I when its margin has a width of 2 cm or less, grade II when it includes up to half of the hemisphere, and grade III when it's larger than half of the hemisphere. In glioblastomas, edema of grades II and III predominated, but no correlation between frequency or grade of edema and specific types of intracranial neoplasms was found. However, mass effect evidenced by ventricular distortion or displacement is noted in all cases (Tchang 1977).

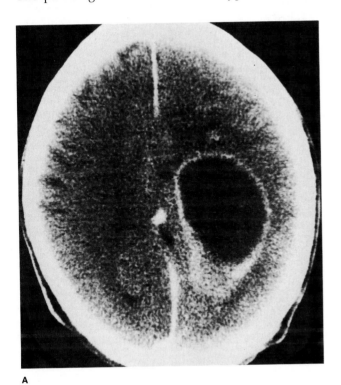

A

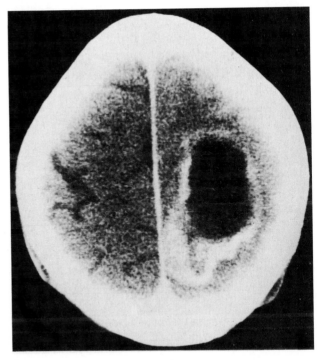

B

Figure 7-20 A and **B.** Glioblastoma with central cystic cavity. CECT **(A)** demonstrates a large oval lesion with a relatively thin enhancing rim and a large central hypodense area. Posteriorly the rim shows an irregular thick wall. At a higher level **(B)** an irregular thick wall is well shown. Surgery revealed a large cyst of a clear yellowish fluid within the tumor. (*Continued on p. 334.*)

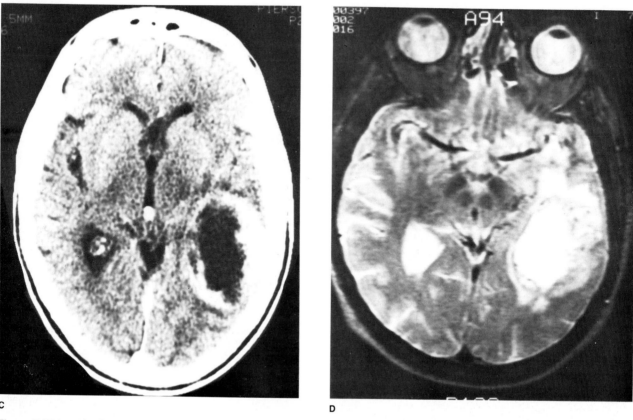

C   D

Figure 7-20 (cont.)   **C** and **D.** Temporooccipital glioblastoma: CECT (**D**) shows a large irregular cavitary tumor with necrotic center. Axial MR (T$_2$ − WI)$_{(E)}$ demonstrates hyperintense necrotic center, thick and irregular tumor at the periphery, and mild peritumoral edema.

Oligodendroglioma

This is a relatively rare brain tumor, making up to 9 percent of all primary intracranial gliomas. Its incidence is predominantly in adult life, most frequently in the fourth and fifth decades, and it is rare in childhood and adolescence. The cerebral hemispheres, especially the frontal lobes, account for the great majority of tumors: rarely they are found in the region of the third ventricle or the cerebellum or within the spinal cord. The cerebral cortex and subcortical white matter are most affected (Russell 1977). Calcification, when present, is related to the intrinsic blood vessels: these deposits are a feature of radiologic importance and are reported to occur in 46.7 percent of cases on skull films (Kalan 1962). Slow clinical evolution is usual.

On NCCT, oligodendroglioma presents as a hypodense lesion associated with slight to moderate mass effect and minimal surrounding edema. Intratumoral calcification on CT occurs in 91 percent of cases (Vonofakos 1979); the calcification may be located at the periphery of the lesion, in its center, or both. Segments of the peripherally located calcifications appear linear or shell-like, with incomplete ring formation, but a nodular type of calcification predominates (Vonofakos 1979) (Fig. 7-22), forming masses of considerable size. The prevalence of this characteristic calcification distinguishes oligodendrogliomas from other tumors.

On CECT thick, irregular enhancement shows at the periphery, completely defining the outer borders of the tumor with calcifications. Areas of nonenhancement within the tumor, concentric or eccen-

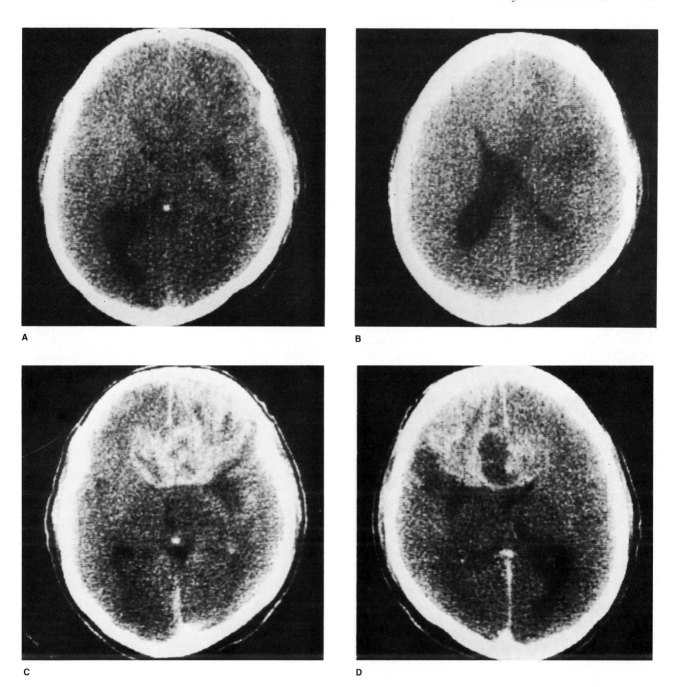

A

B

C

D

Figure 7-21   Glioblastoma multiforme involving the corpus callosum.   **A** and **B.** On NCCT, a large area of mixed density (iso- and hypodensity) in the frontal lobes. Frontal horns are effaced and compressed.   **C.** On CECT, a heterogeneous enhancement pattern represents solid and necrotic tumor tissues. The tumor involves the corpus callosum and extends into both frontal lobes.   **D.** On CECT, at a higher level, the tumor shows a central area of necrosis, a variegated thick wall, and surrounding edema in the white matter. (*Continued on p. 336.*)

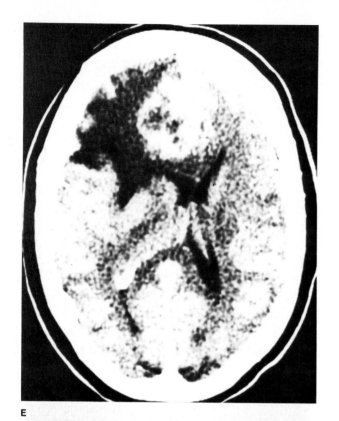

E

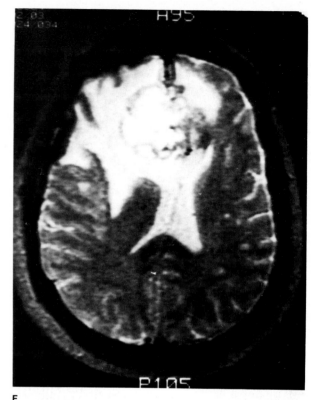

F

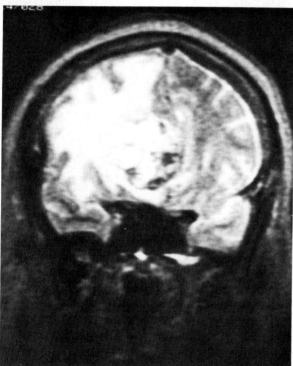

G

Figure 7-21 (*cont.*)   **E, F, G**: Another case of frontal glioblastoma involving the corpus callosum: **E** (Axial CECT), **F** Axial MRI (T$_2$-WI), and **G** coronal MRI (T$_2$-WI) demonstrate clearly the tumor, intratumoral tissue characteristics, tumor extension and peritumoral edema. Differential diagnosis from metastatic tumor is difficult because of extensive peritumoral edema.

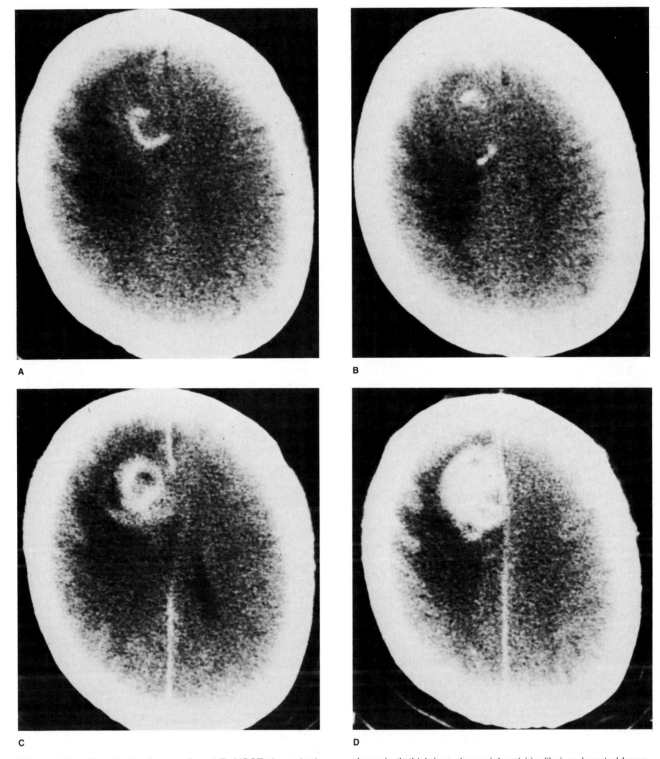

Figure 7-22 Oligodendroglioma. **A** and **B.** NCCT shows both shell-like and nodular calcifications at the periphery of the tumor. Surrounding white matter edema is prominent. **C** and **D.** CECT shows both thick irregular peripheral (ringlike) and central homogeneous enhancement. Areas of nonenhancement represent foci of necrosis and cystic degeneration.

tric, are frequently observed and represent foci of necrosis and cystic degeneration (Fig. 7-22). Rarely, intratumoral fluid-fluid levels indicating a cystic component are noted. Vonofakos et al. (1979) claim that all the cases with contrast enhancement and definitive evidence of a cystic component (fluid-fluid level) on CT proved to be malignant histologically. Spontaneous intratumoral hemmorrhage, metastasis by way of the CSF, or remote extracranial metastasis may occur.

Choroid Plexus Papilloma

Papillomas of the choroid plexus are uncommon lesions which constitute 0.5 to 0.6 percent of all intracranial tumors and 2 percent of the glioma group. They occur usually in the first decade, with slight male predominance. The fourth, lateral, and third ventricles are affected, in that order of frequency. Choroid plexus papilloma of the fourth ventricle is commonly seen in adults, whereas in children it occurs more commonly in the lateral and third ventricles. Those tumors in the lateral ventricles show a remarkable preference for the left side (Russell 1977). Macroscopically, the tumor is readily identified as a globular mass with a round irregular surface. Occasionally it is heavily calcified and rarely undergoes ossification.

On NCCT, the tumor presents as a well-defined, smoothly marginated mass of increased density. Focal dense areas of calcification may be detected (Fig. 7-23). Local expansion of the involved ventricle and generalized hydrocephalus are common. The hydrocephalus in choroid plexus papillomas is due to overproduction of CSF and intermittent hemorrhage with blockage of the arachnoid granulations. On CECT, all these tumors enhance intensely and almost all of them homogeneously (Figs. 7-23, 7-24). Occasional demonstration of low-density areas, concentric or eccentric, within the tumor probably represents the choroid plexus itself or areas of intratumoral necrosis and infarction (Zimmerman 1979c).

Other lesions of the choroid plexus derived from the mesenchymal stromal layer are meningioma and vascular malformations such as cavernous angioma and hemangioma; those derived from the ependymal layer are carcinoma and papilloma. They present as high-density lesions prior to contrast injection and enhance homogeneously after injection. CT features such as calcification, transgression of adjacent ventricular wall and invasion of the parenchyma, absence of generalized hydrocephalus, and intratumoral hemorrhage, association with other entities—namely, neurofibromatosis and Sturge-Weber disease—are helpful in the differential diagnosis if the patient's age and sex and the clinical course are also considered.

Ganglioglioma

An uncommon brain tumor in children and young adults, the ganglioglioma occurs under the age of 30 in 60 percent of reported cases (Anderson 1942; Garrido 1978). Presenting symptoms usually relate to the location of the tumor and its protracted course, usually presenting with a long-standing history of seizures or headaches. This neoplasm is commonly found in the cerebral hemispheres, most often the temporal lobe, less frequently in the parietal lobe, the brainstem and cerebellar hemispheres, thalamic and pineal region (Dorne 1986). No site in the central nervous system is exempt, however. The tumors are usually single masses, but a few have been multiple.

Macroscopically, the lesion is small, firm, and well circumscribed, with a finely granular gray surface. It may contain one large cyst or multiple cysts. Calcified foci are frequent. Some tumors contain capillary vessels in a marked telangiectatic pattern (Russell 1977). CT findings generally reflect the varied macroscopic appearances.

On CT, the tumor is usually well circumscribed, often isodense, but frequently hypodense with areas of increased density due to calcification (Fig. 7-25). Foci of calcifications are detected by CT in more than one-third of the lesions (Dorne 1986). On CECT, single or multiple cysts with mural nodules may be seen. Contrast enhancement is observed in the majority (Fig. 7-25). Although the CT characterization is not specific, a mixed hypodense, partially calcified, contrast-enhancing tumor with or without cysts

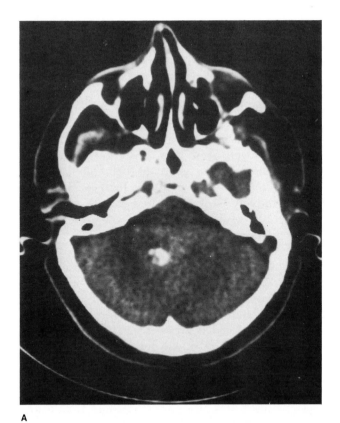

A

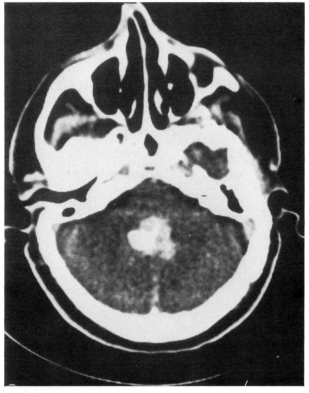

B

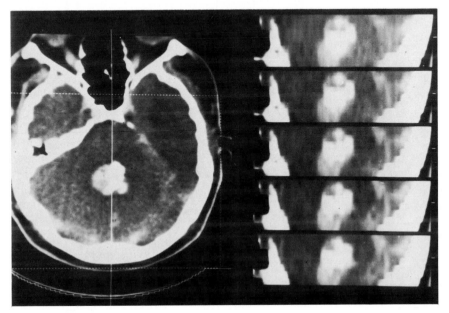

C

Figure 7-23 Choroid plexus papilloma of the fourth ventricle.   **A.** NCCT: Slightly hyperdense lesion with poor demarcation is noted in the region of the fourth ventricle. Mutliple calcifications are eccentrically located within the lesion.   **B.** CECT: Intense contrast enhancement of the tumor manifests as a mottled appearance with sharp, irregular margins.   **C.** Sagittal reformation images confirm the tumor within the fourth ventricle.

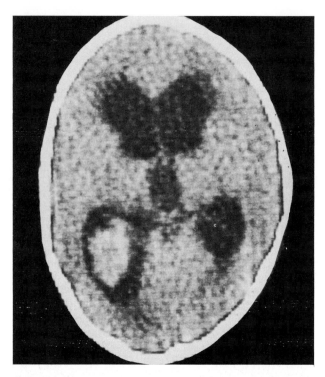

Figure 7-24   Choroid plexus papilloma of the lateral ventricle. On CECT, a large, well-demarcated tumor within the trigone of the lateral ventricle shows intense homogeneous contrast enhancement. Hydrocephalus is due to overproduction of CSF by the tumor and intermittent hemorrhage into the ventricles and subarachnoid space.

in a young patient with a prolonged clinical history should raise the question of ganglioglioma. Histologic confirmation to establish the benign nature of the tumor is important prior to instituting any aggressive therapeutic modalities.

Colloid Cyst

This entity accounts for 0.5 to 1 percent of all intracranial tumors (Guner 1976). Very few colloid cysts are seen in infancy and childhood, with most being found in early adult life. Males and females are about equally affected. It is thought that most colloid cysts are generated from the ependymal pouches (Ariens-Kappers 1955). Mucoids or dense hyaloid material is surrounded by a smooth, spherical, fibrous wall, and the cyst is attached to the collagenous stroma

of the choroid plexus. Within the third ventricle the cyst is notorious for obstructing the foramen of Monro and causing hydrocephalus, since it can grow to as much as 3 cm in size. If the mass is somewhat pendulous and movable, intermittent obstruction becomes a possibility (Guner 1976).

Common symptoms and physical findings are headache, gait disturbance, and papilledema (Little 1974). Although these tumors are benign and can be completely removed early in their course, Guner et al. (1976) report a mortality as high as 53 percent postoperatively. It is presumed that this figure is high because of the surgical approach and the complex regional anatomy.

NCCT shows a smooth, spherical or ovoid lesion of homogeneously high density (45 to 75 HU) in the anterior third ventricle in front of or behind the foramen of Monro (Fig. 7-26). Uncommonly, the lesion is isodense, and rarely, a central hypodensity within the lesion is noted (Ganti 1981). The high density on NCCT is probably due to desquamative secretory products from the cyst wall, hemosiderin, and possibly microscopic foci of calcification, although the latter are not apparent on CT. Only mild enhancement has been shown on CECT (Osborn 1977; Ganti 1981), but absence of contrast enhancement is not unusual (Fig. 7-26). The presence of blood vessels in the wall or even inside the cyst, as well as diffusion of contrast media into the cavity, may account for the enhancement. Hemorrhage is rare (Malik 1980). Although hydrocephalus, minimal to moderately severe, is present in all cases, its degree is not always proportional to the size of the cyst. In the authors' experience, the anterior portion of the third ventricle is not well visualized, and the posterior third ventricle is usually collapsed. Widening of the septum pellucidum and separation of the posteromedial aspects of the frontal horns are demonstrated in most cases on axial and coronal sections (Ganti 1981). Intraventricular ependymoma, glioma, meningioma, choroid plexus papilloma, arteriovenous malformation, craniopharyngioma, teratomatous tumors, tuberous sclerosis, and cysticercosis should be considered in the differential diagnosis. Occasionally, contrast ventriculography or cisternography may be necessary to localize the lesion

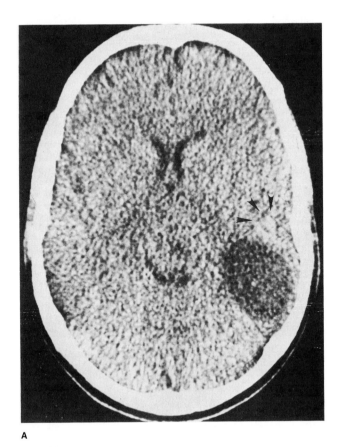

A

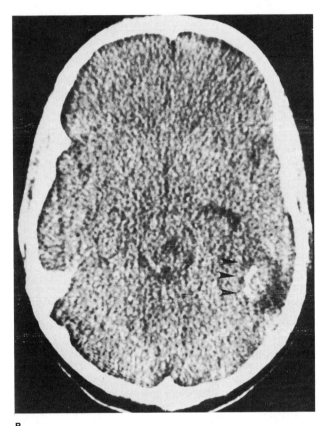

B

Figure 7-25 Ganglioglioma. **A.** A well-circumscribed hypodense lesion in the posterior temporal lobe contains multiple calcifications at the periphery (arrowheads). Minimal mass effect is evidenced by obliteration of the ipsilateral quadrigeminal cistern. **B.** CECT shows minimal contrast enhancement on the medial side of the lesion where calcifications are present (arrows). Slight dilatation of the left temporal horn is due to proximal compression.

within the third ventricle. However, the need for additional study has greatly diminished since the availability of high-resolution CT scanners with multiplanar reformation capabilities and the recent introduction of MRI. When atypical and unusual contrast enhancement is present, the possibility of aneurysm or ectatic vessels should be strongly considered and investigated by cerebral angiography (Fig. 7-27).

Meningiomas

These represent 15 percent of all intracranial tumors in adults; a lower incidence of 3 to 4 percent is noted in the pediatric population. Meningiomas manifest a clear female predominance (3:2), with most tumors detected near midlife and reaching a peak in the seventh decade.

Macroscopically, meningiomas are usually spherical or globular but may be flat and platelike. They are well circumscribed, demarcated, and readily separated from the adjacent brain tissue. All meningiomas arise from meningoendothelial cells. Microscopically, they may be classified as syncytial, transitional, fibroblastic, angioblastic, or sarcomatous. The diversity of types of meningioma reflects the adaptive potential of these cells (Russell 1977).

The common sites of intracranial meningiomas

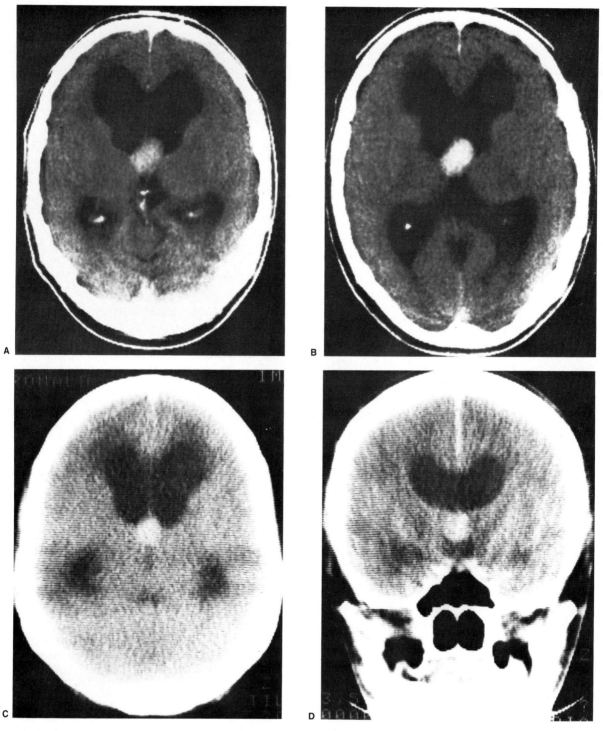

Figure 7-26 Colloid cyst of the third ventricle. **A.** NCCT shows an oval hyperdense lesion in the region of the third ventricle with separation of the posteromedial sides of the frontal horns. **B.** Axial CECT demonstrates mild CE. Noncommunicating hydrocephalus is apparent. Angiogram prior to surgical intervention is necessary to rule out aneurysm. **C** and **D.** Another case: axial NCCT (**C**) presents a colloid cyst as a round hyperdense lesion at the foramen of Monro. (**D**) Coronal CECT demonstrates obstructive hydrocephalus at the foramen. Minimal contrast enhancement is noted.

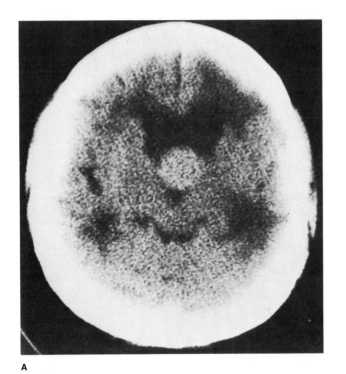

A

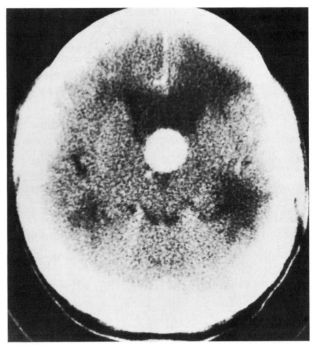

B

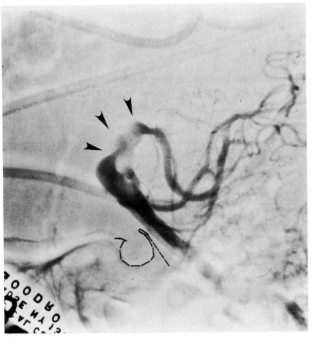

C

Figure 7-27 Basilar artery aneurysm simulating third ventricular colloid cyst. **A.** On NCCT, slightly hyperdense round lesion in the region of the anterior third ventricle. Note visualization of the posterior third ventricle, which is usually collapsed in colloid cyst. Hydrocephalus is present. Periventricular hypodensity may represent transventricular absorption. **B.** CECT shows intense homogeneous enhancement, not a characteristic feature of colloid cyst. **C.** Vertebral angiogram demonstrates a large, partially thrombosed (after surgery) aneurysm of the basilar artery (arrowheads) projecting into the third ventricle.

are the parasagittal and lateral convexities (43 percent), sphenoid ridge (7 percent), olfactory groove (10 percent), suprasellar region (8 percent), posterior fossa (7 percent), and other rare sites (15 percent) such as the falx-tentorial junction, the intracerebral, intraorbital, and pineal regions, and the intraventricular region (Baker 1973).

CT characteristically demonstrates a rounded, sharply delineated, isodense or hyperdense tumor (16 to 35 HU) in a juxtadural location with intense homogeneous contrast enhancement. Mass effect is almost a constant CT feature of meningiomas large enough to obliterate CSF pathways (cisterns) or alter the shape of the ventricular system (Claveria 1977a). Another compressive phenomenon on CT, the inward "buckling" of the white matter, if present, helps to confirm the extraaxial location of the tumor (George 1980). In addition, other CT features, such as the broad base of the tumor abutting the dura and adjacent bone changes, hyperostotic or destructive, may be of assistance in the diagnosis of meningioma.

Hyperdensity on NCCT is attributed to the compactness of the tumor cells, the presence of psammoma bodies within the tumor, and the hypervascularity of the tumor (Fig. 7-28). Calcifications are usually punctate and may be conglomerate, peripheral, or central. They are present on CT in 20 percent of meningiomas (Claveria 1977a) (Fig. 7-29). Transitional and fibroblastic tumors are frequently seen with visible calcium aggregates (39 percent), a feature that characterizes a nonaggressive meningioma (Vassilouthis 1979; Ambrose 1975a). Isodense meningiomas on NCCT (Mani 1978; Amundsen 1978) are difficult to distinguish from the surrounding normal brain tissue; however, on CECT intense, persistent opacification is a usual finding. Occasion-

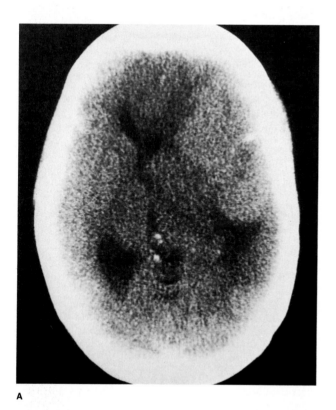

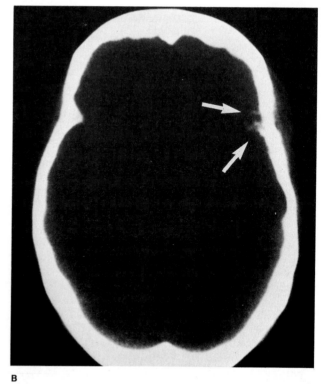

A

B

Figure 7-28 Pterional meningioma. **A.** NCCT shows a large, well-demarcated, lobulated, hyperdense mass with compression and displacement of the adjacent brain tissue and the ventricle.

B. On bone settings, hyperostosis of the pterion, involvement of the calvarium, and extension into the scalp are well demonstrated (arrows). (*Continued on p. 345.*)

Figure 7-28 (*cont.*) **C.** CECT delineates the well-marginated, homogeneously enhancing tumor abutting the inner table of the skull. **D** and **E.** MRI: **D** (T_1-coronal image) and **E** (T_2-axial image) demonstrate a meningioma (arrows) with mild signal intensity change and minimal mass effect in another patient.

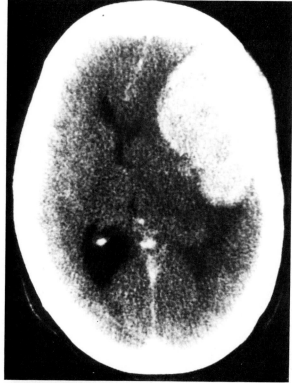

C

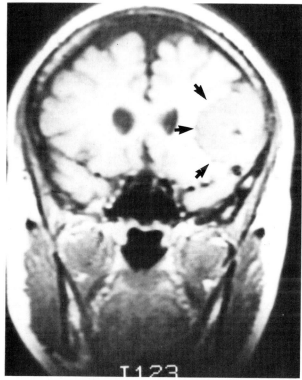

D

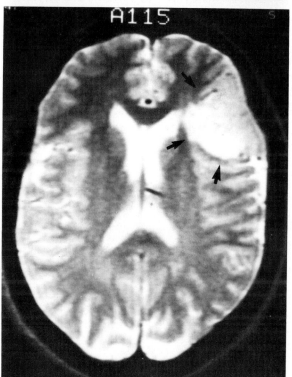

E

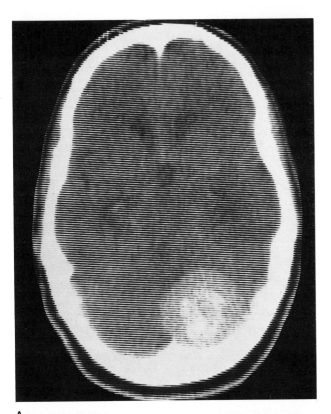

A

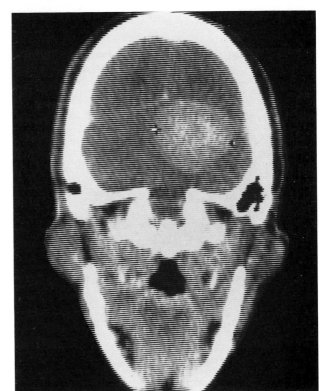

B

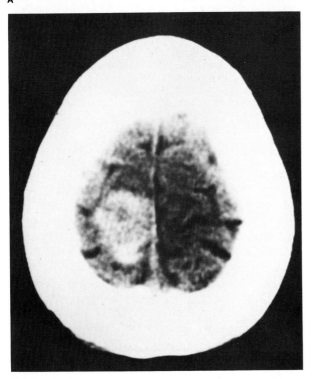

C

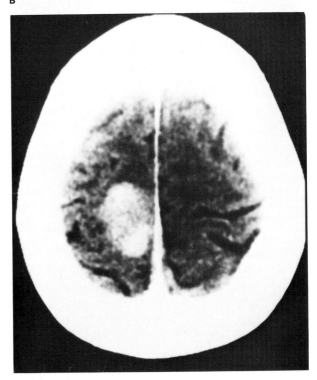

D

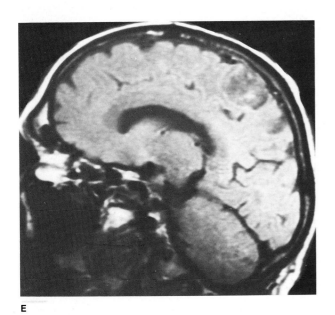

E

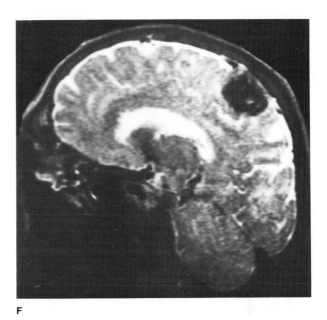

F

Figure 7-29   Posterior fossa meningioma with calcifications. **A.** Axial view shows large, well-marginated, hyperdense tumor containing multiple calcifications.   **B.** Coronal view shows tumor attachment to the tentorium cerebelli.   Parasagittal meningioma:

C (NCCT) and **D** (CECT) in another patient demonstrate a calcified, mildly enhancing meningioma on the right parasagittal convexity. MRI: **E** (sagittal T$_1$) and **F** (sagittal T$_2$) show the meningioma with signal void phenomenon due to calcifications.

ally an isodense area may represent subacute hemorrhage within the tumor. Hypodensity within the tumor on NCCT is a rare finding and may represent tumor necrosis, old hemorrhage, cystic degeneration, or lipomatous transformation (Russell 1980; Vassilouthis 1979). These areas of hypodensity exhibit minimal or no contrast enhancement (Fig. 7-30). Cystic formation on CT may be located centrally or peripherally within the tumor or around the tumor (peritumoral cyst) and is difficult to differentiate from the edematous brain (Rengachary 1979).

Intratumoral hemorrhage is rare and presents on CT as a focal area of high density in the acute phase (Vassilouthis 1979) (Fig. 7-31). Intratumoral hemorrhage occurs mostly in fibroblastic and meningoendotheliomatous meningiomas, and less frequently in angioblastic variant (Russell 1980). Its exact mechanism is not known, although a constant association of hemorrhage with large and small thin-walled endothelial channels has been noted (Modesti 1976), and the onset of bleeding has been attributed to

acute pressure changes (Vassilouthis 1979). Extremely rare coexistence of hemorrhage and necrosis within a tumor may present as a mixed-density lesion. Bleeding into subarachnoid or subdural spaces may rarely occur.

The consistency of meningiomas may be of surgical importance when the tumors are in close relation to vital structures. According to Kendall (1979), 90 percent of hard meningiomas, excluding those showing diffuse calcification, are hyperdense, and the other 10 percent are of the same density as brain. Of the soft meningiomas, 49 percent, excluding those showing marked cystic or necrotic changes, are hyperdense, but compared to the brain 35 percent are isodense and 16 percent are hypodense. The Kendall (1979) study, however, found no relationship between the degree of contrast enhancement and the consistency or the vascularity of the tumor as estimated by the surgeon or histologist.

CT features have been considered helpful in predicting the histology and aggressiveness of the tumor (Vassilouthis 1979). Less aggressive types such

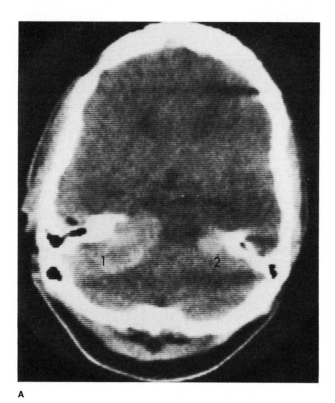

A

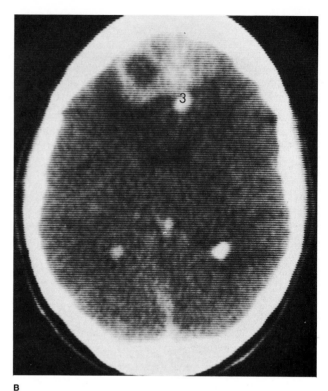

B

Figure 7-30 Coexistent acoustic neuroma, neurofibroma, and meningioma in a patient with neurofibromatosis. **A.** CECT demonstrates bilateral enhancing lesions in the cerebellopontine angles representing meningioma (1) and acoustic neuroma (2).

B. At a higher level, a large frontal meningioma (3) with a cystic cavity is seen. (*Courtesy of William A. Buchheit, M.D., Temple University Hospital, Philadelphia, Pennsylvania.*)

as transitional variants are well defined, with more or less regular shapes, and contain visible calcium aggregates. Most of the tumors (92 percent) are surrounded by edema of varying degrees, and the edema is not considered a specific feature except in the fibroblastic type, where it is almost invariably moderate. Tumor density on NCCT has not been considered specific in predicting histologic types, but a homogeneous density distribution on CECT suggests the transitional type. Marked edema, absence of visible calcium aggregates, and nonhomogeneous contrast enhancement, with nonenhancing low-density components and poorly defined irregular borders, point to aggressive or invasive characteristics, more commonly found in the angioblastic and syncytial variants (Shapir, 1985).

Intraventricular meningiomas arise from either the choroid plexus or the tela choroidea. They represent 17 percent of meningiomas in children and

1.6 percent in adults. An association between intraventricular meningioma and neurofibromatosis is well known. CT demonstrates a homogeneous, well-marginated, isodense or slightly hyperdense mass in the ventricle, particularly in the region of the choroid plexus, most often within the atrium of the lateral ventricle. Intense, homogeneous contrast enhancement is almost always present on CECT, as well as ipsilateral, contralateral, or bilateral ventricular dilatation (Fig. 7-32). Differentiation from other intraventricular lesions such as papilloma, carcinoma, vascular malformation, cavernous angioma, hemangioma, and astrocytoma may be possible on the basis of age, location, density differences with contrast enhancement characteristics, and associated systemic mesenchymal abnormalities (Zimmerman 1979c).

The occurrence of multiple meningiomas is uncommon (Fig. 7-33) apart from an association with

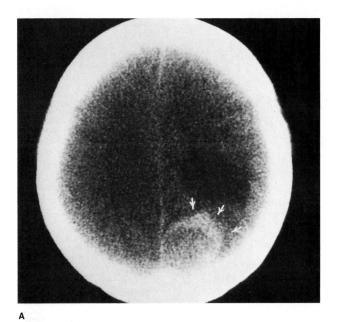

A

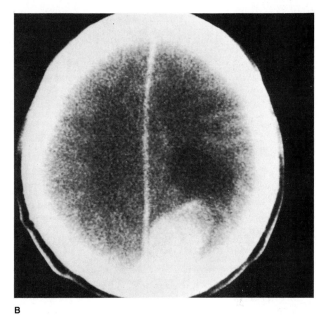

B

Figure 7-31 Meningioma with intratumoral hemorrhage. **A.** NCCT demonstrates an area of hyperdensity on the anterolateral portion of the tumor (arrowheads) with a mass effect. Increased density in the interhemispheric fissures represents subarachnoid hem-

morhage. **B.** On CECT, an eccentric intense enhancement of the posteromedial portion of the meningioma is seen. At surgery, the hyperdensity in the anterolateral portion was found to be due to hemorrhage within the tumor.

neurofibromatosis (Fig. 7-30). Association of meningioma with other types of primary neoplasm such as glioblastoma multiforme or pituitary adenoma (Brenner 1977) is probably coincidental.

Miscellaneous Tumors

Hemangioblastoma

These are histologically benign, true neoplasms of vascular structure. They constitute from 1.1 to 2.5 percent of all intracranial tumors and approximately 7 percent of posterior fossa tumors (Olivercrone 1952). They occur at any age, but young and middle-aged adults are most frequently affected. The most frequent site is the cerebellum, commonly in the paramedian hemisphere. Macroscopically, the tumor is usually well circumscribed without a capsule, and approximately 60 percent are cystic, with a mural

nodule. The tumor may be associated with erythrocytosis and is the primary feature of Hippel-Landau disease (Russell 1977).

CT may demonstrate a solid, homogeneous, isodense mass with distinctive contrast enhancement after intravenous contrast injection. More characteristically, cystic tumor with solid mural nodules is demonstrated (Figs. 7-4*A*, 7-34). The mural nodules are enhanced homogeneously and may be solitary or multiple (Adair 1978). The central low-density areas in the cyst range from 4 to 23 HU and show no contrast enhancement. The margin of a cyst, when isodense with no demonstrable contrast enhancement, represents gliosis and compressed cerebellum; areas that are hyperdense with contrast enhancement correspond to a highly vascular tumor. Rarely, central low density in a tumor suggesting a cyst may prove to be a solid tumor. Angiography not only confirms the presence of hypervascular mural nodules but also increases the detection rate for multiple lesions (Seeger 1981). Rare cases of su-

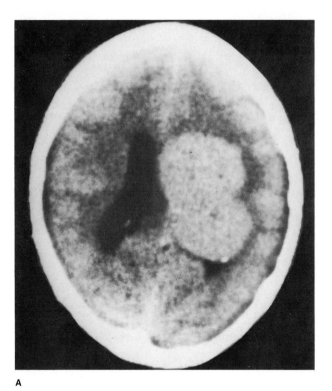

A

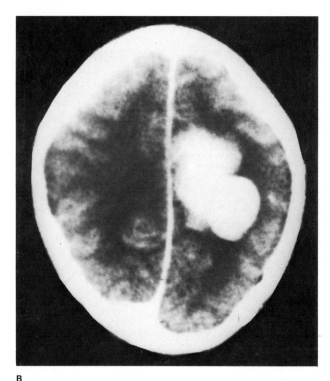

B

Figure 7-32 Intraventricular meningioma. **A.** On NCCT, a large, slightly lobulated, hyperdense tumor with clear margination is situated within the lateral ventricle. A small, calcified choroid plexus is markedly displaced posteriorly. Hydrocephalus is present. Note the absence of density changes in the adjoining brain tissue. **B.** On CECT, intense, homogeneously enhancing tumor is well demonstrated.

pratentorial hemangioblastoma have been recorded (Wylie 1973; Bachmann 1978).

Primary Intracranial Lymphoma

Tumors of the lymphoreticular system may be primary lesions of the brain or metastatic lesions as part of generalized lymphomatous diseases. Primary malignant lymphoma of the brain is a relatively rare tumor, with incidence ranging from 0.8 percent (Jellinger 1975) to 1.5 percent (Zimmerman 1975) of all intracranial tumors.

The cells of origin of these tumors within the brain are not clearly defined; the confusion regarding cells of origin is well reflected in the literature by the multiplicity of synonyms describing this tumor, such as reticulum cell carcinoma, histiocytic lymphoma, microglioma, round cell carcinoma, lymphosarcoma, perithelial sarcoma, adventitial sarcoma, and malignant reticulohistiocytic encephalitis (Tadmor 1978; Kazner 1978).

The clinical presentation of these tumors is varied and nonspecific, and most cases run a fulminating course if left untreated, with 3 to 5 months' survival after the first symptoms. A higher incidence of primary CNS lymphoma is noted in patients with AIDS and immunosuppression. This course may be altered by radiotherapy, and early diagnosis assumes major importance. Grossly, no uniform patterns of involvement by primary cerebral lymphoma are recognizable; the tumors range from solitary or multiple circumscribed nodules to diffuse infiltration or widespread distribution. A mixed pattern is rather frequent. There is a predilection for the basal ganglia, thalamus, periventricular white matter, and corpus callosum, but the tumors may occur in the cerebellar hemispheres, vermis, brainstem, and meninges as well.

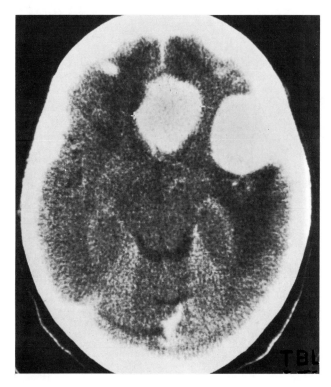

Figure 7-33 Multiple meningiomas. CECT shows two large meningiomas, one originating from the planum sphenoidale, the other from the pterion. A third one is in the frontopolar region.

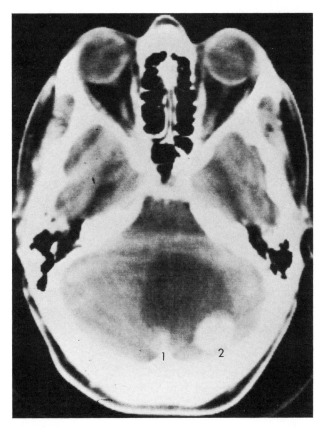

Figure 7-34 Hemangioblastoma. On CECT, a large, cystic posterior fossa tumor is noted in the left cerebellum. Two round, homogeneously enhancing tumor nodules (1, 2) are present at the posterolateral wall of the cyst. Absence of enhancement of the cyst wall itself is characteristic.

Jack (1985) reviewed 28 cases and summarized CT findings as follows: hyperdensity on NCCT (63 percent), contrast enhancement (100 percent) with homogeneous enhancement (71 percent) and prominent peritumoral edema zone (87 percent) (Fig. 7-35). All primary and secondary lymphoma lesions are in contact with either the ventricular ependyma or the superficial subarachnoid space (Holtås 1984). Occasionally a heterogeneous area with mixed enhancement is noted, particularly in the diffuse infiltrating type. Tadmor (1978) emphasized absence of conspicuous mass effect or ventricular enlargement. The tumor margins are invariably poorly defined and irregular, probably because of the characteristic perivascular and vascular infiltration pattern of the tumor cells. This was seen in 50 percent of cases and was thought to be an important diagnostic clue (Kazner 1978), although well-defined tumor

margins are noted in 85 percent of 27 lesions according to Jack (1985). Multicentricity (43 percent) and infiltration into the adjoining tissue and across the midline, with no respect for the normal anatomic boundaries, are frequently observed. Contrast enhancement of the subarachnoid space due to leptomeningeal involvement occurs but cannot be detected on CT (Enzmann 1979). Cerebral angiogram may demonstrate a meningioma-like pattern, i.e., homogeneous vascular stain in the late arterial or early venous phase, and MRI shows nonspecific hyperintense signal on T_2 images (Jack 1985).

The most common site for secondary lymphoma involvement is the cerebral meninges which are rarely

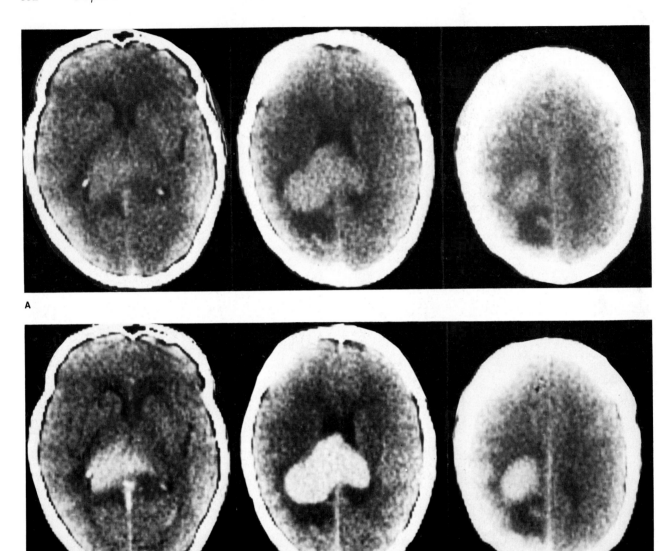

A

B

Figure 7-35   Primary malignant lymphoma.   **A** (upper) and **C.** On NCCT, slightly hyperdense, homogeneous, poorly marginated lesions are found in the thalamus, the splenium of the corpus callosum, and the deep parietal white matter. Note relative absence of mass effect and of hydrocephalus in spite of the extensive tumor involvement.   **B** (lower). On CECT, the tumor shows homogeneous, intense enhancement. The margins are indistinct, particularly in the deep white matter, indicative of infiltration pattern. Multicen-tricity, without respect for the normal anatomic boundaries and with infiltration into the adjoining tissue and across the midline, is characteristic.   **C.** Another case with involvement of the basal ganglia and deep white matter and surrounding edema. Intense, homogeneous CE is characteristic.   **D.** The same patient as in **C** exhibits almost complete disappearance of tumors after x-ray therapy.

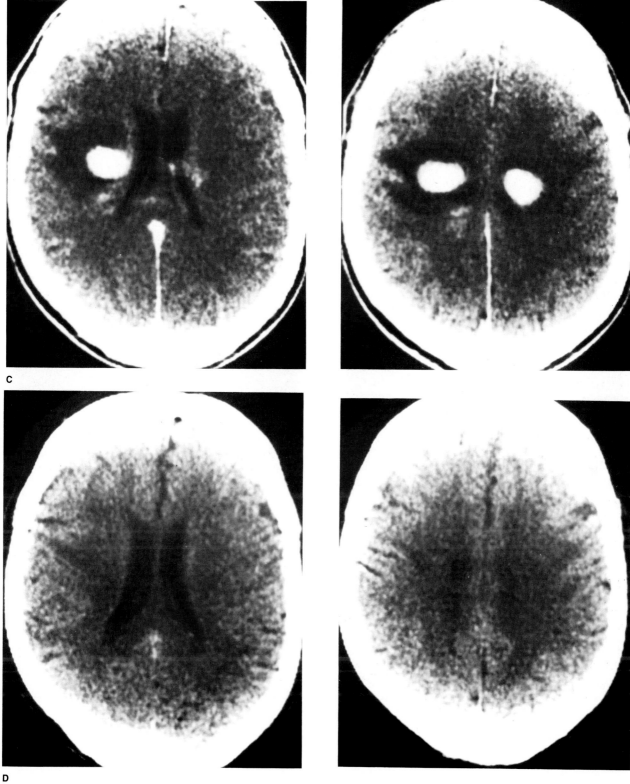

C

D

detectable by CT (Brant-Zawadzki 1978; Pagani 1981). Parenchymal involvement of the brain by systemic lymphoma and by primary malignant lymphoma of the brain are indistinguishable on CT (Brant-Zawadzki 1978). Differentiation from glioma, metastasis, melanoma, meningioma, or progressive multifocal leukoencephalopathy may be difficult.

Unusual Features

HEMORRHAGE   A variety of vascular changes can occur within a tumor, resulting in infarction, necrosis, and hemorrhage. Massive hemorrhage into a brain tumor may eventuate in rapidly deteriorating neurologic deficits and death. Intratumoral hemorrhage is not as rare as is usually believed. Mauersberger (1977) believes it occurs in 4 to 7 percent of all gliomas,

especially in glioblastomas, medulloblastomas, and metastases. The overall incidence detected by CT is 3.6 percent of all intracranial tumors (Zimmerman 1980a). It occurs in a variety of primary cerebral neoplasms, such as glioblastoma, chromophobe adenoma (pituitary apoplexy: see Chapter 10), grade I astrocytoma, medulloblastoma, central neuroblastoma, histiocytic lymphoma, oligodendroglioma, and hemangiopericytoma (Little 1979; Zimmerman 1980a; Post 1980). Less frequently, ependymoma, choroid plexus papilloma, and hemangioblastoma have been associated with intratumoral hemorrhage, and rarely, meningioma (Modesti 1976; Russell 1980). High-grade malignancy and extensive, abnormal vascularity have been thought to be predisposing factors. Analysis of the CT appearance of tumoral hemorrhage led Zimmerman (1980a) to classification of various patterns: central

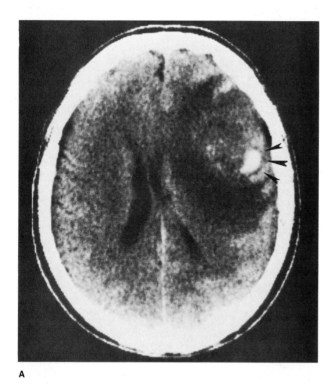

A

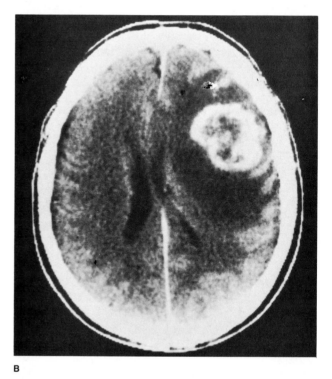

B

Figure 7-36 Intratumoral hemorrhage in glioblastoma multiforme. **A.** NCCT demonstrates an area of hemorrhage (arrowheads) within a mixed-density tumor in the frontoparietal lobe. Note the surrounding edema.   **B.** CECT shows nonhomogeneous enhancement of the entire tumor with central necrosis. The intratumoral hemorrhage is completely obscured by contrast enhancement.

hemorrhage pattern was most commonly observed in glioblastomas and astrocytomas, and other patterns, such as solid hemorrhage and hemorrhagic infarction, were most frequent in patients with metastasis. Little (1979) noted CT findings in 13 patients that include a neoplastic core (high or low density); small multifocal hemorrhage, usually at the margin of the tumor (Fig. 7-31); and surrounding, often extensive, edema (Fig. 7-36). Enhancement of tumor tissue on CECT has a peripheral distribution in proximity to the site of the hemorrhage (Fig. 7-36).

Intramural hemorrhage may dissect into the adjacent compressed and edematous brain (peritumoral hematoma) and extend through the cortex into the subarachnoid space (subarachnoid hemorrhage) (Fig. 7-31) or deep through the white matter and ependyma into the ventricle (intracerebral and intraventricular hematoma) (Mandybur 1977). Differentiation from atypical intracranial hemorrhage from various causes, such as aneurysm, vascular malformation, trauma, or hypertension, may be difficult, since most of these lesions demonstrate a mass consisting of a hematoma and concentric or eccentric contrast enhancement, almost indistinguishable from intratumoral hemorrhage. Angiography is helpful when tumor vascularity is demonstrated. The diagnosis of intratumoral hemorrhage should be considered whenever patients with certain types of tumor with a propensity for hemorrhage exhibit an intracerebral hematoma that is atypical in relation to the clinical history, age of patient, location, or CT appearance.

MULTICENTRIC TUMORS These are uncommon and account for 2.5 percent of all gliomas (Batzdorf 1963). The multicentricity is most frequently demonstrated in glioblastomas and primary malignant lymphoma, rarely in anaplastic astrocytoma. The tumors may be widely separated, occupying different lobes of the same hemisphere or opposite hemispheres. Although the diagnosis of multicentric tumors is usually obtained at autopsy because of their nonspecific clinical presentation, in vivo recognition adds significantly to the management of the patient. CT, with its high sensitivity, can easily visualize multi-

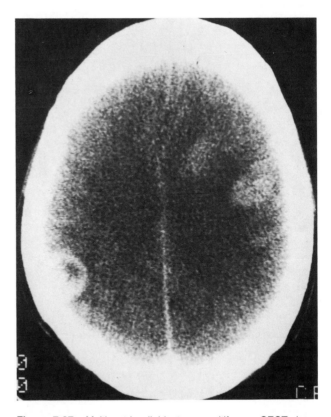

Figure 7-37 Multicentric glioblastoma multiforme. CECT demonstrates multiple enhancing lesions involving both hemispheres. Relative absence of edema is conspicuous. Differential diagnosis with metastic lesions may be extremely difficult.

centric patterns such as bihemispheric involvement (Fig. 7-37) and satellite foci of a tumor (Altemus 1977). However, differentiation from infiltrating primary tumors with microscopic or macroscopic connections as well as multiple metastatic foci may be extremely difficult on the basis of CT findings alone (Rao 1980) and even with MRI.

CONCURRENT TUMORS The concurrence of histologically different intracranial tumors is well documented in dysgenetic syndromes such as tuberous sclerosis, Lindau's syndrome, neurocutaneous melanosis, and neurofibromatosis. Other associations of multiple tumors, such as meningioma and glioblastoma or acoustic neurinoma, or glioblastoma and sarcoma, may be coincidental. In these collision or

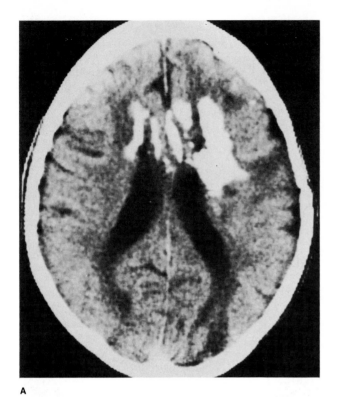

A

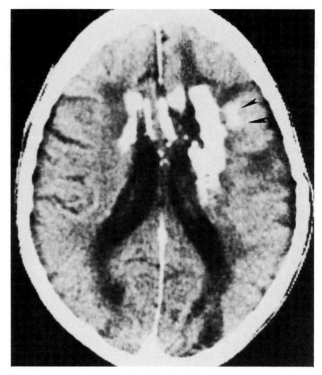

B

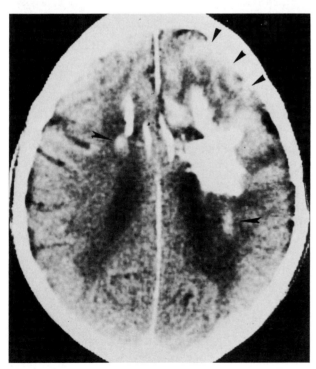

C

Figure 7-38 Mixed glioma (oligodendroglioma and astrocytoma).
A. NCCT exhibits multiple thick, bandlike calcifications in both frontal lobes. Frontal horns are compressed.   **B** and **C.** On CECT, multiple small scattered areas of contrast enhancement (arrowheads) are intermixed with calcifications. On histologic examination, mixed glioma (oligodendroglioma and astrocytoma) was found.

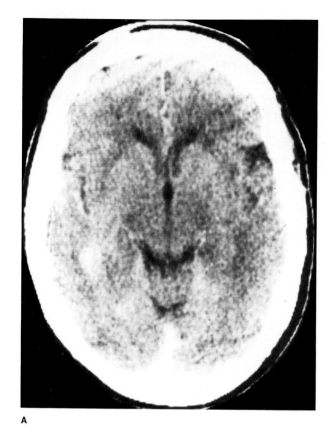

A

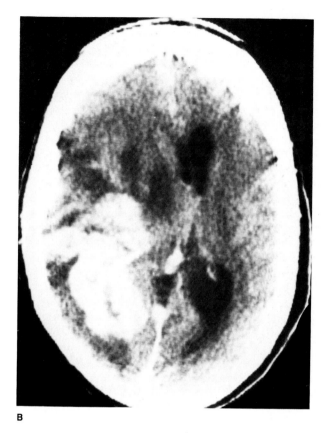

B

Figure 7-39 Rapid growth of glioma: initial CT **(A)** revealed a small CE lesion in the right temporooccipital lobe. CECT three months later **(B)** showed rapid, aggressive growth with a marked mass effect and surrounding edema.

tandem tumors, CT demonstrates multiplicity of lesions (Fig. 7-30), but histologic diagnosis should rely on the CT characteristics and location of each tumor (Brenner 1977). The rare occurrence of mixed gliomas such as mixed oligodendroglioma and astrocytoma may render CT diagnosis difficult. Unfortunately, CT distinction between the two histologically different tumor components may not be possible, although the characteristic CT features of one tumor component may predominate (Fig. 7-38).

RAPID GROWTH OR ALTERATION Rapid growth or morphologic alteration of gliomas may present as false negative CT scans initially, presumably because of the infiltrating nature of the lesions. They

become positive 14 to 17 days later (Tenfler 1977; Rao 1979) and present as mass lesions, probably because of sudden vascular changes and rapid necrosis or rapid growth of tumors (Fig. 7-39).

METASTASIS Local spread beyond the confines of a primary tumor by direct infiltration into the immediately adjacent meninges and ependymal surface is sufficiently known, although this feature bears little relation to the intrinsic malignancy of the tumor. Of greater concern is the manner in which this ependymal infiltration leads to metastasis via the CSF. Dissemination to distant points, in either the ependyma or the meninges, is noted in glioblastoma multiforme, medulloblastoma, ependymoma, tera-

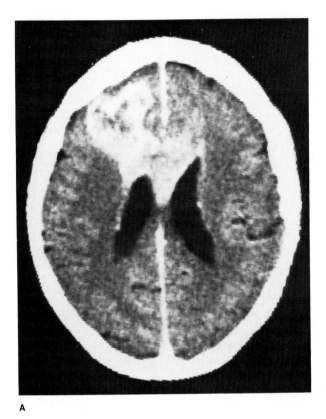

A

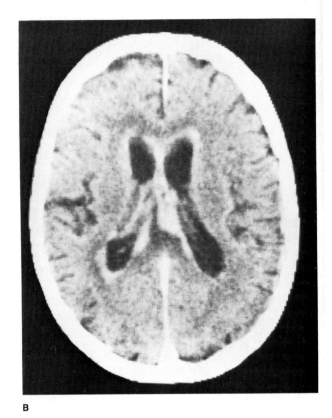

B

Figure 7-40 Local and distant metastasis **A.** Frontal glioblastoma with direct ventricular invasion with ependymal infiltration. **B.** Subependymal dissemination of high-grade glioma presents as contrast enhancement along the ventricular margins. (*Courtesy of Dr. Douglas Yock, Minneapolis, Minnesota.*)

toma, and pinealblastoma. These diffuse or nodular metastases via CSF pathways are easily detectable in the ependymal and subependymal layers of the ventricles on CECT (Fig. 7-40) (Osborn 1978*a*), but meningeal spread is difficult to detect on CT (Enzmann 1978; Pagani 1981).

Remote metastasis of a primary tumor may occur when the tumor cells obtain access to the lymphatics or to veins outside the central nervous system. Such metastasis is recorded in glioblastoma, medulloblastoma, ependymoma, and oligodendroglioma, in order of frequency. All the patients had had one or more previous operations, and this mechanical access to the hematolymphatic system must play a decisive role in the process.

Bibliography

ADAIR LB, ROPPER AH, DAVIS KR: Cerebellar hemangioblastoma: CT, angiographic and clinical condition in seven cases. *CT: J Comput Tomogr* **2**(4):281–294, 1978.

AFRA D, NORMAN D, LEVIN CA: Cysts in malignant glioma identification by CT. *J Neurosurg* **53**:821–825, 1980.

ALDERSON PO et al: Optimal utilization of computerized cranial tomography and radionuclide brain imaging. *Neurology* **26**:803–807, 1976.

ALDERSON PO, GADO MH, SIEGAL BA: CCT and RN imaging in the detection of intercranial mass lesions. *Semin Nucl Med* **VII**:161–174, 1977.

ALTEMUS LR, RADVANY J: Multifocal glioma visualized by contrast enhanced computed tomography: Report of a case with pathologic correlation. *J Maine Med Assoc* **68**:324–327, 1977.

AMBROSE J, GOODING MB, RICHARDSON AE: An assessment of the accuracy of computerized transverse axial scanning (EMI scanners) in the diagnosis of intracranial tumor: A review of 366 patients. *Brain* **98**:569–582, 1975a.

AMBROSE J, GOODING MB, RICHARDSON AE: Sodium iothalamate as an aid to diagnosis of intracranial lesions by computerized transverse axial scanning. *Lancet:* 669–674, 1975b.

AMENDOLA MA et al: Preoperative diagnosis of a ruptured intracranial dermoid cyst by computerized tomography: Case report. *J Neurosurg* **48**:1035–1037, 1978.

AMUNDSEN P, DUGSTAD G, SYVERTSEN AH: The reliability of computer tomography for the diagnosis and differential diagnosis of meningiomas, gliomas, and brain metastasis. *Acta Neurochirurgica* **41**:177–190, 1978.

ANDERSON FM, ADELSTEIN LJ: Ganglion cell tumor in the third ventricle. *Arch Surg* **45**:129–139, 1942.

ARIENS-KAPPERS J: The development of the paraphysis cerebri in man with comments on its relationship to the intercolumnar tubercle and its significance for the origin of cystic tumors in the third ventricle. *J Comp Neurol* **102**:425, 1955.

BAKER HL, HOUSER OW, CAMPBELL JK: National Cancer Institute Study: Evaluation of CT in the diagnosis of intracranial neoplasms: I. Overall Results. *Radiology* **136**:91–96, 1980.

BAKER AB, BAKER LH: *Clinical Neurology.* Hagerstown, Md. Harper & Row, 1973.

BACHMANN K, MARKWALDER R, SEILER RW: Supratentorial hemangioblastoma: Case report. *Acta Neurochirurgica* **44**:173–177, 1978.

BANERJEE T, KRIGMAN MR: Intracranial epidermoid tumor: discussion of four cases. *Southern Med* **7**(6):1977.

BATZDORF U, MALMUD N: The problem of multicentric gliomas. *J Neurosurg* **20**:122–136, 1963.

BECKER D, NORMAN D, WILSON CB: Computerized tomography and pathological correlation in cystic meningiomas: Report of two cases. *J Neurosurg* **50**:103–105, 1979.

BODIAN M, LAWSON D: The intracranial neoplastic diseases of childhood. *Brit J Surg* **40**:368, 1953.

BRANT-ZAWADZKI M, ENZMANN DR: Computed tomographic brain scanning in patients with lymphoma. *Radiology* **129**:67–71, 1978.

BRAUN IE et al: Dense intracranial epidermoid tumors. *Radiology* **122**:717–719, 1977.

BRENNER TG, RAO KCVG, ROBINSON W, ITANI A: Tandem lesions: Chromophobe adenoma and meningioma. *CT: J Comput Tomogr* **1**:517–520, 1977.

BUELL U, NIENDORF HP, KAZNER E et al: CAT and cerebral serial scintigraphy in intracranial tumors: Rates of detection and tumor-type identification. (Concise communication) *J Nucl Med* **19**:476–479, 1977.

BUTLER AR, HORRI SC, KRICHEFF II, SHANNON MB, BUDZILOVICH GN: Computed tomography in astrocytomas: A statistical analysis of the parameters of malignancy and the positive contrast-enhanced CT scan. *Radiology* **129**:433–439, 1978.

CAMINS MB, TAKEUCHI J: Normotopic plus heterotopic atypical teratomas. *Child's Brain* **4**:151–160, 1978.

CHAMBERS AA et al: Cranial epidermoid tumors: Diagnosis by computed tomography. *Neurosurgery* **1**:276–280, 1977.

CLAVERIA LE, SUTTON D, TRESS BM: The radiological diagnosis of meningiomas, the impact of EMI scanning. *Brit J Radiol* **50**:15–22, 1977a.

CLAVERIA LE, KENDALL BE, DUBOULAY GH: CAT in supratentorial gliomas and metastasis, in Du-Boulay GH, Moseley IF (eds): *CAT in Clinical Practice,* Heidelberg, Springer-Verlag, 1977b, p 85.

CLIFFORD JR, CONNOLLY ES, VOORHIES RM: Comparison of radionuclide scan with computer assisted tomography in diagnosis of intracranial disease. *Neurology* **26**:1119–1123, 1976.

CORNELL SH, GRAF CJ, DOLAN KD: Fat-fluid level in intracranial epidermoid cyst. *Am J Roentgenol* **128**:502–503, 1977.

DAVIS KR et al: Theoretical considerations in the use of contrast media for computed cranial tomography. *Neurosurgery* **1**:9–12, 1976a.

DAVIS KR, TAVERAS JM: Diagnosis of epidermoid tumor by computed tomography. *Radiology* **119**:347–353, 1976b.

DAVIS JM, DAVIS KR, NEWHOUSE J, PFISTER RC: Expanded high iodine dose in computed cranial tomography: A preliminary report. *Radiology* **131**:373–387, 1979.

DECK MDF, MESSINA AV, SACKETT JR: Computerized tomography in metastatic disease of the brain. *Radiology* **119**:115–120, 1976.

DORNE HL, O'GORMAN AM, MELANSON D: CT of intracranial gangliomas. *Am J Neuroradiology* **7**:281–285, 1986.

DORSCH JA, WADSENHEIM A: Density of intracranial masses in computed tomography. *J Belge Radiol* **61**:292–296, 1978.

ENZMANN DR et al: CT in primary reticulum cell sarcoma of the brain. *Radiology* **130**:165–170, 1979.

ENZMANN DR, TOKYE KC, HAYWARD R: CT in leptomeningeal spread of tumor. *J Comput Assist Tomogr* **2**:448–455, 1978 (abstract).

EVENS RG, JOST RG: The clinical efficacy and cost analysis of cranial computed tomography and the radionuclide brain scan. *Semin Nucl Med* **VII**:129–136, 1977.

FAWCITT RA, ISHERWOOD I: Radiodiagnosis of intracranial pearly tumors with particular reference to the value of CT. *Neuroradiology* **11**:234–242, 1976.

FUTRELL NN, OSBORNE AQ, CHESON BD: Pineal region tumors: CT-pathologic spectrum. *Am J Neuroradiol* **2**:415–420, 1981.

GADO MH, PHELPS ME, COLEMAN RE: An extravascular component of contrast enhancement in cranial computed tomography. *Radiology* **177**:589–593, and 595–597, 1975.

GANTI SR, ANTUNES JL, LOUIS KM, HILAL SK: CT in the diagnosis of colloid cysts of the third ventricle. *Radiology* **138**:385–391, 1981.

GANTI SR, HILAL SK, STEIN BM, SILVER AJ, MAWAD M, SANE P: CT of pineal region tumors: *Am J Neuroradiol* **7**:97–104, 1986.

GARDEUR D, SABLAYROLLES JL, KLAUSZ R, METZGER J: Histographic studies in computed tomography of contrast enhanced cerebral and orbital tumors. *J Comput Assist Tomogr* **1**(2):231–240, 1977.

GARRIDO E, BECKER LF, HOFFMAN HJ et al: Gangliogliomas in children. *Child's Brain* **4**:339–346, 1978.

GAWLER J et al: Computer assisted tomography (EMI scanner): its place in investigation of suspected intracranial tumors. *Lancet* **2**:419–423, 1979.

GEORGE AE, RUSSELL EJ, KRICHEFF II: White matter buckling: CT sign of extra-axial intracranial mass. *Am J Neuroradiol* **1**:425–430, 1980.

GHOSHHAJRA K, BHAGAI-NAINI P, HAHN HS: Spontaneous rupture of a pineal teratoma. *Am J Neuroradiol* **17**:215–217, 1979.

GILBERTSON EL, GOODING CA: Roentgenographic signs of tumors of the brain. *Am J Roentgenol* **76:**226, 1956.

GROSS SW: Radiographic visualization of an intracranial dermoid cyst. *J Neurosurg* **2:**72–75, 1945.

GUNER M, SHAW M: Computed tomography in the diagnosis of colloid cyst. *J Neurosurg* **2:**72–75, 1976.

HANDA J, HANDA H: Radiolucent intracranial dermoid cyst, case report. *Neuroradiology* **17:**211–214, 1979.

HAYMAN LA, EVANS RA, HINCK V: Rapid high dose cranial CT: a concise review of normal anatomy. *J Comput Assist Tomogr* **3**(20):147–154, 1979.

HAYMAN LA, EVANS RA, HINCK VC: Delayed high iodine dose contrast computed tomography: cranial neoplasms. *Radiology* **136:**677–684, 1980.

HILAL SK, CHANG CH: Specificity of computed tomography in the diagnosis of supratentorial neoplasms: Consideration of metastasis and meningiomas. *Neuroradiology* **16:**537–539, 1978.

HILAL SK, CHANG CH: Sensitivity and specificity of CT in supratentorial tumors. *J Comput Assist Tomogr* **2:**511, 1978.

HOLTÅS S, NYMAN U, CRONQUIST S: CT of malignant lymphoma of the brain. *Neuroradiology* **26:**33–38, 1984.

HUCKMAN MS: Clinical experience with the intravenous infusion of iodinated contrast material as an adjunct to CT. *Surg Neurol* **4**(3):297–318, 1975.

HUCKMAN M, ACKERMAN L: Use of automated measurements of mean density as an adjunct to computed tomography. *J Comput Assist Tomogr* **1**(1):37–42, 1977.

JACK CR, REESE DF, SCHEITHAUER BW: Radiographic findings in 32 cases of primary CNS lymphoma. *AJNR* **6:**899–904, 1985.

JELLINGER K, RADSKIEWICZ T, SLOWIK F: Primary malignant lymphomas of the central nervous system in man. *Acta Neuropath,* Suppl VI: 95–102, 1975.

KALAN C, BURROWS EH: Calcification in intracranial gliomata. *Br J Radiol* **35:**589–602, 1962.

KAZNER E, WILSKE J, STEINHOFF H, STOCHDORPH O: Computer assisted tomography in primary malignant lymphomas of the brain. *J Comput Assist Tomogr* **2:**125–134, 1978.

KENDALL B, PULLICINO P: Comparison of consistency of meningiomas and CT appearance. *Neuroradiology* **18:**173–176, 1979.

KENDALL BE: Difficulties in diagnosis of supratentorial gliomas by CAT scan. *J Neurol Neurosurg Psych* **42:**485–492, 1975.

KRAMER RA, JANETOS GP, PERLSTEIN G: An approach to contrast enhancement in computed tomography of the brain. *Radiology* **16:**641–647, 1975.

KUSHNET MW, GOLDMAN RL: Lipoma of the corpus callosum associated with a frontal bone defect. *Am J Roentgenol* **131:**517–518, 1978.

LASTER DW, MOODY DM: Epidermoid tumors with intraventricular and subarachnoid fat: Report of two cases. *Am J Roentgenol* **128:**504–507, 1977.

LATCHAW RE, GOLD LHA, TORRIJE EJ: A protocol for the use of contrast enhancement in cranial computed tomography. *Radiology* **126:**681–687, 1978a.

LATCHAW R, PAYNE JT, GOLD LH: Effective atomic number and electron density as measured with a computed tomography scanner: Computation and correlation with brain tumor histology. *J Comput Assist Tomogr* **2:**199–208, 1978b.

LATCHAW R, PAYNE JT, LOEWENSON RB: Predicting brain tumor histology: Change of effective atomic number with contrast enhancement. *Am J Neuroradiol* **1:**289–294, 1980.

LEE SH, DELGADO TE, BUCHEIT WA: Intracranial dermoid tumor: Diagnosis by computed tomography, a case report. *Neurosurgery* **1**:281–283, 1977.

LEWANDER R, BERGSTROM M, BERGVALL U: Contrast enhancement of cranial lesions in computed tomography. *Acta Radiolog* **19**:529–552, 1978.

LITTLE JR et al: Brain hemorrhage from intracranial tumor. *Stroke* **10**(3):283–288, 1979.

LITTLE JR, MACCARTY CS: Colloid cysts of the third ventricle. *J Neurosurg* **40**:230–235, 1974.

MALIK GM et al: Colloid cysts. *Surg Neurol* **13**(1):73–77, 1980.

MANCES P, BABIN E, WACKENHEIM A: Contribution of histograms to the computer tomographic study of brain tumors. *J Belge Radiol* **61**(4):297–312, 1978.

MANDYBUR TI: Intracranial hemorrhage caused by metastatic tumors. *Neurology* **27**:650–655, 1977.

MANI RL et al: Radiographic diagnosis of meningioma of the lateral ventricle. Review of 22 cases. *J Neurosurg* **49**:249–255, 1978.

MAUERSBERGER W, CUEVAS-SOLORZANO JA: Spontaneous intracerebellar hematoma during childhood caused by spongioblastoma of the fourth ventricle. *Neuropädiatrie* **8**:443–450, 1977.

MCCORMACK TJ, PLASSCHE WM, LIN SR: Ruptured teratoid tumors in the pineal region. *J Comput Assist Tomogr* **2**:499–501, 1978.

MIKHAEL MA, MATTAR AG: Intracranial pearly tumors: the role of CT, angiography and pneumoencephalography. *J Comput Assist Tomogr* **2**:421–429, 1978.

MODESTI LM, BINET EF, COLLINS GH: Meningiomas causing spontaneous intracranial hematomas. *J Neurosurg* **45**:437–441, 1976.

NAIDICH TP et al: Evaluation of sellar and parasellar masses by computed tomography. *Radiology* **120**:91–99, 1976.

NAUTA HJW et al: Xanthochromic cysts associated with meningioma. *J Neurol Neurosurg Psychiat* **42**:529–535, 1979.

NEUWELT EA et al: Malignant pineal region tumors. *J Neurosurg* **51**:597–607, 1979.

NEW PFJ, SCOTT WR, SCHNUR JA, DAVIS DR, TAVERAS TM, HOCHBERG FH: Computed tomography with the EMI scanner in the diagnosis of primary and metastatic intracranial neoplasms. *Radiology* **114**:75–87, 1975.

NORMAN D et al: Quantitative aspects of contrast enhancement in cranial computed tomography. *Radiology* **129**:683–688, 1978.

NOSAKA Y et al: Primary intracranial epidermoid carcinoma. *J Neurosurg* **50**:830–833, 1979.

OI S, WETZEL N: Gliomas in computerized axial tomography, correlation with tumor malignancy in 100 cases. *Neurosurgery (Jap)* **7**(8):759–763, 1979.

OLIVERCRONE H: The cerebellar angioreticulomas. *J Neurosurg* **9**:317–330, 1952.

OSBORN AG: Diagnosis of descending transtentorial herniation by cranial computed tomography. *Radiology* **123**:93–96, 1977.

OSBORN AG, HEASTON DK, WING SD: Diagnosis of ascending transtentorial herniation by cranial computed tomography. *Am J Roentgenol* **130**:755–760, 1978*a*.

OSBORN AG et al: The evaluation of ependymal and subependymal lesions by cranial computed tomography. *Radiology* **127**:397–401, 1978*b*.

PAGANI JJ et al: Cranial nervous system leukemia of lymphoma: CT manifestations. *Am J Neuroradiol* **2**:397–403, 1981.

PATEL AN: Lipoma of the corpus callosum: A nonsurgical entity. *NC Med J* **26**:328–335, 1965.

PAXTON R, AMBROSE J: The EMI scanner: A brief review of the first 650 patients. *Brit J Radiol* **47**:530–565, 1974.

PENDERGRASS HP, MCKUSICK KA, NEW PFJ: Relative efficacy of radionuclide imaging and computed tomography of the brain. *Radiology* **116**:363–366, 1975.

PENMAN J, SMITH MC: *Intracranial gliomata*, Spec Rep Series, No. 284, Med Res Council, HM Stationary Office, London, 1954.

POST JD, NOBLE JD, GLASER JS, SAFRAN A: Pituitary apoplexy: diagnosis by CT. *Radiology* **134**:665–670, 1980.

RAO KCVG, GOVINDAN S: CAT in rapidly growing brain tumors. *Comput Tomog* **3**:9–13, 1979.

RAO KCVG, LEVINE H, ITANI A, SAJOR E, ROBINSON W: CT findings in multicentric glioblastoma. Diagnostic-pathologic correlation. *CT: J Coput Tomogr* **4**:187–192, 1980.

REEVES GI, MARKS JE: Prognostic significance of lesion size for glioblastoma multiforme. *Radiology* **132**:469–471, 1979.

RENGACHARY S et al: Cystic lesions associated with intracranial meningiomas. *Neurosurgery* **4**:107–114, 1979.

RUSSELL DS: Meningeal tumors: a review. *J Clin Path* **3**:191, 1950.

RUSSELL DS, RUBINSTEIN LJ: Pathology of tumors of the nervous system. 4th ed., Baltimore, Williams and Wilkins, 1977.

RUSSELL EG, GEORGE AJ, KRICHEFF II, BUDZILOVICH G: Atypical CT features of intracranial meningioma: radiological-pathological correlation in a series of 131 consecutive cases. *Radiology* **135**:673–682, 1980.

SEEGER JF et al: CT and angiographic evaluation of hemangioblastomas. *Radiology* **138**:65–73, 1981.

SHAFFER KA, HAUGHTON VM, WILSON CR: High resolution CT of the temporal bone. *Radiology* **134**:409–414, 1980.

SHAPIR J, COBLENTZ C, MALANSON D et al: New CT findings in aggressive meningioma. *Am J Neuroradiol* **6**:101–102, 1985.

STEINHOFF H, AVILES C: Contrast enhancement response of intracranial neoplasms: its validity for the differential diagnosis of tumors in CT, in Lanksch W, Kazner E (eds): *Cranial Computerized Tomography*, New York, Springer-Verlag, 1976, pp 151–161.

STEINHOFF H, KAZNER E, LANKSCH W, GRUMME T, MEESE W, LANGE S, AULICH A, WENDE S: The limitations of computerized axial tomography in the detection and differential diagnosis of intracranial tumours: A study based on 1304 neoplasms, in Bories J (ed): *The Diagnostic Limitations of Computerized Axial Tomography*, New York, Springer-Verlag, 1978, pp 40–49.

STEINHOFF H et al: CT in the diagnosis and differential diagnosis of glioblastomas. *Neuroradiology* **14**:193–200, 1977.

STOVRING J: Contralateral temporal horn widening in unilateral supratentorial mass lesions: a diagnostic sign indicating tentorial herniation. *J Comput Assist Tomogr* **1**:319–323, 1977.

TADMOR R, DAVIS K, ROBERSON G, KLEINMAN G: Computed tomography in primary malignant lymphoma of the brain. *J Comput Assist Tomogr* **2**:135–140, 1978.

TADMOR R, TAVERAS JM: Computed tomography in extradural epidermoid and xanthoma. *Surg Neurol* **7**:371–375, 1977.

TAKEUCHI J, HANDA H, NAGAT I: Suprasellar germinoma. *J Neurosurg* **49**:41–48, 1978.

TAKEUCHI J et al: Neuroradiological aspects of suprasellar germinoma. *Neuroradiology* **17**:153–159, 1979.

TANS J, DE JONGH IE: Computed tomography of supratentorial astrocytoma. *Clin Neurol, Neurosurg* **80**:156–168, 1978.

TCHANG S et al: Computerized tomography as a possible aid to histological grading of supratentorial gliomas. *J Neurosurg* **46**:735–739, 1977.

TENFLER RL, PALACIOS E: False negative CT in brain tumor. *JAMA* **238**:339–340, 1977.

THOMSON JLG: Computerized axial tomography and the diagnosis of glioma: A study of 100 consecutive histologically proven cases. *Clin Radiol* **27**:431–441, 1976.

TOGLIA JU et al: Epithelial tumors of the cranium: their common nature and pathogenesis. *J Neurosurg* **23**:384–393, 1965.

VASSILOUTHIS J, AMBROSE J: Computerized tomography scanning appearance of intracranial meningiomas. *J Neurosurg* **50**:320–327, 1979.

VONOFAKOS D, HACKER H: CT histogram in the pathologic definition of supratentorial brain tumors. *Neuroradiology* **16**:552–555, 1978.

VONOFAKOS D, MARCU H, HACKER H: Oligodendrogliomas: CT patterns with emphasis on features indicating malignancy. *J Comput Assist Tomogr* **3**(6):783–788, 1979.

WENDE S et al: A German multicentric study of intracranial tumors, in duBoulay GH, Moseley IF (eds): *Computerized Axial Tomography in Clinical Practice.* Heidelberg, Springer-Verlag, 1977.

WYLIE IG, JEFFREYS RV, MACLAINE GN: Cerebral hemangioblastoma. *Br J Radiol* **46**:472–476, 1973.

ZETTNER A, NETSKY MG: Lipoma of the corpus callosum. *J Neuropathol Exp Neurol* **19**:305–319, 1960.

ZIMMERMAN HM: Malignant lymphomas of the nervous system. *Acta Neuropath,* Suppl VI: 69–74, 1975.

ZIMMERMAN RA, BILANIUK LT: Cranial computed tomography of epidermoid and congenital fatty tumors of maldevelopment origin. *J Comput Assist Tomogr* **3**(1):40–50, 1979a.

ZIMMERMAN RA, BILANIUK LT: CT of intracerebral gangliogliomas. *J Comput Assist Tomogr* **3**(1):24–29, 1979b.

ZIMMERMAN RA, BILANIUK LT: Computed tomography of choroid plexus lesions. *J Comput Assist Tomogr* **3**(2):93–102, 1979c.

ZIMMERMAN RA, BILANIUK LT: Computed tomography of acute intratumoral hemorrhage. *Radiology* **135**:355–359, 1980a.

ZIMMERMAN RA et al: CT of pineal, parapineal and histologically related tumors. *Radiology* **137**:669–677, 1980b.

PRIMARY TUMORS IN CHILDREN

Charles R. Fitz

Krishna C.V.G. Rao

It is perhaps unnecessary to emphasize the obvious—that is, the changes that CT has brought about in the diagnosis and management of brain tumors in children. Before CT, children in most hospitals underwent a two- or three-stage investigative diagnostic study consisting of radionuclide brain scan, arteriogram, and/or air ventriculogram or air encephalogram. This meant one or two anesthetics for the procedure, shunting of the ventricles when hydrocephalus was present, and often a 2-day interval between procedures to recover from previous anesthesias. With increasing utilization of MRI, the diagnostic route may be one or two stages whether or not both CT and MRI are available. MRI offers an unparalleled view in the sagittal plane similar to pneumoencephalography, with the added advantage of evaluating tissue densities. MRI shows the

extent of the abnormal tissue changes better than CT, as well as the amount of edema (Peterman 1984). Since calcification and necrosis within a tumor can be helpful in determining the histologic type, CT is still a recommended procedure at this time. In some cases angiography may still be necessary, since it is helpful for comparing vascular anatomy with CT anatomy so that normality or abnormality of the underlying brain can be predicted. Angiography is also useful in defining lesions which may mimic a neoplasm because of their location or enhancing pattern (Fig. 8-1). It has become the philosophy to recommend angiography when a tumor on CT appears unusual or has an appearance unusual for a tumor in its particular location. A brainstem tumor with considerable enhancement would be such an example.

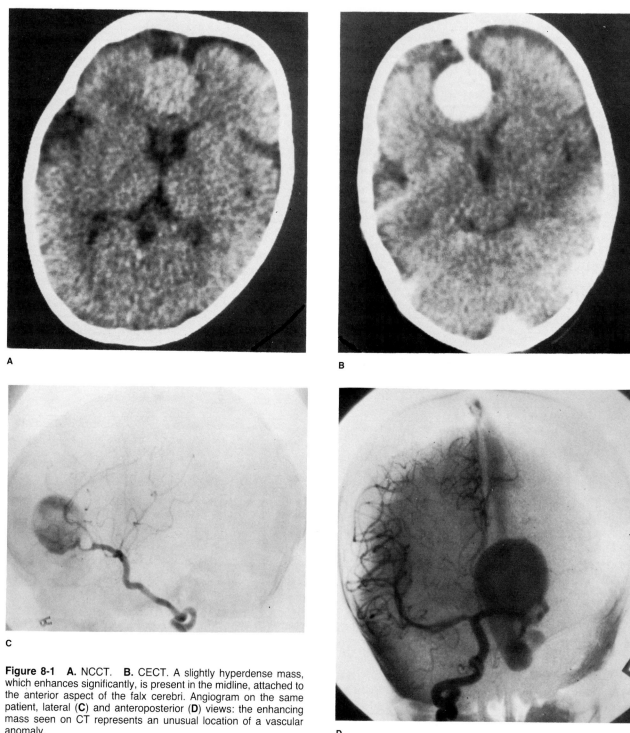

Figure 8-1   A. NCCT.   **B.** CECT. A slightly hyperdense mass, which enhances significantly, is present in the midline, attached to the anterior aspect of the falx cerebri. Angiogram on the same patient, lateral (**C**) and anteroposterior (**D**) views: the enhancing mass seen on CT represents an unusual location of a vascular anomaly.

With the availability of MRI, it is considered more sensitive and superior imaging modality in evaluating posterior fossa tumors (Lee 1985; Kucharczyk 1985).

The skull x-ray is now a neglected part of tumor workup even in pediatric centers, but the authors believe this is an error. Relative head size is more easily recognized on skull x-ray than on CT. A child's skull responds rapidly to changes in intracranial pressure, and this part of the workup should not be neglected. The authors prefer a full skull series during the initial workup. After treatment, skull x-ray is helpful in seeing shunt tubing outside the calvarium, and in defining operative defects. Repeated routine skull x-rays are not necessary unless changes in the calvarium or changes in the shunt external to the calvarium occur.

Because of the rapidity with which tumors are diagnosed with CT, shunting of hydrocephalus is less commonly needed, especially as a procedure separate from tumor exploration.

CT Technique

Even with the faster scanners, sedation still remains necessary in most children below age 5. The sedation schedule followed by the authors is given in Table 8-1. Pentobarbital is the sedative most commonly used. Usually the child will fall into a heavy sleep in 20 to 30 minutes, and this will last 20 to 30 minutes. Approximately one-third of children sedated with pentobarbital will require resedation with a smaller dose, and this will suffice in most cases. In children who require heavier sedation, such as retarded or deaf children, or in children in whom pentobarbital has previously been unsuccessful, a three-drug mixture (meperidine HCl, promethazine HCl, and chlorpromazine) is used. Valium is used only in the occasional older patient who is very nervous and needs calming rather than sedation. Use of these three medications takes care of about 98 percent of children who need sedation. Others have reported good results with rectal thiopental (White 1979). Chloral hydrate is a reasonable alternative to Nembutal. The ease of oral administration is balanced by the child who spits out or vomits the drug. This is especially a problem when a second dose needs to be given.

When intravenous contrast is used, it is given in a dose of 3 ml/kg of 60% meglumine diatrizoate (282 mg/ml of iodine). Contrast is usually given in a single bolus. Specialized contrast-injection techniques such as a very rapid bolus or infusion tend to be impractical in younger children and are generally not used in infants.

Cisternography (water-soluble) when utilized, is done by lumbar injection at a dose of 2–5 ml of 170 mg/ml iodine, depending on age. The patient is usually put in a 15 to 20° Trendelenberg position for approximately 5 minutes after the injection.

Table 8-1   Sedation for CT or MRI in Children 5 Years and Younger

Drug	Initial dose	Route of administration	Supplementary dose
Pentobarbital (Nembutal)	6 mg/kg of body weight for children up to 15 kg; 5 mg/kg for children over 15 kg; maximum of 200 mg	IM 20 to 30 minutes before CT	1 to ½ hour later if initial dose not effective, 2 mg/kg for children over 15 kg; maximum of 100 mg
Diazepam (Valium)	0.4 mg/kg body weight, maximum of 12 mg	IV, slowly, 5 to 10 minutes before CT	½ hour later if initial dose not effective
Demorol compound (Meperdine HCL 25 mg/ml) (Chlorpromazine 6.25 mg/ml) (Promethazine 6.25 mg/ml)	0.1 ml/kg up to a maximum of 2 ml	IM 10 to 20 minutes before study	No supplementary dose given
Chloral hydrate	60 mg/kg to a maximum of 2500 mg	Oral	30 mg/kg, 45 minutes later

CT itself is usually done in the conventional 20° semiaxial position both before and after contrast enhancement of the entire head on any initial examination. Usually the thicker 10-mm section thickness available on most equipment is sufficient, because the tumors are relatively large and easily seen through two or more slices. When symptoms are strongly in favor of a posterior fossa tumor, or other information such as calcification on the skull x-ray has already localized the lesion, the cuts before contrast enhancement may be limited to the posterior fossa. The authors believe that the precontrast views are helpful in determining tumor types, though not essential for localization.

Thinner, 5-mm sections are occasionally done, especially to better see the brainstem or extraaxial lesions. Very thin sections of 1.5 to 2 mm are of limited value in children. The heat buildup of the x-ray tubes causes long delays between slices. Sick children and small children, even if sedated, usually are not able to hold still long enough to provide

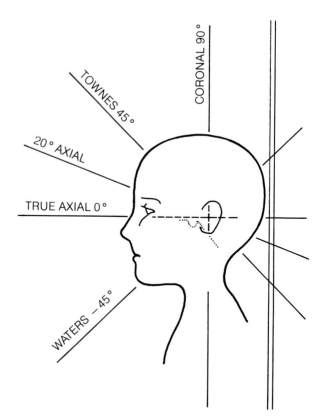

Figure 8-3 Patient positioning for Towne's view. The Towne's view can be obtained by angling the gantry and extending the patient's head backward to achieve the appropriate position.

images that can be reconstructed in other planes without movement between slices.

Additional views are usually necessary when the extent of a tumor or parts of its intrinsic character require better definition. The most common is the clival perpendicular or Water's view (Fitz 1978a). As the slices are perpendicular to the tentorium, clivus, and brainstem, they show the posterior fossa in what may be considered its coronal projection. The clival perpendicular view is easier to obtain than the true coronal, requiring only a moderate extension of the neck and forward angulation of the gantry (Fig. 8-2).

This view is most helpful to examine the extension of a tumor into the cerebellar hemispheres, displacement of the fourth ventricle by branstem or

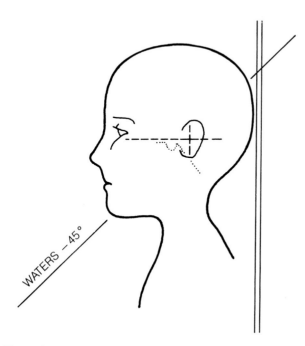

Figure 8-2 Patient positioning for clival perpendicular (Water's) view. This can be achieved by angling either the gantry or the table top, depending on the type of scanner.

cerebellar tumors, or the cross-sectional size of either the fourth ventricle or the brainstem.

The clival parallel, or Towne's, view is easily obtained by flexing the patient's neck and angling the gantry back (Fig. 8-3) (Byrd 1978). Being at 90° to the clival perpendicular view, the slices are through the axis of the brainstem. This view is most helpful in visualizing the fourth ventricle and brainstem through their length and often shows extraaxial masses to best advantage. Both accessory views are usually done in 5-mm slices through the regions determined from the standard examination.

The incidence of primary intracranial neoplasms in children is less than that of the adult population (Wilson 1975). Metastatic tumors are also less common than in adults. In the past, infratentorial neoplasms were thought to constitute more than 50 percent of all neoplasms in children. Utilizing CT, the incidence of neoplasms in the supratentorial compartment in children is almost the same as or slightly higher than that in the adult population (Table 8-2). The change in ratio is probably due to the earlier utilization of CT as a diagnostic modality, whereas in the past, neoplasms were either missed or did not undergo diagnostic studies, because of their invasive nature, until late in the course of the disease. The histological characteristics of neoplasms in children are also different from those in adults. In general, tumors such as meningiomas and pituitary adenomas are less common in children. Certain cell types of tumors, however, have a greater predilection for the younger age group—e.g., primitive neural ectodermal tumor, hypothalamic and optic glioma, and rhabdomyosarcoma.

Certain tumors, such as malignant astrocytoma, are more often found in the supratentorial compartment. Similarly, choroid plexus papilloma or its malignant version, choroid plexus carcinoma, should

Table 8-2 Incidence of Intracranial Neoplasm in Pediatric Age Group (Up to 15 Years)

Type	U. of Md. Hospital (76 tumors)		Hosp. for Sick Children (269 tumors)	
	No. of cases	% of total	No. of cases	% of total
Infratentorial	30	39.5	113	42
Astrocytoma	14	18.4	46	17.1
Medulloblastoma	7	9.2	39	14.5
Ependymoma	5	6.7	16	5.9
Miscellaneous	4	5.3	12	4.5
Supratentorial	46	60	156	58
Gliomas	18*	23.7	41	15.2
Neuroblastoma	4	5.3	3	1.1
Craniopharyngioma	6	7.9	23	8.5
Teratoma/pinealoma/ectopic pinealoma	6	7.9	13	4.8
Ganglioglioma/cytoma	4	5.3	12†	4.5
Ependymoma	3	3.9	1	0.4
Choroid plexus papilloma/carcinoma	2	2.6	3	1.1
Optic nerve glioma			22‡	8.2
Miscellaneous	3	3.9	38§	14.1

* Includes three optic nerve gliomas, two giant cell astrocytomas.
† Includes three cases of hamartoma.
‡ Includes eleven cases of intraorbital optic nerve glioma.
§ Includes four cases of lipoma, pituitary adenoma, and meningioma; eight cases of leukemia; two schwannomas of the fifth nerve; seven meningeal neoplasms; and eight other neoplasms without specific histologic findings.

be suspected when an enhancing mass is encountered in the trigone of the lateral ventricle in a child, whereas such a mass is more likely to be a meningioma when encountered in the older population.

A few tumors, such as craniopharyngioma, appear to have two peaks, the majority of these neoplasms being encountered either in children under 15 years or in adults beyond their fifth decade.

Although the CT appearance may not be dissimilar in neoplasms common to both the pediatric and the adult population, a combination of the CT appearance, the tumor location, the age of the patient, and attenuation characteristics (Probst 1979) provides a reasonable diagnostic clue to the type of tumor.

For descriptive purposes, neoplasms in the pediatric population are grouped in this chapter into the following major regional categories: (1) infratentorial, or posterior fossa, neoplasms; and (2) supratentorial neoplasms.

INFRATENTORIAL TUMORS

Incidence

The overall incidence of supratentorial and infratentorial tumors in children remains similar to the proportions described earlier by Harwood-Nash and Fitz (1976). Since 1976, 113 children with primary benign and malignant tumors in the posterior fossa have been examined at the Hospital for Sick Children.

These represent 42 percent of all intracranial tumors found on CT. Biopsy confirmation was available for the majority of the infratentorial tumors, except when their location precluded securing adequate tissue samples. These were primarily brainstem gliomas. At the University of Maryland Hospital, posterior fossa tumors represented 40 percent of 76 cases reported. Overall, some shifts were noted in the major categories of infratentorial neoplasms, compared to the larger series, primarily before CT, that was reported by Harwood-Nash and Fitz in 1976. Ten percent of the infratentorial tumors were in children under 2 years of age. This probably reflects earlier diagnosis because of CT (Tadmor 1980). Some shift in tumor cell type was also noted, with medulloblastoma making up 35 percent of all posterior fossa tumors (Table 8-3).

Types of Tumor

Medulloblastoma

With CT, medulloblastomas have shown a slight "stretching" of age incidence, with 16 percent of the patients being less than 2 years of age and 49 percent 8 years of age or older; of the latter, nearly 50 percent were 12 years or older (Table 8-4). Medulloblastomas, though having a generally characteristic appearance (Zimmerman 1977), tend to have more variable CT findings than other posterior fossa tumors. The usual location of medulloblastoma is in the midline. Most often it is smoothly ovoid or spherical in shape. It tends to be slightly greater in

Table 8-3   Incidence of Posterior Fossa Tumors in Children

Histologic type	Number of cases		Percent of posterior fossa tumors	
	Hospital for Sick Children	U. of Md. Hospital	Hospital for Sick Children	U. of Md. Hospital
Astrocytoma	46	14	41	47
Medulloblastoma	39	7	35	23
Ependymoma	16	5	14	17
Miscellaneous	12	4	10	13

Table 8-4   Posterior Fossa Tumors Diagnosed by CT at Hospital for Sick Children

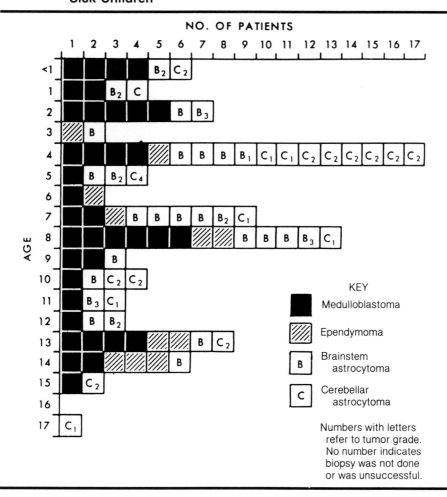

density than the surrounding cerebellum and has a rim of edema (Fig. 8-4) or compressed white matter. In the authors' experience, medulloblastomas have nearly always shown enhancement on CECT, with a 5 percent incidence of no visible enhancement as reported by Woodrow (1981). The density of the contrast enhancement is usually uniform throughout its extent, though the contrast enhancement is not always homogeneous. Small "cystic" areas are visible in about 10 percent of cases. On pathologic study, these represent true cysts rather than regions of necrosis within the neoplasm.

Calcification within the neoplasm can be detected by CT in 25 percent of medulloblastomas. The calcification is usually small and homogeneous, eccentric in location, and rarely visible on skull x-ray. Hemorrhage within the tumor is also unusual, and the small punctate calcifications may be mistaken for hemorrhages (Fig. 8-5).

As the tumor is most commonly located in the vermis, the fourth ventricle is usually compressed and displaced anterosuperiorly. Moderate to severe hydrocephalus is common.

Medulloblastoma with unusual CT patterns has

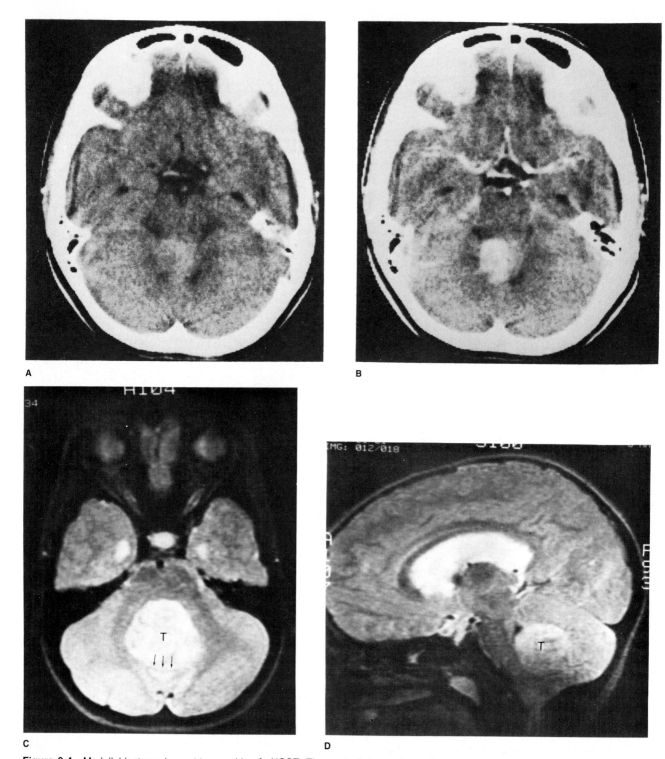

A

B

C

D

Figure 8-4 Medulloblastoma in an 11-year-old. **A.** NCCT: The centrally located vermian tumor is slightly denser than the cerebellum and has a rim of decreased density surrounding it. **B.** CECT: There is enhancement throughout nearly all of the tumor. The enhancement is relatively homogeneous. **C** and **D.** Medulloblastoma on MRI. A large hyperintense Mass (T) on T_2-WI compresses on the fourth ventricle (arrowheads). (*Courtesy of Dr. W. Cunningham, Robert Wood Johnson Hospital, N.J.*)

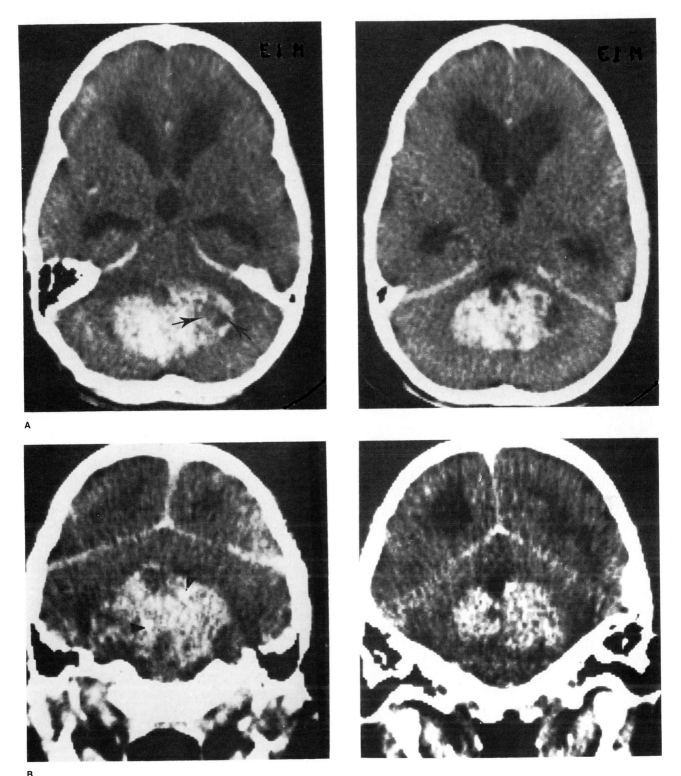

Figure 8-5 Medulloblastoma in an 9-year-old. **A.** Axial CT. **B.** Coronal CT. The enhancing tumor surrounds the fourth ventricle. It consists of regions of calcification (arrowheads), as well as unusual necrotic or cystic components (arrows).

more often been noted in children over 8 years old. Perhaps because of its invasive quality, medulloblastoma is more likely to be mistaken for a brain-stem or hemispheric astrocytoma than other tumors and more likely to be uncharacteristic in appearance, with features such as a large cyst, an irregular, lumpy border, or an eccentric location (Fig. 8-6). Very rarely, enlargement of the fourth ventricle, typical of ependymoma, may be seen. Metastasis at the time of diagnosis is common (North 1985). Stanley et al. (1983) reported an incidence of 90 percent on myelography. The authors' experience in the past 2 years has been approximately 50 percent.

Ependymoma

Ependymomas are mostly seen in older children: in the series analyzed in Table 8-4, 8 out of 15 were 8

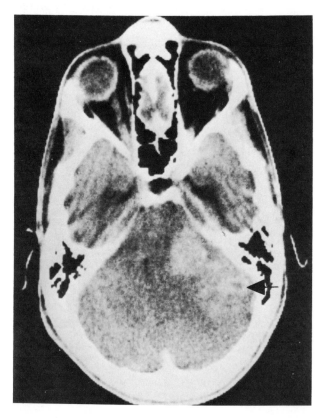

Figure 8-6 Medulloblastoma in a 13-year-old, primarily hemispheric in location and with irregular borders. Small cyst (arrow), confirmed at surgery, also visible.

years of age or more, and 4 were under 4. This also is slightly different from the larger series (Harwood-Nash 1976).

Ependymomas, because they arise in the wall or, particularly, the floor of the fourth ventricle, are occasionally nearly identical to medulloblastoma (Fig. 8-7), though sometimes visibly more inferior in location and closer to the foramen magnum. One characteristic that is nearly diagnostic but occurs in only about 10 percent of cases is the desmoplastic extension of the tumor through the fourth-ventricle foramina down over the medulla and upper cervical cord (Fig. 8-8). On ventriculography and pneumoencephalography before CT, it was noted that this tumor very often allowed or caused the fourth ventricle to enlarge and surround it as though the tumor were invaginating a balloon. This appearance is less visible on CT but, when noted, is usually a sign of ependymoma (Fig. 8-9). Ependymoma typically has the highest incidence of calcification among posterior fossa tumors (45%); however, since they are less common in occurrence than astrocytoma and medulloblastoma, it cannot be said that a calcified posterior fossa tumor is most likely to be an ependymoma. The calcification is somewhat characteristic and is more likely to be punctate and distributed throughout much or several portions of the tumor, as compared with other posterior fossa masses (Fig. 8-9A).

The tumor is of variable density before contrast enhancement, but the density tends to be equal to or slightly greater than that of the surrounding cerebellum (Figs. 8-7, 8-9). As in medulloblastomas, a ring of edema is fairly common. Contrast enhancement is present in *nearly* all tumors, tending to be somewhat nonhomogeneous in both area and density. Moderate hydrocephalus is common in ependymoma and relates to size and location of the tumor.

Cerebellar Astrocytoma

Astrocytoma is the most common tumor in the posterior fossa. Variable in age incidence, with a sharp peak at 4 years (Table 8-4), the tumor shows several relatively common characteristics. It is more often cystic than other posterior fossa tumors, and the

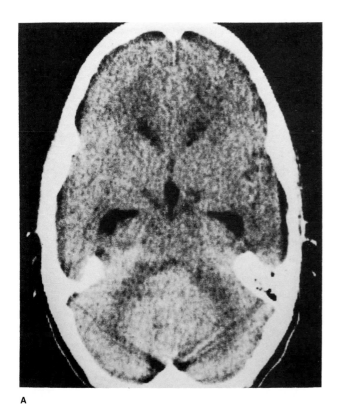
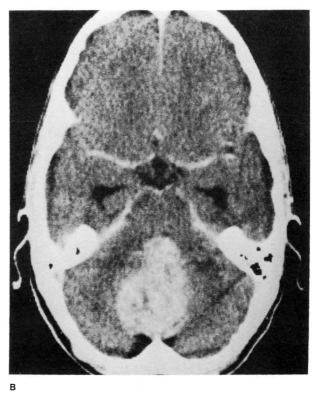

A   **B**

Figure 8-7 Ependymoma in a 14-year-old. **A.** NCCT shows rim of edema in large ependymoma and density equal to or just greater than surrounding cerebellum **B.** On CECT, much of the tumor shows a blush of uniform density. Irregular, nonenhancing, central areas of necrosis are visible.

cysts are frequently large and single. Whether the tumor is solid or cystic, the solid portion is typically lower in density than the surrounding cerebellum on the NCCT (Fig. 8-10). The cyst is of higher density than the CSF but may be difficult to distinguish from surrounding edema if the cyst wall does not show contrast enhancement.

Contrast enhancement of the solid portion and cyst wall of the cerebellar astrocytomas is variable. Particularly in the lower-grade tumors, only a portion of the solid part of the tumor may enhance (Fig. 8-11). The enhancement is frequently nonhomogeneous, with small cysts or necrotic areas of tumor within the enhancing portion of the mass. This is particularly true in those tumors without large peripheral cysts. The tumor may or may not show contrast enhancement in the cyst wall. This is most often the case in grade 1 cystic tumors (Naidich 1977*b*).

Enhancement of the cyst wall and tumor nodularity is often present in malignant glioma and astrocytoma of grade 2 and over (Fig. 8-12) (Zimmerman 1978*a*). It is generally thought that enhancement of the cyst wall indicates that the wall is made of tumor cells (Goi 1963). It has also been noted that delayed scanning will show leakage or excretion of contrast into the cyst itself (Kingsley 1977). Although enhancing tumor nodules are the rule in the cystic tumor, they may occasionally be too small to be seen at CT.

Calcification is less common in astrocytomas (20 percent). No characteristic features of the calcification can be described. Although the tumor often appears to be centrally located on CT, the larger tumors in particular are more likely than other posterior fossa tumors to involve one of the cerebellar hemispheres and cause some lateral displacement

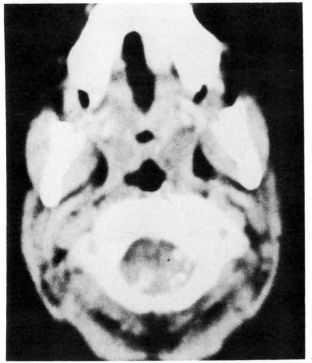

Figure 8-8   A. (Opposite, left) Ependymoma in a 4-year-old. CECT slice through C2 level shows several calcified and enhancing lesions in the spinal canal from extension of an ependymoma out of the fourth ventricle.   **B.** CECT in another 6-year-old child with ependymoma arising from the lateral recess of the fourth ventricle. The enhancing mass is projecting into the cerebellopontine angle cistern and extends down to the level of the foramen magnum. Like any other mass in the cerebellopontine angle there is resultant widening of the cistern on the ipsilateral side.   **C.** Coronal reformatted image demonstrates the tumor relationship to the brainstem and the cistern.

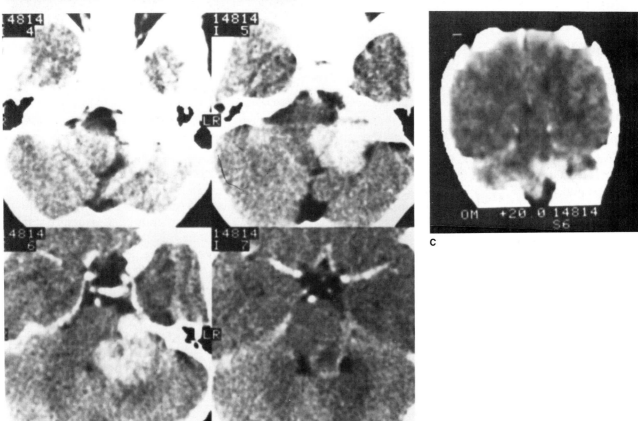

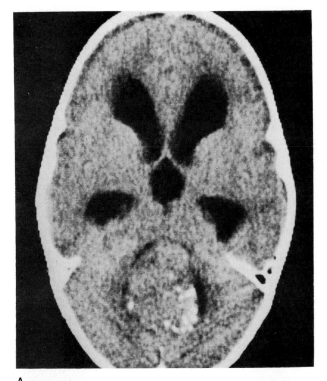

A

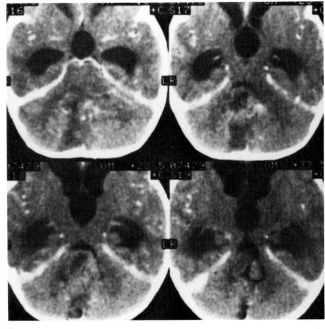

B

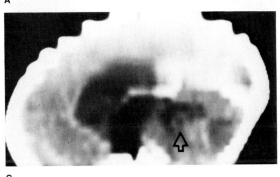

C

Figure 8-9 Ependymoma: **A.** NCCT shows multiple calcifications scattered throughout the tumor. The tumor has invaginated the fourth ventricle, which surrounds it almost like a horseshoe. **B.** Serial axial sections and (**C**) coronal reformatted image demonstrates another child with ependymona (⟳) invaginating into the fourth ventricle with apparent dilatation of the ventricle. Because of obstruction of the CSF pathway there is resultant hydrocephalus.

of the fourth ventricle. Moderate or severe hydrocephalus is the rule with cerebellar astrocytomas.

Brainstem Tumor

This is a difficult group to analyze, since in many cases biopsy proof is not available for confirmation, although biopsy may have been attempted and the location is at least visually confirmed. In the Table 8-4 series, the ages of the patients with confirmed and with unconfirmed tumors were not significantly different.

Brainstem tumors are the most homogeneous in appearance of all the posterior fossa masses. They are typically of low density throughout (Fig. 8-13). Cysts are relatively uncommon. Contrast enhancement is usually present in 50 percent, and is usually less intense. Enhancement may occur in only a small portion of the tumor. Prominent contrast enhancement tends to occur in the eccentric portion of tumors protruding into the fourth ventricle or cerebellar pontine angle (Fig. 8-14). Contrast enhancement is not a reliable indicator of tumor grade (Fig. 8-15). As brainstem gliomas are usually slow-growing, the

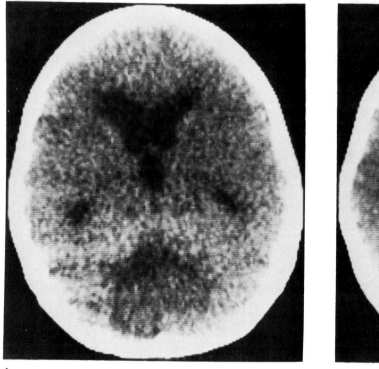
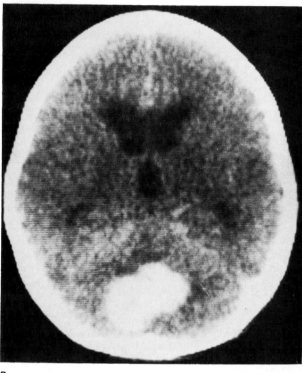

A   B

Figure 8-10 Astrocystoma, grade II, in a 9-year-old. **A.** NCCT slice shows large solid tumor of lower density than surrounding cerebellum. A thin anterior rim of edema, possibly averaged with the fourth ventricle, is visible. **A.** CECT shows fairly homogeneous enhancement throughout the tumor.

fourth ventricle and aqueduct are usually stretched over the tumor and remain open (Fig. 8-15). Hydrocephalus is uncommon in brainstem tumors. Zimmerman et al. (1980) described a method which can be used to measure the subtle anteroposterior displacement of the fourth ventricle on axial CT. The reliability of these measurements depends on precise positioning of the patient's head in relation to the x-ray beam. If a brainstem glioma is eccentric, the lateral recess of the fourth ventricle on the ipsilateral side will be displaced backward (Hayman 1979). On the other hand, in symmetrically enlarged brainstem gliomas, not only may both lateral recesses be spread apart, but the floor of the fourth ventricle is convex backward. A medullary tumor can displace the fourth ventricle forward (Fig. 8-14). Although thin-section CT following intrathecal water-soluble contrast may be used to identify subtle dis-

placement of the fourth ventricle, sagittal MR is reliable and sensitive in detection and follow-up of these tumors (Lee 1985) (Figs. 8-13 and 8-15).

Acoustic Neuroma

In children and adolescents, most acoustic neuromas are associated with neurofibromatosis (Jacoby 1980). Because of this association, the tumor is relatively large compared with that usually seen in adults. A mild contrast enhancement of the rim of the entire mass (Fig. 8-16) and an enlarged internal auditory canal are present in most cases. Bilateral acoustic neuromas may be seen in neurofibromatosis. Schwannomas without neurofibromatosis although rare are not uncommon (Hernanz-Shulman 1986; see also Chap. 10).

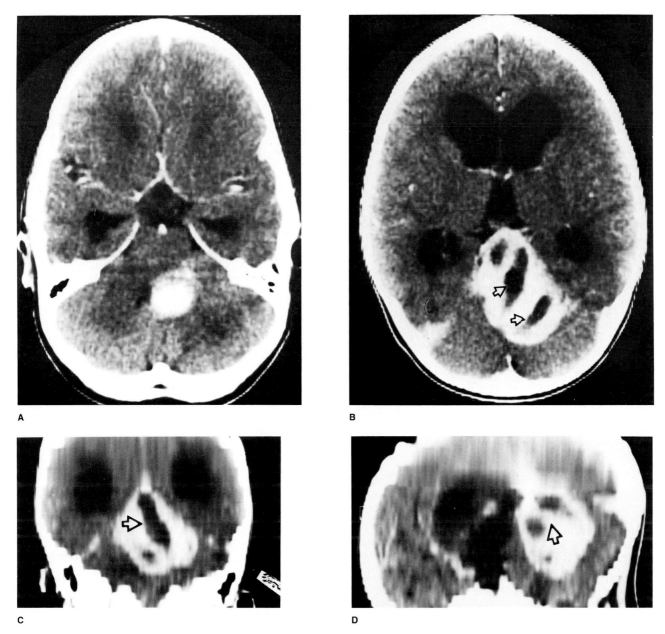

Figure 8-11   Astrocytoma in a 7-year-old.   **A** and **B.** CECT adjacent axial section demonstrates the enhancing tumor with cystic components. **C.** Coronal and (**D**) sagittal reformation clearly demonstrate tumor location.

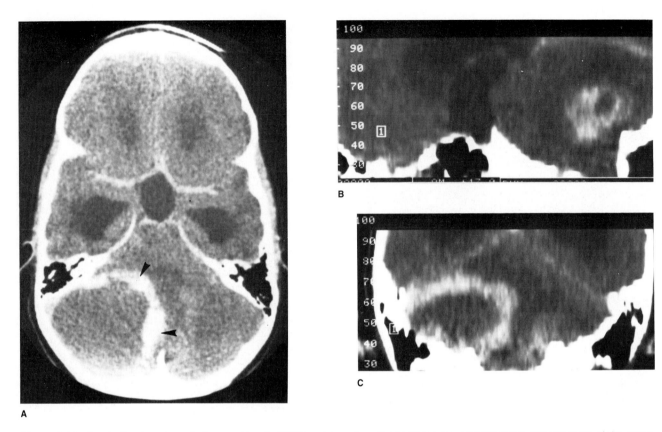

Figure 8-12   Grade II astrocytoma in 9-year-old.   **A.** CECT, axial section demonstrates the peripheral rim enhancement of the tumor (▲). The density within the tumor is slightly less hypodense than adjacent parenchyma.   **B.** Sagittal and (**C**) coronal reformatted image helps in better definition of the relationship of tumor in the posterior fossa.

Miscellaneous Tumors

HEMANGIOBLASTOMA   Hemangioblastoma is rare in children below 15 years. On CT the tumor is visible as a cyst with a small nodule visible at its periphery (Fig. 8-17). The diagnosis is best made by angiography, which shows the extremely vascular nodule to advantage. Angiography is recommended as a confirmatory examination when this tumor is suspected on CT. The CT finding of a small enhancing nodule within a large cyst is characteristic, though solid tumors also occur (Naidich 1977*b*) (see Chapter 7). A cystic astrocytoma can have a similar appearance on CT but does not show the intense vascular blush on angiography.

CAVERNOUS HEMANGIOMA   Although rare, cavernous hemangioma can occur in the posterior fossa. Calcification may be present and may enhance significantly. The calcification is multifocal and quite dense. This may be a significant diagnostic finding (Fig. 8-18), although noncalcified cavernous hemangiomas have also been described (Tera 1979). Diagnostic distinction from other posterior fossa lesions on the basis of CT alone is difficult (see Chapter 13).

GANGLIOGLIOMA   The CT appearance is often similar to a low-grade tumor related to other gliomas. Calcification may occasionally be present within the tumor. The tumor shows some surrounding edema

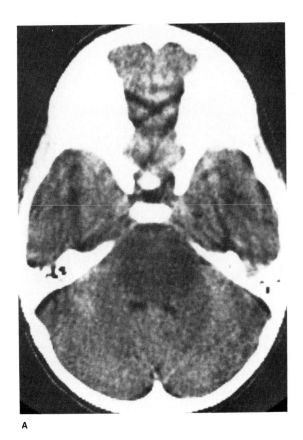

A

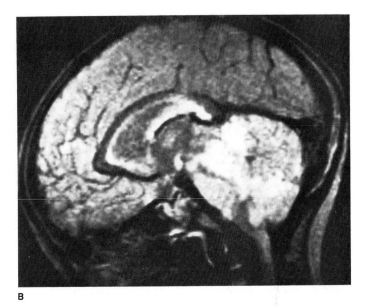

B

Figure 8-13 Brainstem glioma in an 8-year-old. CECT shows enlarged midbrain with the floor of the fourth ventricle displaced backward (arrow). The tumor is hypodense. MRI 3 months following radiation; sagittal view clearly demonstrates the tumor (increased signal intensity) as well as the postradiation charges involving the cerebellar hemisphere.

and slight diffuse contrast enhancement. They are rare in the posterior fossa (see Chapter 7).

RHABDOSARCOMA   Although frequently arising in the middle ear, rhabdosarcoma uncommonly invades the posterior fossa. Next to retinoblastoma, they are the most common extradural intracranial tumors in children (Scotti 1982). They usually present as extraaxial posterior fossa mass. Adjacent bone erosion as well as extracranial extension is common (Fig. 8-19). Seeding into the subarachnoid space, although extremely rare, has been reported (Zimmerman 1978*b*). Homogeneous enhancement of both intracranial and extracranial portions of rhabdosarcomas is common. Extension into the posterior fossa is not uncommon, even among rhabdosarcomas originating in the middle ear. Rarely, primary rhabdosarcoma may occur in the posterior fossa and cannot be distinguished from other tumors. Most often, it mimics medulloblastoma.

CHORDOMA   Chordomas typically occur in older children. Combined erosion and reactive thickening of the clivus is seen on CT. The tumor mass is visible as an enhancing extradural mass over the clivus (Fig. 8-20) and is often calcified. The extracranial component of the tumor is variable but can be quite extensive. CT following intrathecal water-soluble contrast, along with reformatted images, is helpful in defining the intraspinal extension of chordoma.

Postoperative Examination

Following operation and x-ray treatment of tumors, those showing recurrence as well as residual tumor undergo morphologic changes. No matter what the pretreatment type, they are more likely to be cystic after treatment. This is probably related to the radiation therapy. Residual tumors may be present

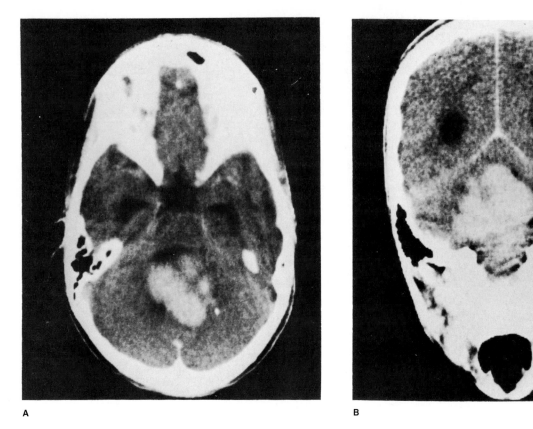

A   B

Figure 8-14   Brainstem glioma in an 8-year-old: **A.** CECT shows enhancing irregular tumor with low-density area anteriorly that resembles fourth ventricle, mimicking a primary cerebellar tumor.   **B.** Clival perpendicular (Waters) view shows the full extent of the tumor from brainstem to near the tentorium, with eccentric growth out into the left hemisphere.

and unchanged for two or three years, then quickly undergo growth for no apparent reason.

SUPRATENTORIAL TUMORS

For purposes of comparison between different histological grades of tumor, the CT findings are discussed on a regional basis. Neoplasms that have no significant differences from the adult variety are mentioned only in passing.

Sellar and Parasellar Tumors

Lesions around the sella account for 20 percent of all intracranial neoplasms in children (Wilson 1975; Harwood-Nash 1976). One of the most common neoplasms encountered in the pediatric age group in this region is craniopharyngioma. Other less common neoplasms in this age group include hypothalamic glioma, optic chiasm and nerve glioma, hypothalamic histiocytosis, hypothalamic hamartoma, arachnoid cyst, and ectopic pinealoma (teratoma, germinoma, embryonal carcinoma, and the rare choriocarcinoma).

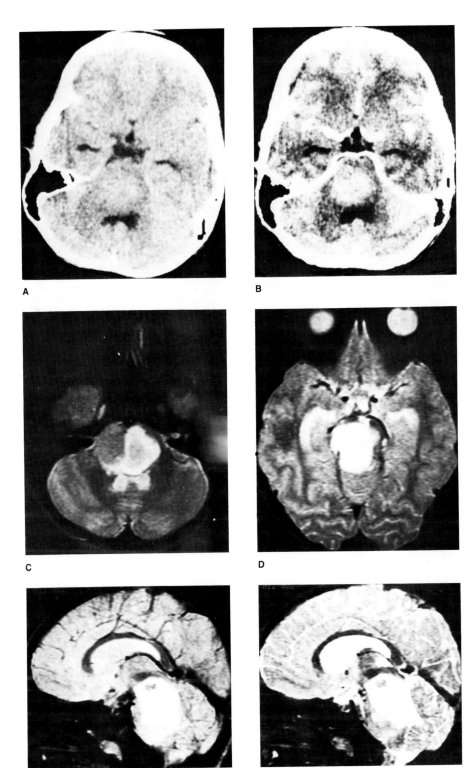

Figure 8-15 Brainstem glioma in a 9-year-old. **A.** NCCT and (**B**) CECT demonstrates a slightly hyperdense enlarged brainstem with marked enhancement of the tumor. The floor of the fourth ventricle is displaced backward. MRI (T$_2$-weighted sequence) clearly demonstrates the extent of the tumor as region of increased signal intensity in the (**C** and **D**) axial as well as in the (**E** and **F**) sagittal plane.

A

B

C

D

E

F

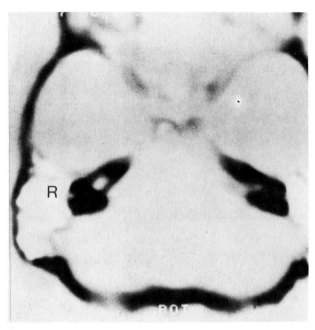

A

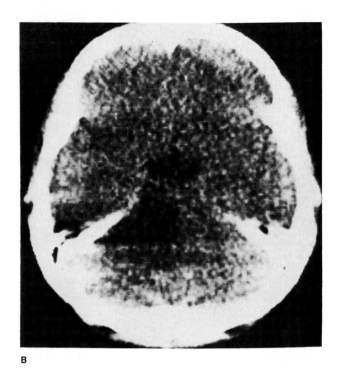

B

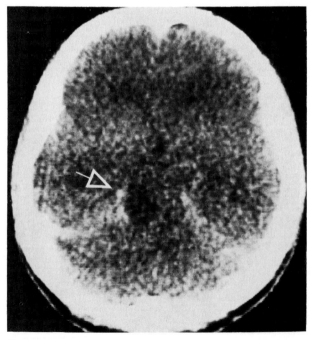

C

Figure 8-16 Acoustic neuroma in a 15-year-old.   **A.** CT section through petrous bone shows enlarged right internal auditory canal (reverse gray scale).   **B.** Higher section without enhancement shows low-density tumor and surrounding edema.   **C.** CECT shows a small rim of enhancement (arrow) adjacent to tentorium along tumor border.

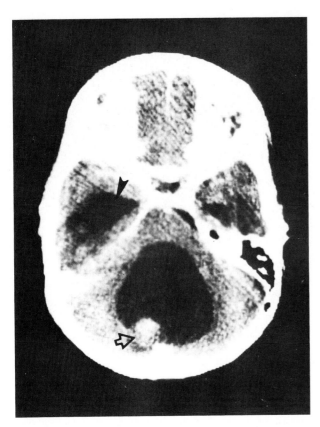

Figure 8-17 Hemangioblastoma in a 10-year-old female. CECT shows an enhancing tumor nodule (arrowhead) with large surronding cyst. The compressed fourth ventricle is not visualized. Hydrocephalus demonstrated by the enlarged temporal horn (arrow).

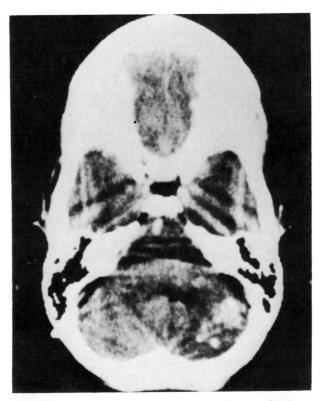

Figure 8-18 Cavernous hemangioma in a 17-year-old. CT shows calcified left cerebellar hemispheric mass that does not enhance. No displacement of the fourth ventricle is present. Lesions also were present in the frontal lobe and thalamus. The child had been misdiagnosed as having a malignant tumor by pneumoencephalogram 8 years earlier at another hospital.

Even after the availability of CT, numerous authors indicated the need for positive contast CT studies or pneumoencephalography to define the presence and location of the lesion within the suprasellar cistern (Strand 1978; Reich 1976; Kishore 1980; Volbe 1978). In most cases, CT not only is diagnostic but shows the extent of the lesion. In occasional cases, CT cisternography with axial and coronal sections may be necessary. MRI will eventually replace the need for CT cisternography.

Craniopharyngioma

This is a relatively common tumor in the pediatric age group, accounting for about 7 percent of all intracranial neoplasms and more than 50 percent of all sellar and parasellar neoplasms (Harwood-Nash 1976). Most often the tumor is suprasellar in location, although in less than 10 percent of children it may be totally intrasellar (Rao 1977). Craniopharyngiomas in children tend to have calcific components either within the tumor or around its rim: calcification is seen in nearly 80 percent of cases, especially by computed tomography.

Cystic components within the tumor are more common in children than in adults, as is enhancement of the tumor on CECT. An isodense, nonenhancing craniopharyngioma is more common in the adult population.

In the majority of craniopharyngiomas, CT dem-

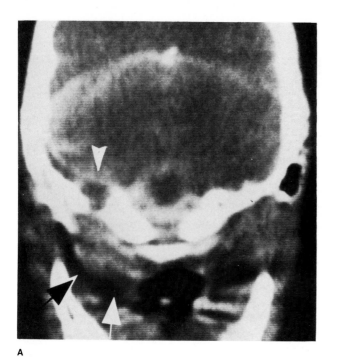

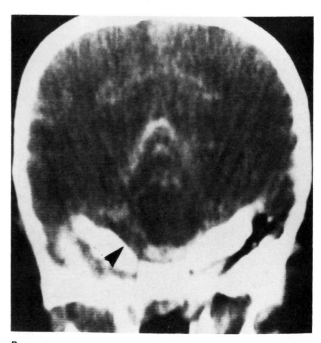

A

B

Figure 8-19 Rhabdosarcoma in a 6-year-old. **A.** Clival perpendicular view with intrathecal metrizamide shows pharyngeal mass (arrows), erosion of medial petrous bone, and extradural posterior fossa extension of tumor (arrowhead). **B.** Same examination at the dorsum shows forward extension of extradural tumor beneath brainstem on the right side (arrowhead).

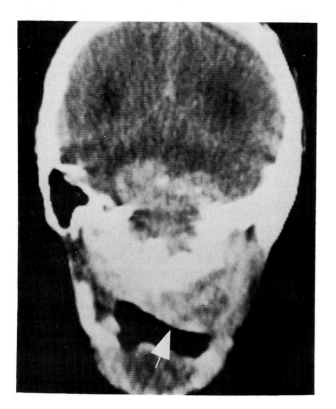

Figure 8-20 Chordoma. CECT, clival perpendicular view: Large recurrent chordoma shows clival erosion and enhanced and calcified bilobed mass extending up from the clivus and a large pharyngeal extension (arrow).

onstrates a calcified mass located in the suprasellar region. The calcification may be along the periphery of the tumor, as in purely cystic forms of craniopharyngioma (Fig. 8-21), or may be present within the tumor as discrete masses (Fig. 8-22). CECT will usually show a variegated pattern, depending on the nature of the calcification as well as cystic components within the tumor. Nonhomogeneous enhancement is thus a common finding, the hypodense regions probably representing cysts containing a mixture of keratin and cholesterol debris. Occasionally the neoplasm is isodense and enhances significantly. In these cases, differentiation from a chromophobe adenoma or even a giant aneurysm may become difficult. Rarely, the tumor may be massive, occupying a large portion of the intracranial compartment (Fig. 8-23) (Lipper 1981), or may be totally within the third ventricle (Fitz 1978*b*).

Craniopharyngioma, or its variant the Rathke's cleft cyst, occasionally may be hypodense (Fig. 8-24) and when small has been missed on routine CT examination (Volbe 1978; Eisenberg 1976).

Coronal CT, either by reformation or in the direct coronal mode, helps in defining the supero-inferior limit of the neoplasm and its relation to the sellar and hypothalamic areas. Metrizamide CT cisternography, in both axial and coronal planes, is occasionally necessary to define the neoplasm and its relation to adjacent structures. This test may not be necessary with wider usage and availability of MRI.

Other neoplasms in this area which should be differentiated from craniopharyngioma include optic chiasm glioma, hamartoma of the tuber ciner-

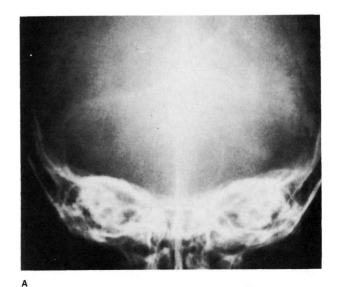

A

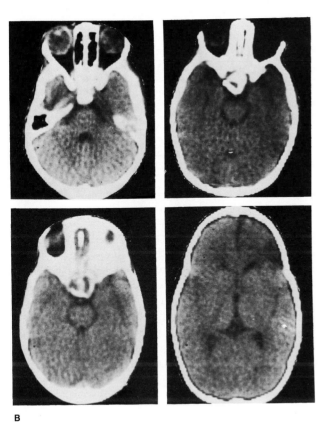

B

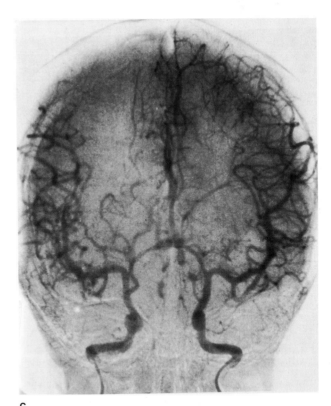

C

Figure 8-21   Craniopharyngioma in a 2-year-old.   **A.** Curvilinear calcification around the rim of tumor identified on skull x-ray. **B.** CT demonstrating calcified mass in the suprasellar cistern. This pattern of calcification is characteristic of craniopharyngioma. **C.** Angiogram (superimposed) anteroposterior view demonstrating the characteristic angiographic appearance of sellar mass with suprasellar extension. (*Continued on p. 388.*)

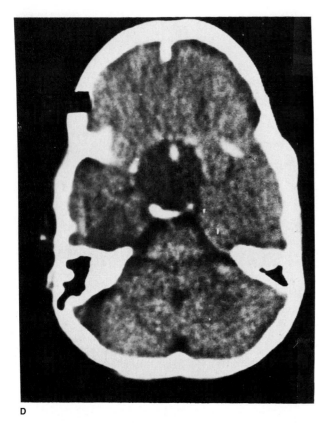
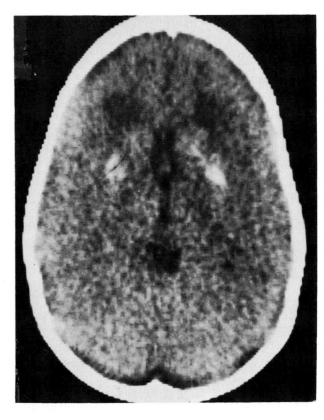

D

Figure 8-21 (*cont.*)   **D.** Cystic craniopharyngioma in a 4-year-old: large cystic craniopharyngioma with marginal calcification. A catheter tip is noted, used for intermittent drainage. In a slightly higher section, calcification of the basal ganglia secondary to radiation therapy is present.

eum, hypothalamic glioma, pituitary adenoma, aneurysm, and arachnoid cyst.

Diagnostic characteristics are the presence of calcifications, usually ringlike; nonhomogeneous enhancement; and the location of the mass. Angiography may be needed if intense homogeneous enhancement and clinical presentation suggest a giant aneurysm (Kokoris 1980) or before surgery.

Hamartoma

Hamartomas are rare neoplasms which are not true tumors (Lin 1978; Mori 1981). They are congenital heterotopic collections of tissue located in normal or abnormal locations. The tissue usually consists of glial cells. Hamartomas can occur anywhere, but when located in the hypothalamic region they are usually close to the tuber cinereum. The presenting clinical history usually includes diabetes insipidus. The tumor is slightly more common in males than in females. The CT characteristics are nonspecific. The mass if large will usually obliterate the suprasellar cistern. Enhancement characteristics are variable, but the majority do not enhance (Lin 1978). The hamartoma may also be multiple (Fig. 8-25). Differentiation from solitary hypothalamic histiocytosis (Miller 1980) by CT may be difficult.

Ectopic Pinealoma

Tumors with histological characteristics similar to those in the pineal region occur in the parasellar

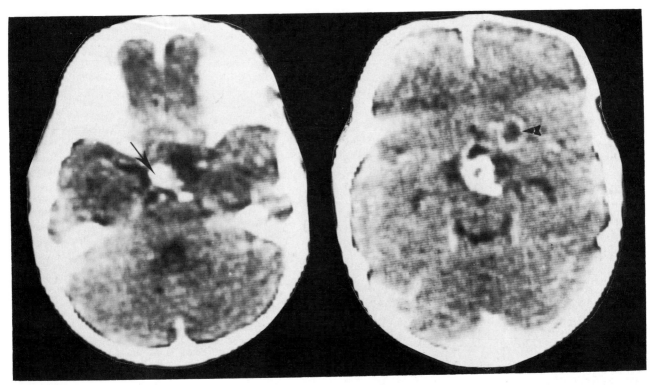

Figure 8-22   Craniopharyngioma in a 12-year-old. The tumor shows areas of calcification (arrow), ring enhancement (arrowhead), and a hypodense area.

region, predominantly in the suprasellar cistern. Their CT appearance and enhancement characteristics are similar to histologically different neoplasms in the pineal region. Embryonal carcinoma and endodermal sinus tumors in the suprasellar hypothalamic region do not demonstrate calcification, unlike those in the pineal region. Primary choriocarcinoma is a rare form of embryonal carcinoma, usually presenting as an isodense mass with intense enhancement. Hemorrhage within this tumor is common. Differentiation from other suprasellar masses may require further diagnostic studies.

Optic Nerve Glioma

Glioma of the optic nerve can be focal, involving either the intraorbital segment of the nerve or the intracranial component. Or the tumor may be diffuse and involve the intraorbital as well as the intra-

cranial component of the optic nerve. The CT features of intraorbital optic nerve glioma and its intracranial extension have been dealt with elsewhere (Chapter 3). Optic glioma is most often seen in children. Since the majority of the neoplasms are low-grade gliomas, on NCCT they appear as isodense masses obliterating the suprasellar cistern. If the glioma involves the intracranial component of the optic nerve, asymmetry of the anterior aspect of the "pentagonal" suprasellar cistern provides a clue to the presence of the optic or perioptic neoplasm (Naidich 1976). On the other hand, in large and bulky chiasmatic gliomas, dilatation of the basal and sylvian cisterns has been noted (Savoiardo 1981). The mechanism is presumed to be similar to projection of extraaxial masses into the cisterns. Enhancement of the glioma is variable but often intense; however, it may occasionally be minimal. Evaluation of the total extent and spread of the neoplasm requires

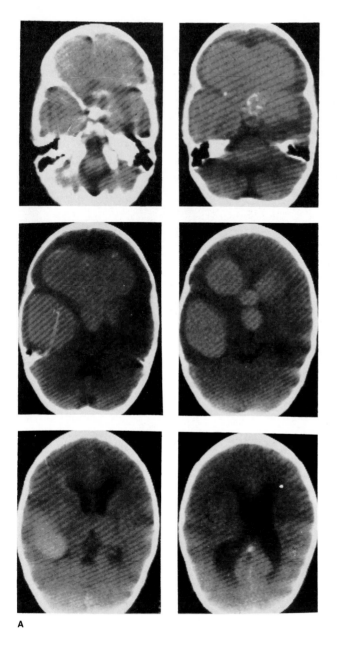

A

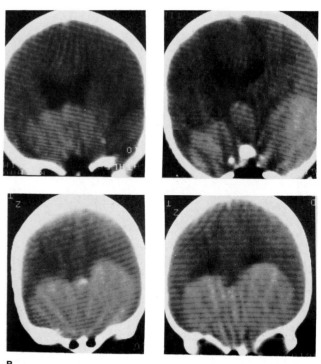

B

Figure 8-23 Craniopharyngioma. Axial (**A**) and coronal enhanced CT (**B**) demonstrating a massive craniopharyngioma extending into both temporal regions, besides its suprasellar extension.

thin CT sections in the axial as well as the coronal plane. Occasionally, in spite of these additional methods of CT examination, differentiation of the enhancing mass from such other suprasellar neoplasms as hypothalamic glioma with extension to the chiasm and optic tract may be difficult. In the past, CT following intrathecal metrizamide, angiography, and pneumoencephalography was necessary to identify the neoplasm. MRI has replaced the need for these studies. Enlargement of the optic chiasm can be clearly demonstrated. In the majority of cases reported (Albert 1986) the tumor can be well delineated by the spin echo technique. MRI in the sagittal plane is optimal in detecting chiasmal enlargement and posterior extent into the optic tract. Coronal and axial sections help in demonstrating the lateral and posterior extension of the tumor (Fig. 8-26).

These additional studies may still be indicated, in the absence of appropriate clinical findings, to define other suprasellar masses discussed in this chapter as well as other less common masses in children, such as pituitary adenoma and giant internal carotid aneurysm. In childhood pituitary adenomas, the sella is often enlarged in association with an

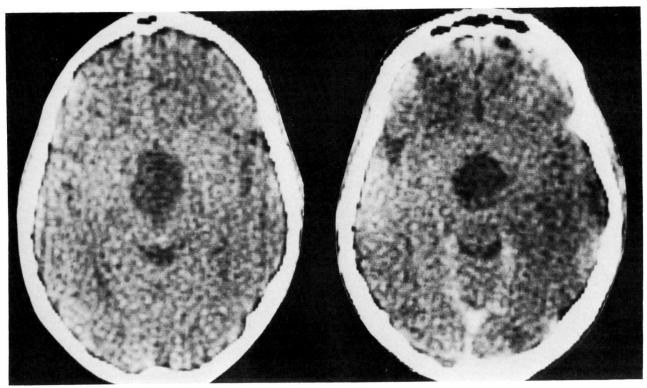

Figure 8-24   Nonenhancing, low-density, suprasellar cystic craniopharyngioma.

enhancing intrasellar mass. In one large series, pituitary adenomas in patients under 20 years of age were most often in females, the majority presenting with delayed puberty (Richmond 1978). In the presence of clinical findings and an enhancing sellar mass, pituitary adenoma should be considered (see Chapter 10). Since calcification rarely occurs in optic gliomas, differentiation from craniopharyngioma may occasionally be difficult.

Arachnoid Cyst

Congenital arachnoid cysts are commonly seen in the temporal region (Fig. 8-27) and in the posterior fossa as extraaxial cysts. Other less common locations of arachnoid cysts are the suprasellar and prepontine regions, the quadrigeminal and circummesencephalic cisterns, and the interhemispheric fissure,

as well as the region adjacent to the lateral ventricles.

Suprasellar arachnoid cysts may occasionally be missed on routine CT studies. They produce a characteristic appearance of focal ballooning of the anterior third ventricle on axial CT (Fig. 8-28). Diagnosis can be suspected on the basis of the CT appearance such as associated dilatation of the basal cistern, loss of the normal pentagonal shape of the suprasellar cistern, and depending on the size and upward extension, the appearance of the third and lateral ventricles. The extent of the cyst can be precisely defined by axial and coronal CT. Large suprasellar arachnoid cysts invaginate the third ventricle and, in some cases, appear to be intraventricular.

Differentiation from other cystic lesions in this region such as ependymal cysts, Rathke's cleft cyst,

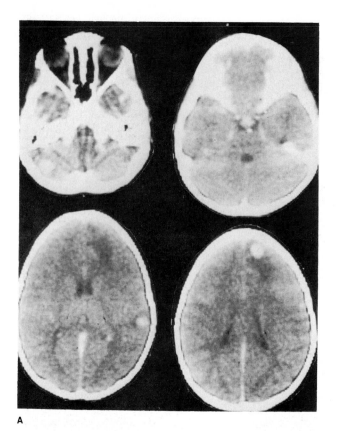

A

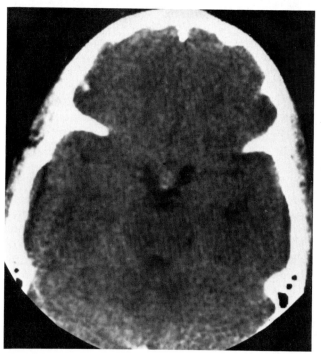

B

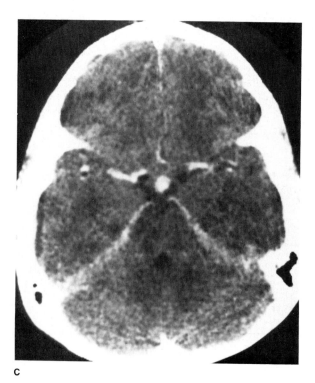

C

Figure 8-25 **A** multiple hamartoma in a 5-year-old male. Multiple enhancing lesions, proved at biopsy to be hamartomas, in a child presenting with diabetes insipidus. **B** NCCT demonstrates a hyperdense mass which enhances significantly on **C** CECT. (*Continued on p. 393.*)

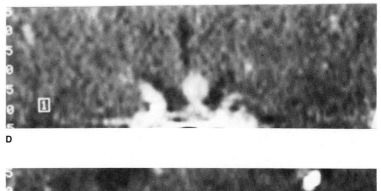

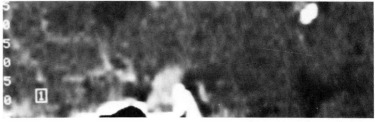

Figure 8-25 (*cont.*) **D** Coronal and **E** Sagittal reformation demonstrates the extent and location of the tumor precisely.

D

E

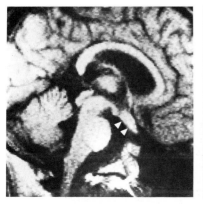

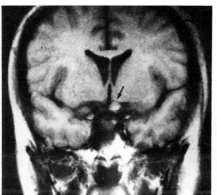

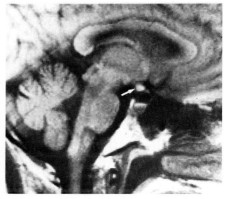

A

B

C

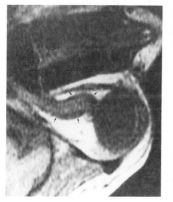

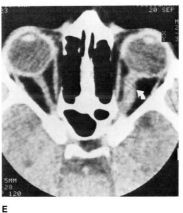

D

E

Figure 8-26 Optic glioma: (**A**) Sagittal MRI (SE 30/500) demonstrates an enlarged optic nerve and chiasm (arrowhead) secondary to optic nerve glioma. (**B**) Coronal MRI (SE 30/500). Another patient with optic glioma (arrow). Note increased signal intensity compared to adjacent normal nerve. (**C**) Sagittal MRI (SE 30/500). In comparison another patient with increased signal intensity due to a hematoma. Tumor and hematoma can not be differentiated. (**D**) Surface coil image of intraorbital glioma. The tumor can be separated from the nerve sheath and the surrounding CSF (arrows) by their decreased signal intensity. (**E**) C.T. at the same level. (Figures A–C courtesy of Dr. B. C. P. Lee, Figure D, E courtesy Dr. D. L. Daniels and AJNR, Vol. 7, 1986.)

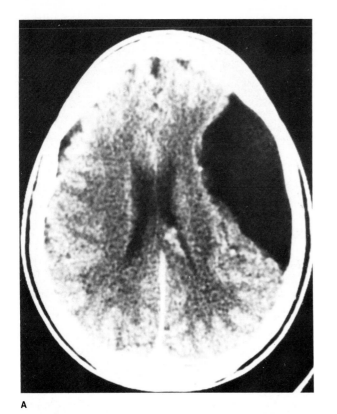

A

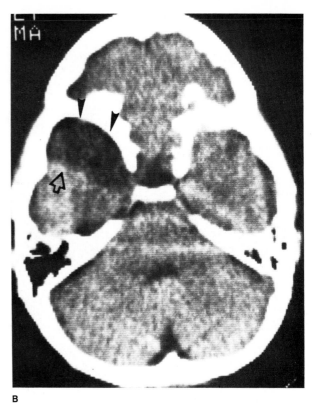

B

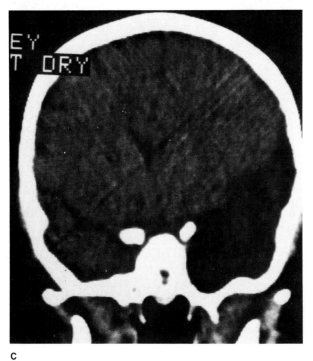

C

Figure 8-27 Arachnoid cyst (**A**). A large CSF density mass in the temporal region displacing the brain parenchyma medially (arrowheads). There is some amount of thinning of the adjacent temporal bone. **B** and **C.** Another patient with arachnoid cyst in the temporal region causing bowing of the greater wing of the sphenoid (arrowheads) and displacement of the temporal lobe (arrow).

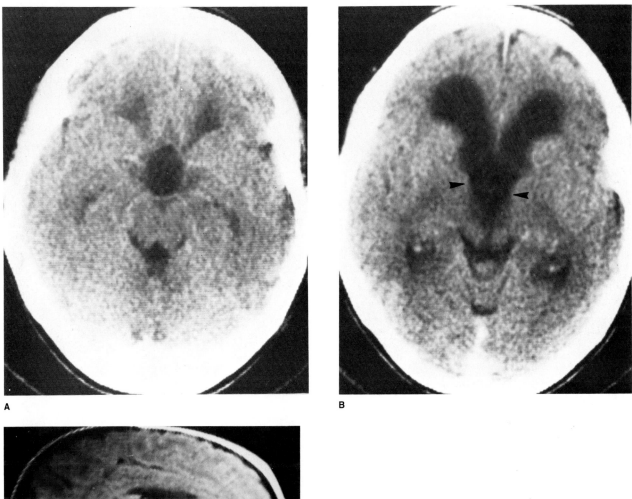

A

B

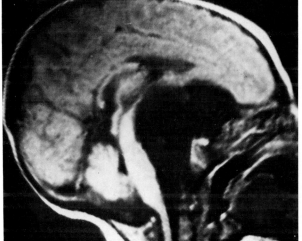

C

Figure 8-28 Suprasellar arachnoid cyst. **A.** The CT appearance is suggestive of a dilated third ventricle projecting into the suprasellar cistern, however at a higher level (**B**) there is lateral displacement of the walls of the ventricle (arrowheads) indicating the cyst compressing the ventricular system along its undersurface. **C.** Sagittal MRI demonstrates large suprasellar arachnoid displacing the brainstem and brain parenchyma, posteriorly and upwards. Signal intensity similar to CSF.

parasitic cysts, and marked enlargement of the third ventricle may occasionally be difficult.

Tumors of the Pineal Region

Tumors of the "pineal region" have in the past commonly been identified as *pinealomas,* whatever their histologic character. Similar tumors occurring in the anterior aspect of the third ventricle, within the suprasellar cistern, have been termed *ectopic pinealomas.* Pineal tumors have been classified according to their behavior, clinical presentation, and histological characteristics into germ-cell tumors, pineal parenchymal tumors, glial tumors, and meningiomas (Rubenstein 1970; Russell 1977). Of these the germ-cell tumors and pineal parenchymal tumors are more common in the pediatric age group.

Pineal and ectopic pineal tumors represent less than 2 percent of all intracranial tumors, although in the series summarized in Table 8-2 they represented 5 to 8 percent of all pediatric-age neoplasms.

In the pineal region, the greatest likelihood of confusion occurs in differentiating the various types of pineal neoplasms from those arising in regions adjacent to the pineal gland, such as astrocytoma involving the splenium of the corpus callosum or the tectum of the midbrain.

Since certain histological types of pineal tumors are radiosensitive (germinoma, pinealcytoma, embryonal cell carcinoma), not only precise localization of the neoplasm but its histological typing by the use of CT have been attempted (Zimmerman 1980*b;* Futrell 1981; Messina 1978). Pursuit of these ends requires evaluation of the CT findings by pre- and postcontrast studies. Occasionally, even with thin-

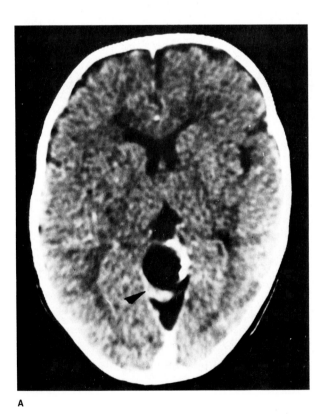

A

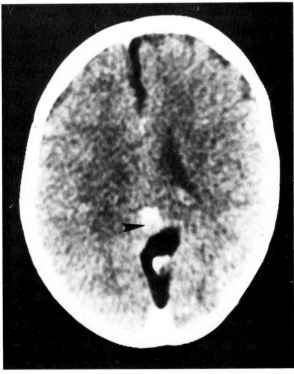

B

Figure 8-29 Pineal germinoma. **A.** CECT demonstrates a hypodense mass with density representing fat surrounded by a densely calcified rim (arrowhead) in the pineal region. **B.** An enhancing component is noted (arrowhead) on the next higher section.

section as well as direct coronal or sagittal and co-ronal multiplanar reformation to localize the origin of the tumor, angiography for tumor stain and vas-cular pattern may be necessary. The most frequent tumors of the pineal region are the germinoma and the teratoma. They occur in older children (over 15) in the second decade and are more frequent in males. Tumors of the pineal cell origin, however—pineal-cytoma and pinealblastoma—have no significant sex predilection although they are slightly more com-mon in females. More recent studies, however, in-dicate a male preponderance in both types of tumor (Ganti 1986). Their biological and clinical features, besides such CT findings as calcification, presence or absence of hemorrhages, and cysts, are helpful in arriving at a CT diagnosis and appropriate treat-ment. The CT characteristics of the major pineal tu-mors are briefly discussed below.

Germinomas are teratomatous tumors com-monly seen in males. On NCCT they appear as hy-perdense or isodense masses, usually deforming and encroaching on the posterior aspect of the third ven-tricle. Punctate calcification within the mass is usu-ally apparent. In the absence of calcification, oblit-eration of the quadrigeminal cistern, as well as deformity of the posterior aspect of the third ven-tricle, should be looked for, since the tumor com-monly infiltrates the adjacent tissues (Fig. 8-29). Often, depending on the size of the tumor, there is noncommunicating hydrocephalus. On CECT, in-tense enhancement of the neoplasm occurs. Occa-sionally these tumors have two components, one in the pineal region and the other an ectopic compo-nent in the anterior third ventricular region.

Teratoma in the pineal region usually appears as a hypodense mass (Fig. 8-30). Calcification within the mass and occasionally other formed elements may be present (Zimmerman 1980b). Fatty compo-nents within the tumor are common. Minimal en-hancement is the rule. In the absence of formed ele-ments such as a tooth or the like, CT differentiation from other lesions in this region, such as epider-moid tumor or quadrigeminal plate arachnoid cyst, may be difficult. Spontaneous rupture of this variety of neoplasm into the ventricular system or the subarachnoid cisterns has also been documented

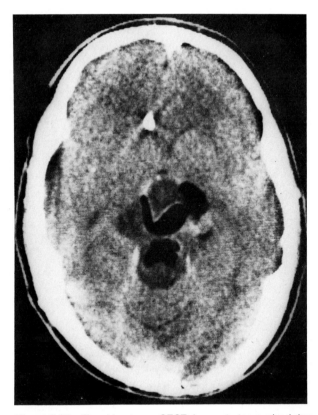

Figure 8-30 Pineal teratoma. CECT demonstrates a mixed den-sity tumor with cystic and fatty areas and associated linear calci-fication. No significant enhancement is seen. Hyperdensity in frontal region represents a shunt catheter tip. (*Courtesy of Dr. S. R. Ganti and AJNR, vol 7, 1986.*)

(Goshhajra 1979; McCormack 1978). Malignant de-generation of the tumor is associated with signifi-cant contrast enhancement.

Embryonal cell carcinoma, as well as endoder-mal sinus, or "yolk sac," carcinoma, are tumors found both in the pineal region and in the suprasellar re-gion (Zimmerman 1980b; Rao 1979). On NCCT they may be hypodense or slightly hyperdense (Fig. 8-31). Calcification has been described in these neo-plasms when located in the pineal region (Zimmer-man 1980b). They are prone to hemorrhage within the neoplasm. Intense enhancement of the tumors is characteristic, although rarely they may not en-hance.

The pinealblastoma has an appearance almost like that of the embryonal cell carcinoma. Calcification

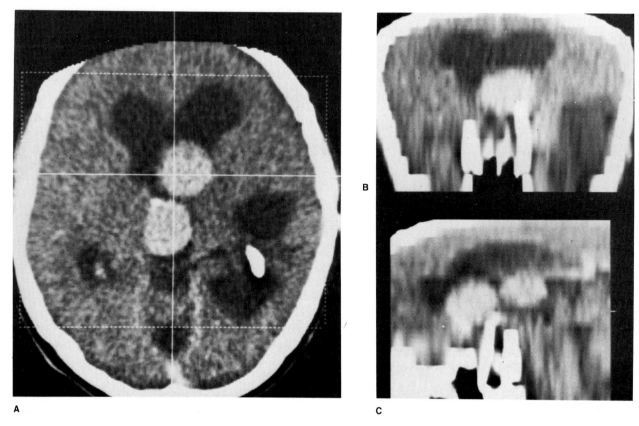

A

B

C

Figure 8-31   Embryonal cell carcinoma. CECT in (**A**) axial plane, (**B**) coronal, and (**C**) sagittal reformatted images. A large enhancing tumor is seen in the pineal region with a satellite lesion in the anterior third ventricular region. There is homogeneous enhancement of both the masses.

within or surrounding the neoplasm is rare. Pineal-cytoma, on the other hand, is associated with dense calcification with mild to moderate enhancement on CECT (Fig. 8-32). In spite of the above features, histological diagnosis on the basis of CT alone is extremely difficult. Spread of tumors along the ependymal surface of the ventricles can be seen not only with dysgerminoma (Osborn 1978) but also with pinealoblastoma, choriocarcinoma, and teratocarcinoma. CT plays an important role after surgery or radiation therapy in follow-up of these tumors.

Ependymal and Intraventricular Tumors

Neoplasms derived from the ependyma include (1) ependymoma, (2) choroid plexus papilloma and its

malignant version, choroid plexus carcinoma, and (3) heterotopias and cysts extending into the parenchyma or within the ventricle, the walls of the cyst being lined by ependymal cells. Parenchymal neoplasms may spread along the ependymal surface. These neoplasms may be primary or secondary and may project into the ventricular cavity due to their location and proximity to the ventricular spaces. In the majority of cases, CT in the axial and coronal plane following contrast enhancement will delineate the exact site of origin of these neoplasms and their extent. From the clinical history, the enhancing pattern, and the location of the neoplasm, the nature of the tumor can often be predicted. Angiography is helpful not only in the evaluation of tumor vascularity and the tumor's histological characteristics but in excluding vascular lesions extending along the ependymal surface (Coin 1977). A majority of neoplasms arising from the ependymal surface or from its derivatives result in hydrocephalus. Thus in children below 5 years, the presenting feature is progressive enlargement of the head size (not rapid). In children over 10 years of age the presenting feature is constant or intermittent headache. Cranial-nerve involvement and ataxia are late findings. Tumors involving the ependyma and its derivatives in general are rare.

Choroid Plexus Papilloma

Choroid plexus papillomas are rare neoplasms making up less than 2 percent of all intracranial neoplasms in children (Table 8-2). Unlike the adult form,

which occurs within the fourth ventricle, the papillomas in the pediatric age group (1 to 12 years) are more common in the lateral ventricle and rarely the third ventricle. In the lateral ventricle location, the tumor is more often seen in the left lateral ventricle than the right. The majority of benign choroid plexus papillomas are detected in children around the age of 2 years. The tumor manifests as prominence of the glomus of the choroid plexus, located in the trigone of the lateral ventricle and having a frondlike appearance. Calcification may be detected within the mass. The hydrocephalus associated with this neoplasm cannot be explained on the basis of obstruction of the CSF pathway, although a large mass in the trigone can result in entrapment of the ipsilateral temporal horn (Fig. 8-33). The hydrocephalus

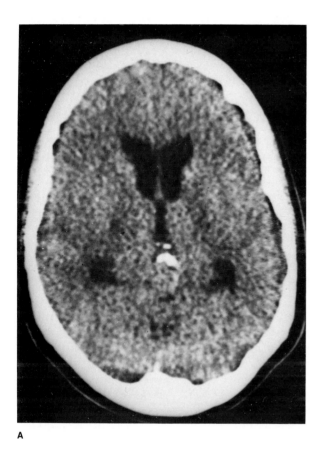

A

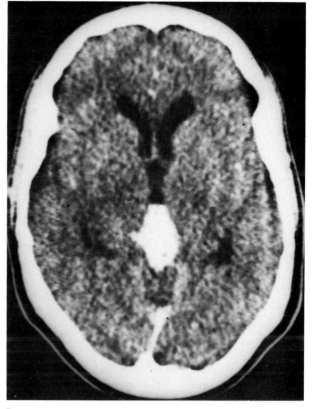

B

Figure 8-32 Pinealocytoma: (A-NCCT/ B-NCCT). **A.** An isodense pineal mass with calcification demonstrates (**B**) homogeneous enhancement of the tumor. (*Continued on p. 400.*)

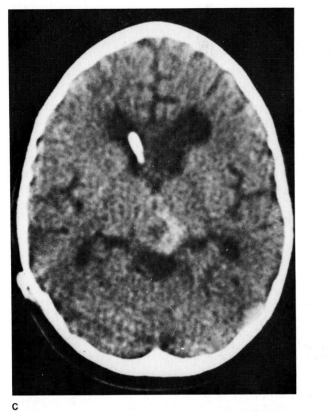

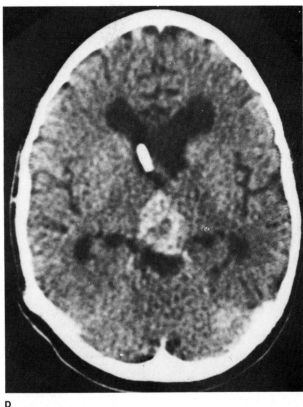

C

D

Figure 8-32 (*cont.*)   Pinealoblastoma: **C.** NCCT demonstrates a slightly hyperdense mass with central lucency. **D.** CECT demonstrates enhancement with minimal enhancement within the central lucent area, most likely representing necrosis. There is dilatation of the ventricles with a shunt catheter tip in the ventricle. (*Courtesy of Dr. S. R. Ganti and AJNR, vol 7, 1986.*)

has been attributed to a variety of factors: (1) elevated intraventricular pulse pressure, (2) diffuse spread along the meninges, (3) decreased CSF absorption by arachnoid granulations from frequent occult bleeding, and (4) increased CSF production. The fact that the hydrocephalus disappears after removal of these neoplasms indicates that the last factor is probably the most important mechanism. On NCCT the tumor is seen as a mass of slight hyperdensity compared to the rest of the parenchyma, due partly to the tumor vascularity and partly to the tumor's location within the CSF space. It enhances significantly on CECT.

Hydrocephalus with an enlarged, enhancing choroid plexus in a child with enlarging head is characteristic of choroid plexus papilloma. On an-

giography, choroid plexus papillomas are noted to be characteristically fed by the choroidal arteries. Intense vascular stain is a frequent finding.

Choroid Plexus Carcinoma

Choroid plexus carcinoma is the malignant form of the papilloma. The malignancy of the tumor can be suspected from the extension of the tumor beyond the confines of the ependymal barrier into the cerebral parenchyma. These neoplasms are less common than choroid plexus papilloma. Like the benign form, the choroid plexus carcinoma is associated with massive hydrocephalus. On NCCT the lesion can be seen, within the ventricle as well as extending into the parenchyma, as an isodense to slightly hy-

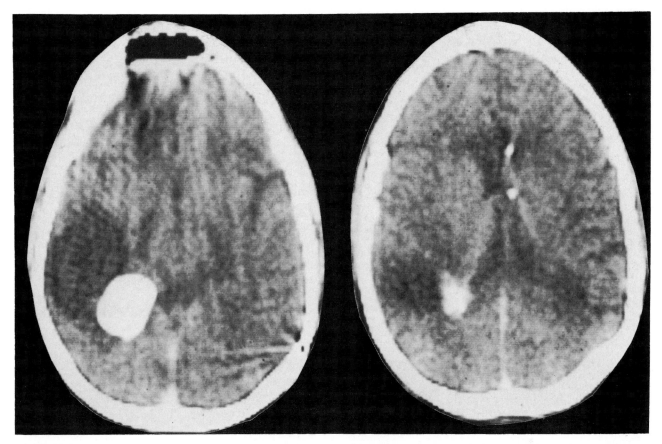

Figure 8-33 Choroid plexus papilloma in a 12-year-old. A large calcified, enhancing mass representing a benign papilloma involving the glomus of the left lateral ventricle. Hydrocephalus controlled by ventricular shunting. Note entrapment of the ipsilateral temporal horn with dilatation.

perdense mass (Fig. 8-34). Intense enhancement on CECT is a common feature.

Since a parenchymal extension or component is common in choroid plexus carcinoma, it may have to be differentiated from other neoplasms such as ependymoma, glioblastoma, and meningioma or, rarely, vascular anomalies.

Glioblastomas and vascular anomalies within the ventricles are rare in children. It is not unusual for even an experienced neuropathologist to call this tumor ependymoma, since the choroid plexus is derived from ependymal cells. However, the CT and the angiographic characteristics are usually helpful in differentiating the two neoplasms.

The choroid plexus carcinoma is always associated with hydrocephalus, which extends distal to the location of the neoplasm. The tumor mass has frondlike projections, almost like a "ball of spaghetti," with areas of hypodensity within it, most often representing old focal hemorrhages or necrosis. These are highly vascular on angiography, although rarely the neoplasm can be avascular (Zimmerman 1979*b*).

Ependymoma

In children, ependymomas are most common in the posterior fossa but can arise from the walls of the

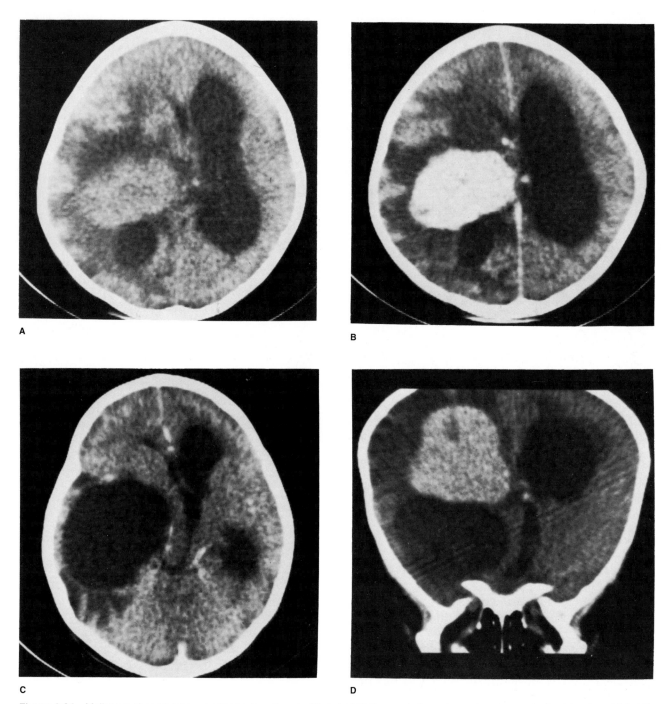

A

B

C

D

Figure 8-34 Malignant choroid plexus papilloma in a 2-year-old. Axial CT demonstrates a hyperdense mass in the lateral ventricle (**A**) with intense enhancement on CECT (**B**) associated with trapped temporal horn (**C**). **D.** Coronal CECT demonstrates the intraventricular as well as parenchymal extension of the neoplasm. The combination of communicating hydrocephalus and an enhancing intraventricular mass with parenchymal extension indicates a choroid plexus carcinoma. (*Continued on p. 403.*)

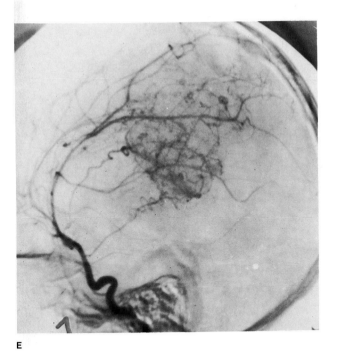

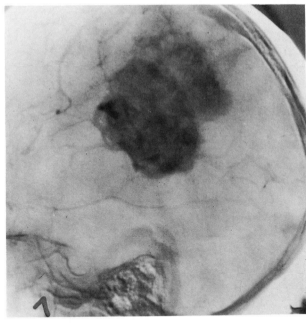

E   **F**

Figure 8-34 *(cont.)*   Arterial (**E**) and capillary (**F**) phases of the angiogram indicating the vascular feeders and intense tumor stain.

third and lateral ventricles and the adjacent white matter. Supratentorial ependymomas often arise from cell rests adjacent to or farther from the ventricular wall. They are common at sites where the ventricles are sharply angled, and posterior to the occipital horns (Swartz 1982). The trigone of the lateral ventricle appears to be a common site (Shuman 1975; Swartz 1982). In the few cases the author has seen, the ependymomas were located in the region of the foramen of Monro (Fig. 8-35). Supratentorial ependymoma is often seen in children or in young adults between the ages of 15 and 25 years.

On NCCT, the tumor is isodense or slightly hyperdense. Punctate calcification within the neoplasm is common, as is enhancement of the neoplasm following CECT. The enhancement, unlike that in choroid plexus carcinoma, is nonhomogeneous to homogeneous. When the tumor arises from the ependymal wall of the ventricles, obstructive hydrocephalus beyond it is common. Ependymoma can be differentiated from choroid plexus carcinoma by the CT characteristics and by angiography.

Ependymoblastoma is a malignant form of ependymal tumor in which the tumor grows rapidly; spread by meningeal seeding is common. The growth of the tumor can be so rapid as to involve the whole ventricular system, almost forming a cast of the ventricle (Fig. 8-36). Although a histological diagnosis cannot be made by CT, this CT finding is associated with a high mortality.

Hamartomas of tuberous sclerosis or other heterotopias along the ependymal surface do not enhance unless malignant transformation takes place.

Subependymal Giant Cell Astrocytoma

This neoplasm is most often seen in children with tuberous sclerosis. It is due to malignant transformation of hamartoma. The astrocytoma is most often located in the region of the foramen of Monro (Fig. 8-37). On NCCT, other hamartomas may be noted along the ependymal wall of the ventricles. Many subependymal, as well as parenchymal, hamartomas show calcification. In the presence of these

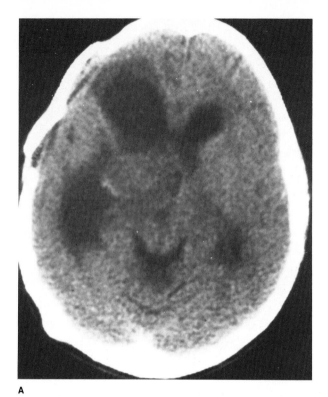

A

Figure 8-35 Ependymoma. (**A**) NCCT demonstrates a large hypodense mass with calcific densities within the mass causing ipsi-

B

lateral obstructive hydrocephalus. **B.** CECT shows intense enhancement of the tumor.

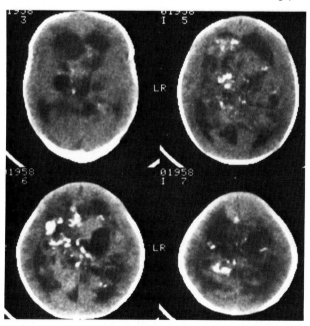

A

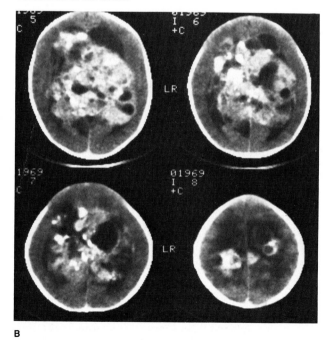

B

Figure 8-36 Ependymoblastoma. **A.** NCCT serial sections (4) demonstrates a large bulky tumor located within the ventricle, with regions of hyperdensity as well as calcifications. **B.** CECT of similar four sections demonstrating intensely enhancing tumor with cystic or necrotic component.

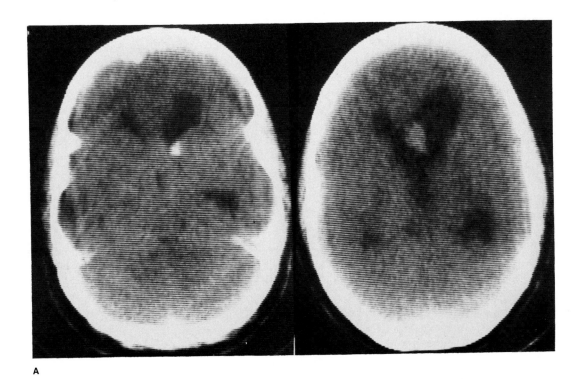

A

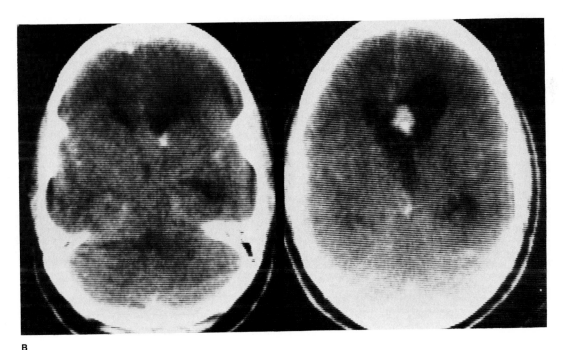

B

Figure 8-37   Subependymal giant cell astrocytoma.   **A.** NCCT shows a soft-tissue mass in the region of the foramen of Monro, with calcification of the ependymal hamartoma.   **B.** CECT shows the enhancing tumor causing unilateral obstruction of the left lateral ventricle.

findings, the CT diagnosis is specific for this neoplasm.

Parenchymal Tumors

Astrocytoma

Astrocytoma is the most common primary neoplasm in the pediatric age group as it is in the adult population. Among the pediatric age group, supratentorial astrocytomas are more common in older children. Unlike astrocytomas in the posterior fossa, which are usually cystic and carry a better prognosis, the supratentorial astrocytomas behave as in adults. The CT findings are also similar to those in the adult population. Low-grade astrocytomas (grades I and II) appear hypodense or isodense and may not show significant enhancement on CECT. They may also appear as cystic tumors on CT even though they may be solid at surgery (Fig. 8-38).

Higher-grade astrocytomas (grades III and IV) will show either homogeneous enhancement or a ring pattern and are often associated with peritumoral edema. When the glioma has the appearance of a ring with a smooth outer and inner wall, which may happen occasionally, differentiation from an abscess may be difficult. Most often a nodular component or an irregular, shaggy inner wall is seen in gliomas (Fig. 8-39). The other CT features are similar to those described for adults (Chapter 7).

Primitive Neuoroectodermal Tumors

Primary cerebral neuroblastoma along with cerebral medulloblastoma and undifferentiated glioma have all similar histological characteristics and were grouped together as primitive neuroectodermal tumors by Hart and Earl (1973). They are relatively rare tumors. The tumor has a slight male preponderance, and from the reported series (Altman 1985; Ganti 1983) is more commonly seen in the age range

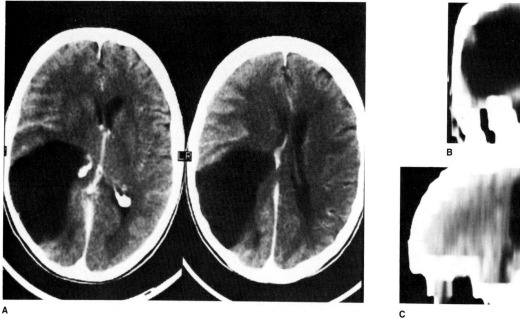

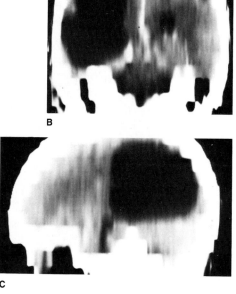

Figure 8-38 Low-grade astrocytoma. CECT (**A**) axial, (**B**) reformatted coronal, and (**C**) sagittal views. A large hypodense lesion with minimal edema and mass effect is seen. Condidered to be a porencephalic cyst and turned out to be a solid low-grade astrocytoma.

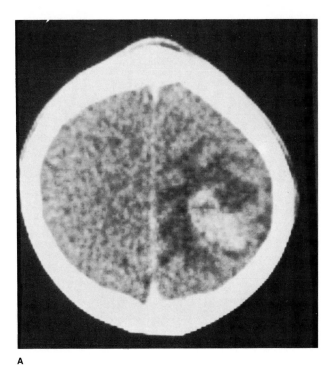

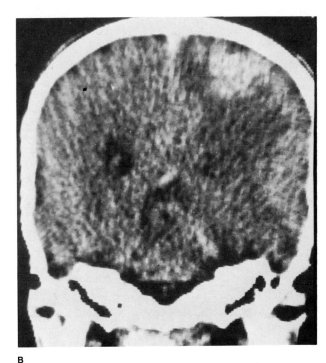

A   B

Figure 8-39 Glioblastoma in 4-year-old. Postcontrast axial CT (**A**) and coronal CT (**B**) in high-grade astrocytoma. Note the volume of edema relative to the tumor volume and the intense enhancement of the neoplasm.

of 3 to 6 years. This is unlike the female preponderance associated with primary cerebral neuroblastomas (Zimmerman 1980a; Chambers 1981). Although the tumor may involve any region of the cerebrum, there is a greater predilection for the frontal lobes. By the time clinical and radiological diagnosis is established, due probably to its location in the frontal lobes, the tumor is large and bulky. They are typically iso- or hypodense on the NCCT. Calcification may be discrete throughout the tumor or may be in clumps. CECT demonstrates heterogeneous intense enhancement with hypodense regions most likely representing cystic or necrotic components (Fig. 8-40). Minimal surrounding edema is almost always seen. Unlike in the past with appropriate treatment presently longer survival periods have been documented (Altman 1985).

The above-described CT findings are helpful in differentiating this tumor from astrocytoma either benign or malignant. When all of the above features are present in a young patient the diagnosis of primitive neuroectodermal tumor should be strongly considered.

Ganglioglioma

Gangliogliomas are relatively benign parenchymal neoplasms most commonly encountered in the younger age group; 60 percent of the tumors have been reported in persons under the age of 30 years (Russell 1977).

The tumor consists of mature ganglion cells and glial tissue. Depending on the predominant cell type, the tumor has been classified as ganglioglioma (astrocytes predominant) or ganglioneuroma (ganglion cells predominant). In the series reported by Zimmerman (1979a), gangliogliomas constituted 14 percent of supratentorial tumors in the pediatric age group. The neoplasm is most common in the cerebral parenchyma, often in the region of the anterior

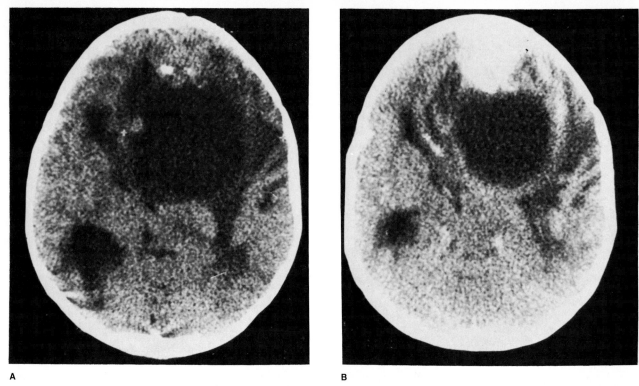

A   **B**

Figure 8-40 Neuroblastoma. **A.** A large, low-density mass with regions of different degrees of hyperdensity representing calcification is present on NCCT. **B.** CECT shows marked enhancement of the hyperdense component of the tumor, demarcating its cystic from its solid component.

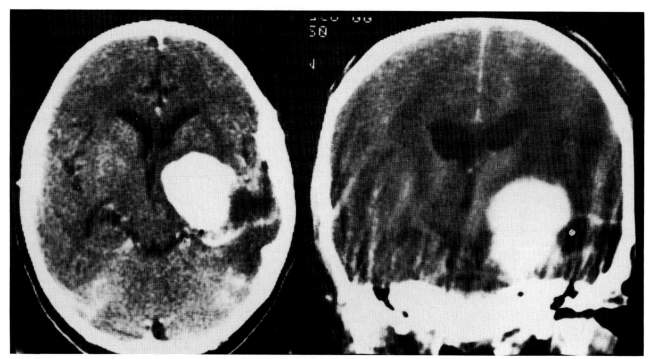

Figure 8-41 Ganglioglioma. Axial (left) and coronal (right) CECT images of a 9-year-old girl. The homogeneous enhancement with minimal surrounding edema is unusual for this tumor. Its location may suggest a meningioma.

third ventricle. It is usually solid, although cyst formation and calcification within it are not uncommon. The tumor appears on CT as an isodense mass with some enhancement (Fig. 8-41). Punctate calcifications within the tumor are often seen (Dome 1986; see also Chapter 7).

Bibliography

ALBERT A, LEE BCP, SAINT-LOUIS L, DECK MDF: MRI of optic chiasm and optic pathways. *Am J Neuroradiol* **7**:255–258, 1986.

ALTMAN N, FITZ CR, CHUANG S et al: Radiologic characteristics of primitive neuroectodermal tumors in children. *Am J Neuroradiol* **6**:15–18, 1985.

ANDERSON FM, SEGALL HD, CATON WL: Use of computerized tomography scanning in supratentorial arachnoid cyst. *J Neurosurg* **50**:33, 1979.

BYRD SE, HARWOOD-NASH DC, FITZ CR, BARRY JF, ROGOVITZ DM: Two projection computed tomography: Axial and Towne projection. *Radiology* **128**:512, 1978.

CHAMBERS EF, TURSKI PA, SOBEL D, WASA W, NEWTON TH: Radiologic characteristics of primary cerebral neuroblastomas. *Radiology* **139**:101–106, 1981.

COIN CG, COIN JW, GLOVER MB: Vascular tumors of the choroid plexus: Diagnosis by computed tomography. *J Comput Assist Tomogr* **1**:146–148, 1977.

DORNE HL, O'GORMAN AM, MELANSON D: Computed tomography of intracranial gangliogliomas. *Am J Neuroradiol* **7**:281–285, 1986.

EISENBERG HM, SARWAR M, SCHOCHET S: Symptomatic Rathke's cleft cysts. *J Neurosurg* **45**:585–588, 1976.

FITZ CR, HARWOOD-NASH DC, CHUANG SH, RESJO IM: The clival-perpendicular or modified Waters' view in computed tomography. *Neuroradiology* **16**:15–16, 1978a.

FITZ CR, WORTZMAN G, HARWOOD-NASH DC, HOLGATE RC, BARRY JF, BOLDT DW: Computed tomography in craniopharyngioma. *Radiology* **127**:687–691, 1978b.

FUTRELL NN, OSBORNE AG, CHESON BD: Pineal region of tumors: CT—pathological spectrum. *Am J Neuroradiol* **2**:415–420, 1981.

GANTI SR, SILVER AJ, DIEFENBACH P et al: Computed tomography of primitive neuroectodermal tumors. *Am J Neuroradiol* **4**:819–822, 1983.

GANTI SR, HILAL SK, STEIN BM et al: CT of pineal region tumors. *Am J Neuroradiol* **7**:97–104, 1986.

GENTRY LR, SMOKER WRK, TURSKI PA et al: Suprasellar arachnoid cysts; 1. C.T. recognition. *Am J Neuroradiol* **7**:79–86, 1986.

GOI A: Cerebellar astrocytomas in childhood. *Am J Dis Child* **106**:21–24, 1963.

GOSHHAJRA K, BHAGAI-NAINI P, HAHN HS: Spontaneous rupture of a pineal teratoma. *Neuroradiology* **17**:215–217, 1979.

HART MN, EARLE KM: Primitive neuroectodermal tumors of the brain in children. *Cancer* **32**:890–897, 1973.

HARWOOD-NASH DC, FITZ CR: *Neuroradiology in Infants and Children.* St. Louis, The C.V. Mosby Company, 1976.

HAYMAN LA, EVANS RA, HINCK VC: Choroid plexus of the fourth ventricle: Useful CT landmark. *Am J Roentgenol* **133**:285–290, 1979.

HERNANZ-SHULMAN M, WELCH K, STRAND R, ORDIA JI: Acoustic neuromas in children. *Am J Neuroradiol* **7**:519–521, 1986.

HORTON BC, RUBENSTEIN LC: Primary cerebral neuroblastoma: Clinicopathological study in 35 cases. *Brain* **99**:735–756, 1976.

JACOBY CG, GO RT, BERAN RA: Cranial CT of neurofibromatosis. *Am J Neuroradiol* **1**:311–315, 1980.

KINGSLEY D, KENDALL BE: Dependent layering of contrast medium in cystic astrocytomas. *Neuroradiology* **14**:107–110, 1977.

KISHORE PRS, RAO KCVG, WILLIAMS JP, VINES FS: The limitations of computerized tomographic diagnosis of intracranial midline cysts. *Surg Neurol* **14**:417–431, 1980.

KOKORIS N, ROTHMAN LM, WOLINTZ AH: CT and angiography in the diagnosis of suprasellar mass lesions. *Am J Ophthalmol* **89**:278–283, 1980.

KUCHARCZYK W, BRANT-ZWADZKI M, SOBEL DF et al: Central nervous system tumors in children: detection by magnetic resonance imaging. *Radiology* **155**:131–136, 1985.

LEE BCP: Intracranial cysts. *Radiology* **130**:667–674, 1979.

LEE BCP, KNEELAND JB, WALKER RW et al: MR imaging of brainstem tumors. *AJNR:* **6**:159–163, 1985.

LEO JS, PINTO RS, HULVAT GF, EPSTEIN F, KRICHEFF II: Computed tomography of arachnoid cysts. *Radiology* **130**:675–680, 1979.

LIN SR, BRYSON MM, GOBIEN RP, FITZ CR, LEE YY: Radiologic findings of hamartomas of the tuber cinereum and hypothalamus. *Radiology* **127**:697–703, 1978.

LIPPER MH, RAD FF, KISHORE PRS, WARD JD: Craniopharyngioma: Unusual computed tomographic presentation. *Neurosurgery* **9**:76–78, 1981.

MCCORMACK TJ, PLASSCHE WM, LIN SR: Ruptured teratoid tumor in the pineal region. *J Comput Assist Tomogr* **2**:499–501, 1978.

MESSINA AV, POTTS DG, SIGEL RM: Computed tomography evaluation of the posterior third ventricle. *Radiology* **119**:581–592, 1978.

MILLER JH, PENA AM, SEGALL HD: Radiological investigation of sellar region masses in children. *Radiology* **134**:81, 1980.

MORI K, HANDA H, TAKEUCHI J, HARAKITA J, NAKANO Y: Hypothalamic hamartoma. *J Comput Assist Tomogr* **5**:519–521, 1981.

NAIDICH TP: Infratentorial masses, in Norman D, Korobkin M, Newton T (eds): *Computed Tomography.* St. Louis, The C.V. Mosby Company, 1977a, pp. 231–242.

NAIDICH TP, LIN JP, LEEDS NP, PUDLOWSKI RM, NAIDICH JB: Primary tumors and other masses of the cerebellum and fourth ventricle: Differential diagnosis by computed tomography. *Neuroradiology* **14**:153–174, 1977b.

NAIDICH TP, PINTO RS, KUSHNER MJ, LIN JP, KRICHEFF II, LEEDS NE, CHASE NE: Evaluation of sellar and parasellar masses by computed tomography. *Radiology* **120**:91, 1976.

NORTH C, SEGALL HD, STANLEY P: Early CT detection of intracranial seeding from medulloblastoma. *Am J Neuroradiology* **6**:11–13, 1985.

OSBORN AG, DAINES JH, WING SK: The evaluation of ependymal and subependymal lesions by cranial computed tomography. *Radiology* **127**:397–401, 1978.

PETERMAN SB, STEINER RE, BYDDER GM: Magnetic resonance imaging of intracranial tumors in children and adolescents. *Am J Neuroradiol* **5**:703–709, 1984.

PROBST FP, LILIEQUIST: Assessment of posterior fossa tumors in infants and children by means of computed tomography. *Neuroradiology* **18**:9–18, 1979.

RAO KCVG, GOVINDAN S: Intracranial choriocarcinoma. *J Comput Assist Tomogr* **3**:400–404, 1979.

RAO KCVG, HARWOOD-NASH DC, FITZ CR: Neurodiagnostic studies in craniopharyngiomas in children. *Rev Interam Radiol* **2**:149–159, 1977.

REICH NE, ZELCH JV, ALFIDI RJ: Computed tomography in the detection of juxtasellar lesions. *Radiology* **118**:333–335, 1976.

RICHMOND IL, WILSON CB: Pituitary disorders in childhood and adoelscence. *J Neurosurg* **49**:163–168, 1978.

RUBENSTEIN I: Tumors of the central nervous system. *Atlas of Tumor Pathology,* 2nd series. Washington DC. AFIP, 269–384, 1970.

RUSH JL, KUSSKE JA, DEFOE DR, PRIBRAM HW: Intraventricular craniopharyngioma. *Neurology* **25**:1094–1096, 1975.

RUSSELL DS, RUBINSTEIN LJ: *Pathology of Tumors of the Nervous System,* 4th ed. Baltimore, Williams & Wilkins, 1977.

SAVOIARDO M, HARWOOD-NASH DC, TADMORE R, SCOTTI G, MUSGRAVE M: Gliomas of the intracranial anterior optic pathways in children: the role of computed tomography, angiography, pneumoencephalography and radionuclide brain scanning. *Radiology* **138**:601–610, 1981.

SCHULLER DE, LAWRENCE TL, NEWTON WA: Childhood rhabdomyosarcomas of the head and neck. *Arch Otolaryngol* **105**:689–694, 1979.

SCOTTI D, HARWOOD-NASH DC: Computed tomography of rhabdomyosarcomas of the skull base in children. *J Comput Asst Tomgr* **6**:33–39, 1982.

SHUMAN RM, ALVORD EC JR, LEECH RW: The biology of childhood ependymomas. *Arch Neurol* **32**:731–739, 1975.

STANLEY P, SENAC MO JR, SEGALL HD: Intraspinal seeding from intracranial tumors in children. *Am J Neuroradiol* **5**:805–809, 1984.

STRAND RD, BAKER RA, IDAHOSA JO, ARKINS TJ: Metrizamide ventriculography and computed tomography in lesions about the third ventricle. *Radiology* **128**:405–410, 1978.

SWARTZ JD, ZIMMERMAN RA, BILANIUK LT: Computed tomography of intracranial ependymomas. *Radiology* **143**:97–101, 1982.

TADMOR R, HARWOOD-NASH DC, SAVOIARDO M, SCOTTI G, MUSGRAVE M, FITZ CR, CHUANG S: Brain tumors in the first two years of life: CT diagnosis. *Am J Neuroradiol* **1**:411–418, 1980.

TAKEUCHI J, HANDA H, OTSUKA S: Neuroradiological aspects of suprasellar germinomas. *Neuroradiology* **17**:153–159, 1979.

TERA H, HORI T, MATSUTANI M, OKEDA R: Detection of cryptic vascular malformations by computed tomography. *J Neurosurg* **51**:546–551, 1979.

VOLBE BT, FOLEY KM, HOWIESON J: Normal CAT scan in craniopharyngioma. *Ann Neurol* **3**:87, 1978.

WHITE TJ, SIEGLE RL, BURCKART GJ, RAMEY DR: Rectal thiopental for sedation of children for computed tomography. *J Comput Assist Tomogr* **3**:286–288, 1979.

WILSON CB: Diagnosis and surgical treatment of childhood brain tumors. *Cancer* **35** (suppl):950–956, 1975.

WOODROW PK, GAJARAWALA J, PINCK RL: Coputed tomographic documentation of a non-enhancing posterior fossa medulloblastoma: An uncommon presentation. *CT: J Comput Tomogr* **5**:41–43, 1981.

ZIMMERMAN RA, BILANIUK LT, PAHLAJANI H: Spectrum of medulloblastomas as demonstrated by computed tomography. *Radiology* **126**:137–147, 1977.

ZIMMERMAN RA, BILANIUK LT, BRUNO L, ROSENSTOCK J: Computed tomography of cerebellar astrocytoma. *Am J Roentgenol* **130**:929–933, 1978a.

ZIMMERMAN RA, BILANIUK LT, RAMEY RB, LITTMAN P: Computed tomography of pediatric craniofacial sarcoma. *CT: J Comput Toogr* **2**:113–121, 1978*b*.

ZIMMERMAN RA, BILANIUK LT: Computed tomography of intracerebral gangliogliomas. *CT: J Comput Tomogr* **3**:24–30, 1979*a*.

ZIMMERMAN RA, BILANIUK LT: Computed tomography of choroid plexus lesions. *CT: J Comput Tomogr* **3**:93–103, 1979*b*.

ZIMMERMAN RA, BILANIUK LT: CT of primary and secondary craniocerebral neuroblastoma. *Am J Neuroradiol* **1**:431–434, 1980*a*.

ZIMMERMAN RA, BILANIUK LT, WOOD JH, BRUCE DA, SCHULTZ A: Computed tomography of pineal, parapineal and histologically related tumors. *Radiology* **137**:669–677, 1980*b*.

ZIMMERMAN RD, RUSSELL EJ, LEEDS NE: Axial CT recognition of anteroposterior displacement of fourth ventricle. *Am J Neuroradiol* **1**:65–70, 1980.

9

INTRACRANIAL TUMORS: METASTATIC

Krishna C.V.G. Rao

J. Powell Williams

AN OVERVIEW

Cancer is the second-leading cause of death in the United States, with 690,000 new cases a year and over 1000 deaths a day (Silverberg 1977). Extensive amounts of money are spent in the detection, palliation, and cure of cancer. Twenty percent of patients who die of systemic cancer harbor intracranial metastases (Posner 1978; Aronson 1964). These figures suggest that more patients present with intracranial metastatic disease than primary glioma, although in clinical practice, metastatic disease, when compared with all brain tumors, as reported in different series (Black 1979; VanEck 1965), constitutes only 7 to 17 percent of the brain tumors seen. This probably reflects selection of clinical material in the different series. In a recent National Cancer Institute study (Baker 1980; Potts 1980) dealing with an evaluation of CT in the diagnosis of intracranial neoplasms, metastatic brain disease accounted for nearly 31 percent (343/1071 patients) of the intracranial lesions by CT.

An important feature of CT in the diagnosis of intracranial metastases is its ability to detect small metastatic foci, especially with the present high-resolution, thin-section CT. To a certain degree the myth of the high incidence of solitary metastases seen in clinical practice as opposed to pathological studies is being resolved by better scanner resolution. Even with the sensitivity of present-generation scanners, a fair number of metastases less than 5 mm in diameter, especially in certain areas of the brain parenchyma, may remain undetected.

Cranial CT plays an important role in the detection of intracranial metastases in patients with extracranial sites of cancer presenting with neurological findings. Because of their location or size presence of asymptomatic or occult intracranial metastases is not uncommon. CT detection of occult or "silent" metastases has been extensively reported (Butler 1979; Jennings 1980; Johnson 1982; Potts 1980), their incidence ranging from 2.8 percent (Johnson 1982) to 21 percent (Jennings 1980). Pretreatment cranial CT thus probably may have an important role in the management of the patient with cancer and overall health care cost.

Metastases to the cranial vault and intracranial contents can occur from any primary source (Table 9-1). The most common primary sites or types with metastases to the brain, in order of frequency, are lung, breast, kidney, and melanoma. Less common are metastases from the gastrointestinal tract (predominantly the colon), thyroid, ovary, and prostate (Ranshoff 1975), and rarely from the pancreas and from sarcomas. In a few series nearly 50 percent of the patients presented with CNS findings as the first manifestation of their malignancy (VanEck 1965; Simionescue 1960; Vieth 1965). However, most patients with intracranial metastases have known primary sites of cancer. This information is extremely helpful in the CT diagnosis. From our experience nearly 14 percent of the metastases detected by CT presented with neurological symptoms as the presenting clinical manifestation without a known primary site of cancer. The probable histologic type was suggested from the CT study and subsequently confirmed by other diagnostic studies. In 4 percent the primary source was not found after extensive diagnostic work-up of the patient, but the histologic type of the metastatic lesion was confirmed by biopsy of the intracranial lesion. Metastases may involve the cranial vault as well as the intracranial contents. Parenchymal metastases, apart from the calvarium and leptomeningeal carcinomatosis, may be solitary or multiple.

The incidence of solitary metastasis detected by various diagnostic modalities is reported to be between 50 and 55 percent (Black 1979; Walker 1973), although in autopsy series the incidence is between 25 and 40 percent (Walker 1973; Posner 1978). The overall incidence of solitary metastasis on the basis of CT studies was 43 percent (Table 9-2). A subsequent analysis of metastatic intracranial deposits utilizing high-resolution CT demonstrated a lower incidence of solitary metastatic deposits, 38 percent. These findings suggest that with improvement in technology and utilization of adequate amounts of contrast (Hayman 1980), the incidence of solitary metastasis will be closer to the results of pathological studies.

Table 9-1   Primary Origin of Intracranial Metastatic Tumors

Organ System	University of Maryland series	Posner's series (1980)	Paiella's series (1976)	National Cancer Institute Study (1980)
Lungs	156	61	55	129
Breast	69	33	26	44
Digestive tract	16	6	16	14
Kidney	8	11	14	4
Bladder	3	—	1	—
Genital tract	6	3	7	—
Skin and mucous membrane	1	0	4	—
Thyroid	2	0	1	—
Other	—	57	45	24
Unknown primary	—	—	—	37
Multiple primary	—	—	—	7

Table 9-2   Frequency of Solitary versus Multiple Intracranial Metastasis

	Solitary, %	Multiple, %
University of Maryland*	38	62
Posner (1980) 225 patients	47	53
Chason (1963) Autopsy series	14	86

* Based on CT-pathological correlation.

CLINICAL AND
PATHOLOGICAL FINDINGS

The clinical presentation in the majority of intracranial metastatic brain tumors is due to the mass effect. These include headache, nausea, vomiting, ataxia, and papilledema (Russcalleda 1978). These manifestations are due to metastatic foci, either single or multiple in the brain parenchyma, leptomeninges, or adjacent calvarium. Occasionally, the clinical presentation will be acute in onset like that of a patient with an infarct or intracerebral hemorrhage. In these patients, a careful history usually reveals episodes of headaches and transient neurological changes prior to the acute episode. Rarely, patients with intracranial metastases may present with a finding of dementia. Absence of focal neurological findings may be as high as 5 to 12 percent (Butler 1979; Jacobs 1977). Although intracranial metastases may occur in any age group, their highest incidence is between the fourth and seventh decade (Vieth 1965). Intracranial metastases, although less common, can also be seen in children. In one large series, postmortem studies demonstrated an incidence of 6 percent in 273 children (Vannucci 1974).

Brain metastases are often circumscribed. Central necrosis is fairly common. A few of them may have discernible calcification (Potts 1964). Parenchymal metastases are most often seen at the junction of the gray and white matter. Edema forms a significant component of the mass seen, even with small metastases. There have been very few reports dealing with the ultrastructural alteration in the brain parenchyma secondary to intracranial metastases, although absence of the tight junctions in the blood vessels of the tumor has been noted (Hirano 1972; Long 1970). Suffice it to say that the vascular architecture within the metastatic deposit is often similar to the cellular-vascular architecture in the primary cancer. Ultrastructural alteration in the form of fenestrated vessels has been reported with metastatic hypernephroma (Hirano 1975; Hirano 1972). Similar changes probably occur in other types of metastases, although no detailed analysis of the vascular anatomy in different types of cerebral metas-

tases is available. The presence of the metastatic deposit within the brain parenchyma probably causes an alteration in the blood-brain barrier associated with varying degrees of edema, as manifested by enhancement on CT scan. The different amounts of edema with different cell types of tumor probably reflect a specific tissue response. The edema seen on CT in different types of intracranial metastases, in association with the enhancement pattern, may thus help indicate the histological cell type.

In our series of 482 metastases detected on CT where histological proof was available in 294 cases (Tables 9-3, 9-4), metastatic tumors which were relatively less vascular demonstrated the maximum amount of edema. This was further confirmed in proven intracranial metastases from different cell types of lung carcinomas. Analysis of the amount of edema on CT shows that usually adenocarcinoma has the maximum surrounding edema, with oat cell carcinoma next and squamous cell carcinoma having the least edema. It has also been noted that edema may increase dramatically coincident with central necrosis in a tumor. The tumors with the poorest blood supply are probably earliest to develop central necrosis. Potts et al. (1980), however, in their anal-

Table 9-3 Frequency of Pathological Confirmation of Source of Intracranial Metastases

Site of tissue	No. of cases	Adeno-	Oat-cell	Squa-mous	Mela-noma	Other
Primary + intracranial	98	38	23	21	8	12
Primary only	182	67	36	36	24	15*
Intracranial only	14	4	3	3	1	3†
TOTAL	294	109	62	60	33	30

Source: Rao 1979.
* Based on 294 of the 482 cases for which pathological confirmation was available from either surgical specimen or autopsy.
† The 15 patients in this category included patients with metastatic tumors which did not fall in the above histological group. Three patients had bladder cancer, three renal cell carcinoma, two thyroid metastasis and one squamous cell carcinoma.
‡ The three patients in this group included two with multicentric glioma and one with coccidioidomycosis.

Table 9-4   Cellular Differentiation from the Various Organs*

Site (or type)	No. of cases	Adeno-	Oat-cell	Squa-mous	Undiffer-entiated
Lungs	156	55	58	37	6
Breast	69	47	—	14	8
Melanoma	33	—	—	—	—
Digestive tract	16	9	—	—	7
Kidney	8	3	—	—	5
Genitourinary tract	3	—	—	—	—
Reproductive system	6	3	—	—	3
Thyroid	2	—	—	—	2
Skin	1	—	—	—	1

* Based on 294 proved cases in authors' series. Categorization was done on the basis of maximum cell population.

ysis of metastatic tumors, did not find this to be a useful feature in analysis of different types of metastases.

THE ROLE OF NEURODIAGNOSTIC STUDY

The detection of intracranial metastases as well as their management has been revolutionized by the availability of CT. There has been a dramatic decrease in the demand for other diagnostic modalities except in unusual circumstances (Table 9-5). *Plain skull views* in metastatic work-up are indicated only when there is suspicion of calvarial metastases on CT, to demonstrate the location of the lesion visualized by CT as well as to search for other smaller calvarial metastatic foci, particularly if they are osteoblastic.

Radionuclide brain scan is rarely indicated with the CT scanner resolution presently available. The complementary role of CT and radionuclide scanning had been the subject of a series of reports in the

Table 9-5   Frequency of Neurodiagnostic Studies—University of Maryland Hospital

Type of study	1975	1980	Change, %
Skull radiography (neuro-related)	740	323	− 56
Radionuclide brain scan	1590	236	− 84
Cerebral angiography	479	421	− 12
Pneumoencephalogram	87	2	− 97
Cranial computed tomogram	1953	5027	+ 257

early days of CT (Gawler 1974; Gado 1975; New 1975; Pendergrass 1975; Bradfield 1977; Fordham 1977). In these reports, although all agreed on the superiority of CT in detecting intracranial pathology, radionuclide scan was felt to be slightly superior to CT in the detection of metastases which were less than 1 cm in size located in the posterior fossa. Factors which decreased the sensitivity of CT studies in these early reports were related to the fixed matrix (80 × 80 or 160 × 160) and slice thickness available in the earlier CT scanner as well as the amount of contrast utilized in those studies. Comparative studies (Table

Table 9-6   Comparison of Radionuclide Brain Scan and Cranial CT

	CT/RN both +	CT + RN −	CT − RN +	CT − RN −
NCI study (Potts et al. 1980), 225 patients	174	43	1	7
Bradfield et al. (1977) 47 patients	44	44		
Pendergrass et al. (1975) 22 patients*	19	3		
Univ. of Maryland Hosp. series 187 patients†	161	23	1	2

* Only patients with metastases were used for comparison.
† Only patients who had both CT and radionuclide brain scans are included in this table.

9-6) made by different authors support the present role of CT as the primary modality of examination for intracranial neoplasms, including metastatic disease. Buell (1978) stated that CT was superior to radionuclide scanning in the detection of intracranial neoplasms: the detection rate (sensitivity) was 99 percent for CT and 91 percent for radionuclide brain scanning. In this series, it was also possible to correctly identify tumor type (specificity) in 76 percent of neoplasms by CT as against 69 percent by radionuclide scanning.

Radionuclide scanning probably has a place in the evaluation of patients who have a definite history of prior allergic reaction to intravenous contrast medium as well as a few patients in whom motion is a problem. In the majority of patients in this group MRI will eventually replace this study.

Cerebral angiography is rarely necessary for evaluation of intracranial parenchymal metastases, but there are some situations in which it is helpful. As an example, when a solitary hemorrhagic lesion is seen on noncontrast CT (NCCT) which appears to accentuate further on contrast-enhanced CT (CECT), in the absence of a known systemic cancer the lesion may be dificult to differentiate from other intracranial pathologic processes such as ruptured vascular malformation, primary intracranial glioma, or abscess. Cerebral angiography is also occasionally helpful in differentiating a primary glioma from a solitary metastasis, but more often it is performed to provide a map of the arteries and superficial veins relative to the neoplasm when surgery is contemplated.

Pneumoencephalography has no place in the evaluation of intracranial metastases.

Computed tomography is today most often the initial study performed when evaluating for intracranial metastases. With the improvement in technology, as well as use of increased amounts of contrast material, the detection rate of metastatic lesions by CT has improved significantly. Most centers have evolved various protocols for CT studies, with guidelines for contrast enhancement (Latchaw 1978*b*; Kramer 1975). The necessity of NCCT in evaluation of intracranial pathology has been the subject of a few reports (Butler 1978; Latchaw 1977). Elimination

of NCCT may result in decreasing the radiation dose to the patient. However, the authors believe that eliminating NCCT may cause the examiners to miss fresh hemorrhage or calcification of a tumor when masked by contrast enhancement. These findings can occasionally be of clinical importance. NCCT followed by CECT may help characterize the tumor histologically and provide the optimum mode of study in screening patients for metastases in the initial work-up. However, for practical purposes, procurement of CECT only in patients with a known primary tumor may suffice in the management of the patient. Occasionally, thin sections (2 to 5 mm) following a high dose of contrast are necessary to demonstrate multiplicity of metastatic lesions (Fig. 9-1), especially when the decision as to the treatment modality of both the primary and intracranial metastases depends on the CT findings.

CT DIAGNOSIS

Calvarial Metastases

The incidence of metastatic involvement of the cranial vault or base is approximately 5 percent (Willis 1973). Calvarial metastases may present as lytic or blastic lesions, although most commonly there is an admixture. The result may be expansion of the inner and outer table, causing compression of the brain parenchyma (Fig. 9-2). When the involvement is predominantly of the inner table, with extension over the surface of the dura or invasion through the dura, determination of a purely epidural or subdural component is difficult (Fig. 9-3). The most common primary cancers associated with calvarial or dural metastases, in the authors' experience as well as those reported in the literature (Naheedy 1980; Deck 1980), are those of the prostate, breast, lung, and kidney. The metastatic lesion may have a crescentic or biconvex appearance. The shape of the lesion is not helpful in distinguishing an epidural from a subdural metastasis (Fig. 9-4). Bony changes can be missed if CT is viewed with a narrow window set-

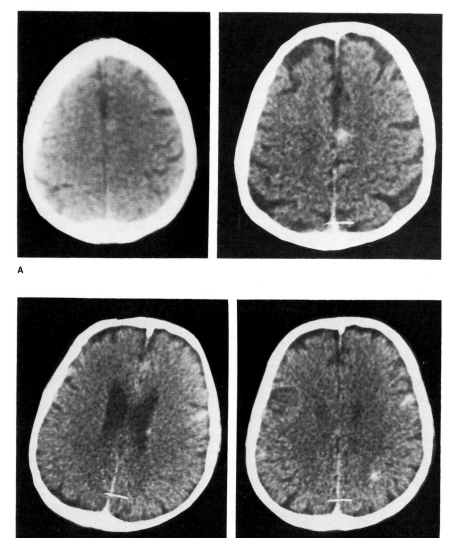

Figure 9-1 **A.** *Left:* Contrast-enhanced CT. Initial CT following 42 g iodine and using 13-mm section thickness demonstrates a single enhancing lesion. *Right:* Following 56 g iodine and using 5-mm section thickness, the enhancing lesion is well visualized. **B.** On this examination, other lesions are also present.

ting. To demonstrate the calvarial lesions, visualization at a very wide window setting is best (Fig. 9-5).

Lytic lesions, particularly in the region of the vertex, may be missed on CT, and coronal views are necessary for best evaluation. Becker (1978) determined that lesions less than 4 mm in diameter may not be detected by CT because of partial-volume averaging. However, with thinner sections and higher kVp this resolution can be improved. In metastatic involvement of the base of the skull, sella, and sphenoid sinus, CT in axial and coronal planes provides better demonstration of the destructive lesion than conventional radiographs (Fig. 9-6).

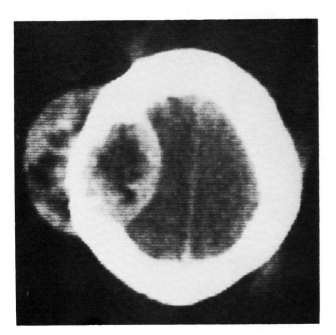

Figure 9-2 Metastases from renal carcinoma involving the calvarium, with expansion of the inner and outer table of the skull.

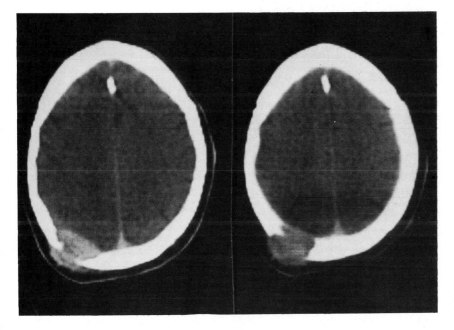

Figure 9-3 Metastases from adenocarcinoma of the kidney involving the calvarium, with epidural extension.

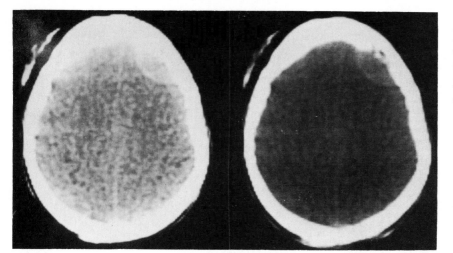

A

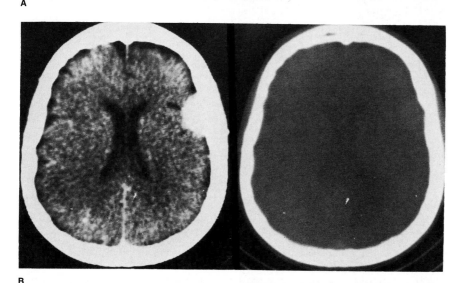

B

Figure 9-4 **A.** Epidural metastases from adenocarcinoma of the breast. The enhancing dura is well defined. At a wider window setting, the destructive process involving the calvarium is well defined. **B.** Another patient with subdural metastases. Lack of inner table involvement excludes epidural metastases.

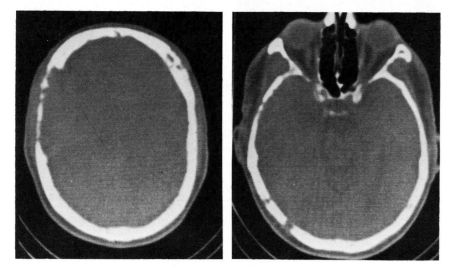

Figure 9-5 Axial CT in a patient with adenocarcinoma of the lung. Extensive calvarial involvement is visualized, with epidural extension.

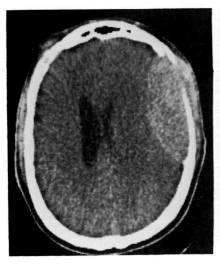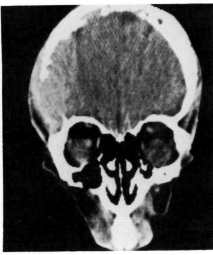

Figure 9-6 Axial and coronal CT are useful in demonstrating the total extent of the disease, as in this patient.

Epidural and Subdural Metastases

Fifteen percent of metastatic foci in the cranial vault or base of the skull extend into the epidural or subdural space (Naheedy 1980). Distinction of subdural or epidural extension from calvarial metastases by CT is difficult (Naheedy 1980; Chirathivat 1980). Subdural or epidural extension of calvarial metastases is diagnosed on the basis of an irregular, moth-eaten appearance of the inner table of the skull in association with a crescent-shaped adjacent lesion, which most often shows enhancement on CECT. Differentiation of subdural metastasis from a subdural hematoma may be difficult, especially in the absence of a known systemic primary cancer. Homogeneous enhancement of the lesion is, however, highly suggestive of subdural metastasis rather than subdural hematoma (Fig. 9-7).

Intracerebral Metastases

CT has revolutionized diagnostic accuracy in intracerebral metastatic disease. It permits an earlier evaluation of patients with primary systemic cancer, providing better localization and more accurate estimation of the number or extent of metastatic deposits, with the least amount of patient morbidity.

On NCCT, metastatic deposits are delineated by change in tissue density and by brain edema. The extent of brain edema is variable but commonly exceeds the tumor volume. Edema is commonly seen involving the white matter, with fingerlike projections into the gray matter, which tends to be spared (Fig. 9-8). The edema may be hemispherical and may be associated with only a single small enhancing lesion on CECT. At other times, when many metastatic deposits are present on CECT, the NCCT may appear completely normal (Fig. 9-9).

The metastatic deposits on NCCT may be hypodense, hyperdense, or similar in density to normal brain tissue. These appearances are related to a variety of factors such as cellular density, tumor neovascularity, and degree of necrosis. Metastases from lung, breast, kidney, and colon and those from lymphoma tend to be hypodense or isodense (Deck 1980). Metastatic lymphoma appears to be isodense or hyperdense. Hyperdensity on NCCT is commonly due to a dense cellular structure, and these metastases appear slightly denser than normal brain tissue but certainly less dense than when there is hemorrhage or calcification, either within or adjacent to the tumor.

It is not uncommon for hemorrhage to occur in metastases (Fig. 9-10), as in some primary gliomas of the brain; 3.7 percent of all gliomas show intra-

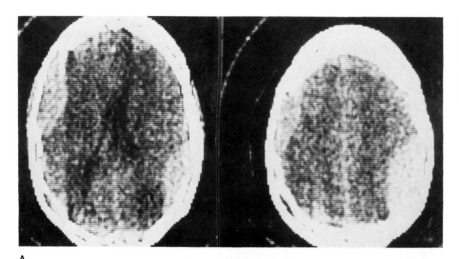

A

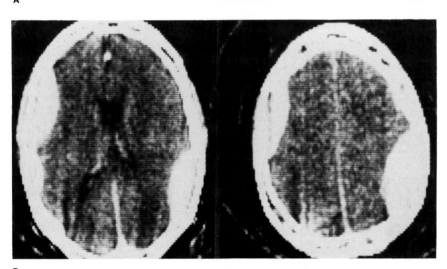

B

Figure 9-7 **(A)** Noncontrast and **(B)** contrast-enhanced CT in a patient with diffuse osteoblastic metastases and associated epidural metastases bilaterally mimicking subdural hematoma. Enhancement of the metastases differentiates them from hematoma.

tumoral or adjacent hematoma (Olderberg 1933). Although similar data are not available for intracerebral metastases, the detection rate by CT of hemorrhage within tumors, primary or metastatic, is probably high (Little 1979).

Among metastatic tumors, intratumoral hemorrhage is most commonly seen with melanoma and choriocarcinoma and less commonly with hypernephroma and lung carcinoma (Deck 1976; Gildersleeve 1977; Solis 1977; Mandybur 1977; Enzmann 1978*b*; Little 1979). A variety of factors have been

implicated to explain hemorrhage within metastatic tumors. Conditions such as hypertension, coagulopathy, and extreme tumor vascularity are predisposing factors. Chemotherapy and radiation therapy may also produce hemorrhage within tumors.

Hemorrhage may be associated with rapid increase in size of a metastatic focus or may be from adjacent damaged brain tissue (Mandybur 1977). Hemorrhage may be the first sign of a previously unsuspected metastatic tumor or other neoplasm (Weisberg 1977). Diagnosis of hemorrhage within a

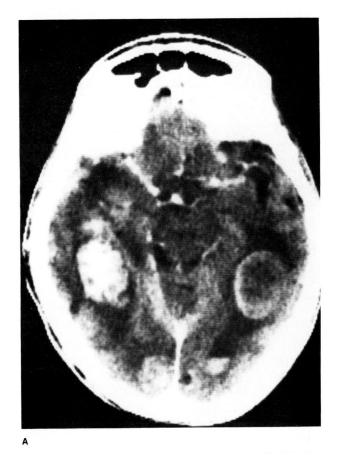

A

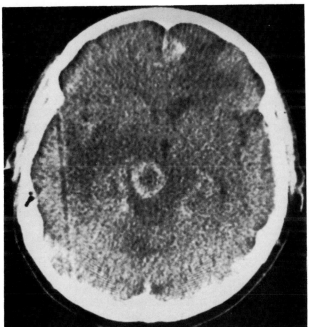

B

Figure 9-8 CECT Multiple mets from cancer of the colon. The enhancing lesions have multifaceted appearance. Some are solid enhancing, others with fluid level due to necrosis. There is also enhancement of the cistern due to meningeal involvement.

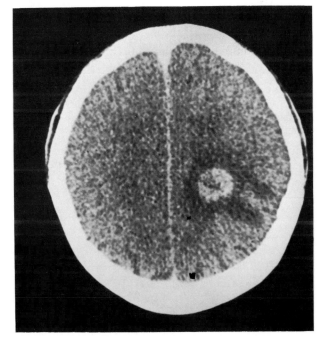

C

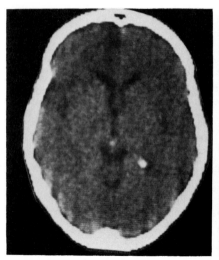
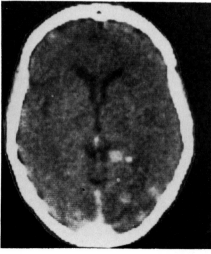

Figure 9-9 Multiple enhancing metastatic foci in an asymptomatic patient with breast carcinoma. The NCCT is normal. Other lesions were also noted at higher levels.

metastatic tumor by CT depends on the time interval between the episode and CT examination, as well as other factors such as location of the hematoma and amount of surrounding edema. Contrast enhancement may or may not be helpful, since hemorrhagic infarcts, unlike solid hematomas, may demonstrate some degree of enhancement, like a neoplasm with hemorrhage. Contrast enhancement may obscure hemorrhage or calcification in tumors, and a preliminary unenhanced scan is important in the diagnosis.

Unlike hemorrhage, calcification within a metastatic tumor is rare, except in metastatic osteogenic sarcoma (Danziger 1979). Although prior to availability of CT, the incidence of calcification within brain metastases was between 5 and 6 percent (Potts 1964), presently utilizing CT their incidence appears to be higher (Anand 1982). The calcification on CT may be punctate, curvilinear, or amorphous. Most often the calcifications tend to be in the necrotic portions of the metastases. Occasionally when such metastases are found adjacent to the calvarium or

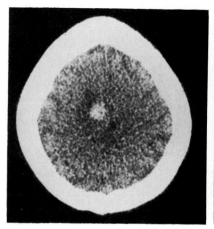
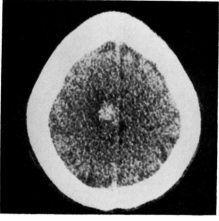

Figure 9-10 Hemorrhage within metastatic foci. Minimal change in density on CECT in a patient with a solitary metastatic melanoma.

the base of the skull but within the parenchyma and the rest of the tumor enhances, differentiation from a meningioma may be difficult.

ENHANCEMENT PATTERN IN METASTASES

Contrast enhancement of metastatic tumors, as in other enhancing lesions, is presumed to be due to the tumor vascularity and blood-brain or blood-tumor barrier defects (Lewander 1978). Most metastatic neoplasms demonstrate enhancement, although the degree of enhancement is variable. In a study in which both CT and radionuclide scans were performed, only one metastatic neoplasm failed to enhance on CT (Bradfield 1977). The degree of enhancement depends on such factors as the initial density of the lesion (on NCCT), the volume of contrast material administered, the elapsed time between contrast infusion and CT study, and the influence of therapeutic drugs, mainly steroids, although radiation and chemotherapy may both cause changes in density and enhancement characteristics. Apart from these general factors, the degree of enhancement in different metastatic tumors depends also on the cellular structure and vascularity.

Intracranial metastasis from choriocarcinoma, melanoma, thyroid tumors, and occasionally hypernephroma demonstrates the maximum degree of enhancement. This probably is related to the highly vascular nature of the metastasis. Although enhancement in metastatic melanoma has been reported in 82 percent of lesions (Enzmann 1978*b*), others have reported low incidence of enhancement of melanoma metastases (Deck 1980; Solis 1977).

Metastatic foci which are relatively denser on NCCT enhance less on CECT than lesions which are hypodense on NCCT (Hilal 1978). In our own experience squamous cell metastases which are relatively denser on NCCT demonstrate the least degree of enhancement; in increasing order of enhancement come adenocarcinoma, oat-cell carcinoma, melanoma, and choriocarcinoma. Similar findings based on time/density curves have also been shown by others (Wing 1980) (Fig. 9-11). The pattern of enhancement is nonspecific, appearing as ring enhancement or as solid density. Purely gyral enhancement, as seen in infarction or occasionally infiltrating gliomas, is rarely seen with metastases.

Metastatic lesions in general have a relatively larger low-density area, probably representing edema, when compared with the size of the enhancing component. Presence of multiple enhancing lesions is highly suggestive of metastatic

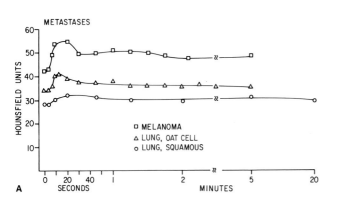

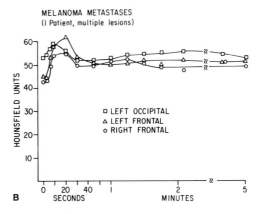

Figure 9-11   A. Time curves of density numbers in three different types of intracranial metastasis. Apart from the initial phase, no change in density is seen with increase in time. The curves also demonstrate the difference in density numbers between the different types of metastasis.   **B.** Time/density curve in multiple melanoma. No changes seen in the curves in spite of the different size and location of the melanoma deposits. (*Courtesy of Dr. S. D. Wing, University of Utah.*)

disease in a patient known to have extracranial primary cancer. However, in the presence of multiple enhancing lesions and absence of a known primary cancer, multicentric or multifocal glioma (Fig. 9-12), as well as abscesses and rarely meningioma should be considered (Rao 1980).

Histological specificity has been attempted, utilizing the commonly seen denominators such as degree of enhancement, relative volume of edema in relation to the enhancing lesion, and density of the lesion on NCCT (Rao 1979). The following features were noted in metastases of different histologic type:

1. In metastatic melanoma (Fig. 9-13), the lesions were denser than the adjacent parenchyma, with minimal edema. Hemorrhage was seen in nearly 30 pecent of cases. There was significant enhancement on CECT.
2. Oat-cell carcinoma (Fig. 9-14) demonstrated lesions isodense with or slightly denser than nor-

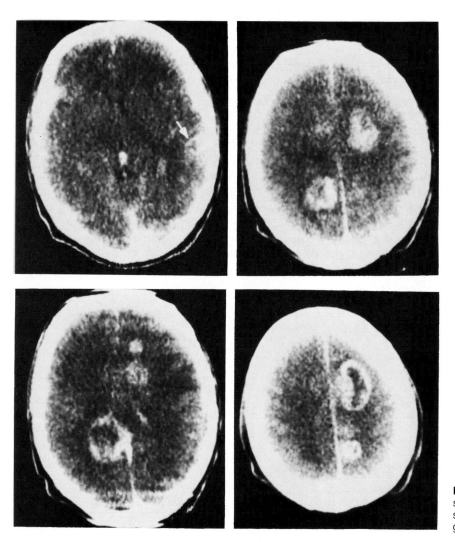

Figure 9-12 Multiple enhancing lesions suggestive of metastatic disease, which was subsequently proved to be multicentric glioma.

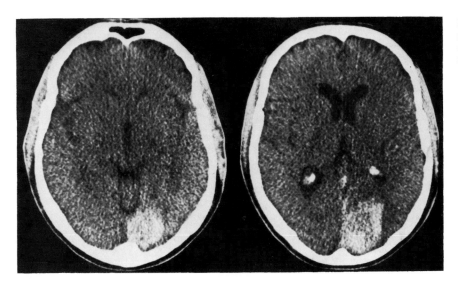

Figure 9-13 Metastatic melanoma. Slightly denser lesion than adjacent parenchyma on NCCT, which enhances significantly on CECT. The amount of edema is minimal.

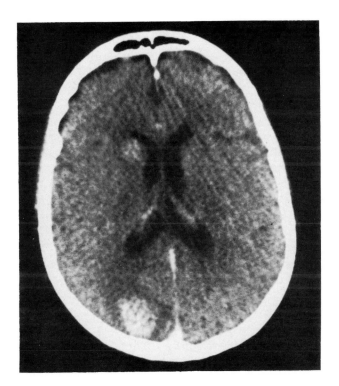

Figure 9-14 Metastasis in a patient with proven oat-cell carcinoma of the lung. The hypodense area, which most often represents edema relative to the enhancing component, is small.

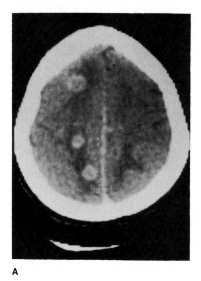
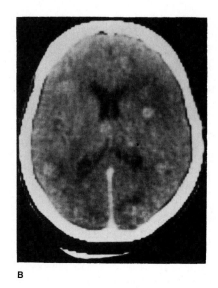
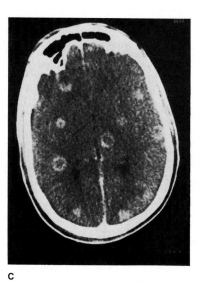

A   B   C

Figure 9-15 Metastatic adenocarcinoma; three examples. **A.** Typical appearance: NCCT demonstrates an isodense or slightly denser area surrounded by a large hypodensity. A ring lesion is seen on CECT.   **B.** Another patient with adenocarcinoma of the colon demonstrates multiple enhancing ring lesion. The ratio of edema (low density) relative to the enhancing metastases is less. **C.** Metastatic adenocarcinoma in a patient treated with steroids. Note the lack of edema around the multiple enhancing ring lesions.

mal brain parenchyma. Most oat-cell metastases showed significant enhancement, with mild to moderate surrounding hypodensity. Although these tumors are histologically prone to central necrosis, a central low-density area in oat-cell carcinoma was less commonly seen.

3. The typical metastatic adenocarcinoma (Fig. 9-15) was usually isodense with or minimally denser than normal brain parenchyma. Edema was more prominent and usually greater than the volume of the enhancing lesion. Ring pattern was a common feature seen in 62 percent of the cases.

4. Squamous-cell metastases (Fig. 9-16) were associated with large low-density areas. Nonhomogeneous enhancement was a common feature. The degree of enhancement was less when compared with other cell types of metastases.

5. Metastatic lymphoma (Fig. 9-17) involving the brain is similar to primary lymphoma. Differentiation from glioma can be difficult (Kazner 1978). These metastases tended to have ill-defined margins with homogeneous enhancement. Periven-

tricular spread of tumor was common (DuBois 1978), although other types of metastasis may also present with homogeneous periventricular enhancement.

Although the above characteristic CT pattern represents the more common source of intracranial metastases, it is not uncommon to encounter metastases from almost any organ in the body as well as occasionally from intracranial extraaxial tumors (Figs. 9-18, 9-19).

MENINGEAL CARCINOMATOSIS

Meningeal carcinomatosis is due to infiltration of the basal cisterns and leptomeninges by the metastatic neoplasm. Leptomeningeal spread may be due to contiguity, perineural, perivascular, and often hematogenous routes. Often they may be associated

Figure 9-16 Metastatic squamous cell carcinoma. A solitary minimally enhancing lesion with significant edema is present. A ring lesion or nonhomogeneous enhancement is not uncommon.

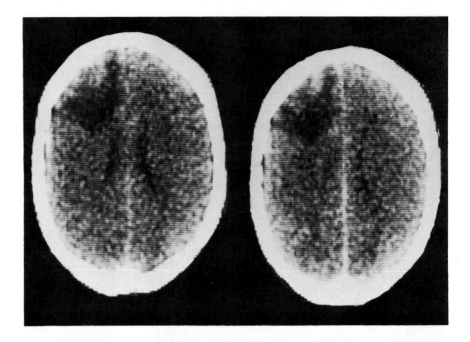

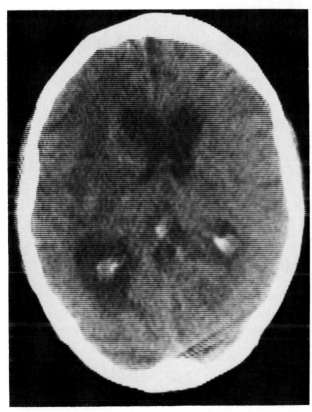

A

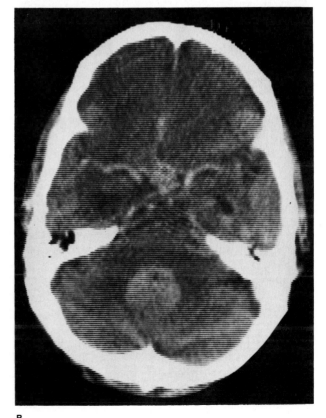

B

Figure 9-17 Metastatic lymphoma. Homogeneous periventricular spread of tumor. Similar spread may also be seen in primary glioma or other types of metastases. **A.** NCCT. **B,** CECT. (*Continued on p. 430.*)

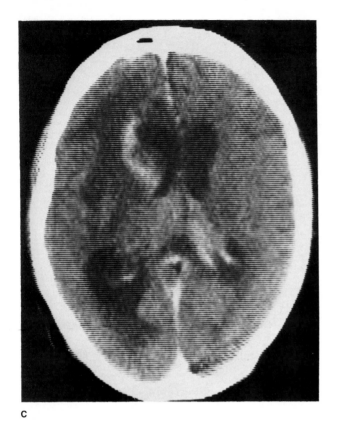
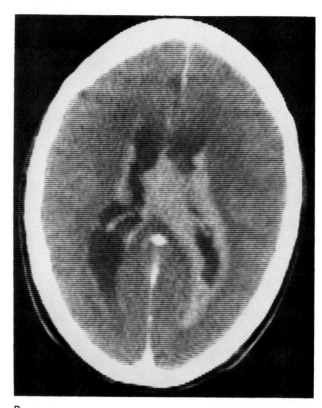

C

D

Figure 9-17 (*cont.*) **C** and **D.** CECT.

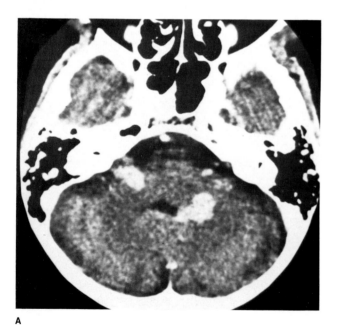
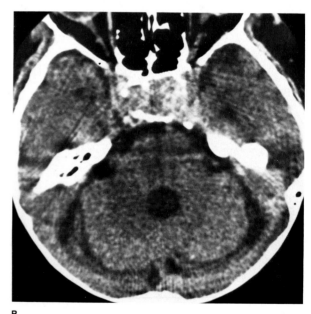

A

B

Figure 9-18 **A–D.** Metastases from prolactin secreting pituitary tumor: Multiple enhancing lesions are present both within the parenchyma as well as in the subarachnoid cisterns. (*Courtesy of Dr. Gunadi, Hagerstown.*) (*Continued on p. 431.*)

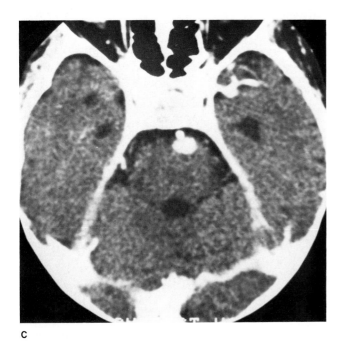

C

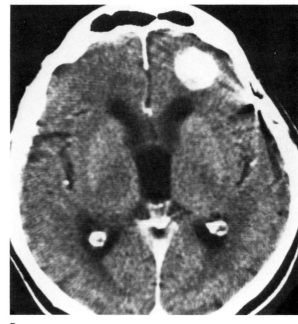

D

Figure 9-18 (*cont.*)

with parenchymal metastases. Based on autopsy reports their incidence is between 8 and 10 percent (Posner 1978). Recent CT studies, however, indicate a higher incidence of leptomeningeal carcinomatosis (Lee 1984). Contrast enhancement is necessary to identify the lesions. On CECT there is usually intense enhancement of the sulci and adjacent cistern (Enzmann 1978a; Lee 1984; Ascherl 1982), as well as along the ependymal-subependymal surface. CT pattern may show enhancement of just the sulci and adjacent cistern (Figs. 9-20, 9-21), or may appear as nodular densities within the cisterns (Figs. 9-18, 9-19, 9-22). It may also involve the ependymal surface of the ventricle (Fig. 9-21). Even though there is always diffuse spread of the neoplastic cells throughout the cisternal CSF, CT may demonstrate focal (Fig. 9-19) or diffuse (Fig. 9-22) lesions. The tentorial region often appears thickened. Hydrocephalus as the only manifestation may be seen in nearly 11 percent of cases (Enzmann 1978a). Even in the absence of meningeal enhancement, a rapid

increase in the size of the ventricles on serial CT (Fig. 9-20) in a patient with known primary cancer is almost pathognomic of leptomeningeal carcinomatosis.

DIFFERENTIAL DIAGNOSIS

An attempt has been made to define the CT pattern in metastatic disease, with some criteria relating to specific histological patterns. A variety of intracranial processes may mimic metastases, including primary brain tumors, meningiomas, infarcts, and abscesses. Other less common entities which may be confused with intracerebral metastases include multiple sclerosis, drug-induced leukoencephalopathy, multifocal leukoencephalopathy, and radiation necrosis.

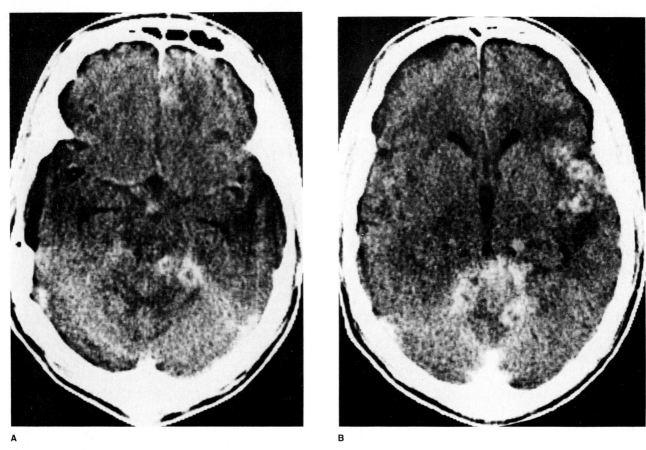

A   B

Figure 9-19   Metastases from nasopharyngeal carcinoma: CECT (**A, B**) demonstrates multiple enhancing lesions within the subarachnoid cisterns and adjacent parenchyma.

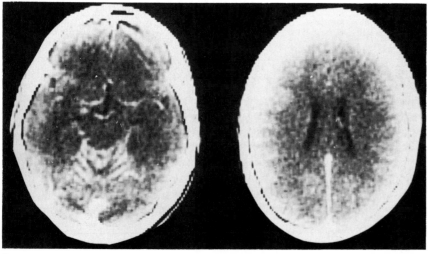

A

Figure 9-20   **A.** CECT in a patient with proven leptomeningeal carcinomatosis. There is significant enhancement of the subarachnoid cisterns. The ventricles are not enlarged. (*Continued on p. 433.*)

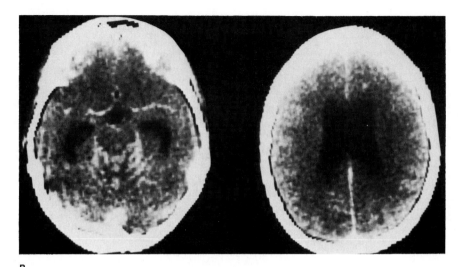

Figure 9-20 (*cont.*)   **B.** CECT in the same patient 3 weeks later. Apart from enhancement of the subarachnoid cisterns, there is enlargement of the ventricular system, indicating communicating hydrocephalus. (*Courtesy of Dr. A.J. Kumar, Johns Hopkins Hospital.*)

B

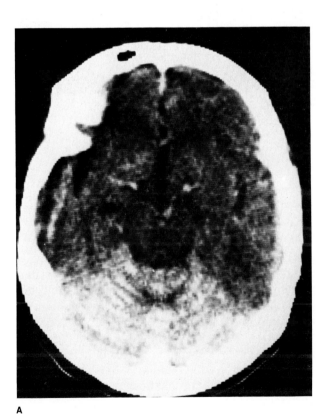

A

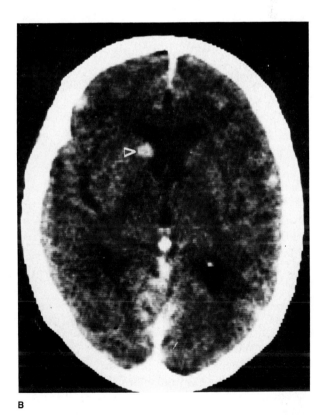

B

Figure 9-21   Leptomeningeal carcinomatosis from lung: sulci from leptomeningeal spread of oat-cell carcinoma. from tumor seeding. (*Continued on p. 432.*)   **A–D.** Selected sections demonstrates diffuse enhancement of the cisterns and **B.** A solitary nodule (arrowhead) along the ependymal surface of the ventricle

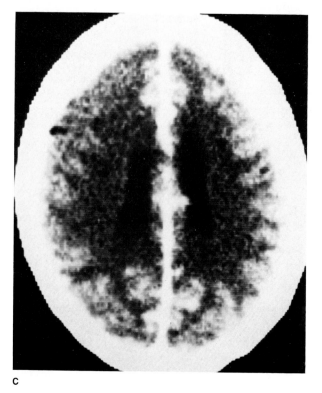

C

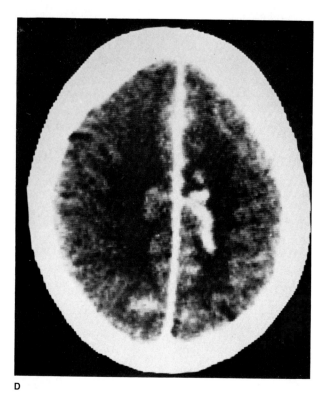

D

Figure 9-21 *(cont.)*

In multiple sclerosis, during the active phase, enhancing lesions with surrounding low density may be seen on CECT (Fig. 9-23) (Cala 1976; Aita 1978; Allen 1978; Sears 1978). They usually disappear spontaneously in a few weeks, unlike metastases, and occur only during an acute exacerbation.

In drug-induced leukoencephalopathy, focal or generalized areas of low density are present. They usually do not show any enhancement. Some amount of ventricular enlargement is a common feature. Differentiation from leptomeningeal carcinomatosis may occasionally be difficult.

Progressive multifocal leukoencephalopathy is commonly seen in patients who have been treated by chemotherapy for systemic cancer and subjected to immunosuppression. Areas of decreased density on CT are common. Most often these are located periventricularly in the frontal or occipital area and are symmetrical. Differentiation from cerebral metastasis is based on the location of these low-density areas and by lack of enhancement (Lane 1978; Norman 1978). Diagnosis of progressive multifocal leukoencephalopathy is by brain biopsy and viral culture.

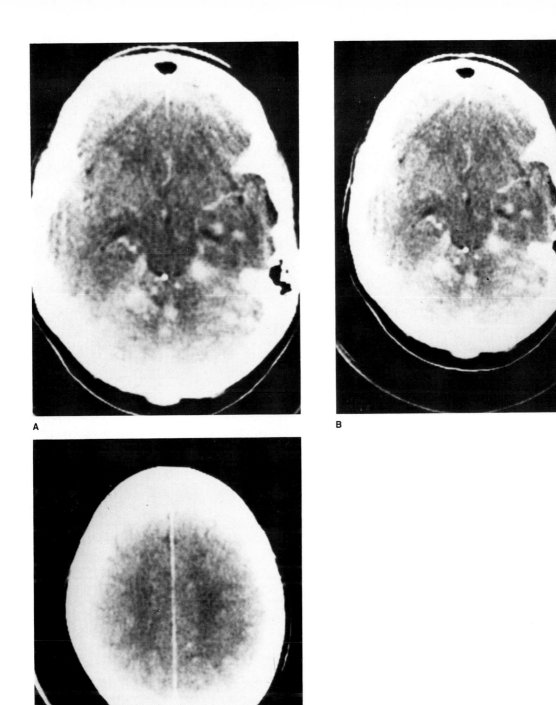

A

B

C

Figure 9-22 Leptomeningeal and parenchymal metastases from lung carcinoma. **A–C.** Multiple enhancing lesions, both infra- and supratentorial in the cisterns as well as in the parenchyma.

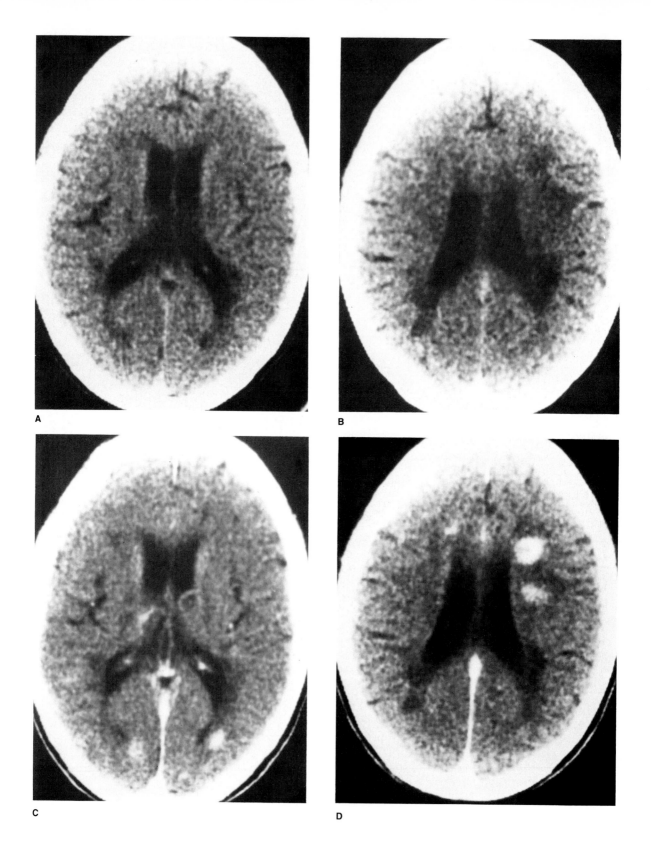

A

B

C

D

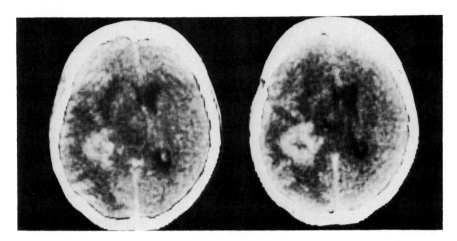

Figure 9-24 Postradiation necrosis. The enhancing ring lesion with surrounding edema could represent either primary or metastic tumor. Mass proved at autopsy to represent postradiation necrosis with sarcomatous changes in a patient who had had surgery for solitary metastasis.

RADIATION NECROSIS

Occasionally in the past prophylactic radiation to the brain was utilized as part of the treatment of systemic cancer. Radiation-induced necrosis of the brain may present as a mass lesion (Fig. 9-24). On CT such lesions are usually hypodense, with some contrast enhancement and surrounding edema (Mikhael 1978). Differentiation from primary or metastatic tumor or abscess by CT alone is difficult (Danziger 1979).

CT FOLLOWING TREATMENT MODALITIES

Following various therapeutic modalities, CT provides an innocuous method of evaluating their ef-

Figure 9-23 Multiple sclerosis: **A, B.** NCCT and (**C, D**) CECT. Noncontrast CT demonstrates a hypodense area adjacent to the occipital horn. The enhanced study demonstrates multiple enhancing lesions involving both hemispheres with minimal edema.

ficacy. The edema-reducing effect of steroids and the dramatic clinical response to them are well known. Steroids may also decrease the degree of enhancement within the metastasis and occasionally may mask metastatic foci. This effect of corticosteroid has been shown both on CT and on radionuclide brain scan (Crocker 1976).

Serial CT studies are also useful in determining the response to various chemotherapeutic agents and radiation therapy (Hyman 1978; Kretzchmar 1978). Most chemotherapeutic agents have not had significant impact in metastatic brain tumors. On the other hand, dramatic response can be observed following radiation therapy, especially in oat-cell carcinoma (Fig. 9-25). Unfortunately, the metastases reappear with both modalities, eventually exceeding their original size. Treatment may increase the density of tumors on NCCT or decrease the density by producing necrosis. Enhancement characteristics may be altered as with steroids.

Delayed effects of radiation therapy include postradiation cerebral atrophy, which may be suggested by CT when there is an increase in the size of the ventricles and sulci. Other complications have been discussed earlier.

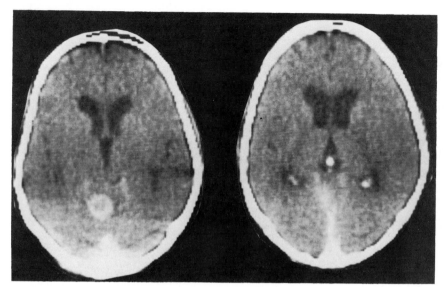

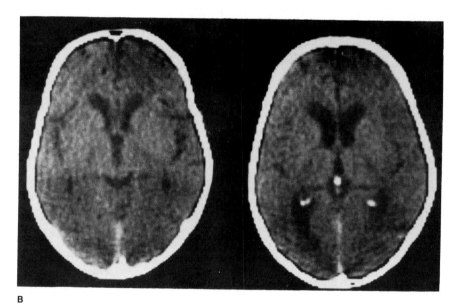

A

B

Figure 9-25 CECT in a patient with metastases from oat-cell carcinoma. **A.** Preradiation. **B.** Postradiation. Demonstrates role of CT in evaluating intracranial metastasis.

SUMMARY

CT in metastatic disease has resulted in the following benefits: (1) earlier evaluation of patients suspected of having intracranial metastases; (2) better determination of the number, size, and location of metastatic foci; (3) noninvasive follow-up of the various treatment modalities; and (4) occasional suggestion of possible primary site or sites when not already known.

Bibliography

ANAND AK, POTTS DG: Calcified brain metastases: demonstration by computed tomography. *Am J Neuroradiol* **3**:527–529, 1982.

ARONSON SM, GARCIA JH, AARONSON BE: Metastatic neoplasms of the brain: Their frequency in relation to age. *Cancer* **17**:558–563, 1964.

AITA JF, BENNETT DR, ANDERSON RE, ZITER F: Cranial CT appearance of acute multiple sclerosis. *Neurology* **28**:251–255, 1978.

ALLEN JC, THALER HT, DECK MDF, ROTHENBERG DA: Leukoencephalopathy following high-dose intravenous methotrexate chemotherapy. Quantitative assessment of white matter attenuation using computed tomography. *Neuroradiology* **16**:46–64, 1978.

ASCHERL GF JR, HILAL SK, BRISMAN R: Computed tomography of disseminated meningeal and ependymal malignant neoplasms. *Radiology* **142**:274–277, 1982.

BAKER HI, HOUSER OW, CAMPBELL JK: National Cancer Institute study: Evaluation of computed tomography in diagnosis of intracranial neoplasms. *Radiology* **136**:91–96, 1980.

BECKER H, NORMAN D, BOYD DP, HATTNER RS, NEWTON TH: Computed tomography in detecting calvarial metastases: A comparison with skull radiography and radionuclide scanning. *Neuroradiology* **16**:504–505, 1978.

BLACK P: Brain metastasis: Current status and recommended guidelines for management. *Neurosurgery* **5**(5):617–631, 1979.

DUBOULAY GH, RADUE EW: Comparison of computerized tomography with other neuroradiologial methods: A plea for a different kind of analysis. *Neuroradiology* **16**:474–476, 1978.

BRADFIELD PA, PASSALAQUE AM, BRAUNSTEIN P, RAGHAUENDRA BN, LEEDS NE, KRICHEFF II: A comparison of radionuclide scanning and computed tomography in metastatic lesions of the brain. *J Comput Asst Tomogr* **1**:315–318, 1977.

BRISMAR J, STROMBLAD LG, SALFORD LG: Impact of CT in neurosurgical management of intracranial tumors. *Neuroradiology* **16**:506–509, 1978.

BUELL U, NIENDORF HP, STEINHOFF H: Validity of serial scintigraphy with 97m Tc-Pertechnetate in comparison with computerized tomography, in Lauksch W, Kazner E (eds): *Cranial Computerized Tomography.* New York, Springer-Verlag 1976, pp 177–182.

BUELL U, NIENDORF HP, KAZNER E, LAUKSCH W, WILSKE J, STEINHOFF H, GAHR H: Computerized transaxial tomography and cerebral serial scintigraphy in intracranial tumors—Rates of detection and tumor type identification: Concise communication. *J Nucl Med* **19**:476–479, 1978.

BUTLER AR, KRICHEFF II: Noncontrast CT scanning: Limited value in suspected brain tumors. *Radiology* **126**:689–693, 1978.

BUTLER AR, LEO JS, LIN JP, BOYD AD, KRICHEFF II: The value of routine cranial computed tomography in neurologically intact patients with primary carcinoma of the lung. *Radiology* **131**:399–401, 1979.

CALA IA, MASTAGLIA FL: Computerized axial tomography in multiple sclerosis. *Lancet* **1**:689, 1976.

CHASON JL, WALTER FB, LANDERS JW: Metastatic carcinoma in the central nervous system and dorsal root ganglia. A prospective study. *Cancer* **16**:781–787, 1963.

CHIRATHIVAT S, POST MJD: CT demonstration of dural metastases in neuroblastoma. *J Comput Assist Tomogr* **4**(3):316–319, 1980.

CONSTANT P: Cerebral metastases—A study of computed tomography. *Comput Tomogr* **1**:84–94, 1977.

CROCKER EF, ZIMMERMAN RA, PHELPS ME, KUHL DE: The effect of steroids on the extra-vascular distribution of radiographic contrast material and technetium pertechnetate in brain tumors as determined by computed tomography. *Radiology* **119**:471–476, 1976.

DANZIGER J, WALLACE S, HANDEL SF, DESANTOS LA: Metastatic osteogenic sarcoma of the brain. *Cancer* **44**:707–710, 1979.

DECK MDF, MESSINA AV, SACKETT JF: Computed tomography in metastatic disease of the brain. *Radiology* **119**:115–120, 1976.

DECK MDF: Computed tomography of metastatic disease of the brain, in Weiss L, Gilbert H, Posner J (eds): *Workshop on Brain Metastasis,* Memorial Sloan-Kettering Cancer Center, 1978. Boston, Hall, 1980.

DICHIRO G, BROOKS RM, KESSLER GS, JOHNSTON EA, HERDT JR, SHERIDAN WT: Tissue signatures from dual energy computed tomography. *Radiology* **124**:99–107, 1977.

DUBAL L, WIGGLE U: Tomochemistry of the brain. *J Comput Assist Tomogr* **1**(3):300–307, 1977.

DUBOIS PJ, MARTINE AJ, MYEROWITZ RL, ROSENBAUM AE: Subependymal and leptomeningeal spread of systemic malignant lymphoma demonstrated by cranial computed tomography. *J Comput Assist Tomogr* **2**:218–221, 1978.

ELKE M et al: The diagnosis of intracranial metastases: The efficiency of CT and scintigraphy in patients investigated by both methods, in Lanksch W, Kazner E (eds): *Cranial Computerized Tomography.* New York, Springer-Verlag, 1976, pp 171–176.

ENZMANN DR, KRICORIAN J, YORKE C, HAYWOOD R: Computed tomography in leptomeningeal spread of tumor. *J Comput Assist Tomogr* **2**:448–455, 1978*a*.

ENZMANN DR, KRAMER R, NORMAN D, POLLOCK J: Malignant melanoma metastatic to the central nervous system. *Radiology* **127**:177–180, 1978*b*.

FORDHAM E: The complementary role of computerized axial tomography and radionuclide imaging of the brain. *Semin Nucl Med* **7**(2):137–159, 1977.

GADO MH, PHELPS ME: The peripheral zone of increased density in cranial computed tomography. *Radiology* **117**:71–74, 1975.

GAWLER J, DUBOULAY GH, BUELL JWD: Computer assisted tomography (EMI scanner): Its place in investigation of suspected intracranial tumors. *Lancet* **2**:419–423, 1974.

GILDERSLEEVE N, KOO AH, MCDONALD CJ: Metastatic tumor presenting as intracerebral hemorrhage: Report of 6 cases examined by computed tomography. *Radiology* **124**:109–112, 1977.

GREITZ T: Computer tomography for diagnosis of intracranial tumors compared with other neuroradiologic procedures. *Acta Radiol* [Suppl] (Stockh) **346**:14–20, 1975.

HAYMAN LA, EVANS RA, HINCK VC: Delayed high iodine dose contrast computed tomography: Cranial neoplasms. *Radiology* **136**:677–684, 1980.

HILAL SK, CHANG CH: Specificity of computed tomography in the diagnosis of supratentorial neoplasms. *Neuroradiology* **16**:537–539, 1978.

HIRANO A, MATSUI T: Vascular structures in brain tumors. *Humam Pathol* **6**:611–621, 1975.

HIRANO A, ZIMMERMAN HM: Fenestrated blood vessels in a metastatic renal carcinoma in the brain. *Lab Invest* **26**(4):465–468, 1972.

HUCKMAN MS, ACKERMAN LV: Use of automated measurements of mean density as an adjunct to computed tomography. *J Comput Assist Tomogr* **1**(10):37–42, 1977.

HYMAN RA, LORING MI, LIEBESKIND AL, NAIDICH JB, STEIN HL: Computed tomographic evaluation of therapeutically induced changes in primary and secondary brain tumors. *Neuroradiology* **14**:213–218, 1978.

JACOBS L, KINKEL WR, VINCENT RG: Silent brain metastasis from lung carcinoma determined by computerized tomography. *Arch Neurol* **34**:690–693, 1977.

JENNINGS EC, AUNGST CW, YATCO R: Asymptomatic patients with primary carcinoma. Computer axial tomography study. *NY State J Med* **80:**1096–1098, 1979.

JOHNSON DH, WINDHAM WW, ALLEN JH, GRECO FA: Limited value of CT brain scans in staging of small cell lung cancer. *Am J Neuroradiol* **3:**649–652, 1982.

KAZNER E, WILSKE J, STEINOFF H, STOCKDORPH O: Computer assisted tomography in primary malignant lymphoma of the brain. *J Comput Assist Tomogr* **2:**125–134, 1978.

KIDO DK, GOULD R, TAASTI F, DUNCAN A, SCHNUR J: Comparative sensitivity of CT scans, radiographs and radionuclide scans in detecting metastatic calvarial lesions. *Radiology* **128:**371–375, 1978.

KRAMER RA, JANETOS GP, PENDSTEIN G: An approach to contrast enhancement in computed tomography of the brain. *Radiology* **116:**641–647, 1975.

KRETZCHMAR K, AULICH A, SCHINDER E, LANGE S, GUMME T, MEESE W: The diagnostic value of CT for radiotherapy of cerebral tumors. *Neuroradiology* **14:**245–250, 1978.

LANE B, CARROLL BA, PEDLEY TA: Computerized cranial tomography in cerebral diseases of white matter. *Neuroradiology* **28:**534–544, 1978.

LATCHAW RE, GOLD LHA, MOORE JS, PAYNE TJ: The nonspecificity of absorption coefficients in the differentiation of solid tumors and cystic lesions. *Radiology* **125:**141–144, 1977.

LATCHAW RE, PAYNE JT, GOLD LHA: Effective atomic number and electron density as measured with a computed tomography scanner: Computation and correlation with brain tumor histology. *J Comput Assist Tomogr* **2**(2):199–208, 1978*a*.

LATCHAW RE, GOLD LHA, TOURJE EJ: A protocol for the use of contrast enhancement of cranial computed tomogrpahy. *Radiology* **126:**681–687, 1978*b*.

LEE YY, GLASS JP, GEOFFRAY A, WALLACE S: Cranial computed tomographic abnormalities in leptomeningeal metastases. *Am J Neuroradiol* **5:**559–569, 1984.

LEWANDER R, BERGSTROM M, BEGVALL U: Contrast enhancement of cranial lesions in computed tomography. *Acta Radiol* [Diagn] (Stockh) **19:**529–552, 1978.

LITTLE JR, DIAL B, BELANGER G, CARPENTER S: Brain hemorrhage from intracranial tumor. *Stroke* **10**(3):283–288, 1979.

LONG DM: Capillary ultrastructure in human metastatic brain tumors. *J Neurosurg* **32:**127–144, 1970.

MANDYBUR TI: Intracranial hemorrhage caused by metastatic tumors. *Neurology* **27:**650–655, 1977.

METZGER J, GARDEUR O, NACHANAKIAN A, MILLARD JC: Comparison des tomodensitometre, cinegammagraphique et angiographique dousé les diagnostics topographique et histologique préoperatives des 300 tumors intracraniennes sustentorielles. *Neuroradiology* **16:**495–498, 1978.

MARSHALL WH, EASTER W, ZATZ LM: Analysis of the dense lesion at computed tomography with dual kVp scans. *Radiology* **124:**87–89, 1977.

MESSINA AV: Cranial computed tomography. *Arch Neurol* **34:**602–607, 1977.

MIKHAEL MA: Radiation necrosis of the brain: Correlation between computed tomography pathology and distribution. *J Comput Assist Tomogr* **2:**71–80, 1978.

NAHEEDY MH, KIDO DK, O'REILLY GV: Computed tomography evaluation of subdural and epidural metastases. *J Comput Assist Tomogr* **4**(3):311–315, 1980.

NEW PFJ et al: Computed tomography with the EMI scanner in the diagnosis of primary and metastatic intracranial neoplasms. *Radiology* **114:**75–87, 1975.

NORMAN D, STEVENS EA, WING SD, LEVINE V, NEWTON TH: Quantitative aspects of contrast enhancement in cranial computed tomography. *Radiology* **129:**683–688, 1978.

OLDERBERG E: The hemorrhage into glioma: A review of eight hundred and thirty-two consecutive verified cases of glioma. *Arch Neurol Psychiatry* **30:**1061–1073, 1933.

PAILLAS JE, PELLET W: Brain metastaess, in Vinken PJ and Bryn GW (eds): *Handbook of Clinical Neurology*, vol. 18. New York, American Elsevier Publishing Co., 1976, pp. 201–232.

PENDERGRASS HP, MCKUSICK KA, NEW PFJ, POTSAID MS: Relative efficacy of radionuclide imaging and computed tomography of the brain. *Radiology* **116**:363–366, 1975.

PEYLAN-RAMU N, POPLACK DG, BLIE LC, HERDT GR, VERMESS D, DECHIRO G: Computed assisted tomography in methotrexate encephalopathy. *J Comput Assist Tomogr* **1**(2):216–221, 1977.

PEYLAN-RAMU N: Abnormal CT scans of the brain in asymptomatic children with acute lymphocytic leukemia after prophylactic treatment of the central nervous system with radiation and intrathecal chemotherapy. *N Engl J Med* **293**:815–818, 1978.

POSNER JB: Brain metastases: A clinician's view, in Weiss L, Gilbert H, and Posner JB (eds): *Brain Metastases,* Boston, G.K. Hall, 1980.

POSNER JB: Diagnosis and treatment of metastases to the brain. *Clin Bull* **4**:47–57, 1974.

POSNER JB, CHERNIK NL: Intracranial metastases from systemic cancer. *Adv Neurol* **19**:575–587, 1978.

POTCHEN EJ: Radiologic approaches to the diagnosis of cerebral metastases. *Int J Radiat Oncol* **2**(1–2):173–178, 1977.

POTTS DG, SVARE GT: Calcification in intracranial metastases. *Am J Roentgenol* **92**:1249–1251, 1964.

POTTS DG, ABBOTT GF, VONSNEIDEN JV: National Cancer Institute Study: Evaluation of computed tomography in diagnosis of intracranial neoplasms: III. Metastatic tumors. *Radiology* **136**:657–664, 1980.

RANSHOFF J: Surgical management of metastatic tumors. *Semin Oncol* **2**:21–27, 1975.

RAO KCVG, KUMAR AJ, FOUAD G: Computed tomography in metastatic disease. Paper presented at 65th Annual Meeting of the Radiological Society of North America, November 1979.

RAO KCVG, LEVINE H, SAJORE, ITANI A, WALKER R: CT in multicentric glioma: Radiological-pathological correlation. *CT: J Comput Tomogr* **4**(3):187–192, September 1980.

ROTHE R, FISHER K: Comparison between computerized tomography and conventional contrast medium methods in the diagnosis of brain tumors, in Lanksche W, Kazner E (eds): *Cranial Computerized Tomography.* New York, Springer-Verlag, 1976, 183–187.

RUSSCALLEDA J: Clinical symptomatology and computerized tomography in brain metastases. *Comput Tomogr* **2**(2):69–77, 1978.

SEARS ES, TINDALL RSA, ZARNOW H: Active multiple sclerosis: Enhanced computerized tomographic imaging of lesions and effects of corticosteroids. *Arch Neurol* **35**:426–436, 1978.

SILVERBERG E: Cancer statistics 1977. *CA* **27**:26–41, 1977.

SIMIONESCUE MD: Metastatic tumors of the brain: A follow-up study of 195 patients with neurosurgical considerations. *J Neurosurg* **17**:361–373, 1960.

SOLIS OJ, DAVIS KR, ADAIR LB, ROBERTSON AR, KLEINMAN G: Intracerebral metastatic melanoma—CT evaluation. *Comput Tomogr* **1**:135–143, 1977.

STEINHOFF H, KAZNER E, LAUKSCH W, GRUMME T, MEESE W, LANGE S, AULICH A, WENDE S: The limitation of computerized axial tomography in the detection and differential diagnosis of intracranial tumors: A study based on 1304 neoplasms, in Bories J (ed): *Diagnostic Limitations of Computerized Axial Tomography.* New York, Springer-Verlag, 1978.

SYLVESTER AH, DUGSTAD G, AMUNDSEN P: Computerized tomography in brain tumors correlated to histology, angiography, gas encephalography, in Lanksch W, Kazner E (eds): *Computerized Cranial Tomography.* New York, Springer-Verlag, 1978, pp 167–170.

VANECK JHM, GO KG, EBELS EJ: Metastatic tumors of the brain. *Neurol Neurochir* **68**:443–462, 1965.

VANNUCCI RC, BATEN M: Cerebral metastatic disease in childhood. *Neurology* **24**:981–985, 1974.

VEITH RG, ODOM GL: Intracranial metastases and their neurosurgical treatment. *J Neurosurg* **23**:375–383, 1965.

WALKER MD: Brain and peripheral nervous system tumors, in Holland JF, Frei E (eds): *Cancer Medicine*. Philadelphia, Lea & Febiger, 1973.

WEISBERG LA, NICE CN: Intracranial tumors simulating the presentation of cerebrovascular syndromes. *JAMA* **63**:517, 1977.

WENDLING LR: Computed tomography of intracerebral leukemic masses. *Am J Roentgenol* **132**(2):217–220, 1979.

WILLIS RA: *The Spread of Tumors in the Human Body*, 3d ed. London, Butterworth, 1973.

WING DS, ANDERSON RE, OSOBORN, AG: Cranial computed angiotomography. Paper presented at the Radiologial Society of North America, Dallas, November 18, 1980.

ZIMMERMAN RA, BILANIUK LT: Computed tomography of acute intratumoral hemorrhage. *Radiology* **135**:355–359, 1980.

10

THE BASE OF THE SKULL: SELLA AND TEMPORAL BONE

David L. Daniels

Katherine A. Shaffer

Victor M. Haughton

The skull base consists of membranous bone and cartilage perforated by nerves, spinal cord, arteries, and veins. The complex anatomic relationships, especially within the sella and temporal bone, are effectively evaluated by CT or MR. CT is optimal for demonstrating the osseous structures and some veins and nerves, MR, the soft tissues, vessels, and nerves. The multitude and complexity of the abnormalities at the base of the skull will be presented in two parts: the sella and the temporal bones.

SECTION A: SELLA

When the appropriate techniques are used, CT provides the most definitive and complete examination of the pituitary fossa and adjacent structures (Reich 1976; Gyldenstein 1977; Belloni 1978; Wolpert 1979; Gardeur 1981). To achieve a high degree of diagnostic accuracy, one must use coronal imaging, thin sections, high radiation flux, and an optimal technique for intravenous contrast administration. With these techniques, CT is sensitive, and accurate in the differential diagnosis.

The role of MR in studying the sella is currently being evaluated (Mark 1984; Pojunas 1986; Daniels 1984a, 1986; Lee 1985; Oot 1984; Bilaniuk 1984). MR demonstrates pituitary adenomas and some microadenomas noninvasively and without x-irradiation but with less sensitivity than CT. With intravenous contrast agents the sensitivity of MR may equal that of CT. The effectiveness of MR in distinguishing actively secreting and inactive adenomas by relaxation times needs evaluation. MR is indicated as a supplement to CT in many cases at the present time.

TECHNICAL ASPECTS

Direct coronal CT images of the sella permit more accurate demonstration of sellar abnormalities and a lower radiation dose to the lens than axial images (Earnest 1981; Taylor 1982). High-quality coronal images with the least movement are obtained if the patient is placed supine or prone on the scanning table with his neck extended in a modified head-holder. A digital localizer image is used so that the plane of section is nearly perpendicular to the sella and without artifacts from dental fillings (Fig. 10-1). Technical factors for CT imaging include: high radiation flux, long scan times to maximize contrast resolution (4 to 10 sec), and thin (for example, 1.5

mm or less) sections to maximize spatial resolution. If the sella is enlarged, 5-mm-thick sections are more practical. If direct coronal sections are not feasible because the patient cannot extend his neck sufficiently, coronal images can be obtained by reformatting multiple, contiguous 1.5-mm axial sections at 1- or 1.5-mm intervals.

An optimal MR study at the pituitary gland requires a homogeneous magnetic field, a slice thickness of 3 mm or less, a fine (256 by 256) matrix, an averaging of signals from two to four excitations, and combinations of pulse sequences. The use of intravenous contrast agents such as Gadolinium DTPA increases the sensitivity, especially of the short TR images. The MR study consists of short TR images (<800 msec) supplemented in some cases with long TR sequences (2000 msec) with multiple echoes (TE 25 to 120 msec).

An MR study is initiated with a sagittal (short TR and TE) image to select the locations for higher-resolution coronal or sagittal images. The coronal images most effectively show the pituitary gland and its upper contour and the cavernous sinuses, with the least artifact from chemical shift misregistration. Coronal images are usually followed by axial and sagittal ones when a large mass is present. The short TR and TE images (T_1 weighted) because of the higher signal to noise ratio demonstrate contrast between sellar structures most effectively. Long TR and TE images, which are T_2 weighted, may help characterize abnormalities found with shorter pulse sequences. Clotted blood, fat, gland, and tumor tissue can be differentiated effectively with a combination of T_1 and T_2 weighted images.

The cavernous sinuses, pituitary gland, and pituitary stalk, because of their incomplete blood-brain barrier, increase substantially in density on CT after the administration of iodinated intravenous contrast medium. This increase in density, "contrast enhancement," may be helpful in characterizing intrasellar or juxtasellar masses. To achieve optimal contrast enhancement, a high plasma concentration of iodinated contrast medium is obtained by infusing 200 ml of 30 percent iodinated contrast medium rapidly into an antecubital vein immediately prior to scanning. To maintain the high plasma iodine con-

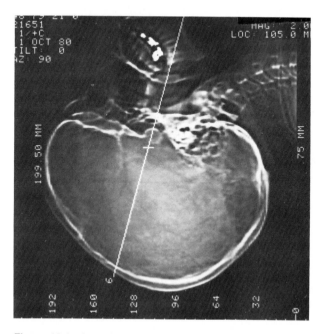

Figure 10-1 Lateral localizer image demonstrating the optimal CT gantry angle (white line) perpendicular to the sellar floor for CT imaging of the sella. (*From Daniels 1985a.*)

centration during scanning, contrast medium is infused during the scanning procedure (an additional 100 ml of 30 percent contrast medium). The same dose of contrast medium (total of 42 g iodine) can be effectively given with different concentrations and volumes. Contrast enhancement facilitates the detection of microadenomas, which enhance to a lesser degree than the normal pituitary gland, and vascular structures in the sella. If scanning is delayed more than 20 minutes after the intravenous injection of contrast medium, the detection of microadenomas may be impaired because the adenoma increases progressively in density while the gland and cavernous sinuses gradually diminish in density (Hemminghytt 1983) (Fig. 10-2).

Contrast enhancement is achieved in MR by administering a paramagnetic compound (e.g., Gadolinium EDPA) intravenously. It shortens the relaxation times of tissues in which it accumulates, increasing the signal intensity of the normal pituitary gland, infundibulum, and cavernous sinuses in T_1-weighted imaging sequences. The risks and side effects are minimal. The conventional dose is 0.1 mmol/kg.

Dynamic scanning, which refers to sequential CT sections obtained at a single level every few seconds after a bolus injection of contrast medium, may be used for evaluation of the sella (Cohen 1982; Pinto 1982; Wing 1980). On such dynamic studies, vascular, glandular, and neoplastic tissues, which have different density vs. time curves, can be effectively detected and differentiated (Fig. 10-3). Aneurysms or normal vessels have a rapid increase and then decrease in density after the bolus injection. Venous structures have a rapid increase and decrease in density which follows the arterial peak by several seconds. Solid tumors within or near the sella, such as pituitary adenomas, have a slow increase in density, and even slower decrease in density. Cystic or avascular or densely calcified tumors, such as craniopharyngiomas, have little change in density with time.

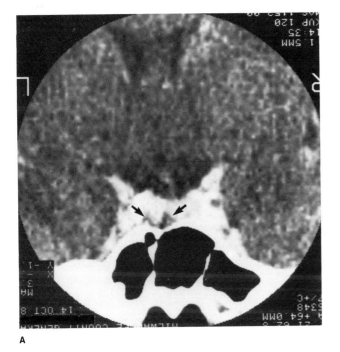
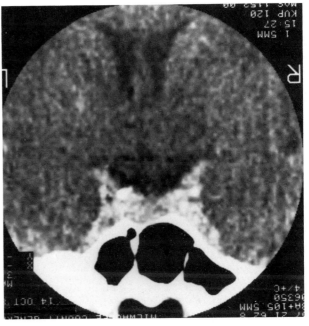

A   **B**

Figure 10-2 Coronal CT scans of a prolactinoma. After intravenous contrast administration the tumor (arrows, **A**) appears as a hypodense area and **(B)** 15 minutes later it is nearly isodense with normal pituitary tissue. (*From Hemminghytt 1983.*)

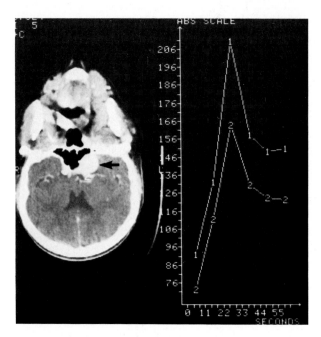

Figure 10-3 Dynamic CT scanning in a parasellar aneurysm (arrow). The aneurysm has almost the same time/density curve (1) as an adjacent artery (2). (*From Daniels 1985a.*)

With dynamic scanning, a small capillary bed in the midline below the upper margin of the pituitary gland may be demonstrated during the arterial phase of dynamic scanning (Fig. 10-4) (Bonneville 1983). Displacement of the capillary bed ("tuft") indicates an expanding intrasellar process such as pituitary adenoma.

Intrathecal contrast agent has few applications in the CT study of the sella except for suspected intra- or suprasellar cysts (Fig. 10-5). It has been used to verify an empty sella when the intravenously enhanced images were suboptimal. Intrathecal enhancement is accomplished with a lumbar puncture, the injection of 5 ml of an intrathecal water-soluble contrast medium such as metrizamide, iohexol, or Iopamidol (170 to 200 mg I/ml), the patient tilted prone and head end down on a fluoroscopic table for 2 minutes, and then CT scanning with the patient supine.

NORMAL ANATOMY

Pituitary Fossa

The sella is a saddle-shaped osseous structure with the following landmarks: anteriorly the tuberculum sella, inferiorly the lamina dura, and posteriorly the dorsum sella. Within the sella is the pituitary gland. Its upper surface is usually straight or very mildly concave or, especially in adolescents or menstruous women, slightly convex (Fig. 10-6) (Wolpert 1984; Gardeur 1982). Its height normally is approximately 2 to 9 mm with an average height of 3.5 mm in men and 4.8 mm in women (Mark 1984; Syvertsen 1979). It appears nearly homogeneous in NCCT or CECT images with a density that is almost the same as that of the cavernous sinuses. It may have a mild degree of nonhomogeneity, especially in menstruous females and adolescents, but without discrete and well-demarcated low-attenuation regions (Swartz 1983; Roppolo 1983*a,b*). The areas of greater density or enhancement may represent more compact glandular or vascular tissue; tiny colloid cysts in the pars intermedia which have a lower density may also contribute to nonhomogeneity.

In short TR and TE MR (T_1-weighted) images, the pituitary gland has a homogeneous signal intensity, without or with intravenous contrast administration, which contrasts to the negligible signal (black) from the cortical bone in the sella and cerebrospinal fluid in the suprasellar cistern (Fig. 10-7). Fat in the marrow of the dorsum sellae and within the postero-inferior pituitary fossa appears in MR images as a region of hyperintense signal. Anterior to the fat in sagittal images a "chemical shift" misregistration artifact may produce a small region of low signal intensity depending on the direction of the frequency encoding gradient. Small venous channels, which have negligible signal because of the flowing blood, are prominent at the lateral part of the pituitary gland. In long TR and TE (T_2-weighted) images, the gland's signal is homogeneous and less intense than that of cerebrospinal fluid, which appears white (Fig. 10-8*B*). The diaphragma sellae, a thin membrane rostral to the gland through

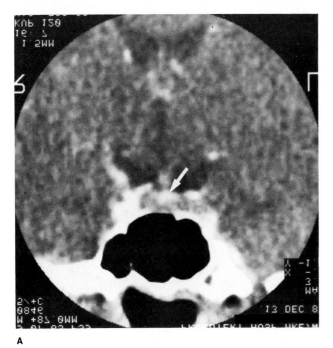

A

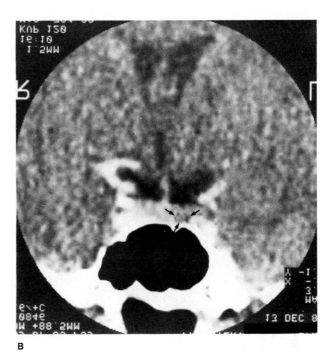

B

Figure 10-4 Arterial phase of coronal dynamic CT sequence showing a normal capillary "tuft" (arrow, **A**) below the surface of a pituitary gland. The tuft is not displaced by a hypodense baso-philic adenoma (small black arrows, **B**) that is demonstrated in a nondynamic coronal CECT study. (*From Daniels 1985a.*)

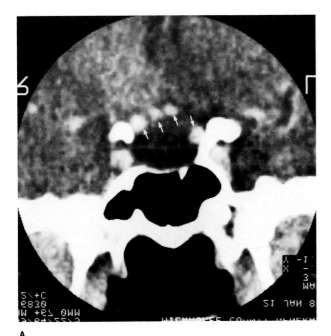

A

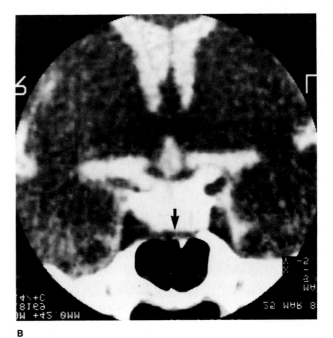

B

Figure 10-5 Empty sella. In intravenously enhanced coronal CT (**A**) it appears as a region of hypodensity in the sella. Enhancing round structures (small white arrows) represent suprasellar blood vessels. In **B** after opacification of the pituitary fossa with intrathecal contrast agent a small gland (black arrow) is demonstrated. (*From Daniels 1985a.*)

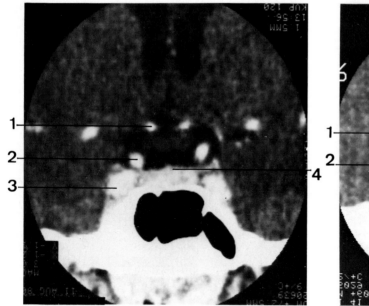

1. anterior cerebral artery 2. supraclinoid internal carotid artery
3. intracavenous internal carotid artery 4. pituitary gland

A

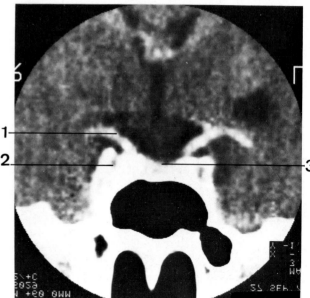

1. supraclinoid internal carotid artery 2. oculomotor nerve 3. pituitary
gland

B

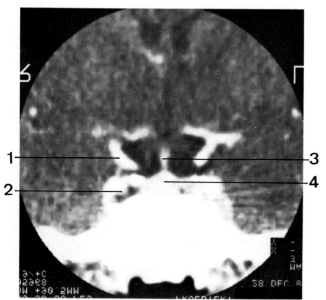

1. supraclinoid internal carotid artery 2. intracavernous internal
carotid artery 3. infundibulum 4. pituitary gland

C

Figure 10-6   Examples of normal pituitary glands in coronal CECT
images. The glands homogeneously enhance and have straight
(A), concave **(B)** or at the attachment point of the infundibulum a
midline convex upper contour **(C)**. (*From Daniels 1985a.*)

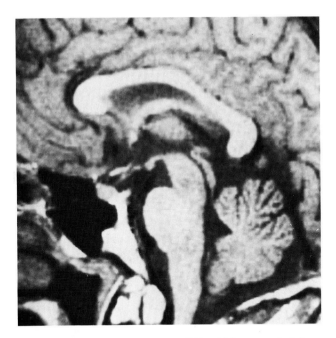

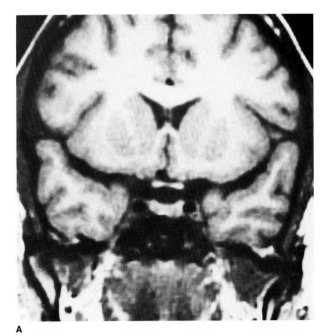

A

Figure 10-7 Sagittal T_1-weighted MRI in which a normal pituitary gland has a nearly straight upper contour and a homogeneous signal that contrasts with the negligible signal (black) from cerebrospinal fluid and cortical bone and the high-intensity signal (white) from fat in the dorsum sellae.

which the infundibulum runs, is commonly demonstrated in coronal, long TR, and short TE images as a transversely oriented thin band having negligible signal (Daniels 1986).

Cavernous Sinuses

The venous structures on either side of the pituitary fossa, the cavernous sinuses, appear nearly triangular in coronal CT and MR sections with a straight or slightly concave lateral wall (Fig. 10-9). The lateral wall is formed by a layer of dura under which is a fenestrated membrane containing cranial nerves III (oculomotor), IV (trochlear), and V_1, V_2 (trigeminal, first and second divisions) (Umansky 1982). Cranial nerve VI (abducens) is contained within the lumen of the cavernous sinus. The Gasserian ganglion lies within Meckel's cave, an invagination along the posterior margins of the cavernous sinus (Figs.

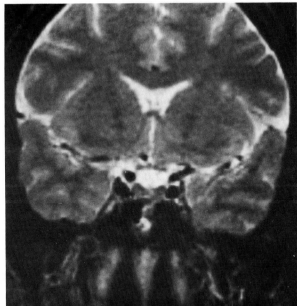

B

Figure 10-8 Coronal T_1-weighted **(A)** and T_2-weighted **(B)** MR images of a normal pituitary gland. The gland has a mildly concave upper contour; the cavernous internal carotid arteries and venous spaces have negligible signal in **A** and **B**. Cranial nerves in the cavernous sinuses are shown in **A**, the lateral wall of the cavernous sinus in **B** with its negligible signal in contrast to the high signal intensity (white) of adjacent cerebrospinal fluid.

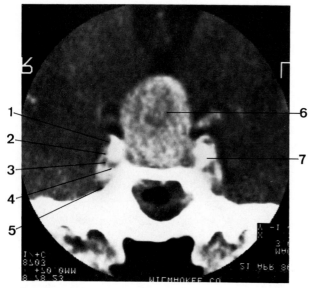

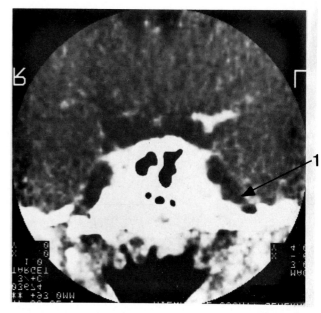

1. oculomotor nerve (III) 2. trochlear nerve 3. ophthalmic nerve (V$_1$)
4. abducens nerve (VI) 5. maxillary nerve (V$_2$) 6. pituitary adenoma
7. internal carotid artery

1. Meckel's cave

Figure 10-9 Coronal CT of a pituitary macroadenoma. The tumor enhances to a lesser degree than the cavernous sinuses. Note cranial nerves III–VI, which appear as filling defects in the enhanced cavernous sinuses. (*From Daniels 1985a.*)

Figure 10-10 Meckel's cave in a coronal CECT through the posterior aspect of the cavernous sinuses. The cave (arrow) has the density of CSF. (*From Daniels 1985a.*)

10-10, 10-11). A portion of the internal carotid artery lies within the cavernous sinus. Cranial nerves, Meckel's cave, and portions of the internal carotid artery can be identified within the enhanced cavernous sinuses in CT, especially when dynamic scanning is used (Kline 1981).

In MR, the anatomy of the cavernous sinus is effectively shown (Daniels 1985). Flowing blood in the cavernous venous sinuses and in the carotid artery has a negligible signal in most T$_1$- or T$_2$-weighted sequences (Fig. 10-8). Meckel's cave is nearly isointense with CSF, that is, hypointense in T$_1$-weighted and hyperintense in T$_2$-weighted images (Fig. 10-11). The dural margin of the sinus has a hypointense signal in either T$_1$- or T$_2$-weighted images. The nerves have a signal intensity similar to white matter in the corpus callosum. After intravenous MR contrast medium injection, the signal intensity (in T$_1$-weighted images) in the cavernous sinuses, nerves, dura, and gland increases.

The suprasellar cistern contains the hypothalamus, optic chiasm, infundibulum, and mammillary bodies (Peyster 1984; Daniels 1980, 1984b). The optic chiasm, because of the surrounding cerebrospinal fluid, can be demonstrated effectively in either axial or coronal CT or MR images (Figs. 10-8, 10-12). In axial images through the lower part of the chiasm and adjacent optic nerves a U-shaped structure is identified. Slightly higher sections showing portions of the chiasm and proximal optic tracts show a boomerang-shaped structure. In a slice intermediate between these two levels, the chiasm has a butterfly shape. In coronal images, the optic chiasm together with the adjacent hypothalamus appear as a U-shaped structure just below the teardrop-shaped optic recess (Fig. 10-12). Coronal sections slightly anterior to this level show a dumbbell-shaped structure representing the junction of the optic nerves and optic chiasm. Immediately posterior to the chiasm in axial images, the infundibulum can be identified

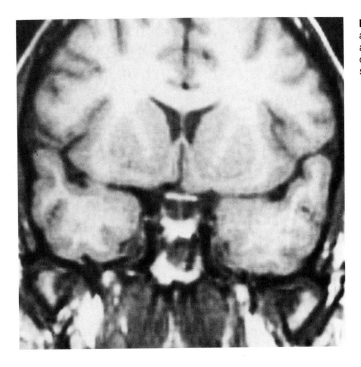

Figure 10-11 Coronal T$_1$-weighted MRI through the posterior aspect of the sella. Meckel's cave, containing neural structures and cerebrospinal fluid, has slightly greater signal intensity than cerebrospinal fluid. Fat in the dorsum sellae has a hyperintense signal, the cavernous internal carotid arteries negligible signal.

as a round structure which enhances with intravenous contrast medium in both CT and MR. Behind the infundibulum are the mammillary bodies. In coronal images the infundibular recess of the third ventricle appears slitlike and pointed inferiorly immediately above the infundibulum. In axial sections the suprasellar cistern appears either pentagonal or hexagonal, depending on whether the section is at the level of the pons or the mesencephalon.

PATHOLOGY

Pituitary Adenomas

The most common intrasellar tumors are pituitary adenomas. They are classified as macroadenomas (larger than 1 cm in diameter) which usually present because of pituitary insufficiency or bitemporal visual field impairment or are found in the evaluation of an incidentally discovered enlarged sella, or as microadenomas (less than 1 cm in diameter) which present as excessively secreting prolactin (amenorrhea and/or galactorrhea), ACTH (Cushing's disease), or HGH (gigantism or acromegaly) (Merritt 1969; Chason 1971; Post 1980). Pituitary adenomas are usually solid, encapsulated tumors that may have necrotic, cystic, hemorrhagic, or calcified regions. The pituitary adenomas which cause hypersecretion are usually diagnosed very accurately by serum assays. However, medications (e.g., alpha methyldopa, reserpine, phenothiazines, butyrophenones, tricyclic antidepressants, oral contraceptives) or diseases that involve the hypothalamus or pituitary gland (e.g., sarcoidosis, histiocytosis, neoplasm, hypothyroidism, renal failure, or severe stress) may cause false-positive elevated serum prolactin levels.

The CT diagnosis of microadenomas is sensitive and precise, if the patients are appropriately selected and if the CT and clinical findings are correlated. The most common microadenoma, the prolactin-secreting adenoma or prolactinoma, typically produces some enlargement of the pituitary gland and a discrete hypodense region within the en-

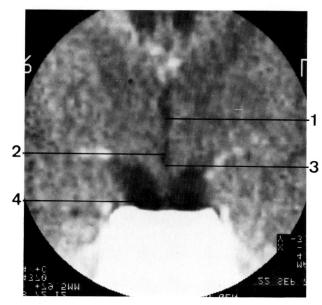

1. third ventricle **2.** infundibular recess **3.** tuber cinereum
4. infundibulum

A

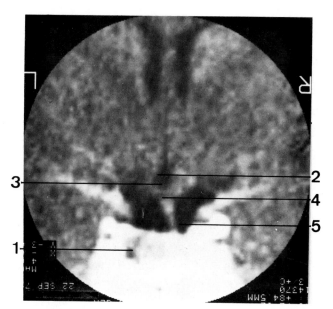

1. pituitary microadenoma **2.** optic recess **3.** hypothalamus **4.** optic
chaism **5.** infundibulum

B

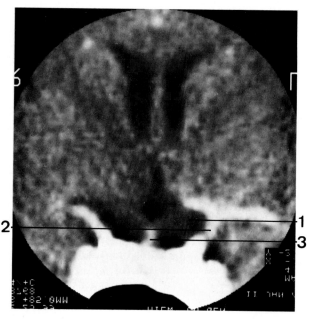

1. optic chaism **2.** internal carotid artery **3.** infundibulum

C

Figure 10-12 Coronal CECT from posterior to anterior through
the optic chiasm and hypothalamus in which **(A)** the tuber cinereum appears conical and the infundibular recess of the third ventricle is thin and inferiorly pointed, **(B)** the optic chiasm and adjacent hypothalamus together appear U-shaped and the optic recess
of the third ventricle has a teardrop shape, and **(C)** the optic chiasm
appears dumbbell-shaped near its attachment point with the optic
nerves. Note that the infundibulum is deviated from the midline in
B owing to a low-density pituitary microadenoma. (*From Daniels
1980.*)

hanced gland (Fig. 10-13). (Hemminghytt 1983; Syvertsen 1979). Usually the upper surface of the gland is convex and the height of the gland is greater than 9 mm. However, a gland may have a normal size and contour and still contain a small prolactinoma appearing as a hypodense area. CT findings which are not specific for intrasellar tumor include thinning or asymmetry of the sellar floor, displacement of the infundibulum from the midline, or displacement of the "capillary tuft" (Bonneville 1983; Syvertsen 1979; Roppolo 1983*b*). Small cysts may simulate prolactin-secreting adenomas; therefore, the diagnosis of prolactinoma should not be made in a patient without evidence of hyperprolactinemia. In adolescents or menstruous females with normal prolactin levels, nonhomogeneity or slight enlargement of the gland should not be interpreted as evidence of a prolactinoma (Wolpert 1984; Gardeur 1982; Swartz 1983). Serial CT imaging may be indicated in patients who are undergoing bromocriptine treatment to demonstrate shrinkage of the adenoma (Fig. 10-14).

HGH- and ACTH-secreting adenomas produce less distinctive CT findings (Figs. 10-15, 10-16). (Hemminghytt 1983). Because the tumors are less well encapsulated and less discrete, hypodense regions within the gland are identified less regularly. Furthermore, the gland may have minimal enlargement. Therefore, in a patient with the appropriate clinical symptomatology and chemical findings, the CT demonstration of a normal-sized and homogeneously enhancing pituitary gland does not exclude the diagnosis of adenoma.

Macroadenomas are reliably and accurately identified by CT (Fig. 10-17). Macroadenomas are isodense or slightly less dense than the cavernous sinuses in CECT (Daniels 1981). A macroadenoma usually enlarges the sella, compresses the sphenoid sinus, or encroaches on the suprasellar cistern and possibly displaces the chiasm or temporal lobes. A solid adenoma enhances homogeneously; cystic or necrotic regions appear as zones of hypodensity within it. In atypical cases calcification is identified in the rim of the tumor, or even less commonly,

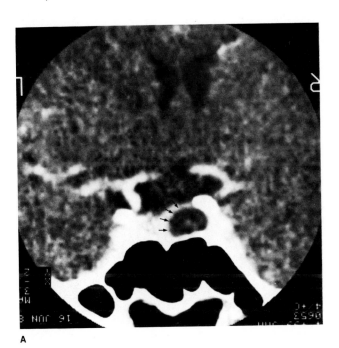 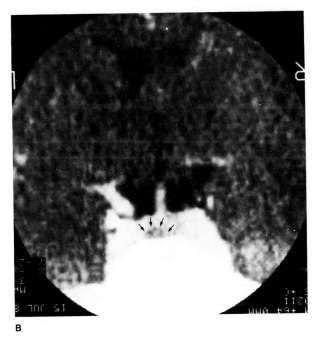

A   B

Figure 10-13 Two examples of prolactinomas (arrows) that appear in coronal CECT as hypodense regions in the gland. The pituitary gland is enlarged in one case (**A**) but not in the other (**B**). (*From Hemminghytt 1983.*)

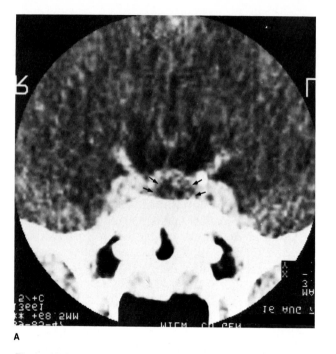

A

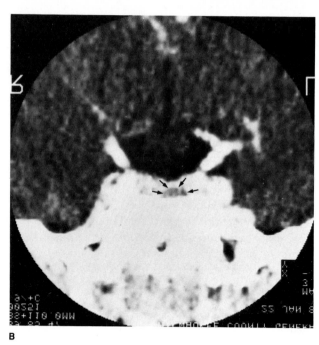

B

Figure 10-14 Effect of bromocriptine on a pituitary microadenoma. Coronal CECT shows a hypodense region (arrows, **A**) that decreases in size during bromocriptine therapy (arrows, **B**). (*From Daniels 1985a.*)

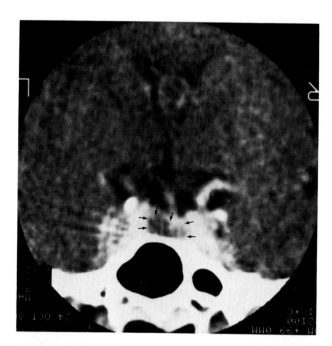

Figure 10-15 ACTH-secreting microadenoma in coronal CECT. The tumor (small black arrows) appears as a hypodense region that displaces the infundibulum. (*From Hemminghytt 1983.*)

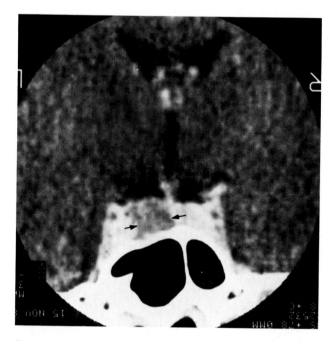

Figure 10-16 HGH-secreting microadenoma. Coronal CECT shows a hypodense region (small black arrows) associated with mild gland enlargement. (*From Hemminghytt 1983.*)

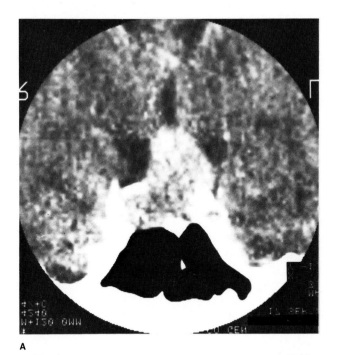

A

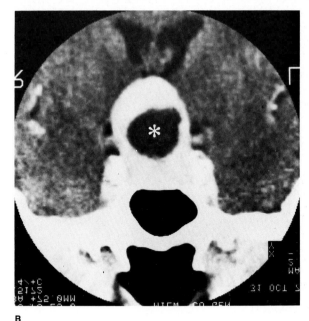

B

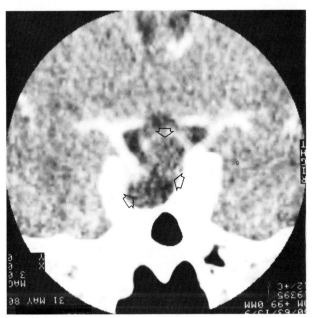

C

Figure 10-17   Examples of pituitary adenomas with solid **(A)** partially necrotic (asterisk * in **B**) and cystic (open arrows in **C**) regions. Necrotic tissue and fluid are not distinguishable with CT. (*From Hemminghytt 1983.*)

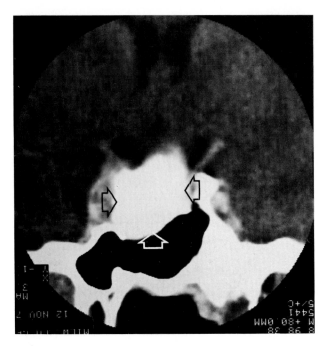

Figure 10-18   Atypical pituitary adenoma that is densely calcified (open arrows) in coronal CT. (*From Daniels 1981.*)

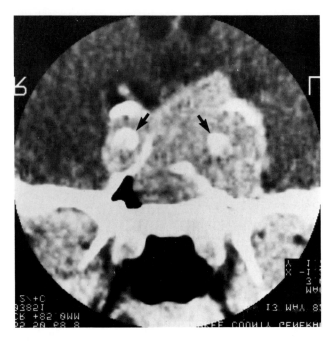

Figure 10-19   Aggressive benign pituitary macroadenoma in coronal CECT. The tumor destroys bone and extends into both cavernous sinuses where it enhances less than the internal carotid arteries (black arrows). (*From Daniels 1985a.*)

homogeneously throughout the tumor matrix (Fig. 10-18) (Gyldenstein 1977; Critin 1977). Rarely pituitary adenomas destroy the skull base or degenerate to carcinoma (Fig. 10-19).

Experience with the MR evaluation of pituitary adenomas is not extensive. However, large solid pituitary adenomas which are effectively demonstrated by MR appear as masses isointense with brain in both T_1-weighted and T_2-weighted images (Lee 1985; Oot 1984; Bilaniuk 1984; Hawkes 1983). Cystic components within the tumor are intermediate in signal intensity between cerebrospinal fluid and tumor. Coronal MR images effectively demonstrate the adenomas which extend upward to the optic chiasm or laterally to obliterate the cavernous sinus (Fig. 10-20). The chiasm when displaced by an adenoma can be identified more effectively by MR than by CT (Bilaniuk 1984). Extension of tumor into the cavernous sinus is characterized by tissue with an intermediate signal replacing the flowing blood in the sinus, by displacement of the cavernous sinus wall, and by encasement of the carotid artery (Daniels

1986). Sagittal MR images are especially useful to demonstrate posterior extension of the tumor and chiasmal compression.

In a small series of prolactin-secreting pituitary microadenomas MR demonstrated the tumors less effectively than did CT (Pojunas 1986). The majority of microadenomas had lesser signal intensity than the normal gland in T_1-weighted images (Fig. 10-21); others with typical CT findings of microadenoma were isointense and a few were hyperintense. The effectiveness of intravenous contrast agents in the MR study of microadenomas has not been measured.

Pituitary tumors occasionally undergo ischemia, necrosis, and hemorrhage since the blood supply to the tumor is impaired as a result of expansion with compression at the opening of the diphragma sellae. The patient shows evidence of a rapidly expanding sellar mass: compression of the third, fourth, and sixth cranial nerves with diplopia (unilateral or bi-

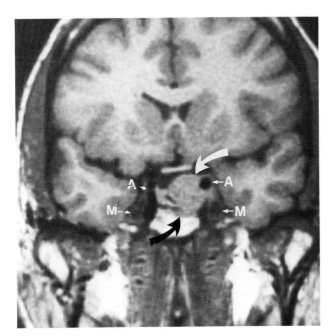

Figure 10-20 A pituitary macroadenoma in coronal T_1-weighted MRI. The tumor (curved arrows) extends to the left cavernous sinus, encases the internal carotid artery **(A)** and deforms Meckel's cave **(M)**.

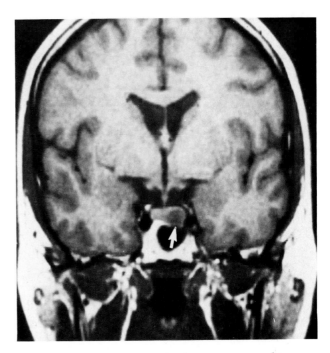

Figure 10-21 Prolactin-producing microadenoma in coronal T_1-weighted MRI. The tumor (arrow) has a signal intensity slightly less than that of normal pituitary gland. The infundibulum is slightly deviated from the midline, and the gland is mildly enlarged.

lateral); optic nerve compression with rapidly decreasing visual impairment; headache; and, occasionally, signs of meningeal irritation (Banna 1976). This apoplectiform attack has been termed *pituitary apoplexy.* The choice of medical or prompt surgical management depends almost exclusively on the status and impending threat to the visual apparatus (Rovit 1985). CT shows evidence of a sellar mass which is either hypodense owing to edema from infarction or shows hyperdensity due to hemorrhage (Fig. 10-22). CT may show only hypodensity in the sella with rim enhancement in a fashion similar to peripheral enhancement seen in cerebral hemorrhages and some infarcts (Post 1980). Pituitary apoplexy may occur spontaneously as indicated but is known to be precipitated by radiotherapy in some instances, presumably as a result of swelling of the mass.

CT study (on new generation scanners) has become the method of choice for complete evaluation of pituitary adenomas of all size. CT provides pre-

cise information and thus is useful in evaluating the results of various treatment modalities not available in the past. Preoperative decision whether the transsphenoidal approach or the intracranial approach can be easily made is based on the size and direction of growth of the adenoma. CT is also useful in demonstrating the amount of residual tumor following surgery, the results of radiation or medical therapy, and in the long-term followup of the patient.

With all the above statements, a word of caution is indicated. Cerebral arteriography, either conventional film-screen or digital subtraction method, is currently the method for reliably detecting the following arterial abnormalities which can considerably complicate pituitary surgery; they are incidental associated internal carotid artery aneurysm, congenital carotid abnormalities including arterial communication between the cavernous portions of the internal carotid arteries, and intrasellar location

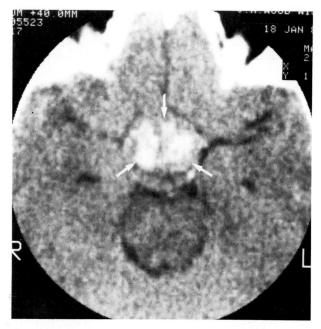

Figure 10-22 Pituitary apoplexy: Hemorrhage (arrows) in a pituitary adenoma is demonstrated in axial NCCT of a patient who suddenly developed right eye blinders. (*From Daniels 1981.*)

of the cavernous portion of the internal carotid artery, intrasellar cavernous carotid aneurysm, and arterial encasement of the tumor. Cerebral arteriography is thus considered by many surgeons to be a necessary component of preoperative evaluation for pituitary adenomas.

Craniopharyngioma

Craniopharyngiomas, which occur at any age, but especially the second and fifth decades of life, are the second most common intrasellar tumor. They are encapsulated, cystic tumors of the sella or the suprasellar region which originate from remnants of Rathke's pouch (Chason 1971). The clinical manifestations are usually hypopituitarism, diabetes insipidus, or hypothalamic or visual symptoms.

The characteristic CT findings of craniopharyngioma are a combination of hypodense areas representing cysts and focal hyperdense areas representing calcifications (Figs. 10-23, 10-24) (Daniels 1981). The cystic components can be extensive, ex-

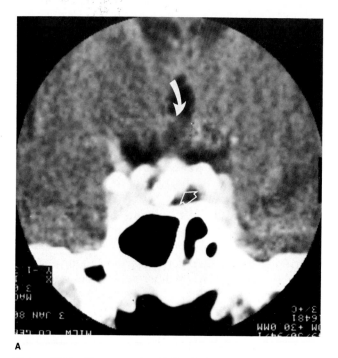

A

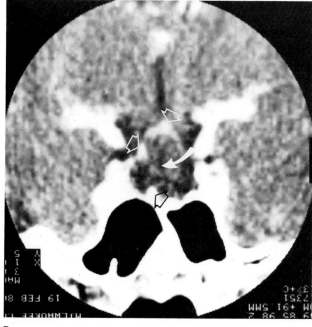

B

Figure 10-23 Two examples (**A,B**) of intra- and suprasellar craniopharyngiomas in coronal enhanced CT. Dense globular calcification (open arrows) and cystic regions (curved arrows) are common. (*From Daniels 1985a.*)

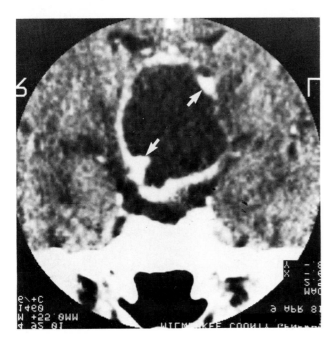

Figure 10-24 Cystic craniopharyngioma in coronal CECT. Rim enhancement and focal rim calcification (straight arrows) are detected. (*From Daniels 1981.*)

tending even into the posterior fossa. Calcification is less common and extensive in adults than in children. Except when the tumors are completely solid and without calcification or cystic areas, they are usually easily distinguished from pituitary adenomas (Fig. 10-25).

MR is unlikely to replace CT for evaluation of craniopharyngioma because MR shows calcification ineffectively. Solid and cystic portions of the tumor may be shown by MR. In some cases, the sagittal images which MR provides complement the study by defining some anatomic relationships effectively.

Meningioma

Meningiomas arise on the dural surface of the anterior clinoic processes, the diaphragma sellae, tuberculum, or dorsum sellae or the cavernous sinuses. Many supra- and parasellar meningiomas have characteristic features which, when detected by CT, permit a specific diagnosis. Globular calcification,

which is less common in parasellar meningiomas than in meningiomas elsewhere, and hyperostotic bone adjacent to the tumor, are common in meningiomas but not in other parasellar neoplasms (Figs. 10-26 to 10-28) (Lee 1976).

With CT meningiomas that lack calcification and hyperostosis are more difficult to distinguish from adenomas and other parasellar tumors (Fig. 10-29). The matrix of a meningioma is usually homogeneous and homogeneously enhancing (Daniels 1981). Rarely meningiomas have cystic, hypodense areas within them (Russell 1980). They may encroach on the suprasellar cistern, displace the brain, invaginate in the temporal lobe, enlarge the cavernous sinus, or very uncommonly, extend through the diaphragma sella into the pituitary fossa. Their margins are always well defined and smoothly marginated. Edema may be present when the brain is compressed. The attachment of the meningioma to the dural surface is usually broad, sessile, and eccentrically located with respect to the sella. Therefore, reformatted sagittal images may help to distinguish adenomas from meningiomas (Fig. 10-30). Angiog-

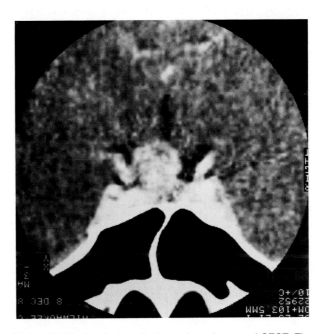

Figure 10-25 Atypical craniopharyngioma in coronal CECT. The tumor homogeneously enhances without calcification of a significant cystic component. (*From Daniels 1985a.*)

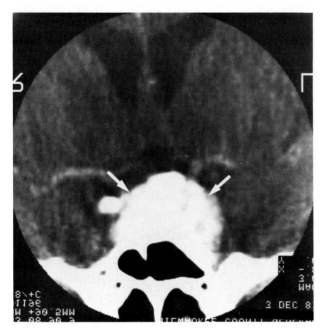

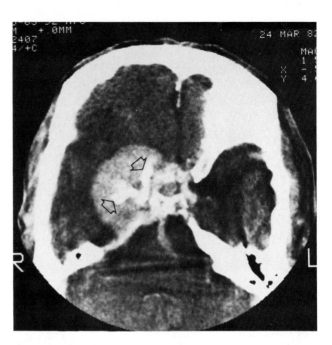

Figure 10-26 Densely calcified meningioma (arrows) in coronal CECT.

Figure 10-27 Axial CECT demonstrates a parasellar meningioma that contains dense globular calcifications (open arrows). (*From Daniels 1985a.*)

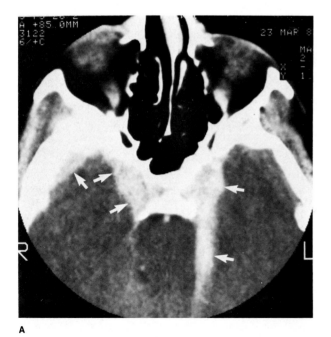

A

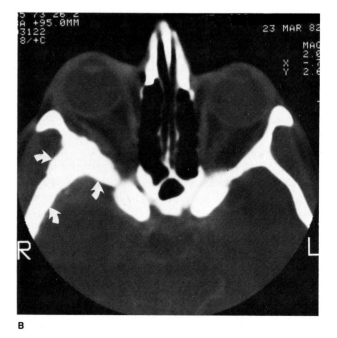

B

Figure 10-28 Parasellar meningioma in axial CT; soft tissue **(A)** and bone **(B)** windows. It spreads along the tentorial reflections and the right sphenoid bone (short arrows in **A**) and has associated sphenoid hyperostosis (curved arrows in **B**). (*From Daniels 1981.*)

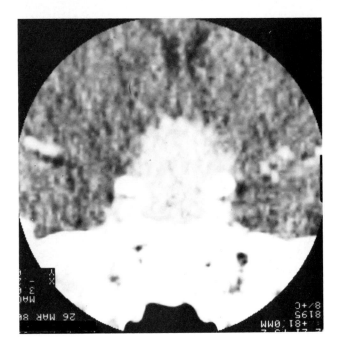

Figure 10-29 Meningioma in coronal CT. Homogeneously enhancing without calcification, the tumor could be mistaken for a pituitary adenoma. (*From Daniels 1985a.*)

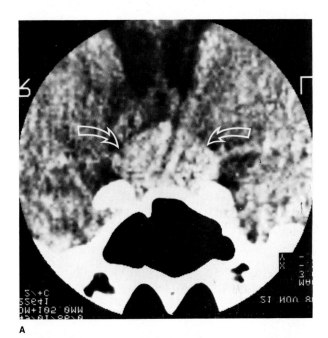

A

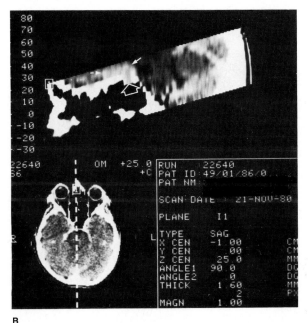

B

raphy may be necessary in questionable cases to identify the characteristic dense stain and dural arterial supply of meningioma from the late faint venous blush and capsular arterial supply of a pituitary adenoma.

Meningiomas which are characteristically nearly isointense with brain in T_1- or T_2-weighted images are not easily detected with MR unless contrast medium is used. After intravenous administration of Gadolinium DTPA, meningiomas have a high signal intensity in T_1-weighted images. Calcification, either globular or psammomatous calcification, may not be recognized in the MR images. Detection of meningiomas and differentiation from adenoma may be difficult. In sagittal images tuberculum sellae meningiomas that are anterior to the sella and pituitary macroadenoma that extends upward and through the diaphragma can be differentiated (Daniels 1986).

Figure 10-30 Example of tuberculum sellae meningioma. The tumor (open curved arrows, **A**) homogeneously enhances and appears somewhat diamond-shaped in coronal CECT. In a sagittal reformatted image **(B)** the tumor (small arrows) is broad-based and centered anterior to a normal-sized sella (open arrow). (*From Daniels 1985a.*)

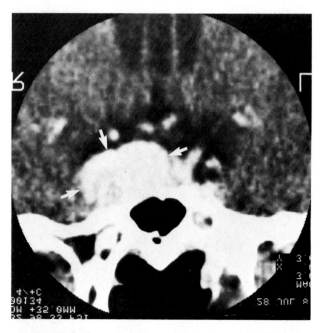

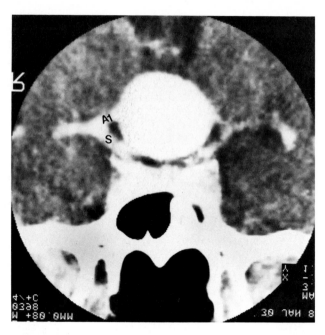

Figure 10-31 Giant aneurysm of the cavernous internal carotid artery (white arrows) with an intrasellar component is demonstrated. Coronal CECT shows intense homogeneous enhancement. (*From Daniels 1985a.*)

Figure 10-33 Anterior communicating artery aneurysm markedly enhances and appears oval-shaped in coronal CECT. S = supraclinoid internal carotid artery; A₁ = A₁ segment of internal carotid artery. (*From Daniels 1985b.*)

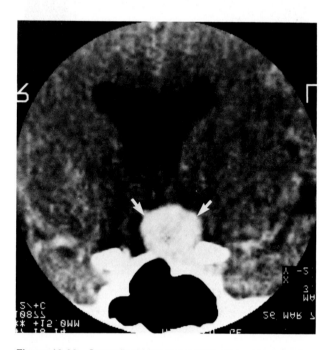

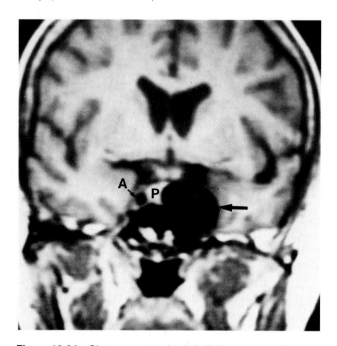

Figure 10-32 Supraclinoid internal carotid artery aneurysm (arrows) in coronal CECT. It has dense homogeneous enhancement. (*From Daniels 1985a.*)

Figure 10-34 Giant aneurysm (arrow) of the cavernous internal carotid artery distorting the pituitary gland (P) in a coronal T₁-weighted MRI. The aneurysm has a hypointense signal with some nonhomogeneity, probably from turbulent blood flow. (A = internal carotid artery.) (*From Daniels 1985a.*)

Aneurysm

Aneurysms are in the differential diagnosis of intra- and parasellar masses (Daniels 1981). The internal carotid artery aneurysms which erode into the sella represent a greater differential diagnostic problem than those that occur in the circle of Willis, especially at the anterior communicating, posterior communicating, internal carotid, and middle cerebral arteries. Especially in coronal images, circle of Willis aneurysms have a characteristic anatomic relationship to the cerebral vessels. In CT the intercavernous and paracavernous ones may appear as homogeneously enhancing rounded or lobulated masses (Figs. 10-31 to 10-33). They may have calcification, especially in the rim, and a nonhomogeneous appearance if organized thrombus enhances less than the lumen and the vessel wall. MR may help characterize juxtasellar aneurysms (Fig. 10-34) (Daniels 1985b). Aneurysms with flowing blood have little signal intensity. Turbulent flow may lead to a nonhomogeneous signal. A thrombosed aneurysm has a higher signal intensity.

Aneurysms present in a number of different ways. They may cause a cranial nerve palsy if they compress the cavernous sinus or visual difficulty if the chiasm is compressed. Severe headache and meningismus is another presentation in those aneurysms that bleed (see Chapter 13).

Chordoma

Chordomas, neoplasm of primitive notochord remnants, are locally invasive, slow-growing neoplasms occurring in the clivus and sphenoid bone. Characteristic CT features are destruction of the adjacent bone in the skull base and a soft tissue mass which is often calcified (Fig. 10-35) (Daniels 1985a). They usually occur in the sixth and seventh decades of life but may occur in the early decades. The degree of CT enhancement and nonhomogeneity is variable. Chordomas are therefore distinctive from most other sellar or parasellar masses except for metastasis. An aggressive pituitary adenoma could conceivably simulate a chordoma.

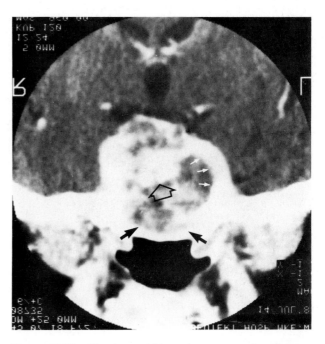

Figure 10-35 Chordoma which nonhomogeneously enhances, has central calcification (open arrow), destroys the skull base (black arrows), and displaces the left cavernous sinus (small white arrows) in coronal CECT.

Metastasis

Metastases to the sellar region are most commonly from lung, breast, kidney, GI tract, or the nasopharynx (Figs. 10-36, 10-37) (Taveras 1976). In CT the metastases, whether primarily to bone or to the pituitary gland, produce a permeative destructive pattern in the sphenoid bone characterized by irregular, indistinct margins. The tumors show a varying degree of enhancement and rarely calcification (Daniels 1981). Differentiation from an aggressive pituitary adenoma and from a chordoma may be difficult. MR effectively demonstrates a malignant tissue invading the pituitary fossa, cavernous sinus, sphenoid sinus, and sellar cortex. Osseous destruction is, however, difficult to demonstrate. Hemorrhagic areas within malignant tumors may appear as hyperintense regions in both T_1- and T_2-weighted images (Gomeri 1985).

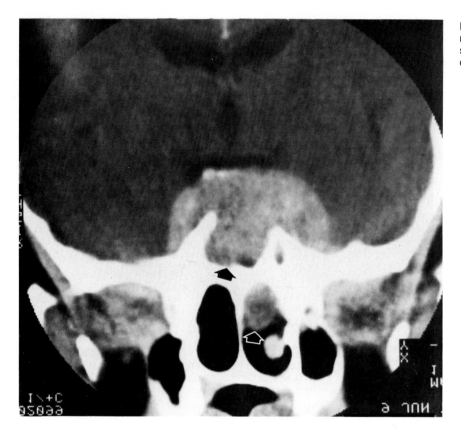

Figure 10-36 Nasopharyngeal carcinoma (open arrow) invades the sphenoid sinus (closed arrow) and sellar region in coronal CECT. (*From Daniels 1985a.*)

Empty Sella

Empty sella is a benign anomaly of the pituitary fossa. Empty sella is associated with incomplete diaphragma sellae either from transient pituitary gland enlargement due to pregnancy or a pituitary tumor, or a congenital weakness of the diaphragma sellae (Taylor 1982). The empty sella usually is an incidental finding, most commonly in women (Taveras 1976). Intrasellar herniation of the optic chiasm has been found with empty sella.

The diagnosis of empty sella may be made in coronal CT or MR images. Although the empty sella is often enlarged, a normal or elongated infundibulum connects the tuber cinereum with the small pituitary gland in the sella. Identification of the infundibulum by CT or MR is facilitated by intravenous contrast administration and thin high-resolution coronal sections (Fig. 10-38) (Haughton 1980). The "infundibulum sign" can be used to differentiate the empty sella from other CSF density processes like a cystic tumor or an intrasellar third ventricle which displaces the infundibulum. In rare cases when the infundibulum cannot be identified in CECT and MR is not available, intrathecally enhanced CT may be used to diagnose empty sella.

Neurinoma

Parasellar neurinomas may arise from cranial nerves III–VI in the cavernous sinus. A neurinoma of cranial nerve V or the Gasserion ganglion characteristically erodes the base of the skull, particularly at the foramen ovale and tip of the petrous pyramid (Fig. 10-39) (Escourolle 1978). These tumors some-

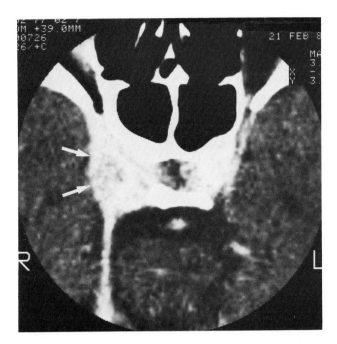

Figure 10-37 Squamosal carcinoma metastatic to the right cavernous sinus is shown by abnormal bulging of the right lateral cavernous sinus margin (long arrows). (*From Daniels 1985a.*)

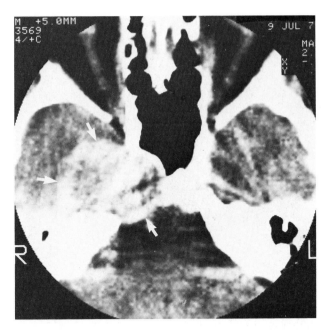

Figure 10-39 Axial CECT of a neurinoma of cranial nerve V (arrows) effaces the skull base by the right petrous apex. It enhances nonhomogeneously.

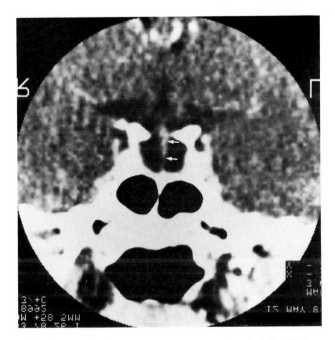

Figure 10-38 Coronal CECT of an empty sella. The infundibulum (arrows) extends to the sellar floor. (*From Daniels 1985a.*)

times show nonhomogeneous enhancement on CECT.

Epidermoid and Dermoid

Epidermoids and dermoids are in the differential diagnosis of suprasellar cystic lesions. Epidermoids have a thin epithelial cyst wall and fluid contents; dermoids have hair, complex dermal elements, calcification, or fat in addition to epithelium (Paul 1972). On CT images, either a dermoid or epidermoid may be isodense with cerebrospinal fluid (5 to 15 HU), like an arachnoid cyst. The presence of calcification or fat in a predominantly cystic lesion suggests a dermoid rather than epidermoid. Intrathecal contrast agent may be required to define the margins of a dermoid or epidermoid that is isodense with CSF. Enlargement of the suprasellar cistern and displacement of the normal cisternal structures such as the chiasm suggest the presence of a cystic suprasellar mass.

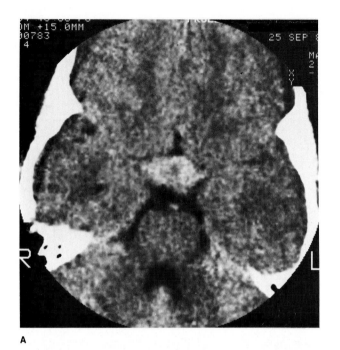

A

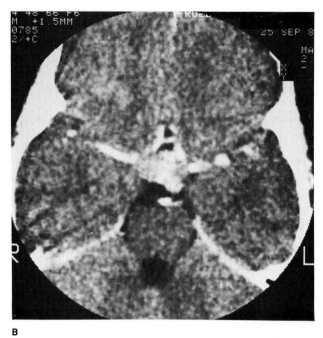

B

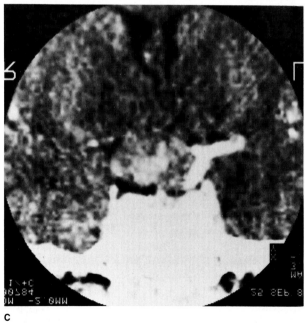

C

Figure 10-40   Chiasmal glioma hyperdense on axial NCCT (**A**) or CECT (**B**) and in coronal (**C**) CECT.

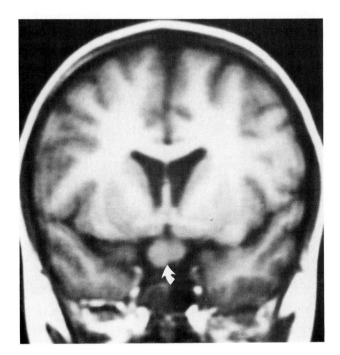

Figure 10-41   Chiasmal glioma (curved arrow) in this coronal T₁-weighted MRI. (*From Daniels 1985a.*)

Chiasmal Glioma

The most common presentation of a chiasmal glioma is in adolescent girls with bilateral visual abnormalities and optic atrophy (Merritt 1969; Miller 1980). Some are associated with neurofibromatosis. In CT or MR, chiasmal gliomas appear as sharply defined globular suprasellar masses (Figs. 10-40, 10-41). Other CT findings of chiasmal gliomas are slightly increased density of the chiasm and sometimes the optic nerves and little contrast enhancement (Daniels 1980). To detect a glioma, the vertical diameter of the chiasm may be measured. A diameter greater than 6 mm indicates a tumor. Optic gliomas must be distinguished from chiasmal neuritis, which has a characteristic clinical picture: the acute onset and rapid progression of visual loss in a young woman. CT shows a normal-sized or slightly enlarged chiasm with variable enhancement. In cases of optic neuritis, vision usually improves after steroid therapy.

Sharply defined contours, globular shape, position below the hypothalamus, and lack of a cystic component and calcification usually distinguish a chiasmal glioma from other suprasellar masses.

Hypothalamic Glioma

Hypothalamic gliomas have a variety of clinical presentations. A hypothalamic astrocytoma in an infant typically produces a syndrome of failure to thrive in spite of adequate caloric intake, unusual alertness, and hyperactivity (Merritt 1969). In a young adult, a hypothalamic glioma usually produces visual symptoms, fever, and altered level of consciousness.

Hypothalamic gliomas typically are large and irregularly contoured masses having markedly enhancing and hypodense regions in CT images (Fig. 10-42). Tumor calcification may be present but difficult to detect in MR images. The cystic components are usually not as large as those associated

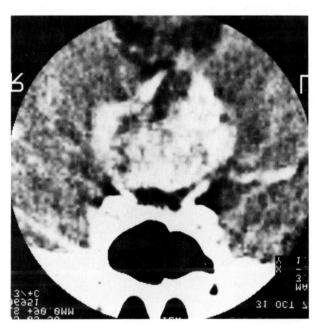

Figure 10-42   Hypothalamic glioma in coronal CECT. It enhances nonhomogeneously. (*From Daniels 1985a.*)

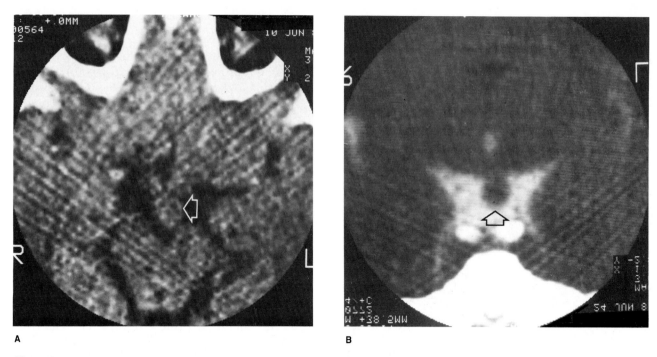

A

B

Figure 10-43 Hamartoma (open arrow) of the tuber cinereum in **(A)** axial NCCT and **(B)** coronal intrathecally enhanced CT.

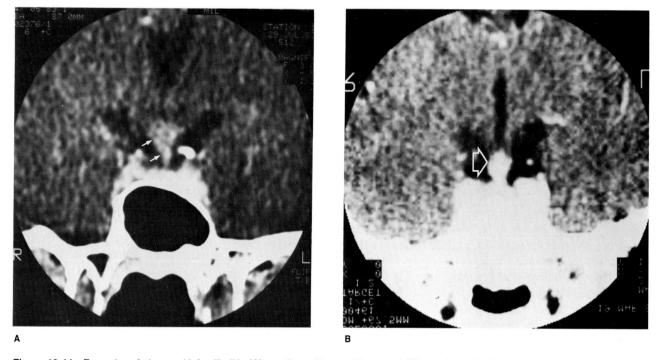

A

B

Figure 10-44 Examples of abnormal infundibuli in **(A)** a patient with sarcoidosis and **(B)** a patient with histiocytosis X. The infundibuli are enlarged and enhanced. (**A** *from Daniels 1985a,* **B** *courtesy of Anne M. Hubbard, M.D. Kansas City.*)

with craniopharyngiomas. A hypothalamic glioma's nonhomogeneity differentiates it from a chiasmal glioma.

Hamartoma of the Tuber Cinereum

A hamartoma of the tuber cinereum is a rare, benign, distinctive lesion with nerve cells similar to those normally present in the tuber cinereum. The tumor presents with precocious puberty, seizures, behavior disorders, or intellectual deterioration (Lin 1978).

On CT it appears as a small mass that is isodense with respect to brain, nonenhancing, sharply defined, smoothly contoured, and attached to the posterior aspect of the hypothalamus between the tuber cinereum and the pons (Fig. 10-43) (Lin 1978). Uncommonly, the mass may be large and densely calcified, resembling a craniopharyngioma.

Infundibular Tumor

Tumors (metastatic carcinoma, especially breast, glioma, lymphoma), histiocytosis X or sarcoid, may involve the infundibulum, causing diabetes insipidus (Chason 1971; Manelfe 1979; Peyster 1984b; Brooks 1982). Involvement of the infundibulum with on of these processes enlarges it to a diameter greater than 4.5 mm or than the basilar artery in axial scans and changes its shape to a cone in coronal CT or MR images (Fig. 10-44). (Peyster 1984a). CT shows an enhancing, usually homogeneous mass. In sarcoid CT may show enhancement of the meningeal granulomas, infiltration of the basal cisterns and leptomeninges, and often hydrocephalus (Chapter 12: Fig. 12-27).

Germ Cell Tumor

Germ cell tumors such as germinomas (atypical teratomas), teratomas, and teratocarcinomas occasionally involve the suprasellar region, sometimes oc-

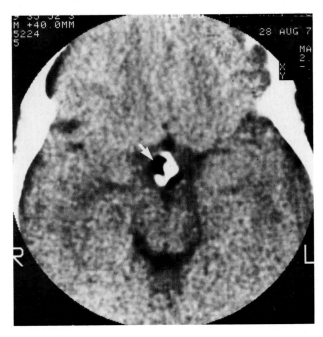

Figure 10-45 Suprasellar teratoma. Axial CT shows fat (arrow) and dense calcification in the tumor. (*From Daniels 1985a.*)

curring as an isolated suprasellar mass and sometimes (germinomas and teratocarcinomas) spreading through the basal cisterns (Futrell 1981).

In CT suprasellar germ cell tumors may be hypodense or hyperdense with respect to brain, homogeneous or nonhomogeneous, enhancing or nonenhancing, and frequently calcified (Figs. 10-45, 10-46) (Futrell 1981).

Solid suprasellar germ cell tumors may resemble glial tumors on CT; a teratoma containing fat or globular calcification may resemble a dermoid or epidermoid.

Arachnoid Cyst

Suprasellar arachnoid cysts may present with hydrocephalus (most commonly in infancy), visual impairment, or endocrine dysfunction (Armstrong 1983). The characteristic CT appearance of these cysts is a CSF density (5 to 15 HU) with no solid or enhancing structures (Gentry 1986a) (Fig. 10-47, 8-28).

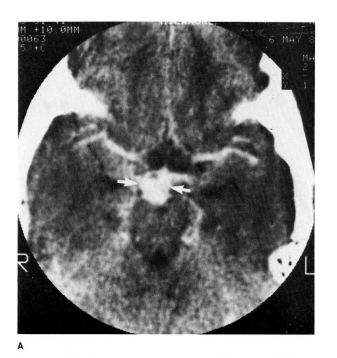

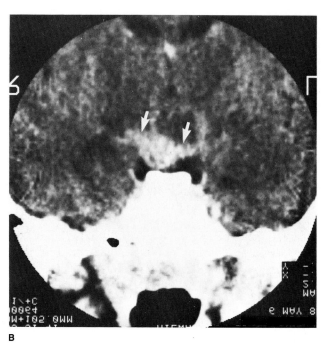

A   B

Figure 10-46   Dysgerminoma (arrows) in **(A)** axial, and **(B)** coronal CECT. The tumor enhances homogeneously. (*From Daniels 1985a.*)

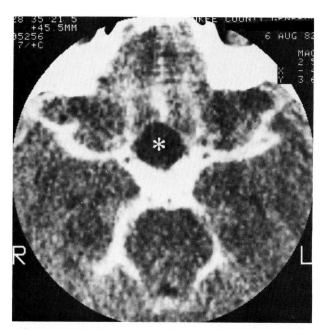

Figure 10-47   Suprasellar epidermoid tumor (asterisk) having hypodensity and a sharply defined contour is shown in axial intrathecally enhanced CT. Preoperatively the differential diagnosis had included arachnoid cyst. (*From Daniels 1985a.*)

Because the capsule is so thin, suprasellar arachnoid cysts are not reliably demonstrated by CT unless intrathecal enhancement is used (Fig. 10-47). Also, investigation of CSF dynamics of cysts by intrathecal contrast CT-cisternography may be valuable in selecting the optimal method of treatment (Gentry 1986*b*). The most important clue to its presence may be an enlarged suprasellar cistern or enlarged pituitary fossa in which no solid tissue or normal structures such as the pituitary stalk or optic chiasm are present. Large arachnoid cysts may be difficult to differentiate from an enlarged third ventricle; small intrasellar arachnoid cysts may suggest an empty sella. An arachnoid cyst can be distinguished from an intraventricular cyst by its location and from a suprasellar epidermoid, a cystic glioma, or a craniopharyngioma by the lack of enhancing or solid or calcified components. Suprasellar epidermoids are rare in infants while arachnoid cysts are not. With intrathecal contrast medium, CT shows the arachnoid cyst as a portion of the suprasellar cistern that fails to opacify and has sharply defined and curvilinear margins (Fig. 10-47).

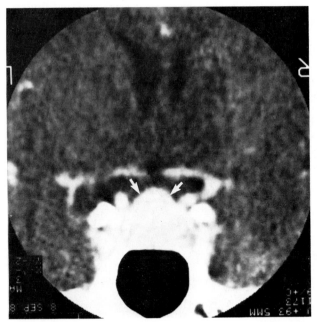

Figure 10-48 Coronal CT study of lymphoid hypophysitis appearing as an enlarged homogeneously enhancing pituitary gland (arrows). The postpartum woman with thyrotoxicosis subsequently had a normal CT study of the pituitary gland. (*From Daniels 1985a.*)

Lymphoid Hypophysitis

Lymphoid hypophysitis is an autoimmune disorder in which lymphocytes infiltrate the pituitary gland. The condition presents usually postpartum with thyrotoxicosis and hypopituitarism.

CT demonstrates an enlarged and homogeneously enhancing pituitary gland, which with treatment, undergoes spontaneous regression (Fig. 10-48) (Hungerford 1982; Quencer 1980; Zeller 1982). The sella is usually normal sized. The CT appearance can simulate a solid pituitary tumor with suprasellar extension.

Pituitary Abscess

Pituitary abscesses are a rare complication of meningitis or sphenoid sinusitis. In the few CT studies of pituitary abscess reported, the abscess has appeared as a hypodense intra- and suprasellar mass having a thin rim of enhancement (Chambers 1982;

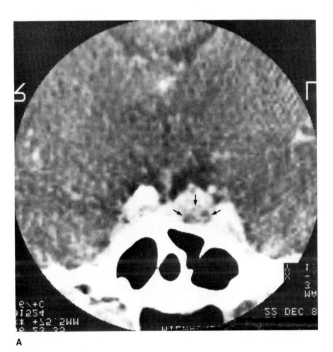

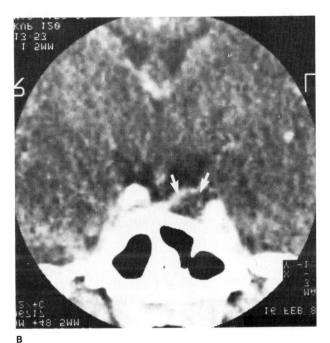

A **B**

Figure 10-49 CECT demonstrates a recurrent prolactinoma. A hypodense region (black arrows in **A**) was proven by transsphenoidal surgery to be a prolactinoma. It recurred (white arrows in **B**).

Enzmann 1983). With radiographic or CT findings alone an abscess cannot be differentiated from other cystic pituitary masses (see Chapter 12).

Postoperative Sella

The bony defect in the sellar floor and soft tissue placed in the sphenoid sinus in transsphenoidal surgery are usually identified with CT.

CT is commonly used to detect residual or recurrent tumor (Fig. 10-49) (Taylor 1982). Fibrotic tissue, muscle, and fat (which may be the result of surgery) have similar densities and degrees of enhancement (Fig. 10-50). They are not usually associated with a convex upward gland contour and contralateral displacement of the infundibulum, which are seen in tumors. Increasing amounts of enhancing intrasellar tissue in sequential CT studies indicate tumor (Waller 1983). CT findings should be correlated with hormonal assays if a hormone-secreting tumor could be present.

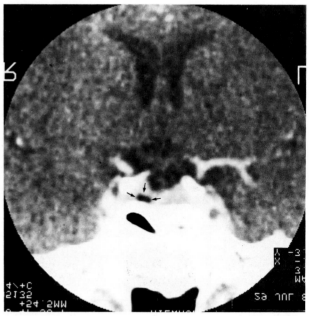

Figure 10-50 Postoperative sella. Fat (black arrows) placed in the sella transsphenoidally after pituitary tumor removal could be confused with a microadenoma if postoperative changes are not recognized.

Bibliography

ARMSTRONG EA, HARWOOD-NASH DCF, HOFFMAN H et al: Benign suprasellar cysts: the CT approach. *Am J Neuroradiol* **4**:163–166, 1983.

BANNA M: Radiology in Hankinson J, Banna M (eds.): *Pituitary and Parapituitary Tumors.* Philadelphia, Saunders, 1976, pp. 135–149.

BELLONI G, BACIOCCO A, BURELLI P et al: The value of CT for the diagnosis of pituitary microadenomas in children. *Neuroradiol* **15**:179–181, 1978.

BILANIUK LT, ZIMMERMAN RA, WEHRLI FW et al: Magnetic resonance imaging of pituitary lesions using 1.0 to 1.5 T field strength. *Radiology* **153**:415, 1984.

BONNEVILLE JF, CATTIN F, MOUSSA-BACHA K et al: Dynamic computed tomography of the pituitary gland: the "tuft sign." *Radiology* **149**:145–148, 1983.

BROOKS BS, GAMMAL TE, HUNGERFORD GD et al: Radiologic evaluation of neurosarcoidosis: role of computed tomography. *Am J Neuroradiol* **3**:513–521, 1982.

CHAMBERS EF, TURSKI PA, LAMASTERS D et al: Regions of low density in the contrast-enhanced pituitary gland: normal and pathologic processes. *Radiology* **144**:109–113, 1982.

CHASON JL: Nervous System and Skeletal Muscle, in Anderson WAD, ed.: *Pathology.* St. Louis, Mosby, pp. 1403–1428, 1796–1799, 1838–1842, 1971.

COHEN WA, PINTO RS, KRICHEFF II et al: Dynamic CT scanning for visualization of the parasellar carotid arteries. *Am J Neuroradiol* **3**:185–189, 1982.

CRITIN CM, DAVIS DO: Computed tomography in the evaluation of pituitary adenomas. *Invest Radiology* **12**:27–35, 1977.

DANIELS DL, HAUGHTON VM, WILLIAMS AL et al: Computed tomography of the optic chiasm. *Radiology* **137**:123–127, 1980.

DANIELS DL, WILLIAMS AL, THORNTON RS et al: Differential diagnosis of intrasellar tumors by computed tomography. *Radiology* **141**:697–701, 1981.

DANIELS DL, POJUNAS KW, PECH P, HAUGHTON VM: Magnetic resonance imaging of the sella and juxtasella region. General Electric Company, 1984*a*.

DANIELS DL, HERFKINS R, GAGER WE, MAYER GA, KOEHLER PR, WILLIAMS AL, HAUGHTON VM: Magnetic resonance imaging of the optic nerves and chiasm. *Radiology* **152**:79–83, 1984*b*.

DANIELS DL: The Sella and Juxtasellar Region, in Williams AL, Haughton VM: *Cranial Computed Tomography: A Comprehensive Text.* St. Louis, Mosby, 1985*a*, pp. 444–511.

DANIELS DL, PECH P, MARK L, POJUNAS K, WILLIAMS AL, HAUGHTON VM: Magnetic resonance imaging of the cavernous sinus. *Am J Neuroradiol* **6**:187–192, 1985*b*.

DANIELS DL, POJUNAS KW, KILGORE DP, PECH P, MAYER GA, WILLIAMS AL, HAUGHTON VM: MR imaging of the diaphragma sellae. *Am J Neuroradiol* **7**:765–769, 1986.

DANIELS DL, PECH P, POJUNAS KW, KILGORE DP, WILLIAMS AL, HAUGHTON VM: Magnetic resonance imaging of the trigeminal nerve. *Radiology* in press.

EARNEST F IV, MCCULLOUGH EC, FRANK DA: Fact or artifact: an analysis of artifact in high-resolution computed tomographic scanning of the sella. *Radiology* **140**:109–114, 1981.

ENZMANN DR, SIELING RS: CT of pituitary abscess. *AJNR* **4**:79–80, 1983.

ESCOUROLLE R, POIRIER J: *Manual of Basic Neuropathology.* Philadelphia, W.B. Saunders, 1978, pp. 48–49.

FUTRELL NN, OSBORN AG, CHASON BD: Pineal region tumors: computed tomographic-pathologic spectrum. *Am J Neuroradiol* **2**:415–420, 1981.

GARDEUR D, NAIDICH TP, METZGER J: CT analysis of intrasellar pituitary adenomas with emphasis on patterns of contrast enhancement. *Neuroradiol* **20**:241–247, 1981.

GARDEUR D, METZGER J: Pathologic sellaire, Ellipses. 1982, Paris, France, p. 10.

GENTRY LR, SMOKER WR, TURSKI PA et al: Suprasellar arachnoid cysts: 1. CT Recognition *AJNR* **7**:79–86, 1986*a*.

GENTRY LR, MENEZES AH, TURSKI PA et al: Suprasellar arachnoid cysts: 2. Evaluation of CSF Dynamics. *AJNR* **7**:87–96, 1986*b*.

GOMERI, JM, GROSSMAN RI, GOLDBERG HI, ZIMMERMAN RA, BILANIUK LT: Intracranial hematomas: imaging by high-field MR. *Radiology* **157**:87–93, 1985.

GYLDENSTEIN C, KARLE A: Computed tomography of infra- and juxta-sellar lesions. A radiological study of 108 cases. *Neuroradiol* **14**:5–13, 1977.

HAUGHTON VM, ROSENBAUM AE, WILLIAMS AL et al: Recognizing the empty sella by CT: The infundibulum sign. *Am J Neuroradiol* **1**:527–529, 1980.

HAWKES RC, HOLLAND GN, MOORE WS, CORSTON R, KEAN DM, WORTHINGTON BS: The application of NMR imaging to the evaluation of pituitary and juxtasellar tumors. *AJNR* **4**:221–222, 1983.

HEMMINGHYTT S, KALKHOFF RK, DANIELS DL et al: Computed tomographic study of hormone-secreting microadenomas. *Radiology* **146**:65–69, 1983.

HUNGERFORD GD, BIGGS J, LEVINE JH et al: Lymphoid adenohypophysitis with radiologic and clinical findings resembling a pituitary tumor. *Am J Neuroradiol* 3:444–446, 1982.

KLINE LB, ACKER JD, POST MJD et al: The cavernous sinus: A computed tomographic study. *Am J Neuroradiol* 2:229–305, 1981.

LEE KF: The diagnostic value of hyperostosis in midline subfrontal meningioma. *Radiology* 119:121–130, 1976.

LEE BCP, DECK MDF: Sellar and juxtasellar lesion detection with MR. *Radiology* 157:143–147, 1985.

LIN S-R, BRYSON MM, GOBLEN RP et al: Radiologic findings of hamartomas of the tuber cinereum and hypothalamus. *Radiology* 127:697–703, 1978.

MANELFE C, LONVEY JP: Computed tomography in diabetes insipidus. *J Comput Assist Tomogr* 3:309–316, 1979.

MARK L, PECH P, DANIELS D, CHARLES C, WILLIAMS A, HAUGHTON V: The pituitary fossa: a correlative anatomic and MR study. *Radiology* 153:453–457, 1984.

MERRITT HH: *A Textbook of Neurology.* Philadelphia, Lee & Febiger, 1969, pp. 243–254, 269–279, 281–282.

MILLER JH, PENA AM, SEGALL HD: Radiological investigation of sellar region masses in children. *Radiology* 134:81–87, 1980.

OOT R, NEW PFJ, BUONANNO FS et al: MR imaging of pituitary adenomas using a prototype resistive magnet: preliminary assessment. *AJNR* 5:131–137, 1984.

PAUL, LW, JUHL H: *The Essentials of Roentgen Interpretation.* Hagerstown, Md., Harper & Row, 1972, pp. 366–372, 375.

PEYSTER RG, HOOVER ED, ADLER LP: CT of the normal pituitary stalk. *Am J Neuradiol* 5:45–47, 1984a.

PEYSTER RG, HOOVER ED: CT of the abnormal pituitary stalk. *Am J Neuroradiol* 5:49–52, 1984b.

PINTO RS, COHEN WA, KRICHEFF II et al: Giant intracranial aneurysms: rapid sequential computed tomography. *Am J Neuroradiol* 3:495–499, 1982.

POJUNAS K, DANIELS D, WILLIAMS A, HAUGHTON V: MR imaging of prolactin-secreting microadenomas. *Am J Neuroradiol* 7:209–213, 1986.

POST MJD, DAVID NJ, GLASEN JS et al: Pituitary apoplexy: diagnosis by computed tomography. *Radiology* 134:665–670, 1980.

QUENCER RM: Lymphocytic adenohypophysitis: autoimmune disorder of the pituitary gland. *Am J Neuroradiol* 1:343–345, 1980.

REICH NE, ZELCH JV et al: Computed tomography in the detection of juxtasellar lesions. *Radiology* 118:333–335, 1976.

ROPPOLO HMN, LATCHAW RE: Normal pituitary gland: 2. microscopic anatomy–**CT** correlation. *Am J Neuroradiol* 4:937–944, 1983a.

ROPPOLO HMN, LATCHAW RE, MEYER JD et al: Normal pituitary gland: 1. macroscopic anatomy—CT correlation. *Am J Neuroradiol* 4:927–935, 1983b.

ROVIT RL: Pituitary apoplexy, in Wilkins RH and Rengachary SS (eds.), *Neurosurgery.* vol. 1. New York, McGraw-Hill, 1985, pp. 879–883.

RUSSELL EJ, GEORGE AE, KRICHEFF II et al: Atypical computed tomographic features of intracranial meningioma: radiological-pathological correlation in a series of 131 consecutive cases. *Radiology* 135:673–682, 1980.

SWARTZ JD, RUSSELL KB, BASILE BA et al: High resolution computed tomographic appearance of the intrasellar contents in women of child-bearing age. *Radiology* 147:115–117, 1983.

SYVERTSEN A, HAUGHTON VM, WILLIAMS AL et al: The computed tomographic appearance of the normal pituitary gland and pituitary microadenomas. *Radiology* 133:385–391, 1979.

TAVERAS JM, WOOD EH: *Diagnostic Neuroradiology.* Baltimore, Williams & Wilkins, 1976, pp. 70, 519–537, 736–749.

TAYLOR S: High Resolution Computed Tomography of the Sella, in Leeds NE, ed.: *Radiologic Clinics of North America,* vol. 20, no. 1. Philadelphia, W.B. Saunders, 1982, pp. 207–236.

UMANSKY F, NATHAN H: The lateral wall of the cavernous sinus with special reference to the nerves related to it. *J Neurosurg* **56**:228–234, 1982.

WALLER RM, HOFFMAN JC, TINDALL GT: CT of the sellar and parasellar regions following transsphenoidal surgery. Scientific exhibit presented at annual meeting of the Radiological Society of North America, Chicago, 1983.

WING SD, ANDERSON RE, OSBORN AG: Dynamic cranial computed tomography: preliminary results. *Am J Neuroradiol* **1**:135–139, 1980.

WOLPERT SM, POOL KD, BILLER BJ et al: The value of computed tomography in evaluating patients with prolactinomas. *Radiology* **131**:117–119, 1979.

WOLPERT SM, MOLITCH ME, GOLDMAN JA et al: Size, shape and appearance of the normal female pituitary gland. *Am J Neuroradiol* **5**:263–267, 1984.

ZELLER JR, CERLETTY JM, RABINOVITCH RA et al: Spontaneous regression of a post-partum pituitary mass demonstrated by computed tomography. *Arch Intern Med* **142**:373–374, 1982.

SECTION B:
THE TEMPORAL BONE

INTRODUCTION

Computed tomography with submillimeter spatial resolution, slice thickness of 2 mm or less, wide CT number range, "bone detail" reconstruction programs, target reconstruction, and high-quality image reformations is effective for evaluating temporal bone pathology (Shaffer 1980; Turski 1982; Shaffer 1985). Compared to pluridirectional tomography CT has superior low-contrast resolution which permits visualization of middle ear muscles, ligaments, and the tympanic membrane, inflammatory disease, and neoplasms (Lufkin 1982; Shaffer 1982; Mafee 1983*a*). There is nearly equivalent bony resolution, resulting in precise evaluation of the ossicles, otic capsule, fractures, and otodystrophies. Conventional pluridirectional tomograms may substitute for CT coronal reformatted scans when direct coronal scans cannot be obtained.

Magnetic resonance (MR) imaging should eventually replace CT and cisternography for evaluating the cerebellopontine angle cisterns and internal auditory canals. Because bone produces negligible MR signal, MR images of the internal auditory canal are minimally affected by partial volume averaging or other artifacts. Therefore, MR can demonstrate the cranial nerves within the internal auditory and the facial nerve canals (Daniels 1984*a,b*, 1985; Reese 1984). MR presently is competitive with CT for imaging acoustic neurinomas (Bydder 1982; Young 1983; New 1985; Kingsley 1985). Intravenous Gadolinium-DTPA increases the sensitivity of MR for cerebellopontine angle and intracanalicular tumors because most of them intensely enhance (Curati 1986).

TECHNICAL ASPECTS

Temporal Bone CT Scanning

Scanning in two planes, usually axial and coronal, is required for optimum demonstration of temporal bone structures. The axial scan plane is parallel to the infraorbitomeatal line to avoid scanning the eyes, and the coronal plane is nearly perpendicular to the axial with the patient supine in a hanging head position. Other gantry angulations for axial and coronal scans have also been suggested to evaluate specific intratemporal structures (Zonneveld 1983; Chakeres 1983). Specialized views, such as semiaxial, sagittal, and Stenvers, must be obtained separately for each ear, and patient positioning is difficult particularly if an angling table is not available.

The technical factors utilized in obtaining CT images depend on the clinical indication for the study. For acoustic neurinoma or other intracranial abnormalities lacking contrast with adjacent tissues, high photon flux is necessary; so high mAs, soft tissue reconstruction algorithm, and narrow windows are used. For osseous pathology or high-contrast structures such as bone and air in the middle ear, low mAs, bone detail reconstruction algorithm and very wide windows are used. If reformatted images are planned because a patient cannot assume the position for coronal scans or because other image planes are needed, then 1.5-mm axial sections at 1-mm intervals provide optimal image detail.

CT Cisternography

CT gas cisternography has replaced Pantopaque cisternography for the diagnosis of small acoustic neurinomas (Sortland 1979; Anderson 1981). Gas CT cisternography is done to diagnose an intracanalicular tumor when a high-resolution contrast-enhanced CT scan suggests tumor or appears negative despite strong clinical evidence of tumor. Gas cisternography is not indicated and not safe in patients with large cerebellopontine angle or intracranial masses; thus it should always be preceded by intravenous CECT.

Several techniques for gas CT cisternography have been described (Pinto 1982; Anderson 1982). A simple and reliable technique is to perform a lumbar puncture with the patient in the lateral decubitus position on a tilt table with his symptomatic side up. After the lumbar subarachnoid space is cannulated with a 22- or 25-gauge needle and the table is tilted approximately 15 to 20 degrees head end up, approximately 5 cm^3 of gas (oxygen, air, CO_2) is

injected. When the gas reaches the cerebellopontine angle cistern, the patient usually reports pressure, pain, buzzing, or popping behind the ear. Subsequently, the patient is positioned horizontally and scanned in the same decubitus position, his head rotated 10 degrees nose up. Several 5-mm-thick scans are used to localize the internal auditory canal and to determine whether adequate gas is present. Then contiguous 1.5-mm-thick scans through the internal auditory canal are obtained, reconstructed with a bone detail algorithm, and viewed at a wide (4000 HU) window width (Fig. 10-51). Gas CT cisternography may be performed on outpatients. The only significant side effect reported has been headache, usually mild to moderate, which nearly all patients experience. Side effects may be minimized by using CO_2, which is more rapidly reabsorbed from the cisternal spaces. Disabling "spinal headaches," which may be treated by epidural blood patch therapy, are rare if large-gauge needles are avoided (Anderson

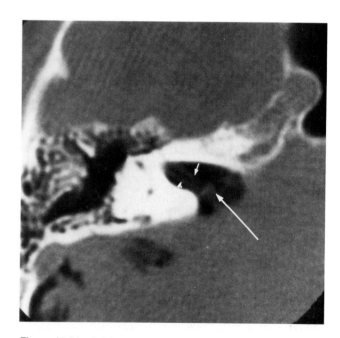

Figure 10-51 Axial scan from a normal air CT cisternogram (oriented similarly to a standard axial scan) with bone detail reconstruction viewed at 4000 HU window. Individual nerves (small arrows) and a probable vascular loop (long arrow) are demonstrated in a mildly widened internal auditory canal. (*From Shaffer 1985.*)

1982; Johnson 1984). Bilateral studies may be obtained without injection of more gas by turning the patient to the opposite decubitus position after images are obtained on the one side (Johnson 1984*a;* Lee 1981).

Temporal Bone MR Imaging

For evaluating the internal auditory canals with a commercial 1.5-T MR system, 3-mm-thick contiguous axial and coronal images through the temporal bones are obtained. A spin echo pulse sequence with a short repetition time (TR) of 600 to 800 msec and a short echo time (TE) of 20 to 25 msec, a 256×256 matrix, and two excitations provides excellent contrast and detail, especially if intravenous Gadolinium-DTPA is used. A spin echo sequence with a long TR (2000 to 2500 msec) and long TE (75 to 100 msec) is sometimes used if Gadolinium is not injected, although the signal to noise ratio is poorer. Head coils are usually used to permit side-to-side comparison. Surface coils provide images with higher spatial resolution of one side. For contrast enhancement, intravenous Gadolinium-DTPA (0.1 mmol/kg) is injected. Acoustic neurinomas, cerebellopontine angle meningiomas, and other benign tumors are enhanced; that is, their signal intensity in T_1-weighted images is increased by 30 to 50 percent.

The cranial nerves are best demonstrated with T_1-weighted MR images (Daniels 1984*a*). In short TR and TE MR images, the cranial nerves are almost isointense with brain in contrast to the hypointense signal from the temporal bone or CSF (Fig. 10-52). In long TR and TE MR (T_2-weighted) images, the nerves are obscured by the hyperintense signal from cerebrospinal fluid (the fluid appears white). The increased resolution provided by surface coil imaging improves the visualization of the individual cranial nerves (Fig. 10-53). (Daniels 1985).

NORMAL ANATOMY

Several articles describe the CT and MR anatomy of the temporal bone in detail (Zonneveld 1983;

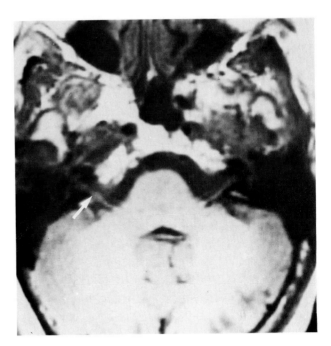

Figure 10-52 The cisternal and intracanalicular segments of cranial nerves VII and VIII (arrow) shown in a T_1-weighted axial MR image.

Chakeres 1983; Swartz 1983*a*). In this chapter, the key landmarks of the temporal bone are emphasized (Figs. 10-54, 10-55).

The temporal bone is composed of the styloid process and tympanic, mastoid, squamous, and petrous portions. The tympanic portion of the temporal bone forms the anterior and inferior walls of the bony external auditory canal. The mastoid portion forms the posterior wall of the external canal and the middle ear, and contains the mastoid air cells and mastoid antrum. The squamous portion superiorly is part of the calvarium, and the petrous portion is a wedge-shaped bone which contains the inner ear.

External Auditory Canal

The shape of the external auditory canal is variable (Virapongse 1983). Its medial two-thirds is bony while

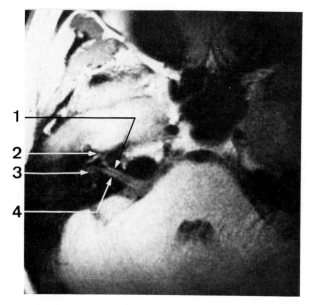

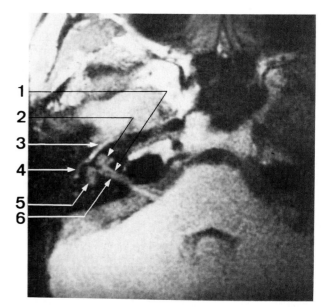

1. facial nerve 2. geniculate ganglion 3. vestibule 4. superior vestibular nerve

1. cochlear nerve 2. cochlea 3. greater superficial petrosal nerve 4. horizontal segment of facial nerve 5. vestibule 6. inferior vestibular nerve

A

B

Figure 10-53 Cranial nerves in the internal auditory canal demonstrated in surface coil MRI. Axial short T_1-WI identify nerves in the upper **(A)** and lower **(B)** parts of the canal.

the rest is cartilagenous. The tympanic membrane forms the sloping medial end of the canal.

Middle Ear

The middle ear is an air-filled chamber which can be subdivided into the epitympanic recess (attic) above the tympanic annulus, the hypotympanum below it, and the mesotympanum medial to it. The eustachian tube provides a communication between the widest (anterior) part of the hypotympanum and the nasopharynx. The epitympanic recess communicates with the mastoid antrum posteriorly via the aditus ad antrum. The mastoid is variably pneumatized depending on hereditary factors and childhood middle ear infections.

The ossicles transmit sound from the tympanic membrane through the middle ear to the oval window. The malleus handle attaches to the tympanic membrane and the head articulates with the body of the incus, which is immediately behind it in the epitympanum. The incus has a long process, which articulates with the stapes, and short process. The malleus and incus appear as an ice cream cone on axial CT scans, with the malleus head representing the ice cream ball and the short process of the incus, the cone (Mancuso 1982). The stapes is the smallest of the ossicles. Its two crura and a footplate in the oval window resemble a stirrup. CT shows the stapedial crura but seldom the obliquely oriented footplate, which is only 0.05 to 0.1 mm thick centrally.

The complex posterior wall of the middle ear including the round window niche, sinus tympani, pyramidal eminence, and facial recess is best visualized in axial CT sections (Swartz 1983). The tensor tympani muscle, stapedius muscle, and ligaments in the posterior middle ear can also often be identified on high-resolution CT scans.

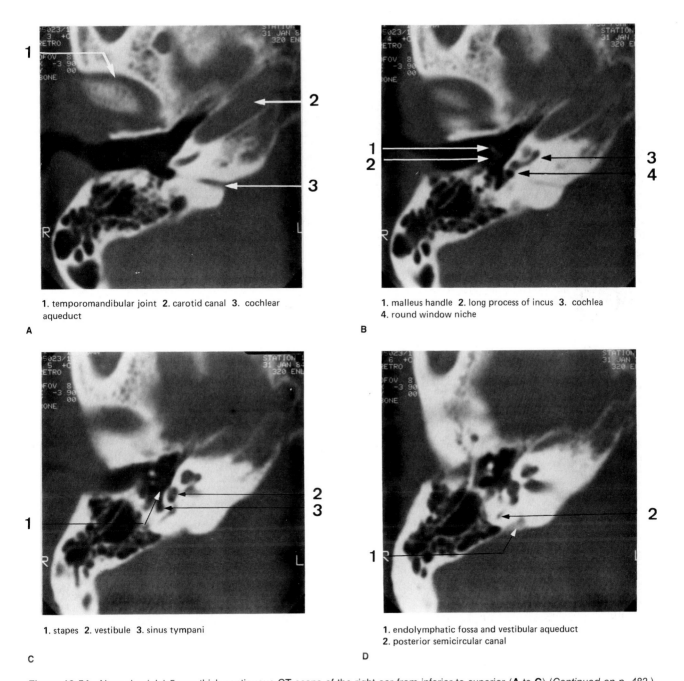

A

1. temporomandibular joint 2. carotid canal 3. cochlear aqueduct

B

1. malleus handle 2. long process of incus 3. cochlea
4. round window niche

C

1. stapes 2. vestibule 3. sinus tympani

D

1. endolymphatic fossa and vestibular aqueduct
2. posterior semicircular canal

Figure 10-54 Normal axial 1.5-mm-thick contiguous CT scans of the right ear from inferior to superior (**A** to **G**) (*Continued on p. 482.*).

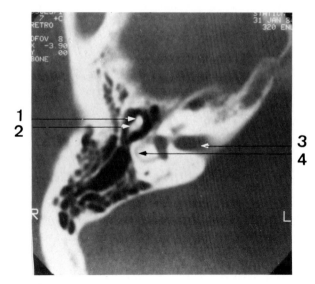

1. malleus head 2. body and short process of the incus
3. internal auditory canal 4. lateral semicircular canal

E

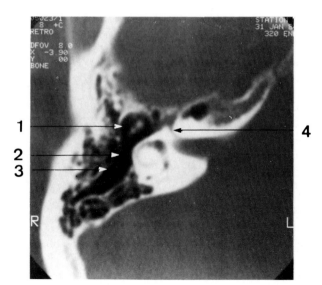

1. attic 2. aditus ad antrium 3. antrum
4. labyrinthine segment of facial nerve canal

F

1. superior semicircular canal 2. common crus between superior
and posterior semicircular canals

G

Figure 10-54 (*cont.*)

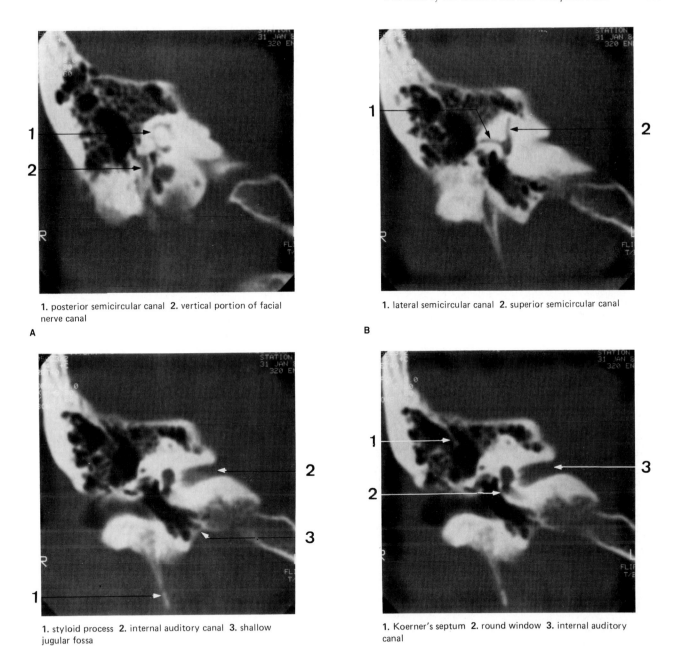

1. posterior semicircular canal 2. vertical portion of facial nerve canal

A

1. lateral semicircular canal 2. superior semicircular canal

B

1. styloid process 2. internal auditory canal 3. shallow jugular fossa

C

1. Koerner's septum 2. round window 3. internal auditory canal

D

Figure 10-55   Normal coronal 1.5-mm-thick contiguous CT scans of the right ear from anterior to posterior (**A** to **G**). (*Continued on p. 484.*)

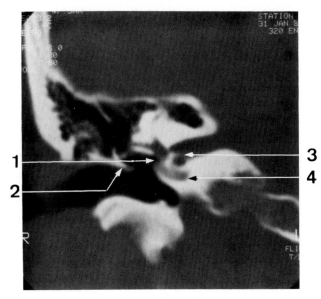

1. oval window **2.** drum spur **3.** falciform crest **4.** basal turn of cochlea

E

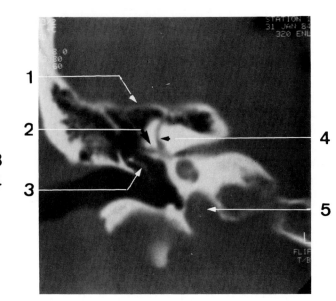

1. tegmen **2.** lateral semicircular canal **3.** incus **4.** superior semicircular canal **5.** carotid canal

F

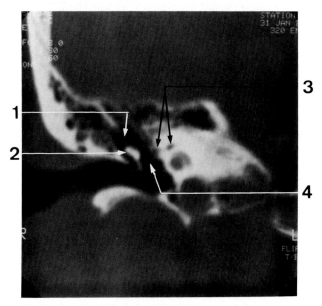

1. attic **2.** malleus **3.** limbs of facial nerve canal **4.** tensor tympani muscle

G

Figure 10-55 *(cont.)*

Labyrinth

The bony labyrinth is located in the inner ear. The membranous labyrinth, containing primarily perilymph and an endolymphatic space surrounded by perilymph in the cochlea, is inside the bony labyrinth. Sound waves, transmitted through ossicular chain, are transferred through the oval window to the perilymph and the organ of Corti in the endolymphatic space to produce the sensation of sound. The cochlea resembles a snail with 2½ to 2¾ turns. The basal turn of the cochlea in the medial wall of the tympanic cavity forms the cochlear promontory in the middle ear. The round window is an opening in the basal turn of the cochlea, covered by a membrane. The cochlear aqueduct, parallel to and below the internal auditory canal, connects the cochlea and the posteromedial surface of the petrous pyramid to equilibrate perilymph with the cerebrospinal fluid. Posterior and slightly superior to the cochlea, the bony inner ear contains lateral, posterior, and superior semicircular canals, which are connected to the vestibule. The semicircular canals are perpendicular to each other. The posterior semicircular canal is parallel to the posterior surface of the petrous pyramid, which is oriented at approximately 45 degrees to the coronal plane.

Internal Auditory Canal

The internal auditory canal is usually oriented in a nearly coronal plane. The porus acousticus is the medial end of the internal auditory canal. The posterior lip of the porus is well defined, while the anterior wall blends with the petrous apex. The internal canal contains the facial (VII) and cochlear (VIII) nerves anteriorly, separated by the falciform crest, and the superior and inferior divisions of the vestibular (VIII) nerve posteriorly.

The vestibular aqueduct, the bony canal for the endolymphatic duct, originates in the vestibule, and curves superiorly, posteriorly, and then inferiorly to the posterior surface of the temporal bone.

The fascial (VII) nerve has a complex course through the temporal bone. It enters in the antero-superior portion of the internal auditory canal, exits from the anterolateral end of the canal, and extends anteriorly to the geniculate ganglion, which is above the cochlea and where the greater superficial petrosal nerve originates. The facial nerve then reverses its course, passing along the medial wall of the middle ear under the lateral semicircular canal. Posterior to the middle ear at the level of the sinus tympani, the nerve turns approximately 90 degrees to exit inferiorly at the stylomastoid foramen and then continues into the parotid gland. The locations of the geniculate ganglion and of horizontal and vertical portions of the facial nerve are easily identified in CT. MR can demonstrate the facial nerve itself within its canal (Reese 1984).

Jugular Foramen

The jugular foramen, posterior to the temporal bone, is divided into a small anteromedial pars nervosa containing the glossopharyngeal (IX) nerve and the inferior petrosal sinus and a large posterolateral pars vascularis which contains the jugular bulb, vagus (X), and spinal accessory (XI) nerves. The right jugular foramen is often larger than the left because the right jugular vein and sigmoid sinus are larger.

CONGENITAL ANOMALIES

Congenital malformations of the ear usually affect the inner ear or the middle and external ear, but not usually both except in a few specific conditions such as maternal ingestion of thalidomide, chromosomal abnormalities, and craniofacial dysplasias (Hanafee 1980). The inner ear forms during the second and third months from the otocyst, which arises from ectodermal thickening on the side of the head. The auricle, ossicles, and external auditory canal develop from the first and second branchial arches and first branchial groove. The endoderm-lined first pharyngeal pouch forms the tympanic cavity and eustachian tube. Pneumatization of the mastoid begins in the seventh to eighth fetal month and may continue into adulthood. The cartilagenous otic capsule ossifies in the fifth fetal month.

External and Middle Ear

Except for the isolated minor soft tissue malformations of the pinna and external auditory canal, bony anomalies usually coexist in the external canal and middle ear. The bony external auditory canal may be partially filled with soft tissue, hypoplastic or nonexistent (Fig. 10-56). The degree of hypoplasia correlates with mastoid pneumatization. Normal mastoid pneumatization generally indicates a less severe anomaly. When the external canal is atretic, the length of the atretic segment correlates with the severity of ossicular malformation. The temporomandibular joint is usually deformed in patients with congenital anomalies of the external ear. The glenoid fossa may be flattened and the distance from the condyle to the tympanic bone markedly increased (Wright 1981). Other middle ear anomalies which occur with external canal atresia are a deformed, fused incus and malleus, complete or partial absence of the ossicles, and aplasia of the middle ear (Bergstrom 1980).

A common CT finding in these anomalies is a bony plate replacing the tympanic membrane. The middle ear cavity is usually smaller than normal and often not pneumatized. CT may show a misshapen bony mass instead of normal ossicles, fusion of the malleus handle to the atresia plate, no osseous covering over the facial nerve in the middle ear, partial absence of the ossicles, or variable mastoid development and pneumatization. The tympanic portion of the temporal bone may be hypoplastic. In less severe anomalies, abnormal soft tissue may be demonstrated in an otherwise normal canal. In more severe malformations, CT shows an abnormal course of the nerve or a bifid canal through the middle ear. The descending portion of the nerve is frequently

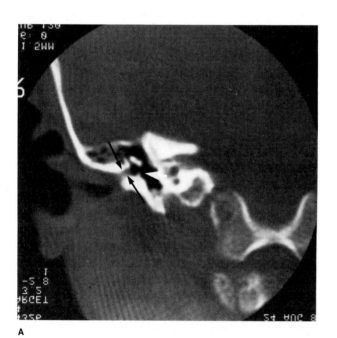

A

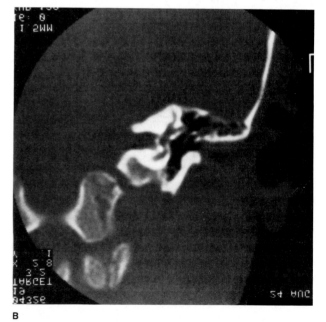

B

Figure 10-56 Congenital atresia of the external auditory canal in coronal CT. In the right ear **(A)**, soft tissue (black arrows) is demonstrated in the narrow bony external auditory canal and the malleus handle may be fused to the atresia plate (white arrow). In the left ear **(B)**, the middle ear and ossicles appear normal, but a similar external canal malformation is present. (*From Shaffer 1985.*)

anteriorly positioned in patients with a contracted tympanic cavity and hypoplastic tympanic bone (Wright 1982; Phelps 1981*a*). The surgeon must know the position of the facial nerve, particularly the vertical portion, before attempting to reconstruct the external auditory canal in a patient with atresia.

Inner Ear

Several malformations of the inner ear, each associated with an eponym, have been described. The rare Michel deformity is total aplasia of the inner ear. The Mondini malformation designates a decreased number of cochlear turns because the apical and intermediate coils are combined as a single cavity, while the Mondini-Alexander malformation includes vestibular abnormalities as well as the cochlear malformation (Fig. 10-57). The Scheibe and Siebenmann-Bing malformations involve the membranous labyrinth only and have no specific CT findings. Another anomaly without an eponym is an abnormally short and broad lateral semicircular canal, which is an incidental finding. Clinical manifestations of severe vestibular and semicircular canal malformations are hearing loss, cerebrospinal fluid leakage into the middle ear, or recurrent episodes of meningitis. The CT findings include enlarged semicircular canals and a sac-shaped cochlea. If CT shows a small internal auditory canal (2 mm or less), eighth nerve atresia should be suspected (Fig. 10-58).

Miscellaneous

A high jugular bulb or aberrant carotid artery may produce a mass in the middle ear (Fig. 10-59). The clinical manifestations include pulsatile tinnitus or hearing loss. The aberrrant internal carotid artery is

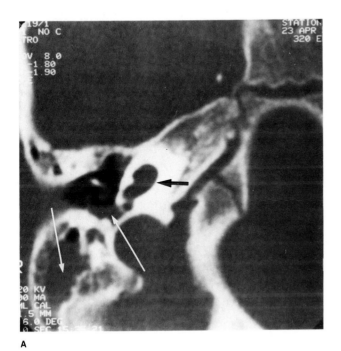

A

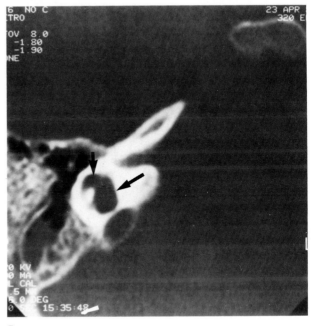

B

Figure 10-57   Mondini-Alexander malformation of the cochlea and vestibule in axial CT. The lower section **(A)** demonstrates fewer cochlear turns than normal (black arrow) and fluid in the middle ear and mastoid (white arrows). In **B** the enlarged vestibule (long arrow) and dilated lateral semicircular canal (short arrow) are identified. (*From Shaffer 1985.*)

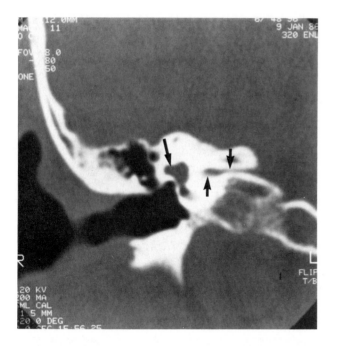

a rare anatomic variant which, if not recognized, may lead to an injudicious attempt at biopsy. Persistance of a primitive vessel, lateral to the normal location of the carotid artery, results in the carotid artery lying within the middle ear. Other anatomic variations, such as a persistent stapedial artery or an aberrant middle meningeal artery, may be associated with these vascular anomalies (Guinto 1972; Damsma 1984; Lo 1985). CT shows a defect in the normal bony covering of the carotid canal or jugular vein. The tissue within the dehiscence and the mass in the middle ear have enhancement similar to that of the carotid artery or jugular vein on dynamic CT scans. If CECT is not confirmatory, angiography should be used to verify the anomaly.

Figure 10-58 Hypoplastic internal auditory canal (short arrows) in a deaf child. Coronal CT also demostrates a bulbous lateral semicircular canal (long arrow).

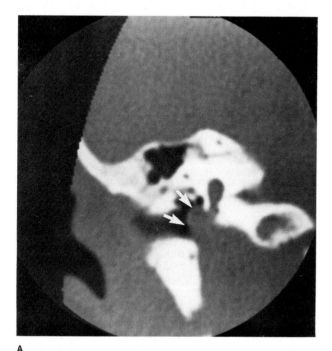

A

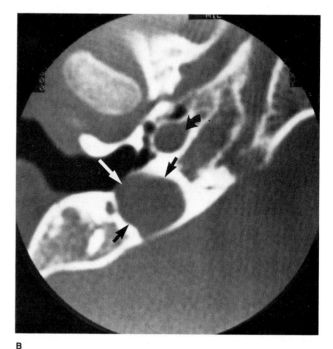

B

Figure 10-59 High jugular bulb (straight arrows) demonstrated in axial **(A)** and coronal **(B)** CT (curved arrow, **A** = carotid canal). In **B**, the bulb lacking a bony covering protrudes into the middle ear. Clinically, it appeared as a bluish mass in the hypotympanum. (*From Shaffer 1985.*)

Axial CT demonstrates the osseous and soft tissue findings in congenital anomalies of the ear as well as or better than tomography. Coronal CT images are necessary to evaluate the bony walls covering the carotid artery and jugular bulb and the vertical portion of the facial (VII) nerve canal.

TRAUMA

Fractures

Thin-section CT is effective for evaluating temporal bone fractures. Temporal bone fractures are classified as longitudinal or transverse by the direction of the major fracture line with respect to the long axis of the petrous pyramid (Kaseff 1969). Fractures may have both longitudinal and transverse components or fit neither classification. The thick (10-mm) CT sections done routinely in nearly all patients with significant head injuries usually fail to detect temporal bone fractures (Holland 1984). To evaluate patients with fractures, more than one scan plane, whether obtained directly or by reformation, is essential (Johnson 1984*b*).

Longitudinal Fractures

Three quarters of temporal bone fractures are longitudinal ones, produced by direct trauma to the temporoparietal region (Fig. 10-60). The longitudinal fracture lines usually pass from the squamous portion of the temporal bone anteriorly and inferiorly through the tegmen tympani, external auditory canal, middle ear, and foramen lacerum. Clinical signs of longitudinal fracture include blood in the external auditory canal, conductive hearing loss, and tympanic membrane tear. The facial nerve is injured in a quarter of cases. Facial weakness or paralysis occurring with some delay after trauma and resolving spontaneously is probably due to edema of the nerve. Paralysis that occurs immediately after trauma suggests a bone fragment in the facial nerve canal or nerve disruption. Temporal bone fractures may

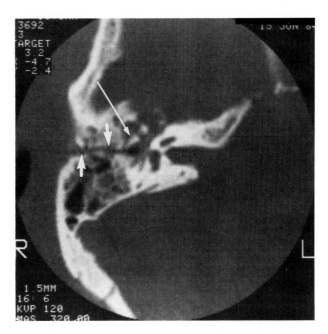

Figure 10-60 Axial CT scan showing longitudinal fracture (short arrows) through the right mastoid. Also noted is dislocation of the incus (long arrow) from the malleus appearing as ice cream cone separated from its scoop. (*From Shaffer 1985.*)

also cause pneumocephalus, cerebrospinal fluid leak manifested as otorrhea, or temporal lobe herniation into the temporal bone if a large defect is produced in the tegmen.

Longitudinal temporal bone fractures may cause ossicular dislocation or fractures. The incus, because of its relatively loose attachments to the malleus and stapes, is dislocated more frequently than the malleus, which is anchored to the tympanic membrane, or the stapes, which is fixed in the oval window. When the malleus or stapes is fractured or dislocated, the incus is usually also involved (Wright 1974).

Longitudinal fractures can be accurately identified on axial CT scans. The tegmen, drum spur, and facial nerve canal are best evaluated on coronal images. The CT findings in longitudinal fractures include fracture lines in the mastoid and fluid or air-fluid levels in the air cells (Fig. 10-60). If the incus is subluxed or dislocated or the ossicular chain is more severely disrupted, the "ice cream cone" shape of the malleus and incus is distorted. The malleus and incus, which are normally equidistant from the medial and lateral attic walls, may be displaced. The stapes is usually obscured in CT sections when blood is present in the middle ear. When facial nerve paralysis is present, the course of the facial nerve should be inspected. Longitudinal fractures commonly injure the facial nerve near the geniculate ganglion (Holland 1984).

Transverse Fractures

Although transverse fractures of the temporal bone are less common than longitudinal ones and are not usually produced by trauma directly to the temporal bone, the clinical manifestations are usually more severe. Transverse fractures, crossing the long axis of the petrous pyramid, usually injure the bony labyrinth and may extend laterally to the middle ear. Clinical findings include vertigo, sensorineural hearing loss, and facial nerve paralysis (approximately 50 percent of patients). Dural tears with cerebrospinal fluid leakage (as rhinorrhea when the tympanic membrane is intact), blood and fluid in the middle ear, and facial nerve paralysis which seldom recovers spontaneously are common.

Transverse fractures are seen equally well on axial or coronal scans, which are perpendicular to the fracture planes. CT findings include fracture lines through the internal auditory canal, cochlea, vestibule, semicircular or facial nerve canals, and occasional opacification of the middle ear or mastoid.

Other Fractures

Trauma to the mandible may fracture the anterior wall of the external auditory canal. This injury usually does not involve the middle ear or inner ear. Bleeding and deformity of the external canal are evident otoscopically. These fractures can be identified on axial and sagittal reformatted CT scans or lateral tomograms. Microfractures in the region of the oval and round windows which are not visible on radiographs may cause hearing loss. Occasionally, a direct blow to the mastoid may produce a localized fracture which does not extend into the remainder of the temporal bone. Isolated styloid process fractures may occur, causing facial nerve paresis.

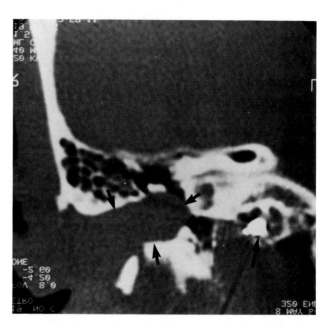

Figure 10-61 Cholesteatoma (short arrows) in the external auditory canal and middle ear in coronal CT. The mass developed after a gunshot wound, one fragment (long arrow) still present near the carotid canal. (*From Shaffer 1985.*)

Foreign Bodies

Foreign bodies such as bullets, slag, and shrapnel are easily seen with CT (Fig. 10-61). Nonopaque foreign bodies may be undetected by CT unless associated with other abnormalities. CT is useful to detect ossicular dislocation by an ear swab or to identify displacement of a stapes prosthesis causing sudden hearing loss or vertigo.

NEOPLASMS

External Ear and Mastoid

Benign Tumor

Exostoses occur in the external auditory canal, especially in people who swim frequently in cold water. Although these bony projections are often multiple and bilateral, they do not extend into the adjacent

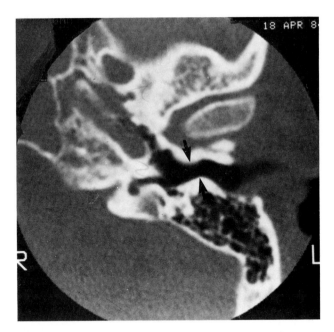

Figure 10-62   Exostoses (arrows) narrow the inferior aspect of the external auditory canal in axial CT. (*From Shaffer 1985.*)

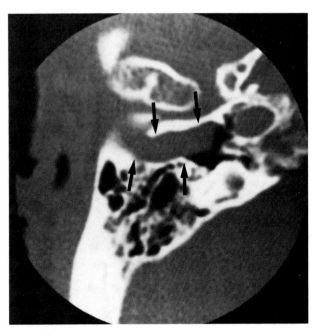

Figure 10-63   Ceruminoma (arrows) in axial CT. A soft tissue mass filling the right external auditory canal does not erode bone. (*From Shaffer 1985.*)

mastoid (Fig. 10-62). Exostoses become significant when they narrow the canal, hindering examination of the tympanic membrane and occasionally obstructing egress of squamous debris from the canal. CT shows multiple uniformly dense ovoid masses blending with the external canal walls. They resemble osteomas, which are, however, usually single.

Oteomas, unlike exostoses, are neoplasms which increase in size and invade adjacent bone. Osteomas in the external auditory canal occur at the junction of the bony and cartilagenous portions of the canal. Osteomas are also common in the mastoid. CT shows an osteoma as a solitary uniformly dense bony mass of variable size.

Gland cell tumors may arise rarely from eccrine, modified apocrine (ceruminous), and sebaceous glands within the external auditory canal skin. Apocrine adenomas (ceruminomas) are the majority of the gland cell tumors (Batsakis 1979). CT shows a ceruminoma as a soft tissue mass in the external auditory canal (Fig. 10-63). If bone destruction is associated with the tumor, malignancy should be suggested.

Primary Malignant Tumor

The most frequent primary malignancies of the external ear are squamous carcinoma, basal cell carcinoma or less frequently adenocarcinoma, adenoid cystic carcinoma, and melanoma of the pinna. Tumors in the external auditory canal are not usually detected as early as the pinna malignancies. Patients who develop external auditory canal carcinomas often have chronic suppurative otitis media, which delays the diagnosis of tumor (Phelps 1981*b*). Malignant tumors usually produce otorrhea, pain, hearing loss, or facial nerve palsy. CT may show only permeative bone destruction which is not easily distinguished from an aggressive infection (Fig. 10-64). Resectability and survival can be predicted by staging of a malignancy of the external auditory canal. Bone destruction and soft tissue extent of disease can only be identified with a combination of axial and coronal CT scans (Bird 1983). Coronal scans or pluridirectional tomograms are necessary to evaluate the tegmen, floor of the middle ear, superior and inferior

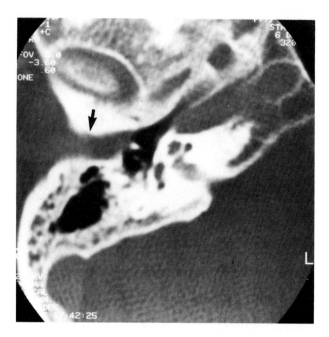

Figure 10-64 Squamous carcinoma in axial CT. Tumor fills right external auditory canal and minimally erodes bone (arrow) but does not invade the middle ear. (*From Shaffer 1985.*)

walls of the external auditory canal, and the carotid and jugular canal roofs. CECT is needed if extension into the brain is suspected. Preferred treatment is surgical extirpation followed by radical irradiation.

Metastasis

Temporal bone metastases are of two types: from hematogenous spread, usually to the marrow spaces, and from direct extension of a local lesion. Neoplasms which commonly metastasize to the temporal bone include carcinoma of the breast, prostate, lung, kidney, and thyroid. Temporal bone metastases usually occur late in the course of malignant disease, so they may not be evaluated radiographically. Neoplasms arising in skin, parotid, nasopharynx, brain, and meninges may invade the temporal bone through foramina and along nerves and fascial planes. Systemic malignancies such as leukemia, lymphoma, and myeloma occasionally affect the temporal bone (Berlinger 1980).

CT shows temporal bone metastases by bone destruction and soft tissue masses. The differential diagnosis includes primary tumor, histiocytosis X, malignant external otitis, and large cholesteatoma. The CT appearance of metastatic disease is not specific.

Histiocytosis X

Idiopathic proliferation of histiocytes characterizes three syndromes called histiocytosis or histiocytosis X. The three, in order of increasing age at onset and decreasing severity, are Letterer-Siwe disease, Hand-Schuller-Christian syndrome, and eosinophilic granuloma. Eosinophilic granuloma usually involves bone whereas Letterer-Siwe disease and Hand-Schuller-Christian syndrome involve viscera. In approximately 15 percent of cases of histiocytosis X the ear is involved. Ear drainage, external otitis, and swelling over the temporal bone are common symptoms (McCaffery 1979). In cases of histiocytosis of the temporal bone, CT shows a soft tissue mass and irregular bone destruction which may be indistinguishable from infection, metastatic disease, or cholesteatoma.

Middle Ear

Glomus Tumor

Glomus tumors, also known as chemodectomas or nonchromaffin paragangliomas, arise from chemoreceptor cells at several sites in the head and neck. Those masses which arise primarily on the cochlear promontory are glomus tympanicum tumors (Fig. 10-65). Glomus jugulare tumors arise in the jugular fossa and may invade the middle ear from below. The symptoms of glomus tumors often are pulsatile tinnitus and hearing loss. The glomus tumor is often visible behind the tympanic membrane. Chemodectomas, although usually benign, are sometimes multiple, and are histologically malignant in about 10 percent of patients (Som 1983). Chemodectomas are more common in women than in men.

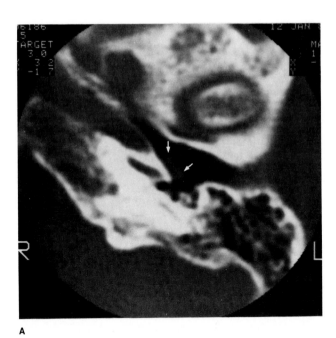

A

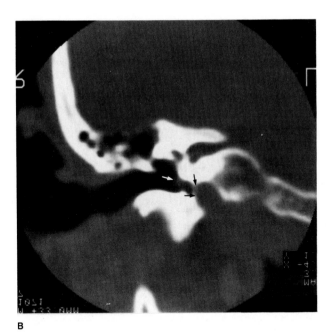

B

Figure 10-65 Two examples of glomus tympanicum tumors (white arrows). In one case axial CT **(A)** demonstrates a mass adjacent to the left cochlear promontory. In the second case **(B)**, coronal

CT shows the normal carotid canal (black arrows) below tumor in the middle ear. (*From Shaffer 1985.*)

The small soft tissue mass produced by a glomus tympanicum tumor is identified on CT scans although it may be missed on pluridirectional tomograms. Dynamic CT scans show that the maximal enhancement of the tumor occurs later than that of the carotid artery and earlier than that of the jugular vein (Mafee 1983b). CT shows bone erosion typically in the roof of the jugular bulb and the septum between the carotid artery and jugular vein in glomus jugulare tumors but seldom in glomus tympanicum tumors. Rarely a glomus tumor may extend intracranially through the jugular foramen (Fig. 10-66).

The differential diagnosis of a middle ear mass with pulsatile tinnitus includes aberrant carotid artery and dehiscence of bone covering the jugular vein. The key CT finding in the vascular anomalies is loss of the osseous margin of the carotid or jugular canals on the coronal CT scans. Angiography may be needed to verify the vascular origin of the middle ear mass. Correct diagnosis prior to surgery is needed to prevent serious complication.

Facial Nerve Neurinoma

In approximately 5 percent of cases of persistent Bell's palsy a facial nerve neurinoma or other tumor is the cause. Neurinomas occur along the intracranial, intratemporal, or extratemporal portions of the facial nerve. A facial nerve neurinoma in the internal auditory canal is indistinguishable from the more common intracanalicular acoustic neurinoma. Elsewhere in the temporal bone, the tumor is identified primarily by its expansion of the facial canal. Detection of abnormality in the vertical portion of the facial nerve canal requires high-quality, direct coronal CT scans or reformatted sagittal images. Identification of extratemporal tumors depends on recognition of tumor enhancement and displacement of normal soft tissue planes (Curtin 1983).

CT shows a uniformly enhancing homogeneous mass, which if located in the facial nerve canal or internal auditory canal, causes pressure erosion. CT may show the middle ear completely filled with soft

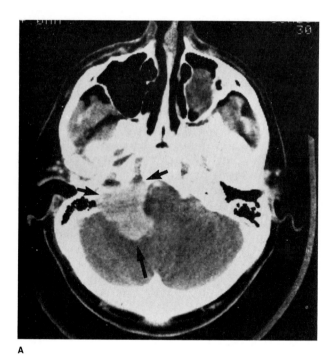

A

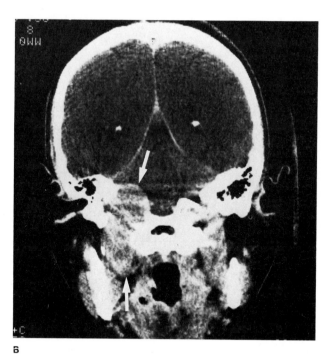

B

Figure 10-66 Large glomus jugulare tumor (long arrow) that erodes the jugular fossa (short arrows) and extends into the right cere- bellar hemisphere in axial CT **(A)**. In coronal CT **(B)**, the tumor's extension below the skull base is demostrated. (*From Shaffer 1985.*)

tissue. Correct diagnosis depends on recognizing that the mass or bone erosion is related to the course of the facial nerve.

Malignant Tumor

When squamous cell carcinoma occurs in the middle ear, it is usually as the result of spread from the external auditory canal (Chen 1978). Adenocarcinomas and their variants are also rare in the middle ear (Adam 1982). The diagnosis of malignant tumor is often delayed since it may masquerade as chronic inflammatory disease. Rhabdomyosarcoma, usually the embryonal type, is the most common soft tissue sarcoma in children, and the ear is the most common site after the orbit and nasopharynx (Fig. 10-67) (Schwartz 1980).

A soft tissue mass in the middle ear destroying bone characterizes most primary middle ear malignancies and some aggressive benign processes such as infection. The primary role of CT in temporal bone malignant tumors is staging rather than differential diagnosis.

Inner Ear

Acoustic Neurinoma

These benign tumors arise from schwann cells, especially those near Scarpa's ganglion of the superior vestibular nerve. The tumors frequently arise in the internal auditory canal and grow medially into the cistern. Expansion of the bony canal, particularly its medial end, is a common feature of most acoustic neurinomas. Most have a cerebellopontine angle mass by the time of diagnosis. Patients who have acoustic neurinomas present with a variety of symptoms, including sensorineural hearing loss with poor discrimination, dizziness or true vertigo, tinnitus, facial nerve paralysis, pain, decreased corneal sensation, or brainstem signs.

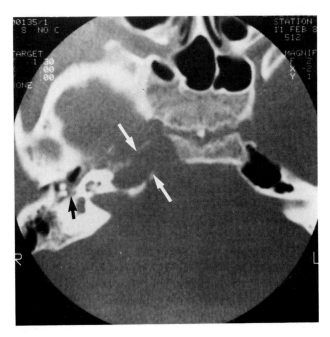

Figure 10-67   Rhabdomyosarcoma in a 12-year-old boy with right hearing loss. The axial CT demonstrates petrous apex destruction (white arrows) and tumor in the middle ear (black arrow). (*From Shaffer 1985.*)

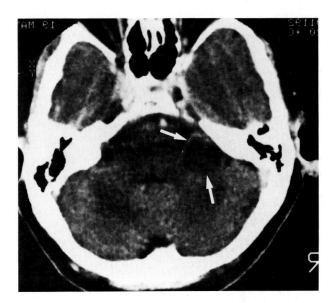

Figure 10-68   Necrotic acoustic neurinoma (arrows) in axial enhanced CT. The central low density with rim enhancement is atypical for acoustic neurinoma. (*From Shaffer 1985.*)

The sensitivity of CT for detecting acoustic neurinomas is high, especially with newer scanners which have improved resolution and thin sections. CT shows acoustic neurinomas as enhancing masses in the internal auditory canal or cerebellopontine angle (Valvassori 1982; Wu 1986). Contrast enhancement is characteristic of acoustic neurinomas because there is no restriction of capillary permeability (blood-brain barrier), although there may be lower-density areas in the tumor (Fig. 10-68). Patients can be scanned immediately after the iodinated contrast agent (42 g iodine) has been administered, or while the last 10 g is infusing.

Completely intracanalicular acoustic neurinomas without enlargement of the canal are difficult to detect on CT scans by their contrast enhancement alone, but identification is easier if the canal is expanded by the tumor (Fig. 10-69). The normal canal contains nerves and CSF which together have a density intermediate between brain and CSF; a tumor after enhancement has a substantially higher density. A comparison of one side with the other usually reveals the tumor. However, a negative CT study in a patient with strong clinical evidence of an acoustic neurinoma should be followed by gas CT cisternography or MR. Thick slices will not identify intracanalicular tumors because of partial volume averaging, which obscures the intracanalicular enhancement.

Large series have shown that CT gas cisternography is a reliable test to diagnose intracanalicular tumors (Salti-Bohman 1984; Robertson 1983). CT demonstration of an internal auditory canal not filled with gas is evidence of an intracanalicular acoustic neuroma if there is a convex surface of the tumor projecting into the cerebellopontine angle (Fig. 10-69). A canal filled with gas excludes tumor. Surface tension between gas and cerebrospinal fluid in the cistern may prevent gas from entering the internal auditory canal; therefore, the patient's head should be shaken gently to dislodge the fluid from the canal if gas fails to fill the canal. When the interface between the gas and the contents of the canal is concave, a technical cause for obstruction to gas, rather than a neoplasm, should be considered. A loop of AICA in the internal auditory canal or thick-

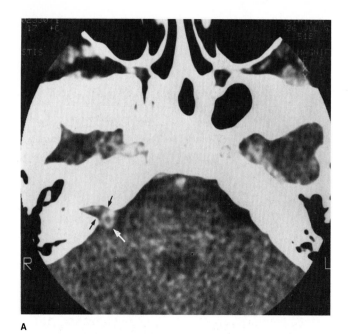

A

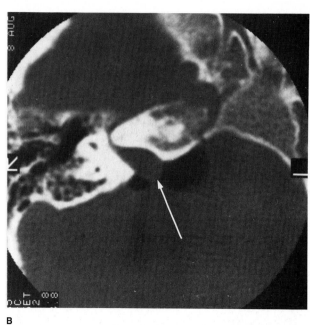

B

Figure 10-69 Acoustic neurinoma with a small extracanalicular component (arrows). The tumor enhances in axial CT **(A)** and dis- places air from the right internal auditory canal in air CT cister- nogram. **(B)**. (*From Shaffer 1985.*)

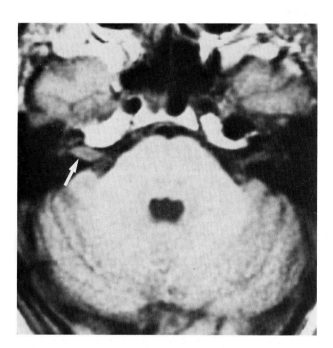

Figure 10-70 Intracanalicular acoustic neurinoma (arrow) in axial T$_1$-weighted MRI. The tumor has an nonhomogeneous signal (darker center) of uncertain etiology with no anatomic correlate found at surgery. (*From Daniels 1984a.*)

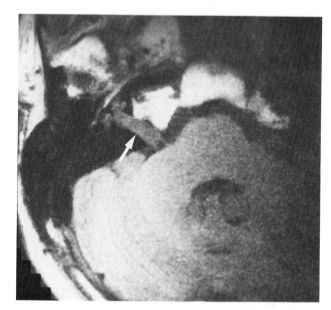

Figure 10-71 Surface coil MR image of a predominantly intra- canalicular acoustic neurinoma (arrow) obscuring the nerves in the right internal auditory canal. (Axial short TR/TE scan). (*From Daniels 1985.*)

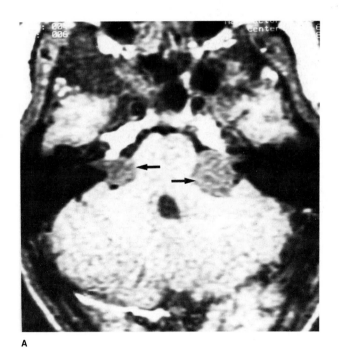

A

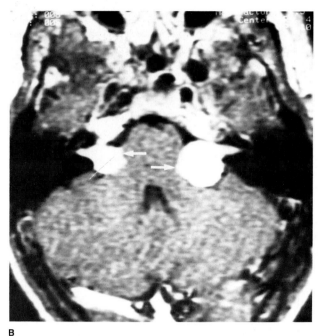

B

Figure 10-72 Bilateral large acoustic neurinomas (arrows) in a patient with neurofibromatosis without **(A)** and with **(B)** intravenous Gadolinium. Axial T₁-WI demonstrates the tumors slightly less hy-

pointense than that of normal brainstem **(A)** and intense enhancement **(B)**.

ened nerves may mimic tiny acoustic neurinomas by preventing gas from entering the canal. In these cases imaging the contralateral ear with gas may be helpful. Intracanalicular tumors as small as 3 mm have been diagnosed by gas CT cisternography (Johnson 1984).

Because MR demonstrates acoustic neurinomas effectively (even small intracanalicular ones) it can replace CT cisternography and contrast-enhanced CT to study patients with sensorineural hearing loss (Figs. 10-70, 10-71). With intravenous Gadolinium-DTPA, the relatively fast T₁-weighted imaging sequences can be used to identify acoustic neurinomas which typically enhance intensely (Figs. 10-72, 10-73). The MR exam is therefore effective, fast, and

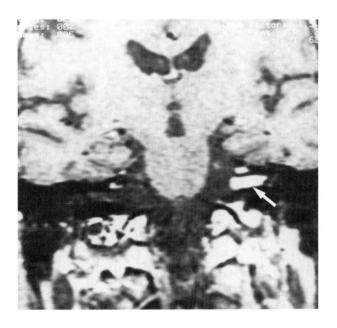

Figure 10-73 Intense enhancement of an intracanalicular acoustic neurinoma (arrow) is demonstrated in coronal T₁-weighted MRI after Gadolinium injection.

safe. CT will be reserved for cases in which visualization of osseous structures is crucial (e.g., congenital anomalies, trauma, otodystrophies, inflammatory disease, and some tumors primarily affecting the temporal bone).

Meningioma

Meningiomas, which arise along the posterior surface of the petrous portion of the temporal bone, must be differentiated from the more common acoustic neurinomas (Valavanis 1981). Less commonly, meningiomas arise from ectopic arachnoid granulations which occur in the temporal bone (Guzowski 1976).

On CT, a meningioma appears as a uniformly enhancing mass in the cerebellopontine angle cistern. Meningiomas resemble acoustic neurinomas only superficially. A meningioma has a sessile broad-based attachment to the petrous bone, atypical of acoustic neurinoma, and they rarely enlarge the internal auditory canal. Frequently, meningiomas cause hyperostosis or have dense focal calcifications (Fig. 10-74). In cases which are not easily differentiated by CT, angiography is indicated to distinguish the characteristic blush and dural blood supply of meningioma from the more subtle changes of acoustic neurinoma.

Epidermoid Tumor

Epidermoid tumors, also called congenital or primary cholesteatomas, arise from ectodermal rests at multiple intracranial sites, including the cerebellopontine angle cistern, the petrous apex, middle ear, or elsewhere in the temporal bone. Epidermoid tumors are the third most common cerebellopontine angle mass. They may produce a variety of symptoms depending on the exact location of the mass and extension to surrounding structures. CT is a reliable way to detect epidermoid tumors since their keratin content gives them lower density than brain on NCCT and CECT. Smooth or scalloped borders are typical (Fig. 10-75).

The differential diagnosis of petrous apex epidermoid includes schwannoma, meningioma, glo-

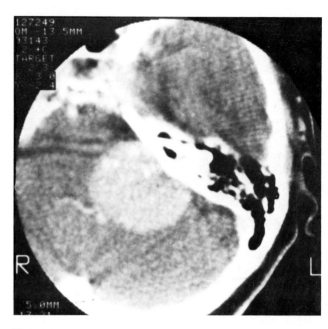

Figure 10-74 A meningioma presents as a homogeneously enhancing, round mass with punctate calcifications in the cerebellopontine angle cistern on CECT.

mus tumor, metastasis, petrositis, histiocytosis, cholesterol granuloma, and mucocele (Gacek 1980). The smooth bone erosion and lack of enhancement differentiate epidermoid tumors from most other masses except mucocele and cholesterol granuloma.

Other Tumors

Neurinomas of the fifth, seventh, ninth, tenth, eleventh, or twelfth cranial nerves may erode bone in the inner ear. Fifth cranial nerve neurinomas characteristically can amputate the petrous apex. Seventh cranial nerve neurinomas arising in the intracanalicular segment of the nerve will expand the internal canal exactly like an acoustic neurinoma. Neurinomas of the ninth, tenth, and eleventh cranial nerves enlarge the jugular fossa like a glomus tumor but without irregular margins. Neurinomas enhance less than glomus tumors, which are extremely vascular.

Cholesterol granuloma is a recently described mass which may be mistaken for an epidermoid tu-

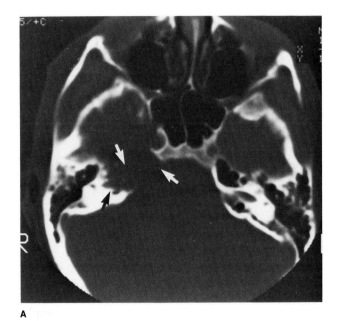 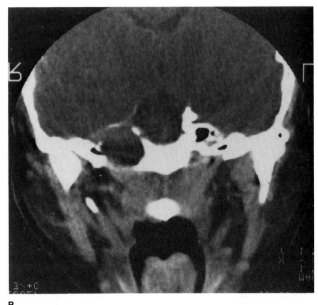

A   **B**

Figure 10-75   Epidermoid in petrous apex erodes the apex and skull base in axial CT **(A)** and does not enhance in coronal CECT **(B)**. (*From Shaffer 1985.*)

mor in the petrous apex, middle ear, or mastoid. It may be caused by obstructed ventilation, poor drainage, and hemorrhage. Cholesterol granulomas, unlike epidermoid tumors, contain cholesterol crystals, giant cells, and dark or yellow material, while epidermoids contain a pale and flaky material. CT shows a mass smoothly eroding bone with a density nearly isodense to the brain, and therefore higher than that of an epidermoid (Lo 1984).

Mucocele is another process like a cholesterol granuloma or epidermoid that destroys bone in the petrous apex. Since it arises in an apex air cell, CT usually shows a pneumatized air cell on the opposite side. Ipsilaterally, the mastoid air cells may be fluid-filled (Osborn 1979).

Hemangiomas are rare tumors which may occur in the internal auditory canal or any portion of the temporal bone. Characteristic features, including spokelike trabeculations or phleboliths, may be demonstrated by CT in some cases.

Fibro-osseous tumors including chondroma and osteoma affect the inner ear as well as other portions of the temporal bone.

Metastatic involvement of the inner ear occurs by direct extension or hematogenous spread of tumor. Tumor can extend directly to the inner ear from a nasopharyngeal carcinoma, meningeal carcinomatosis, or an adjacent intracranial malignancy. Hematogenous metastasis to the temporal bone usually occurs late in the course of disease. Most cases arise from tumors which commonly metastasize to bone, such as carcinoma of the breast, prostate, lung, and kidney. The petrous apex contains marrow spaces which may trap circulating tumor cells, but the otic capsule and well-pneumatized bone are often not involved (Schuknecht 1968).

INFLAMMATORY DISEASE

External Ear

Except for the so-called malignant form, otitis externa is seldom evaluated radiographically. The malignant appellation refers to the aggressive course of *Pseudomonas aeruginosa* infection in elderly diabetics or immunosuppressed patients. Malignant external otitis is divided into an early stage, characterized by soft tissue changes without bone destruction, and the advanced stage characterized by spread of infection and bone destruction (Mendez 1979). Pain, drainage from the ear, impaired hearing, and granulation tissue in the external auditory canal occur in both stages. Facial nerve paralysis, other cranial nerve palsies, and temporomandibular joint involvement occur late. Long-term systemic antibiotic therapy and local surgical debridement are needed.

CT findings in malignant external otitis include normal soft tissue in the external auditory canal, middle ear, and mastoid; destruction of the bone in the external canal and skull base; and mass in the nasopharynx and subtemporal space (Fig. 10-76). The CT findings of malignant external otitis are not specific. The nasopharyngeal inflammatory mass may be mistaken radiographically for malignant tumor since the infection crosses fascial planes. Only with the typical clinical findings are the CT abnormalities easily interpreted. In these patients, CT is effective to evaluate bone destruction as well as the soft tissue spread in the ear and subtemporal space. Nuclear scanning more effectively defines the extent of active infection in patients being treated for malignant external otitis. Technetium 99m bone scanning is more sensitive for detecting bony involvement than either CT or pluridirectional tomography. Gallium 67 citrate scans can determine activity of an infection under treatment (Strashun 1984).

Middle Ear

Temporal bone cholesteatoma, an epithelium-lined cyst filled with keratin debris, is usually a complication of inflammatory disease, but rarely is a congenital neoplasm arising from epithelial rests. Congenital cholesteatoma in the middle ear appears as a pearly mass behind an intact tympanic membrane in patients with no history of middle ear inflammatory disease.

Acquired cholesteatomas usually occur in patients with a history of otitis media. Retraction of the pars flaccida portion of the tympanic membrane, tympanic membrane perforation, and migration of epithelial cells into the middle ear cause most acquired cholesteatomas (Nager 1977; Swartz 1984). Eustachian tube dysfunction, poor pneumatization of the mastoid, and hereditary factors are contributory. The epithelial cells produce a cyst which accumulates keratin debris. Bone destruction results in most cases because of collagenase activity of the cholesteatoma or associated inflammatory disease.

CT is the most accurate means for determining the extent of disease prior to planning surgical treatment. CT demonstrates the soft tissue mass in the middle ear, air-fluid levels, erosion of the tegmen and lateral semicircular canal, and the posterior wall of the middle ear more accurately than pluridirectional tomography (Fig. 10-77) (Shaffer 1984). Characteristically CT shows bone erosion, particularly involving the drum spur (scutum) and the long process

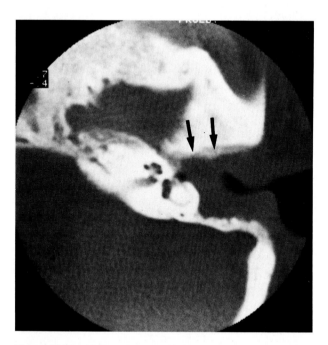

Figure 10-76 Malignant external otitis in a diabetic woman with a history of a left mastoidectomy. In axial CT, soft tissue filling the surgical defect destroys bone anteriorly (arrows). *Pseudomonas aeruginosa* was cultured from the ear. (*From Shaffer 1985.*)

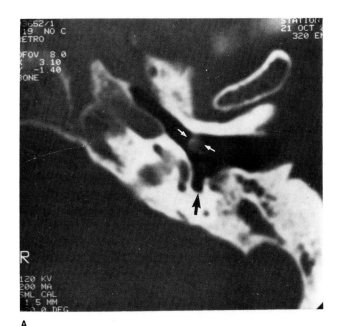

A

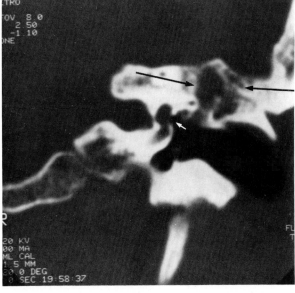

B

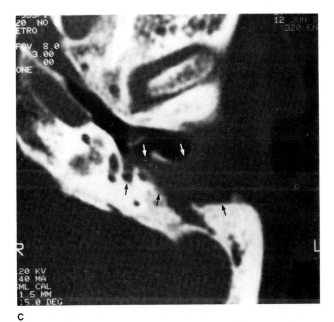

C

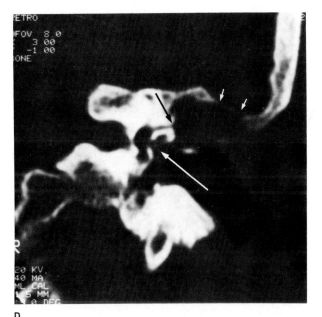

D

Figure 10-77 Cholesteatoma in axial **(A)** and coronal **(B)** CT scans. Soft tissue mass (white arrows) is small in **A** sparing the sinus tympani (black arrow). Mastoid antrum opacification (long black arrows) and a clear oval window (white arrow) are shown in **B**. In follow-up study 7 months after modified radical mastoidectomy, increase in size of the cholesteatoma is demonstrated in axial **(C)** and coronal **(D)** CT. Cholesteatoma (arrows, **C**) is present in the surgical cavity extending into the sinus tympani, In **D**, cholesteatoma is identified that erodes the bone over the lateral semicircular canal (black arrow) and fills the oval window niche (long white arrow). Thinning of the tegmen (small white arrows) is probably secondary to surgery. (*From Shaffer 1985.*)

of the incus. In an extensive cholesteatoma, there may be erosion of the lateral semicircular canal, the lateral attic wall, and occasionally the tegmen tympani. In the partially opacified middle ear and mastoid, movement of fluid between axial and coronal scans and air-fluid levels helps distinguish fluid from mass. Granulation tissue from chronic infection, which often coexists with cholesteatoma, cannot be differentiated reliably from cholesteatoma by CT numbers. CT may show calcification (tympanosclerosis) or retraction of the tympanic membrane (Swartz 1983*b*, 1984*a*).

In the patient previously operated on for cholesteatoma it is difficult to determine which abnormalities are the result of disease, which were due to surgery, and which developed afterward. In the modified radical mastoidectomy, a mastoidectomy cavity is created with or without an intact canal wall. CT in the postoperative patient is useful to identify recurrent cholesteatoma or granulation tissue and to evaluate ossicular reconstruction. Baseline axial CT scans 3 to 6 months after surgery may be helpful in patients who have residual cholesteatoma or an intact canal wall mastoidectomy, and therefore have a higher risk of developing a recurrent cholesteatoma (Johnson 1984*c*).

Inner Ear

Labyrinthitis ossificans, bone filling the inner ear, which often produces a "dead" ear, is most commonly due to suppurative labyrinthitis but may result from trauma, severe otosclerosis, surgery, or tumors (Hoffman 1979). Labyrinthitis ossificans has a characteristic appearance with decreased luminal size and sclerosis of affected tumor ear structures (Fig. 10-78). Acute labyrinthitis is a clinical diagnosis without radiographic findings.

Petrositis is infection of petrous apex air cells secondary to middle ear and mastoid infection. The majority of individuals, without air cells in the petrous apices, do not develop petrositis. The classical clinical presentation of petrositis is pain along the fifth

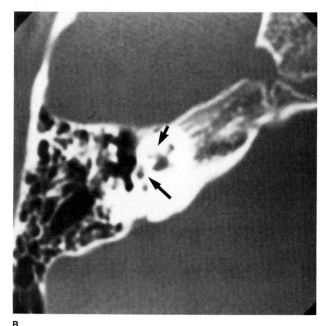

A   **B**

Figure 10-78 Postinfectious labyrinthitis ossificans in a deaf 8-year-old boy. Axial CT (**A,B**) demonstrates bone that obliterates most of the cochlear turns (short arrow, **A**), vestibule (long arrow, **A**) and semicircular canals (arrows, **B**). (*From Shaffer 1985.*)

cranial nerve distribution and sixth cranial nerve palsy (Gradenigo's syndrome). Air-cell opacification, middle ear disease, and bone destruction are important CT findings in patients with petrositis. Infection in any portion of the temporal bone may cause meningitis, lateral sinus thrombosis, and epidural, subdural, or brain abscess (Chapter 12).

OTODYSTROPHIES

Otosclerosis

Otosclerosis, a disease of unknown etiology, is responsible for hearing loss and tinnitus particularly in young Caucasian women. The dense enchondral layer of the bony labyrinth is replaced by foci of thick, vascular bone. Otosclerosis may be hereditary and is frequently bilateral. Stapedial otosclerosis, the more common form, fixes the stapes in the oval window, causing conductive hearing loss. CT shows lytic (spongiotic) changes early, and sclerotic reparative changes later. CT may show bone obliterating the oval window niche (Fig. 10-79) (Swartz 1984*b*; Mafee 1985*a*). Small otosclerotic foci may produce hearing loss without radiographic abnormalities. When otosclerosis involves the otic capsule and cochlea in addition to the stapes, sensorineural as well as conductive hearing loss may be present (mixed hearing loss).

The CT diagnosis of otosclerosis is not precise. The semiaxial projection perpendicular to the plane of the oval window provides the best view of the stapes footplate. However, with this projection each ear must be scanned separately. CT demonstrates replacement of the oval or round windows with bone in moderately advanced cases. The improved contrast resolution of CT compared to pluridirectional tomography identifies lytic foci in the otic capsule more accurately. Advanced cochlear otosclerosis has been demonstrated on CT as a lucent halo around the cochlea. The CT appearance of cochlear otosclerosis is quite specific, except for differentiation from osteogenesis imperfecta. (Mafee 1985*b*). Other

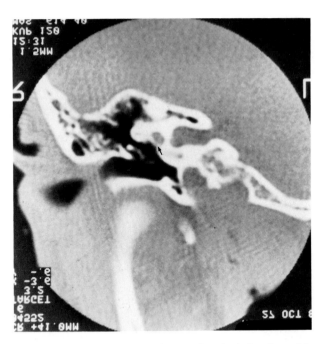

Figure 10-79   Otosclerotic reclosure of oval window (arrow) in coronal CT. The patient had a history of stapedectomy and wire loop prosthesis. (*Courtesy of Kedar N. Chintapalli, M.D., Milwaukee.*)

processes such as tumor, infection, and Paget's disease produce lucent areas in the petrous portion of the temporal bone but do not affect the otic capsule primarily.

CT is also useful to study the poststapedectomy ear when there has been sudden or progressive hearing loss. Ankylosis of the prosthesis in the oval window or posttraumatic dislocation can be identified. Dislocation is demonstrated as a displacement of the prosthesis away from the oval window or protrusion into the vestibule, producing vertigo.

Paget's Disease

Paget's disease produces chronic progressive changes in the skeleton of middle-aged and elderly adults. A lytic phase characterized by loss of bone is followed by a sclerotic phase characterized by coarse thickened trabeculae. The skull, and less frequently

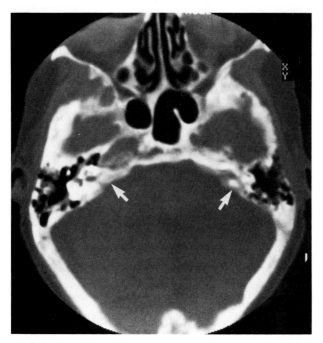

Figure 10-80 Paget's disease causing bilateral mixed hearing loss in a middle-aged woman. Demineralized petrous apices (arrows) and normal otic capsule density are shown in axial CT. (*From Shaffer 1985.*)

the temporal bones, may be affected. Temporal bone involvement usually causes conductive hearing loss if the stapes becomes fixed in the oval window or sensorineural hearing loss if the cochlea is involved. Temporal bone Paget's disease usually is accompanied by severe skull involvement.

In Paget's disease, temporal bone changes are usually lytic (Petasnick 1969). Demineralization begins medially in the petrous pyramid and progresses laterally. The dense otic capsule bone is the last to be affected (Fig. 10-80). The diagnosis of Paget's disease is made by identifying calvarial changes in association with the lytic changes in the temporal bone. Alone, the lytic areas in the temporal bone cannot be distinguished from otosclerosis, metastases, or luetic osteitis.

Fibrous Dysplasia

Fibrous dysplasia is a congenital osseous disorder of unknown etiology in which cancellous bone is replaced by fibrous tissue that erodes and expands normal cortical bone from within. It has monostotic and polyostotic types. There is a variable amount of metaplastic bone formation; so fibrous dysplasia can have a cystic, a dense, or a "ground glass" appearance depending on the mix of bony and soft tissue elements. The temporal bone is involved less frequently than the skull (Nager 1982). When fibrous dysplasia occurs in the sinuses or temporal bones, the lesion usually is osteomatoid, appearing as a uniformly dense region of expanded bone. Patients often present with mastoid prominence and hearing loss due to narrowing of the external auditory canal or middle ear.

On CT, fibrous dysplasia of the temporal bone is usually characterized by homogeneous dense thickened bone which may narrow the external auditory canal and middle ear (Fig. 10-81). The uncom-

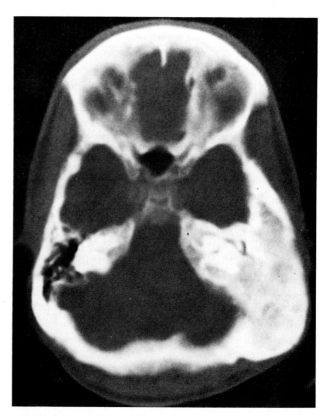

Figure 10-81 Fibrous dysplasia markedly enlarging the left temporal bone in axial CT. (*From Shaffer 1985.*)

mon lucent foci due to fibrosis have an expanded cortex. Differential diagnosis includes metastasis, meningioma, Paget's disease, osteosarcoma, ossifying fibroma, and osteopetrosis.

Bibliography

ADAM W, JOHNSON JD, PAUL DJ, CLAUSEN K, SCHULLER DE: Primary adenocarcinoma of the middle ear. *AJNR* **3**:674–676, 1982.

ANDERSON R, DIEHL J, MARAVILLA K, FANCHER J, SCHAEFER S: Computerized axial tomography with air contrast of the cerebellopontine angle and internal auditory canal. *Laryngoscope* **91**:1083–1097, 1981.

ANDERSON R, OLSON J, DORWART R, MERKLE M, SCHAEFER S: CT air-contrast scanning of the internal auditory canal. *Ann Otol Rhinol Laryngol* **91**:501–504, 1982.

BATSAKIS JG: *Tumors of the Head and Neck*, 2d ed., Baltimore, Williams & Wilkins, 1979.

BERGSTROM L: Pathology of congenital deafness—present status and future priorities. *Ann Otol Rhinol Laryngol* **89**: Suppl 74, 31–42, 1980.

BERLINGER NT, KOUTROUPAS S, ADAMS G, MAISEL R: Patterns of involvement of the temporal bone in metastatic and systemic malignancy. *Laryngoscope* **90**:619–627, 1980.

BIRD CR, HASSO AN, STEWART EC, HINSHAW DB JR, THOMPSON JR: Malignant primary neoplasms of the ear and temporal bone studied by high-resolution computed tomography. *Radiology* **149**:171–174, 1983.

BYDDER GM, STEINER RE, YOUNG IR et al: Clinical NMR imaging of the brain: 140 cases. *AJNR* **3**:459–480, 1982; *AJR* **139**:215–236, 1982.

CHAKERES DW, SPIEGEL PK: A systematic technique for comprehensive evaluation of the temporal bone by computed tomography. *Radiology* **146**:97–106, 1983.

CHEN KTK, DEHNER LP: Primary tumors of the external and middle ear. I. Introduction and clinico-pathologic study of squamous cell carcinoma. *Arch Otolaryngol* **104**:247–252, 1978.

CURATI WL, GRAIF M, KINGSLEY DPE, NIENDORF HP, YOUNG IR: Acoustic neuromas: Gd-DTPA enhancement in MR imaging. *Radiology* **158**:447–451, 1986.

CURTIN HD, WOLFE P, SNYDERMAN N: The facial nerve between the stylomastoid foramen and the parotid: Computed tomographic imaging. *Radiology* **149**:165–169, 1983.

DAMSMA H, MALI WPTM, ZONNEVELD FW: CT diagnosis of an aberrant internal carotid artery in the middle ear. *J Comput Assist Tomogr* **8**:317–319, 1984.

DANIELS DL, HERFKINS R, KOEHLER PR, MILLEN SJ, SHAFFER KA, WILLIAMS AL, HAUGHTON VM: Magnetic resonance imaging of the internal auditory canal. *Radiology* **151**:105–108, 1984*a*.

DANIELS DL, PECH P, HAUGHTON VM: Magnetic resonance imaging of the temporal bone. Milwaukee: General Electric Systems Group, 1984*b*.

DANIELS DL, SCHENCK JF, FOSTER T, HART H JR, MILLEN SJ, MEYER GA, PECH P, SHAFFER KA, HAUGHTON VM: Surface-coil magnetic resonance imaging of the internal auditory canal. *AJNR* **6**:487–490, 1985.

GACEK RR: Evaluation and management of primary petrous apex cholesteatoma. *Otolaryngol Head Neck Surg* **88**:519–523, 1980.

GUINTO FC JR, GARRABRANT EC, RADCLIFFE WB: Radiology of the persistent stapedial artery. *Radiology* **105**:365–369, 1972.

GUZOWSKI J, PAPARELLA MM, RAO KN, HOSHINO T: Meningiomas of the temporal bone. *Laryngoscope* **84**:1141–1146, 1976.

HANAFEE WN, BERGSTROM L: Radiology of congenital deformities of the ear. *Head Neck Surg* **2**:213–221, 1980.

HOFFMAN RA, BROOKLER KH, BERGERON RT: Radiologic diagnosis of labyrinthitis ossificans. *Ann Otol Rhinol Laryngol* **88**:253–257, 1979.

HOLLAND B, BRANT-ZAWADZKI M: High-resolution CT of temporal bone trauma. *AJNR* **5**:291–295, 1984; *AJR* **143**:391–395, 1984.

JOHNSON DW: Air cisternography of the cerebellopontine angle using high-resolution computed tomography. *Radiology* **151**:401–403, 1984a.

JOHNSON DW, HASSO AW, STEWART CE, THOMPSON JR, HINSHAW DB JR: Temporal bone trauma: High-resolution computed tomographic evaluation. *Radiology* **151**:411–415, 1984a.

JOHNSON DW: CT of the postsurgical ear. *Radiol Clin North Am* **22**:67–76, 1984c.

KASEFF LG: Tomographic evaluation of trauma to the temporal bone. *Radiology* **93**:321–327, 1969.

KINGSLEY DPE, BROOKS GB, LEUNG AW-L, JOHNSON MA: Acoustic neuromas; evaluation by magnetic resonance imaging. *AJNR* **6**:1–5, 1985.

LEE SH, LEWIS E, MONTOYA JH, SEELAUS JF: Bilateral cerebellopontine angle air-CT cisternography. *AJNR* **2**:105–106, 1981.

LO WEM, SOLTI-BOHMAN LG, BRACKMANN DE, GRUSKIN P: CT diagnosis of cholesterol granuloma of the petrous apex. Presented at the American Society of Head and Neck Radiology Annual Meeting, San Antonio, TX, May 3–6, 1984. Accepted for publication in *Radiology*.

LO WEM, SOLTI-BOHMAN L, MCELVEEN JT JR: Aberrant carotid artery: radiologic diagnosis with emphasis on high-resolution computed tomography. *Radiographics* **5**:985–993, 1985.

LUFKIN R, BARNI JJ, GLEN W, MANCUSO A, CANALIS R, HANAFEE W: Comparison of computed tomography and pluridirectional tomography of the temporal bone. *Radiology* **143**:715–718, 1982.

MCCAFFREY TV, MCDONALD TJ: Histiocytosis X of the ear and temporal bone: Review of 22 cases. *Laryngoscope* **89**:1735–1742, 1979.

MAFEE MF, KIMAR A, YANNIAS DA, VALVASSORI GE, APPLEBAUM EL: Computed tomography of the middle ear in the evaluation of cholesteatomas and other soft tissue masses: Comparison with pluridirectional tomography. *Radiology* **148**:465–472, 1983a.

MAFEE MF, VALVASSORI GE, SHUGAR MA, YANNIAS DA, DOBBEN GD: High resolution and dynamic sequential computed tomography: use in the evaluation of glomus complex tumors. *Arch Otolaryngol* **109**:691–696, 1983b.

MAFEE MF, HENDRICKSON GC, DEITCH RL et al: Use of CT in stapedial otosclerosis. *Radiology* **156**:709–714, 1985a.

MAFEE MF, VALVASSORI GE, DEITCH RL et al: Use of CT in the evaluation of cochlear otosclerosis. *Radiology* **156**:703–708, 1985b.

MANCUSO AA, HANAFEE WN: *Computed Tomography of the Head and Neck,* Baltimore, Williams & Wilkins, 1982, pp. 244–287.

MENDEZ G JR, QUENCER RM, POST MJD, STOKES NA: Malignant external otitis: A radiographic-clinical correlation. *AJR* **132**:957–961, 1979.

NAGER GT: Cholesteatoma of the middle ear: Pathogenesis and surgical indication in *Cholesteatoma First International Conference,* McCabe BF, Sade J, Abramson M, eds., Aesculapius Publishing Company, Birmingham, AL, 1977, pp. 193–203.

NAGER GT, KENNEDY DW, KIPSTEIN E. Fibrous dysplasia: a review of the disease and its manifestations in the temporal bone. *Ann Otol Rhinol Laryngol* (Suppl) **92**:5–52, 1982.

NEW PFJ, BACHOW TB, WISMER GL, ROSEN BR, BRADY TJ: MR imaging of acoustic nerves and small acoustic neuromas at .6T: Prospective study. *AJNR* **6**:165–170, 1985.

OSBORN AG, PARKIN JL: Mucocele of the petrous temporal bone. *AJR* **132**:680–681, 1979.

PETASNICK JP: Tomography of the temporal bone in Paget's disease. *AJR* **105**:838–843, 1969.

PHELPS PD, LLOYD GAS: Course of the facial nerve in congenital ear deformities. *Acta Radiologica Diagn* **22**(fasc. 4):475–583, 1981*a*.

PHELPS PD, LLOYD GAS: The radiology of carcinoma of the ear. *Br J Radiol* **54**:103–109, 1981*b*.

PINTO RS, KRICHEFF II, BERGERON RT, COHEN N: Small acoustic neuromas: Detection by high resolution gas CT cisternography. *AJR* **139**:129–132, 1982.

REESE DF, HARNER SG, KIPERT DB, BAKER HL JR: Magnetic resonance display of the internal auditory canal, cochlea, vestibular apparatus and facial nerve. Presented at the annual meeting of the American Society of Neuroradiology, Boston, June 1984.

ROBERTSON HJ, HATTEN HP JR, KEATING JW: False-positive CT gas cisternogram. *AJNR* **4**:474–477, 1983.

SCHUKNECHT HF, ALLAM AF, MURAKAMI Y: Pathology of secondary malignant tumors of the temporal bone. *Ann Otol Rhinol Laryngol* **77**:5–22, 1968.

SCHWARTZ RH, MOROSSAGHI N, MARION ED: Rhabdomyosarcoma of the middle ear: A wolf in sheep's clothing. *Pediatrics* **65**:1131–1132, 1980.

SHAFFER KA, VOLZ DJ, HAUGHTON VM: Manipulation of CT data for temporal-bone imaging. *Radiology* **137**:825–829, 1980.

SHAFFER KA, LITTLETON JT, DURIZCH ML, CALLAHAN WP: Temporal bone anatomy: comparison of computed tomography and complex motion tomography. *Head Neck Surg* **4**:296–300, 1982.

SHAFFER KA: Comparison of computed tomography and complex motion tomography in the evaluation of cholesteatoma. *AJNR* **5**:303–306, 1984; *AJR* **143**:397–400, 1984.

SHAFFER KA: The Temporal Bone, in Williams AL and Haughton VM, eds.: *Cranial Computed Tomography: A Comprehensive Text,* St. Louis, Mosby, 1985.

SOLTI-BOHMAN LG, MAGARAM DL, LO WWM, WADE CT, WITTEN RM, SHIMIZU FH, MCMONIGLE EM, RAO AKR: Gas-CT cisternography for detection of small acoustic nerve tumors. *Radiology* **150**:403–407, 1984.

SOM PM, REEDE DL, BERGERON RT, PARISIER SC, SHUGAR JM, COHEN NL: Computed tomography of glomus tympanicum tumors. *J Comput Assist Tomogr* **7**:14–17, 1983.

SORTLAND O: Computed tomography combined with gas cisternography for the diagnosis of expanding lesions in the cerebellopontine angle. *Neuroradiology* **18**:19–22, 1979.

STRASHUN AM, NEGATHEIM M, GOLDSMITH SJ: Malignant external otitis: Early scintigraphic detection. *Radiology* **150**:541–545, 1984.

SWARTZ JD: High resolution computed tomography of the middle ear and mastoid. Part I: Normal radioanatomy including normal variations. *Radiology* **148**:449–454, 1983*a*.

SWARTZ JD, GOODMAN RS, RUSSELL KB, MARLOWE FI, WOLFSON RJ: High resolution computed tomography of the middle ear and mastoid. Part II: Tubotympanic disease. *Radiology* **148**:455–459, 1983*b*.

SWARTZ JD: Cholesteatomas of the middle ear: Diagnosis, etiology and complications. *Radiol Clin North Am* **22**:15–36, 1984*a*.

SWARTZ JD, FAERBER EN, WOLFSON RJ, MARLOWE FI: Fenestral otosclerosis: significance of preoperative CT evaluation. *Radiology* **151**:703–707, 1984*b*.

TURSKI P, NORMAN D, DEGROOT J, CAPRA R: High-resolution CT of the petrous bone: Direct vs. reformatted images. *AJNR* **3**:391–394, 1982.

VALAVANIS A, SCHUBIGER O, HAYEK J, POULIADIS G: CT of meningiomas on the posterior surface of the petrous bone. *Neuroradiology* **22**:111–121, 1981.

VALVASSORI GE, MAFEE MF, DOBBEN GD: Computerized tomography of the temporal bone. *Laryngoscope* **92**:562–565, 1982.

VIRAPONGSE C, SARWAR M, SASAKI C, KIER EL: High resolution computed tomography of the osseous external canal. 1. Normal anatomy. *J Comput Assist Tomogr* **7**:486–492, 1983.

WRIGHT JW JR: Trauma of the ear. *Radiol Clin North Am* **12**:527–532, 1974.

WRIGHT JW JR: Polytomography and congenital external and middle ear anomalies. *Laryngoscope* **91**:1806–1811, 1981.

WRIGHT JW JR, WRIGHT JW III, HICKS G: Polytomography and congenital anomalies of the ear. *Ann Otol Rhinol Laryngol* **91**:480–484, 1982.

WU E-R, TANG Y-S, ZANG Y-T et al: CT in diagnosis of acoustic neuromas. *Am J Neuroradiol* **7**:645–650, 1986.

YOUNG IR, BYDDER GM, HALL AS et al: The role of NMR imaging in the diagnosis and management of acoustic neuroma. *AJNR* **4**:223–224, 1983.

ZONNEVELD FW, VAN WAES PFGM, DAMSMA H, RABISCHONG P, VIGNAUD J: Direct multiplanar computed tomography of the petrous bone. *RadioGraphics* **3**:400–449, 1983.

11

TRAUMA: CRANIOCEREBRAL AND CRANIOFACIAL

Pulla R. S. Kishore

Krishna C.V.G. Rao

Maurice H. Lipper

Kalyanmay Goshhajra

SECTION A: CRANIOCEREBRAL TRAUMA

Perhaps the greatest impact of CT in the evaluation of patients with neurological disease has been in the diagnosis and management of head injury. The unique ability of CT to detect subtle differences in tissue density in a noninvasive manner in a short period of time has proved valuable in the detection of various traumatic intracranial lesions, especially hematomas. It has virtually replaced other radiologic investigations in suspected neurologic dysfunction secondary to head injury (Ambrose 1974; French 1977; Koo 1977; Merino-deVillasante 1976; Roberson 1979; Svendsen 1976; Zimmerman 1978a).

TECHNICAL AND CLINICAL FACTORS

Before attempting to evaluate the role of CT in head trauma, the following factors must be considered.

Partial Volume Effect

A brief discussion of this phenomenon with respect to various traumatic lesions will facilitate understanding of the contents of this chapter (see also Chaps. 1 and 16). Partial volume effect results from scanning a structure or a lesion which occupies only part of the CT slice (Brooks 1976; McCullough 1976). Since the density at any point of the CT image is a result of the average attenuation of the entire slice

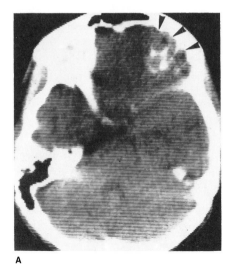

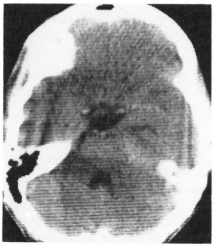

Figure 11-1 Artifact simulating confusion. **A.** A nonhomogeneous high-density zone is present in the frontal region (arrowheads), suggestive of an intracerebral contusion. **B.** An additional overlapping CT slice performed on the same patient reveals no abnormality. The "confusion" was thus an artifact caused by normallly occurring bony irregularity on the floor of the anterior cranial fossa

thickness at that point, it does not contribute its full density to the image. As a result of this effect, an extracerebral subdural hematoma over the convexity measuring half or less of a slice thickness may merge with the bony calvarium and may not be detected on the CT image. This partial volume effect may also be the reason for the nonvisualization of small hematomas reported in some series (Levander 1975; Svendsen 1976). This phenomenon may also explain the experience of encountering a larger hematoma at surgery than expected from the CT image (French and Dublin 1977). A small intracerebral hematoma may be missed for the same reason.

Another area where partial volume effect may cause confusion is the region of the inferior frontal lobe, where the irregular floor of the anterior fossa projecting into the normal brain may simulate contusions (Fig. 11-1). To counteract this effect, one may scan with thinner overlapping slices or use a different angle.

Motion Artifact

Patient motion can produce artifacts which may obscure significant intracranial lesions (Fig. 11-2). Motion artifacts are accentuated by the presence of me-

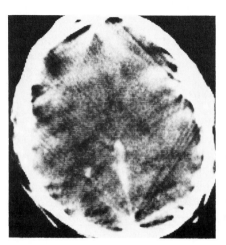

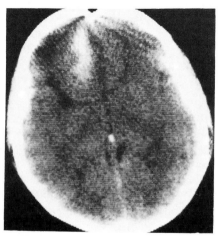

Figure 11-2 Artifact obscuring intracerebral hematoma. **A.** CT showing artifact caused by patient motion with no obvious lesion demonstrated. **B.** The same CT slice performed on the same patient after sedation reveals a frontal high-density zone compatible with an intracerebral hematoma.

tallic fragments associated with missile injuries. Although this may be less of a problem with faster scanners, adequate immobilization is essential. This may be achieved by the use of restraining devices or sedation. The necessity of motion-artifact–free CT in trauma cannot be overemphasized, because a significant hematoma—especially an extracerebral one—can go undetected.

Multiple Injuries

Associated multiple injuries, especially those involving the cervical spine, must be considered. Although the incidence of cervical spine injury associated with head injury varies in the literature, as many as 17 percent of fatal head trauma victims are known to have high spinal cord injury (Alcker 1978). Extreme care should be exercised in moving or manipulating the patient during the CT examination. A transtable lateral radiograph of the cervical spine should be obtained prior to CT to determine whether immobilization of the cervical spine is necessary if there is even a remote possibility of cervical spine trauma. In addition, when other severe life-threatening organ injuries are suspected, a limited CT examination may be performed to exclude the presence of a large intracranial lesion before the patient undergoes a major surgical procedure for injury of other organs.

Traumatic lesions demonstrable on CT include the following:

1. Edema: focal and diffuse
2. Contusion, laceration
3. Hematomas
   a. Intracerebral, acute and delayed
   b. Intraventricular
   c. Cortical and subcortical
   d. Extracerebral, subdural and epidural
4. Subarachnoid hemorrhage
5. Subdural hygroma
6. Fractures, displaced bone fragments, soft-tissue contusion, subgaleal hematoma, foreign bodies, and pneumocephalus

7. Posttraumatic
   a. Ischemic infarction
   b. Acute or delayed hydrocephalus
   c. Atrophy
   d. Abscess formation

CT FINDINGS IN HEAD INJURY

The incidence of traumatic cerebral lesions demonstrated on CT varies considerably, depending on patient selection, the severity of trauma, the interval between injury and CT, and the accessibility of a CT scanner. As few as 37 percent of the patients had CT abnormalities in one series (Baker 1974). In another series, 73 percent were reported to be abnormal (Paxton 1974). In one report on a series of 316 patients, 51 percent had an abnormal CT, with 38 percent having more than one detectable lesion (French 1977). Perhaps a more important observation is that only 13 percent of the neurologically intact patients demonstrated CT abnormalities, while 50 percent of the patients with a focal neurological deficit demonstrated lesions. Merino-de Villasante and Taveras in their retrospective study (1976) found that 75 percent of the patients with lateralized findings had discernible CT abnormalities. However, the above-mentioned reports were results of CT conducted at varying time intervals after different degrees of severity of trauma. An accurate assessment and understanding of traumatic CT lesions can be achieved only by studying patients with well-defined neurological deficit immediately following injury and sequentially thereafter, if necessary (Roberson 1979).

In patients with severe head injury associated with significant neurological deficits (Table 11-1), nearly 60 percent will demonstrate different forms of hemorrhagic lesions. In the authors' series 26 percent had intracerebral hematoma or contusion, 30 percent had extracerebral hematoma (subdural, epidural, subarachnoid), and 14 percent had combined hemorrhagic lesions (Kishore 1981). In nearly 30 percent of cases the CT may fail to demonstrate any

**Table 11-1   Initial CT Findings in 150
            Consecutive Patients
            with Severe Head Injury**

Normal	47
Edema	13
Extracerebral hematoma	.30
Intracerebral hematoma contusion	39
Combined intracerebral and extracerebral hematoma	21

lesions on the initial study. In the remaining 9 to 10 percent edema may be the only CT finding. The specific traumatic craniocerebral lesions demonstrable on CT are discussed in greater detail in the following sections.

Edema

The CT appearance of edema is that of low-density zones with attenuation value of 10 to 14 Hounsfield units (HU), less than that of white matter (22-36 HU). This may be focal, multifocal, or diffuse (Fig. 11-3). The last may be difficult to diagnose because of the lack of normal brain density for comparison. Edema may be associated with mass effect leading to compression, distortion, and displacement of the adjacent ventricles. Generalized edema may manifest only as generalized compression and decrease in size of the ventricles. The compression may be so severe as to cause nonvisualization of the ventricular system and subarachnoid cisterns (Auh 1980) (Fig. 11-4).

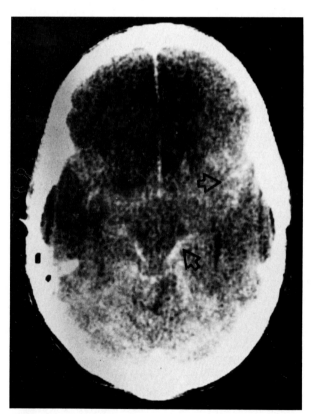

Figure 11-3 Posttraumatic diffuse cerebral edema. This appears as areas of hypodensity involving both frontal and temporal lobes. The cisterns appear as hyperdense regions due to associated blood products in the subarachnoid cisterns.

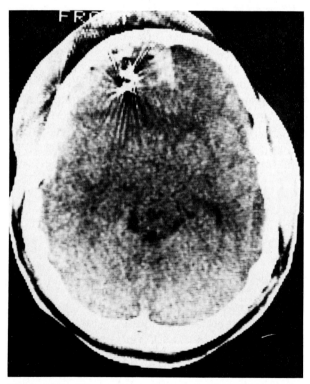

Figure 11-4 Excessively small ventricles. CT following gunshot wound to head. The ventricles are compressed due to edema. A hemorrhagic component is present in the frontal region, hyperdense in appearance. Adjacent to it toward the left a markedly dense region with streak artifact is seen due to the fragments of the metallic density within the brain parenchyma.

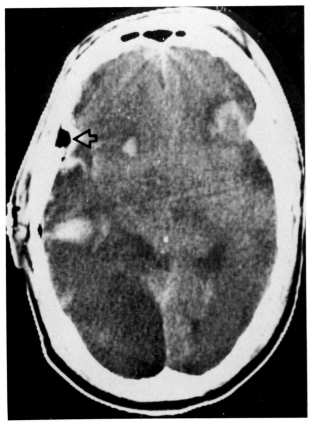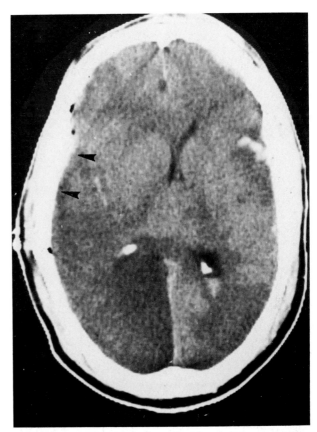

Figure 11-5 Posttraumatic infarction. CT demonstrates diffuse hemorrhagic contusions involving both cerebral hemispheres. In addition there is pneumocephalus (⬧) as well as a thin subdural collection (⭡) on the left side. Due to the significant trauma there is an infarct involving the posterior temporal, occipital region on the left side which is hypodense in appearance.

Adding confusion to the diagnosis of posttraumatic edema on CT is the fact that low-density areas may be due to causes other than edema. Low-attenuation substances such as lipids or cavitation and necrosis in subacute traumatic lesions may blend with small adjacent areas of hemorrhage, resulting in low-density zones. Conversely, edema may not be evident as low density if a simultaneous decrease in the lipid content counterbalances any decrease in attenuation caused by increased cerebral water content.

Finally, the hypodensity on the CT may not represent true posttraumatic edema and may be a result of ischemic infarction (Fig. 11-5), which does not have the same connotation as edema in terms of management and outcome (Miller 1980).

Contusion

Contusions, which may be single or multiple, occur usually in the anterior frontal and temporal lobes (Fig. 11-6). They appear as areas of nonhomogeneous high-density zones with attentuation values of 50 to 67 HU. This appearance is due to the presence of multiple small areas of hemorrhage within the brain substance interspersed with areas of edema and tissue necrosis. Contusions may have varying proportions of high- and low-density areas, depending on the extent of hemorrhage, degree of edema, and time elapsed since injury. During the first 24 hours, increased density predominates; but with resolution of the hemorrhage, the amount of low density increases progressively until an ap-

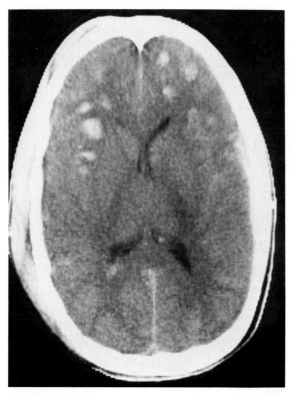

Figure 11-6 Multiple contusions with edema. Multiple bilateral frontal, temporal, and deep nonhomogeneous high-density zones with surrounding low density and ventricular compression. These features represent multiple contusions with surrounding edema.

pearance similar to that of edema is seen. On CT done several hours or days after injury, the contusions may be misinterpreted (Fig. 11-7) (French 1977).

A contusion usually has a poorly defined margin, often surrounded by a low-density zone representing edema. These areas are single or multiple and often demontrate a mass effect with ventricular compression, distortion, and displacement. The initial high density and size of the contusion generally decrease, and CT resolution of the contusion is usually complete by 6 weeks, leaving no residual changes or changes similar to porencephaly or focal atrophy, seen as CSF density; but occasionally the contusion may get larger as hemorrhage increases.

It may occasionally be difficult to differentiate between contusion and an extracerebral hematoma with intracerebral extension, especially in frontal and inferior temporal regions (Fig. 11-8). Approximately 15 percent of patients with severe head injury can be expected to have both extra- and intracerebral hemorrhages.

Intracerebral Hematoma

This is seen as a well-circumscribed, homogeneous, high-density zone with an attenuation of 70-90 HU, usually surrounded by areas of low density due to edema (Fig. 11-9). A recent lesion as small as 0.5 cm

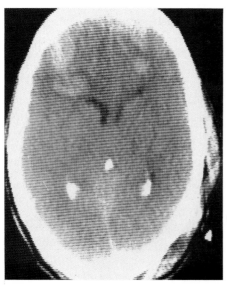

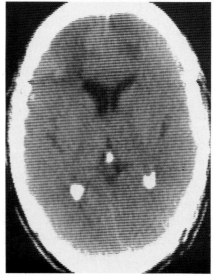

Figure 11-7 Contusion with resolution. **A.** Bilateral frontal nonhomogeneous high-density zones with surrounding edema and ventricular displacement compatible with contusions. **B.** CT performed 6 days later demonstrating almost complete resolution of the bifrontal contusions, with residual hypodense areas which may simulate edema.

A   **B**

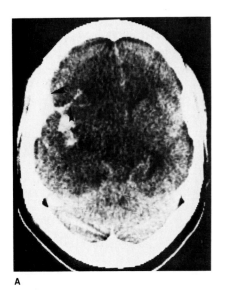
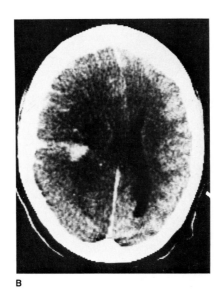

A   B

Figure 11-8 Contusion with intracerebral and subdural hematoma. A hemorrhagic contusion involving the insula and extending into the white matter is seen on the left side. Linear hyperdensity (↓) in (**A**) relates to blood products in the subarachnoid cisterns. There is also an associated subdural hematoma (↓).

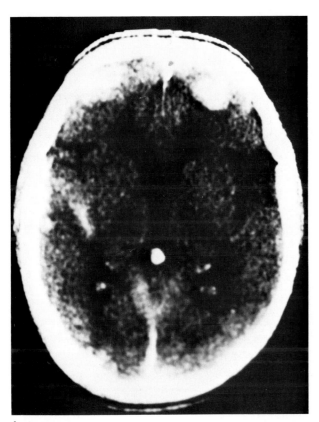
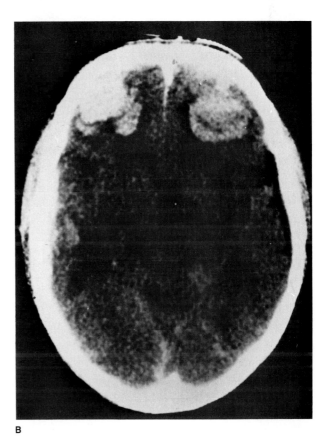

A   B

Figure 11-9 Intracerebral hematoma: bifrontal intracerebral hematoma, homogeneously hyperdense with surrounding edema. Hyperdensity in the left insula represents block in the subarachnoid cisterns. Punctate hemorrhage is also seen in both hemispheres posteriorly.

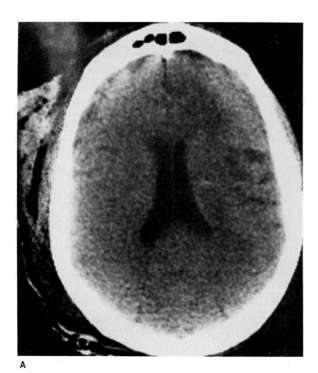

A

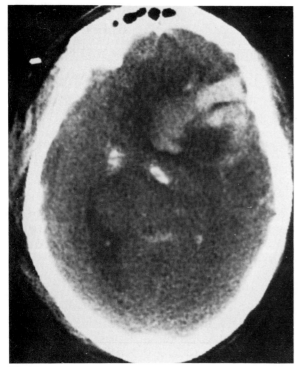

B

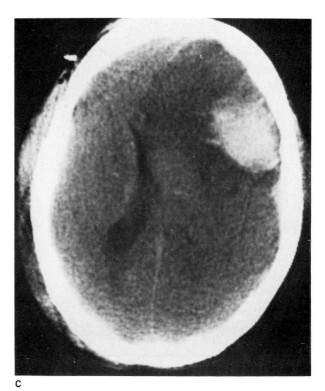

C

Figure 11-10   Traumatic intracerebral hematoma.   **A**. Initial CT demonstrates mild generalized edema with mild compression of the body of right lateral ventricle.   **B** and **C**. Twenty-four hours later CT demonstrates a large hemorrhagic component with surrounding edema and obliteration of the cisterns. The right lateral ventricle is compressed with dilatation of the contralateral ventricle due to the hematoma and associated edema.

in diameter may be detected on CT because of the contrast between the high attenuation of the hematoma and the surrounding low-density brain tissue. The high attenuation value of a recent hematoma is attributed to clot retraction and the high absorption coefficient of the globin molecule of hemoglobin. This high density diminishes gradually because of disintegration of the blood components. During this resolution, a certain point in time is reached, usually 2 to 4 weeks after injury, when the attenuation is similar to that of the adjacent brain and the hematoma is termed *isodense,* being undetectable to the naked eye. At this stage the hematoma may be completely missed unless attention is paid to mass effect. It is important to be aware that a hematoma may be present intracerebrally, even in a patient with an apparently normal CT (Messina 1975). Contrast enhancement may assist in visualizing such isodense lesions (Zimmerman 1977). With further resolution an area of density similar to that of porencephaly may result.

Traumatic intracerebral hematomas may differ from those resulting from hypertension, aneurysms, or arteriovenous malformations in that the traumatic lesions are frequently of irregular contour. They tend to be poorly demarcated, with no uniformity of density. They may often be multiple and are usually located in the frontal or anterior temporal lobes, although they may occur in any intracranial location.

Although the majority of intracerebral hematomas develop immediately after head injury, they may show a delay in appearance (Fig. 11-10). Prior to the advent of CT, the time period for the development of delayed traumatic intracerebral hematomas was believed to be as late as several weeks after trauma (Baratham 1972). With increasing use of CT, however, it appears that most delayed hematomas occur during the first week after injury (Brown 1978; Diaz 1979). The authors, in their experience using serial CT, found that the majority (11 out of 12) developed during the first 48 hours following injury (Gudeman 1979). Delayed hematoma is usually associated with poor outcome (Gudeman 1979), with 50 percent of the patients dying subsequently. Although 50 percent of the delayed hemorrhages develop following

decompression surgery, they may develop in patients with normal initial CT. A repeat CT at 48 hours or earlier should be obtained to detect the lesions in patients who undergo decompressive surgery or those who do not show improvement, even if they had a normal CT on admission.

Confusion may arise when an intracerebral hematoma located near the brain surface mimics an extracerebral hematoma. This may be distinguished by the relationship of the medial margin of the hematoma to the inner table. With an intracerebral hematoma, this margin usually forms an acute angle with the inner table, whereas with an extracerebral hematoma the angle is obtuse (Koo 1977).

Subdural Hematoma

Acute subdural hematomas usually appear as peripheral zones of increased density following the surface of the brain and having a concave inner margin and a convex outer margin adjacent to the inner table of the skull (Fig. 11-11). Although there is an occasional overlap in the appearance of the two types of extracerebral hematoma, the typical subdural lesion tends to be more diffuse than the epidural one. The extension of the latter is limited by the firm attachment of the dura mater to the calvarium. A subdural hematoma with a depth of as little as 5 mm is usually clearly demonstrable on CT. Thinner collections and occasionally even larger hematomas occurring along the high convexity may be missed because of the partial volume effect. Sometimes the only clue to the presence of a large lesion may be the mass effect. A high convexity lesion may be more easily detected if the scanning is performed with the x-ray beam perpendicular to the affected region; this may be accomplished by tilting the patient's head or placing the patient in a lateral decubitus position (Svendsen 1976).

Although hematomas can sometimes be classified as acute, subacute, or chronic on the basis of the CT attenuation values, absolute reliance on such a classification may lead to an inaccurate diagnosis. Scotti et al. (1977) found a high degree of correlation between the CT density and the age of the hema-

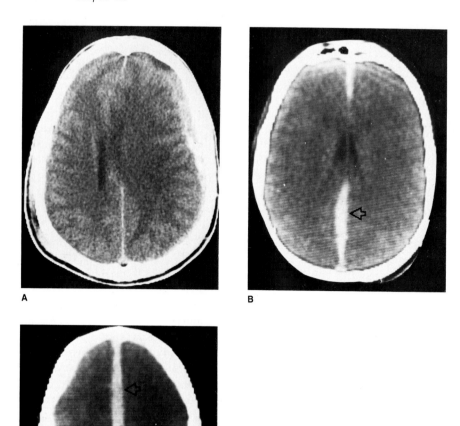

A

B

C

Figure 11-11 Acute subdural hematoma: Typical acute subdural hematoma as demonstrated by a peripheral zone of increased density following the surface of the brain, having a concave inner margin with obliteration of the right lateral ventricle. **B** and **C**: Another patient with acute interhemispheric subdural hematoma on the left side. The sharp margin on the right side (◁) of the hyperdense zone demonstrates the rigid falx in the midline.

toma: 100 percent of acute (within 7 days following injury) subdural hematomas showed as areas of increased density, 70 percent of the lesions classified as subacute (7 to 21 days) were isodense, and 76 percent of the chronic subdural hematomas (more than 22 days) were of decreased density. On the basis of this classification, a mistaken diagnosis of subacute or chronic subdural hematoma may be made if recent hemorrhage occurs into a chronic subdural collection, with resultant isodense appearance (Fig.

11-12). Similarly, in patients with a low hematocrit, an acute hematoma may have relatively low attenuation because of the low hemoglobin level and may mimic subacute or chronic lesions (New 1976; Smith 1981).

Because of the foregoing reasons, it is probably best to describe extracerebral lesions as hyper- or hypodense and to specify the size unless one is certain of all clinical factors. It is important to remember that the management of the patient with intra-

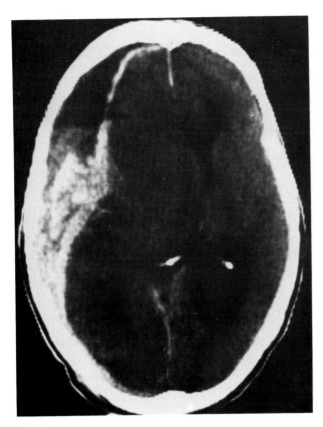

Figure 11-12 Acute on chronic subdural hematoma. A large extracerebral collection with resulting mass effect is seen involving the left cerebral hemisphere. The fluid collection has a hypodense component in the top and a hyperdense component in the bottom. This represents the different components of the blood products. Similar appearance can also be seen in an acute subdural hematoma due to layering of blood products.

cranial hematoma depends on the clinical condition, the size of the lesion, and the resultant brain compression rather than the "acute" or "chronic" nature of the lesion as determined by CT density. For therapeutic purposes, an acute lesion, especially if there is sufficient brain compression, requires decompressive surgery.

A subdural hematoma is usually associated with mass effect, which is seen as compression of the brain with obliteration of gyral markings over the affected hemisphere and midline displacement. If midline displacement away from the side of the lesion is not present or is less than expected, one must

suspect lesions on the contralateral side. Approximately 40 percent of extracerebral hematomas are associated with other traumatic lesions such as cerebral contusions or hematomas in patients with severe head injury (Kishore 1981).

As with intracerebral hematomas, the attenuation value of a subdural lesion decreases gradually over a period of weeks; this is dependent on the initial size and whether or not low-attenuation fluids such as CSF are mixed with the clot. When the hematoma reaches the isodense stage, it may not be visualized on CT unless a significant mass effect is present. Findings such as effacement of the sulci over the affected side and distortion of the ipsilateral ventricle should alert one to the presence of such a lesion (Fig. 11-13). Contrast-enhanced CT (CECT) may be of value in visualizing such lesions by causing enhancement of the membrane around the subdural hematoma or enhancement of the subdural collection itself as a result of seepage of the contrast material into the collection (Messina 1976) (Fig. 11-14). If isodense subdural hematoma is suspected and not resolved by CT, MRI would be an alternative imaging modality because of lack of bone artifacts and excellent soft-tissue anatomy visualization (Moon 1984). Isodense subdural hematomas tend to have shorter T_1 and longer T_2 values. It has also been shown that as many as 40 percent of isodense subdural hematomas may be enhanced after 4 to 6 hours on a delayed CECT (Amendola 1977). The lesion may also be demonstrated by utilizing alteration in window and center settings, digital filtering techniques, and subtraction techniques (Larson 1977). Contrast infusion has been shown to demonstrate the isodense hematoma by visualizing the displacement of cortical veins and/or brain (Hayman 1979; Kim 1978). Also, CECT is extremely helpful in detection of bilateral isodense subdural hematomas. The absence of focal enhancement within the parenchyma on the CECT in a patient with midline shift and a history of recent trauma should suggest the presence of an extracerebral lesion.

Further changes in the appearance of the subdural hematoma are probably due to absorption of fluid across the membrane, with a resultant decrease in attenuation value until it reaches that of

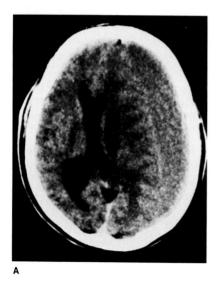
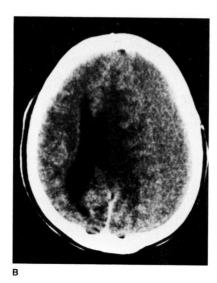

Figure 11-13 Isodense subdural hematoma. This illustrates the features of an isodense subdural hematoma with effacement of the sulci over the affected side and distortion of the ipsilateral ventricle.

A

B

CSF. The membrane's rich vascularity leads to its visualization on CECT. A chronic subdural hematoma is usually seen on CT as a biconvex low-density zone. A subdural hygroma developing acutely may also resemble a chronic subdural hematoma in appearance but does not have the biconvex configuration or enhancement of the membrane on CECT.

Occasionally a subdural hematoma may be seen in which sedimentation of corpuscular elements into the dependent portion of the hematoma has occurred, giving rise to the appearance of a low-attenuation zone in the supernatant area with increased density in the dependent portion. A subdural hematoma usually passes from an initial hyperdense value through the isodense stage into the CSF density stage within a space of 3 to 6 weeks (Bergstrom 1977).

A diagnostic problem may arise in patients with focal atrophy, in which the dilated subarachnoid space may resemble a chronic subdural hematoma. On careful screening, one may see the CSF density extending into the enlarged sulci, thus differentiating it from a compressive lesion (Fig. 11-15). The CT image of a patient with hemiatrophy may be similar to that of an isodense hematoma. A relatively small lateral ventricle and absent or normal sulci over the convexity on the normal hemisphere, with midline shift to the atrophic side harboring a large ventricle in the case of hemiatrophy, can be mistaken for a hematoma on the normal side. However, wide windowing will permit the diagnosis of hemiatrophy by demonstrating a thicker bony calvarium on the side of the atrophy (Zilkha 1980). Additional findings such as enlarged sinuses and petrous bone associated with a small middle cranial fossa may be seen on the affected side.

Delayed Subdural Hematoma

Subdural hematomas, like intracerebral hematomas, may develop in a delayed manner either ipsilaterally or contralaterally following evacuation of a preexisting intracranial lesion (Fig. 11-16) (Lipper 1979). The delayed development of subdural hygromas occurs in the frontal and temporal area. The hygromas are frequently bilateral. These are found to occur at varying time intervals following injury, usually between 6 and 46 days (French 1977). The authors' own experience with sequential CT of severe head injury patients indicates that 5 percent develop frontal hygromas. All the hygromas developed during the first 2 weeks after injury. These collections may

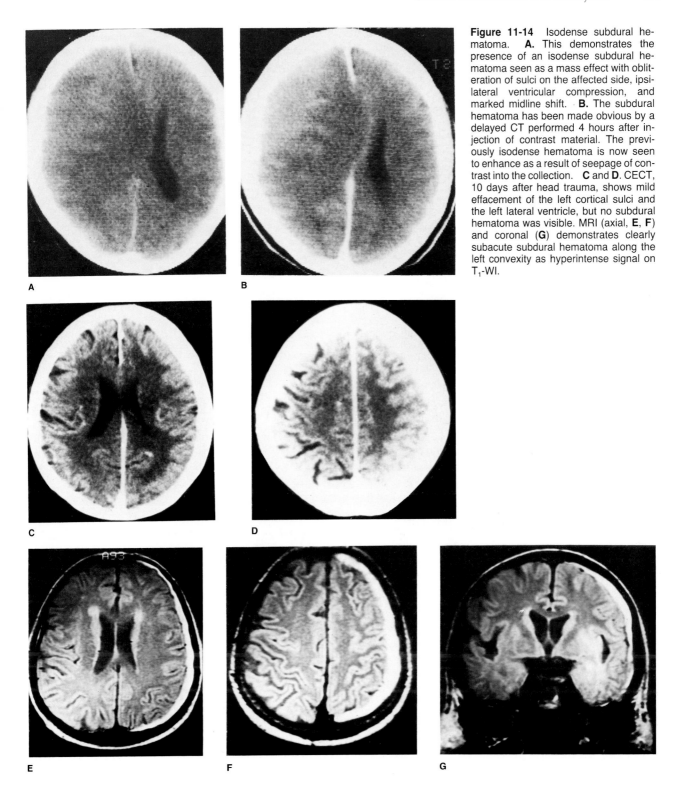

Figure 11-14 Isodense subdural hematoma. **A.** This demonstrates the presence of an isodense subdural hematoma seen as a mass effect with obliteration of sulci on the affected side, ipsilateral ventricular compression, and marked midline shift. **B.** The subdural hematoma has been made obvious by a delayed CT performed 4 hours after injection of contrast material. The previously isodense hematoma is now seen to enhance as a result of seepage of contrast into the collection. **C** and **D.** CECT, 10 days after head trauma, shows mild effacement of the left cortical sulci and the left lateral ventricle, but no subdural hematoma was visible. MRI (axial, **E**, **F**) and coronal (**G**) demonstrates clearly subacute subdural hematoma along the left convexity as hyperintense signal on T$_1$-WI.

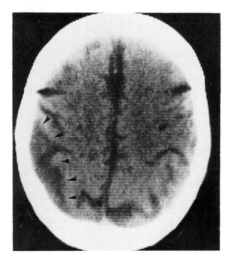

Figure 11-15 Cortical atrophy mimicking subdural hematoma. CT of an 89-year-old patient with cerebral atrophy which may suggest the presence of a posterior parietal chronic subdural collection (arrowheads). However, the extension of the peripheral low density into the sulci should confirm the presence of an enlarged subarachnoid space as seen in atrophy, rather than a collection.

disappear spontaneously by 3 months and probably do not require surgical evacuation (Fig. 11-17) (Lipper 1979).

Epidural Hematoma

On CT, an acute epidural hematoma is usually seen as a biconvex peripheral high-density lesion (Fig. 11-18*A*). Epidural hemorrhage in the majority of cases is due to arterial bleed, with stripping of the dura. Occasionally epidural hematoma could also be due to rupture of the venous sinuses, which lie adjacent to the inner table of the skull. The majority of the arterial epidural hematomas are thus located where branches of the meningeal artery are situated, the most frequent site being the temporal or frontal region. The mass effect and cerebral edema are most manifest with arterial epidural hematomas. Venous epidural hematomas are usually small, commonly associated with a fracture which has not crossed a

Figure 11-16 Delayed subdural collection.   **A.** Initial CT after trauma demonstrating a left temporal contusion and subdural hematoma (arrowheads).   **B.** A CT performed 14 days later, after surgical evacuation of the hematoma, demonstrates a right frontoparietal peripheral low-density zone (arrowheads), consistent with a delayed contralateral extracerebral lesion.

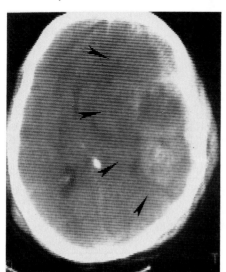

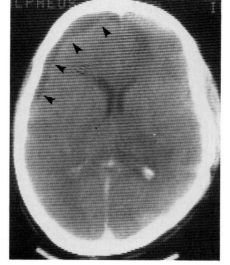

A   **B**

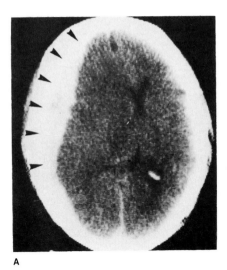 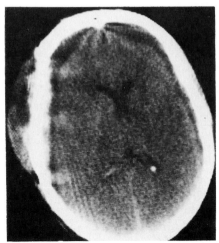

A   B

Figure 11-17 Subdural hygromas. **A.** A large right acute subdural hematoma (arrowheads). **B.** CT on day 14 following evacuation of the hematoma shows bifrontal peripheral low-density zones representing bilateral hygromas.

meningeal artery. Larger venous epidural hematomas are more common and should be suspected when the epidural hematoma straddles over the cerebral hemisphere, pushing the falx downward (Fig. 11-18 *BCD*). They occur when a major dural sinus has been torn. Similar epidural can also be seen in the region of the torcula and may dissect between the two leaves of the dura forming the tentorium. The biconvex appearance is caused by the firm dural adherence to the inner table. This lesion is usually denser on CT than a subdural hematoma because it is less likely to mix with CSF or brain. Occasionally, when associated with a large subdural hematoma on the contralateral side, a small epidural hematoma may not be seen in the initial scan, and may enlarge rapidly following surgical evacuation of the subdural hematoma (Fig. 11-18) (Nelson in press). This emphasizes the necessity of postoperative CT in these cases. Acute isodense epidural hematomas are rare compared to acute isodense subdural hematomas.

Although epidural and subdural hematomas can be differentiated by CT appearance, as described above, it may not always be possible to localize hematomas exactly to one or the other space. Approximately 20 percent of patients show blood in both spaces at surgery or autopsy (Jamieson 1968).

Delayed Epidural Hematoma

Delayed epidural hematoma may manifest on the ipsilateral or contralateral side following removal of either an epidural or a subdural hematoma (Nelson 1982). Usually it manifests itself within 24 hours. Occasionally delayed epidural hematoma may also occur following decrease in the cerebral edema (Fig. 11-18*E, F*). The epidural hematoma is due to release of the tamponade effect caused by the decrease in the cerebral edema. In the majority of cases the hematoma is due to a venous bleed rather than a torn artery, although occasionally this may be arterial. If the hematomas are small, they are usually followed utilizing CT, as long as there is no significant mass effect or associated neurological deficit.

Intraventricular Hemorrhage

Intraventricular hemorrhage appears as high density within the ventricles (Fig. 11-19). The increased density disappears relatively quickly in comparison with intracerebral, subdural, and epidural hematomas. The return to CSF density in the ventricles occurs within days, and clot density is rarely present after 1 week (Fig. 11-19). As with intracerebral hem-

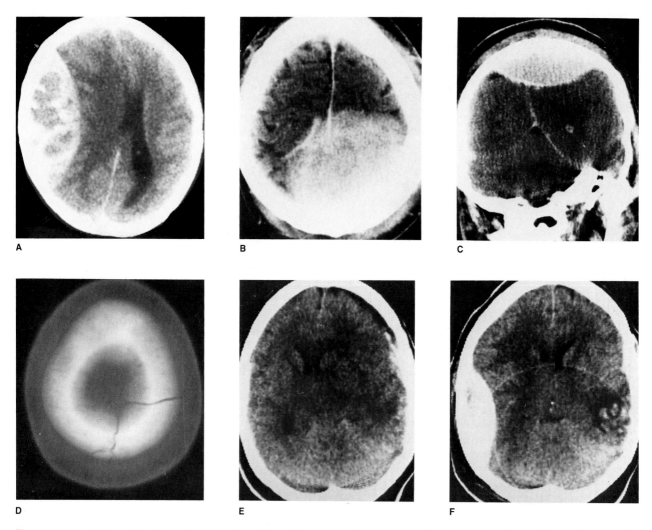

Figure 11-18 Acute epidural hematoma. **A.** A peripheral biconvex nonhomogeneous hyperdense hematoma. The nonhomogeneity is due to admixture of clotted and nonclotted blood products. **B–D.** Another patient with high-convexity epidural hematoma associated with skull fracture. The epidural hematoma in coronal view (**C**) is in the midline displacing the dura and the sinus from the calvarium. **D**. Bone window setting demonstrates the skull fracture. **E,F.** Delayed epidural hematoma: **E**. Initial NCCT demonstrates diffuse cerebral edema with a thin subdural hematoma (arrowhead) and associated cerebral contusion (arrow). There is a shift of midline structures to the left. **F**. NCCT 24 hours later demonstrates a large delayed hematoma (arrow) on the left side, and the region of cerebral contusion now appears as an area of hemorrhagic infarct (arrow).

orrhage, nonvisualization of hematoma in the ventricles may not imply total resolution of the clot. Occasionally sedimentation of the corpuscular elements occurs in the dependent portion of the ventricles, giving rise to some increased density in the dependent portion sharply demarcated from a CSF density in the uppermost portion (Fig. 11-20). This is frequently associated with intraparenchymal

hemorrhage and appears to be more common than was realized before the advent of CT (French 1977; Roberson 1979; Zimmerman 1978*a*). Five percent of patients with severe head injury can be expected to have intraventricular hemorrhage (Roberson 1979). These reports indicate that intraventricular hemorrhage does not imply as grave a prognosis as was previously thought. Perhaps early CT recognition of

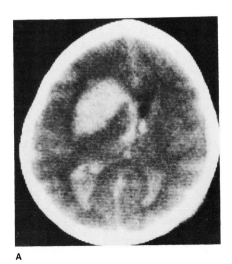

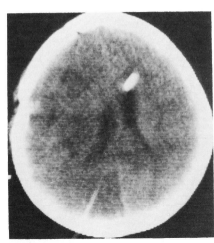

A   B

Figure 11-19 Intracerebral hematoma with intraventricular hematoma. **A.** A large traumatic hematoma in the right basal ganglion region with intraventricular hemorrhage seen as high density within the lateral ventricles on day 1 CT. **B.** NCCT performed after 4 days shows almost complete resolution of the intraventricular hematoma. (The basal ganglion hematoma has been surgically removed and a ventriculostomy tube is present in the lateral ventricle.)

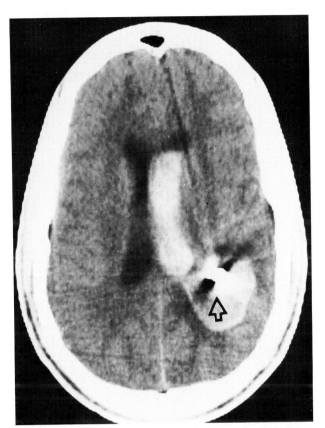

Figure 11-20 Traumatic intraventricular hemorrhage. Sedimentation of the corpuscular elements of the blood has resulted in a sharp demarcation between the blood in the most dependent portion of the ventricle and the CSF density in upper portion. Hematoma surrounding a metallic density is present in the adjacent brain parenchyma (⇧).

ventricular enlargement, resulting in prompt therapeutic measures such as ventricular drainage, has improved the prognosis.

Other Acute Traumatic Lesions

Subarachnoid hemorrhage (SAH), frequently found in patients with head injury, is seen as zones of increased density in the basal cisterns, sylvian fissures, interhemispheric fissure, and sulci (Fig. 11-21). As may be expected, SAH is often present with other intracranial hematomas (Dolinskas 1978). The increased density on CT due to SAH rarely lasts more than a few days. The high density of the falx in older patients should not be mistaken for SAH, and caution should be exercised in making the diagnosis of SAH on CT if there is high density only in the falcial region, not in any other subarachnoid space (Osborn 1980). (See Chapter 17.)

Fractures with displaced bone fragments (Fig. 11-22), soft-tissue contusions, foreign bodies, and pneumocephalus are also easily recognizable on CT (Fig. 11-23). CT is also extremely valuable in the demonstration of lesions caused by gunshot wounds. Bone and bullet fragments are well demonstrated, as is the hemorrhagic track of the missile (Fig. 11-24). In patients with shearing injury, CT clearly demonstrates hemorrhage into the deep white matter, especially the corpus callosum (Fig. 11-29). These

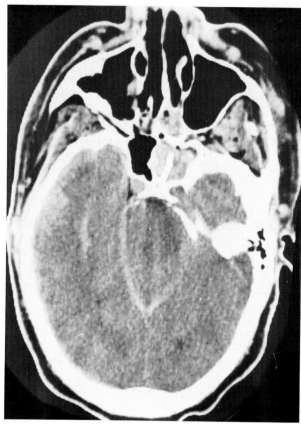

Figure 11-21   Traumatic subarachnoid hemorrhage. Increased density in the basal cisterns, sylvian fissure denotes presence of blood in these spaces due to traumatic subarachnoid hemorrhage.

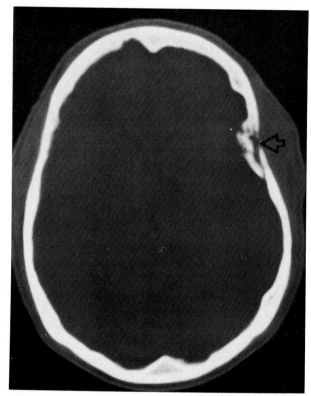

Figure 11-22   Depressed skull fracture. CT in bone window setting demonstrates inward projection of the portion of the inner table (◄).

small hemorrhages are most often seen in the corpus callosum, internal capsule, upper brainstem, and corticomedullary junctures. The gross CT manifestations of shearing injury are often unimpressive and may be misleading relative to the much greater underlying gray and white matter damage (Zimmerman 1978*b*).

DELAYED SEQUELAE

Communicating *hydrocephalus* may develop following trauma as a result of blood in the subarachnoid space causing obstruction to the CSF pathways. Less

commonly, noncommunicating hydrocephalus may develop acutely secondary to hemorrhage within the ventricular system or around the aqueduct, obstructing the ventricular pathways. The latter type of hydrocephalus develops more rapidly compared to the one resulting from extraventricular obstruction.

The diagnosis of communicating hydrocephalus can be made on CT if there is a distended appearance of enlarged frontal horns, associated with dilatation of the temporal horns and the third and fourth ventricles. The absence of sulcal enlargement, and periventricular low density if present, are further evidence of hydrocephalus (Fig. 11-25) (Mori 1977). (See Chapter 5.)

Serial CT evaluation of 200 consecutive severe head injuries revealed that hydrocephalus, if it is to

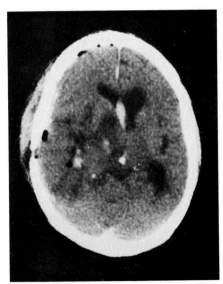

Figure 11-23 Multiple injury. There is a fracture, associated with intraventricular blood, punctate hemorrhagic contusion, with surrounding edema and intracranial air in subarachnoid space.

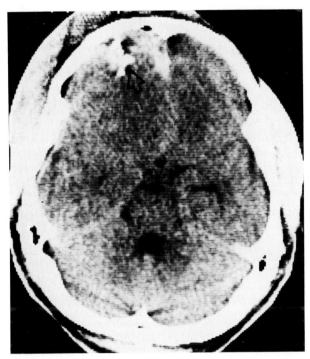

Figure 11-24 High-velocity missile injury. A hyperdense area adjacent to the falx represents a frontal hematoma. To the left of the hematoma are bone fragments (△), thus absence of the streak artifact.

develop, will do so by the end of the second post-trauma week in a majority (82 percent). Approximately 5.5 percent of all patients, or 8 percent of the survivors at 3 months after severe head injury, will have hydrocephalus (Gudeman 1981).

Posttraumatic atrophy appears to be a more common cause of ventricular enlargement following severe head injury and can be distinguished from hydrocephalus by associated sulcal enlargement (Fig. 11-26). It may be seen in as many as 30 percent of severe head injury survivors (Gudeman 1981). It is important not to confuse with ventricular enlargement the return of the ventricles to normal size following compression by brain swelling due to edema or hematomas in the immediate posttraumatic period.

Acute ischemic infarction, appearing as low-density areas, may be detectable within 24 hours of onset and by 7 days in over 60 percent of patients (Norton 1978). Ease of detection depends on the size of the lesion. The diagnostic yield is improved by nearly 15 percent by contrast infusion, with enhancement occurring most frequently between 1 and 4 weeks (Fig. 11-27) (Wing 1976; Yock 1975).

Posttraumatic abscess, occurring as the result of a penetrating injury or fracture or as a complication of surgery, takes the form of a low-density zone surrounded by a ring of enhancement following contrast infusion, usually associated with a large surrounding area of low density due to edema. Ventricular compression and displacement are also usually present. (See Chapter 13.)

VALUE OF CT IN HEAD INJURY

Although the prognostic significance of CT in head injury needs further documentation, certain conclusions can be drawn from the various studies that have been conducted so far. Needless to say, a patient with normal initial CT following head injury can be expected to have a good outcome unless secondary complications supervene, whether in the brain or other organs, especially pulmonary problems (Domingues de Silva, in press). Secondary

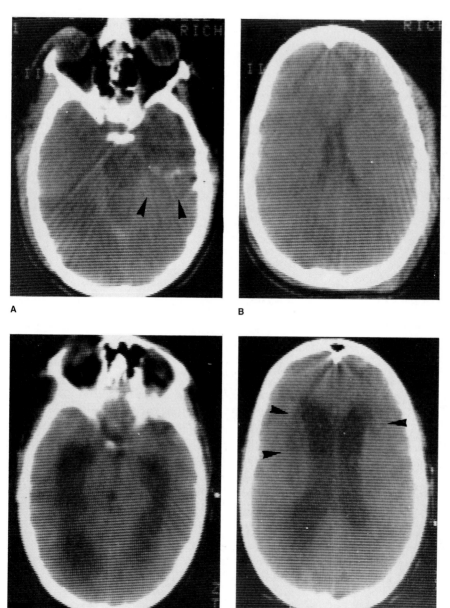

A

B

C

D

Figure 11-25 Communicating hydrocephalus. **A** and **B**. Initial CT performed on a 15-year-old male following head trauma reveals left frontal and temporal nonhomogeneous high-density zones (arrowheads) consistent with contusion associated with blood in the subarachnoid spaces. **C** and **D**. Study performed 1 month later reveals the features of communicating hydrocephalus as seen from the dilated ventricles, including enlargement of the frontal and temporal horns and third ventricle with periventricular low density (arrowheads) and the absence of sulcal enlargement.

complications in the brain, as mentioned earlier, include the development of delayed extra- and intracerebral hemorrhage, transtentorial herniation, edema, and intracranial hypertension (Clifton 1980; Cooper 1979a; Gudeman 1979; Lipper 1979; Miller 1980; Tsai 1978).

Although attempts to correlate CT findings and intracranial pressure have led to conflicting reports (Auer 1980; Sadhu 1979), patients with normal initial CT can be expected to have normal intracranial pressure in 98 percent of cases during the first 24 hours (Kishore 1981). Furthermore, only 17 percent

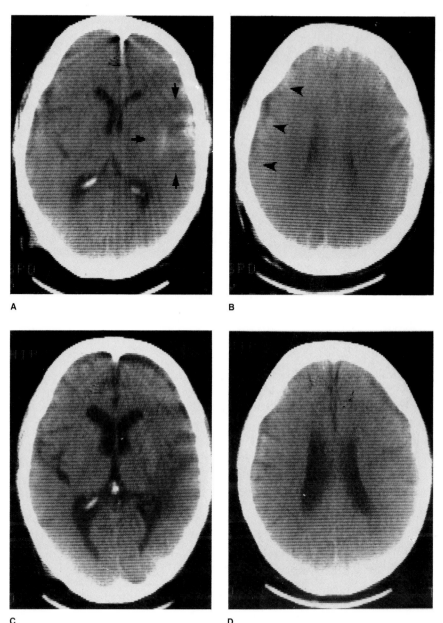

Figure 11-26 Posttraumatic atrophy. **A** and **B**. Admission CT on a male aged 55 showing a left temporal contusion (arrows) and low-density right frontotemporal extraaxial collection (arrowheads). **C** and **D**. Repeat study performed after 3 months shows, in comparison with the above, enlargement of the lateral ventricles and cortical sulci, features consistent with posttraumatic atrophy.

A   B

C   D

of patients may develop intracranial hypertension subsequently; and at least 91 percent of patients with normal initial CT have normal pressure during the first 48 hours following injury. On the other hand, 55 to 66 percent of patients with hemorrhagic lesions are likely to have intracranial hypertension.

An increased incidence of poor outcome is noted in patients with contusions and increased intracranial pressure (Miller 1979).

Patients who develop delayed lesions on CT are more likely to have a poor outcome whether or not they had a normal initial CT (Cooper 1979*a*; Gude-

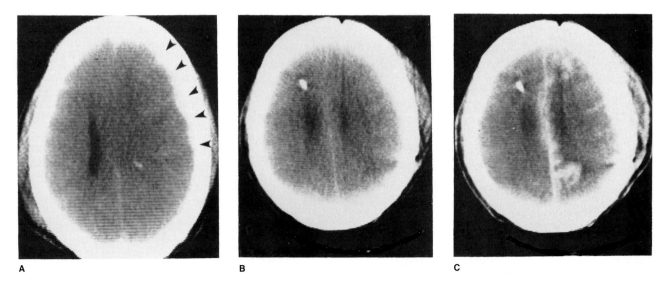

A   B   C

Figure 11-27   Traumatic cortical infarct.   **A.** Initial CT demonstrating a thin acute left subdural hematoma (arrowheads) with hemispheric edema, ventricular compression, and ventricular shift to the contralateral side.   **B.** Study performed 2 weeks later shows a left frontoparietal craniotomy with ill-defined low density over the left parietal region.   **C.** CECT shows extensive high parietal enhancement following the gyral pattern, typical of a parietal infarct.

man 1979; Lipper 1979). It is also well documented that a majority (75 percent) of patients with bilateral hemorrhagic lesions on CT during the first week end up in a persistent vegetative state or die (Sweet 1978); and 67 percent of patients with both intra- and extraaxial hemorrhagic lesions on initial CT can be expected to have a poor outcome, i.e., severe disability or worse (Kishore 1981). A case for repeat CT during the first week, preferably by the third day, is thus made in some reports (Clifton 1980; Cooper 1979a; Gudeman 1979; Kishore 1981). In one series (Clifton 1980), two thirds of patients who deteriorated after the first 48 hours had a new lesion on CT.

The location of the lesion in the brain as seen on CT is also important for prognosis. For example, it is well documented that patients with lesions involving the brainstem (Cooper 1979b; Tsai 1978) have poor outcome. Approximately 25 percent of those with primary brainstem injury survive in a permanent vegetative state (Tsai 1978). Unfortunately, a majority of brainstem lesions are not detectable on conventional CT because of artifacts in this region and because only 20 percent of brainstem lesions

are hemorrhagic, although partial or complete obliteration of the quadrigeminal cistern is frequently observed in patients with brainstem compression (Auh 1980). Cooper et al. (1979b) documented a similar poor outcome with brainstem injuries. Thus, if a brainstem hemorrhage is demonstrated on CT (Fig. 11-28), a poor outcome can be expected.

Shearing injuries involving the corpus callosum, if demonstrated on CT, indicate a poor outcome (Fig. 11-29). Seven of the eight patients with deep white-matter injuries involving the corpus callosum reported by Zimmerman et al. (1978b) ended up in a persistent vegetative state or died; they also noted a mortality rate of 40 percent in patients who had intraventricular in addition to intracerebral hemorrhage, as opposed to a 19 percent mortality for intracerebral hemorrhage alone.

Correlation has also been shown between atrophic changes seen on delayed CT (at the end of 3 months or 1 year) in surviving patients and the outcome (Gudeman 1981; Kishore 1978; Van Dongen 1980; Levin 1981). Although these correlations should be studied over an extended period of time, it is fair to assume that patients with documented atrophic changes on a

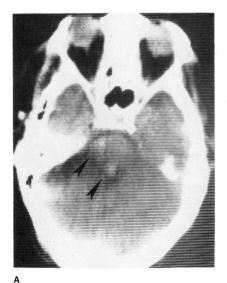
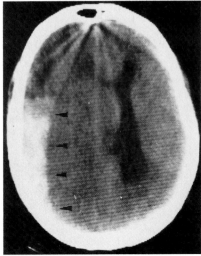

A   B

Figure 11-28 Brainstem hemorrhage. **A.** CT showing high-density zones in the pons and immediately anterior to the fourth ventricle (arrowheads). The presence of a brainstem hemorrhage was confirmed at autopsy. **B.** A large right subdural hematoma is also seen.

3-month or 1-year CT scan can be expected to demonstrate corresponding neurological deficit.

In summary, (1) patients with normal CT can be expected to have a good outcome unless secondary complications supervene; (2) patients with lesions involving areas such as the brainstem, corpus callosum, and basal ganglia can be expected to have a poor outcome; (3) patients with bilateral hemorrhagic lesions or both intracerebral or intraventricular and extracerebral hemorrhages can be expected to have a worse outcome in a majority of instances; and finally, (4) patients who develop delayed lesions during the first week can be expected to have a poor outcome.

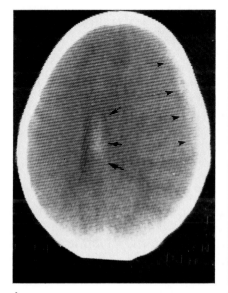
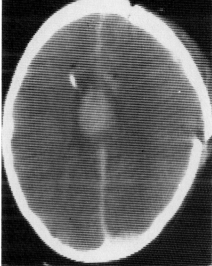

A   B

Figure 11-29 Hemorrhage in the corpus callosum. **A.** CT performed immediately following trauma reveals a high-density zone in the midline in the region of the corpus callosum (arrows). A thin left subdural hematoma (arrowheads) is present. **B.** CT performed 4 days later, following evacuation of the subdural hematoma, demonstrates marked increase in size of the corpus callosum hemorrhage.

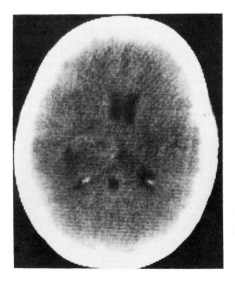 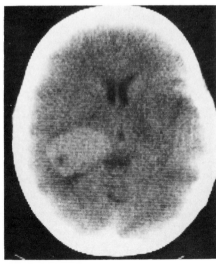

Figure 11-30 Differential diagnosis of resolving hematoma. An ill-defined mixed high- and low-density zone is present in the right posterior temporal region with resultant ventricular compression and displacement. CECT reveals enhancement of this region extending beyond the high-density zone previously noted. On NCCT this could easily be mistaken for a resolving hemorrhage, but CECT establishes the diagnosis of neoplasm (astrocytoma).

RADIOLOGIC WORKUP OF PATIENTS WITH HEAD INJURY

Contrast-Enhanced CT in Acute Head Injury

Although some authors have recommended the routine use of contrast enhancement in acute head injury (Tsai 1978), this is probably not necessary (French 1977). If NCCT reveals appropriate lesions (extra- or intracerebral hemorrhages) to account for a patient's neurological status, CECT may not provide additional pertinent information. However, if a patient presents with a history of recent trauma and no significant lesion is evident on CT, CECT should be performed if the patient's clinical status permits. Contrast enhancement may help in visualizing isodense lesions (Amendola 1977). CECT is essential if there is a mass effect as evidenced by ventricular compression or midline shift in the absence of mass lesions demonstrable on NCCT. Even if there is no evidence of mass effect on NCCT but the patient has a neurological deficit, CECT should be performed, because an isodense lesion, whether extra- or intracerebral, may be seen on CECT only, and this may obviate further invasive procedures such as angiography.

Not infrequently, a clear history is not available

in patients with trauma (Figs. 11-13, 11-14). A patient may be harboring an isodense lesion from an apparently trivial trauma and present to the emergency room with recent injury and neurological deficit. CECT is helpful in bringing out the isodense lesion in such instances. It is important to remember that not all acute traumatic subdural hematomas present as hyperdense lesions on CT. A patient may rebleed into a low-density chronic subdural hematoma, and the admixture of recent clots and chronic low-density collection may appear isodense on CT. If two different densities are seen on CT, as shown in Fig. 11-12, there is no need for CECT. However, even when a somewhat dense lesion is evident on CT following recent trauma, CECT is helpful in demonstrating the true nature of a lesion such as meningioma, as demonstrated by French (1978), thus differentiating an apparent hematoma from a tumor by enhancing additional areas beyond the high-density zones seen on NCCT (Fig. 11-30).

Value of Repeat CT During the First Week

As indicated earlier, a repeat CT during the first week, preferably on the third day if not earlier, should be obtained in all patients who do not show improvement in neurological status, whether they had a normal CT or had undergone surgery for an initial hemorrhagic lesion, because of the incidence of new lesions detected on CT in patients who show deterioration. Although the outcome for patients developing new lesions is poor, it should be kept in mnd that these lesions may develop before detectable neurological deterioration or intracranial hypertension occurs. It has also been documented that decompressive surgery is beneficial in improving the outcome in some of these patients (Brown 1978; Diaz 1979).

Skull Radiography

The role of skull films in the evaluation of brain disorders has been debated since the advent of CT (Cumming 1980; DeSmet 1979; Masters 1980; Weinstein 1977). It has been shown that even before the advent of CT, skull series did not affect the management of patients with head injury (Roberts 1972), even though it is known that 80 percent of fatal head injury patients have skull fracture at autopsy (Adams 1975). Basal skull fractures, not detectable on CT, may be demonstrated by skull radiography. However, with the present high-resolution CT a majority of the basal skull fractures can be demonstrated. CT should be the diagnostic examination of choice for initial evaluation of virtually every patient with significant head trauma, with plain skull films obtained after CT if critical to decision making in patient management.

Angiography

As indicated in the beginning of the chapter, CT has virtually replaced angiography as the preferred method of investigation in head injury patients. Nevertheless, in spite of recent advances in CT technology facilitating "dynamic computed tomography," angiography remains the only means to detect vascular lesions resulting from head injury. Traumatic vascular lesions such as intimal tear of the internal carotid artery, occlusion, traumatic aneurysm, and arteriovenous fistula can be accurately evaluated only by angiography. Angiogaphy may also be necessary following CT study to detect an underlying aneurysm as a cause of intracerebral hematoma rather than trauma (Fig. 11-31). Finally, arterial spasm following trauma can be evaluated only by angiography. Venous thrombosis also can be best evaluated by angiography, although CT signs consisting of increased density on CECT or high density due to thrombosis in the sinus area on NCCT have been reported (Buonanno 1978; Patronas 1981; Wendling 1978). In summary, angiography may be necessary when isodense or vascular lesions are suspected. This study can be performed by means of digital subtraction mode if so desired.

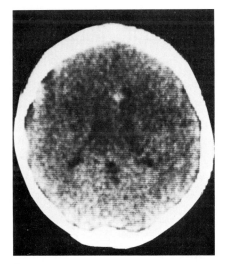

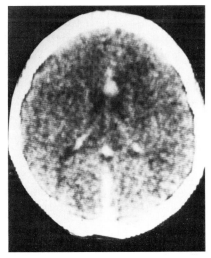

Figure 11-31 Posttraumatic aneurysm. **A.** NCCT demonstrates a punctate hyperdensity in the midline overlying the corpus collusum. **B.** CECT demonstrates increase in the intensity of the density as well as size. (*Continued on* *p. 534.*)

A   B

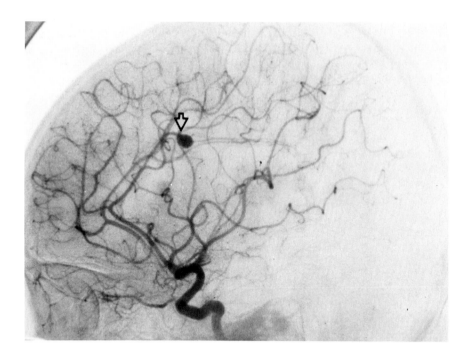

Figure 11-31 (*Cont.*) **C.** Lateral view angiography performed two weeks later indicating a posttraumatic aneurysm of the pericallosal artery from the shearing effect.

Magnetic Resonance Imaging

With greater availability of MRI, its application in head trauma is still being evaluated. Based on limited experience its usage in the acute stage of head trauma will be limited to those groups of patients who present with head injury without any other organ injuries, and are not in need of life support systems. In the majority of acute head injuries, since the patient is restless, MRI, due to its longer scanning time and resulting motion artifact, cannot replace CT. CT is the optimal imaging modality in patients with acute head injury. In the majority of cases it will more often be utilized in the subacute or later stages when CT findings are equivocal and MRI may provide the diagnostic information (Fig. 11-32) (Zimmerman 1986).

Figure 11-32 MRI in trauma. Posttraumatic resolving hematoma ▶ involving the frontal lobe (⇨) detected on CT and associated hematoma of the optic chiasm (⬆) as well as adjacent hypothalamus not visualized on CT study. (*Continued on p. 535.*)

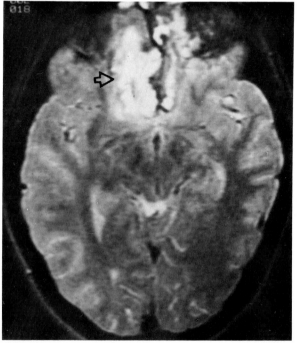

A

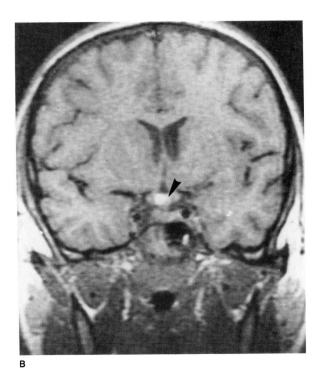

B

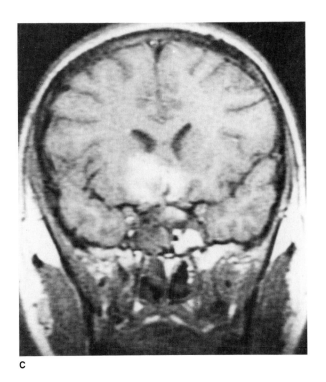

C

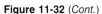
Figure 11-32 (*Cont.*)

SECTION B:
CRANIOFACIAL TRAUMA

Until recently the standard radiological examination for craniofacial injury was a plain radiograph of the skull and face followed by tomography (Taveras 1976; Fischgold 1973; Ratzen 1973). The yield of a plain radiograph in the evaluation of craniofacial trauma is very low (Masters 1980). Although a depressed or comminuted fracture may be recognized on skull roentgenograms, it often requires an additional tangential view of the skull. Computed tomography, in addition to demonstrating the depressed fracture, is helpful in demonstrating the associated extracerebral or intracerebral hemorrhage. A fracture at the base of the skull is rarely visualized in a plain film of the skull because of overlapping densities. Since many patients who come with craniofacial trauma have an associated craniocerebral trauma it appears appropriate that all information can be obtained from a CT study without having the need to move the patient to obtain the different views necessary when evaluating plain skull or facial x-rays. Presently the high-resolution thin-section CT has replaced the standard radiological examination such as plain skull x-rays and pluridirectional tomography in evaluation of acute craniofacial injuries (Cooper 1983; Brant-Zwadzki 1982; Kreipke 1984). The images are not only complementary but are superior to tomography. The associated soft-tissue injury and hemorrhage are often visualized better on the CT study.

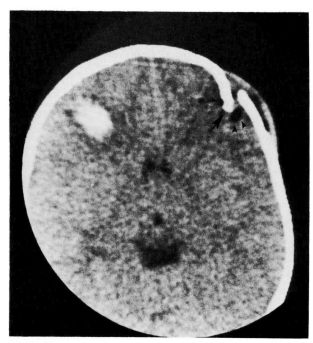

Figure 11-33 Axial CT scan through the cranial vault in a 1-year-old boy shows a depressed fracture (arrow) with presence of air (arrowheads) at the fracture site and left frontal lobe contusion.

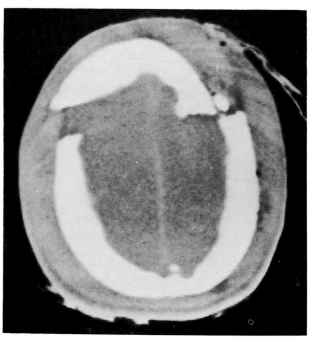

Figure 11-34 Displaced fracture of the vault of the skull. Axial CT scan through the cranial vault shows a displaced fracture involving the right frontal bone, with diffuse scalp swelling.

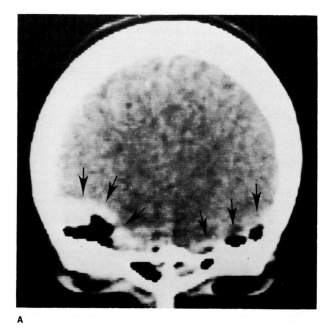

A

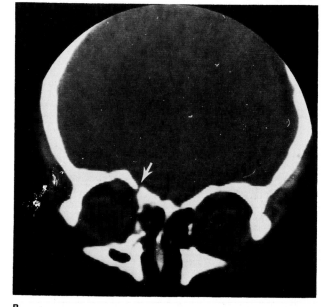

B

Figure 11-35 Fracture of the roof of the orbit.   **A.** Coronal section through the anterior cranial fossa shows a bilateral subfrontal dural collection of air and blood (arrows).   **B.** At bone window, the fracture of the roof of the right orbit (arrow) is seen.

TECHNICAL ASPECTS

In evaluating craniofacial trauma there is a need for three-dimensional projection of the images in case reconstructive surgery is being planned. This can be obtained either by reformatted sagittal or coronal images or if it is possible for the patient to move his head in obtaining true coronal projections. Although a gross fracture of the vault of the skull can easily be detected by standard axial CT scan in soft-tissue window settings (Figs. 11-33, 11-34), the evaluation of bony injury requires adjustment of the window settings to a wider width (Fig. 11-35). When viewing in soft-tissue setting, the thin rim of an acute extracerebral hemorrhage can often blend with the adjacent skull as the same density as bone; moreover, a linear or diastatic fracture may not be seen at a normal window setting. Therefore, it is imperative to examine the images at different window settings for the evaluation of intracranial hemorrhage as well as the associated bony injury. When a fracture of the base of the skull is suspected in the axial CT, it may become necessary to reexamine the patient in coronal projection or obtain thin axial sections such that coronal and sagittal reformatted images can be obtained.

ANTERIOR CRANIAL FOSSA

Injury to the floor of the anterior cranial fossa may involve the inner table of the frontal sinus, orbital roof, and cribriform plate (Figs. 11-36, 11-37, 11-38). Fractures of the planum sphenoidale may extend to the floor of the sella turcica (Figs. 11-38, 11-39). A depressed fracture of the orbital roof can compress the orbital contents. Fractures of the ethmoid sinuses, cribriform plate, and planum sphenoidale are often associated with recurrent cerebrospinal fluid (CSF)

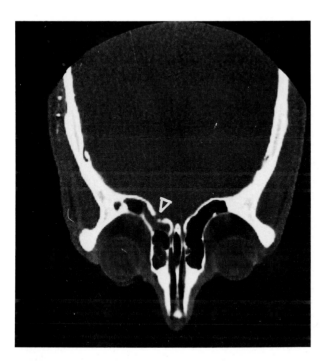

Figure 11-36 Fracture of the frontal sinus. Coronal CT scan through the anterior cranial fossa with intermittent CSF rhinorrhea following head injury shows a depressed fracture (arrow) through the right anterior cranial fossa extending into the frontal sinus. Right frontal sinus is opacified with CSF.

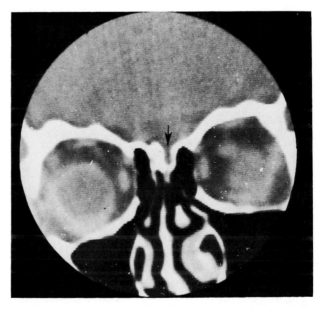

Figure 11-37 Fracture of the cribriform plate. Coronal CT scan through the anterior cranial fossa of 20-year-old woman with previous head injury and intermittent CSF rhinorrhea shows diastatic fracture of the left cribriform plate (arrow).

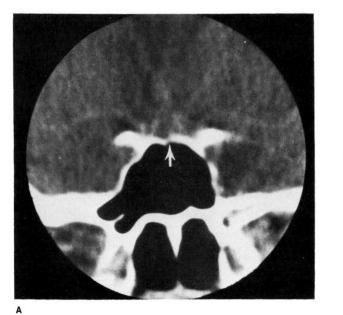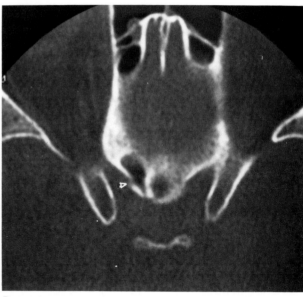

A   **B**

Figure 11-38   A fracture of the planum sphenoidale. Coronal CT scan at the level of the chiasmatic floor shows fracture of the planum sphenoidale (arrow) with slight depression. This fracture was not seen in plain skull radiography.   **B.** Axial CT in bone window setting clearly demonstrates fracture involving the medial wall of the optic canal (arrowhead).

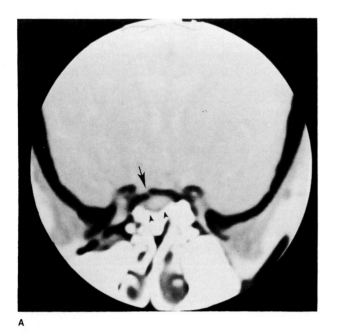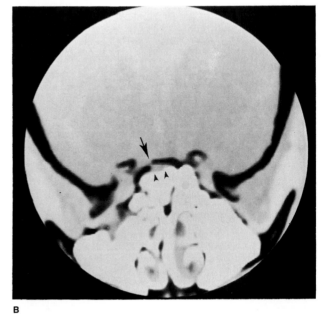

A   **B**

Figure 11-39   Fracture of the planum sphenoidale with herniation of subarachnoid space.   **A.** Coronal CT scan through the planum sphenoidale shows a slightly depressed fracture (arrow) on the right side of the planum sphenoidale, with herniation of subarachnoid space into the sphenoid sinus (arrowheads).   **B.** Repeat coronal CT scan after 2 months shows marked decrease in subarachnoid space herniation (arrowheads).

rhinorrhea. Ascending infection from paranasal sinuses may cause meningitis, cerebritis, and abscess formation (Taveras 1976; Zatzkin 1965). If untreated, the fracture may widen, causing herniation of the subarachnoid space and brain (Figs. 11-39, 11-50, 11-52). A fracture of the cribriform plate may cause injury to the olfactory nerves, with transient or permanent loss of the sense of smell.

MIDDLE CRANIAL FOSSA

Fractures involving the planum sphenoidale and the floor of the sella turcica are not uncommon (Figs. 11-38, 11-39). A cribriform plate fracture may extend posteriorly to the planum sphenoidale and floor of the sella turcica (Fig. 11-50). Fractures involving the planum sphenoidale (Fig. 11-39*A*) or the bony optic canal (Fig. 11-38*B*) can result in visual defects (Guyon 1984). Injury to the pituitary gland may cause panhypopituitarism or diabetes insipidus (Dublin 1976; Young 1980). Traumatic hemorrhage involving the pituitary gland can be seen on high-resolution CT (Tsai 1980). CSF rhinorrhea and leptomeningeal cyst formation through these structures are common (Figs. 11-50, 11-52). Fracture through the basisphenoid can result in involvement of the cavernous sinus and its contents. When an air fluid level in the sphenoid sinus is seen in the axial CT or in upright or cross-table lateral skull film, further examination of the area is required with coronal CT. Cavernous sinus thrombosis may result as a delayed complication of trauma in this region. Proptosis and ophthalmoplegia are highly suggestive of carotid cavernous fistula. CT will demonstrate the fractures, prominent cavernous sinus, and ophthalmic vein. Confirmation, however, requires angiographic studies (Rao 1980).

POSTERIOR FOSSA

The temporal bone shares the boundaries of both middle and posterior cranial fossa. For convenience of description it is included in this paragraph. The most common type of fracture involving the temporal bone occurs in the petromastoid region. A fracture of the tegmen tympani may involve the horizontal portion of the facial canal, causing facial nerve paralysis (Jongkees 1965). When the fracture involves the middle ear, it may cause hemotympanum and CSF otorrhea via the ruptured tympanic membrane (Figs. 11-40, 11-41). Fractures of the middle ear may result in CSF rhinorrhea via the eustachian tube when the tympanic membrane remains intact. It may cause ossicular disruption and thereby severe impairment of hearing. Pluridirectional tomography has been successfully utilized in the evaluation of such fractures (Jongkees 1965; Davis 1971). High-resolution CT scan in axial and coronal projection will delineate these structures well (Holland 1984). High-resolution CT with bone algorithm has also resulted in excellent osseous resolution and thus is helpful in defining fracture of the ossicular structures (Shaffer 1980). Opacification of the mastoid air cells and soft-tissue injury are also well seen by CT (Figs. 11-40, 11-41, 11-42). Fractures of the petrous apex and internal auditory canals are rare and when they occur may cause seventh and eighth nerve injury. Fractures of the cochlea and vestibule are uncommon. Fractures involving the clivus and the foramen magnum region are rarely seen, probably because they are usually fatal. A fracture of the jugular foramen and hypoglossal canal should be suspected when ninth, tenth, eleventh, or twelfth cranial nerve palsy occurs after a head injury. Axial and coronal CT sections will delineate these fractures well.

ORBIT

A fracture involving the superior rim of the orbit is not uncommon. It normally occurs with a direct blow around the orbit. The most common trauma involving the orbit is a blowout fracture. When a blowout fracture is suspected by clinical examination or plain radiography, the patient should be reexamined by coronal CT of the orbit (Ghoshhajra 1980*b*). The coronal CT is ideal, as sections are taken at right an-

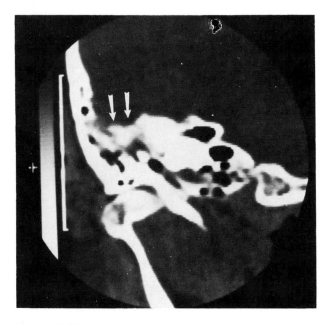
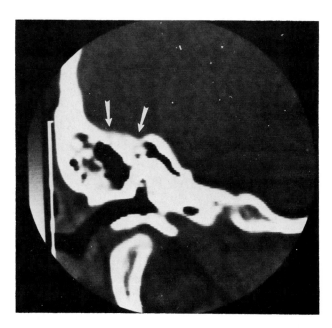

Figure 11-40 Fracture of the temporal bone. Coronal CT shows depressed fracture of the petromastoid region (arrow) with partial opacification of mastoid air cells. At surgery, the facial nerve was seen to be transected.

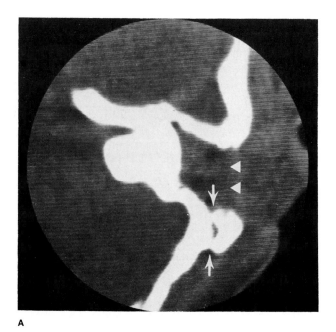
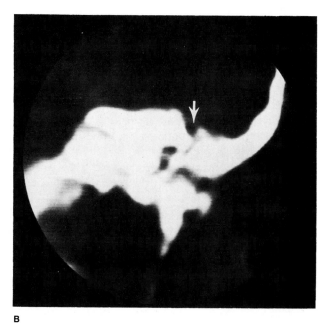

A

B

Figure 11-41 Fracture of the temporal bone. **A.** Axial section through external auditory meatus shows opacification of the left external auditory canal (arrowheads), with fracture in the posterior wall (arrow). **B.** Section through the tegmen shows a depressed fracture (arrow) extending into the middle ear. (*Continued on p. 541.*)

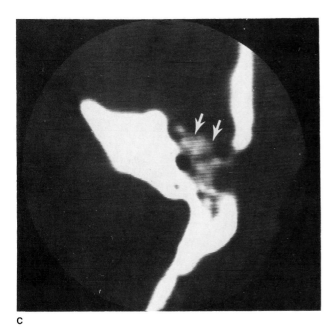

C

Figure 11-41 (*Cont.*) **C.** Section through the petromastoid junction shows the depressed fracture extending inferiorly (arrow). (*Courtesy of H. Curtin, M.D., University of Pittsburgh.*)

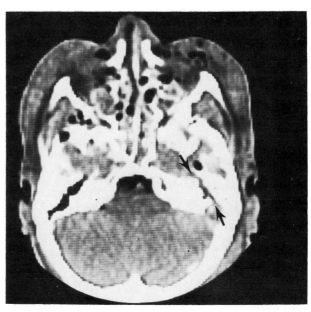

Figure 11-42 Fractures of the temporal bone and paranasal sinus. Axial CT scan through the face and temporal bones shows a fracture through the left petrous bone (arrow). There were also multiple fractures involving paranasal sinuses, with soft-tissue swelling of the face.

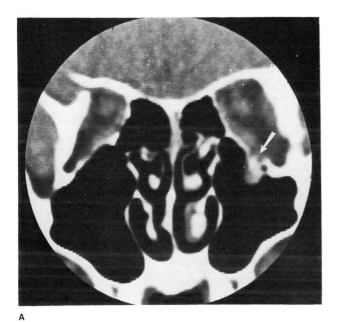

A

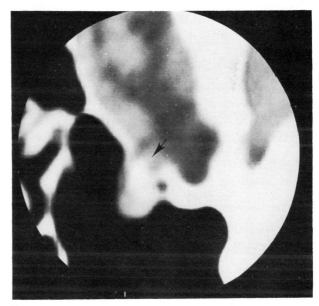

B

Figure 11-43 Blowout fracture of the orbit. **A.** Coronal CT scan of the orbit shows fracture involving the floor of the left orbit, with entrapment of the inferior rectus muscle (arrow). **B.** Magnified view of the left orbit shows a fractured bony fragment with muscle entrapment (arrow).

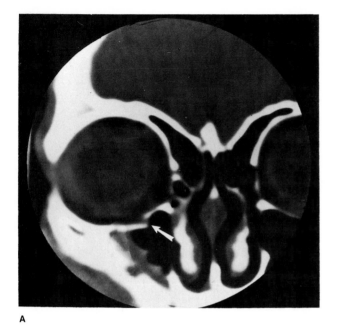

A

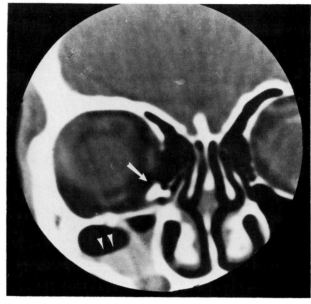

B

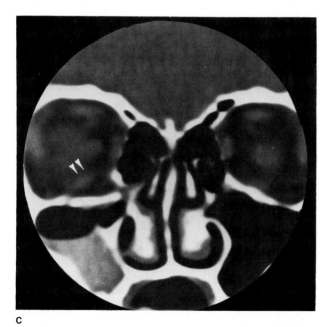

C

Figure 11-44 Blowout fracture of the orbit.   **A,B.** Serial coronal sections through the right orbit show a fracture through the floor of the right orbit extending to the medial wall (arrow). The right maxiliary sinus shows an air-fluid level (arrowheads).   **C.** There is, in addition, superolateral displacement of the inferior rectus muscle (arrowheads) by a hematoma.

gles to the floor of the orbit. Although the previous method of examination by pluridirectional tomography has been successful in demonstration of blowout fracture (Fuerger 1966; Dodick 1969), it fails to demonstrate entrapment of the orbital muscles and associated injury to the eyeball. Orbital or ocular hemorrhage can be easily diagnosed by CT. Blowout fracture involving the floor of the orbit is frequently associated with entrapment of the inferior rectus muscles causing diplopia (Fig. 11-43). Fracture of the medial orbital wall is not uncommon (Davidson 1965; Prasad 1975), occurring separately or as an extension of the inferior wall fracture (Fig. 11-44). The limitation of movement is due either to entrapment of the orbital muscles or to intraorbital hematoma. A fracture may also involve the supraorbital region (Fig. 11-35). Fracture of the lateral wall is often associated with fracture of the zygoma. Posteriorly, injury to the orbit may fracture the greater or lesser wing of the sphenoid bones (Figs. 11-45, 11-46). These fractures may compromise the optic canal and superior orbital fissure. Injury to the optic nerves will cause loss of vision (Fig. 11-45). Compromise of the superior orbital fissure may cause superior orbital fissure syndrome.

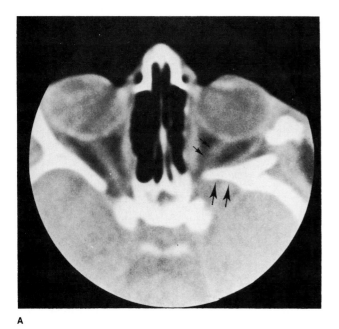

A

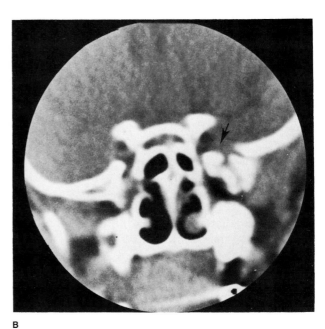

B

Figure 11-45   Fracture of the sphenoid wing with injury to the optic nerve.   **A.** Axial CT scan through the orbit shows a fracture involving the lateral orbital wall (arrows), with anterior displacement of the sphenoid wing and impingement on the optic nerve (small arrows). **B.** Coronal section through the orbital cone shows comminuted fragments (arrow) at the optic foramen. (*Courtesy of Z. L. Deeb, M.D., University of Pittsburgh.*)

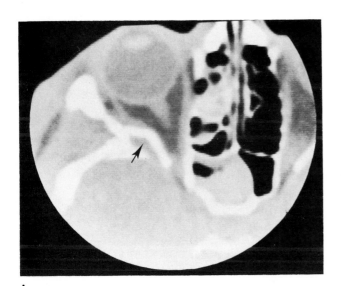

A

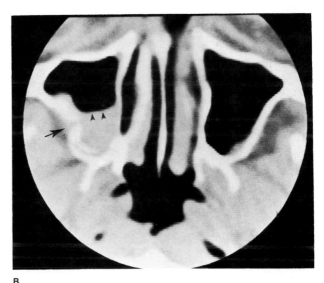

B

Figure 11-46   Fractures of the sphenoid wing and maxilla. **A.** Axial CT scan of the orbit shows a fracture of the greater wing of the sphenoid on the right (arrow). The optic canal is not compromised. There is also opacification of the right ethmoid sinuses.   **B.** Section through the maxillary sinus shows depressed fracture (arrow) of the right lateral maxillary wall, with the air-fluid level within the maxillary sinus (arrowheads). (*Courtesy of Z.L. Deeb, M.D., University of Pittsburgh.*)

FACIAL BONES

The most common facial injury involves the nasal bones. Nasal bone fractures are easily diagnosed by plain radiography. Other facial bone injuries commonly involve the orbital rim, floor of the maxillary sinus, and zygoma. Fractures involving the nasal septum and pterygoid plates, though not uncommon, are often associated with other facial bone fractures. Fractures involving the zygomatic arch and mandible are probably best evaluated by plain radiography. CT provides a three-dimensional projection of the fracture involving the facial bones and thus helps in the planning of surgery.

MAXILLARY AND ZYGOMATIC BONES

CT is excellent when evaluating simple or complex facial fractures involving the maxillary and zygomatic bones in both the axial and coronal projections

(Figs. 11-46, 11-47). Fractures as well as soft-tissue abnormalities, especially the obstruction of nasal passages, are easily delineated by CT. Coronal views (Fig. 11-47) are ideal when evaluating fractures involving the pterygoid plates and zygoma. High-resolution thin CT sections are useful such that reformatted images in any plane can be obtained and displacement of the bony fragments can be clearly delineated. Because of the anatomic configuration and location, fractures involving the nasal bones, mandible, and zygomatic arch are best evaluated by standard plain radiography.

CEREBROSPINAL FLUID FISTULA

When a fracture of the base of the skull accompanies an injury to the meninges, a communication of the intracranial subarachnoid space with the paranasal sinuses or middle ear occurs, resulting in cerebrospinal fluid (CSF) rhinorrhea or otorrhea. The clinical presentations of rhinorrhea or otorrhea are quite

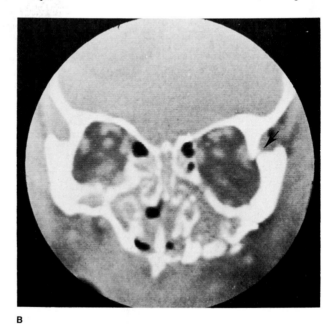

A   **B**

Figure 11-47   Fractures of maxilla and zygoma.   **A.** Axial CT scan shows multiple fractures (arrows) involving the walls of both maxillary sinuses, with obliteration of the right nasal passage.   **B.** Coronal section through the zygoma shows a fracture of the left zygoma (arrow). Again, multiple fractures involving both maxillae, with obliteration of air passage, are well demonstrated. (*Continued on p. 545.*)

variable. There may be leakage of CSF or of blood mixed with CSF through the nose, postnasal space, or middle ear, depending on the location of the fistula. Severe cerebral injury in these patients may often be associated with fractures of the base of the skull. A CSF leakage may stop spontaneously. This is commonly seen when fracture of the petrous bone is involved. Occasionally CSF rhinorrhea, and rarely otorrhea, is precipitated by stress such as coughing or sneezing. Once the communication is established with the paranasal sinuses or middle ear, the incidence of recurrent meningitis or intracranial abscess formation from ascending infection is quite high. The diagnosis and accurate anatomic localization of these fistulas are thus imperative for proper medical and surgical management.

The accurate localization of the site of the fistula has always been a diagnostic challenge. Although isotope cisternography has been the procedure of choice for tracing CSF leakage, it lacks precise anatomic definition (DiChiro 1968). Other procedures, such as positive contrast (Pantopaque) and isotope ventriculography, have been utilized with some success in demontrating the fistula tract (Allen 1972). Outlining of a CSF fistula with air during pneumoencephalography has been reported (Marc 1973). The presence of intracranial air bubbles close to the fracture site and air within the fistulous tract during CT examination has occasionally been successful in identifying the site of leak (Fox 1979; Levy 1978). With the availability of water-soluble contrast media for intrathecal use, CT cisternography is the ideal method for successful localization of the site of CSF leakage (Drayer 1977; Manelfe 1977). High-resolution CT has further improved the precise localization of the site of CSF leakage utilizing CT cisternography (Ghoshhajra 1979; Hilal 1980; Ghoshhajra 1980c; Naidich 1980; Manelfe 1982). Intermittent CSF rhinorrhea is a common manifestation of traumatic CSF leakage. Traumatic CSF otorrhea frequently stops spontaneously without intervention (Davis 1971; Frey 1973; Raaf 1967).

When symptoms of rhinorrhea or otorrhea persist, accurate anatomic demonstration of the fistula tract is imperative for surgical treatment. The conventional CT study may demonstrate the presence of intracranial air, and sections through the base of the skull will often demonstrate opacification or air fluid level either in the paranasal sinuses or in the middle ear. For precise anatomic demonstration of the fistula tract, CT cisternogaphy using a water-soluble contrast appears to be the ideal modality at the present time.

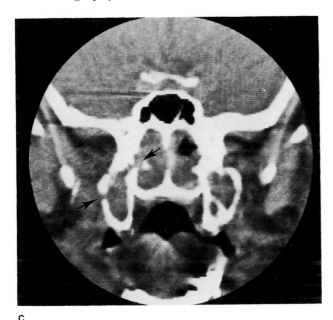

c

Figure 11-47 (*Cont.*) **C.** Coronal section through the pterygoid processes shows extension of the fracture through the pterygoid plates (arrows).

TECHNICAL ASPECTS

CT cisternography with water-soluble intrathecal contrast is a relatively simple procedure. Successful demonstration of the fistula tract depends on the presence and severity of the rhinorrhea or otorrhea during the examination. If the rhinorrhea or otorrhea is infrequent, the patient should be placed in a head-down position with frequent coughing, 24 hours prior to the examination, so that active leakage can be reproduced at the time of the examination. The patient should be well hydrated prior to the examination by adequate oral fluid. A 10-mg dose of diazepam is given orally for premedication. Intrathecal administration of water-soluble contrast at a dose of 5 to 6 cc in a concentration of 190 to 200 mg of iodine per milliliter is used by a lumbar route or C1-2 cisternal puncture. A slightly higher concentration and larger dose should be used when the leakage of CSF is profuse. The patient is then placed in a 60-degree Trendelenburg's position for 1 to 2 minutes. If no CSF leakage occurs in this position, the patient is asked to cough for induction of CSF leakage (Ghoshhajra 1980*a*). Actual leakage of CSF during the examination is a prerequisite for success in localizing a fistula tract. The water-soluble contrast solution is injected under fluoroscopic control on a tilting table to direct the flow of the contrast agent into the head. If the patient has profuse CSF leakage, water-soluble contrast can be introduced on the CT scanner.

Once the patient is taken to the CT room, a systematic approach to the scanning technique should be followed. Study in the axial plane is often complemented by further evaluation in the coronal or lateral decubitus position. The coronal or lateral decubitus views should be perpendicular to the axial plane. Often this may necessitate tilting the gantry or the table top and hyperextension of the patient's neck. Although this can be achieved in most cases, in patients with short necks or other physical problems these maneuvers may not be possible. In these patients, sagittal or coronal reformation, although less desirable, should be attempted. The tracing of a CSF leak is a tedious and time-consuming procedure. Four to six thin axial CT sections through the base of the skull will demonstrate distortions of the interhemispheric fissure or subfrontal sulci, suggesting the possible site of the fracture. The collection of CSF mixed with water water-soluble contrast can be seen in the paranasal sinus. Occasionally a Valsalva maneuver or sneezing may open the site of the leak and help demonstrate the fistula tract. If the leakage is profuse and yet water-soluble contrast mixed with CSF is not seen in any of the sinuses during the examination, further evaluation should be done by lateral decubitus coronal sections or supine coronal sections. A high-resolution CT technique should be employed, using a 4- to 5-mm col-

limation of the x-ray beam with a 1-mm overlapping of the images or contiguous 1.5-mm thin sections.

A $2\times$ to $3\times$ magnification of the reconstructed image will adequately demonstrate the delicate anatomy of the subarachnoid space as well as the site of the fracture. Approximately four to six sections in coronal projection may be necessary, depending on the extent of the fracture and its location. All images are visualized in the standard as well as reverse mode, if available simultaneously, using dual television monitors. In the standard mode it is sometimes difficult to differentiate an enhanced subarachnoid space from the adjacent bony structures. A reverse mode will differentiate the enhanced subarachnoid space (light-gray density) from the dark bony edges. The images are examined for deformity and distortion of subarachnoid spaces, cerebral herniation, bony defects, and the presence of water-soluble contrast in the paranasal sinuses.

CSF rhinorrhea is most often secondary to fracture of the base of the skull constituting the anterior cranial fossa, although rarely it can be spontaneous or postsurgical. The most common site of leakage is the fractured cribriform plate. Such a fracture may extend anteriorly or posteriorly toward the planum sphenoidale. CSF leakage may also occur through the fractured frontal sinus. The other common site of CSF leakage is a fracture involving the floor of the sella turcica. CSF leak through a fractured posterior fossa is relatively uncommon. When it occurs, it commonly involves the petromastoid junction, causing otorrhea or rhinorrhea depending on the status of the tympanic membrane. When multiple fractures are present, with CSF rhinorrhea especially disrupting the sphenoid and ethmoid sinuses, accurate localization becomes difficult (Fig. 11-51). Opacification of the involved sinuses with water-soluble contrast is seen, which may be due to multiple sites of leakage or to disruption of the wall of the sinuses.

Axial CT sections will often demonstrate distortion of the anterior interhemispheric fissure and subfrontal sulci indicating the possible site of the fracture and leakage (Figs. 11-48, 11-50). Anteroposterior extension of the fracture may often be demonstrated in these views (Fig. 11-50). Once the

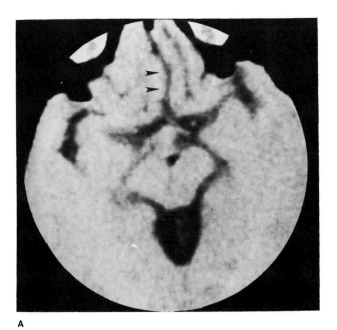

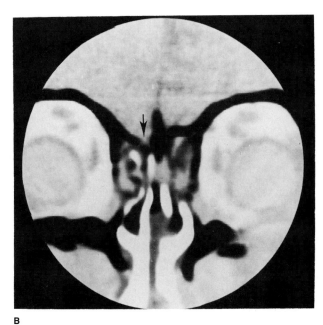

A   B

Figure 11-48   Depressed fracture of cribriform plate with CSF rhinorrhea.   **A.** Axial section in metrizamide CT cisternography of a 56-year-old man with injury to the base of the skull and CSF rhinorrhea shows distortion of the anterior interhemispheric fissure (arrowheads). **B.** Coronal section in the prone position shows a fracture through the cribriform plate (arrow) with CSF leakage.

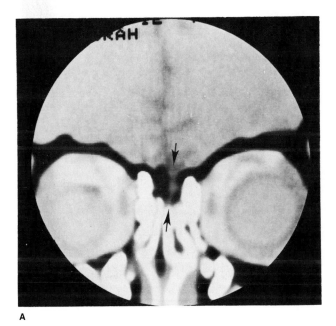

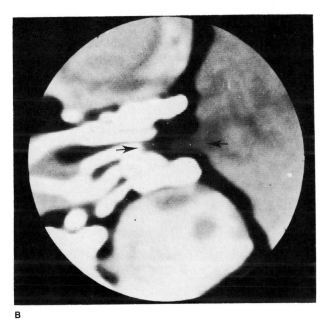

A   B

Figure 11-49   Diastatic fracture of cribriform plate with CSF rhinorrhea.   **A.** Metrizamide CT cisternography in a coronal section (patient prone) of a 20-year-old woman with recurrent CSF rhinorrhea shows a diastatic fracture of the left cribriform plate with leakage of metrizamide (arrows).   **B.** The metrizamide-mixed CSF leakage is best delineated in the left coronal decubitus view (arrows).

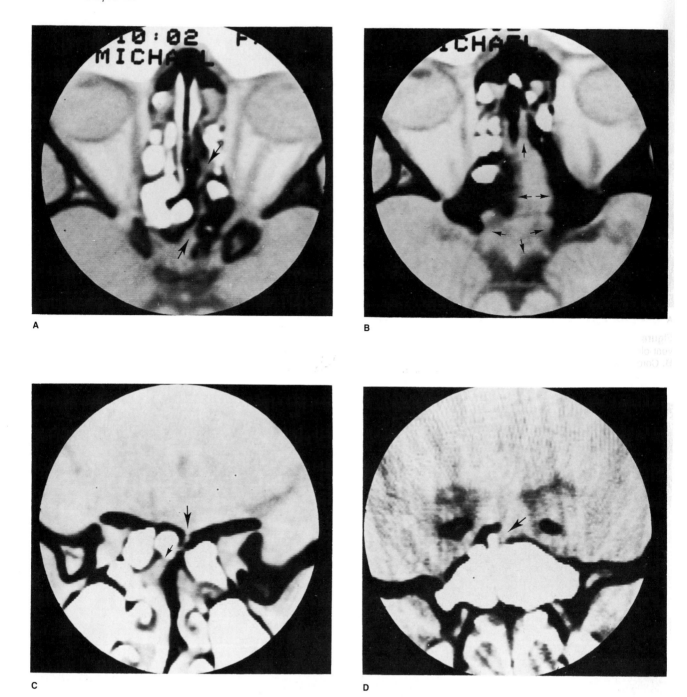

Figure 11-50   CSF rhinorrhea and cerebral herniation.   **A.** Axial section of a metrizamide CT cisternogram shows a fracture extending from the planum sphenoidale to the cribriform plate (arrows).   **B.** Axial section just above **A** shows cerebral herniation (arrows). **C,D.** Prone coronal sections show the fracture of the planum sphenoidale and the floor of the sella turcica (arrow), with leakage of CSF (small arrow). (*Continued on p. 549.*)

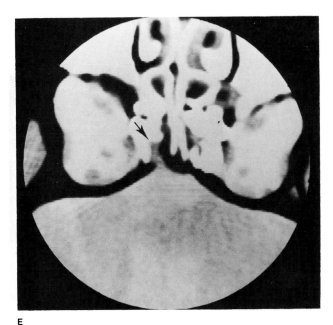

site of the fracture is identified or suspected on axial sections, further evaluation should be carried out by prone coronal projection (Figs. 11-48, 11-53). When profuse CSF leakage occurs during the examination, instead of prone coronal projection, supine coronal sections and occasionally lateral decubitus coronal sections may be helpful in demonstrating the accumulation of water-soluble contrast with CSF at the site of the fracture (Figs. 11-49, 11-50).

Herniation of the brain or leptomeninges is rarely seen immediately after trauma. Widening of the fracture with herniation of leptomeninges may rarely occur as a delayed complication of trauma. Patients may present with intermittent or continuous CSF rhinorrhea. This cannot be differentiated from congenital encephalocele or meningocele purely on the basis of CT findings. The herniation of the brain or leptomeninges with extension of the subarachnoid space can easily be demonstrated in the axial as well as coronal CT (Figs. 11-50 to 11-53).

E

Figure 11-50 (*Cont.*) **E.** Supine coronal section through the anterior cranial fossa gives excellent demonstration of leakage through the fracture site (arrow).

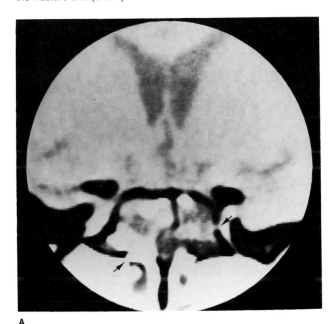

A

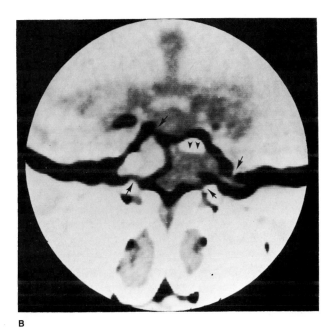

B

Figure 11-51 CSF rhinorrhea through multiple fractures.   **A,B.** Metrizamide CT cisternography in coronal projections (patient prone) shows multiple fractures (arrows) involving the roof as well as the floor of the sphenoid sinuses. The concentration of metrizamide is higher in the left sphenoid sinus (arrowheads) than in the right because of profuse leakage through the fractured floor of the right sinus. (*Continued on p. 550.*)

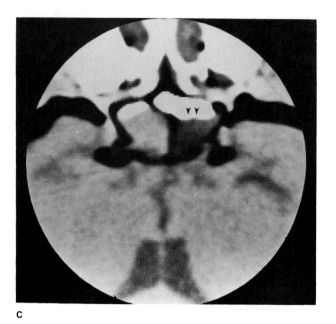

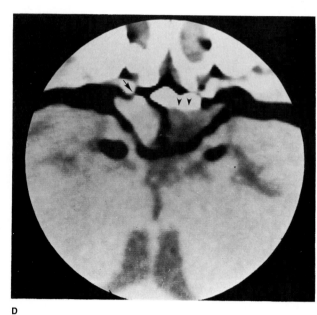

C

D

Figure 11-51 (*Cont.*) **C,D.** Supine coronal sections through the sphenoid sinus again demonstrate a higher concentration of metrizamide in the left sphenoid sinus (arrowheads).

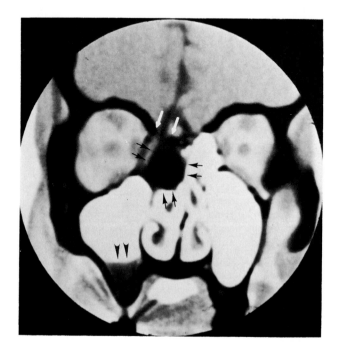

CT cisternography is a relatively simple procedure with minimum morbidity, and it can be repeated when necessary. Incidence of headache, nausea, vomiting, and occasional seizures seen in water-soluble myelography is lower, probably because of the low dose and the faster clearance of the water-soluble contrast from the subarachnoid space due to CSF leakage.

Figure 11-52 Leptomeningeal cyst with CSF rhinorrhea. Coronal section of metrizamide CT cisternography demonstrates a diastatic fracture (white arrows) of the roof of the right ethmoid sinus, with herniation of the subarachnoid space (black arrows) and leakage of metrizamide-mixed CSF into the right maxillary sinus (arrowheads). This patient had sustained a fracture of the base of the skull 12 years earlier. (*Courtesy of R.M. Desai, M.D., and V.S. Rishi, M.D., West Penn Hospital, Pittsburgh.*)

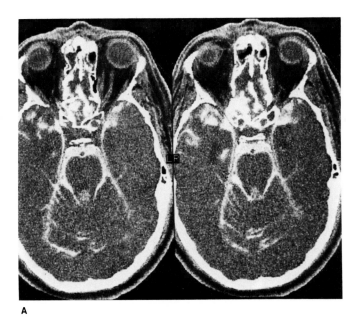

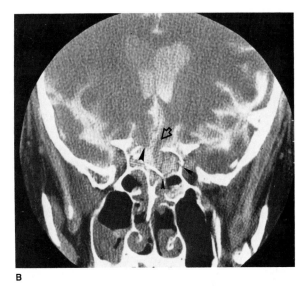

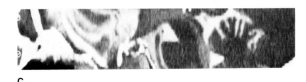

Figure 11-53   CSF. Rhinorrhea through multiple fractures: (**A**) axial (**B**) coronal and (**C**) reformatted saggital study demonstrates contrast leakage into the sinuses through multiple fracture sites (arrowheads). In coronal view (**B**) there is deviation of the inter-hemispheric fissure and herniation of the brain tissue. This is also clearly demonstrated in the saggital reformatted view.

Bibliography

ADAMS JH: The neuropathology of head injuries, in Vinken PJ, Bruyn GW (eds): *Handbook of Clinical Neurology*, vol. 23, *Injuries of the Brain and Skull*. Amsterdam, Oxford, North-Holland Publishing Company, 1975, pp 35–65.

ALCKER GJ et al: High cervical spine and craniocervical junction injuries in fatal traffic accidents. *Orthop Clin North Am* **9**:1103–1110, 1978.

ALLEN BM et al: Fistula detection in cerebrospinal fluid leakage. *J Neurol Neurosurg Psychiatry* **35**:664–668, 1972.

AMBROSE J: Computerized x-ray scanning of the brain. *J Neurosurg* **40**:679–695, 1974.

AMENDOLA MA, OSTRUM BJ: Diagnosis of isodense subdural hematomas by computed tomography. *Am J Roentgenol* **129**:693–697, 1977.

AUER L et al: Relevance of CAT-scan for the level of ICP in patients with severe head injury, in Shulman K et al (eds): *Intracranial Pressure IV*. Berlin, Springer-Verlag, 1980, pp 45–47.

AUH YH, LEE SH, TOGLIA JU: The excessively small ventricle on cranial computed tomography: Clinical correlation in 75 patients. *J Comput Assist Tomogr* **4**:325–329, 1980.

BAKER HL et al: Computer assisted tomography of the head: An early evaluation. *Mayo Clin Proc* **49**:17–27, 1974.

BARATHAM G, DENNYSON WG: Delayed traumatic intracerebral hemorrhage. *J Neurol Neurosurg Psychiatry* **35**:698–706, 1972.

BERGSTROM M et al: Computed tomography of cranial subdural and epidural hematomas: Variation of attenuation related to time and clinical events such as rebleeding. *J Comput Assist Tomogr* **1**:449–455, 1977.

BRANT-ZWADZKI MN, MINAGI H, FEDERLE MP, ROWE LD: High resolution CT with image reformation in maxillofacial pathology. *AJNR* **3**:30–37, 1982.

BROOKS RA, DICHIRO G: Principles of computer assisted tomography (CAT) in radiographic radioisotope imaging. *Phys Med Biol* **21**:689–732, 1976.

BROWN FD, MULLAN S, DUDA EE: Delayed traumatic intracerebral hematomas: Report of 3 cases. *J Neurosurg* **48**:1019–1022, 1978.

BUONANNO FS, MOODY DM, BALL MR, LASTER DW: Computed cranial tomographic findings in cerebral sinovenous occlusion. *J Comput Assist Tomogr* **2**(3):281–290, 1978.

CLIFTON GL, GROSSMAN RG, MAKELA ME, MINER ME, HANDEL S, SADHU V: Neurological course and correlated computerized tomography findings after severe closed head injury. *J Neurosurg* **52**:611–624, 1980.

COOPER PR, MARVILLA K, MOODY S, CLARK WK: Serial computerized tomographic scanning and the prognosis of severe head injury. *Neurosurgery* **5**(5):566–569, 1979a.

COOPER PR, MARAVILLA K, KIRKPATRICK J, MOODY SF, SKLAR FH, DIEHL J, CLARK WK: Traumatically induced brainstem hemorrhage and the computerized tomographic scan: Clinical pathological and experimental observations. *Neurosurgery* **4**(2):115–124, 1979b.

COOPER PW, KASSEL EE, GRUSS JS: High resolution CT scanning of facial trauma. *AJNR* **4**:495–498, 1983.

CUMMINS RO: Clinicians' reasons for overuse of skull radiographs. *Am J Neuroradiology* **1**(4):339–342, 1980.

DAVIDSON TM, OBSEN RM, NAHUM AM: Medial orbital wall fracture with rectus entrapment. *Arch. Otolaryngol* **101**:33–35, January 1965.

DAVIS DO, RAUMBAUGH CL: Temporal bone, in Newton TH, Pott DG (eds): *Radiology of the Skull and Brain*, vol. 1, *The skull.* St. Louis, Mosby, 1971, pp 431–436.

DESMET AA, FRYBACK DG, THORNBURY JR: A second look at the utility of radiographic skull examination for trauma. *Am J Roentgenol* **132**:95–99, 1979.

DIAZ FG, YOCK DH JR, LARSON D, ROSKWOLD GL: Early diagnosis of delayed posttraumatic intracerebral hematomas. *J Neurosurg* **50**:217–223, 1979.

DICHIRO CG et al: Isotope cisternography in the diagnosis and follow-up of cerebrospinal fluid rhinorrhea. *J Neurosurg* **28**:522–529, 1968.

DODICK JM, GALIN MA, BERRETT A: Radiographic evaluation of orbital blowout fracture. *Can J Ophthalmol* **4**:370, 1969.

DOLINSKAS CA, ZIMMERMAN RA, BILANIUK LT: A sign of subarachnoid bleeding on cranial computed tomograms of pediatric head trauma patients. *Radiology* **126**:409–411, 1978.

DOMINGUES DA, SILVA AA, KISHORE PRS, BECKER DP: Delayed CT changes and correlation with outcome in patients with normal initial CT (in press).

DRAYER BP et al: Cerebrospinal fluid rhinorrhea demonstrated by metrizamide CT cisternography. *Am J Roentgenol* **129**:149–151, 1977.

DUBLIN AB: Fracture of the sella turcica. *Am J Roentgenol* **127**:969–972, 1976.

FISCHGOLD H, METZGER J: Tomography of the base of the skull, in Berrett A, Brunner S., Valvassori GE (eds): *Modern Thin Section Tomography.* Springfield, Ill, Charles C Thomas, 1973.

FORBES GS et al: Computed tomography in the evaluation of subdural hematomas. *Radiology* **126**:143–148, 1978.

FOX JL, SCHIEBEL FG: Intracranial air bubbles localizing cerebrospinal fluid fistula. *J Comput Assist Tomogr* **3**:832–833, 1979.

FRENCH BN, DUBLIN AB: The value of computerized tomography in the management of 1000 consecutive head injuries. *Surg Neurol* **7**:171–183, 1977.

FRENCH BN: Limitations and pitfalls of computed tomography in the evaluation of craniocerebral injury. *Surg Neurol* **10**(6):395–401, 1978.

FREY KW: Diagnosis of trauma of the temporal bone, in Berrett A, Brunner S, Valvassori GE (eds): *Modern Thin Section Tomography.* Springfield, Ill., Charles C Thomas, 1973, pp 78–79.

FUERGER GE, MILANSKAS AT, BRITTON W: The roentgenologic evaluation of blowout injuries. *Am J Roentgenol* **97**:614, 1966.

GHOSHHAJRA K: High resolution metrizamide CT cisternography for diagnosis and accurate localization of CSF rhinorrhea. Presented at the 65th Scientific Assembly and Annual Meeting of the Radiological Society of North America at Atlanta, Ga. November 1979.

GHOSHHAJRA K: Diagnosis and accurate localization of CSF rhinorrhea by high resolution CT cisternography. Presented at the International Symposium and Course on Computed Tomography, Las Vegas, 1980*a*.

GHOSHHAJRA K: Fracture of the base of the skull and its complications. *CT: J Comput Tomogr* **4**(4):271–276, December 1980*b*.

GHOSHHAJRA K: Metrizamide CT cisternography in CSF rhinorrhea. *J Comput Assist Tomogr* **4**(3):306–310, 1980*c*.

GUDEMAN SK, KISHORE PRS, MILLER JD, GIREVENDULIS AK, LIPPER MH, BECKER DP: The genesis and significance of delayed traumatic intracerebral hematoma. *Neurosurgery* **5**:309–313, 1979.

GUDEMAN SK, KISHORE PRS, BECKER DP, LIPPER MH, GIREVENDULIS AK, JEFFRIES BF, BUTTERWORTH J: Computerized tomography in the evaluation of incidence and significance of post-traumatic hydrocephalus. *Radiology* **141**:597–402, 1981.

GUYON JJ, BRANT-ZWADZKI M, SEIFF SR: CT demonstration of optic canal fractures. *AJNR* **5**:575–578, 1984.

HAYMAN LA, EVANS RA, HINCK VC: Rapid-high-dose contrast computed tomography of isodense subdural hematoma and cerebral swelling. *Radiology* **131**:381–383, 1979.

HEINZ RE, WARD A, DRAYER BP, DUBOIS PJ: Distinction between obstructive and atrophic dilatation of ventricles in children. *J Comput Assist Tomogr* **4**(3):320–325, 1980.

HILAL SK: CSF leaks. Presented at the International Symposium and Course on Computed Tomography, Las Vegas, 1980.

HOLLAND BA, BRANT-ZWADZKI M: High resolution CT of temporal bone trauma. *AJNR* **5**:291–296, 1984.

JAMIESON KG, YELLAND JDN: Extradural hematoma: Report of 167 cases. *J Neurosurg* **29**:13–23, 1968.

JONGKEES LB: Facial paralysis complicating skull trauma, *Arch Otolaryngol* **81**:518–522, 1965.

KIM KS, HEMMATI M, WEINBERG PE: Computed tomography in isodense subdural hematoma. *Radiology* **128**:71–74, 1978.

KISHORE PRS, LIPPER MH, BECKER DP, DOMINGUES DE SILVA AA, NARAYAN RK: The significance of CT in the management of patients with severe head injury: Correlation with ICP. *Am J Neuroradiology* **2**:307–311, 1981.

KISHORE PRS, LIPPER MH, MILLER JD, GIREVENDULIS AK, BECKER DP, VINES FS: Post-traumatic hydrocephalus in patients with severe head injury. *Neuroradiology* **16**:261–265, 1978.

KOO AH, LAROQUE RL: Evaluation of head trauma by computed tomography. *Radiology* **123**:345–350, 1977.

KREIPKE DL, MOSS JJ, FRANCO JM, MAVES MD, SMITH DJ: Computed tomography and thin section tomography in facial trauma. *AJNR* **5**:185–190, 1984.

LANTZ EJ, FORBES GS, BROWN ML, LAWS ER: Radiology of cerebrospinal fluid rhinorrhea. *Am J Neuroradiology* **1**:391–398, 1980.

LARSON GN et al: Computer processing of CT images: Advances and prospects. *Neurosurgery* **1**:78–79, 1977.

LEVANDER B, STATTIN S, SVENDSEN P: Computer tomography of traumatic intra and extracerebral lesions. *Acta Radiol.* [Suppl. 346] *(Stockh)* pp 107–118, 1975.

LEVIN HS, MEYERS CA, GROSSMAN RG, SARWAR M: Ventricular enlargement after closed head injury. *Arch Neurol* **38**:623–629, 1981.

LEVY JM, CHRISTENSEN FK, NYKAMP PW: Detection of a cerebrospinal fluid fistula by computed tomography. *Am J Roentgenol* **131**:344–345, August, 1978.

LIPPER MH, KISHORE PRS, GIREVENDULIS AK, MILLER JD, BECKER DP: Delayed intracranial hematoma in patients with severe head injury. *Radiology* **133**:645–649, 1979.

LOFSTROM JE: Injuries of the cranial vault and brain. *Radiol Clin North Am* **4**:323–340, 1966.

MANELFE C, GUERAUD B, TREMOULET M: Diagnosis of CSF rhinorrhea by computerized cisternography using metrizamide (letter). *Lancet* **2**:1073, 1977.

MANELFE C et al: Cerebrospinal fluid rhinorrhea *Am J Neuroradiology* **3**:25–30, 1982.

MARC JA, SCHECTER MM: The significance of fluid-gas displacement in the sphenoid sinus in post-traumatic cerebrospinal fluid rhinorrhea. *Radiology* **108**:603–606, September 1973.

MASTERS SG: Evaluation of head trauma: Efficacy of skull films. *Am J Neuroradiology Res* **1**:329–337, July/August 1980.

MCCULLOUGH EC et al: Performance evaluation and quality assurance of computed tomography scanners, with illustrations from the EMI, ACTA, and Delta scanners. *Radiology* **120**:173:1976.

MERINO-DE VILLASANTE J, TAVERAS JM: Computerized tomography (CT) in acute head trauma. *Am J Roentgenol* **126**:765–778, 1976.

MESSINA AV, CHERNICK NL: Computed tomography: The "resolving" intracerebral hemorrhage. *Radiology* **118**:609–613, 1975.

MESSINA AV: Computed tomography: Contrast media within subdural hematomas. *Radiology* **119**:725–726, 1976.

MILLER JD, GUDEMAN SK, KISHORE PRS, BECKER DP: CT, ICP and early neurological evaluation in the prognosis of severe head injury. *Acta Neurochir* [Suppl] *(Wein)* **28**:86–88, 1979.

MILLER JD, GUDEMAN SK, KISHORE PRS, BECKER DP: Post-traumatic brain edema on CT. *Adv Neurol* **28**:413–422, 1980.

MOON KL JR, BRANT-ZWADZKI M, PITTS LH, MILLS CM: NMR imaging of CT isodense subdural hematomas. *AJNR* **5**:319–322, 1984.

MORI D, MARATA T, NAKANO Y, HANDA H: Periventricular lucency in hydrocephalus on computerized tomography. *Surg Neurol.* **8**:337–340, 1977.

NAIDICH TP: Trauma, in Korbkin M, Newton TH (eds): *Computed Tomography 1977.* St. Louis, Mosby, 1977.

NAIDICH TP, MORAN CJ: Precise anatomic localization of atraumatic sphenoethmoidal cerebrospinal fluid rhinorrhea by metrizamide CT cisternography. *J Neursurg* **53**:222–228, 1980.

NELSON AT, KISHORE PRS, LEE SH: Development of delayed epidural hematoma. *Am J Neuroradiology* **3**:583–585, 1982.

NEW PF, ARONOW S: Attenuation measurements of whole blood and blood fractions in computed tomography. *Radiology* **121**:635–640, 1976.

NORTON GA, KISHORE PRS, LIN J: Contrast enhancement in cerebral infarctions on CT. *Am J Roentgenol* **131**:881–885, 1978.

OSBORN AG, ANDERSON RE, WING SD: The false falx sign. *Radiology* **134**:421–425, 1980.

PATRONAS NJ, DUDA EE, MIRFAKHRAEE M, WOLLMAN RL: Superior sagittal sinus thrombosis diagnosed by computed tomography. *Surg Neurol* **15**(1):11–14, 1981.

PAXTON R, AMBROSE J: The EMI scanner: A brief review of the first 650 patients. *Br J Radiol* **47**:530–565, 1974.

PRASAD SS: Blow-out fracture of the medial wall of the orbit. *Mod Probl Ophthalmol* **14**:493–505, 1975.

RAAF J: Post-traumatic CSF leaks. *Arch, Surg* **95**:648–655, 1967.

RAO KCVG: The role and limitation of CT in craniocerebral trauma. *CT: J Comput Tomogr* **4**:253–260, 1980.

RATZEN E: Paranasal sinuses, in Berrett A, Brunner S, Valvassori GE (eds): *Modern Thin Section Tomography.* Springfield, Ill, Charles C Thomas, 1973, pp 214–218.

REED D, ROBERTSON WD: Acute subdural hematomas: Atypical C.T. findings. *Am J Neuroradiology* **7**:417–421, 1986.

ROBERSON FC, KISHORE PRS, MILLER JD, LIPPER MH, BECKER DP: The value of serial computerized tomography in the management of severe head injury. *Surg Neurol* **12**:161–167, 1979.

ROBERTS F, SHOPFNER CE: Plain skull roentgenograms in children with head trauma. *Am J Roentgenol* **114**:230–240, 1972.

SADHU VK, SAMPSON J, HAAR FL, PINTO RS, HANDEL SF: Correlation between computed tomography and intracranial pressure monitoring in acute head trauma patients. *Radiology* **133**:507–509, 1979.

SCOTTI G et al: Evaluation of the age of subdural hematomas by computerized tomography. *J Neurosurg* **47**:311–315, 1977.

SHAFFER KA et al: Manipulation of CT data for temporal bone imaging. *Radiology* **137**:825–829, 1980.

SMITH WP JR, BATNITZKY S, RENGACHARY SS: Acute isodense subdural hematomas: A problem in anemic patients. *Am J Neuroradiol* **2**(1):37–40, 1981.

SVENDSEN P: Computed tomography of traumatic extracerebral lesions. *Br J Radiol* **49**:1004–1012, 1976.

SWEET RC et al: Significance of bilateral abnormalities on the CT scan in patients with severe head injury. *Neurosurgery* **3**:16–21, 1978.

TAVERAS JM, WOOD EH: *Head Injuries and Their Complications*, vol 2, *Diagnostic Neuroradiology.* Baltimore, Williams & Wilkins, 1976, pp 1047–1090.

TSAI FY et al: Pituitary gland injury. Presented at the American Society of Neuroradiology, 18th Annual Meeting at Los Angeles, Calif., March 1980.

TSAI FY, HUPRICH JE, GRADNER FC, SEGALL HD, TEAL JS: Diagnostic and prognostic implications of computed tomography of head trauma. *J Comput Assist Tomogr* **2**:323–331, 1978.

VAN DONGEN KJ, BRAAKMAN R: Later computed tomography in survivors of severe head injury. *Neurosurgery* **7**:14–22, 1980.

WEINSTEIN MA, ALFIDI RJ, DUCHESNEAU PM: Computed tomography versus skull radiography. *Am J Roentgenol* **128**:873, 1977.

WENDLING LR: Intracranial venous sinus thrombosis: Diagnosis suggested by computed tomography. *Am J Roentgenol* **130**:978–980, 1978.

WING SD et al: Contrast enhancement of cerebral infarcts in computed tomography. *Radiology* **121**:89–92, 1976.

YOCK DH, MARSHALL WH: Recent ischemic brain infarcts at computed tomography: Appearances pre- and post-contrast infusion. *Radiology* **117**:599–608, 1975.

YOUNG HA, OLIN MS, SCHIDEK H: Fracture of the sella turcica. *Neurosurg* **7**(1):23–29, 1980.

ZATZKIN HR: Injuries to the Head, in *The Roentgen Diagnosis of Trauma*. Chicago, Year Book 1965, pp 57–94.

ZILKHA A: CT of cerebral hemiatrophy. *Am J Neuroradiology* **1**:255–258, 1980.

ZIMMERMAN RA, BILANIUK LT, GENNARELLI T, BRUCE D, DOLINSKAS C, UZZELL B: Cranial computed tomography in diagnosis and management of acute head trauma. *Am J Roentgenol* **131**:27–34, 1978*a*.

ZIMMERMAN RA, BILANIUK LT, GENNERALLI T: Computed tomography of shearing injuries of the cerebral white matter. *Radiology* **127**:393–396, 1978*b*.

ZIMMERMAN RD, LEEDS NE, NAIDICH TP: Ring blush associated wth intracerebral hematoma. *Radiology* **122**:707–711, 1977.

ZIMMERMAN RA, BILANIUK LT: Computed tomographic staging of traumatic epidural bleeding. *Radiology* **144**:809–812, 1982.

ZIMMERMAN RA, BILANIUK LT, HACKNEY DB et al: Head injury: Early results of comparing CT and high-field MR. *Am J Neuoradiol* **7**:757–764, 1986.

12

INFECTIOUS DISEASES

Seungho Howard Lee

GENERAL CONSIDERATIONS

Central nervous system infections represent a group of life-threatening diseases that present a formidable challenge to physicians. Despite the development of effective antimicrobial agents and modern surgical techniques, significant mortality and morbidity with CNS infections persist. Since the introduction of computed tomography, there is evidence of a marked decrease in mortality among patients with brain abscesses, although the morbidity has not changed significantly (Rosenbaum 1978). CT correlation with pathology of the various CNS infections may aid in earlier diagnosis and bring about further decrease in morbidity and mortality.

The brain and spinal cord are well protected from direct spread of infectious disease processes by osseous and membranous coverings. However, once infection has involved the central nervous system, the brain is more sensitive to infection than other tissues. Microorganisms with weak pathogenic properties are capable of producing a fatal outcome when the central nervous system is involved. CNS infection may be a manifestation of a systemic disease (tuberculosis), or may be an independent process (meningococcal meningitis, encephalitis), or may be localized to a focal area (brain abscess). Possible reasons for the peculiar CNS response to microorganisms include certain structural peculiarities of the brain and its coverings, such as the absence of true lymphatics; differences in vascular supply in gray and white matter; the absence of capillaries in the subarachnoid space; intercommunication between intra- and extracranial venous systems via facial and emissary veins; and the presence of perivascular arachnoid space around the veins as well as around the large vessels (Virchow-Robin spaces) and the perivascular glial membrane. Cerebrospinal fluid also is an excellent culture medium for bacterial growth (Harriman 1984).

Infections reach the brain or meninges mainly by two routes: (1) hematogenous dissemination from a distant infective focus to the meninges, cortico-medullary junction, and choroid plexus; (2) direct extension by bony erosion from an adjacent focus of suppuration (otitis, mastoiditis, sinusitis), by transmission along anastomotic veins from the face, scalp, and orbits, and by transmission along cranial nerves following neurosurgery or traumatic cranio-cerebral wounds. Certain external factors serve to enhance the risk of intracranial infections, such as radiation; immunosuppressive or steroid therapy; cyanotic congenital heart disease; systemic illness such as diabetes mellitus, alcoholism, or cirrhosis; leukemia, lymphoma, or agammaglobulinemia; severe body stress; midline bony fusion defects; surgical or traumatic craniocerebral injury; and pulmonary or other systemic infections (Moore 1974).

BACTERIAL INFECTION

Epidural Empyema

Extension of infection from the paranasal sinuses or mastoid is the most frequent route of infection of the skull and epidural space. The infectious process is localized outside the dural membrane and beneath the inner table of the skull. The frontal region is most frequently affected, probably because of its close relationship to the frontal sinuses as well as the ease with which the dura can be stripped from the bone. Infection of the diploe (osteomyelitis) may spread through the inner table of the skull to produce an epidural abscess or may break through the outer table to produce a subgaleal or subperiosteal abscess.

On NCCT, epidural infection appears as a poorly defined area of low density adjacent to the inner table of the skull. On CECT the low-density lentiform collection displaces the dura inward; if the collection lies in the midline, the attachment of the falx is displaced inward and separated from the adjacent skull, thus identifying its extradural location (Lott 1977; Kaufmann 1977). Thick smooth-walled enhancement on the convex inner side represents inflamed dural membrane. The membrane enhancement is usually thicker in epidural than in subdural abscesses (Figs. 12-1, 12-2, 12-3) although Mosley (1984) could not find clear distinguishing CT features between sub- and epidural empyemas at any stage in his own material. The underlying brain tissue appears normal (unless concomitant cerebritis is present), but there may be significant displacement of brain parenchyma if the epidural abscess is large. When the epidural abscess is situated on the convexity of one hemisphere, differentiation from a subdural empyema may be difficult on the basis of CT appearance alone. Associated findings such as underlying bone destruction, subgaleal soft-tissue mass, or air collection may provide a clue (Figs. 12-2, 12-3). In addition, CT may demonstrate evidence of paranasal sinus or mastoid infection (fluid, soft-tissue thickening) and may complement skull radiography in demonstration of associated osteomyelitis. Occasionally angiography may be necessary to differentiate between epidural and subdural empyema (Handel 1974) (Fig. 12-1), and sometimes CECT in the coronal plane provides additional information by demonstrating inward displacement and/or thrombosis of the adjacent venous sinuses. Often epidural abscess is silent clinically, but focal seizures or neurologic deficits may result from compression or irritation of the underlying cerebral cortex. At surgery, the integrity of the dura is usually preserved because of its prophylactic role as a relatively impermeable barrier protecting the underlying brain.

Subdural Empyema

Subdural infection accunts for about 13 to 20 percent of all cases of intracranial bacterial infection and rep-

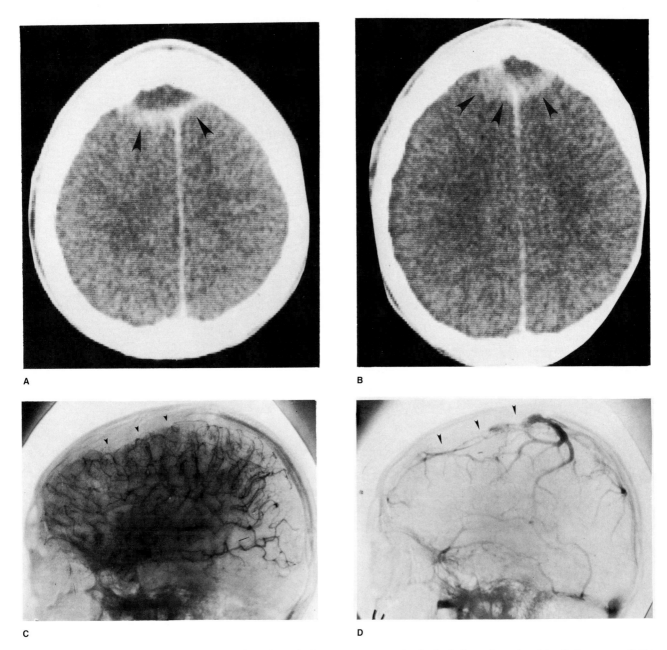

A

B

C

D

Figure 12-1 Epidural abscess. **A.** Biconvex hypodense lesion with contrast-enhanced dural margin (arrowheads) crosses the falx. **B.** Thick, irregular, nonhomogeneous membrane displaces the falx away from the inner table of the skull (arrowheads). **C.** Lateral cerebral angiogram, arterial phase, demonstrates avascular mass compressing the brain tissue (arrowheads). **D.** On venous phase, detachment of the superior sagittal sinus from the inner table of the skull (arrowheads) confirms its extradural location. Also note sinus thrombosis.

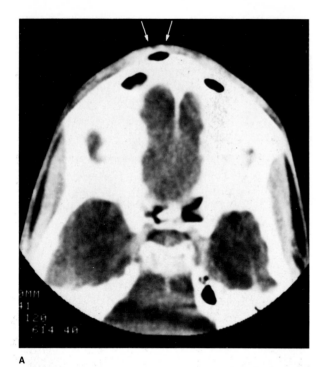

A

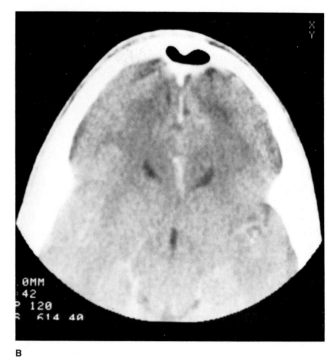

B

C

Figure 12-2 Epidural abscess in an 11-year-old with pansinusitis. **A.** Frontal soft-tissue swelling with air collection (arrows). **B.** Frontal epidural collection with air-fluid level. **C.** Slightly higher level than **B**, a thick membrane crossing the anterior interhemispheric dura is characteristic of epidural abscess which was confirmed at surgery. Of interest was absence of bony dehiscence at surgery.

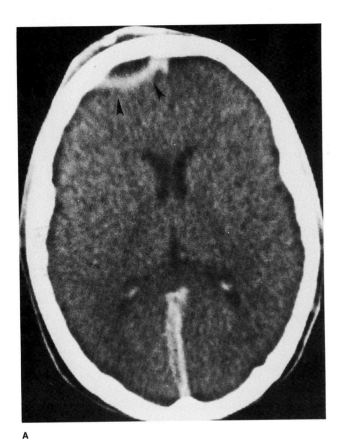

A

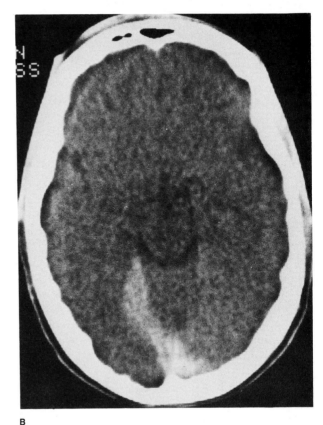

B

Figure 12-3 Frontal epidural abscess associated with subgaleal abscess and subdural empyema. Twenty-eight-year-old drug abuser sustained scalp infection following a minor head trauma. On NCCT (not shown), a hypodensity area in the frontal region was noted with no apparent mass effect or surrounding edema. **A.** On CECT, hypodense, lenticular epidural collection (arrow-

heads) is contiguous with the subgaleal abscess. Enhanced convex margin of the epidural abscess represents inflamed dural membrane. Enhancement of the posterior interhemispheric fissure represents subdural empyema. **B.** CECT at lower level shows enhancement along the tentorium cerebelli, which indicates extension of subdural empyema.

resents 5.1 percent of the space-occupying lesions in the subdural space (Weinman 1972; Galbraith 1974). It can be associated with epidural abscess (Fig. 12-3) and usually presents a fulminating clinical course and an emergent neurosurgical condition. CT findings in acute subdural empyema may be subtle and not apparent initially (Rinaudin 1985). It carried a mortality rate as high as 40 percent in the pre-CT era (Bhardari 1970; Weinman 1972; LaBeau 1973). Whenever progressive neurological deterioration coexists with systemic manifestation of infection, this diagnosis should be strongly considered. The most common cause of subdural empyema is paranasal

sinusitis (Kaufman 1977; Carter 1983). In Zimmerman's (1984) series of 49 patients, frontal sinusitis was the most common cause of empyema; more than 40 percent had preceding frontal sinusitis. Less frequently, subdural empyema may be secondary to otitic infection, a penetrating wound of the skull, craniectomy, or osteomyelitis of the skull. The mechanism of subdural infection may be twofold: progressive retrograde thrombophlebitis or (less likely) direct spread following penetration of the dura. The most common location of a subdural empyema is over the convexity of one or both hemispheres (80 percent), and bilateral involvement is frequent

(Kaufmann 1977), although all lesions were unilateral in Zimmerman's series (1984). Interhemispheric empyema is the next most frequent (12 percent), often occurring as an extension of the convexity collection. Convexity or combined convexity-interhemispheric empyemas or both have a predilection for the anterior aspects of the cranial cavity near the frontal lobes, while isolated interhemispheric collection tends to be more posteriorly and superiorly (Zimmerman 1984). Rarely, the empyema may occur at the base of the brain or beneath the tentorium (Weinman 1972; Grinelli 1977) (Fig. 12-3).

NCCT demonstrates a crescentic or, more frequently, lentiform-shaped area of low density (0 to 16 HU) adjacent to the inner border of the skull, representing pus in the early stages of suspected subdural empyema, frequently subjacent mass effect with hypodense white matter may be more prominent rather than the subtle, minimal extracerebral collection and contrast enhancement (Fig. 12-4). This could be due to edema, cerebritis, or infarction of the white matter (Enzmann 1984). On CECT, a narrow zone of enhancement of relatively uniform thickness separates the hypodense extracerebral collection from the brain surface (Fig. 12-4). This curvilinear enhancement is due to granulation tissue formation at the boundary of the empyema on its leptomeningeal surface and perhaps inflammation in the subjacent cerebral cortex (Grinelli 1977) (Fig. 12-5). The margins of the enhanced zone may show varying degrees of irregularity and thickness (Stephanov 1979; Sadhu 1980; Zimmerman 1984) which, in association with the underlying gyral enhancement due to venous thrombosis or cerebritis, may be of great help in differentiating the subdural empyema from chronic subdural hematoma and uncomplicated epidural abscess. Frequently, septic venous thrombosis leads to edema, hemorrhage, infarction, cerebritis, or brain abscess, resulting in a poor prognosis: these concomitant findings can be demonstrated on CT (Chap. 14). In the author's limited experience with MRI, this new technology seems to be extremely sensitive and noninvasive in the detection of venous thrombosis and concomitant parenchymal alterations (Fig. 12-6).

The spindle shape of an interhemispheric sub-

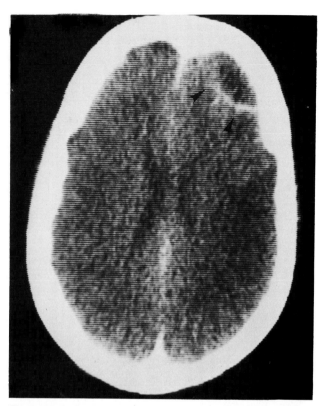

Figure 12-4 Frontal convexity subdural empyema with early cerebritis. CECT shows a thin, convex marginal enhancement outlining a lentiform hypodense collection in the frontal region (arrowheads). The marginal enhancement on the brain surface is usually uniformly thinner than that of the epidural abscess membrane but may be irregular (arrows), depending on the degree of inflammatory reaction in the leptomeninges and subjacent cerebral cortex. Regional hypodense area in the parietal lobe with compression of ipsilateral ventricle represents mass effect due to early cerebritis, infarction, or edema.

dural empyema is determined by the rigid falx cerebri medially and a combination of neovascularization in the abscess membrane and the inflamed leptomeninges and possible disruption of the adjacent cortex laterally (Figs. 12-5, 12-7). Occasionally an interhemispheric subdural empyema may appear crescentic in shape (Joubert 1977; Sadhu 1980). When definite enhancement of the borders of an extracerebral fluid collection cannot be identified on CT as encountered early in the course of the disease despite substantial clinical evidence (Dunker 1981), angiography should be performed. Angiographic findings are enlarged inflammatory meningeal arteries, vasospasm of the large arteries at the base of the brain, and multiple cortical arterial occlusions, spasm, or prolonged flow (Rao 1978; Kim 1976; Sadhu 1980; Luken 1980). Persistence of contrast enhancement long after eradication of active infection does not always indicate persistence of infection (Mosley 1984). The role of MRI in the diagnosis of extracerebral empyema has not been clearly established yet.

Meningitis

Haemophilus influenzae and *Escherichia coli* in neonates and young children and meningococci and pneumococci in adolescents and adults account for the majority of instances of suppurative meningitis. The leptomeninges offer comparatively little re-

sistance to infection, and the common initial response to these invading organisms is meningeal vascular congestion, edema, and minute hemorrhages. The underlying brain and its ependymal surfaces remain intact. CT may be normal at this stage (Claveria 1976; Zimmerman 1976) and may continue to be normal if treatment is instituted promptly and adequately. Once infection progresses, however, the subpial cortex of the brain and the ependymal lining of the ventricles show evidence of inflammatory reaction. On NCCT, increased density in the basal cistern, interhemispheric fissure, and choroid plexuses frequently simulates contrast enhancement, probably because of a combination of hypervascularity in the acutely inflamed leptomeninges and choroid plexuses and fibrinous or hemorrhagic exudate in the subarach-

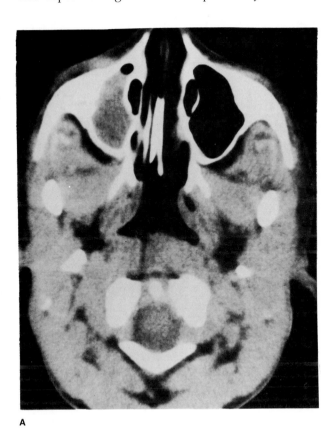

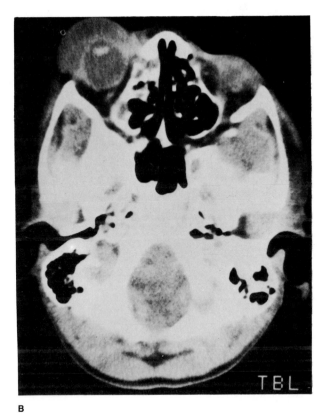

A

B

Figure 12-5 Subdural empyema associated with leptomeningitis and cerebritis. Right maxillary sinusitis **(A)** extends into the right orbit **(B)**. *(Continued on p. 564.)*

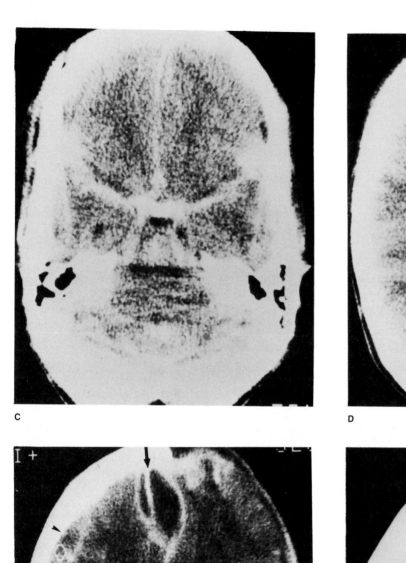

C

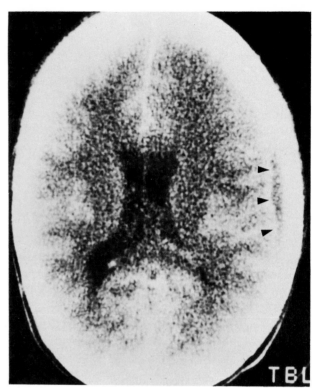

D

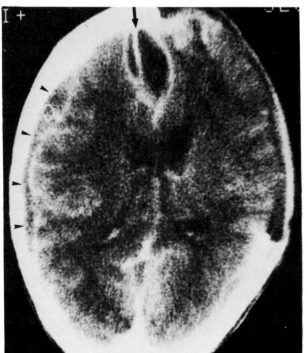

E

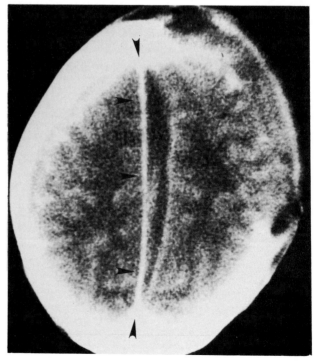

F

Figure 12-5 (*cont.*) CECT at the base **(C)** shows marked contrast enhancement at the basal cistern representing extensive leptomeningitis. **D.** A thin, crescentic, left hemispheric subdural empyema (arrowheads) with marked contrast enhancement of the underlying gyri and of the interhemispheric fissure (leptomeningitis, cerebritis, and/or venous thrombosis). **E.** CECT following surgical evacuation of the left subdural empyema demonstrates occurrence of the right subdural empyema with underlying cerebritis (arrowheads). Frontal interhemispheric subdural empyema can be seen on both sides of the falx cerebri (arrow). **F.** On CECT, convexity level shows a large interhemispheric subdural empyema delineated by a thick falx cerebri on the medial side (arrowheads) and an early membrane formation on the lateral side. Note also gyral contrast enhancement on both hemispheres.

noid space in the interhemispheric fissure and/or the basal cistern. The lateral and third ventricles are symmetrically compressed and extremely small (Auh 1980), perhaps because of diffuse brain swelling representing both cortical congestion and edematous white matter. The cortical congestion is often less severe than in encephalitis. Focal areas of low density representing focal edema may be seen on CT. Abnormal contrast enhancement of bandlike or gyral configuration in the leptomeningeal and cortical zones may be observed, resulting from the vascular

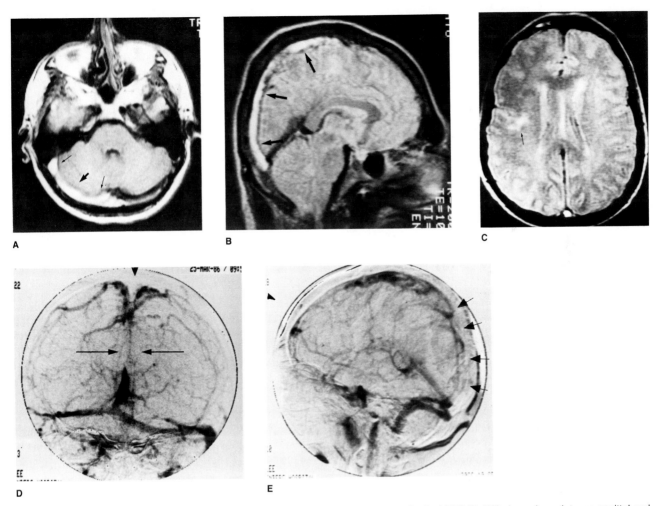

Figure 12-6 Sagittal sinus thrombosis due to sinusitis: **A.** Axial MRI (T$_1$-WI). **B.** Sagittal MRI (T$_2$-WI) shows hyperintense sagittal and right transverse sinuses (arrows). **C.** Axial MRI (T$_2$-WI) demonstrates white matter infarct (arrow). Note thrombosed hyperintense posterior sagittal sinus. **E.** AP and lateral carotid DSA confirm the diagnosis of thrombosis of sinuses (arrows). (*Case courtesy of Drs. Y. Oh and C. Salvati, Edison, N.J.*)

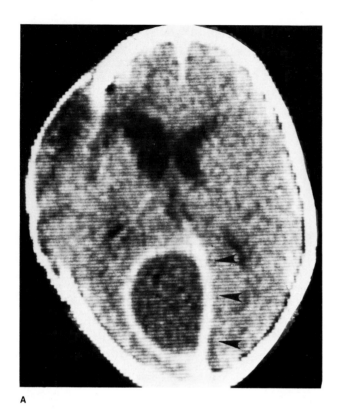

A

B

Figure 12-7 Interhemispheric subdura empyema in 8-year-old boy following surgery for otitis media.   **A.** On CECT, the biconvex pus collection is clearly delineated by enhanced falx cerebri medially (arrowheads) and enhanced membrane laterally. The central low density (10 to 20 HU) represents pus collection, and the shift of the falx cerebri is due to the expansible force of the abscess under increased pressure. Operative defect is noted in the temporal region.   **B.** CECT at the high convexity level in the same patient demonstrates further extension of the subdural empyema. In addition, septation due to membrane formation within the empyema is shown by midline horizontal linear enhancement.

congestion of the meninges and also from disruption of the blood-brain barrier (Figs. 12-5, 12-8).

CT is useful in the early detection of complications of meningitis following subsidence of the acute inflammatory phase. Arterial or venous vasculitis or thrombosis may lead to areas of cerebral infarction. In such cases CT demonstrates diffuse or localized areas of low density within the brain parenchyma, usually conforming to the distribution of the involved vessels (Fig. 12-9). Focal dilatation of the ventricles may be noted adjacent to an area of encephalomalacia as a late sequel of this chain of events. The low-density areas of encephalomalacia and/or atrophy show a predilection for the frontal regions and are most frequently observed with *H. influenzae*

meningitis (Cockrill 1978). Purulent exudate may collect at the base of the brain, particularly in the basal cisterns and convexities, causing communicating hydrocephalus as a result of impaired absorption of CSF from the subarachnoid space (Figs. 12-8, 12-10). Ependymal inflammation in the ventricles may result in hydrocephalus from obstruction of the fourth ventricle or secondary to intraventricular septation and compartmentalization (Schultz 1973). Consequently, a portion of the ventricles—temporal horn or fourth ventricle—can be trapped and may present as an expanding mass lesion (Zimmerman 1978) (Fig. 12-11). Focal areas of periventricular calcification may evolve in neonates during the initial weeks following onset of severe bacterial

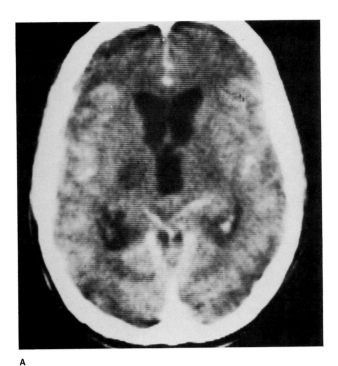

A

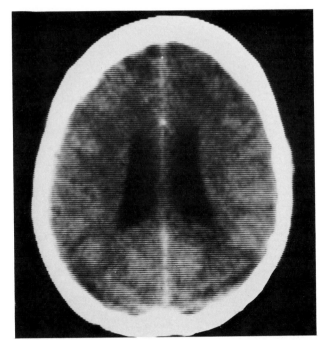

B

Figure 12-8 Extensive meningitis with cortical involvement. **A.** CECT at the level of the third ventricle demonstrates extensive cortical enhancement following gyral pattern of temporal and occipital lobes due to disruption of the blood-brain barrier. The old infarct of the right basal ganglia is visible. **B.** CECT at the level of the bodies of the lateral ventricles again demonstrates a gyral pattern of diffuse cortical enhancement. Hydrocephalus is due to obstruction of the basal cistern.

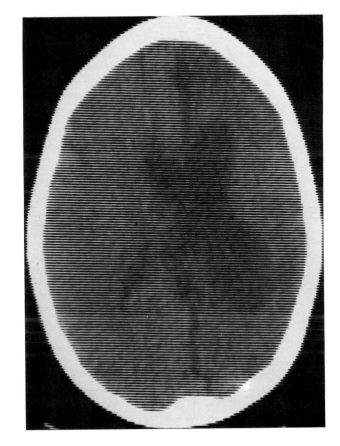

Figure 12-9 Hemispheric infarct following meningitis. Eight-year-old girl with congenital hypothyroidism presented with seizure and hemiparesis. At 2 years of age she suffered severe *Shigella* meningoencephalitis resulting in carotid artery occlusion at the basal cistern. CT discloses an infarct. (*Courtesy of Dr. Raymond Truex, St. Christopher's Hospital, Philadelphia, Pa.*)

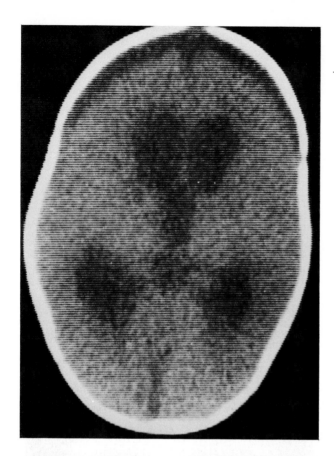

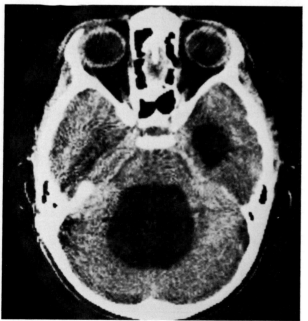

A

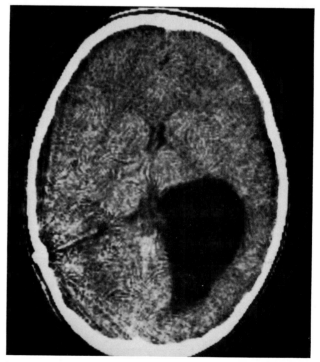

B

Figure 12-10 Subdural effusion following meningitis. Three-month-old infarct with pneumococcal meningitis developed into hydrocephalus and frontal subdural effusion bilaterally.

Figure 12-11 (Below) Trapped ventricles. Four-year-old child with history of tuberculosis meningitis. A shunt was placed for hydrocephalus. A. The trapped fourth ventricle shows a rounded appearance and may present as an expanding mass. Dilated temporal horn is noted. B. In this CT, taken at a higher level, the trapped trigone of the lateral ventricle is also seen.

meningitis complicated by ventriculitis (Kotagal 1981).

Development of subdural effusion is a common and well-recognized complication of leptomeningitis. Loculations of fluid between the thickened meninges occur over the base of the brain and on the surfaces of the cerebral hemispheres (Fig. 12-10). Subdural empyema may develop from a preexisting postmeningitis subdural effusion. Another late result of postmeningitic subdural effusion is calcification in the walls of the effusion (Nelson 1969; Claveria 1976).

Cerebritis

Cerebritis is initially manifested by an area of low density in the white matter with poorly defined bor-

ders and regional (Fig. 12-4) or widespread (Fig. 12-12) mass effect reflecting vascular congestion and edema. There may be little or no contrast enhancement at this early stage. Further progression of the inflammatory process leads to cerebral softening and petechial hemorrhage, reflecting progressive damage to the blood-brain barrier. At this stage, CECT reveals mottled irregular areas of enhancement, mostly in the regional gray matter (New 1980) (Figs. 12-5, 12-8). The appearance of contrast enhancement often simulates the gyral patterns of cerebral infarction. Patchy, irregular enhancement of the white matter may also be noted (Fig. 12-13). Experimental studies of the evolution of brain abscess following direct inoculation of organisms have demonstrated ring enhancement in the cerebritis stage (Enzmann 1979). The degree and extent of the mass effect is evidently out of proportion to that of the gyral en-

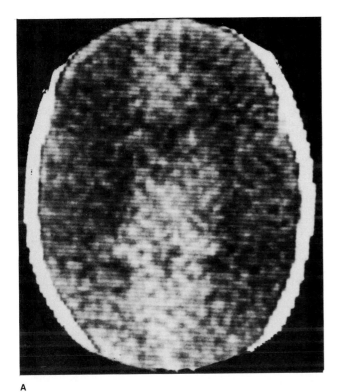

A

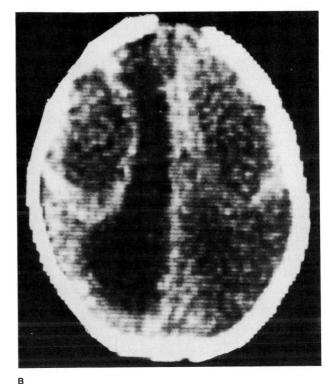

B

Figure 12-12 Diffuse cerebritis involving both hemispheres. **A.** NCCT shows diffuse extensive hypodensity of both hemi-

spheres involving both white and gray matter. **B.** Follow-up CT demonstrates multiple abscess formation.

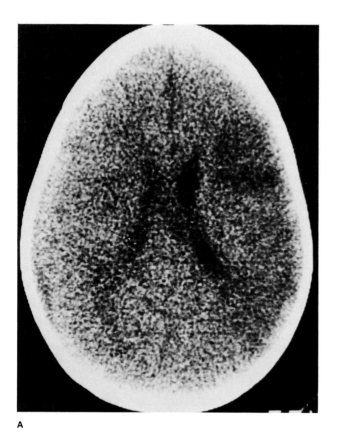

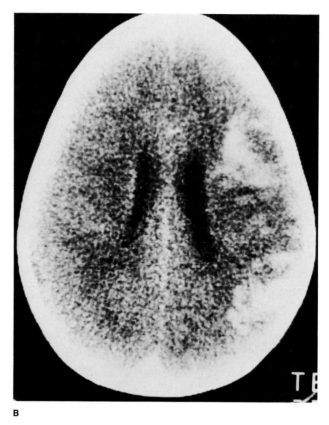

A

B

Figure 12-13 Cerebritis involving both gray and white matter. **A.** NCCT shows poorly defined regional hypodense areas in the left frontal and parietal lobes. **B.** CECT exhibits intense patchy enhancement in the white matter of the frontal lobe and gyral enhancement in the parietal lobe.

hancement. This finding may be of aid in the differential diagnosis from cerebral infarction when clinical findings are equivocal.

Aneurysms of inflammatory origin may be bacterial, syphilitic, or mycotic. Although all are termed mycotic, a bacterial etiology is the most common. These aneurysms originate mainly as an embolic complication of bacterial endocarditis, but less commonly aneurysms form as a complication of cardiac surgery, meningitis, cavernous sinus thrombophlebitis, or osteomyelitis. The most frequent location is at peripheral branches of the middle cerebral artery, followed by the anterior cerebral artery, the internal carotid artery, and the basilar artery. Progressive weakening of the elastica and the media of the aneurysm wall may result in rupture, with hemorrhage into the adjacent cortex or into the subarachnoid or subdural spaces. CT clearly demonstrates the results of aneurysm rupture, but the aneurysm itself is demonstrated only occasionally. Meningitis, cerebral abscess, or cerebral infarction may be associated with mycotic aneurysms.

Abscesses

Development of a brain abscess as a complication of leptomeningitis is unusual, but development of leptomeningitis secondary to an underlying brain abscess is common (Butler 1974). Brain abscesses typically occur as a result of preceding extracerebral infection. The extracerebral sources of infection can be divided into local (otitis media, mastoiditis, paranasal sinusitis, facial cutaneous infection, dental abscess, penetrating skull injury) and systemic (pulmonary infection, bacterial endocarditis, osteomyelitis, and congenital cyanotic heart disease with right-to-left shunt). Most venous-blood–borne abscesses are situated in subcortical white matter and appear on gross inspection as ill-defined areas of infected encephalomalacia (suppurative cerebritis). Arterial-blood-borne abscesses often commence in gray matter rather than in white matter and are located in the distribution of the middle cerebral artery, with a strong tendency toward multiplicity (disseminated microabscesses). In about one-quarter of cases of brain abscess, the source of the infection is uncertain (Kerr 1958) and sterile abscesses on smear and culture are not uncommon. Anaerobic organisms are isolated in the majority of abscesses, but multiple organisms are frequently found. Overall, the most commonly cultured organism currently is *Streptococcus*.

The center of cerebral softening in cerebritis may undergo necrosis and liquefaction, resulting in an abscess. On CT, mass effect on the ventricular system or the midline structures is noted in more than 80 percent of brain abscesses (Nielson 1977). On NCCT, an ill-defined, low-density area is almost always seen (Claveria 1976; Nielsen 1977; Stevens 1978). Frequently a ring of slightly high density surrounding a central area of low density is noted (Paxton 1974; Joubert 1977; Stevens 1978; Whelan 1980). Attenuation values within the central low-density area may vary between 4 and 28 HU. According to Mauersberger (1981), the average density value for the contents of an abscess was 11 HU, while the necrotic center of a glioblastoma revealed an average value of 23 HU. The high-density ring represents the abscess capsule and enhances densely following intravenous contrast injection (Figs. 12-14, 12-16, 12-20). Whelan (1980) reported several examples of dense nodules with further enhancement on CECT and suggested that this pattern was due to hemorrhagic infarction associated with vascular thrombosis and embolism in patients with sepsis. Visualization of gas within the abscess cavity usually indicates that the abscess was caused by gas-forming organisms (New 1976; Nielsen 1977), and

frequently persistent extracranial communications are present (Young 1984). Complete surgical excision is preferred to aspiration and antibiotics alone in these cases. The presence of gas collections within the brain with no antecedent history of penetrating craniocerebral trauma or surgical intervention (Fig. 12-15) may permit a specific diagnosis of abscess.

On CECT, the central low-density area in the cavity does not change in appearance or CT number. Oval or circular peripheral ringlike contrast enhancement is an almost constant finding, delineating the formation of an abscess capsule. The degree of contrast enhancement of the capsule is reported to vary from 11.6 to 74 HU (Nielsen 1977; New 1976). The wall is usually thin (3 to 6 mm) and of uniform thickness (Figs. 12-16, 12-20). Not infrequently, however, an irregularly thick wall of an abscess cavity measuring up to 12 to 15 mm may mimic the wall of a glioblastoma (Figs. 12-14, 12-15).

Pathologically the abscess capsule consists of three layers: an inner layer of granulation tissue, a relatively thick middle layer of collagen, and an outer layer of reactive glial tissue. The collagen layer plays a major role in encapsulation of the infected brain tissue and is derived from fibroblasts which can be found in the meninges and in the walls of neophyte vessels (Waggener 1974; Moore 1974). Thinning of the medial margin of the capsule is frequently observed and is thought to be due to the relatively poor vascular supply of the white matter. This may account for the tendency of abscesses to rupture into the ventricular system and to form daughter abscesses in the white matter. Delay in capsule formation on the deep medial side of the abscess makes the wall less firm than on the side adjacent to the gray matter. Although medial thinning of the abscess wall on CT has been reported in 48 percent of cerebral abscesses (Stevens 1978), increased thickness of the medial wall of the capsule has also been frequently found (Fig. 12-17). The smoothness of the innermost layer of the cavity wall on CT is thought to be strongly suggestive of abscess diagnosis (Stevens 1978). The innermost layer of the wall, on the other hand, is irregular on pathological specimens because it contains uneven layers of necrotic debris and inflammatory granulation tissue (Harriman 1984).

Inasmuch as the simmering infection serves as

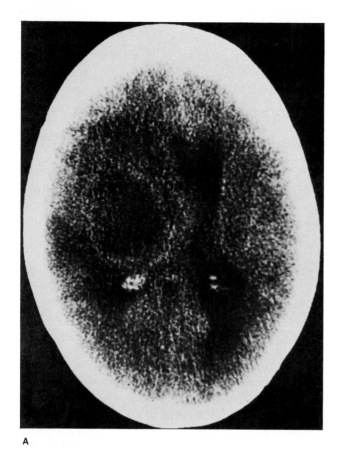

A

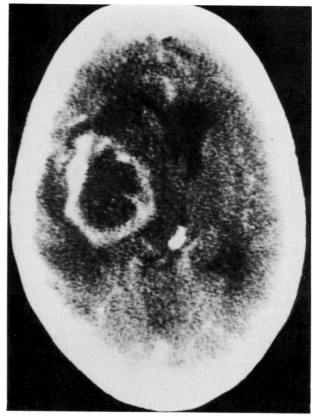

B

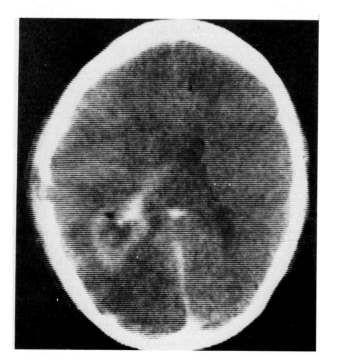

Figure 12-14 Temporal lobe abscess with thick, irregular capsule. **A.** NCCT shows a round, ringlike, hyperdense capsule differentiated from central low density (pus) and marked surrounding edema in the white matter. The compressed ipsilateral ventricle has shifted. **B.** On CECT, densely enhanced abscess capsule is evident. The irregular, thick wall of the capsule is not usual in pyogenic abscess. Central low density represents pus collection and does not change after IV contrast injection. The differentiation from glioblastoma may be extremely difficult in this case.

Figure 12-15 Postsurgical abscess cavity with air and ventriculitis. A small amount of gas present within the abscess cavity is the result of surgical intervention. Contrast enhancement within the ventricle represents ependymitis due to extension of infection from the abscess. Although presence of gas within the abscess produced by gas-forming organisms is diagnostic of a pyogenic abscess, its CT detection is extremely rare.

an ongoing stimulation to vascular proliferation, leakage of protein-containing fluid from neophyte capillaries in an abscess wall is a constant feature and represents a major source of the accompanying edema (Waggener 1974). Edema in the white matter around the lesion is almost a constant finding (80 to 90 percent) on CT (Paxton 1974; Nielsen 1977). The volume of the surrounding edematous white matter is often greater than that of the abscess and is therefore responsible for much of the mass effect (Fig. 12-14).

The varying CT features of cerebral abscess described above are probably a reflection of different stages in the evolution of the abscess (Nahser 1981) and also a function of the host's reaction to infection. If all the parameters of the abscess ring, such as thickness variability, patient's age, outside diameter, average value of CT numbers in the center, maximum wall thickness, and edema-to-ring ratio

are considered, the correct diagnosis of abscess can be made with 84 percent accuracy (Coulan 1980).

Cerebellar abscesses constitute 2 to 18 percent of all brain abscesses (Fig. 12-16*A* and *B*). They are less likely to be encapsulated but have a better prognosis than supratentorial abscesses if recognized early and treated surgically, prior to the onset of irreversible brainstem damage (Morgan 1975).

Pituitary or intrasellar abscess should be suspected if the radiological and clinical features of a rapidly expanding mass in the sella are combined with a history of recurrent episodes of meningitis and rhinorrhea. Preoperative radiologic diagnosis of intrasellar abscess was considered impossible prior to the CT era (Lindholm 1973; Rudwan 1977). CECT demonstrates a focal area of intense contrast enhancement within the sella (Fig. 12-18). Solid or ring CE, sella remodeling in association with adjacent sinusitis may be diagnostic, but differential diag-

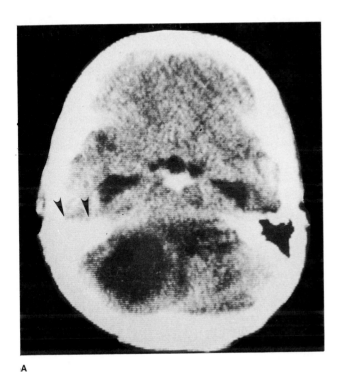

A

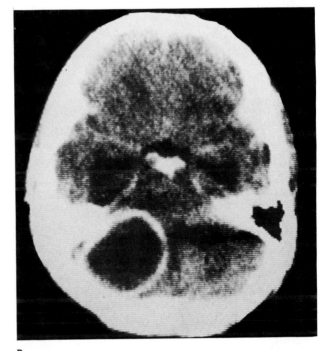

B

Figure 12-16 Cerebellar abscess. Eighteen-year-old with mastoiditis developed cerebellar abscess. **A.** NCCT shows the right mastoid is dense and without air cells (arrow) in comparison with the opposite side. A large, round, low density in the right cerebellar hemisphere displaces the fourth ventricle to the contralateral side. **B.** CECT shows a ringlike abscess cavity, well demarcated by a thin wall of uniform thickness contiguous to the petrous bone. (*Continued on p. 575.*)

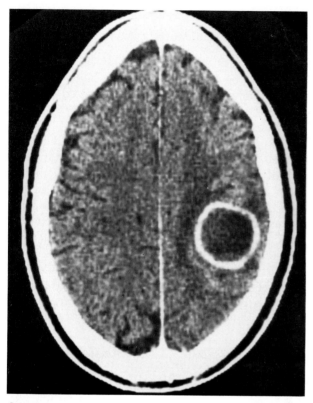

C

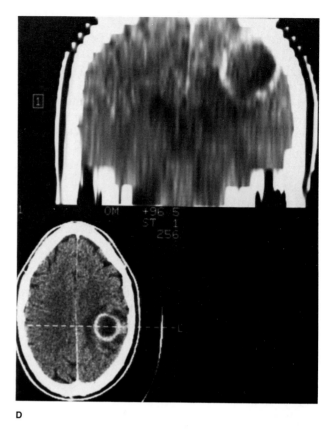

D

Figure 12-16 *(cont.)*   **C** and **D:** CECT shows staphylococcal abscess of the parietal lobe in subacute bacterial endocarditis patient. A thin wall of uniform thickness is associated with peripheral edema and central hypodensity.

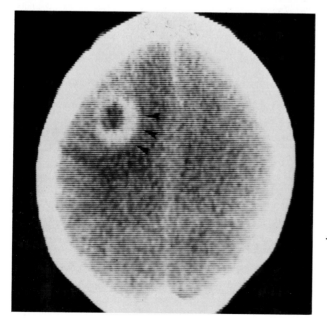

◀ **Figure 12-17**   Frontal abscess. Twenty-four-year-old woman with pneumococcal abscess of the lung developed posterior frontal abscess. On CECT, thick and irregular capsule, especially on the medial side adjacent to the white matter (arrowheads), is noted; this is contrary to the usual pathological finding of thinner, less-firm capsule toward the white matter because of its poor vascularity.

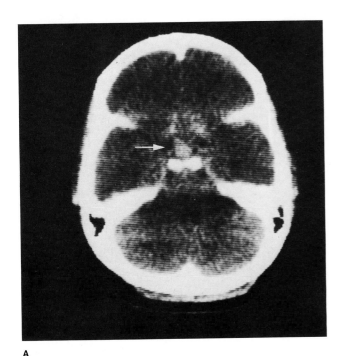

A

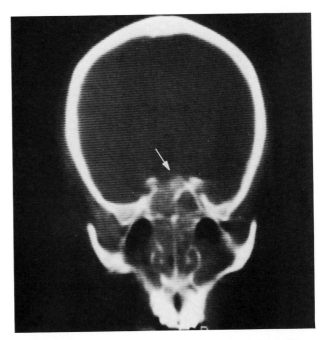

B

Figure 12-18 Intrasellar abscess. **A.** CECT demostrates a triangular enhancement in the sella (arrow). **B.** Coronal view discloses pansinusitis with opacification and fluid levels. Opacified sphenoid sinus with infected mucocele communicates with the intrasellar abscess (arrow) by way of the destroyed floor of the sella. Complete resolution of intrasellar abscess occurred following surgery and vigorous antibiotic therapy.

nosis with a wide variety of intrasellar cysts or tumors can be difficult (Enzmann 1983, 1984). Abscess may also develop in an intrasellar tumor, in which circumstance the prognosis is grave (Zorub 1979).

Detection of septation within an abscess cavity (Fig. 12-19) or of development of daughter abscesses, either contiguous or noncontiguous, or of multiple abscesses (Fig. 12-20) is of utmost importance in surgical or medical management. Of particular interest to surgeons is the fact that a ring pattern on CECT does not necessarily imply a firm capsule at surgery or in pathological specimens; firmness of the capsule wall appears to be a time-dependent phenomenon seen in patients with clinical symptoms lasting more than 2 weeks (Whelan 1980). The duration of symptoms is thus helpful in predicting the firmness of the capsule in association

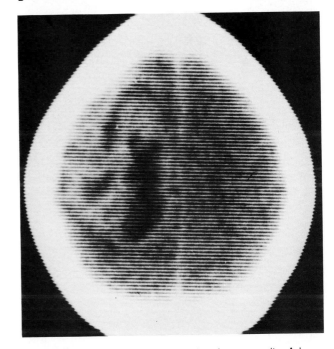

Figure 12-19 Multiseptation within the abscess cavity. A large abscess cavity with irregular nonuniform wall contains multiple thick septations. Satisfactory surgical results can be expected after total excision of all the compartments within the cavity.

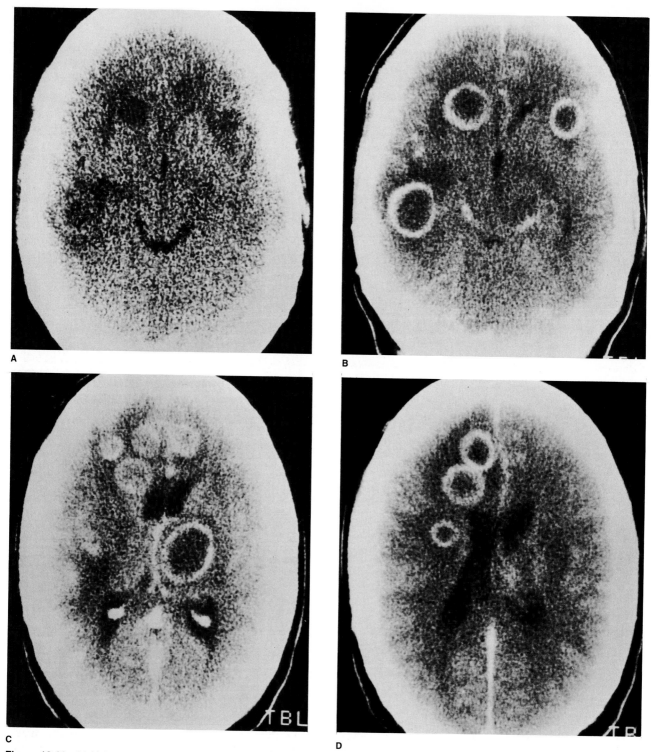

A

B

C

D

Figure 12-20 Multiple abscesses (staphylococcal) of unknown origin in 25-year-old man. **A.** NCCT shows multiple round, hypodense areas in both hemispheres. Faint ringlike hyperdense capsules are visible. **B.** CECT reveals multiple abscesses in the white matter. **C** and **D.** At the higher level, numerous cavities in the white matter, corticomedullary junction of both frontal lobes, and deep gray matter are present.

with ring enhancement on CT. CT is also helpful in the follow-up of multiple abscesses during medical and surgical treatment and in the selection of patients who would benefit from surgical intervention (Kobrine 1981).

Clinical improvement with medical therapy has been correlated with a decrease in both the degree of contrast enhancement of the ring and the amount of surrounding edema (Robertheram 1979; Kamin 1981). Persistence of ring enhancement following surgical drainage may signify a poor result with recurrence of the abscess (Claveria 1976), but prolonged enhancement in the postoperative period without clinical deterioration has been reported to resolve spontaneously within 3 to 4 months (Robertheram 1979). Delayed postsurgical contrast enhancement may be due to vascular granulation tissue present about the circumference of the previous abscess and may not represent persistence of the abscess capsule. Steroids may help reduce the inflammatory edema associated with brain abscesses (Wallenfang 1981) but can also suppress the contrast enhancement completely. The CT diagnosis may then be quite difficult in spite of strong clinical evidence suggesting an abscess. Also, withdrawal of steroids may result in a rebound increase in degree of enhancement (Robertheram 1979).

The greatest dangers for the patient with an abscess are raised intracranial pressure (with the risk of cerebral herniation due to mass effect) and rupture of the abscess into the ventricle. It is thus extremely important to determine the severity of the associated edema as well as the accurate size of an abscess, and CT is certainly the least invasive and perhaps the best diagnostic modality in distinguishing surrounding edema from abscess cavity. Demonstration of coexisting contrast-enhanced ring and contrast enhancement of the adjacent ventricular wall indicates rupture of an abscess into the ventricle with ependymitis (Figs. 12-15, 12-21). The prognosis in this situation is usually poor.

MRI exhibits greater sensitivity in detection of the early cerebritis and brain abscess (Enzmann 1984; Chap. 17), but precise correlation of MR signal changes and pathological findings may be improved with the utilization of MR contrast agent. [See Chapter 17]

Ependymitis

Spread of infection to the ventricles may follow leptomeningitis (usually resulting from retrograde extension of the infection via the lateral recesses of the fourth ventricle) or may follow spontaneous or iatrogenic rupture of an abscess cavity directly into the ventricles. Acute bacterial ependymitis shows distinct thin contrast enhancement along the ventricular wall regionally or more diffusely (Zimmerman 1976; Nielsen 1977) (Figs. 12-15, 12-21). Intraventricular septations and compartmentalization due to organization of intraventricular exudate and debris (Schultz 1973) and blockage of intraventricular foramina by purulent exudate lead to noncommunicating hydrocephalus. The loculated infection in the ventricles acts as a reservoir of infected material. CT not only precisely depicts the size and shape of the ventricles but also may suggest the presence of intraventricular septations and compartmentalization (Fig. 12-21). Trapping of the fourth ventricle because of obstruction of outlets and the aqueduct may ensue as a result of ependymitis following diffuse meningitis or shunt infection. This can act as an expanding mass in the posterior fossa which may require direct shunting procedure (Zimmerman 1978) (Figs. 12-11, 12-22). Occasionally, ventricular instillation of low-dose, low-concentration water-soluble contrast is necessary to demonstrate intraventricular compartmentalization or ventricular trapping (Fig. 12-22). Subependymal gliosis in chronic fungal or tuberculous ependymitis may show marked irregularity of ventricular margins with contrast enhancement (Fig. 12-37).

GRANULOMATOUS INFECTION

Tuberculous Infection

Tuberculous meningitis results from the hematogenous dissemination of bacilli from a primary lesion in the thorax, abdomen, or genitourinary tract. Small granulomas located in the cerebral cortex or in the meninges may rupture into the subarachnoid space, initiating a widespread meningeal infectious process. The very young and the very old are mainly af-

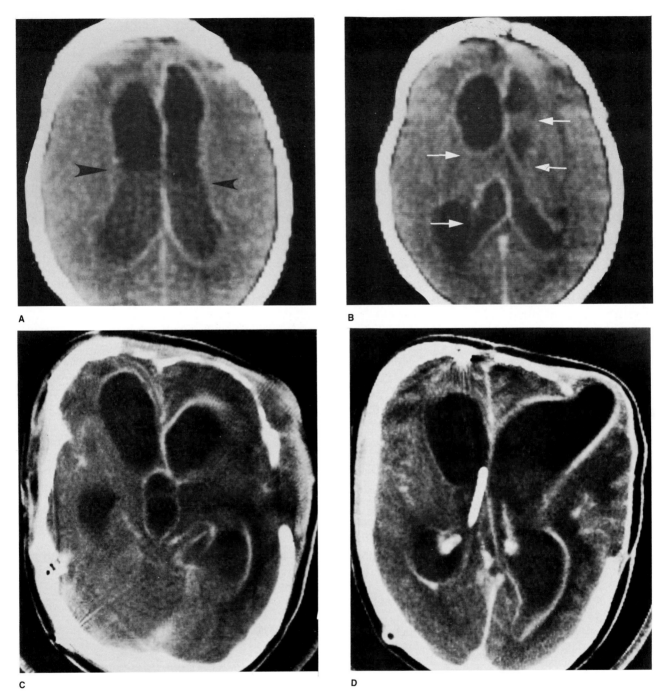

A

B

C

D

Figure 12-21 **A** and **B.** Ependymitis with septations following surgery for frontal sinusitis and abscess. On CECT (**A**) extensive ependymitis shows as a thin contrast enhancement along the ventricular wall. CSF levels in the ventricles (arrowheads) are due to layering of pus in the dependent posterior halves of the bodies of dilated lateral ventricles. Frontal craniotomy defect is the result of surgery for frontal abscess secondary to frontal sinusitis. CECT at lower level (**B**) demonstrates intraventricular septations (arrows) resulting in multiple compartmentalization. Note again extensive enhancement of the inflamed ventricular wall.   **C** and **D.** A young man sustained multiple craniofacial fractures following a gas-tank explosion. Postsurgical evacuation of the extracerebral collection was complicated by the wound infection and drainage of pus in the shunt tube. CECT demonstrates intense linear contrast enhancement along the walls of the ventricular system. Pus-CSF fluid levels are also noted in the lateral ventricles. Noncommunicating hydrocephalus is evident.

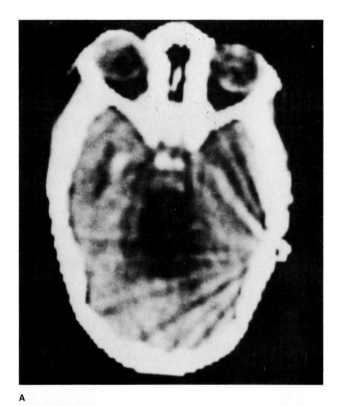

A

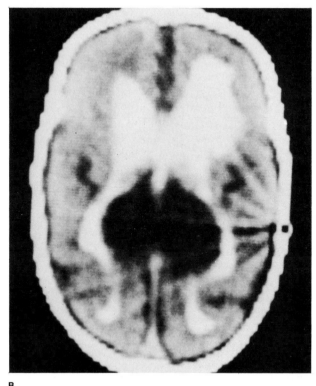

B

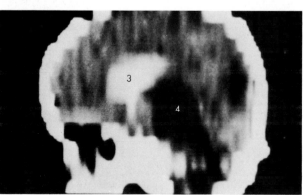

C

Figure 12-22   Fourth ventricle trapping following postshunt infection.   **A.** The large midline cavity of CSF density represents the fourth ventricle, which is markedly dilated. Although they are not shown, the lateral and third ventricles were also greatly dilated; however, this in itself is not diagnostic of a trapped fourth ventricle. **B.** Opacified lateral and third ventricles on instillation of metrizamide reveal noncommunication with the fourth ventricle.   **C.** Sagittal reformation in the midline clearly demonstrates marked dilatation of the fourth ventricle (4) extending supratentorially with no communication with the opacified third ventricle (3).

fected, with the highest incidence in the first 3 years of life (Pfuetze 1966). The fibrinous pachymeningitis is associated with a purulent exudate accompanied by a vascular inflammatory response and formation of granulation tissue, which can result in communicating hydrocephalus with obstruction at the level of the basal cistern. Constriction of the major vessels at the base of the brain and in the sylvian fissures is seen in response to direct insult by the infecting organism (vasculitis) and as a result of the surrounding meningeal inflammation. Cerebritis, caseous granuloma formation (tuberculoma), and arterial or venous infarctions are further complications seen in association with tuberculous meningitis. True tuberculous abscess of the brain, as opposed to tuberculoma, is very rare.

On NCCT, the basal cisterns may be partially obscured by the presence of inflammatory tissue and exudate. Obliterated and asymmetrical suprasellar and basal cisterns may be identified (Fig. 12-23). On CECT, the involved cisterns are uniformly and intensely enhanced, with an appearance that may resemble that of subarachnoid hemorrhage on NCCT or the images obtained with subarachnoid metrizamide (Enzmann 1976) (Fig. 12-23). The basal cisterns are most frequently affected, although frequently the sylvian cisterns and other subarachnoid spaces are involved (Armitsu 1979; Casselman 1980). Hydrocephalus secondary to blockage of the basal cisterns is a common sequela of tuberculous meningitis and is usually persistent, without progression or improvement in spite of antituberculous therapy (Price 1978; Stevens 1978). Calcification of the meninges at the base of the brain has been demonstrable 18 months to 3 years after the onset of the disease in 48 percent (Lorber 1958). Calcification within tuberculoma is not so common and ranges from 1 to 13 percent (Lorber 1958).

Cerebral *tuberculoma* is a rare manifestation of tuberculosis in the United States. The infrequency of the disease often results in diagnostic oversight. Definitive diagnosis may be particularly difficult since 42 percent of patients with intracranial tuberculomas have no evidence of extracranial disease (Mayers 1978). The clinical features of intracerebral tuberculoma are rarely distinguishable from other space-occupying intracranial lesions (Anderson 1975). A tuberculoma is composed of a caseous center surrounded by a ring of granulomatous tissue and may be spherical or multiloculated and single or multiple. Tuberculomas are found in any part of the cerebral or cerebellar tissue and in the epidural, subdural, and subarachnoid spaces (Harriman 1984). On NCCT, varying image patterns have been reported: a tuberculoma may be isodense (Welchman 1979) or hyperdense or occasionally of mixed density (Lee 1979). After contrast injection, ringlike enhancement (Fig. 12-24) is commonly seen (Welchman 1979); but homogeneous enhancement (Claveria 1976; Peatfield 1979), irregular heterogeneous enhance-

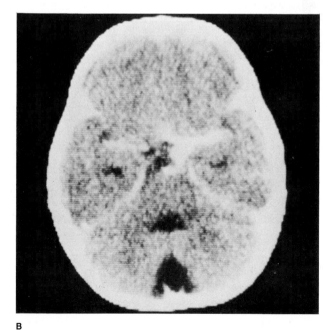

A

B

Figure 12-23 Tuberculous meningitis. Two-year-old child with choreoathetoid movement of face and arms. Cerebral angiogram demonstrated narrowing of the supraclinoid internal carotid arteries (not shown). **A.** NCCT demonstrates partial obliteration of supra- sellar cistern. **B.** CECT demonstrates marked enhancement at the basal cisterns extending into both sylvian fissures and tentorial margins and mimicking subarachnoid hemorrhage or intrathecal contrast.

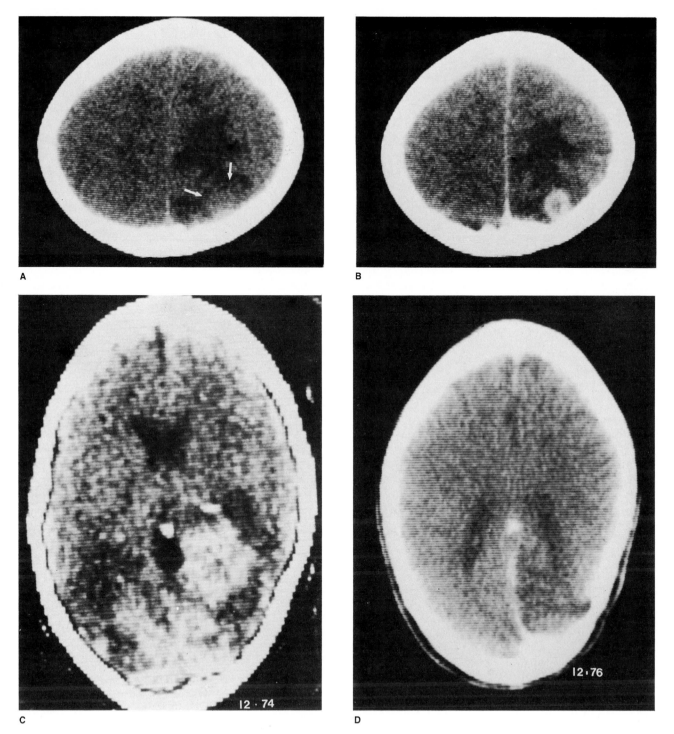

A

B

C

D

Figure 12-24 **A** and **B** Tuberculoma. **A.** NCCT shows edema in the white matter and an isodense round cortical lesion (arrows). **B.** CECT shows a thick, ringlike lesion in the cortex. The center of the lesion remains isodense, with no change on contrast injection. (*Courtesy of J. H. Suh, M.D., Severance Hospital, Yonsei University, Seoul, Korea.*) **C** amd **D.** Tuberculoma. On NCCT, mixed irregular density in the occipital lobes (not shown) was noted. **C.** CECT shows nonhomogeneous enhancement mimicking malignant glioma. Cerebral angiogram (not shown) demonstrated avascular mass. Culture and smear of the surgical specimen disclosed the correct diagnosis. **D.** Two years later, following surgery and antituberculous medical therapy, repeat CECT shows almost complete resolution.

ment (Price 1978; Lee 1979) (Fig. 12-24), or absence of enhancement have also been described. The ring, when it is present, tends to be unbroken and is usually of uniform thickness (Hirsh 1978). It may be smooth or irregular in outline. This ringlike enhancement is attributed to enhancement of the capsule as well as the surrounding gliotic tissue. The density of the tissue within the ring is similar to that of the surrounding brain (Welchman 1979) (Fig. 12-24), in contradistinction to the central low density of pyogenic bacterial abscess cavities. Tuberculomas may spontaneously become cystic, fibrous, or calcified, but their chief risk lies in their liability to spill into the meninges. The "target sign" described by Welchman (1979) represents a central ni-

dus of calcification or contrast enhancement surrounded by a ring of enhancement and is strongly suggestive of tuberculoma. Disproportionate surrounding edema and mass effect are usual but not prominent findings.

Tuberculomas may be predominantly extracerebral in location and attached to the dura (Welchman 1979) (Fig. 12-25). These en plaque tuberculomas closely resemble meningiomas, both clinically and operatively. Multiple tubercules may be found within the brain at the corticomedullary junction and in the paraventricular regions, because of extensive hematogenous spread, usually from miliary tuberculosis of the lungs. On NCCT, the nodules may not be identified because of their isodensity, but on CECT,

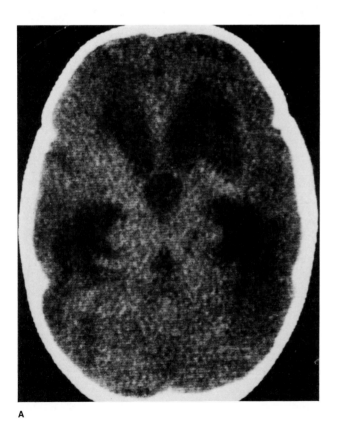

A

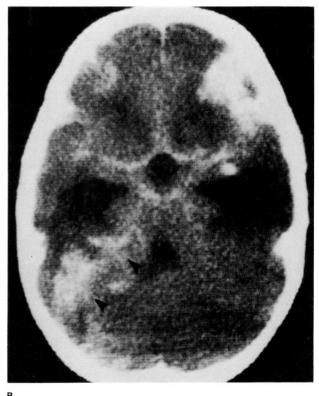

B

Figure 12-25 Tuberculomas, intracerebral and extracerebral. **A.** NCCT shows obliteration of the basal cistern and slightly increased density along the tentorial margins. Noncommunicating hydrocephalus (third and lateral ventricles) is due to obstruction at the level of the basal cistern.   **B.** CECT demonstrates extradural

granulomas (en plaque tuberculomas) along the right tentorial margin (arrowheads) and in the basal subarachnoid cistern. Irregular, mixed contrast-enhancing lesion in the left frontal lobe represents intracerebral tuberculoma.

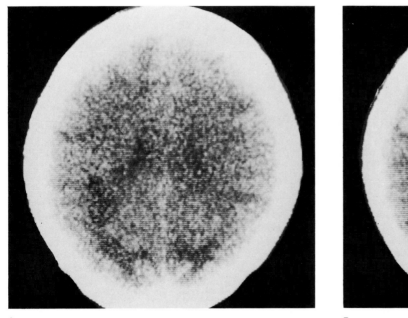
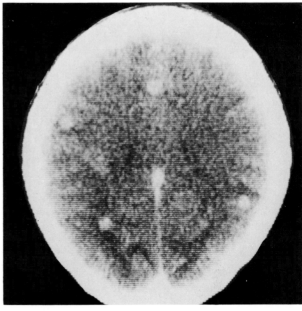

A

B

Figure 12-26   Multiple tuberculomas. Hematogenous dissemination in 24-year-old with miliary tuberculosis and tuberculous peritonitis. **A.** NCCT shows mild ventricular compression bilaterally, but no apparent density changes are noted.   **B.** CECT shows numerous discrete nodules in the cortex and corticomedullary junction. No apparent edema is present. Complete resolution was noted following vigorous antituberculosis therapy.

numerous small, round discrete nodules are readily detected (Witham 1979) (Fig. 12-26). Occasionally, centrally decreased density within the nodule may be visualized, but edema adjacent to the tubercle is not a common finding (Whelan 1981). Midline shift and ventricular compression are not usual or prominent findings, most probably because of the relative paucity of edema and diffuse involvement of both hemispheres. These tuberculous nodules may undergo complete resolution after antituberculosis therapy. CT is essential both in establishing the diagnosis of tuberculous meningitis and tuberculomas and in monitoring the response of the tuberculous lesions and the associated hydrocephalus to therapy.

Intracranial Sarcoidosis

Involvement of the central nervous system is a rare occurrence in systemic sarcoidosis. Although 4 to 7 percent of patients with sarcoidosis present with neurological manifestations, the incidence of intracranial involvement in patients with known sarcoidosis is about 15 percent (Silverstein 1965; Weiderholt 1965). Rarely, CNS involvement may be the only manifestation of this disease (Cahill 1981; Griggs 1973). Sarcoid may present at any age (Robert 1948) but is most common in the third and fourth decades, usually in females. Two patterns of intracranial involvement have been identified: (1) as a granulomatous leptomeningitis, and (2) as an intracerebral mass. Granulomatous leptomeningitis may occur diffusely or as a circumscribed process at the skull base, involving the optic chiasma, pituitary gland, floor of the third ventricle, and hypothalamus. Communicating hydrocephalus is a common result. The second pattern of CNS sarcoid, less commonly seen, consists in noncaseating granulomas either scattered diffusely in the brain parenchyma or as a single large mass which mimics a brain neoplasm

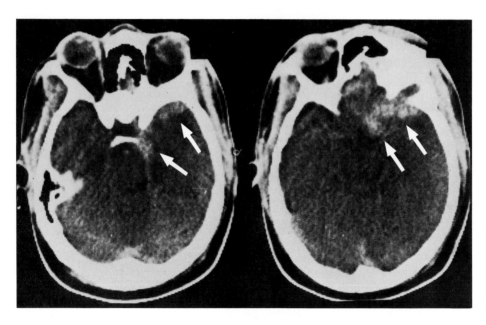

Figure 12-27 Leptomeningeal sarcoid granulomas. On CECT, extensive granulomas present as nonhomogeneous densities in the temporal fossa along the sphenoid bone (arrows) and in the parasellar region (arrows).

(Saltzman 1958; Silverstein 1965; Robert 1948; Griggs 1973).

On CT, sarcoidosis may thus present as hydrocephalus secondary to leptomeningitis (Morehouse 1981) (Fig. 12-27) or an obstructing mass lesion (Bahr 1978; Kendall 1978; Kumpe 1979) (Fig. 12-28). Dif-

ferentiation from other causes of communicating hydrocephalus may be difficult unless the patient has proved pulmonary sarcoidosis. Recent review of 32 patients with neurosarcoidosis by Ketonen (1986) demonstrated normal CT in 60 percent. One of the common abnormalities was hypodense white

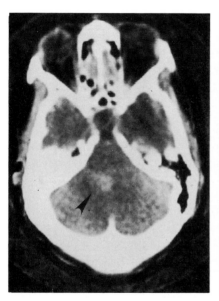
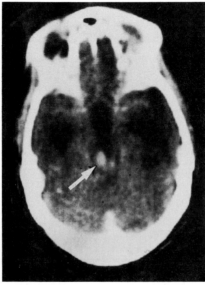

Figure 12-28 Parenchymal sarcoid granulomas. CECT demonstrates sarcoid granulomas in the brainstem (arrowhead) and midbrain (arrow).

matter lesions, which was attributed to small-vessel involvement. Mirfakharee (1986) reported that CT appearance of linear or nodular meningeal CE extending deep into the parenchyma is highly suggestive of meningeal infiltrative process with secondary parenchymal extension through the Virchow-Robin space, i.e., another path of spread in neurosarcoidosis. Granulomatous masses usually appear as a hyperdense area on NCCT, with further homogeneous enhancement on CECT. In a patient with known sarcoidosis, the intracranial mass may be suspected to represent sarcoid granulomas. When there is no evidence of peripheral sarcoidosis, differentiation from a meningioma or other hyperdense contrast-enhancing intracranial neoplasm may be difficult unless CSF analysis or biopsy is performed. Differentiation from other pathological entities, such as carcinomatous metastases or multiple intracerebral granulomas following other chronic infectious processes, is not possible on CT alone. However, unlike most metastases, sarcoid granulomatous masses within the parenchyma rarely demonstrate surrounding edema. Sarcoid granulomas decrease in size following treatment with steroids.

VIRAL INFECTION

Manifestations of viral diseases of the CNS on CT differ from those of bacterial or fungal etiology by their tendency to diffuse parenchymal involvement and the frequent absence of distinctive gross alterations in the involved parenchyma. An exception to this statement is herpes encephalitis.

Herpes simplex virus, type 1, is the most common cause of sporadic viral encephalitis in the United States. Herpetic encephalitis is characterized by a fulminant necrotizing encephalitis with petechial hemorrhages, with early involvement of the subfrontal and medial temporal regions. Mortality is high (in the vicinity of 70 percent). The success of treatment depends on early diagnosis and prompt institution of therapy. Even in the presence of char-

acteristic CT findings strongly suggestive of herpes infection, definitive diagnosis must be based on positive fluorescein antibody staining or culture of virus from brain biopsy.

The most commonly noted CT findings in herpes infection are a poorly marginated hypodense area (63 to 64 percent), mass effect (50 to 52 percent) and nonhomogeneous contrast enhancement (50 to 57 percent) (Davis 1978; Leo 1978). The earliest and predominant CT finding is the low-density abnormality in the temporal and frontal lobes, which are also characteristic sites of involvement in gross pathologic specimens (Davis 1978; Leo 1978) (Fig. 12-29). The hypodense area may later extend to involve the deep frontal or occipital lobes, but isolated frontal or occipital lobe involvement is uncommon (Ketonen 1980). The hypodensity in the early period probably represents a combination of tissue necrosis and focal brain edema. Abrupt transition to normal density at the lateral margin of the lenticular nucleus has been considered characteristic (Zimmerman 1980) (Figs. 12-29, 12-30).

The mass effect is manifested either as a midline shift or as a focal mass causing compression of the ventricles or sylvian cisterns. This is usually concomitant with a hypodense area and persists for more than a month (Davis 1978). Occasionally there may not be a midline shift owing to bilateral balanced involvement (Fig. 12-30).

The pattern of contrast enhancement may be gyral (Davis 1978), linear streaks at the periphery of the hypodense lesion (Enzmann 1978) (Fig. 12-30), patchy (Fig. 12-29), or multiple ringlike (Ketonen 1980) (Fig. 12-30). Occasionally, the location of the enhancement does not correspond to the areas of hypodensity (Davis 1978). The wide variation in appearance of the enhancement pattern may be due to the nonspecificity of the compromised blood-brain barrier in the area of rapid progressive hemorrhagic necrosis. Subarachnoid enhancement suggestive of meningeal involvement on CECT and intracerebral hemorrhage depicted on NCCT as a well-defined mass (Zegers de Beyl 1980) or as ill-defined linear streaks of increased density (Enzmann 1978) are uncommon findings. These CT abnormalities are usually not seen in the initial 5 to 7 days after onset of

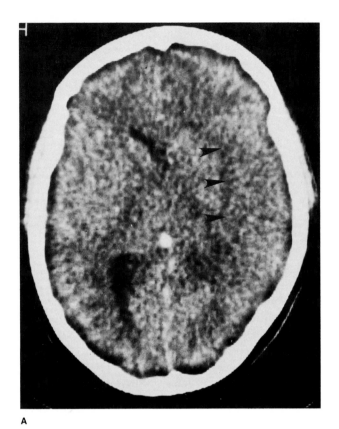

A

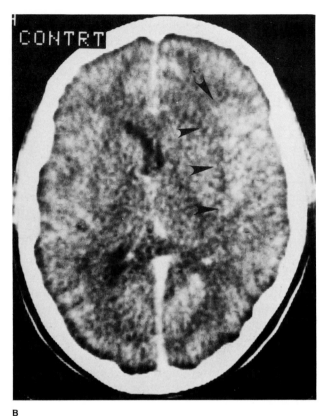

B

Figure 12-29   Herpes simplex (type 1) encephalitis.   **A.** NCCT exhibits poorly defined mixed-density area in the temporal lobe (arrowheads), with effacement of the ipsilateral ventricle.   **B.** On CECT, patchy areas of enhancement involve the temporal and frontal lobes (arrowheads).

illness (Zimmerman 1980; Greenberg 1981) although the earliest recorded occurrence of contrast enhancement was at 3 days after the onset of signs and symptoms (Davis 1978). Contrast enhancement may be detectable until 2½ months after disease onset (Ketonen 1980). Thus, a normal CT in the initial symptomatic period does not exclude the diagnosis of herpes simplex encephalitis. Radionuclide brain imaging, with dynamic and static delayed scintiscans, or MRI may be of value in detecting early changes in the initial period.

Late follow-up CT typically demonstrates widespread hypodensity (encephalomalacia) involving the temporal and frontal lobes, indicating extensive involvement of the brain, which is often not appreciated early in the course of the disease.

The primary role of CT in the evaluation of herpes simplex encephalitis is to confirm the clinical diagnosis and to indicate the best site for biopsy as well as to exclude the presence of an abscess or tumor. Early definitive diagnosis is essential prior to treatment with antiviral agents because of their known toxicity.

Infection with *herpes simplex virus, type 2,* in the newborn infant may be acquired transplacentally or during delivery, presumably secondary to genital and perineal infection in the mother. Early intrauterine infection with type 2 virus is known to have marked neurotrophic teratogenic potential and has been associated with microcephaly, micrencephaly, intracranial calcification, microphthalmia, and retinal dysplasia (South 1969; Whitley 1980). Dissemi-

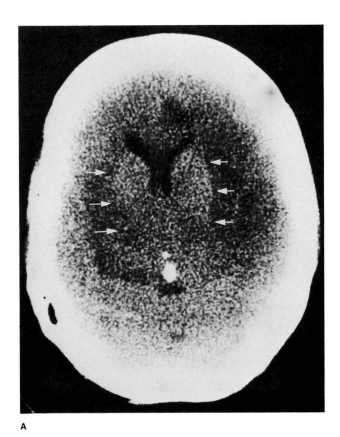

A

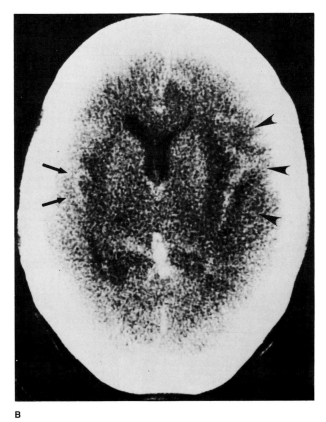

B

Figure 12-30 Herpes simplex (type 1) encephalitis. **A.** On NCCT, extensive low-density lesions in both temporal lobes, more on the left than the right, are clearly demarcated by the lateral margin of the basal ganglia (arrowheads). **B.** CECT shows different pat-

terns of contrast enhancement: linear streaks (arrowheads) on the left and ringlike figures (arrows) on the right. Absence of midline shift is due to bilateral, balanced involvement.

nated encephalitis in infants may produce widespread calcifications conforming to an atrophic cerebral hemisphere.

On initial NCCT (2 to 30 days), a gyral pattern of cortical hyperdensity which probably represents hemorrhage is noted. These usually are accentuated by diffuse decrease in white matter density (Sage 1981; Herman 1985). Subsequently (more than 30 days), extensive cerebral destruction, multicystic encephalomalacia and calcifications are manifest by diffuse hypodensity cystic areas throughout the cerebral hemispheres interspersed with scattered calcifications (Herman 1985) (Fig. 12-31).

Microcephaly with grossly dilated ventricles and

thin cortical mantle are also noted. Masses of calcifications are scattered throughout white and gray matter and may have a periventricular distribution (Dublin 1977).

Other causes of congenital calcification of the brain include toxoplasmosis, rubella, and cytomegalovirus. Toxoplasmosis and rubella calcifications are evenly distributed in necrotic brain substance but may be compressed by hydrocephalus and thus mimic the periventricular subependymal calcifications of cytomegalovirus. Occasionally, cortical and subcortical white-matter calcification is found in cytomegalovirus infection (Harwood-Nash 1970; Malloy 1963).

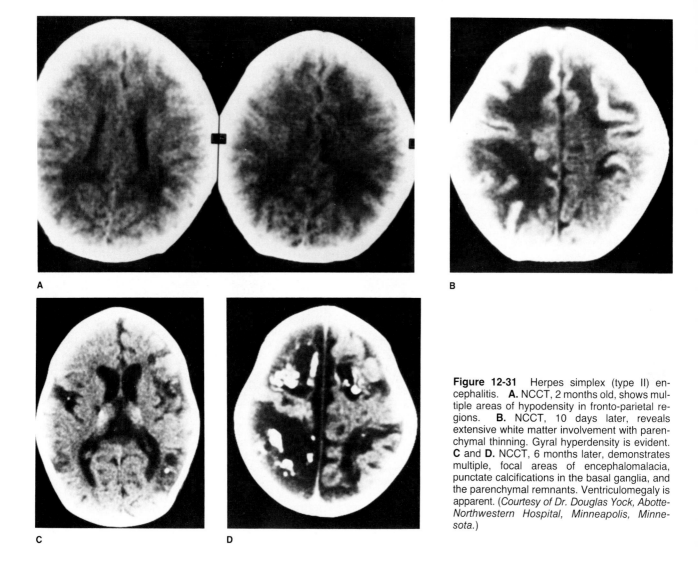

Figure 12-31 Herpes simplex (type II) encephalitis. **A.** NCCT, 2 months old, shows multiple areas of hypodensity in fronto-parietal regions. **B.** NCCT, 10 days later, reveals extensive white matter involvement with parenchymal thinning. Gyral hyperdensity is evident. **C** and **D.** NCCT, 6 months later, demonstrates multiple, focal areas of encephalomalacia, punctate calcifications in the basal ganglia, and the parenchymal remnants. Ventriculomegaly is apparent. (*Courtesy of Dr. Douglas Yock, Abotte-Northwestern Hospital, Minneapolis, Minnesota.*)

Acquired Immune Deficiency Syndrome (AIDS)

In acquired immune deficiency syndrome (AIDS) patients, inversion of the normal ratio of helper to suppressor T-cell lymphocytes results in the alteration of immunity. Virus (HTLV-III/LAV) is thought to be a causative organism. Homosexual men and intravenous drug abusers are more frequently affected, and the mortality approaches 100 percent.

Neurological signs and symptoms occur in 30 to 70 percent of cases and can attribute to the following: (1) opportunistic infections, e.g., toxoplasmosis, cryptococosis, Papovirus, Candidiasis, cytomegalovirus, M. Tuberculosis and Intracellurae, and Aspergillosis; (2) neoplasms such as primary and secondary lymphoma, plasmocytoma, and Kapposi's sarcoma; (3) thrombocytopenia predisposing to cerebral hemorrhage and nonbacterial thrombotic endocarditis resulting in cerebral infarction (Elkin 1985).

The response of the brain to pathogens in AIDS

patients differs from that in individuals with normal cell-mediated immune system. Because of the atypical reaction, the usual CT criteria for intracranial lesions may be altered and not diagnostically pathognomic. Despite its relative lack of specificity, CT abnormalities do localize disease for possible biopsy of mass lesion in AIDS patients (Levy 1984). Many patients with neurological symptoms may have a normal CT scan (Levy 1986).

Toxoplasmosis is by far the most common infection of the brain parenchyma in AIDS patients (Whelan 1983; Post 1985; Levy 1986). CT findings consist of multiple intraparenchymal lesion with ring or nodular contrast enhancement and hypodense

area preferably involving the white matter, corticomedullary junction and basal ganglia (Post 1983; Whelan 1983; Elkin 1985; Bursztyn 1984) (Fig. 12-32).

Common CT findings of cytomegalovirus (CMV) are diffuse cortical atrophy and mild hydrocephalus ex vacuo. Widespread white matter disease with diffuse subependymal contrast enhancement, smooth and regular in outline around the lateral ventricles, is also present (Fig. 12-33). CT is not very sensitive for the detection of CMV encephalitis (Post 1986a).

CT observations in other fungus infections, progressive multifocal leukodystrophy (PML), tuberculosis infection, and lymphoma are described in

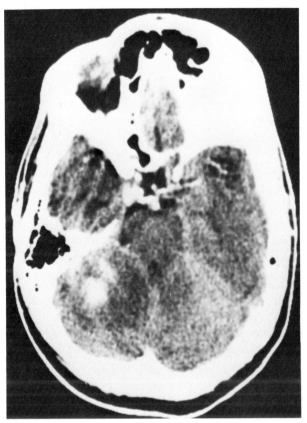

A

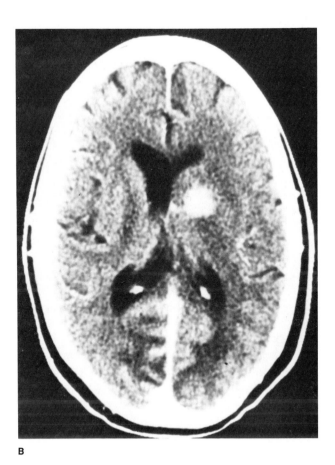

B

Figure 12-32 AIDS patients with toxoplasmosis: CECT of the posterior fossa (**A**) shows multiple nodular enhancing lesions in the right cerebellum. Mild edema is present. Left basal ganglia mass and abnormal gyral enhancement of the occipital lobes are noted (**B**). (*Continued on p. 590.*)

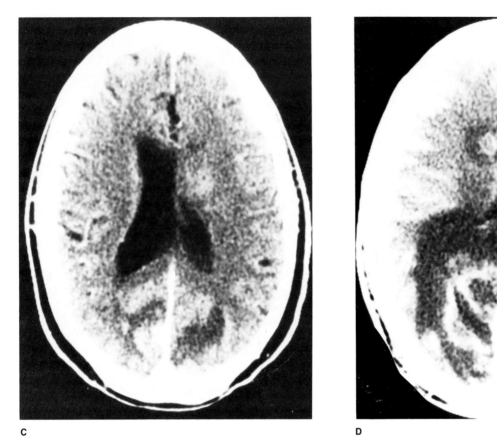

C   D

Figure 12-32 (*cont.*)   At higher level (**C**), irregular hypodense lesions of the parieto-occipital lobes are associated with irregular nodular enhancing lesions.   (**D**). Another patient with peripheral enhancement in right frontal and occipital lobes.

other sections. All AIDS patients should be studied with CT or MR if available when they develop an altered mental status, fever associated with seizures, and/or focal neurologic deficits (Post 1986*b*).

Navia (1986) established AIDS dementia complex as a distinct clinical and pathological entity which is caused by direct LAV/HTLV-III brain infection. CT and MRI showed a variable degree of cortical atrophy frequently accompanied by ventricular dilatation, and diffuse white matter and structural abnormality, with relative sparing of the cortex. Bursztyn (1984) stated that the presence of cerebral atrophy on CT is usually indicative of a fatal outcome within a few months.

FUNGAL INFECTION

Fungal infections represent nontuberculous granulomatous diseases which may be acute and fulminant. Infection may be meningeal, parenchymal (fungal "abscess"), or both. In most instances, the primary portal of entry is the lungs, but fungal osteomyelitis or lymphadenitis may precede brain involvement. The frequency of CNS fungus infection has increased significantly in recent years, because of opportunistic organisms in patients receiving steroids or immunosuppressive drugs (Britt 1981).

Although a variety of opportunistic organisms may involve the central nervous system, not all of

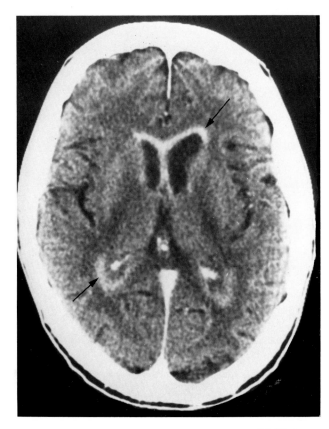

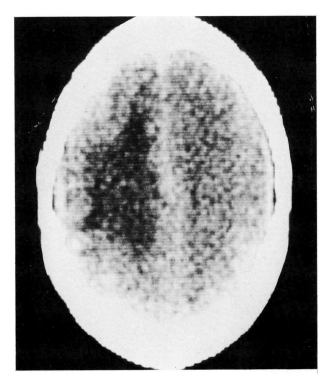

Figure 12-34 Cryptococcal granuloma. CT shows poorly margin-ated, extensive, hypodense lesion in the white matter with no contrast enhancement.

Figure 12-33 AIDS with cytomegalovirus (CMV). CECT shows marked, diffuse periventricular enhancement denoting ependymal and subependymal involvement (arrows). [*From Post (1985) with permission.*]

the entities have a characteristic pattern that suggests the diagnosis purely on the basis of CT findings. Most often CT is useful in demonstrating and localizing the parenchymal or meningeal involvement and confirmation as to the specific fungus involved is based on a variety of CSF studies, most often the CSF culture.

CT features of fungus infection are varied and nonspecific (Enzmann 1980). In general, ringlike contrast enhancement in fungal infection, frequently observed in patients free of additional systemic derangements, probably reflects the host's ability to wall off the organisms, with a better prognosis.

Cryptococcal (torular) meningitis is perhaps the most

common fungal infection of the brain. A thick, immobile exudate is noted at the base of the brain, topographically similar to a tuberculous exudate. Large parenchymal granulomatous "abscesses" (torulomas) also simulate tuberculomas. CT may show poorly marginated hypodense lesions in the white matter with minimal or no contrast enhancement (Fig. 12-34). Intraparenchymal torulomas may exhibit ringlike (Long 1980; Arrington 1984) or focal homogeneous contrast-enhanced areas with or without circumferential edema (Fujita 1981). Long (1980) and Cornell (1982) reported a variety of nonspecific CT changes such as ventricular dilatation, cortical atrophy, focal ischemic changes, meningeal opacification, and cerebritis. Calcification may be present on follow-up studies. In immunosuppressed organ-transplant recipients (Britt 1981), cryptococcal and *Listeria* infections are more fre-

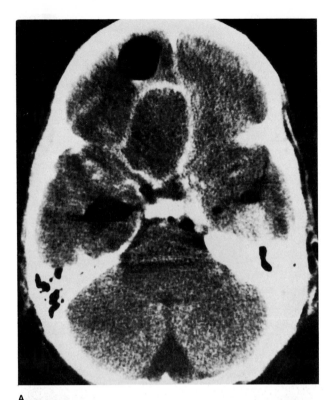

A

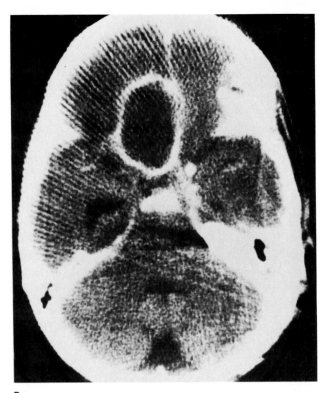

B

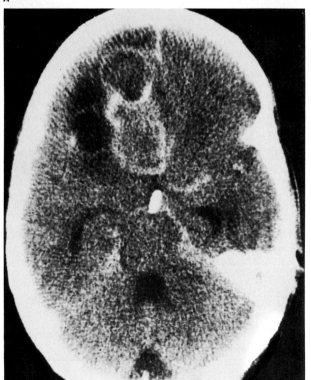

C

Figure 12-35 *Candida* granuloma. Eighteen-year-old involved in severe motor vehicle accident who sustained multiple basal skull fractures.   **A.** Basal skull CECT shows multiple pneumocephalus and left temporal lobe hemorrhage. A large cavity in the right frontal lobe contains an isodense center and irregular wall. Aspiration and culture grew *Candida albicans.*   **B** and **C.** Follow-up CT, after treatment with amphotericin B, demonstrates thicker cavity wall and development of a daughter cavity. Resorption of temporal lobe hematoma and pneumocephalus is noted.

quently seen as meningitis than intraparenchymal granulomas. Basal cisterna contrast enhancement or latent development of subdural hygroma may be seen.

Coccidioides imitis is a dust-borne fungus endemic to the southwestern part of the United States, especially the San Joaquin Valley of California, as well as portions of Mexico and central South America (Fraser 1978). It is spread by inhalation of the spore, which is present in soil. Only 0.02 to 0.2 percent of cases progress to the disseminated form involving the brain, meninges, and other systemic organs (Einstein 1974). Pathologically, CNS coccidioidomycosis is characterized by thickened, congested leptomeninges with multiple granulomas, which are especially prominent in the basal cisterns and result in communicating hydrocephalus. Vasculitis also occurs, but occlusions are rare. Ependymitis and periventricular diffuse focal white-matter and deep gray-matter lesions (focal granulomas without calcification) are also seen (McGahan 1981). The most common CT findings are hydrocephalus (86 percent) and abnormal basal or convexity cisternal contrast enhancement (71 percent) (Dublin 1980; Enzmann 1976).

Candida albicans is increasingly associated with nervous system infection, particularly in patients with diabetes mellitus or those with altered immune status caused by immunosuppressive or cytotoxic drugs or broad-spectrum antibiotics or steroids (Lipton 1984). Candidiasis of the CNS is characterized by scattered granulomatous microabscesses, leptomeningitis, and numerous thrombosed vessels. CT demonstrates areas of poorly circumscribed low density without contrast enhancement in immunosuppressed patients (Enzmann 1980). Cavity formation of various thicknesses with an isodense or slightly hypodense center may be encountered in patients with no predisposing systemic illness (Fig. 12-35). Noteworthy is the central density, which is higher than that of bacterial abscesses except for tuberculosis.

Aspergillus fumigatus usually appears as an opportunistic infection and reaches the brain in most cases by hematogenous dissemination from a primary focus in the lung or by direct extension from the ear, nose, or paranasal sinuses. Solitary brain abscess, thrombosis with hemorrhagic necrosis, and massive subarachnoid and intracranial hemorrhage are known to occur (Visudhiphan 1973). Enzmann (1980) and Grossman (1981) reported nonspecific, poorly circumscribed areas of subtle hypodensity with little or no contrast enhancement and mass effect. However, a ring configuration representing a well-formed, thick, and regular abscess capsule has been noted on CECT (Claveria 1976). Compared to neuropathologic findings, the CT findings generally underestimated the extent of involvement.

Nocardia asteroides infection may demonstrate multiple extensive hypodense lesions on NCCT, with ringlike appearance on CECT (Fig. 12-36). A rare case of *Cladosporium trichoides* following a penetrating craniocerebral injury has been reported (Kim 1981). CT showed a round lesion in the edematous frontal white matter above the original site of injury. The center of the lesion showed near-isodensity with no contrast enhancement. Intense contrast enhancement was present in the walls of the cavity and the ventricles. The ependymitis along the ventricular wall was thick, irregular, and not contiguous (Fig. 12-37). At surgery, a firm subcortical mass, with extensive granulomatous inflammation, was found. No fluid was present within the cavity. *Toxoplasma gondii* infection may exhibit either nonspecific low density or ringlike enhancement on CT (Enzmann 1980).

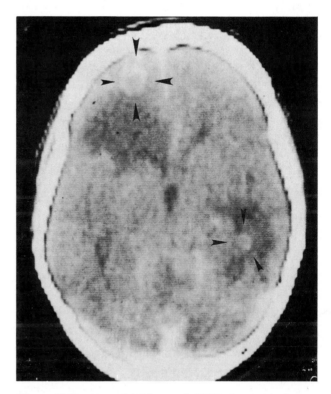

Figure 12-36 Nocardial "abscess." CECT shows two discrete round lesions in the right frontal and left temporal lobes. Peripheral contrast enhancement (arrowheads) and extensive surrounding edema are present.

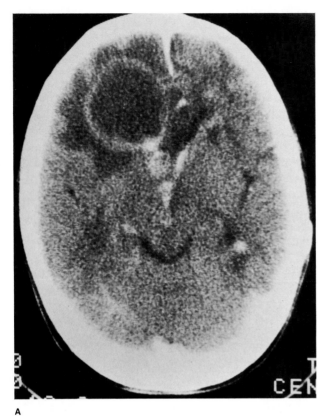

A

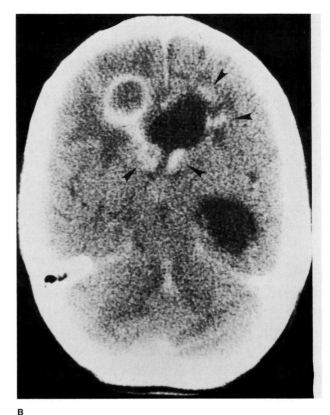

B

Figure 12-37 *Cladosporium* granuloma. **A.** CECT shows a large, thin, ringlike cavity in the frontal lobe with surrounding white matter edema. Thick, irregular enhancement in the ventricular wall represents ependymitis. **B.** CECT, following surgical and medical treatment, demonstrates marked decrease in the size of the cavity and the extent of edema. Dilatation of the left lateral ventricle is due to obstruction of the foramen of Monro by ependymal granulomas (arrowheads). (*Courtesy of Dr. Ronald C. Kim, University of California, Irvine, CA.*)

PARASITIC INFECTIONS

Cysticercosis

Cysticercosis is one of the most common parasitic diseases to affect the brain. Humans serve as the intermediate hosts of *Taenia solium,* the pork tapeworm, in this disease, which is prevalent in parts of Asia, India, Africa, Europe, and Latin America. There appears to be a recent increase in the incidence of cysticercosis in the United States, perhaps due to an increase in travel to and from endemic areas. The central nervous system is the most frequently infected organ system, with reported incidence of CNS involvement as high as 92 percent of cases (Dixon 1961). Classification by anatomic localization include meningeal (39 percent), intraventricular (17 percent), parenchymal (20 percent), mixed (23 percent), and intraspinal (1 percent) (Carbajal 1977).

Meningeal involvement is manifested by extracerebral cysts, arachnoiditis, vasculitis, or a combination of these. Since the walls of subarachnoid cysts are not visible on CT before or after contrast injection and the density of the fluid contents of these cysts is identical to that of CSF, the detection of these cysts is based on focal areas of apparent enlargement of the subarachnoid spaces. Breakdown of these systems provokes an arachnoiditis which may exhibit focal contrast enhancement, and occurrence of one or more cysts in the basal cisterns may

obstruct cerebrospinal fluid pathways, with resultant communicating hydrocephalus. Vasculitis associated with the meningeal cysticercal infestation
may cause arterial narrowing, with thrombosis and
resultant cerebral infarction.

Solitary or multiple intraventricular cysts may be
attached to the ventricular walls or may be free-
floating. Larger cysts may cause focal expansive deformities of the affected ventricle. A large cyst or
cluster of cysts within the fourth ventricle and its
expansion may simulate entrapment of the fourth
ventricle (Fig. 12-38). Noncommunicating hydrocephalus due to obstruction of the foramen of Monro,
unilateral or bilateral, or of the fourth ventricle is a
common finding (Zee 1984). Uniform enhancement
in an isodense cyst in the anterior third ventricle
(Jankowski 1979) and ringlike enhancement in the
fourth-ventricle cyst (Zee 1980) are rare findings and
may not represent enhancement of the cyst wall.
Usually, cysts are not identified on CT because of
their thin walls, approximately CSF-equivalent cyst
contents, and lack of contrast enhancement (Carbajal 1977; Benson 1977). Measurements of the density of the cyst fluid range from 0 to 10 HU. Large
cysts often appear slightly lower in density than the
CSF.

In the acute encephalitic phase of neurocysticercosis, CT manifests multiple, diffuse nodular CE (85
percent) or localized CE (15 percent) commonly in
the cerebral cortex (Rodriguez-Carbajal 1983).

Living larvae create parenchymal masses up to
2 or 3 cm in diameter within the substance of the
brain. On CT, these appear as rounded cystic structures of CSF-equivalent density (Fig. 12-39). Rarely,
isodense or hyperdense masses are noted (Sim 1980).
Since there is little reaction of the surrounding brain
prior to the death of the larva, contrast enhancement or focal edema around the cyst is rarely observed in association with living cysticerci. This lack
of inflammatory reaction about cysticercus cysts is
a striking feature of the disease and is probably related to poor antigenicity of the wall of the parasite
and inaccessibility of cysticercal antigens within the
CNS because of an intact blood-brain barrier (Biagi
1974).

However, at the termination of cohabitant status
with the brain parenchyma, ringlike or nodular con-

trast enhancement occurs, often accompanied by
surrounding focal edema (Fig. 12-40). The exact
mechanism of the acute inflammatory reaction in
the presence of dying cysticerci but not with living
larvae is not known. Perhaps when antigenic stimulation from cysticerci ceases and the immunologi-
cal balance is disrupted, the brain may then react to
dead foreign bodies, resulting in acute inflammation.

Calcifications are a manifestation of dead larvae.
They can appear as early as 8 months after acute
phase (Rodriguez-Carbajal 1983) or may require 10
years or more to develop (Dixon 1961). Calcifications are seen only with the parenchymal form, not
with ventricular or cisternal cysts. Usually they are
located in the gray matter or near its junction with
the white matter, but they are sometimes seen in
the basal ganglia and occasionally in the midst of
the white matter (Santin 1966) (Fig. 12-41). Calcification may involve both the wall and contents of
the cyst. It typically appears round or slightly oval
and is from 7 to 16 mm in size (Carbajal 1977). These
wholly or partially calcified spheres frequently contain an eccentric small nodular calcification measuring 1 to 2 mm in diameter which represents the
scolex of the erupted larva (Jankowski 1979). Both
dead larvae with calcifications and living larvae may
coexist in cases of reinfestation (Fig. 12-41). Vasculitis may develop in the vicinity of these lesions and
lead to cortical arterial occlusion and infarction.

Suss (1986) described MR characteristics of neurocysticercosis consisting of a hypointensity signal
(similar to CSF) focus and a conspicuous hyperintense mural nodule containing the scolex on both
T_1 and T_2-WIs. MRI was more sensitive than CT in
the recognition of parenchymal and subarachnoid
cysts, perifocal edema, and internal changes indicative of cyst death. CT is superior in demonstration
of calcification and blood-brain barrier breakdown
in the absence of MR contrast agent. MR may replace invasive ventriculography in the evaluation of
the CSF pathway neurocysticercosis.

The differentiation of meningeal cysticercosis from
arachnoid cyst and intradural epidermoid cyst, as
well as the differentiation of intraventricular cysticercosis from colloid cyst, ependymal cyst, or
intraventricular epidermoid depends frequently on

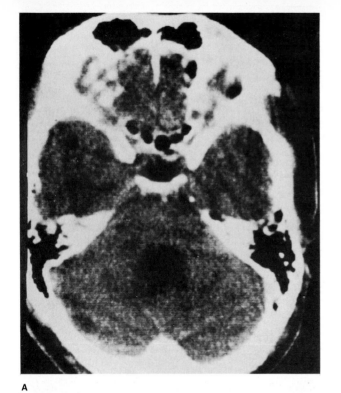

A

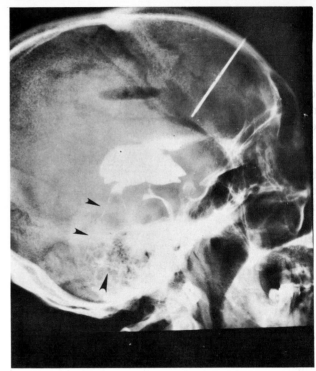

B

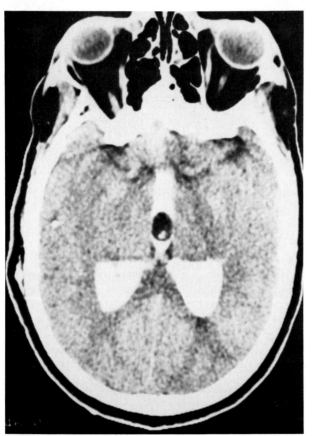

C

Figure 12-38 **A** and **B:** Cysticercosis in the fourth ventricle. **A.** Apparent dilatation of the fourth ventricle and obstructive hydrocephalus. On close inspection, the density within the fourth ventricle is slightly lower than that of cerebrospinal fluid. **B.** On positive-contrast ventriculogram, the fourth ventricle is faintly outlined (arrows). At surgery, multiple cysts were delivered from the fourth ventricle. (*Courtesy of Man Chung Han, M.D., Seoul National University Hospital, Seoul, Korea.*) **C.** Third ventricular cysticercosis with a scolex in another patient—on positive-contrast ventriculogram.

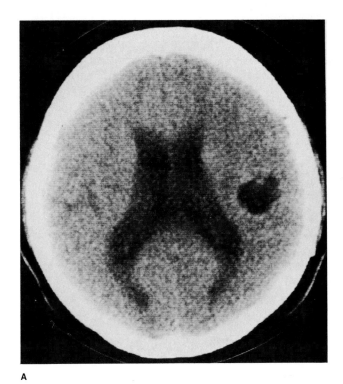

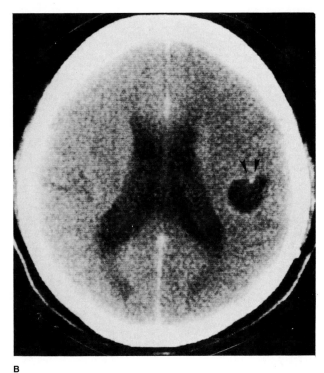

A

B

Figure 12-39 Living intraparenchymal cysticercus.   **A.** NCCT demonstrates a rounded cystic structure of CSF-equivalent density in the white matter of the parietal lobe. No surrounding edema is present. **B.** CECT shows no contrast enhancement around the cyst, but the scolex (arrowheads) is slightly enhanced, indicating the living cysticercus. Note also the absence of adjacent edema or mass effect. (*Courtesy of Dr. S. Y. Kim, Kyung Hee University Medical School, Seoul, Korea.*)

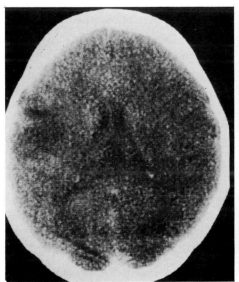
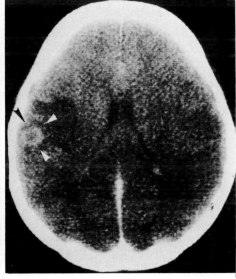

A   **B**

Figure 12-40 Dying intraparenchymal cysticercus.   **A.** NCCT shows ill-defined low-density lesion in the parietal lobe.   **B.** CECT demonstrates ringlike enhancement around the cyst and surrounding edema.

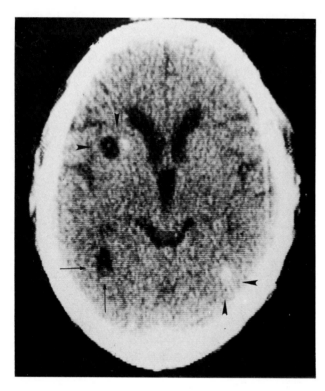

Figure 12-41 Coexistence of dead and living larvae of cysticercosis. NCCT exhibits a rounded, low-density living larva (arrows) in the right occipital lobe and calcified cysts (arrowheads) in the right basal ganglia and the left occipital lobe. Calcification is a manifestation of dead larvae, occurring usually after 10 years and seen only with parenchymal forms.

appropriate clinical information. Parenchymal cysticercosis can simulate primary or metastatic neoplasm, pyogenic abscess, and fungal infection. Cerebral infarctions must be considered in the differential diagnosis when enhancement around the cyst wall exists on CECT.

Hydatid Disease

Hydatid disease due to *Echinococcus granulosus* is usually manifested by cysts in the liver and lungs. Only 2 percent of hydatid infestations involve the CNS (Dew 1934).

Hydatid cysts of the brain are usually large and solitary, lying just a few millimeters below the cor-

tex. Extradural cysts have been reported (Ozgen 1979). Multiple cysts are rare, but daughter cysts are not infrequent after inadvertent rupture or intentional puncture of a solitary cyst (Adams 1984).

On CT, a hydatid cyst appears as a large intraparenchymal cystic lesion, spherical in shape, with sharply defined borders. The density of the cyst contents is similar to that of water or CSF (Ozgen 1979) (Fig. 12-42). Severe distortion and shift of the ventricular system and hydrocephalus due to partial obstruction of cerebrospinal fluid pathways are usual findings. The lack of contrast enhancement at the periphery and of edema surrounding the cyst (Abbassioun 1978) serves to differentiate this lesion from cerebral abscess. Primary extradural hydatid cyst can occur, and differentiation of an extracerebral hydatid cyst from arachnoid cyst may not be possible by CT alone (Ba'assiri 1984).

Paragonimiasis

Paragonimus westermani was endemic in the Far East but recently has been decreasing in incidence. The freshwater crawfish is the intermediary. Owing to its common infestation of the lung, the ova of this fluke are commonly disseminated hematogenously and deposited in the brain parenchyma, meninges, and ventricles (Kim 1955).

Three forms of reaction of CNS tissue to paragonimiasis, namely, chronic arachnoiditis, granuloma, and encapsulated abscess, have been described (Kim 1961). On CT, isodense or mixed-density masses with ringlike or nodular contrast enhancement and perilesional edema are noted in early infestation of brain parenchyma (Figs. 12-43, 12-44). Differential diagnosis from other infectious diseases or even primary or metastatic tumors on the basis of CT findings alone at this stage is extremely difficult without appropriate clinical information. Intraventricular cysts show approximately CSF-equivalent density with no contrast enhancement (Fig. 12-45). Shell-like conglomerate calcification in the later stages is characteristic (Sim 1980), although spotty calcifications have also frequently been observed (Fig. 12-45).

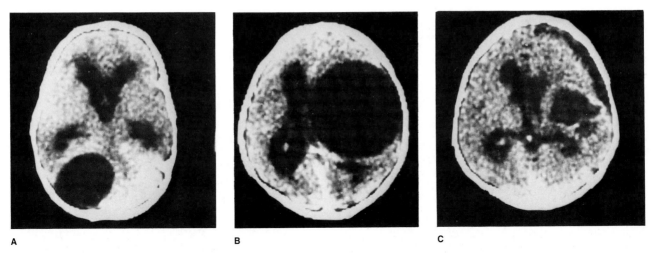

A   B   C

Figure 12-42 Hydatid cysts.   **A.** A large cyst in the occipital lobe with no contrast enhancement of the capsule or perifocal edema. **B.** A large supratentorial hydatid cyst compressing the ipsilateral ventricle.   **C.** Postsurgery view of *B* demonstrates reexpansion of the lateral ventricle. Marked decrease in size of the cyst with minimal rim enhancement. (*Reprinted with permission from Abbassioun et al., J Neurosurg 49:408–411, 1978.*)

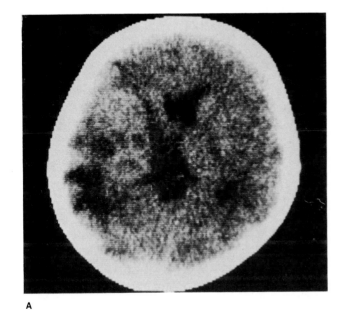

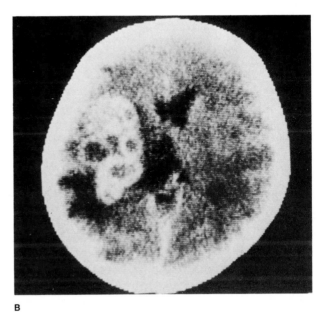

A   B

Figure 12-43 Paragonimiasis: intraparenchymal. **A.** On NCCT, irregular mixed-density lesion in the temporoparietal lobe is as-sociated with focal edema. **B.** On CECT, multiple ova are clearly demonstrated as ringlike enhancement.

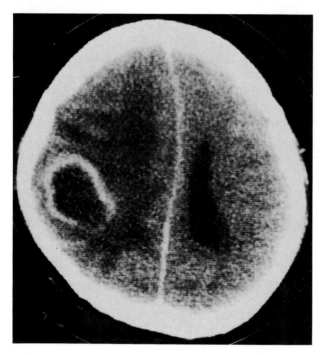

Figure 12-44   Paragonimiasis: intraparenchymal abscess. CECT shows a rounded lesion with peripheral enhancement and extensive edema, which represents encapsulated abscess.

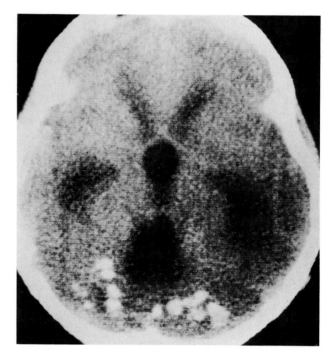

Figure 12-45   Paragonimiasis: intraventricular and intraparenchymal. Fourth and third ventricles are dilated and filled with multiple cysts. Shell-like calcifications in the cerebellum are late manifestations of dead ova.

Bibliography

ABBASSIOUN K et al: CT in hydatid cyst of the brain. *J Neurosurg* **49**:408–411, 1978.

ADAMS H: *Greenfield's Neuropathy.* Chicago, Year Book, 1984, p. 317.

ANDERSON JM, MACMILLAN JJ: Intracranial tuberculoma: An increasing problem in Britain. *J Neurol Neurosurg Psychiatry* **38**:194–201, 1975.

ARMITSU T et al: CT in verified cases of tuberculous meningitis. *Neurology* **29**:384–386, 1979.

ARRINGTON JA, MURTAGH FR, MARTINEZ CR et al: CT of multiple intracranial cryptococcoma. *Am J Neuroradiol* **5**:472–473, 1984.

AUH YH, LEE SH, TOGLIA JU: Excessively small ventricles on cranial CT: Clinical correlation in 75 patients. *CT: J Comput Tomogr* **4**:325–329, 1980.

BA'ASSIRI A, HADDAD F: Primary extradural intracranial hydatid disease: CT appearance. *Am J Neuroradiol* **5**:474–475, 1984.

BAHR AL, KRUMBHOLZ A, KRISTT D, HODGES FJ: Neuroradiological manifestations of intracranial sarcoidosis. *Radiology* **127**:713–717, 1978.

BENSON JR et al: CT in intracranial cysticercosis. *J Comput Assist Tomogr* **1**(4):464–471, 1977.

BHARDARI T, SARKAN N: Subdural empyema: A review of 37 cases. *J Neurosurg* **32**:35–39, 1970.

BIAGI F, WILLIAMS K: Immunologic problems in the diagnosis of human cysticercosis. *Ann Parasitol Hum Comp* **49**:509–513, 1974.

BRITT RH, ENZMANN DR, REMINGTON JS: Intracranial infection in cardiac transplant recipients. *Ann Neurol* **9**:107–119, 1981.

BURSZTYN EM, LEE BCP, BAUMAN J: CT of AIDS. *Am J Neuroradiol* **5**:711–714, 1984.

BUTLER IJ, JOHNSON RT: Central nervous system infection. *Pediatr Clin North Am* **21**(3):649–668, 1974.

CAHILL DW, SALCUMAN M: Neurosarcoidosis—A review of the rare manifestation. *Surg Neurol* **15**(3):204–211, 1981.

CARBAJAL JR et al: Radiology of cysticercosis of the CNS, including CT. *Radiology* **125**:127–131, 1977.

CARTER BL, BANKOFF MS, FISK JD: CT detection of sinusitis responsible for intracranial and extracranial infections. *Radiology* **147**:739–742, 1983.

CASSELMAN ES et al: CT of tuberculous meningitis in infants and children. *J Comput Assist Tomogr* **4**(2):211–216, 1980.

CLAVERIA LE, DU BOULAY GH, MOSELEY IF: Intracranial infections: Investigations by C.A.T. *Neuroradiology* **12**:59–71, 1976.

COCKRILL HH et al: CT in leptomeningeal infections. *Am J Roentgenol Radium Ther Nucl Med* **130**:511–515, 1978.

CORNELL SH, JACOBY CG: The varied CT appearance of intracranial cryptococcosis. *Am J Neuroradiol* **143**:703–707, 1982.

COULAN CN, SESHUL M, DONALDSON J: Intracranial ring lesions: Can we differentiate by CT? *Invest Radiol* **15**(2):103–112, 1980.

DAVIS JM et al: CT of herpes simplex encephalitis with clinicopathological correlation. *Radiology* **129**:409–417, 1978.

DEW HR: Hydatid disease of the brain. *Surg Gynecol Obstet* **59**:312–319, 1934.

DIXON HBF, LIPSCOMB FM: *Cysticercosis: An Analysis and Followup of 450 Cases.* Privy Council, Medical Research Council Report, no. 229, London, Her Majesty's Stationery Office, 1961, pp. 1–57.

DUBLIN AB, MERTEN DF: CT in the evaluation of herpes simplex encephalitis. *Radiology* **125**:133–134, 1977.

DUBLIN AB, PHILLIPS HE: CT of disseminated cerebral coccidioidomycosis. *Radiology* **135**:361–368, 1980.

DUNKER RO, KHAKOO RA: Failure of computed tomographic scanning to demonstrate subdural empyema. *JAMA* **246**(10):1116–1118, 1981.

EINSTEIN HE: Coccidioidomycosis of the CNS. *Adv Neurol* **6**:101–105, 1974.

ELKIN CM, LEON E, GRENELL SL, LEEDS NE: Intracranial lesions in the AIDS; radiologic (CT) features. *JAMA* **253**(3):393–396, 1985.

ENZMANN DR: CT of pituitary abscess. *Am J Neuroradiol* **4**:49–80, 1983.

ENZMANN DR, BRANT-ZAWADZKI M, BRITT RH: Computed tomography of central nervous system infections in immunosuppressed patients. *Am J Neuroradiol* **1**:239–243, 1980.

ENZMANN DR, BRITT RH, YEAGER AS: Experimental brain abscess evolution: Computed tomographic and neuropathologic correlation. *Radiology* **133**:113–122, 1979.

ENZMANN DR et al: CT of herpes simplex encephalitis. *Radiology* **129**:419–425, 1978.

ENZMANN DR, NORMAN D, MAIN J, NEWTON TH: CT of granulomatous basal arachnoiditis. *Radiology* **120**:341–344, 1976.

ENZMANN DR: *Imaging of Infections and Inflammations of the Central Nervous System: CT, US and MRI.* New York, Raven Press, 1984.

FEELY MP, DEMSEY PJ: Assessment of the post-operative course of excised brain abscess by computed tomography. *Neurosurgery* **5**(1):49–52, 1979.

FRASER RG, PARE JAP: *Diagnosis of Diseases of the Chest,* 2d ed. Philadelphia, Saunders, 1978, vol. 2, pp. 778–787.

FUJITA NK et al: Cryptococcal intracerebral mass lesions: The role of CT and non-surgical management. *Ann Intern Med* **94**:382–388, 1981.

GALBRAITH JG, BARR VW: Epidural abscess and subdural empyema. *Adv Neurol* **6**:257–267, 1974.

GREENBERG SB et al: CT in brain biopsy-proven herpes simplex encephalitis: Early normal results. *Arch Neurol* **38**:58–59, 1981.

GRIGGS RC, MANESBERRY WR, CONDEMI JJ: Cerebral mass due to sarcoidosis: Regression during corticosteroid therapy. *Neurology* **23**:981–989, 1973.

GRINELLI VS, BENTSON JR, HELMER E, WINTER J: Diagnosis of interhemispheric subdural empyema by CT. *J Comput Assist Tomogr* **1**(2):99–105, 1977.

GROSSMAN RI et al: CT of intracranial aspergillosis. *J Comput Assist Tomogr* **5**(5):646–650, 1981.

HANDEL SF, KLEIN WC, KIM YU: Intracranial epidural abscess. *Radiology* **111**:117–120, 1974.

HARRIMAN DGE: *Greenfield's Neuropathology.* Chicago, Year Book, 1984, pp. 236–259.

HARWOOD-NASH DC et al: Massive calcification of the brain in a newborn infant. *Am J Roentgenol* **108**:528–532, 1970.

HERMAN PE, CLEVELAND RH, KUSHNER DC, TAVERAS JM: CT of neonatal herpes encephalitis. *Am J Neuroradiology* **6**:773–775, 1985.

HIRSH LF, LEE SH, SILBERSTEIN SD: Intracranial tuberculomas and the CAT scan. *Acta Neurochir (Wien)* **45**:155–161, 1978.

JANKOWSKI R, ZIMMERMAN RD, LEEDS NE: Cysticercosis presenting as a mass lesion at the foramen of Monro. *J Comput Assist Tomogr* **3**(5):694–696, 1979.

JOUBERT MD, STEPHANOV S: CT and surgical treatment in intracranial suppuration. *J Neurosurg* **47**:73–78, 1977.

KAMIN M, BIDDLE D: Conservative management of focal intracerebral infection. *Neurology* **31**:103–106, 1981.

KAUFMANN DM, LEEDS NE: CT in the diagnosis of intracranial abscesses. *Neurology* **27**:1069–1073, 1977.

KENDALL BE, TATELER GLV: Radiological findings in neurosarcoidosis. *Br J Radiol* **51**:81–92, 1978.

KERR FWL, KING RB, MEAGHER JN: Brain abscess: A study of 47 consecutive cases. *JAMA* **168**:868–872, 1958.

KETONEN L, KOSKINIEMI ML: CT appearance of herpes simplex encephalitis. *Clin Radiol* **31**:161–165, 1980.

KETONEN L, OKSANEN V, KUULIALA I et al: Hypodense white matter lesions in computed tomography of neurosarcoidosis. *J Comput Assist Tomogr* **10**(2):181–183, 1986.

KIM KS, WEINBERG PE, MAGIDSON M: Angiographic features of subdural empyema. *Radiology* **118**:621–625, 1976.

KIM RC et al: Traumatic intracerebral implantation of *Cladosporium trichoides. Neurology* **31**:1145–1148, 1981.

KIM SK: Cerebral paragonimiasis. *J Neurosurg* **12**:89–94, 1955.

KIM SK, WALKER AE: Cerebral paragonimiasis. *Acta Psychiatr Neurol Scand* **36**:153, 1961.

KOBRINE A, DAVIS DO, RIZZOLI HV: Multiple abscesses of the brain: Case report. *J Neurosurg* **54**:93–97, 1981.

KOTAGAL S, TANTANASIRIVONGSE S, ARCHER C: Periventricular calcification following neonatal ventriculitis. *J Comput Assist Tomogr* **5**(5):651–653, 1981.

KUMPE DA, RAO KCVG, GARCIA JH, HECK AF: Intracranial neurosarcoidosis. *J Comput Assist Tomogr* **3**(3):324–330, 1979.

LABEAU J et al: Surgical treatment of brain abscess and subdural empyema. *J Neurosurg* **38**:198, 1973.

LEE SH, KUMAR ARV, LORBER B: Tuberculosis of the CNS presenting as mass lesions: Diagnostic dilemma. *Pa Med* **82**:36–38, 1979.

LEO JS et al: CT in herpes simplex encephalitis. *Surg Neurol* **10**:313–317, 1978.

LEVY RM, PONS VG, ROSENBLUM ML: Central nervous system mass lesions in AIDS. *J Neurosurg* **61**:9–16, 1984.

LEVY RM, ROSENBLOOM S, PERRETT LV: Neuroradiological findings in AIDS: A review of 200 cases. *Am J Neuroradiol* **7**:833–839, 1986.

LINDHOLM J, RAMUSSEN P, KORSGAARD O: Intracellar or pituitary abscess. *J Neurosurg* **38**:616–626, 1973.

LIPTON SA, HICKEY WF, MORRIS JH, LOSCALZO J: Candidal infection in the CNS. *Am J Med* **76**:101–108, 1984.

LONG JA et al: Cerebral mass lesion in torculosis demonstrated by CT. *J Comput Assist Tomogr* **4**(6):766–769, 1980.

LORBER J: Intracranial calcification following tuberculous meningitis in children. *Acta Radiol* **50**:204–210, 1958.

LOTT T et al: Evaluation of brain and epidural abscess by CT. *Radiology* **122**:371, 1977.

LUKEN MG, WHELAN MA: Recent diagnostic experience with subdural empyema. *J Neurosurg* **52**:764–771, 1980.

MALLOY PM, LEYMAN RM: The lack of specificity of neonatal paraventricular calcification. *Radiology* **80**:98–102, 1963.

MAUERSBERGER W: The determination of absorption values as an aid in CT differentiation between cerebral abscess and glioblastoma. *Adv Neurosurg* **9**:36–40, 1981.

MAYERS MM, KAUFMANN DF, MILLER MM: Recent cases of intracranial tuberculomas. *Neurology* **28**:256–260, 1978.

MCGAHAN JP: Classic and temporary imaging of coccidioidomycosis. *Am J Roentgenol* **136**:393–404, 1981.

MIRFAKHRAEE M, CROFFORD M, GUINTO FC et al: Virchow-Robin space: A path of spread in neurosarcoidosis. *Radiology* **158**:715–720, 1986.

MOORE GA, THOMAS LM: Infections including abscesses of the brain, spinal cord, intraspinal and intracranial lesions. *Surg Ann* **6**:413–417, 1974.

MOREHOUSE H, DANZIGER A: CT findings in intracranial neurosarcoid. *Comput Tomogr* **4**:267–270, 1981.

MORGAN H, WOOD MW: Cerebellar abscesses: A review of 7 cases. *Surg Neurol* **3**:93–96, 1975.

MOSLEY IF, KENDALL BE: Radiology of intracranial empyemas, with special reference to computed tomography. *Neuroradiology* **26**:333–345, 1984.

NAHSER HC et al: Development of brain abscesses—CT compared with morphological studies. *Adv Neurosurg* **9**:32–35, 1981.

NAVIA BA, JORDAN BA, PRICE RW: The AIDS dementia complex: I. clinical features. *Ann Neurol* **19**:517–524, 1986.

NAVIA BA, CHO E-S, PETITO CK et al: The AIDS dementia complex: II. neuropathology. *Ann Neurol* **19**:525–535, 1986.

NELSON JD, WATTS CC: Calcified subdural effusion following bacterial meningitis. *Am J Dis Child* **117**:730–733, 1969.

NEW PFJ, DAVIS KR: The role of CT scanning diagnosis of infections of the central nervous system, in Remington J, Swartz M (eds): *Current Clinical Topics in Infectious Diseases*. New York, McGraw-Hill, 1980, pp. 1–33.

NEW PFJ, DAVIS KR, BALLANTINE HT: Computed tomography in cerebral abscess. *Radiology* **121**:641–646, 1976.

NIELSEN H, GLYDENSTADT C: CT in the diagnosis of cerebral abscess. *Neuroradiology* **12**:207–217, 1977.

ÖZGEN T et al: The use of CT in the diagnosis of cerebral hydatid cysts. *J Neurosurg* **50**:339–342, 1979.

PAXTON R, AMBROSE J: The EMI scanner: A brief review of the first 600 patients. *Br J Radiol* **47**:530–565, 1974.

PEATFIELD RC, SHAWDON HH: Five cases of intracranial tuberculoma followed by serial CT. *J Neurol Neurosurg Psychiatry* **42**:373–379, 1979.

PFUETZE KH, RADNER DB (eds): *Clinical Tuberculosis: Essentials of Diagnosis and Treatment*. Springfield, Charles C Thomas, 1966.

POST MJD, HENSLEY GT, MOSKOWITZ LB, FISCHL M: Cytomegalic inclusion virus encephalitis in patients with AIDS: CT, clinical, and pathological correlation. *AJNR* **7**:275–280, 1986*a*.

POST MJD, SHELDON JJ, HENSLEY GT et al: CNS disease in AIDS: Prospective correlation using CT, MRI, and pathologic studies. *Radiology* **158**:141–148, 1986*b*.

POST MJD, KURSUNOGLU SJ, HENSLEY GT et al: Cranial CT in acquired immunodeficiency syndrome: spectrum of diseases and optimal contrast enhancement technique. *AJNR* **6**:743–754, 1985.

POST MJD, CHAN JC, HENSLEY G et al: Toxoplasma encephalitis in Haitian Adults with AIDS. A clinical-pathologic-CT correlation. *Am J Neuroradiology (AJNR)* **4**:155–162, 1983.

PRICE HI, DANZIEGER A: CT in cranial tuberculosis. *Am J Roentgenol* **130**:769–771, 1978.

RAO KCVG, WILLIAMS JP, BRENNAN TG, KOSNIK E: Interhemispheric subdural empyema. *Child Brain* **4**:106–113, 1978.

RINAUDIN JW: Cranial epidural abscess and subdural empyema in neurosurgery, in Wilkins and Rengachary (eds.) *Neurosurgery*, New York: McGraw-Hill, 1985, pp. 1961–1963.

ROBERT F: Sarcoidosis of the central nervous system. *Brain* **71**:451–475, 1948.

ROBERTHERAM EB, KESSLER LA: Use of computerized tomography in nonsurgical management of brain abscess. *Arch Neurol* **36**:25–26, 1979.

RODRIGUEZ-CABAJAL J, SALZADO P et al: The acute encephalitic phase of neurocysticercosis: CT manifestations. *Am J Neuroradiol* **4**:51–55, 1983.

ROSENBAUM ML et al: Decreased mortality from brain abscesses since advent of CT. *J Neurosurg* **49**:659–668, 1978.

ROVIRA M, ROMERO F, TORRENT O, IBARRA B: Study of tuberculosis by CT. *Neuroradiology* **19**:137–141, 1980.

RUDWAN MA: Pituitary abscess. *Neuroradiology* **12**:243–248, 1977.

SADHU VK, HANDEL SF, PINTO RS, GLASS TF: Neuroradiologic diagnosis of subdural empyema and CT limitation. *Am J Neuroradiol* **1**:39–44, 1980.

SAGE R, DUBOIS J, OAKS S et al: Rapid development of cerebral atrophy due to perinatal herpes simplex encephalitis. *J Comput Assist Tomogr* **5**:763–766, 1981.

SALMON JH: Ventriculitis complicating meningitis. *Am J Dis Child* **124**:35–40, 1972.

SALTZMAN GF: Roentgenologic changes in cerebral sarcoidosis. *Acta Radiol [Diagn] (Stockh)* **50**:235–241, 1958.

SAMSON DS, CLARK K: A current review of brain abscess. *Am J Med* **54**:201–210, 1973.

SANTIN G, VARGAS J: Roentgen study of cysticercosis of CNS. *Radiology* **86**:520–528, 1966.

SCHULTZ P, LEEDS NE: Intraventricular septations complicating neonatal meningitis. *J Neurosurg* **38**:620–626, 1973.

SILVERSTEIN A, FEUER MM, SILTZBACH LE: Neurologic sarcoidosis: Study of 18 cases. *Arch Neurol* **12**:1–11, 1965.

SIM BS: CT findings of parasitic infestations of the brain in Korea. *J Korean Neurosurg Soc* **9**(1):7–18, 1980.

SOUTH MA et al: Congenital malformation of the CNS associated with genital type (type 2) herpes virus. *J Pediatr* **75**:13–18, 1969.

STEPHANOV S et al: Combined convexity and parafalx subdural empyema. *Surg Neurol* **11**:147–151, 1979.

STEVENS EA et al: CT brain scanning in intraparenchymal pyogenic abscesses. *Am J Roentgenol* **130**:111–114, 1978.

SUSS RA, MARAVILLA KR, THOMPSON J: MR imaging of intracranial cysticercosis: comparison with CT and anatomicopathologic features. *Am J Neuroradiol* **7**:235–242, 1986.

VISUDHIPHAN P et al: Cerebral aspergillosis: Report of 3 cases. *J Neurosurg* **38**:472–476, 1973.

WAGGENER JD: The pathophysiology of bacterial meningitis and cerebral abscesses: An anatomical interpretation. *Adv Neurol* vol. 6, 1974.

WALLENFANG TH, REULEN JG, SCHURMANN K: Therapy of brain abscess. *Adv Neurosurg* **9**:41–47, 1981.

WEIDERHOLT WC, SIEKERT RG: Neurological manifestations of sarcoidosis. *Neurology* **15**:1147–1154, 1965.

WEINMAN D, SAMARASHINGHE HHR: Subdural empyema. *Aust N Z J Surg* **41**:324, 1972.

WELCHMAN JM: CT of intracranial tuberculomata. *Clin Radiol* **30**:567–573, 1979.

WHELAN MA, HILAL SK: Computed tomography as a guide in the diagnosis and followup of brain abscesses. *Radiology* **135**:663–671, 1980.

WHELAN MA, STERN J: Intracranial tuberculoma. *Radiology* **138**:75–81, 1981.

WHELAN MA, KRICHEFF II, HANDLER M et al. Acquired immunodeficiency syndrome: cerebral CT manifestations. *Radiology* **149**:477–484, 1983.

WHITLEY J et al: Adenine arabinoside therapy of biopsy-proven herpes simplex encephalitis. *N Engl J Med* **287**:289–294, 1977.

WHITLEY RJ, NAHMIAS AJ, VISTINE AM, FLEMING CL, CLIFFORD CA: The natural history of herpes simplex virus infection of mother and newborn. *Pediatrics* **66**:489–494, 1980.

WITHAM RR, JOHNSON RH, ROBERTS DL: Diagnosis of miliary tuberculosis by cerebral CT. *Arch Intern Med* **139**:479–480, 1979.

YOUNG RF, FRAZEE J: Gas within intracranial abscess cavities: an indication for surgical excision. *Ann Neurol* **16**:35–39, 1984.

ZEE CS et al: Unusual neuroradiological features of intracranial cysticercosis. *Radiology* **137**:397–497, 1980.

ZEE CS, SEGALL HD, APUZZO MLJ et al: Intraventricular cysticercal cysts: Further neuroradiologic observations and neurosurgical implications. *Am J Neuroradiol* **5**:727–730, 1984.

ZEGERS DE, BEYL D, NOTERMAN J, MARTELART A, FLAMENT-DURAND J, BALERIAUX D: Multiple cerebral hematoma and viral encephalitis. *Neuroradiology* **20**:47–48, 1980.

ZIMMERMAN RA, PATEL S, BILANIUK LT: Demonstration of purulent bacterial intracranial infections by computed tomography. *Am J Roentgenol* **127**:155–165, 1976.

ZIMMERMAN RA, BILANIUK LT, GALLO E: CT of the trapped fourth ventricle. *Am J Roentgenol* **130**:503–506, 1978.

ZIMMERMAN RD et al: CT in the early diagnosis of herpes simplex encephalitis. *Am J Roentgenol* **134**:61–66, 1980.

ZIMMERMAN RD, LEEDS NE, DANZIGER A: Subdural empyema: CT findings. *Radiology* **150**:417–422, 1984.

ZORUB DS et al: Invasive pituitary adenoma with abscess formation: Case report. *Neurosurgery* **5**(6):718–722, 1979.

13

CEREBRAL VASCULAR ANOMALIES

Karel TerBrugge

Krishna C.V.G. Rao

Seungho Howard Lee

Cerebral vascular anomalies, which comprise aneurysms and vascular malformations, commonly present with a history of subarachnoid hemorrhage. Frequently with aneurysm there are a variety of clinical findings, such as transient ischemic attacks or signs of cranial nerve involvement. On the other hand, with vascular malformations seizures may be the presenting clinical symptom. CT is the first modality of examination providing an approach to selecting the patients as well as the time when the definitive study, cerebral angiography, should be performed.

INTRACRANIAL ANEURYSMS AND SUBARACHNOID HEMORRHAGE

An aneurysm is an abnormal focal enlargement of an artery. Aneurysms can be classified according to their appearance as saccular or fusiform. The etiological classification of aneurysms includes congenital, arteriosclerotic, mycotic, and dissecting. By far the most common type is the congenital, or so-called berry, aneurysm, which is thought to be due to a defect in the tunica media (Crawford 1959; Crompton 1966). With advancing age, arteriosclerotic changes are thought to cause further weakening of the already defective tunica media, and this may result in enlargement or rupture of the aneurysm (Crompton 1966; Richardson 1941; Nystrom 1963; DuBoulay 1965; Sarwar 1976a).

The incidence of intracranial aneurysms in the general population is approximately 3 percent (Chason 1958; Housepian 1958). The aneurysm involves the carotid system in 95 percent and the vertebral basilar system in 5 percent of the cases (Locksley 1966). The anterior communicating artery is the single most common site (30 percent), followed by the posterior communicating artery (25 percent) and the middle cerebral artery (20 percent), according to Locksley (1966). Approximately 20 percent of patients with an intracranial aneurysm have more than one aneurysm demonstrated at angiography (McKissock 1964; Locksley 1966; Kendall 1976b). The great majority of the aneurysms are small in size (diameter less than 1 cm) and present with subarachnoid hemorrhage (DuBoulay 1965; Locksley 1966). The large-size (diameter between 1 and 2.5 cm) and giant-size (diameter greater than 2.5 cm) aneurysms usually do not present with subarachnoid hemorrhage but with clinical symptoms related to their localized mass effect and pressure upon the adjacent brain and cranial nerves (Bull 1969; Morley 1969; Sarwar 1976a,b; Scotti 1977; Nadjmi 1978; Deeb 1979; Pinto 1979; Thron 1979).

The *CT appearance* of intracranial aneurysms depends on whether the entire lumen of the aneurysm is patent or whether there is a partial or complete thrombosis of the aneurysm. If the entire lumen of the aneurysm is patent, the lesion can be seen on CT as a rounded or elongated area of slightly increased density (Fig. 13-1) (Scotti 1977; Handa 1978; Pinto 1979). After intravenous injection of contrast material the lumen of the aneurysm will show homogeneous enhancement and the margin of the lesion will be well defined (Scotti 1977; Handa 1978; Pinto 1979; Yock 1980). This appearance is easily explained on the basis of a hyperdense blood pool which is subsequently opacified by circulating iodine contrast material (Pressman 1975b; Pinto 1979; Yock 1980).

Partially thrombotic aneurysms have a different ap-

pearance, which is related to the presence of the thrombus and the degree of patency of the lumen within the aneurysm. On NCCT they show as a central or eccentric hyperdense region within an isodense or calcific area. The lesions are rounded or lobulated in appearance, and the margins are well defined. The central and peripheral zones are enhanced by contrast material, while the isodense zone is not (Fig. 13-2) (Lukin 1975; Sarwar 1976a; Scotti 1977; Perrett 1977; Handa 1978; Nadjmi 1978; Babu 1979; Pinto 1979; Thron 1979; Schubiger 1980). The CT appearance of a partially thrombotic aneurysm is due to a central or eccentric patent lumen of the aneurysm which enhances following contrast infusion. This lumen is surrounded by thrombotic material which is isodense on CT. The peripheral wall of the aneurysm consists of fibrous tissue, which is hyperdense on CT and often calcified. This rim of tissue contains increased vascularity, which is thought to be a meningeal response to the enlarging aneurysm, and enhancement of this tissue may be a phenomenon similar to the dural enhancement in other locations (Pinto 1979).

The *completely thrombosed aneurysm* exhibits a central area of isodensity or slightly decreased density and a peripheral rim of increased density and often calcific density (Fig. 13-3). The peripheral rim of increased density may show enhancement after contrast infusion (Nadjmi 1978; Pinto 1979). The central area of isodensity represents thrombus within the aneurysm, while the peripheral ring enhancement is thought to be due to increased microvascularity within the tissue along the wall of the aneurysm similar to dural enhancement (Pinto 1979). Recent blood clot formation in the acute stage of a thrombosing aneurysm will show as an area of increased density on the NCCT (Fig. 13-3). Meningioma or malignant glioma may mimic giant aneurysms (larger than 1 cm), but the lack of edema in aneurysms should rule out the tumors (Pinto 1979).

Ectasia of the intracranial arteries, and in particular the basilar artery, can be diagnosed on CT (Peterson 1977; Scotti 1978; Deeb 1979; Smoker 1986). The ectatic basilar artery may be seen crossing the prepontine cistern toward a cerebellopontine angle cistern as an elongated band-like structure of increased density on the NCCT. Homogeneous en-

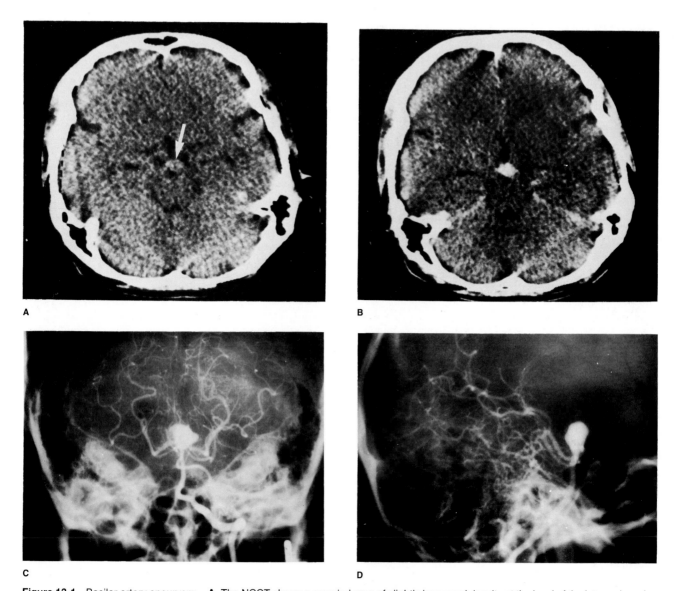

Figure 13-1 Basilar artery aneurysm. **A**. The NCCT shows a rounded area of slightly increased density at the level of the interpeduncular cistern (arrow). **B**. Enhancement occurs on CECT. **C, D**. Angiograms disclose a large aneurysm arising from the tip of the basilar artery.

hancement occurs after contrast infusion (Fig. 13-4). Tortuous vertebral-basilar arteries may be associated with cranial nerve syndromes and may result in hydrocephalus resulting from transmitted pulsation of the ectatic fusiform dilated vertebral basilar artery. CT has proved excellent for screening such cases, possibly obviating angiography (Deeb 1979), and if angiography is necessary, digital subtraction technique is preferred to conventional methods in order to minimize possible complications (Smoker 1986) (Fig. 13-4).

The *differential diagnosis* of lesions which may mimic a small aneurysm consists mainly of variations from the normal vascular anatomy, such as looping of vessels or prominent veins. Depending on the clinical situation, angiography is often nec-

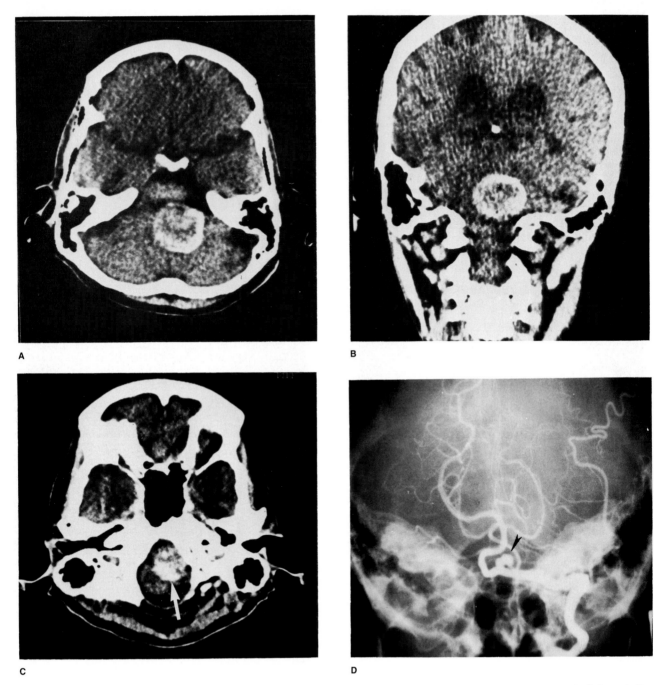

A

B

C

D

Figure 13-2 Posterior inferior cerebellar artery (PICA) aneurysm. **A**. The NCCT shows a rounded lesion adjacent to the left cerebello-pontine angle cistern with a peripheral rim of calcification. **B**. The coronal CT shows the lesion to the left of the midline, superior to the foramen magnum. A central hypodense area is present with a rim of calcification. **C**. The CECT at the level of the foramen magnum shows the lesion to be extraaxial in location, and there is eccentric enhancement in part of the lesion (arrow). **D**. Angiogram shows the PICA aneurysm on the left side, consisting of a large thrombosed part and a small patent lumen.

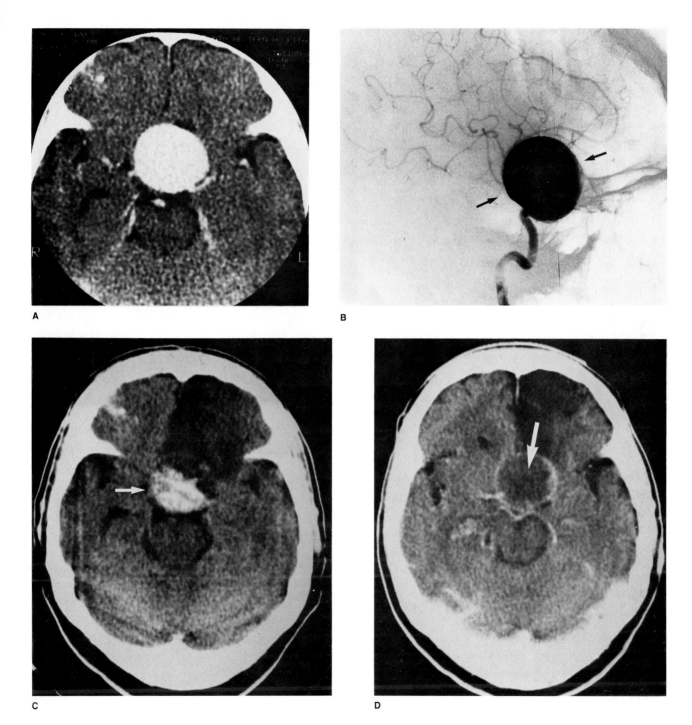

Figure 13-3 Giant patent internal carotid artery aneurysm with acute thrombosis following balloon detachment. **A**. The transaxial CECT shows a large rounded suprasellar lesion with homogeneous enhancement. **B**. The carotid angiogram shows giant-size aneurysm of the cavernous segment of the internal carotid artery (arrrows). **C**. The NCCT 2 days following balloon detachment in the internal carotid artery shows acute clot formation within the aneurysm as an area of increased density (arrow). **D**. The CECT 2 months following sacrifice of the ICA shows complete thrombosis of the aneurysm (arrow) and enhancement along the wall of the aneurysm.

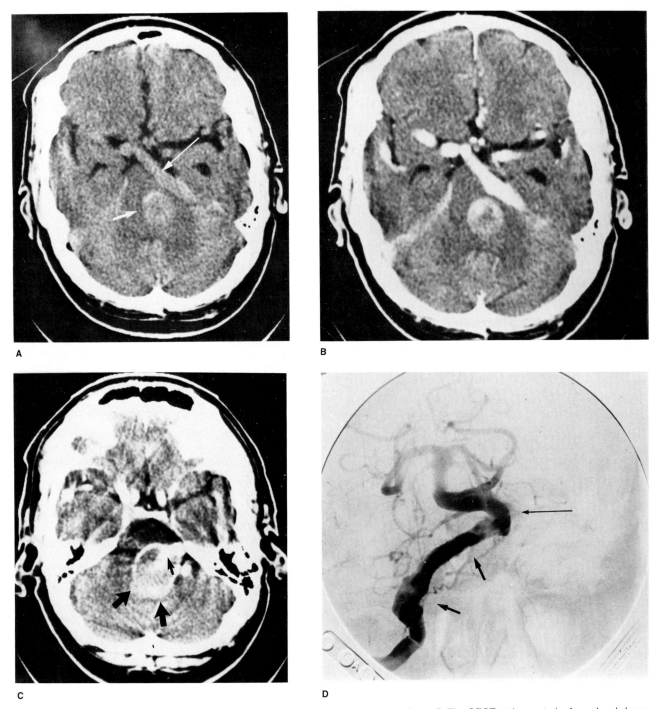

Figure 13-4 Fusiform aneurysmal dilatation of the basilar artery:
A. The NCCT shows an elongated band of increased density at
the level of the ambient and suprasellar cisterns (large arrow) as
well as a rounded density representing the dome of the aneurysm
(small arrow).   **B**. The CECT shows enhancement of the basilar
artery as well as the distal internal carotid and proximal middle
cerebral arteries.   **C**. The CECT at the posterior fossa level shows
a partially thrombosed aneurysm (arrows) with an eccentric patent
lumen (small arrow).   **D**. Angiogram shows elongated and ectatic
basilar artery (large arrow) and irregular outline of the opacified
lumen (small arrows) at the site of the aneurysm shown on CT.

essary to sort out these diagnostic problems. The CT appearance of large and giant aneurysms may be mimicked by a number of disease processes and depends to a certain degree on the location of the lesion. In the posterior fossa, large aneurysms may simulate intra- and extraaxial lesions (Handa 1978; Thron 1979). The extraaxial lesions which most often mimic an aneurysm are acoustic neuromas and meningiomas. Epidermoid tumors and chordomas may occasionally exhibit a CT pattern similar to large aneurysms. Intraaxial tumors which sometimes have a CT appearance mimicking large aneurysms are gliomas, medulloblastomas, ependymomas, choroid plexus papillomas, and metastatic disease (Byrd 1978). Para- and suprasellar lesions which may have a CT appearance similar to large aneurysms include pituitary adenomas, meningiomas, craniopharyngiomas, third ventricular tumors, and metastatic disease (Fig. 13-5) (Perrett 1977; Handa 1978; Babu 1979). Important features of large aneurysms on CT are the absence of surrounding edema and the presence of curvilinear peripheral calcifications. These characteristics are extremely uncommon in neoplastic disease, with the exception of craniopharyngiomas. In such cases, rapid sequence (dynamic) CT scanning following intravenous bolus injection may be of help in distinguishing an aneurysm from a tumor (Fig. 13-6).

The advent of CT has led to postponement of invasive neuroradiological methods such as angiography. Past experience has indicated that many large and giant-size aneurysms were diagnosed on CT as neoplastic disease, and the possibility of a vascular abnormality was often not considered (Lukin 1975; Perrett 1977; Handa 1978; Nadjmi 1978; Babu 1979; Pinto 1979; Thron 1979). Therefore, awareness of the CT appearance of the large aneurysms is important, and angiography is indicated if the possibility of such an aneurysm cannot be excluded on CT. *Angiography* will generally establish the diagnosis but demonstrates only the part of the aneurysm with circulating blood. The mass effect related to the thrombus in the partially thrombotic aneurysm is often much better appreciated with CT. Angiography may be frankly misleading in the totally thrombosed aneurysm, which may show only as a nonvascular mass lesion (Fig. 13-7) (Nadjmi 1978; Pinto 1979; Thron 1979). Aneurysms may increase in size, and further growth of the aneurysm can be correctly diagnosed by means of CT, while a change in the patent lumen part of the aneurysm is better demonstrated by means of angiography (Fig. 13-7). CT can also be used to assess the postoperative status of an aneurysm, and it is the method of choice to investigate the status of the remaining lumen of giant unclippable aneurysms which have been treated by balloon detachment or proximal ligation of the parent vessel (Fig. 13-3) (Handa 1978).

The *CT detection* of intracranial aneurysms is greatly dependent on the size and location of the aneurysm. Since most aneurysms are small and located along the base of the skull, their detection has so far been limited by the spatial resolution of the CT system. A good-quality scan with thin slices and overlapping cuts along the base of the skull will detect an aneurysm larger than 5 mm in diameter, but at present angiography remains the method of choice to detect the small aneurysm with a diameter less than 5 mm.

The advent of CT has significantly changed the method of investigation and management of patients with *subarachnoid hemorrhage* (Kendall 1976b; Liliequist 1977; Scotti 1977; Weir 1977; Modesti 1978). The mortality of patients with subarachnoid hemorrhage is high in the first few days after the ictus and is related to the mass effect of an intracranial hematoma (Weir 1977; Weisberg 1978). CT has proved to be the method of choice in the demonstration of subdural, subarachnoid, and intracerebral or intraventricular hemorrhage (Hayward 1977) (Fig. 13-8). Approximately 75 percent of patients with subarachnoid hemorrhage have a ruptured aneurysm and 5 percent an arteriovenous malformation; in 15 percent no cause for bleeding is identified, based on angiography (Bjorkesten 1965).

In the first few days after the ictus, CT identifies blood in the subarachnoid space in approximately 80 percent of cases. The accuracy of detection of recently extravasated blood in the subarachnoid space declines with time, and generally no blood can be demonstrated 1 week after the ictus (Scotti 1977; Weir 1977; Modesti 1978). A false negative CT scan is not

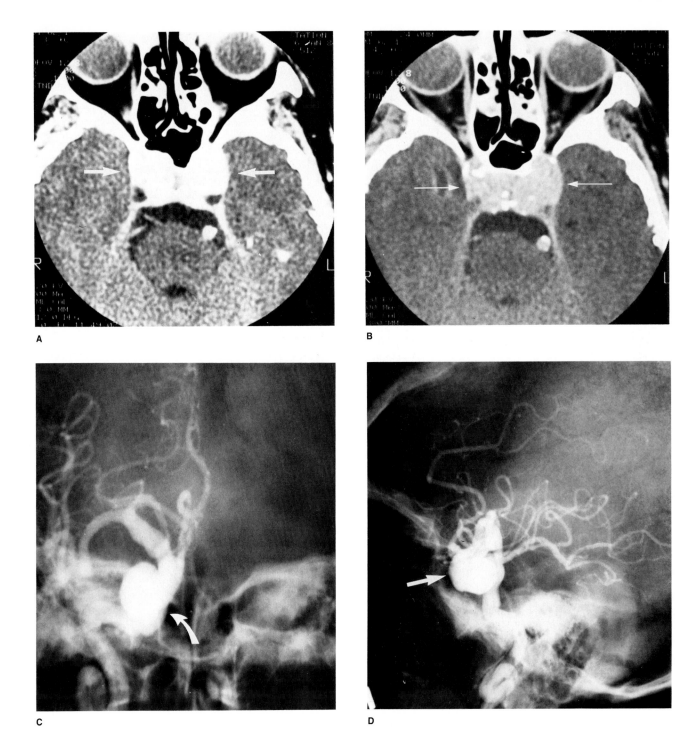

Figure 13-5 Bilateral internal carotid artery aneurysms. **A**. The CECT at the level of the floor of the sella shows homogeneous enhancement of two rounded lesions (arrows) just anterior to the location of the trigeminal ganglia. **B**. The CECT at the level of the pituitary fossa shows obliteration of the parasellar cisterns by enhancing mass lesions (arrows) which may simulate pituitary adenoma or meningioma. **C** and **D**. Angiograms reveal evidence of bilateral aneurysms at the level of the cavernous segment of the internal carotid artery (arrow).

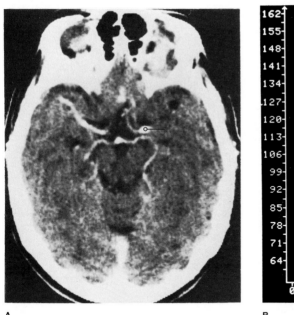

A

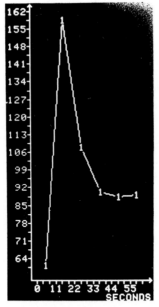

B

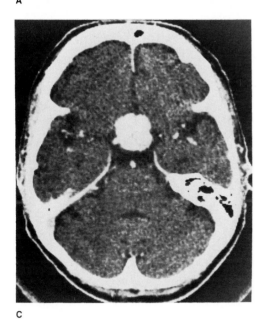

C

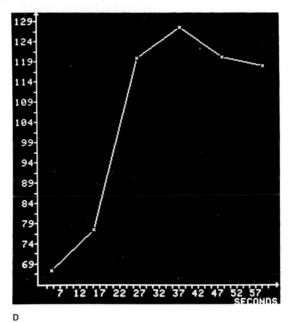

D

Figure 13-6 Dynamic CT scanning. **A**. CECT reveals a round area of hyperdensity (small circle) in the left side of the circle of Willis. **B**. Rapid-sequence CT scanning of the same region with a cursor was performed following intravenous bolus injection of contrast material. A time-density curve shows a rapid initial rise and fall, indicating the vascular structure. Angiography confirmed the presence of an aneurysm arising from the distal end of the internal carotid artery. This curve may be compared with the slow rise-and-decline curve, characteristic of a tumor, seen in a case of tuberculum sellae meningioma (**C, D**).

uncommon in patients with good neurological grades and therefore probably indicates a relatively small amount of blood in the subarachnoid space. This phenomenon is, however, not necessarily associated with a better clinical outcome (Weir 1977).

Various patterns can be recognized on CT in patients with subarachnoid hemorrhage, depending on the location of the ruptured aneurysm (Scotti 1977; Modesti 1978; Yock 1980). The anterior communicating artery aneurysm tends to bleed into the in-

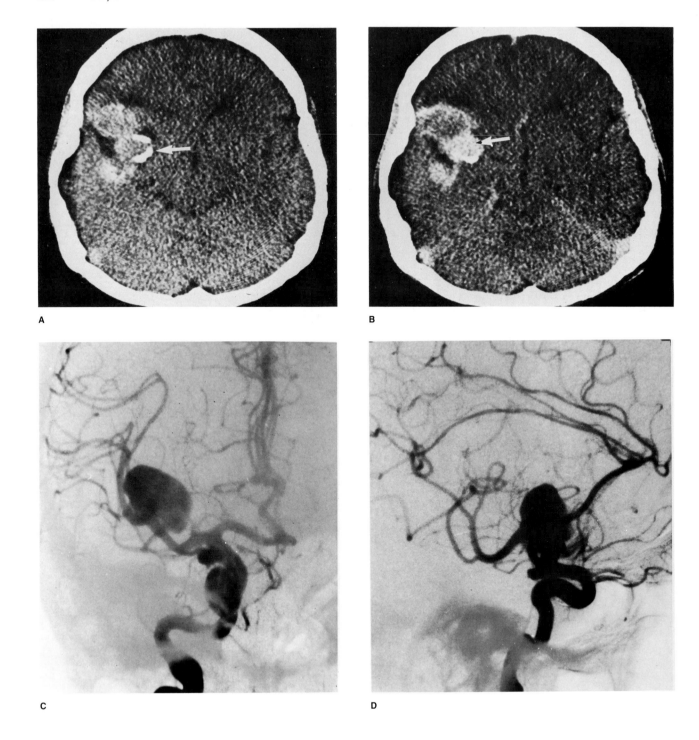

A

B

C

D

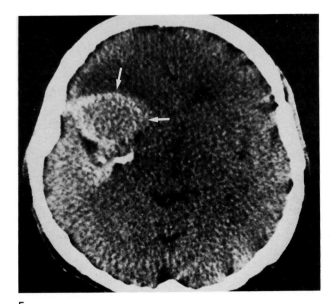

E

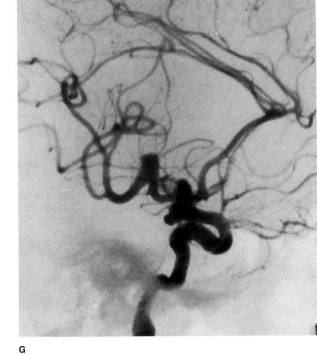

G

F

Figure 13-7   Giant middle cerebral artery aneurysms.   **A**. The nonenhanced scan shows a lobulated lesion within the right sylvian fissure with rimlike calcification (arrow).   **B**. After contrast infusion, eccentric enhancement is present (arrow). **C, D**. Angiogram in frontal and lateral projection shows a giant middle cerebral artery aneurysm. **E**. One-year follow-up without specific treatment shows increase in size of the thrombosed aneurysm (arrows). **F, G**. Angiogram shows that the patent lumen of the aneurysm has diminished dramatically since the initial examination.

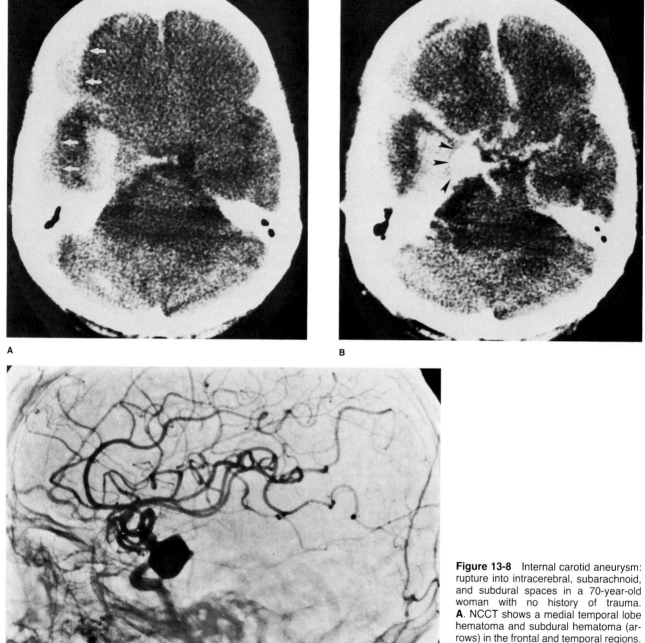

A

B

C

Figure 13-8 Internal carotid aneurysm: rupture into intracerebral, subarachnoid, and subdural spaces in a 70-year-old woman with no history of trauma. **A**. NCCT shows a medial temporal lobe hematoma and subdural hematoma (arrows) in the frontal and temporal regions. **B**. CECT shows a large aneurysm (arrowheads) originating from the internal carotid artery. **C**. Lateral cerebral angiogram confirms the location and origin of the bleeding aneurysm.

terhemispheric fissure and suprasellar cistern. The cingulate and callosal gyri are often outlined by blood. Frequently blood is also present around the brainstem and in the sylvian fissure (Fig. 13-9). Asymmetrical presence of blood in the sylvian fissure has been shown to occur with ruptured anterior communicating artery aneurysms and does not exclude that possibility (Yock 1980). The internal carotid and posterior communicating artery aneurysm tend to bleed into the suprasellar cistern and adjacent sylvian fissure. Blood is less frequently present within the interhemispheric fissure. Middle cerebral artery aneurysms invariably bleed into the sylvian fissure

and adjacent suprasellar cistern. Aneurysms arising from the tip of the basilar artery bleed into the interpeduncular cistern around the brainstem and the suprasellar cistern, while bleeding into the sylvian and interhemispheric fissure is uncommon. Ruptured aneurysms arising from the posterior inferior cerebellar artery are often associated with false negative findings on the CT unless the bleeding is massive. In most cases, blood can be seen outlining the brainstem.

Care should be taken to distinguish the *normal falx* from recently extravasated blood into the interhemispheric fissure (Lim 1977). The posterior or

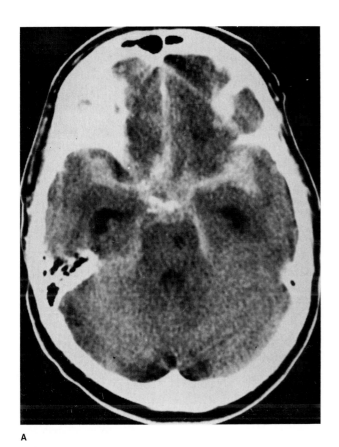

A

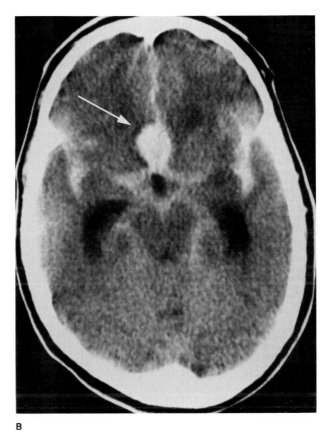

B

Figure 13-9 Subarachnoid hemorrhage following rupture of the anterior communicating artery aneurysm. **A**. The hyperdense recently extravasated blood outlines the prepontine and suprasellar cisterns, the first segment of the sylvian fissures, and the interhemispheric fissure. **B**. The NCCT shows hemorrhage in the interpeduncular cistern, the ambient and suprasellar cisterns, as well as the sylvian fissures. A localized hematoma is present at the level of the interhemispheric fissure (arrow). Note ventricular enlargement.

retrocallosal aspect of the falx can be visualized in 88 percent of normal patients, while the anterior aspect is visualized on CT in 38 percent of patients without subarachnoid hemorrhage (Zimmerman 1982). When the increased density in the interhemispheric fissure does not extend into the paramedian sulci or does not show any change from previous CT, the diagnosis of normal falx is established (Osborn 1980).

The ability to localize the ruptured aneurysm by means of CT is greatly improved if localized *hematoma* is present. Aneurysms arising from the anterior cerebral arterial complex tend to bleed into the adjacent frontal lobes and the septum pellucidum. A septal hematoma is present in 30 percent of ruptured anterior communicating artery aneurysms and invariably indicates the particular location of the aneurysm (Fig. 13-10) (Hayward 1976; Scotti 1977; Yock 1980), although the authors have seen such a hematoma from a ruptured pericallosal artery aneurysm and a posterior communicating artery aneurysm. Temporal lobe and basal ganglia hematomas occur with middle cerebral, posterior communicating, and internal carotid artery aneurysms (Fig. 13-8). The comma-shaped sylvian fissure hematomas are characteristic of ruptured middle cerebral artery aneurysm and are easily distinguishable from the external-capsule hematomas which occur in primary intracerebral hemorrhage in patients with hypertension (Fig. 13-11). Hayward (1976) reported 90 percent accuracy in the ability of CT to distinguish primary intracerebral hemorrhage from intracerebral hematoma caused by a ruptured intracranial aneurysm.

CT is of limited value in identifying, in cases of *multiple intracranial aneurysms,* which one has bled if a nonspecific CT pattern is encountered. However, when localized hematoma is present in addition to the subarachnoid hemorrhage, the accuracy of CT may approach 100 percent (Aalmaani 1978).

Depending on the location of the aneurysm, contrast enhancement will allow for direct visualization of the aneurysm in 30 to 76 percent of the cases of subarachnoid hemorrhage and is therefore recommended (Ghoshhajra 1979; Yock 1980). When subarachnoid hemorrhage is associated with intra-

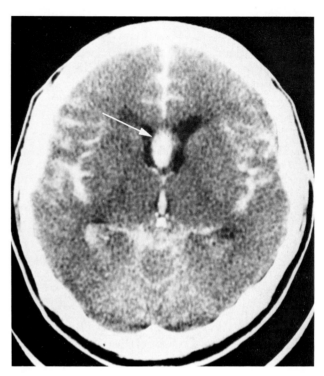

Figure 13-10   Septal hematoma caused by anterior communicating artery aneurysm rupture. On NCCT, recent subarachnoid hemorrhage is noted at the level of both sylvian fissures, the interhemispheric fissure as well as a localized hematoma at the level of the septum pellucidum (arrow).

cerebral or *subdural hematomas,* without a history of trauma, subdural hematoma of arterial origin (aneurysm or arteriovenous malformation) should be considered (Rengachary 1981). In such cases, CECT is indicated to elicit the source of bleeding (Fig. 13-8).

The advent of CT has greatly changed the role of angiography in the investigation and follow-up of patients with subarachnoid hemorrhage. The need for emergency angiography is diminished, and angiography can be delayed until the patient's condition stabilizes and surgery is contemplated. Angiography should be directed primarily toward detailed demonstration of the vessels adjacent to the abnormality shown on CT.

The frequency of neurological deterioration of patients with subarachnoid hemorrhage is well known. CT has a definite role in the follow-up of

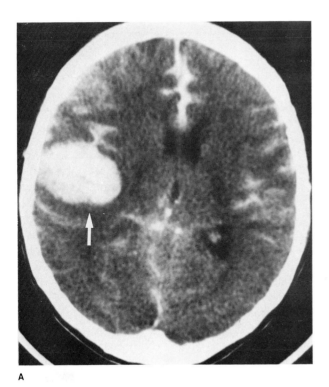

A

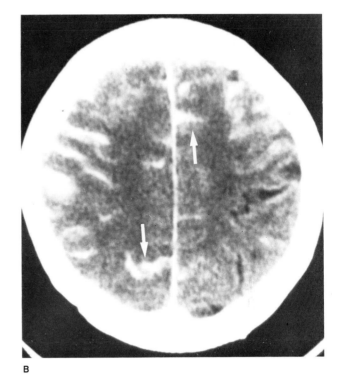

B

Figure 13-11 Sylvian fissure hematoma caused by middle cerebral artery aneurysm rupture. **A**. NCCT shows recent subarachnoid hemorrhage at the level of the interhemispheric fissure and a localized hematoma expanding the right sylvian fissure (arrow). **B**. Extravasated blood is also noted within cortical sulci over the convexity of the brain and adjacent to the falx (arrows).

these patients. Rebleeding of the aneurysm and ventricular enlargement are readily shown on CT. The development of *ventricular enlargement* appears to be a much more common phenomenon than previously realized and occurs in the first few days after the ictus in up to 60 percent of cases of subarachnoid hemorrhage (Modesti 1978). However, in contrast to the preliminary study by Davis et al. (1980), the CT findings in patients with *vasospasm* are not as impressive in the author's experience. Although CT may show cerebral edema and infarction, it often fails to show any change in patients with angiographic evidence of severe vasospasm (Liliequist 1977; Ghoshhajra 1979). A negative CT, however, might be useful in such cases, since it would exclude rebleeding and ventricular enlargement and therefore might indirectly indicate vasospasm in a patient who is clinically deteriorating, although consistent cor-

relation between vasospasm and clinical deterioration has not been proved.

CT should be the first investigative procedure in patients with possible subarachnoid hemorrhage. The study should be done as early as possible after the ictus and, if clinically indicated, should be done as an emergency procedure. CT accurately diagnoses, in addition to the subarachnoid hemorrhage, a significant intracranial hemorrhage or ventricular enlargement which may require immediate neurosurgical intervention. In cases where, in addition to the subarachnoid hemorrhage, a small localized hematoma is present, cerebral angiography and surgery may be postponed until the condition of the patient stabilizes. A negative CT scan does not exclude the possibility of recent subarachnoid hemorrhage, and in these circumstances a lumbar puncture is warranted. If the lumbar puncture reveals evidence of subarachnoid hemorrhage, angiography, digital subtraction or conventional, is indicated when the condition of the patient stabilizes.

INTRACRANIAL VASCULAR MALFORMATION

Vascular malformations are developmental malformations of the vascular bed. They are classified into four groups: capillary telangiectasis, cavernous angioma, arteriovenous malformation, and venous malformation. An increase in the size of the malformation may occasionally be demonstrated, and progressive destruction of the adjacent brain tissue may occur, but there is no evidence of neural tissue proliferation and therefore no evidence of neoplastic disease (Russell 1977).

Capillary Telangiectasis

These lesions are composed of dilated capillary blood vessels which vary greatly in caliber; the vessels are separated by normal neural tissue. The lesions are a relatively common incidental finding at autopsy but are rarely symptomatic. They are uncommonly associated with hemorrhage. In the hereditary form, called Rendu-Osler-Weber disease, multiple cutaneous and mucosal lesions are present. This form is often symptomatic and may be associated with other vascular anomalies such as cavernous angiomas and arteriovenous malformations of the brain (Sobel 1984). The lesions of telangiectasis are most often located in the pons, but other sites include the cerebral cortex and subcortical white matter. Angiographically a blush may be demonstrated in the capillary phase within the malformation, but most often the angiogram is negative (Poser 1957; Roberson 1974). Patients frequently present with focal areas of hemorrhage. The CT may demonstrate cerebellar atrophy in capillary telangiectasis (Assencio-Ferreira 1981), although actual CT demonstration of the lesion itself has, to our knowledge, not been reported.

In one case of telangiectasia pathologically confirmed, NCCT demonstrated two hyperdense lesions with slight enhancement on CECT (Fig. 13-12). These findings are nonspecific.

Cavernous Hemangioma

Cavernous hemangiomas are composed of large sinusoidal vascular spaces which are closely clustered together; the vessels are not separated by normal neural tissue. Hemangiomas represent the rarest form of vascular malformation but are clinically important because they are often symptomatic, causing seizures. They are commonly within the intracerebral hemispheres, particularly in the subcortical region. Calcification is present in 30 pecent of cases. Angiography is frequently normal (Savoiardo 1983), although prolonged injection angiography may demonstrate feeding arteries, a capillary blush, and abnormal draining veins (Numaguchi 1979). CT findings consist of a hyperdense and often partially calcified lesion which shows fairly homogeneous enhancement of minimum degree (Fig. 13-13A) or no enhancement (Fig. 13-13B) depending on whether they are partially or completely thrombosed. The lesion is not associated with mass effect or surrounding edema except when recent hemorrhage is present (Bartlett 1977; Ito 1978; Numaguchi 1979; Ramina 1980). Rarely, cavernous hemangiomas may coexist with other types of vascular malformations within the lesion. These complex malformations show histologically evidence of recent or old hemorrhage, but no specific CT characteristics are manifest (Ahmadi 1985). Occasionally the CT appearance may be indistinguishable from a meningioma (Ishikawa 1980), but the location of the lesion is often intracerebral.

Arteriovenous Malformation

This is a vascular malformation in which there is an intimate topographic admixture of arteries and veins. It represents the most common form of vascular malformation. It is clinically important because it is often symptomatic. According to LeBlanc (1979), 55

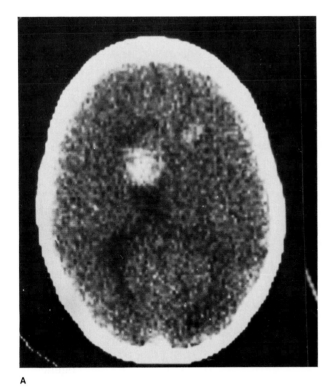

A

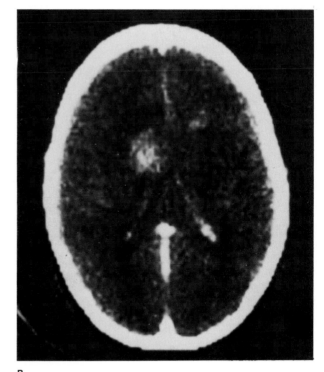

B

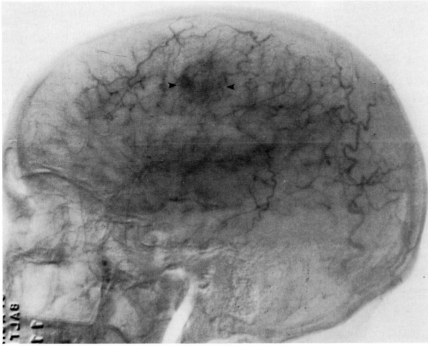

C

Figure 13-12 Telangiectasia. **A**. Two small hemorrhagic areas are seen on NCCT. **B**. No change in density on CECT. **C**. A capillary blush is noted on angiography (arrows). Subsequently proved following surgery. (*Courtesy of Dr. A. J. Kumar, Johns Hopkins Hospital.*)

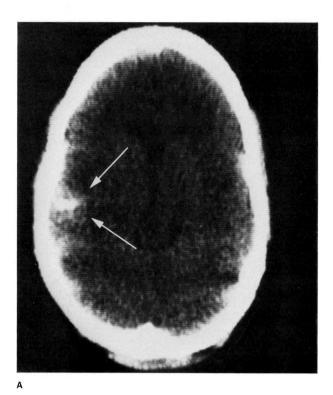

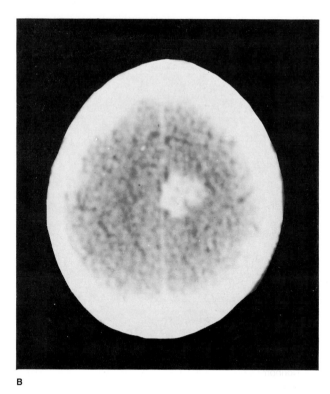

A   **B**

Figure 13-13   Cavernous hemangioma.   **A**. NCCT shows calcified lesion in the temporal lobe in a 33-year-old woman with seizures. CT number measures 90 HU. CECT (not shown) failed to demonstrate obvious enhancement, but, on measurement, increase of 60 to 150 HU in the same area was noted. At surgery, partially thrombosed cavernous hemangioma with dystrophic calcification with old and recent hemorrhages were found.   **B**. Another cavernous hemangioma. CECT shows a calcified parasagittal lesion without evidence of contrast enhancement or surrounding edema. Angiography failed to show any vascular abnormality, but a cavernous hemangioma was proved at surgery. (*Courtesy Dr. G. Wortzman, Toronto General Hospital.*)

percent of arteriovenous malformations present with intracranial hemorrhage, 36 percent with a seizure disorder, and 9 percent with headaches and progressive neurological deficit. Approximately 12 percent of patients with subarachnoid hemorrhage were found to have an underlying arteriovenous malformation (Hayward 1976). The lesions may occur in all parts of the central nervous system but are commonly located in the distribution of the middle cerebral artery along the cortex of the brain. The brain parenchyma adjacent to an arteriovenous malformation shows destructive and atrophic changes (TerBrugge 1977; Russell 1977). Calcifications are often present within the vascular channels as well as in the adjacent brain parenchyma (Fig. 13-14).

The angiographic appearance of an arteriove-nous malformation is that of abnormally dilated and tortuous feeding arteries and a racemose tangle of increased vascularity, which drains early into tortuous and elongated veins. Occasionally the malformation may become partially or completely thrombosed, and angiography may fail to show any evidence of it.

The CT appearance of intracranial arteriovenous malformation, when not associated with recent hemorrhage, is fairly characteristic (TerBrugge 1977; Pressman 1975; Kendall 1976*a*; Kumar 1984). The lesion most commonly presents on NCCT as an area of mixed density. Focal areas of hyperdensity are interspersed with areas of decreased density. The margins of the lesions are poorly defined and irregular in outline. After contrast infusion, the lesion

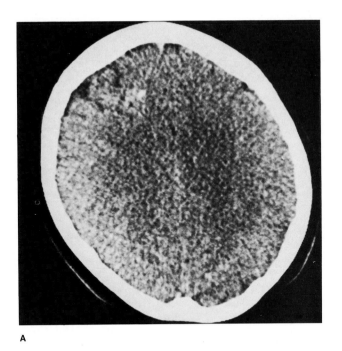

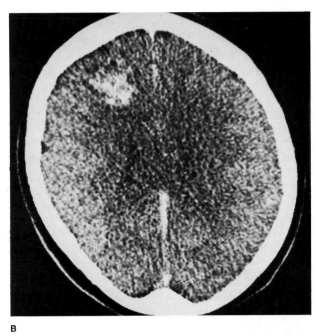

A

B

Figure 13-14   Arteriovenous malformation (AVM).   **A**. A focal area of cortical atrophy is noted on NCCT, with minute calcifications. **B**. Nonhomogeneous enhancement is present on CECT. The margins are poorly defined, without evidence of edema, in this angiographically proved AVM.

will show nonhomogeneous enhancement (Figs. 13-14, 13-18, 13-22). Feeding arteries and draining veins may be recognized on CT. The lesion may be associated with focal atrophy (Fig. 13-14) and localized mass effect (Fig. 13-17), but surrounding edema is extremely uncommon (LeBlanc 1979; TerBrugge 1977; Kumar 1985).

A significant number of arteriovenous malformations will not show an abnormality on NCCT and become apparent only after contrast infusion, which is therefore a mandatory part of the examination (TerBrugge 1977). CECT will show nonhomogeneous enhancement and poorly defined margins of the lesion (Fig. 13-15).

One may observe areas of increased density, usually in the range of 40 to 50 HU, on NCCT (Michels 1977). Postulated explanations for this baseline increased density implicate the presence of local gliosis and hemosiderosis (New 1975), mural thrombus or calcification, or an increased blood pool (Pressman 1975). CECT demonstrates enhancement

of the central angiomatous mass and visualization of adjacent vessels (Figs. 13-15, 13-17).

A small number of arteriovenous malformations exhibit a predominantly hyperdense appearance and are heavily calcified (Fig. 13-16). Enhancement may be difficult to detect in such angiographically occult arteriovenous malformations with CT number measurements (Kramer 1977; Golden 1978; Sartor 1978; Bell 1978; Teraco 1979; LeBlanc 1981; Chin 1983). Delayed high-dose CT scanning is of little value in the evaluation of patients with angiographically occult, thrombosed arteriovenous malformations (Hayman 1981). Contrast enhancement of these calcified, thrombosed arteriovenous malformations, as mentioned earlier under cavernous hemangiomas, probably depends on the degree and extent of thrombosis.

Unusual patterns of arteriovenous malformation on CT have been described in which a well-defined area of decreased density was a prominent feature (Fig. 13-18). These cases frequently reflect patients

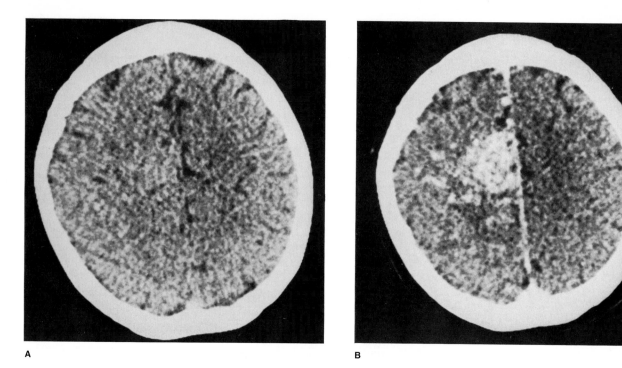

A

B

Figure 13-15 Arteriovenous malformation. **A**. NCCT shows slightly increased density. **B**. On CECT there is nonhomogeneous enhancement of the lesion with poorly defined margins representing central angiomatous mass. Multiple peripheral dotlike enhancement sites represent adjacent enlarged vessels.

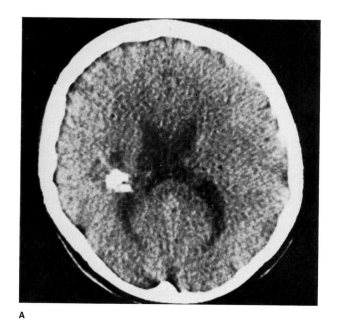

A

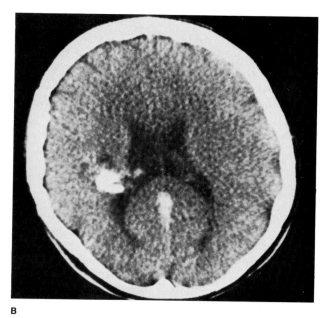

B

Figure 13-16 Thrombosed arteriovenous malformation (AVM). **A**. NCCT shows a small, predominantly calcified lesion adjacent to the trigone of the right lateral ventricle. **B**. CECT shows subtle enhancement detectable only by CT number measurements. Angiogram proved to be normal. A thrombosed AVM was proved at surgery.

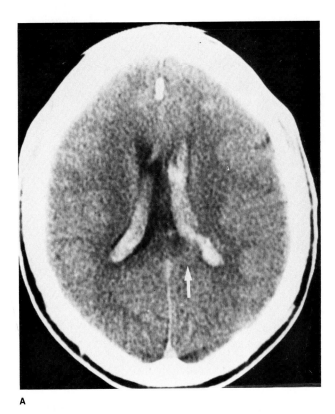

A

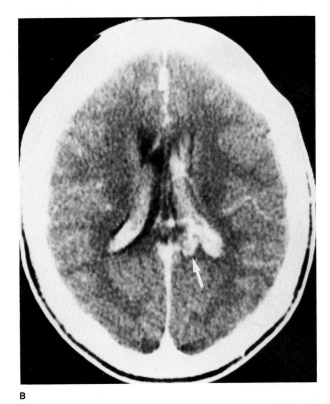

B

Figure 13-17 Arteriovenous malformation with interventricular hemorrhage. **A**. NCCT shows recent intraventricular hemorrhage and a small isodense mass lesion (arrow) indenting the left lateral ventricle. **B**. CECT shows evidence of enhancement of this lesion (arrow) which at angiography proved to be a small arteriovenous malformation in that location.

who have had previous episodes of hemorrhage associated with the arteriovenous malformation with subsequent resolving hematoma and "cyst" formation (Daniels 1979; Britt 1980). On careful inspection, a partial curvilinear enhancement at the margin of the cystlike lesion, without surrounding edema or mass effect, may give a clue as to the presence of underlying arteriovenous malformation (Fig. 13-18). Occasionally, in rupture of arteriovenous malformations, extravasation of blood into the preexisting cystic cavities presents as intraparenchymal blood-fluid levels (Richmond 1981). Spontaneous closure of the arteriovenous malformation of the basal ganglia is demonstrated on CT as nonenhancing, well-demarcated hypodensity with focal dilatation of adjacent lateral ventricle (Sartor 1978).

A characteristic but rare form of arteriovenous malformation has been described in the midbrain associated with ipsilateral angiomatosis of the retina and presence of a cutaneous nevus in the distribution of the trigeminal nerve, called *Wyburn-Mason syndrome* (Wyburn-Mason 1943). CECT usually demonstrates a nonhomogeneous density of varying size, most commonly in the midbrain (Fig. 13-19). The orbital component of the vascular malformation around the optic nerve, which is always on the same side as the retinal angiomas and the intracranial AVM, may not be detected by CT unless high-resolution thin sections are obtained or the orbital vascular component is very large. The extent of the orbital as well as intracranial vascular anomaly can be confirmed by angiography.

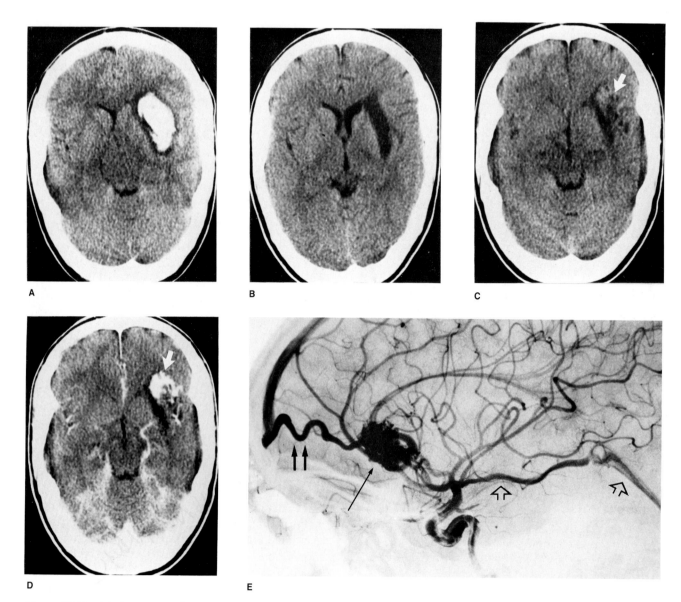

A

B

C

D

E

Figure 13-18   Arteriovenous malformation associated with intracerebral hemorrhage.   **A**. Acute intracerebral hemorrhage deep within the left frontal lobe.   **B**. NCCT 6 weeks later shows a resolved hematoma cavity.   **C**. The NCCT shows an area of mixed density (arrow) adjacent to the inferior aspect of the cavity.

D. CECT shows nonhomogeneous enhancement of a lesion along the anterior aspect of the insular cortex (arrow).   **E**. Angiogram done at the time of the initial hemorrhage shows a moderate-size AVM (arrow) fed by branches of the MCA with early superficial (double arrows) and deep venous drainage (open arrows).

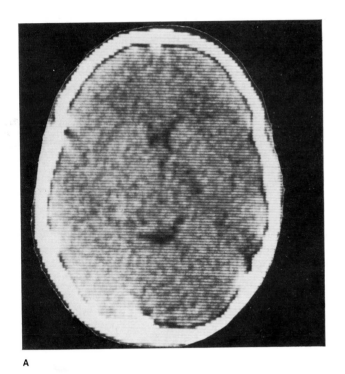

A

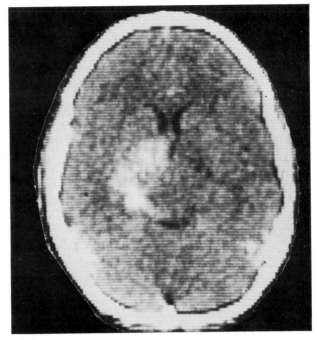

B

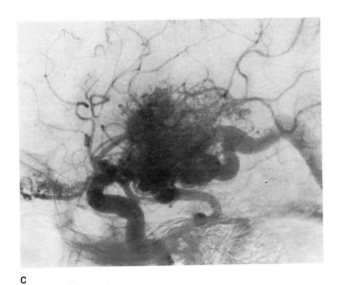

C

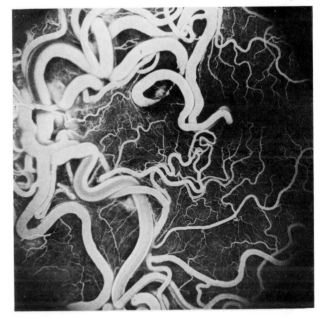

D

Figure 13-19 Wyburn-Mason syndrome. NCCT **(A)** and CECT **(B)** show a nonhomogeneous enhancing lesion in the midbrain and thalamus.   **C**. Angiogram demonstrates the vascular malfor-mation, with extension of vascular anomaly along the optic nerve into the orbit.   **D**. Racemose retinal angiomatosis shown by fluo-rescein angiography.

Another variant of the AVM is the so-called *aneurysm of the vein of Galen*. The venous ectasia in this condition is usually caused by increased flow through a deep-seated arteriovenous shunt in the presence of a dural venous obstacle downstream from the vein of Galen aneurysm (Lasjaunias 1986b). Aneurysmal dilatation of the vein of Galen may cause compression of the midbrain and aqueduct. The CT findings in patients with aneurysm of the vein of Galen are fairly characteristic (MacPherson 1979; Spallone 1979). A well-defined, hyperdense, rounded or triangular mass lesion in the region of the vein of Galen is noted on NCCT. Homogeneous enhancement occurs after contrast infusion (Fig. 13-20). Hydrocephalus is invariably present. CT is of great value in the postoperative assessment of these patients. Ventricular size and possible subdural effusions can be demonstrated readily (Diebler 1981). Advances in therapeutic angiography have allowed for endovascular treatment of these lesions (Lasjaunias 1986a). CT may be helpful in showing

the presence of embolic material within the shunt and the development of thrombosis within the varix (Lasjaunias 1986b).

The accuracy of CT in the detection of pial and mixed pial and dural type of arteriovenous malformation is reported to be as high as 100 percent when good-quality scans are done with and without contrast enhancement (TerBrugge 1977). Pure dural arteriovenous malformations differ from brain arteriovenous malformations in that they represent an acquired condition. They are often associated with previous head injury or inflammatory disease. Venous drainage may be into dural sinuses or into cortical veins. The presence of cortical venous drainage may account for central nervous system symptomatology and indicates a higher incidence of associated intracranial hemorrhage (Lasjaunias 1986c). Dural arteriovenous malformations along the anterior cranial fossa and tentorium are frequently associated with subarachnoid and intracerebral hemorrhage (Fig. 13-21). Although the nidus of the lesion

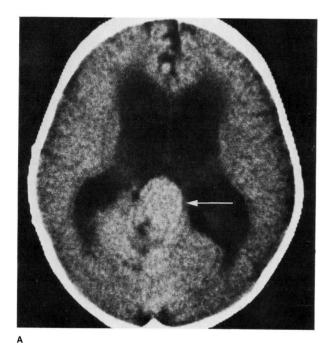

A

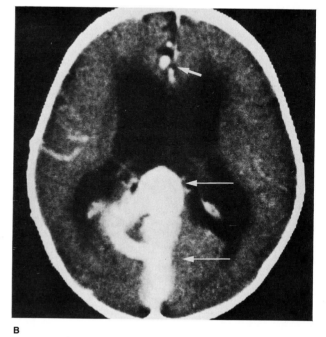

B

Figure 13-20 Midline arteriovenous malformation (AVM) with aneurysmal dilatation of inferior longitudinal sinus and vein of Galen. **A**. An elongated area of slightly increased density is present at the level of the vein of Galen (arrow). **B**. CECT. Enhancement outlines the enlarged anterior cerebral arteries (small arrow) and the engorged vein of Galen and straight sinus (large arrows).
(Continued on p. 631.)

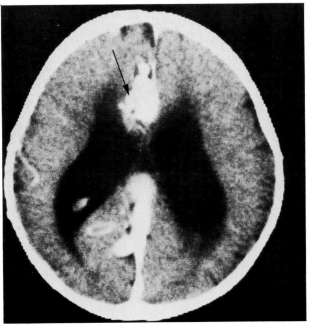

C

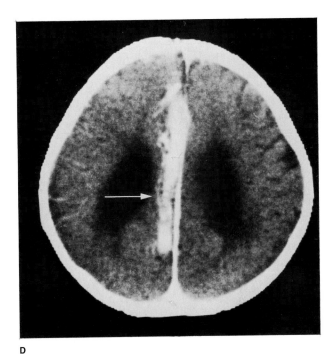

D

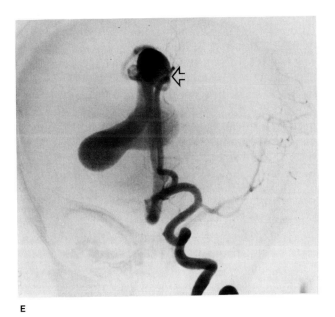

E

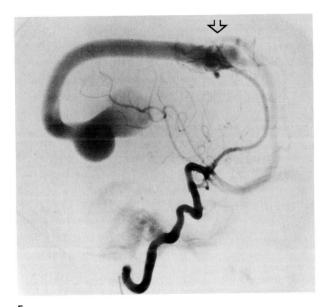

F

Figure 13-20 (*cont.*)   **C, D**. Enhancement of the vascular malformation along the anterior-superior aspect of the corpus callosum (black arrow) and the ectatic inferior longitudinal sinus (white arrow).   **E, F**. Angiogram in the frontal and lateral projection shows a midline AVM (arrow) with secondary enlargement of the inferior longitudinal sinus and vein of Galen. (*Courtesy of Dr. D. Harwood-Nash, Toronto Hospital for Sick Children.*)

is rarely shown on CT, abnormally prominent venous drainage channels may indicate secondary evidence of such a lesion (Fig. 13-22). False negative CT results in pure dural arteriovenous malformations are therefore common, and frequently only the associated complications are apparent on CT.

Approximately 50 percent of patients with an arteriovenous malformation present with intracranial hemorrhage (LeBlanc 1979). Bleeding often occurs into the subarachnoid space or into the ventricular system, less often into the brain parenchyma (Figs. 13-17, 13-18), and rarely into the subdural space (Rengachary 1981). Intracranial hemorrhage may occasionally obscure arteriovenous malformation on initial CT. Therefore, follow-up CT, subsequent to resorption of hemorrhage, may be necessary to demonstrate the underlying AVM. Furthermore, whenever a cortical hematoma is identified in a young patient who is normotensive, an underlying vascular malformation should be strongly suspected and angiography should be done (Solis 1977; Cone 1979). Angiography should include selective visualization of the ascending pharyngeal, occipital, and middle meningeal branches of the external carotid system in order to demonstrate the presence of a dural AVM.

Angiography remains the definitive method of diagnosis of arteriovenous malformation and will certainly be required to demonstrate the detailed anatomy of the malformation before treatment is planned.

Venous Angioma

This vascular malformation is composed solely of veins. The abnormality consists either of an enlarged single vein with many tributaries or a compact group of such veins. They represent the rarest type of vascular malformation. They occur in both the cerebrum and cerebellum, but the most frequent site is the spinal cord and its meninges. They are clinically often asymptomatic, but they may be associated with subarachnoid or intracerebral hemorrhage or with seizures (Wendling 1976; Rothfus 1984). Cerebellar venous angiomas are more prone to bleed, resulting in spontaneous, subacute, recurrent hemorrhage (Rothfus 1984).

The angiogram shows a normal arterial and capillary phase with multiple venules draining in an umbrella-type pattern toward an engorged draining vein, which is often positioned perpendicular to the cortex (transcerebral) (Wendling 1976). NCCT is normal in the majority of cases, although sometimes a rounded hyperdense area is noted. CECT shows a rounded or linear area of enhancement which is not associated with mass effect or surrounding edema (Michels 1977; Fierstein 1979) (Fig. 13-23). Dynamic rapid sequence CT scanning can be a suitable method for the evaluation of venous angioma (Lotz 1983). MRI shows enlarged transcerebral draining veins manifested by hyperintense on T_2-WI and hypointense on T_1-WI without mass effect (Lee 1985; Augustyn 1985).

A variant of venous malformation is the encephalofacial angiomatosis of *Sturge-Weber disease*. This rare condition consists in the association of an extensive capillary-venous malformation affecting one cerebral hemisphere with a homolateral cutaneous nevus or port-wine stain in the trigeminal nerve distribution, together with contralateral hemiparesis and Jacksonian epilepsy. Plain skull films may show characteristic "tram line" type calcification along the cortical gyri. The affected brain is atrophied, and the overlying leptomeninges are thickened. The angiogram shows a decrease in number or a complete absence of cortical superficial veins and enlargement of the deep cerebral venous system (Bentson 1971). On NCCT there is cortical atrophy with superficial cortical calcification (Welch 1980). Enhancement of the involved cortex occurs after contrast infusion (Fig. 13-24). The ipsilateral cranial vault is thickened and the hemicranium is most often smaller in size as compared with the normal opposite side. Ipsilateral enlargement of the hemicranium is uncommon (Enzmann 1977).

The value of CT in *embolization* of cerebral AVM rests on detection of complications, mainly infarction and hemorrhage, following interventional procedure. On CT, tantalum powders mixed with embolizing materials give rise to metal artifacts, but silicone spheres do not (Fig. 13-25). Dynamic scanning with fast scanning time may be of assistance in evaluation of the dynamic changes of blood flow associated with embolization of AVM.

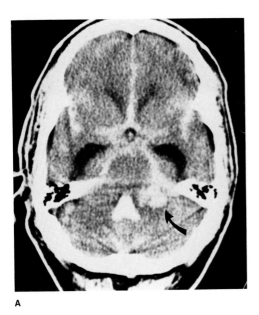

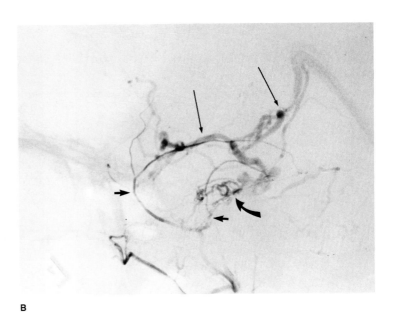

A   **B**

Figure 13-21 Dural AVM with SAH and IVH. **A**. NCCT shows evidence of recent subarachnoid and interventricular hemorrhage with a localized hematoma at the cerebellar/pontine junction (arrow). **B**. Selective angiography revealed evidence of supply from the middle meningeal artery (small arrows) toward a tentorial dural AVM (curved arrow) which drains into the deep venous system (large arrows).

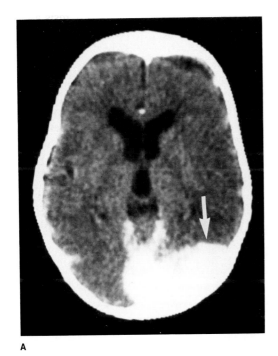

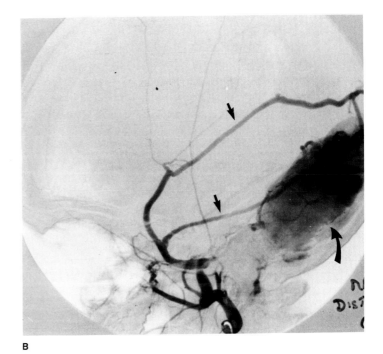

A   **B**

Figure 13-22 Dural arteriovenous malformation. **A**. CECT shows an enlongated area of enhancement at the level of the transverse sinus (arrow). **B**. Selective angiography shows branches of the middle meningeal artery (arrows) supplying a dural AVM which drains into an enlarged transverse sinus (curved arrow). Its outflow further downstream showed a partial block. (*Courtesy of Dr. P. Lasjaunias, Paris, France.*)

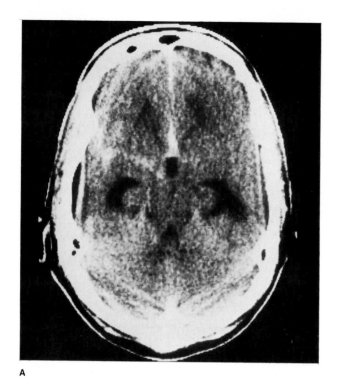

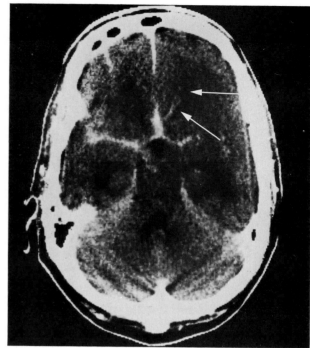

A

B

C

Figure 13-23 Venous angioma. **A**. NCCT shows no abnormality. **B**. CECT shows linear enhancement along the medial border of the frontal horn (arrows), representing draining veins. No surrounding edema or mass effect is noted. **C**. Angiogram reveals irregular vessels in medusa-like pattern, converging into the draining vein (arrows). No arterial or capillary abnormality is noted.

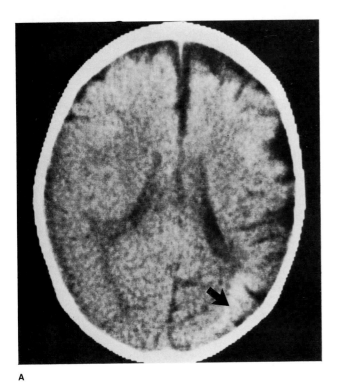
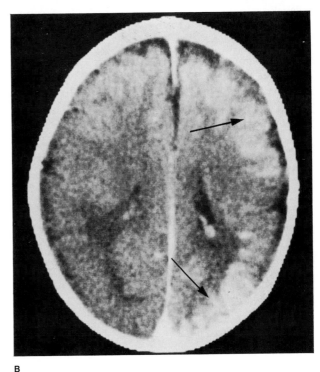

A   **B**

Figure 13-24   Sturge-Weber syndrome.   **A**. NCCT shows cortical atrophy with calcification along the cortex (arrow) in 1-year-old child. **B**. Enhancement after contrast infusion along the cortex of the left frontal and parietal lobe (arrow). (*Courtesy Dr. D. Harwood-Nash, Toronto Hospital for Sick Children.*)

CT should be the first investigation in patients with possible vascular malformations. Both NCCT and CECT are mandatory in the investigation of patients with intracranial vascular malformations. The degree of accuracy in the detection of an abnormality in such patients is high, although frequently angiography may be necessary to establish the definitive diagnosis. CT is superior to angiography in the demonstration of completely thrombosed vascular malformations and in the diagnosis of intracranial hemorrhage, which is frequently a complication associated with intracranial vascular malformation.

Magnetic Resonance Imaging

Present information indicates that CT and MRI are equally effective in detecting angiographically de-

monstrable vascular malformations (Fig. 13-26). It is doubtful that MRI will replace angiograms at this time in the evaluation of vascular malformation. MRI may be more sensitive than CT in the detection of angiographically occult vascular malformations histologically consisting of AV malformations, cavernous angiomas, unclassified or mixed malformations frequently associated with small hemorrhagic foci, calcifications, thrombosis, or abnormal vessels (Lee 1985; New 1986; Gomori 1986; Lemme-Plaghos 1986; Kucharczyk 1985). On the other hand, CT has proved to be more sensitive than MRI in the detection of small calcified malformations (Lemme-Plaghos 1986; Kucharczyk 1985). Further studies to evaluate the role of MRI and CT in the demonstration of intracranial vascular malformations will be necessary (see Chapter 17 also).

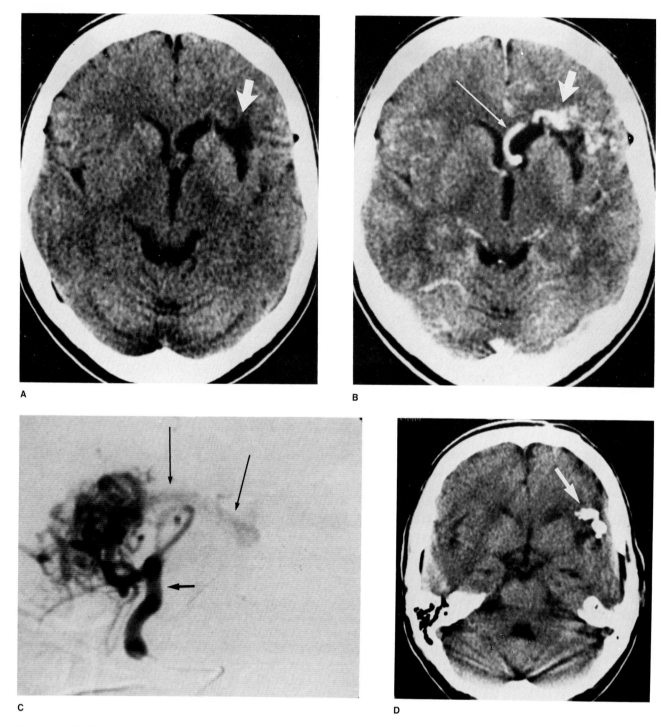

A

B

C

D

Figure 13-25 Endovascular treatment of brain AVM with isobutylcyanoacrylate. **A**. The NCCT shows evidence of focal enlargement of the lateral ventricle as well as a cavity related to a previous hemorrhage (arrow). The CECT shows nonhomogeneous enhancement of a lesion located along the left frontal opercular cortex (arrrow) and a prominent draining vein (large arrow). **C**. Superselective angiogram through a calibrated leak balloon microcatheter shows the main feeder of the AVM to be a middle cerebral artery branch (small arrow). Note the early draining vein (large arrow). **D**. Deposition of IBCA into part of the nidus of the AVM is shown on NCCT (arrow).

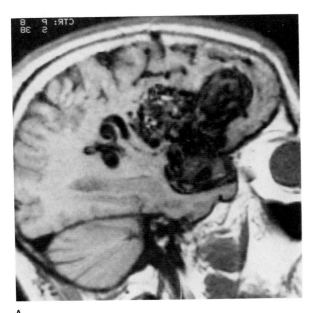
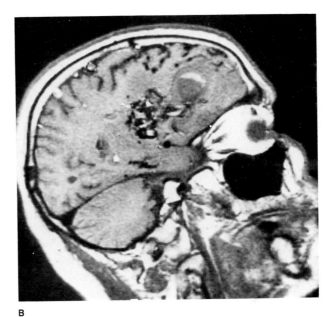

A   **B**

Figure 13-26   T₁-weighted MRI of AVM before **A** and after **B** embolization with bucrylate. See also Chapter 17.

Bibliography

AALMAANI WS, RICHARDSON AE: Multiple intracranial aneurysms: Identifying the ruptured lesion. *Surg Neurol* **9**:303–305, 1978.

AHMADI J, MILER CA, SEGALL HD et al: CT patterns in histologically complex cavernous hemangiomas. *AJNR* **6**:389–393, 1985.

ASSENCIO-FERREIRA VJ et al: Computed tomography in ataxia-telangiectasia. *J Comput Assist Tomogr* **5**(5):660–661, 1981.

AUGUSTYN GT, SCOTT J, OLSON E et al: Cerebral venous angiomas: MR imaging. *Radiology* **156**:391–395, 1985.

BABU VS, EISEN H: Giant aneurysm of anterior communicating artery simulating third ventricular tumor. *Comput Tomogr* **3**:159–163, 1979.

BARTLETT JE, KISHORE PRS: Intracranial cavernous angioma. *Am J Roentgenol Radium Ther Nucl Med* **128**:653–656, 1977.

BELL BA, KENDALL BE, SYMON L: Angiographically occult A-V malformations of the brain: *J Neurol Neurosurg Psychiatr* **41**:1057–1064, 1978.

BENTSON JR, WILSON GH, NEWTON TH: Cerebral venous drainage pattern of Sturge-Weber syndrome. *Radiology* **101**:111–118, 1971.

BJORKESTEN G, HALONEN V: Incidence of intracranial vascular lesions in patients with subarachnoid hemorrhage investigated by four-vessel angiography. *J Neurosurg* **23**:29–32, 1965.

BRITT RH, SILVERBERG GD, ENZMANN DR, HANBERRY JW: Third ventricular choroid plexus arteriovenous malformation simulating a colloid cyst. *J Neurosurg* **52**:246–250, 1980.

BULL JWD: Massive aneurysms at the base of the brain. *Brain* **92**:535–570, 1969.

BYRD SE, BENTSON JR, WINTER J, WILSON GH, JOYCE PW, O'CONNOR L: Giant intracranial aneurysms simulating brain neoplasms on computed tomography. *J Comput Assist Tomogr* **2**:303–307, 1978.

CHASON JL, HINDMAN WM: Berry aneurysms of the circle of Willis: Results of a planned autopsy study. *Neurology* **8**:41–44, 1958.

CHIN D, HARPER C: Angiographically occult cerebral vascular malformations with abnormal computed tomography. *Surg Neurol* **20**(2):138–142, 1983.

CONE JD, MARAVILLA KR, COOPER PR, DIEHL JT, CLARK WK: Computed tomography findings in ruptured arteriovenous malformation of corpus callosum. *J Comput Assist Tomogr* **3**:478–482, 1979.

CRAWFORD T: Some observations on the pathogenesis and natural history of intracranial aneurysm. *J Neurol Neurosurg Psychiatry* **22**:259–266, 1959.

CROMPTON MR: Mechanism of growth and rupture in cerebral berry aneurysm. *Br Med J* **1**:1138–1142, 1966.

DANIELS DL, HAUGHTON WM, WILLIAMS AL, STROTHER CM: Arteriovenous malformation simulating a cyst on computed tomography. *Radiology* **133**:393–394, 1979.

DAVIS JM, DAVIS KR, CROWELL RM: Subarachnoid hemorrhage secondary to ruptured intracranial aneurysm: prognostic significance of cranial CT. *Am J Neuroradiol* **1**:17–21, 1980.

DEEB ZL, JANETTA PJ, ROSENBAUM AE, KERBER CW, DRAYER BP: Tortuous vertebro-basilar arteries causing cranial nerve syndromes: Screening by computed tomography. *J Comput Assist Tomogr* **3**:774–778, 1979.

DIEBLER C et al: Aneurysms of the vein of Galen in infants aged 2 to 15 months. Diagnosis and natural evolution. *Neuroradiology* **21**:185–197, 1981.

DUBOULAY GH: Some observations on the natural history of intracranial aneurysms. *Br J Radiol* **38**:721–757, 1965.

ENZMANN DR, HAYWARD RW, NORMAN D, DUNN RP: Cranial computed tomographic scan appearance of Sturge-Weber disease: Unusual presentation. *Radiology* **122**:721–724, 1977.

FIERSTEIN SB, PRIBRAM HW, HIESHIMA G: Angiography and computed tomography in the evaluation of cerebral venous malformations. *Neuroradiology* **52**:246–250, 1979.

GHOSHHAJRA K, SCOTTI L, MARASCO J, BAGHAINAIINI P: C.T. detection of intracranial aneurysms in subarachnoid hemorrhage. *Am J Roentgenol Radium Ther Nucl Med* **132**:613–616, 1979.

GOLDEN JB, KRAMER RA: The angiographically occult cerebrovascular malformation. *J Neurosurg* **48**:292–296, 1978.

GOMORI JM, GROSSMAN RI, GOLDBERG HI et al: Occult cerebral vascular malformations: High-field MR imaging. *Radiology* **158**:707–713, 1986.

HANDA J, NAKANO Y, AII J, HANDA H: Computed tomography with giant intracranial aneurysms. *Surg Neurol* **9**:257–263, 1978.

HAYMAN LA, FOX AJ, EVANS RA: Effectiveness of contrast regimens in CT detection of vascular malformations of the brain. *AJNR* **2**:421–425, 1981.

HAYWARD RD: Intracranial arteriovenous malformations. *J Neurol Neurosurg Psychiatry* **39**:1027–1033, 1976.

HAYWARD RD, O'REILLY GVA: Intracerebral hemorrhage. *Lancet* **1**:1–4, 1977.

HOUSEPIAN EM, POOL JL: A systemic analysis of intracranial aneurysms from the autopsy file of the Presbyterian Hospital, 1914–1956. *J Neuropathol Exp Neurol* **17**:409–423, 1958.

ISHIKAWA M et al: Computed tomography of cerebral cavernous hemangiomas. *J Comput Assist Tomogr* **4**(5):587–591, 1980.

ITO J, SATO I, TANIMURA K: Angiographic and computed tomography findings of a convexity cavernous hemangioma. *Jpn J Clin Radiol* **23**:204–205, 1978.

KENDALL BE, CLAVERIA LE: The use of computed axial tomography for the diagnosis and management of intracranial angiomas. *Neuroradiology* **12**:141–160, 1976a.

KENDALL BE, LEE BCP, CLAVERIA E: Computerized tomography and angiography in subarachnoid hemorrhage. *Br J Radiol* **49**:483–501, 1976b.

KRAMER RA, WING SD: Computed tomography of angiographically occult cerebral vascular malformations. *Radiology* **123**:649–652, 1977.

KUCHARCZYK W, LEMME-PLAGHOS L, USKE A et al: Intracranial vascular malformations: MR and CT imaging. *Radiology* **156**:383–389, 1985.

KUMAR AJ, FOX AJ, VINUELA F, ROSENBAUM AE: Revisited old and new C.T. findings in unruptured larger arteriovenous malformations of the brain. *J Comput Assist Tomogr* **8**(4):648–655, 1984.

KUMAR AJ, VINUELA F, FOX AJ, ROSENBAUM AE: Unruptured intracranial arteriovenous malformations do cause mass effect. *AJNR* **6**(1):29–32, 1985.

LASJAUNIAS P, TERBRUGGE K, CHIU M: A coaxial balloon-catheter device for endovascular treatment of newborns and infants. Submitted and accepted for publication in *Radiology* 1986a.

LASJAUNIAS P, TERBRUGGE K, LOPEZ L, CHIU M, FLODMARK O, CHUANG S: Vein of Galen ectasia, associated dural sinus anomalies. Submitted for publication in *Journal of Neurosurgery* 1986b.

LASJAUNIAS P, CHIU M, TERBRUGGE K, TOLIA A, HURTH M, BERNSTEIN M: Spontaneous intracranial dural arteriovenous malformations (D AVM): Neurological manifestations. Submitted and accepted for publication in *Journal of Neurosurgery* 1986c.

LEBLANC R, ETHIER R: The CT appearance of angiographically occult arterio-venous malformation of the brain. *Canad J Neuroscience* **8**:7–13, 1981.

LEBLANC R, ETHIER R, LITTLE JR: Computerized tomography findings in arteriovenous malformations of the brain. *J Neurosurg* **51**:765–772, 1979.

LEE BCP, HERZBERG L, ZIMMERMAN RD, et al: MR imaging of cerebral vascular malformations. *Am J Neuroradiol* **6**:863–870, 1985.

LEMME-PLAGHOS L, KUCHARCZYKI W, BRANT-ZAWADZKI M et al: MR imaging of angiographically occult vascular malformation. *Am J Neuroradiol* **7**:217–222, 1986.

LILIEQUIST B, LINDQUIST M, VALDIMARSSON E: Computed tomography and subarachnoid hemorrhage. *Neuroradiology* **14**:21–26, 1977.

LIM ST, SAGE DJ: Detection of subarachnoid blood clot and other thin flat structures by computed tomography. *Radiology* **123**:79–84, 1977.

LOCKSLEY HB: Report on the cooperative study of intracranial aneurysms and subarachnoid hemorrhage. *J Neurosurg* **25**:219–239, 1966.

LOTZ PR, QUISLING RG: CT of venous angiomas of the brain. *AJNR* **4**:1124–1126, 1983.

LUKIN RR, CHABERS AA, MCLAURIN R, TEW J: Thrombosed giant middle cerebral aneurysms. *Neuroradiology* **10**:125–129, 1975.

MCKISSOCK W, RICHARDSON A, WALSH L, OWE E: Multiple intracranial aneurysms. *Lancet* **1**:623–626, 1964.

MACPHERSON P, TEASDALE GM, LINDSAY KW: Computed tomography in diagnosis and management of aneurysm of the vein of Galen. 1979.

MICHELS LG, BEAVSON JR, WINTER J: Computed tomography of cerebral venous angiomas. *J Comput Assist Tomogr* **1**:149–154, 1977.

MODESTI LM, BINET EF: Value of computed tomography in the diagnosis and management of subarachnoid hemorrhage. *Neurosurgery* **3**:151–156, 1978.

MORLEY TP, BARR HWK: Giant intracranial aneurysms: Diagnosis, course and management. *Clin Neurosurg* **16**:73–94, 1969.

NADJMI M, RATZKA M, WODARZ M: Giant aneurysms in C.T. and angiography. *Neuroradiology* **16**:284–286, 1978.

NEW PFJ, SCOTT WR: *Computed Tomography of the Brain and Orbit (EMI Scanning).* Baltimore, Williams & Wilkins, 1975, pp 317–331.

NEW PJ, OJEMANN RG, DAVIS KR et al: MR and CT of occult vascular malformations of the brain. *Am J Neuroradiol* **7**:771–779, 1986.

NUMAGUCHI Y, KISHIKAWA T, FUKUI M, SAWADA K, KITAMUZA K, MATSUURA K, RUSSELL WJ: Prolonged injection angiography for diagnosis of intracranial cavernous hemangiomas. *Radiology* **131**:137–138, 1979.

NYSTROM SHM: Development of intracranial aneurysms as revealed by electron microscopy. *J Neurosurg* **20**:329–337, 1963.

OSBORN AG, ANDERSON RE, WING SD: The false falx sign. *Radiology* **134**:421–425, 1980.

PEACH B: Arnold-Chiari malformation. *Arch Neurol* **12**:613–621, 1965.

PERRETT LV, SAGE MR: Computerized tomography and giant intracranial aneurysms. *Aust Radiol* **21**:308–312, 1977.

PETERSON NT, DUCHESNEAU PM, WESTBROOK EL, WEINSTEIN MA: Basilar artery ectasia demonstrated by computed tomography. *Radiology* **122**:713–715, 1977.

PINTO RS, KRICHELL II, BUTLER AR, MURALI R: Correlation of computed tomographic angiographic and neuropathological changes in giant cerebral aneurysms. *Radiology* **132**:85–92, 1979.

POSER CM, TAVERAS JM: Cerebral angiography in encephalotrigeminal angiomatosis. *Radiology* **68**:327–336, 1957.

PRESSMAN BD, KIRKWOOD JR, DAVIS DO: Computerized transverse tomography of vascular lesions of the brain: I. Arteriovenous malformations. *Am J Roentgenol Radium Ther Nucl Med* **124**:208–215, 1975.

PRESSMAN BD, GILBERT GE, DAVIS DO: Computerized transverse tomography of vascular lesions of the brain: II. Aneurysms *Am J Roentgenol Radium Ther Nucl Med* **124**:215–219, 1976*b*.

RAMINA R, INGUNZA W, VONOFAKOS D: Cystic cerebral cavernous angioma with dense calcification. *J Neurosurg* **52**:259–262, 1980.

RENGACHARY SS, SZYMANSKI DC: Subdural hematomas of arterial origin. *Neurosurgery* **8**(2):166–172, 1981.

RICHARDSON JC, HYLAND HH: Intracranial aneurysms: Clinical and pathological study of subarachnoid and intracerebral hemorrhage caused by berry aneurysms. *Medicine* **20**:1–83, 1941.

RICHMOND T et al: Intraparenchymal blood fluid levels: new CT sign of arteriovenous malformation: rupture. *Am J Neuroradiol* **2**:577–579, 1981.

ROBERSON GH, KASE CS, WOLPOW ER: Telangiectases and cavernous angiomas of the brain stem: "Cryptic" vascular malformations. *Neuroradiology* **8**:83–89, 1974.

ROTHFUS WE, ALBRIGHT AL, CASEY KF et al: Cerebellar venous angioma: "Benign" entity? *Am J Neuroradiol* **5**:61–66, 1984.

RUSSELL DS, RUBINSTEIN LJ: Pathology of tumors of the nervous system, 4th ed. E. Arnold, Edinburg, 1977, pp. 126–145.

SAITO I, SHIGENU T, ARITAKE K, TANISHIMA T, SANO K: Vasospasm assessed by angiography and computerized tomography. *J Neurosurg* **51**:*466–475,* 1979.

SARTOR K: Spontaneous closure of cerebral arteriovenous malformation demonstrated by angiography and computed tomography. *Neuroradiology* **15**:95–98, 1978.

SARWAR M, BATNITZKY S, SCHECHTER MM: Tumorous aneurysm *Neuroradiology* **12**:79–97, 1976*a*.

SARWAR M, BATNITZKY S, SCHECHTER MM, ZIMMER AE: Growing intracranial aneurysms. *Radiology* **120**:603–607, 1976*b*.

SAVOIARDO M, STRADA L, PASSERINI A: Intracranial cavernous hemangiomas: Neuroradiologic review of 36 operated cases. *Am J Neuroradiol* **4**:945–950, 1983.

SCHUBIGER O, VALAVANIA A, HAYEK J: Computed tomography in cerebral aneurysms with special emphasis on giant intracranial aneurysms. *J Comput Assist Tomogr* **4**:24–32, 1980.

SCOTTI G, ETHIER R, MELANCON D, TERRBRUGGE KG, TCHANG S: Computed tomography in the evaluation of intracranial aneurysms and subarachnoid hemorrhage. *Radiology* **123**:85–90, 1977.

SCOTTI G, DEGRAND C, COLOMBO A: Ectasia of the intracranial arteries diagnosed by computed tomography. *Neuroradiology* **15**:183–184, 1978.

SMOKER WRK, CORBETT JJ, GENTRY LR et al: High-resolution CT of the basilar artery: 2. vertebrobasilar dolichoectasia: Clinicopathologic correlation and review. *Am J Neuroradiol* **7**:61–72, 1986.

SOBEL D, NORMAN D: CNS manifestations of hereditary hemorrhagic telangiectasia. *AJNR* **5**(5):569–573, 1984.

SOLIS OJ, DAVIS KR, ELLIS GT: Dural arteriovenous malformation associated with subdural and intracerebral hematoma: A C.T. scan and angiographic correlation. *Comput Tomogr* **1**:145–150, 1977.

SPALLINE A: Computed tomography in aneurysms of the vein of Galen. *J Comput Assist Tomogr* **3**:779–782, 1979.

TERACO H, HOZI T, MATSUTANI M, OKEDA R: Detection of cryptic vascular malformation by computerized tomography. *J Neurosurg* **51**:546–551, 1979.

TERBRUGGE KG, SCOTTI G, ETHIER R, MELANCON D, TCHANG S, MILNER C: Computed tomography in intracranial arteriovenous malformations. *Radiology* **122**:703–705, 1977.

THRON A, BOCKENHEIMER S: Giant aneurysms of the posterior fossa suspected as neoplasms on computed tomography. *Neuroradiology* **18**:93–97, 1979.

WEIR B, MILLER J, RUSSELL D: Intracranial aneurysms: A clinical, angiographic and computerized tomographic study. *Can J Neurol Sci* **4**:99–105, 1977.

WEISBERG LA, NICE C, KATZ M: *Cerebral Computed Tomography: A Text-Like Atlas.* Philadelphia, Saunders, 1978, pp. 87–105.

WELCH K, NAHEEDY MH, ABROMS IF, STRAND RD: Computed tomography of Sturge-Weber syndrome in infants. *J Comput Assist Tomogr* **4**:33–36, 1980.

WENDLING LR, MOORE JS, KIEFFER SA, GOLDBERG HI, LATCHOW RE: Intracerebral venous angioma. *Radiology* **119**:141–147, 1976.

WYBURN-MASON R: The Vascular Abnormalities and Tumors of the Spinal Cord and Its Membranes, Kingston, London, 1943.

YOCK DH, LARSON DA: Computed tomography of hemorrhage from anterior communicating artery aneurysms, with angiographic correlation. *Radiology* **134**:399–407, 1980.

ZIMMERMAN RD, YURBERG E, LEEDS NE: The falx and interhemispheric fissure on axial computed tomography: I. Normal anatomy. *Am J Neuroradiol* **3**:175–180, 1982.

14

STROKE

Herbert I. Goldberg

Seungho Howard Lee

Stroke is the third of the leading causes of death in the United States, exceeded only by heart disease and cancer (*Report to the President* 1964–65). It kills over 200,000 people each year in this country (Kurtzke 1980) and affects close to 400,000 (Whisnant 1971). The incidence rate and death rate from stroke increase dramatically with age (Eisenberg 1964). About 15 to 35 percent of patients will die with each episode of cerebral infarction (Eisenberg 1964; Matsumoto 1973); a much higher mortality—60 to 80 percent—occurs with cerebral hemorrhage (Whisnant 1971). Those who survive are usually left with permanent disability. With the increasing mean population age in this country, stroke will become an even greater medical and social problem. Accurate and early diagnosis may improve the morbidity and mortality rates in the future as newer and more ef-

fective therapies currently being tested are instituted.

The advent of computed tomography (CT) in the early 1970s greatly facilitated the diagnosis and management of stroke and added significantly to our understanding of the pathophysiologic brain alterations it causes in humans. With CT it is now possible for the first time to noninvasively and reliably diagnose and distinguish between stroke resulting from cerebral infarction and that resulting from cerebral hemorrhage. In addition, other brain lesions that at times may clinically present as stroke-like syndromes, such as primary or metastatic brain tumor, brain abscess, or subdural hematoma, can usually be clearly differentiated by the CT examination. In most instances it is no longer necessary to perform cerebral angiography to exclude a possible surgical lesion in patients in whom the clinical diagnosis of stroke may have been in doubt. In some strokes the initial CT findings are of uncertain etiologic significance; however, follow-up scans between 1 and 3 weeks will usually demonstrate a characteristic evolution of the CT alterations, establishing the correct diagnosis.

The high spatial- and density-resolution capabilities of CT result in one of the most accurate methods available for identifying and localizing an infarction within the brain. Ischemic infarction, hemorrhagic infarction, and intracerebral hematoma are usually readily differentiated. CT also permits identification of the acute and chronic sequelae that may develop after an ischemic event. These include, in the acute phase, brain swelling and conversion of a bland into a hemorrhagic infarct and in the chronic phase, cystic parenchymal change, cortical atrophy, and focal ventricular dilatation.

In CT evaluation of stroke, additional and frequently valuable information may be gained when CT scans are performed both before and after the intravenous administration of contrast material. Contrast-enhanced CT greatly aids recognition of other types of brain lesions that may present clinically as stroke and permits detection of up to 13 percent of infarcts which are invisible on noncontrast CT scans (Masdeu 1977; Wing 1976). Although the underlying nature of the vascular pathology causing an infarction is not directly revealed by CT, frequently distinguishing pathophysiologic alterations will be evident on CECT which, in combination with the alterations seen on NCCT, will suggest the correct diagnosis between two major causes of infarction—embolism and primary cerebral vasoocclusive disease. In this differentiation, follow-up NCCT and CECT scans are frequently valuable during the first 2 to 3 weeks, as distinctive differences in the temporal evolution of these two conditions may be revealed. The differentiation of these two varieties of infarction has important therapeutic implications.

Besides diagnosing large-artery, atherosclerotic, or embolic occlusive disease, the CT may reveal alterations which suggest involvement of smaller arteries and other etiologies for the stroke. Hypertensive vascular disease which primarily affects small penetrating arteries (arteriolosclerosis) usually shows ischemic change in the deep gray masses and in the periventricular white matter. In some cases of primary and secondary arteritis the CT patterns of ischemia, in conjunction with other CT alterations and the patient's age, sex, and clinical history, will suggest the correct diagnosis. Cerebral sinovenous thrombosis will frequently demonstrate unique CT changes.

Although intracerebral hematomas all appear relatively similar on CT regardless of their etiology, presenting as circumscribed homogeneous regions of increased density, their various causes may be suggested by the location of the hemorrhage and associated changes which may be revealed on pre- or postcontrast scans. This frequently permits differentiation of hematomas caused by hypertension, trauma, tumor, venous thrombosis, arteriovenous malformation, and aneurysm.

Stroke may be classified as being caused by decreased circulation to the brain (infarction) or by intracerebral hemorrhage. The former produces brain injury from ischemic necrosis, while the latter causes brain damage by compression necrosis and vascular disruption. The incidence of the major causes of stroke, based on a communitywide survey of diagnoses in Rochester, Minn., during the years 1955 through 1969, before the introduction of CT, was as follows: for cerebral infarction, 79 percent, with embolism at 8 percent included in this group; for intracerebral hemorrhage, 10 percent; for subarachnoid hemorrhage, 6 percent; and ill-defined causes, 5 percent (Matsumoto 1973). Kinkel (1976), utilizing CT, found a much higher incidence of intracerebral hemorrhage as a cause for supratentorial stroke (26 percent). In this series a high percentage of cases were clinically misdiagnosed as to the type of stroke: 43 percent with cerebral hemorrhage were clinically thought to have cerebral infarction, and 14 percent with cerebral infarction were diagnosed as having cerebral hemorrhage. A recent clinical survey by Mohr (1980), from the records of the Harvard Cooperative Stroke Registry, in which all appropriate laboratory aids were employed, including CT, four-vessel cerebral angiography, and CSF examination, found cerebral embolism to account for 31 percent of all strokes, atherosclerotic thrombosis 33 percent, and lacunar infarcts 18 percent. Hypertensive intracerebral hemorrhage caused 11 percent of the strokes, and hemorrhage from ruptured aneurysm and vascular malformation 7 percent. The high incidence of cerebral embolism (31 percent) in this clinical series is in agreement with an autopsy study of Fisher and Adams (Mohr 1980), in which cerebral embolism caused 32 percent of the strokes.

Transient ischemic attacks (TIA) are acute neurological deficits which clear completely within 24 hours. These attacks are caused by a short period of reduced blood flow to the eye or brain which does not result in permanent tissue damage. The reduced circulation may result from either small emboli or severe cerebrovascular occlusive disease, the latter usually in association with a transient reduction in arterial pressure (Ruff 1981).

Recovery from a TIA occurs because of the rapid return of normal arterial perfusion pressure to the affected brain tissue. When the TIA is related to a severe vascular stenosis, either a rise in blood pressure or return to a normal cardiac rate and rhythm, depending on the inciting cause, could reestablish the normal perfusion pressure; when caused by emboli, either rapid clot lysis or the rapid establishment of adequate collateral blood flow could account for complete clearing of the ischemic symptom. A TIA is an important warning sign of a possible subsequent major stroke. The CT scan is usually normal after a TIA (Kinkel 1976; Bradac 1980). There have, however, been reports of CT abnormalities with TIAs such as focal low densities in up to 20 percent of the cases (Buell 1979; Ladurner 1979; Perrone 1979). These abnormalities may be related to previous small silent infarcts and not to the current TIA episodes (Bradac 1980).

Tables 14-1 and 14-2 list the major causes of cerebral infarction and nontraumatic intracerebral hemorrhage.

Although cerebral angiography is the only technique short of pathologic examination that may specifically localize and indicate the nature of the vascular disease in some of the categories in Tables 14-1 and 14-2, not infrequently CT alterations are apparent which may be strongly suggestive of many of them. The use of intravenous contrast material after NCCT and the obtaining of follow-up studies

Table 14-1   Causes of Cerebral Infarction

Arterial occlusive disease
  Atherosclerotic occlusion
  Embolism
  Hemodynamic ischemia
  Arteriolosclerosis (lacunar disease)
  Vasculitis
  Moyamoya disease
Anoxic ischemia
Venous thrombosis

in many instances significantly aids in determination of the correct vascular etiology of the stroke, as does correlation of the CT changes with the patient's age, sex, history, and neurological findings.

CEREBRAL INFARCTION

Ischemic stroke has been reported to result in a positive CT scan in from 66 to 98 percent of cases (Bradac 1980; Buell 1979; Campbell 1978; Kinkel 1976). The percentage that becomes positive increases if follow-up CT scans are performed (Campbell 1978; Inoue 1980) and if CT is performed both before and after intravenous contrast administration (Norton 1978; Weisberg 1980; Wing 1976). The CT may become faintly positive as early as 3 hours after the onset of symptoms, but usually a low-density abnormality will become evident between 24 and 72 hours (Inoue

Table 14-2   Causes of Intracerebral Hemorrhage

Hypertensive vascular disease (arteriolosclerosis)
Aneurysm
Vascular malformation
Hemorrhagic arterial and venous infarction
Mycotic aneurysm
Amyloid angiopathy
Premature neonatal germinal matrix
Hemorrhagic hematologic disorders

1980). The size and location of the infarct, along with the degree of patient motion, significantly influences the time at which the lesion will first be detected. Small lesions that are usually not associated with significant edema may not become evident until very late, when necrotic tissue absorption has produced a well-demarcated, hypodense cystic lesion. Infratentorial infarcts (cerebellum and brainstem) have a lower incidence of detection, with focal abnormality apparent in from 31 to 44 percent of cases (Campbell 1978; Kingsley 1980). Brainstem infarcts are usually not identified, because they are frequently very small and because of the inherent large spatial artifacts in this region produced by the dense petrous ridges.

Newer-generation fast CT scanners result in increased early detection of cerebral infarction because of the improved spatial and contrast resolution. Detection rates of only 40 to 50 percent were found for ischemic strokes within 48 hours utilizing the slower early-model scanners (Davis 1975). Recently Inoue et al. (1980) reported that approximately 90 percent of supratentorial infarcts that eventually became positive on sequential CT scanning were evident by 24 hours. All scans obtained between 25 and 35 days after the ictus revealed a focal abnormality in this series. Wall et al. (1981) demonstrated subtle mass effects and/or focal areas of hypodensity within gray matter corresponding to regions of clinical deficit in 79 percent. Of particular note is the fact that of all the positive scans, 65 percent were obtained at or less than 12 hr after infarction. Early CT evaluation of suspected cerebral infarction is clinically important not only in establishing a specific diagnosis but also in excluding hemorrhage, neoplasm, and other significant pathologic entities.

Whereas CT will frequently reveal abnormality during the first week after an infarction, the radionuclide scan usually does not become positive until the second week (Blahd 1971; Di Chiro 1974). The detection rates for both types of studies are approximately equal during the second week for both supra- and infratentorial infarctions, but CT provides a much greater specificity (Campbell 1978; Masdeu 1977; Lewis 1978; Chiu 1977).

The CT alterations that develop and evolve over time with ischemic infarction reflect the pathologic changes that are occurring in the brain tissue. In the first few hours after a large cerebral artery occlusion, widespread tissue damage can be recognized microscopically, involving the gray and white matter. In the central regions of the infarct, coagulation necrosis may develop in all tissue elements. At the periphery of the infarction, where damage is less severe, there is disintegration of nerve cells, myelin sheaths, and oligodendroglia, along with varying lesser degrees of damage to the astrocytes; the microglia and blood vessels are preserved. The small blood vessels and tissues are infiltrated with polymorphocytic leukocytes, which reach their maximum concentration at 3 days and then begin to decline. They are replaced by phagocytic mononuclear cells, which become evident by the fifth day. These cells continue to increase through the fourth week, removing the products of enzymatic digestion of neuronal and myelin disintegration. Beginning around Day 5, proliferation of capillary endothelial cells becomes evident at the margins of the infarct. During the next several weeks these new capillaries greatly increase in number. They first grow into cortex and deep gray areas of infarction and later into the white-matter regions. As the process of tissue breakdown continues, the phagocytes become fat-laden and then degenerate, leaving cystic spaces filled with yellowish fluid. Astrocytes also undergo hypertrophy and hyperplasia, laying down collagen fibers which contribute to tissue repair at the infarct margins. After several months the necrotic tissue has been replaced by cystic spaces containing fluid and a variable number of fat-filled phagocytes. The margin between the infarct and the adjacent normal brain tissue is sharply defined during all stages of the infarct evolution.

Arterial Occlusive Diseases

Large-Artery Thrombotic Infarction (Atherosclerotic Occlusion)

Between 8 and 24 hours after the onset of ischemic symptoms, the NCCT may reveal a poorly marginated, mottled region of slight hypodensity involving both the cortex and the underlying white matter down to the ventricular surface (Figs. 14-1, 14-4*A*) (Baker 1975; Davis 1975; Yock 1975). The hypodensity becomes more distinct after a few days and assumes a triangular or wedge-shaped configuration with its base on the brain surface. The low density is confined within the vascular territory of the occluded artery (Figs. 14-2, 14-3). When the internal carotid artery or the proximal segment of the middle cerebral artery is occluded, the low density may extend into the basal ganglia and the internal capsule region (Figs. 14-3, 14-4, 14-20). This initial low-density pattern represents tissue necrosis with intracellular edema (cytotoxic edema) (Alcala 1978). Little or no mass effect is evident during the initial 24

hours of the infarct. Detection of infarct changes during the first 24 hours is dependent on the size of the infarct, the degree of the ischemic insult, and the availability of scans of high contrast resolution with minimal artifacts from patient motion.

Between the third and the fifth day the region of infarction becomes a more homogeneous low-density area with sharper margins. Its hypodensity increases over that of earlier scans (Figs. 14-2*A*, 14-4*B*) (Davis 1975; Inoue 1980). Pathologically, tissue necrosis and intracellular edema reaches its maximum at this time. This results in a variable degree of mass effect which depends on the size and degree of infarction. Swelling may be mild to severe, with the CT revealing either focal or diffuse

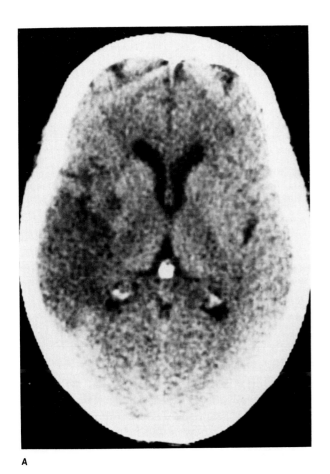

A

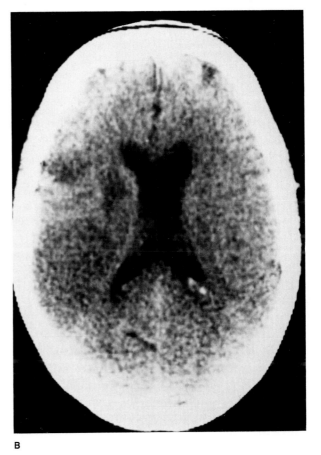

B

Figure 14-1 Early infarct, middle cerebral artery territory. Poorly defined areas of nonhomogeneous hypodensity involving right temporal region with patchy extension to adjacent cortex and white matter on NCCT, less than 2 days old.

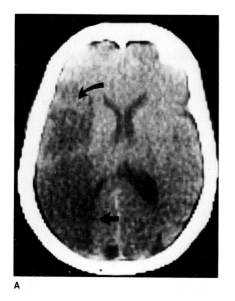

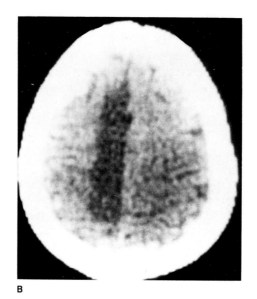

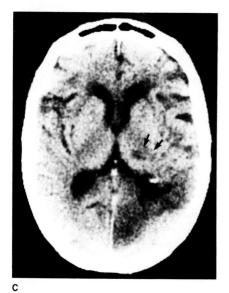

Figure 14-2 Major cerebral infarct territories in 3- to 5-day-old infarcts. **A.** Peripheral middle cerebral artery territory infarct: well-defined homogeneous hypodensity involving cortex and underlying white matter in right posterior temporal and lateral occipital region. The basal ganglia region is normal, indicating that the proximal middle cerebral artery segment from which the lenticulostriate supply arises is not occluded. Linear demarcation at watershed between infarct hypodensity in middle cerebral artery territory and normal tissue density of posterior cerebral artery territory (straight arrow). Hypodensity of cortex and white matter in anterior temporal region is nonhomogeneous, suggesting incomplete infarction in this region (curved arrow). Right lateral ventricle is compressed and shifted slightly to left of midline. **B.** Anterior cerebral artery territory infarct: rectangular, well-defined, homogeneous hypodensity involving the cortex and underlying white matter in the superior medial aspect of the right hemisphere. There is sharp margination of the hypodensity at the watershed region with the middle cerebral artery territory laterally and the posterior cerebral artery territory posteriorly. The hypodensity extends inferiorly on lower sections to the level of the roof of the lateral ventricle. **C.** Posterior cerebral artery territory infarct. Hypodensity involving posterior thalamus on the left (arrow) along with sharply defined cortical and white-matter lesion in the medial posterior occipital region.

compression of the ventricular system and midline shift (Figs. 14-2*B*, 14-3, 14-4*B*). With large infarcts, early signs of tissue swelling may become evident before 24 hours. At this time there may be obliteration or effacement of sulci and the sylvian fissure on the side of the infarct, and the ipsilateral ventricle may be slightly smaller (Fig. 14-4). Mass effect of some degree is reported in from 21 to 70 percent of infarcts (Masdeu 1977; Wing 1976; Yock 1975) and is most marked between the third and fifth days. With large hemispheric infarctions brain swelling may be considerable, with the development of a marked midline shift. This may result in posterior cerebral artery occlusion with occipital lobe infarction from transtentorial herniation. With small infarcts there may be no mass effect or only slight focal ventricular

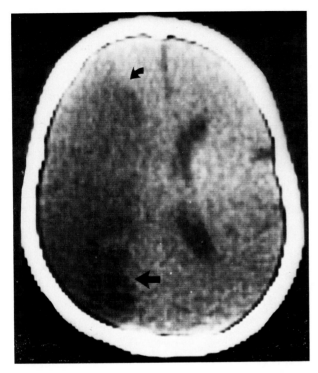

Figure 14-3 Four-day-old complete right middle cerebral artery territory infarction. Obliteration of right lateral ventricle and marked midline shift to the left. Homogeneous hypodensity involving lateral basal ganglia and all cortical white-matter regions of peripheral middle cerebral artery distribution. Sharp linear margination anteriorly at junction with anterior cerebral artery territory (curved arrow) and posteriorly with posterior cerebral artery territory (straight arrow).

involved or to the watershed or border zone between major arterial distributions (Fig. 14-2). This sharp localization is due to the hypodensity representing cellular necrosis and edema, which is mainly intracellular (cytotoxic), in contrast to the vasogenic form of edema, which is extracellular and spreads along white matter tracts and is commonly associated with brain tumor and inflammatory disease.

The low-density pattern associated with infarction can usually be differentiated from that seen with tumor and inflammatory disease. With infarction the region of decreased density usually involves both the gray and the white matter, while with tumor and inflammation it is mainly situated within the white matter, although it may extend to the cortex. With infarction the margins of the hypodensity are sharply demarcated, with a square or wedge-shaped configuration, and are located within or between arterial distributions, whereas with tumor and abscess the low density tends to spread diffusely within the white matter in a pseudopod-like manner, has ill-defined rounded margins, and is usually not limited to an arterial division or to adjacent arterial branches.

During the second and third weeks, isodense to slightly hyperdense curvilinear bands and nodular regions frequently develop within hypodense areas of the infarct (Inoue 1980). They are located mainly in gray matter and result from hyperemia related to new capillary ingrowth and improved collateral circulation in thrombotic infarcts while some of the hyperdensity may be caused by petechial hemorrhage in embolic infarct. The hyperdensity appears most commonly as slightly hyperdense bands in the expected location of the cortical ribbon which are most prominent at the margins of the infarct (Fig. 14-5). They may also occur in cortical regions, more centrally in the infarct, and in the deep gray masses. They tend to produce a mottled appearance at the margins of the infarct, which then become less sharply defined than on earlier poststroke scans. The infarcted white matter usually does not show any density increase and remains hypodense. As the edema resolves in the white matter between the second and the fourth weeks, its low density becomes even more marked than previously, owing to the

distortion. Brain swelling begins to decrease after the first week and usually completely resolves in 12 to 21 days.

With embolic infarcts, considerable further brain swelling may develop, predominantly vasogenic in nature, when antegrade circulation is reestablished following clot lysis. This frequently occurs, usually between the second and fourteenth day after the infarction, and results in the leakage of increased amounts of fluid from the ischemically damaged capillary bed when exposed to the high reperfusion pressure.

The low density of infarction remains strictly confined to the distribution of the arterial system

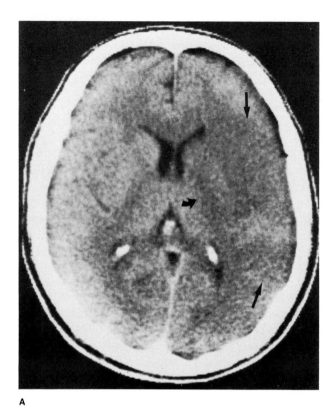

A

B

Figure 14-4 **A.** Early signs of mass effect with large cerebral artery territory infarct: CT obtained at about 12 hours after stroke. Poorly defined region of slight hypodensity involving basal ganglia (curved arrow) and frontotemporal region (straight arrows) on left side. The cortical sulci and sylvian fissure are obliterated on the left side and there is slight compression of the left frontal horn. **B.** Marked mass effect and increased left middle cerebral artery territory hypodensity approximately 2 days after **A.** (*Courtesy of Robert G. Peyster, M.D., Hahnemann Medical College.*)

accumulation of abundant fat-laden phagocytes in the infarct tissue at this time.

Starting at about 4 to 5 weeks and continuing for the next 2 to 3 months, the infarct region becomes more sharply outlined on CT, with its hypodensity becoming more homogeneous and approaching that of cerebral spinal fluid (Davis 1975; Inoue 1980). The isodense cortical bands usually convert to low-attenuation zones. Pathologically there is cystic cavitation of the necrotic infarcted brain tissue, prominent lipid content, and gliosis (Yates 1976). The cystic change predominantly affects the white matter and the region of the basal ganglia, where tissue necrosis is generally most severe. The infarct appears smaller because of absorption of necrotic tissue and

contraction from gliosis (McCall 1975). The adjacent portion of the lateral ventricle dilates and extends toward the region of infarction. A shift of the brain midline to the side of the infarct may also develop with large lesions. The overlying cortex frequently reveals atrophic change, with enlargement of adjacent sulci and cisterns (Fig. 14-6). With some cortical infarcts, sulcal enlargement may be the only long-term abnormality (Fig. 14-7). The chronic brain changes usually become stable by the end of the third month.

CONTRAST ENHANCEMENT CECT has been of great value in the diagnosis and characterization of infarcts. A significant percentage of infarcts reveal

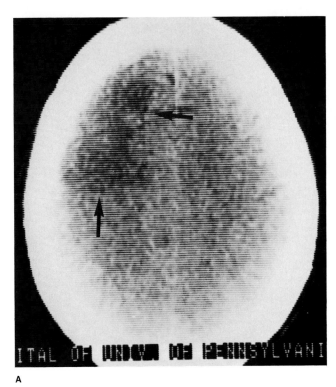

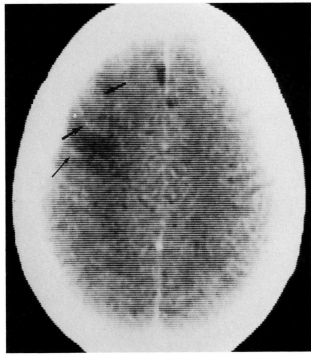

A

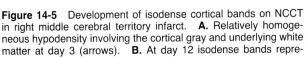

B

Figure 14-5 Development of isodense cortical bands on NCCT in right middle cerebral territory infarct. **A.** Relatively homogeneous hypodensity involving the cortical gray and underlying white matter at day 3 (arrows). **B.** At day 12 isodense bands representing the infolded cortical ribbon (arrows) extend down into white matter hypodensity. Infarct appears smaller with indistinct margins because cortex at periphery of infarct has become isodense.

contrast enhancement, which usually first appears during the second week after the onset of symptoms (Fig. 14-8). Early studies reported contrast enhancement in only about 60 percent of cerebral infarcts (Wing 1976; Masdeu 1977); recent studies have observed enhancement in upward of 82 to 88 percent of infarcts evaluated between the second and fourth weeks (Pullicino 1980; Lee 1978). In a study of supratentorial infarcts with serial CT examinations, 93 percent of those which developed an abnormality showed contrast enhancement between the second and third week (Inoue 1980). There has been a wide range in the reported incidence of enhancement occurring during the first week of the infarct, from zero to 62 percent (Weisberg 1980; Lee 1978). This large variation probably reflects differences in infarct etiology in these series. Those series which have

a high percentage of embolic and hemodynamic infarcts (see next section) reveal a high incidence of early enhancement because these infarcts are reperfused early at systemic arterial pressure levels which will reveal blood-brain barrier abnormalities not evident in persistently anemic infarcts. Hayman et al. (1981), employing high-dose contrast infusion (80 g iodine) along with immediate and delayed (3 hours) CT scans, had a 72 percent incidence of enhancement (13 of 18) within the first 28 hours. Most of the patients with early enhancement had embolic infarcts. In addition, these authors found that enhancement which occurred predominantly on the 3-hour-delayed scans had a grave prognostic implication; four of seven patients with this type of enhancement subsequently developed hemorrhagic infarcts and died. None of the patients with only

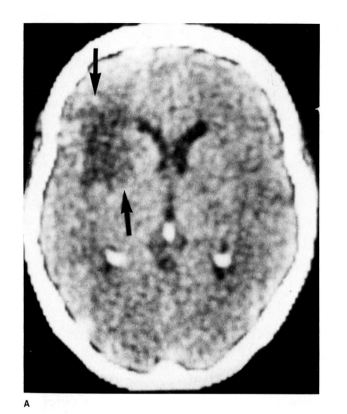

A

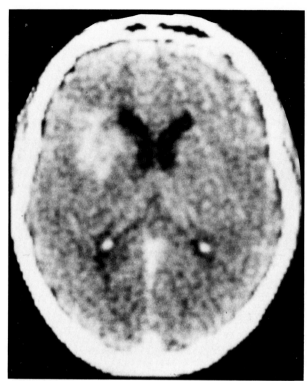

B

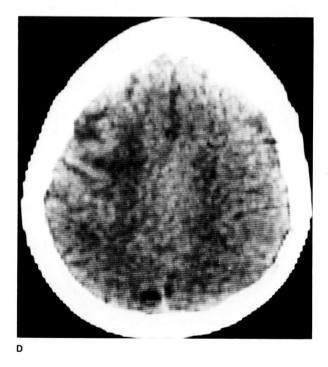

C

D

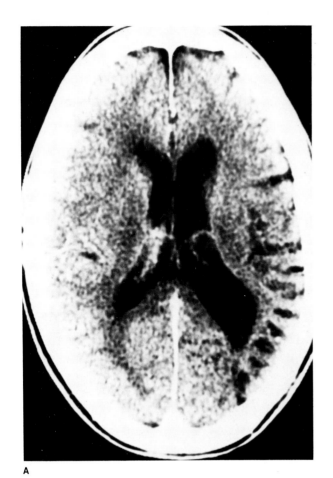

A

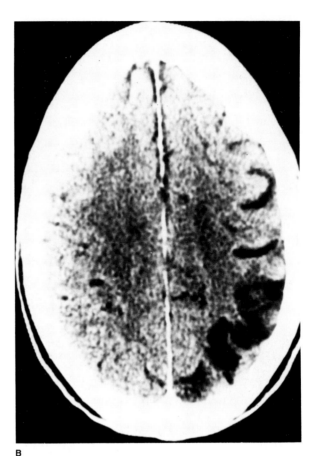

B

Figure 14-6 Infarct evolution to chronic phase.
A. NCCT at 3 days: hypodensity in anterior basal
ganglia and frontal middle cerebral territory (arrows); compression of frontal horn. **B.** CECT at
10 days: enhancement throughout infarct region;
lack of frontal horn compression. **C.** NCCT at 4
months: more marked and well-defined infarct hypodensity; enlargement of right frontal horn and
sylvian fissure with midline shift to right. **D.** CT
at higher level: enlargement of cortical sulci on
right with white-matter hypodensity.

⟵————————————————

Figure 14-7 Dilated cortical sulci from an old
cortical infarct: axial CECTs (**A** and **B**) show dilated left parietal sulci with normal white matter
density. On lower sections (not shown) the ipsilateral sylvian fissure is dilated. Ap digital subtraction angiogram (**C**) discloses complete occlusion of left internal carotid artery with spontaneous
interhemispheric cross filling.

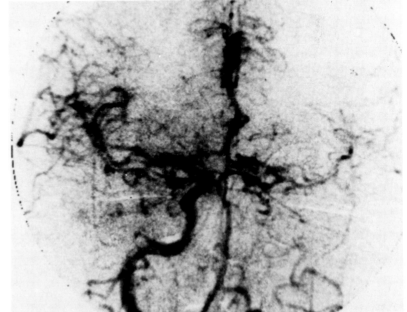

C

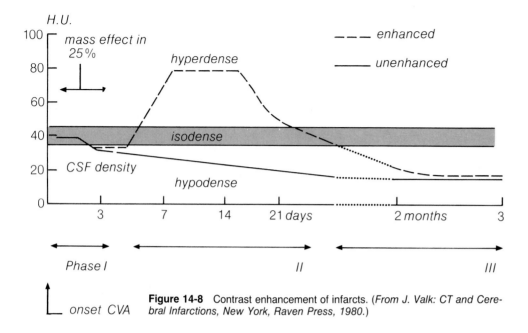

H.U.

Figure 14-8   Contrast enhancement of infarcts. (*From J. Valk: CT and Cerebral Infarctions, New York, Raven Press, 1980.*)

immediate enhancement on high-dose scans had this sequela.

Contrast administration either at high dose (Hayman 1981) or by rapid injection (Heinz 1979; Norman 1981) during the first 24 hours of an infarct or later may reveal characteristic nonenhancing abnormalities in an otherwise normal CT. With both these techniques the cotical gyri and deep gray matter in the infarct region may demonstrate a deficiency in contrast blush of the capillary bed which will be evident in the surrounding uninvolved gray matter and in homologous regions of the opposite hemisphere. With the high-dose technique advocated by Hayman et al. (1981), routine scanning methods which may utilize slow scanning times will demonstrate this change. With the rapid-injection technique (dynamic CT), however, 40–50 ml of contrast must be injected in about 5 seconds and four to six fast scans (5 seconds or less) obtained in rapid sequence, that is, 2 to 3 seconds apart (Fig. 14-9) (Norman 1981). This latter technique requires CT equipment with these special capabilities.

The intensity of enhancement begins to decline after the third week. It will usually persist for 6 to 7 weeks and with large infarcts up to 12 weeks (Weisberg 1980; Pullicino 1980). It may rarely last for as long as 9 months (Norton 1978).

The amount of radiographic contrast injected greatly influences the intensity of enhancement. Weisberg (1980) observed that only 5 percent of 100 patients with infarction demonstrated contrast enhancement after injection of a 50-ml bolus of a 60 percent iodinated contrast agent (14 g of iodine), whereas enhancement occurred in 65 percent of 100 patients after a drip infusion of 300 ml of a 30 percent contrast agent (42 g of iodine).

The mechanism of CT contrast enhancement appears to be identical to that producing delayed uptake in a radionuclide brain scan and is related to abnormality in the blood-brain barrier. Anderson et al. (1980), in a cat stroke model, found a strong positive correlation between tissue concentrations of ^{99m}Tc, sodium pertechnetate, and methylglucamine iothalamate in the area of infarct and the surrounding brain tissues at all time intervals, indicating a similarity in the temporal profile in these two studies. The radionuclide, however, revealed a consistently higher brain-blood ratio than the iodinated contrast material. This probably accounts for the slightly higher incidence of positive nuclide scans

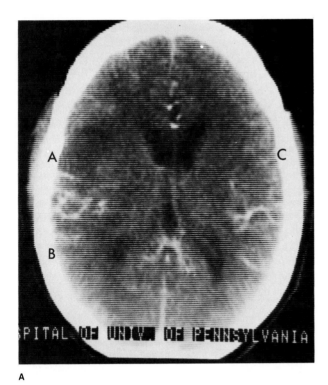

A

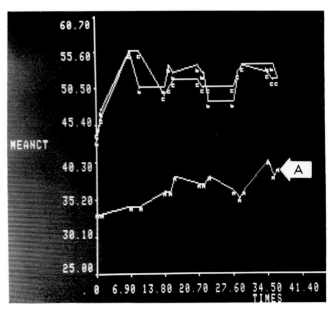

B

Figure 14-9 Ischemic changes on rapid-sequence CT: 2-day-old right middle cerebral territory infarct. **A.** High-speed CT scan (2.4-second scan time) 12 seconds after rapid intravenous injection of 40-ml contrast. Absence of surface vessels and cortical gyral blush in right posterior frontal region (*A*; normal cortical blush in regions *B* and *C*). **B.** Time-density curves following bolus contrast injection in region *A* (area of infarct) and regions *B* and *C* (normal cortical regions) in **A.** Time in seconds displayed on horizontal axis and CT density (H units) on vertical axis. Curves *B* and *C* (upper) display a rapid rise and decline of contrast density, reflecting normal initial circulation of the contrast bolus through the brain. The subsequent fluctuations in the curves reflect to a large extent recirculation of the bolus. Curve *Z* over the infarct indicates a slow circulation probably in association with a defective blood-brain barrier. It seems likely that some of the slow density increase of the infarct results from leakage of contrast from poorly filled, damaged capillaries.

than of standard-dose CECT scans. Depending on the dose of contrast given, at some time periods its brain-blood ratio may be below the level of tissue concentration that can be resolved on CT. Masdeu et al. (1977), in a study in humans, found a slightly higher incidence of positive radionuclide brain scans with infarction when compared with CECT at 2 weeks (72 percent versus 63 percent), using a standard contrast dose. Gado et al. (1975) have shown in human studies that CT contrast enhancement is primarily a result of contrast material in the extracellular space. Only a small degree of contrast enhancement can be explained by tissue hypervascularity, except perhaps when large blood pools are present, as with arteriovenous malformation.

The pathophysiologic abnormality that permits passage of contrast material into the extravascular space is a breakdown in the blood-brain barrier mechanisms of the capillary endothelium (Fishman 1975; Anderson 1980). Brain capillaries, unlike those in other parts of the body, restrict the passage of most large molecules through their walls because of tight endothelial cell junctions. Ischemic insult to the brain damages the blood-brain barrier, permitting large molecules to leak into the extravascular space. Although animal studies have shown that after infarction produced by a permanent arterial occlusion, capillary leakage may become evident at about 4 hours (O'Brien 1974), the CECT or the isotope brain scan will usually not become positive until after the first week (Blahd 1971; Inoue 1980). This appears to be related to persistent severe ischemia of the infarct region during the first week due to limited collateral or antegrade circulation. As a result of this low flow, insufficient contrast is delivered to the infarct for enhancement to be demonstrated even in the presence of a severely disturbed blood-brain barrier. By 7 to 10 days brain swelling is less, and this improves collateral circulation and results in sufficient leakage of contrast from infarct capillaries to be visualized. Concomitantly, considerable neovascular capillary proliferation is occurring around areas of necrosis, and these vessels have an incompetent blood-brain barrier (Dudley 1970; Yamaguchi 1971; Hayman 1980; Anderson 1980). This neovascularity is responsible for persistence of contrast enhancement during the next 4 to 8 weeks as the reparative process is completed.

Contrast enhancement may develop before the usual 7 to 10 days if perfusion at the infarct increases significantly (Hayman 1980). Large-molecule leakage at a disturbed blood-brain barrier varies directly with the systemic blood pressure level (Klatzo 1972). Contrast enhancement tends to occur early with embolic infarcts (after clot lysis) and with hemodynamic infarcts.

Contrast enhancement develops primarily in the cortex and deep gray masses (Inoue 1980). The gray matter is considerably more vascular than white matter. The cortex at the margins of the infarct tends to show enhancement earliest, since collateral circulation is initially more adequate to this region (Fig. 14-10). Delayed scans may demonstrate enhancement extending into the underlying white matter. This may be caused either by diffusion of contrast material leaked from the more numerous cortical

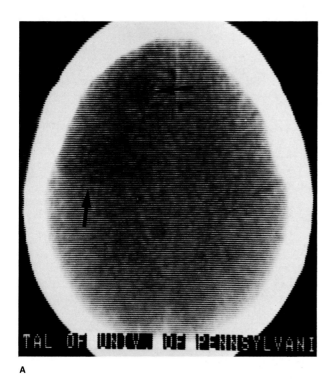

A

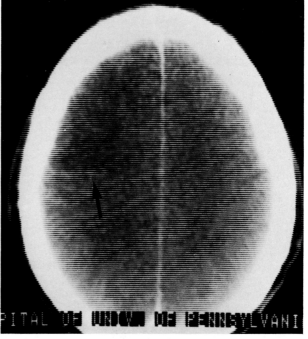

B

Figure 14-10   Marginal enhancement in 3-day-old infarct. **A.** NCCT demonstrating wedge-shaped hypodensity involving the cortex and white matter within the right middle cerebral artery territory (arrows).   **B.** CECT reveals slight linear enhancement at posterior margin of the infarct (arrow), most probably in the cortex of the infolded convolution. (See Figure 14-12 for progression of enhancement at day 12.)

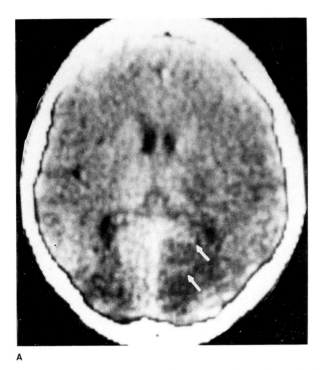

A

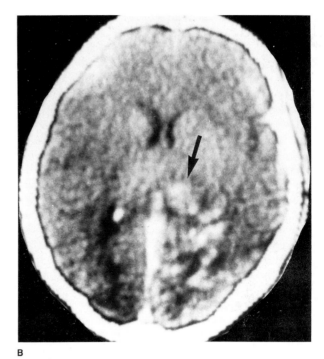

B

Figure 14-11 Heterogeneous enhancement of posterior cerebral artery territory infarct at day 10. **A.** NCCT reveals poorly defined hypodensity in left occipital and posterior thalamic region which contains bands and nodules of isodensity (arrows). **B.** CECT re-veals linear and nodular regions of enhancement roughly corresponding in location to the isodense areas within the infarct in **A.** Homogeneous region of enhancement in posterior thalamus (arrows).

capillaries or by its slower buildup in white matter related to lower blood flow in this tissue. Vasogenic edema fluid accumulates primarily in white matter, which may further decrease its circulation (Klatzo 1972).

The pattern of infarct enhancement usually has a heterogeneous appearance, which may be related to avascular regions of coagulation necrosis or to variability in the degree of collateral recirculation to different portions of the infarct (Fig. 14-11). At times the enhancing pattern is homogeneous, suggesting incomplete tissue necrosis and more uniform reper-fusion of the infarct (Fig. 14-6). With both these pat-terns the cortical ribbon and basal ganglia are the regions that predominantly enhance when imme-diate scans are obtained; with delayed scans after contrast (30 minutes to 3 hours), both homogeneous and heterogeneous enhancement may also develop in the white matter (Fig. 14-12). Norton (1978) re-ported that the patterns of enhancement were ho-mogeneous in 22 percent and heterogeneous in 59 percent of infarcts.

Infarct enhancement may also show a multifocal linear, bandlike configuration or central, peripheral, or ring patterns (Norton 1978; Pullicino 1980). The linear bandlike and the central patterns usually rep-resent different regions of enhancement in the cor-tical ribbon within and surrounding the area of in-farction (Fig. 14-12). Since the cortical ribbon extends into the depth of the brain a variable distance around the sulci, a region of cortical enhancement may ap-pear at times to be situated within white matter. The central pattern may also represent enhancement in the deep gray masses (Fig. 14-6). Differences in these enhancement patterns probably occur because of variations in collateral reperfusion and in the degree of necrosis in different regions of the infarct.

The peripheral enhancing pattern appears as a

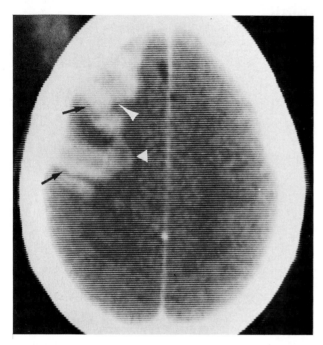

Figure 14-12 CECT: cortical ribbon (gyriform) enhancement (arrows) right middle cerebral artery territory at day 12. Some enhancement of white matter (arrowheads) on delayed CECT at 45 min. See NCCT, Figure 14-5, for isodense bands corresponding to the regions of cortical ribbon enhancement.

rim of enhancement which assumes a roughly hemispheric configuration about the lateral gray matter and deep white-matter margins of the infarct. This pattern would tend to develop about areas of hemispheric infarction when there is necrosis in both gray and white matter as indicated by homogeneous hypodensity in both these regions on NCCT.

The ringlike enhancing pattern is most commonly seen around necrotic infarcts in the basal ganglia (Fig. 14-13) but may also develop around those in the white-matter portion of a hemispheric infarct when there is incomplete nonnecrotic involvement of the overlying cortex. Basal ganglia infarcts may be small, resulting from a single lenticulostriate artery occlusion (Fig. 14-13), or large, when multiple lenticulostriate arteries are blocked secondary to proximal middle cerebral artery occlusion. With the latter, associated infarction may be present in the peripheral middle cerebral artery territory (Fig.

Figure 14-13 Ring enhancement in 9-day-old infarct in basal ganglia–anterior capsule region. **A.** NCCT reveals hypodensity involving left anterior capsule–basal ganglia region (arrow) with compression of adjacent frontal horn. CT was normal 7 days before. **B.** CECT demonstrates ring enhancement within outer margin of hypodensity (arrow).

14-14). Central coagulation necrosis commonly develops with basal ganglia infarcts because of inadequate collateral channels to this territory. Ring enhancement develops from the rich neovascular ingrowth in surrounding unaffected portions of the basal ganglia. When the ring pattern surrounds a necrotic white-matter infarct, the ring results from a combination of overlying cortical and peripheral deep white-matter neovascular ingrowth.

In most cases contrast enhancement will elevate a low-density region to one of higher-than-normal tissue density. Occasionally a zone of hypodensity becomes isodense with the surrounding brain on CECT (Fig. 14-15), and the infarction may not be recognized if only CECT is obtained. Wing et al. (1976) noted this postcontrast normalization phenomenon occurring in about 5 percent of recent infarcts. Conversely, they also observed that in 11 percent of the infarcts that enhanced, the NCCT was normal (Fig. 14-16).

The central, peripheral, and ring enhancement patterns present an appearance which may strongly resemble that of tumor or abscess. With infarction, however, most of the mass effect has usually resolved when enhancement appears, and the entire lesion (low density and area of enhancement) is confined to the territory of one vascular distribution in a wedge-shaped or rectangular pattern. There is usually also involvement of cortex. The combination of these changes, which are generally not present

Figure 14-14 Left basal ganglionic, middle cerebral artery, and right anterior ganglionic infarct at day 16, secondary to bilateral middle cerebral artery emboli from cardiomyopathy (subsequent autopsy confirmation). **A.** NCCT: hypodensity of left basal ganglionic and presylvian region (arrows) with compression of frontal horn. **B.** CECT demonstrates irregular ring enhancement of left basal ganglia (arrow) along with patchy enhancement in the left cortex (arrowhead) and in the right anterior basal ganglia.

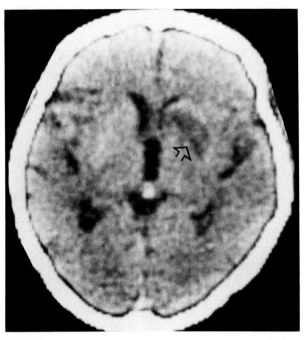

A

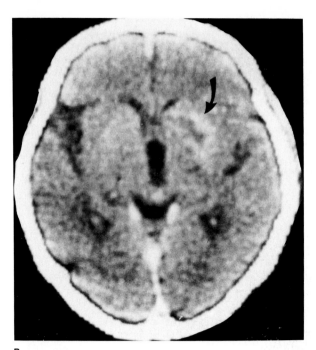

B

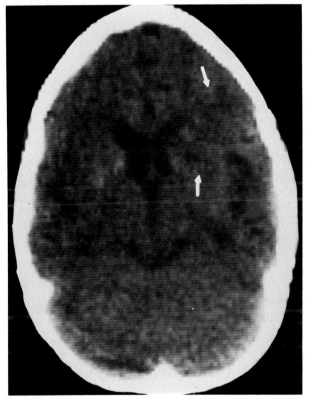

A

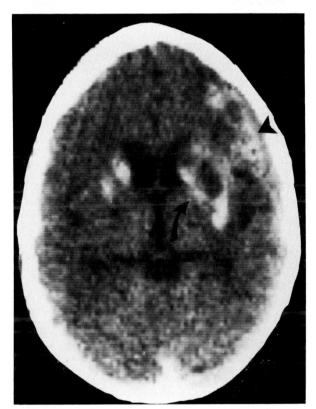

B

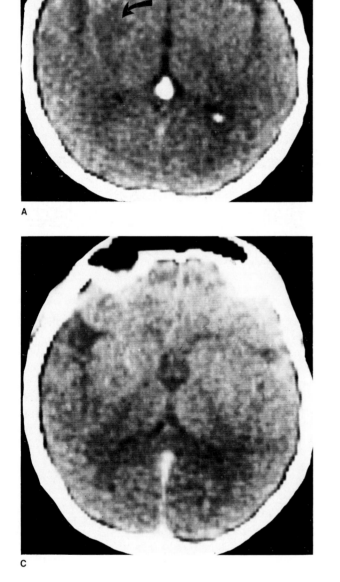

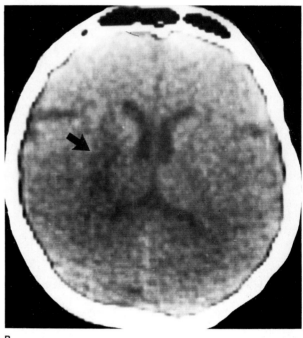

Figure 14-15   Masking of recent infarct with enhancement. **A** and **B.** NCCT, contiguous sections: large right basal ganglia–capsular hypodensity (arrows).   **C.** CECT: region of infarct hypodensity in **A** and **B** isodense after enhancement. Similar change was noted on adjacent sections.

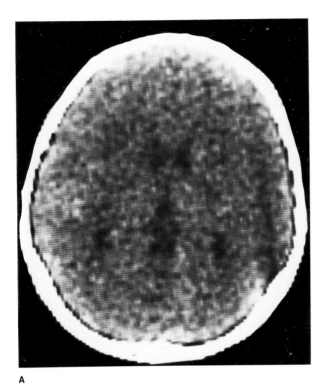

A

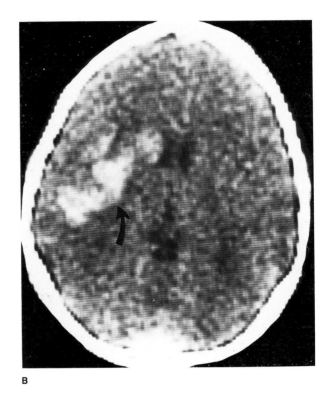

B

Figure 14-16 Enhancement of isodense middle cerebral artery territory infarct. **A.** NCCT: no definite abnormality evident. **B.** CECT: extensive enhancement in basal ganglia and parasylvian region.

with tumor or inflammatory disease, should in most cases reliably differentiate these conditions. If the diagnosis is still uncertain, follow-up CT study should clearly differentiate infarction from the other conditions. With infarction the enhancement usually disappears or markedly decreases in 3 to 4 weeks and atrophic changes develop over the next 1 to 3 months, as evidenced by focal ventricular dilatation and enlargement of overlying cortical sulci.

Weisberg (1980) observed that patients in whom the infarct showed enhancement had a better prognosis than those without enhancement: there were no deaths in a group of 50 patients who had enhancement, whereas 5 of 35 patients without enhancement died after their cerebral infarction. Functional recovery from motor, sensory, visual, and language disturbances was better for patients who showed enhancement and whose follow-up scans showed no residual low-density area, indicating ab-

sence of brain necrosis. These findings are in contrast to those of Pullicino and Kendall (1980), who recently reported that enhancing infarcts in their series had a significantly *poorer* prognosis than those without enhancement. They also found that enhancement was more common with larger infarcts and in those that had mass effect. These two factors would probably account for the more adverse prognosis associated with enhancement in their series.

Embolic Infarction

Embolic infarction is probably much more frequent than concluded on clinical grounds. Adams and Vander Eecken (1953) indicate that it is responsible for 50 percent of infarcts. Lhermitte et al. (1970) found in an autopsy study that 68 percent of middle cerebral artery occlusions were embolic in origin. Cerebral emboli frequently originate from heart disease and from atheromatous disease in the aorta or the carotid or vertebral arteries.

Yock (1981) recently identified emboli on NCCT in the middle and anterior cerebral arteries. They appeared as a focal hyperdensity at the usual location near major bifurcations in these vessels. The emboli had peak attenuation values of 84 to 214 HU, which indicated that most consisted of calcific material with or without thrombus. Those with a density of less than 95 HU may represent only dense clot.

With embolic infarction, the temporal evolution of early CT changes is different from those seen with atherosclerotic thrombotic infarcts. Whereas atherosclerotic occlusion usually results in a relatively permanent arterial obstruction, the embolic occlusion frequently fragments and undergoes lysis between the first and fifth day, resulting in reestablishment of normal antegrade circulation. This exposes the infarcted brain tissue to a much higher perfusion pressure than was present before clot lysis, when circulation depended on the adequacy of collateral channels. The hemodynamic consequences of clot lysis are responsible for the differences in the CT alterations with embolic infarction. The CT scan performed prior to lysis of an embolus will be similar to that present with an atherosclerotic occlusion, except that there may be infarcts in more than one vascular distribution of approximately the same age (Fig. 14-17). After fragmentation and dissolution of the embolus, the rise in perfusion pressure results in a marked increase in blood flow in and around the infarcted tissue, which frequently becomes higher than normal, and increased breakdown of the blood-brain barrier. This hyperemia develops because there is a loss of normal autoregulatory control of blood flow in the infarct region.

Autoregulation is a unique intrinsic property of normal cerebral vasculature which maintains blood flow at a constant level over a wide range of arterial pressures. This control is located mainly in the arterioles, which constrict with rising pressure and dilate with falling pressure. In the normal person the limits of autoregulation extend over a mean arterial pressure ranging from about 50 mmHg to 140 mmHg. The control of this mechanism appears to

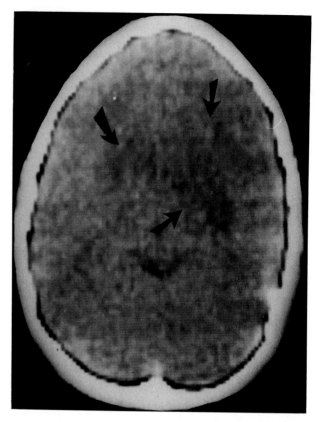

Figure 14-17   Bilateral embolic middle cerebral artery territory infarctions at 36 hours (same patient as in Figure 14-14). Large, poorly defined hypodensity involving basal ganglia and posterior frontal region on left (arrows). Similar but smaller area of hypodensity on right (arrowhead).

be mediated through an intrinsic myotonic stretch reflex in the arteriolar wall. In addition, changes in blood and tissue chemical factors such as carbon dioxide, lactic acid, and molecular oxygen concentrations may alter arteriolar diameter and affect autoregulation. Increased carbon dioxide and lactic acid concentrations and decreased oxygen tension cause vasodilation. Vessels with loss of autoregulation may lose their response to these chemical regulators. Infarction, as well as other conditions which cause brain injury such as trauma, infection, subarachnoid hemorrhage, and tumor, results in loss of normal autoregulation and varying degrees of vasoparalysis in the vascular bed of the affected region.

Loss of autoregulation may persist for several weeks following infarction; its duration is dependent on the severity of the ischemic injury. During this time circulation in these regions passively follows changes in perfusion pressure, as the arterioles no longer have the capacity to dilate or constrict in response to blood pressure change. The local tissue acidosis which develops within the area of infarction due to buildup of acid metabolites causes vasoparalysis (Myer 1957; Lassen 1966; Kassik 1968). This results in arteriolar dilatation, with blood flow becoming markedly increased with the reestablishment of normal perfusion pressure. Lassen (1966) has characterized this hyperemia as "luxury perfusion," because blood flow to the tissues is above its normal metabolic requirements. The *hyperemic (luxury perfusion) reaction* associated with loss of autoregulation becomes evident only after the return of normal perfusion pressure to the region of infarction, as will occur after lysis of an embolic occlusion. With persistent arterial occlusion this reaction is not seen, except possibly at the margins of the infarct, which could be supplied by antegrade flow through nonoccluded vessels. Not infrequently some degree of hypertension develops after infarction, which produces further arteriolar dilatation, resulting in a higher rate of blood flow. Cerebral angiography in the first few weeks after dissolution of an embolus usually reveals dilated cortical arterioles and gyral hyperemia associated with early filling of regional draining veins (Fig. 14-18) (Cronqvist 1967, 1968; Ferris 1966; Irino 1977*a*, 1977*b*; Leeds 1973; Pitts 1964). Concomitantly the radionuclide brain scan will demonstrate a region of high activity in the dynamic flow sequence (Yarnell 1975; Soin 1976). Focal elevation of cerebral blood flow may also be revealed with the Xe 133 technique (Cronqvist 1967, 1968; Hoedt-Rasmussen 1967; Paulson 1970).

Continued development and recent refinement of the stable xenon inhalation method utilizing CT, since its introduction in 1978, have made this technique an advanced and clinically useful method for measuring cerebral blood flow. It has been utilized in ischemia from cerebrovascular diseases, vasoregulatory alterations, and secondary to aneurysm bleed (Fig. 14-19). It also is useful in coma state, brain

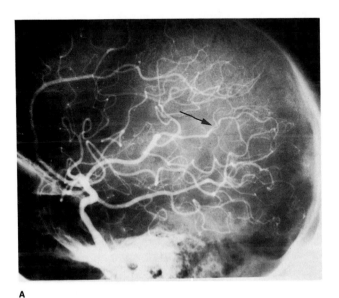 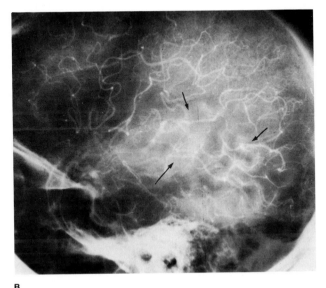

A   **B**

Figure 14-18 Embolic infarction reactive hyperemia (luxury perfusion) at day 5 following major clot lysis and reestablishment of antegrade circulation. **A.** Lateral right carotid angiogram, mid-arterial phase, revealing small embolic fragment partially occluding the angular gyrus artery distally (arrow). **B.** Lateral right carotid angiogram, late arterial phase, revealing early appearance of a prominent gyriform capillary blush (reactive hyperemia) in the posterior temporal–inferior parietal region (arrows). (*Continued on p. 664.*)

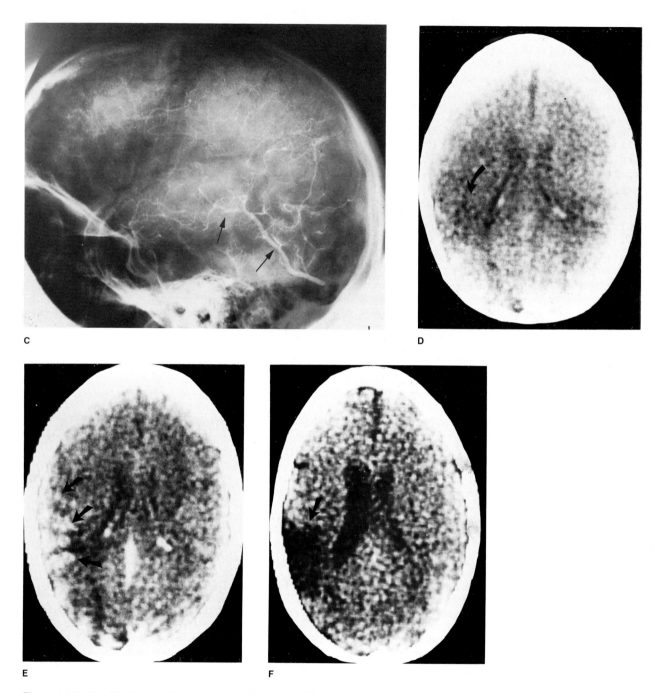

Figure 14-18 (*Cont.*)   **C.** Lateral right carotid angiogram, capillary phase, revealing early venous filling (luxury perfusion) in the posterior temporal–inferior parietal region (arrows).   **D.** NCCT at time of angiogram. Suggestion of ill-defined slight hypodensity in right posterior temporal–parietal region (arrow).   **E.** CECT: gyriform enhancement in right posterior temporal–parietal region (arrows).   **F.** NCCT 4 months after stroke. Well-defined region of marked hypodensity involving cortex and underlying white matter (arrow) in the right posterior temporal–parietal region, associated with ventricular dilatation.

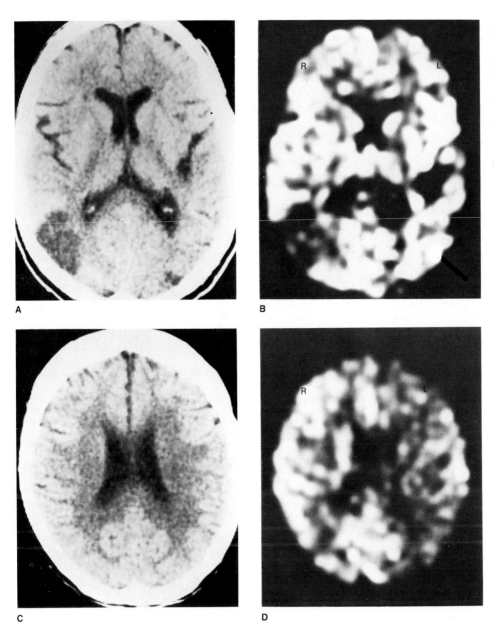

Figure 14-19 Xe/CT cerebral blood flow: **A** (NCCT) and **B** (Xe/CT) show an old right occipital infarct and hyperperfusion on the left frontotemporal lobe representing "luxury perfusion" for recent infarct. **C** (NCCT) and **D** (Xe/CT) demonstrate normal CT and decreased left hemispheric blood flow due to vasospasm and vasculitis. (*Courtesy of GE Co. Medical Systems, Milwaukee, Wisconsin.*)

death, in closed head injury or seizure disorders, and in degenerative syndromes such as acute progressive dementia, Alzheimer's disease, and multiple sclerosis (Wolfson 1985). This technique, although limited, has promise of widespread clinical applications because of its relatively high anatomical resolution, low cost, and ease of procedure.

Infarct hyperemia (luxury perfusion) generally causes some regions which were hypodense on CT obtained before revascularization to become isodense or slightly hyperdense on NCCT (Fig. 14-20). This change develops mainly in the cortex and deep gray matter because these regions have a large capillary bed which passively dilates after reperfusion.

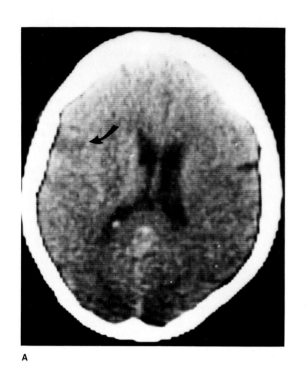

A

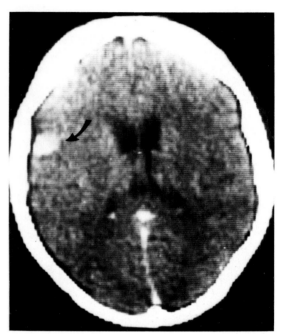

B

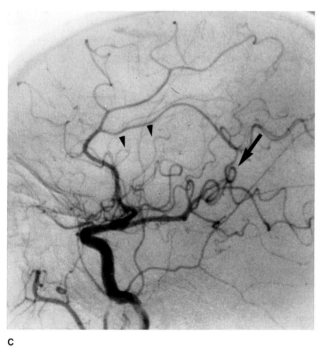

C

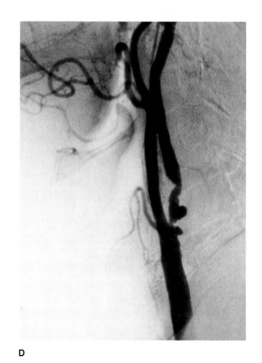

D

Rapid-sequence CT scanning after bolus contrast injection may demonstrate the luxury perfusion reaction (Fig. 14-21). Besides the elevation in blood volume, some of the cortical density increase may be the result of the petechial hemorrhages (Inoue 1980). Because of its much lower capillary volume, the white matter does not appreciably contribute to the hyperemic reaction. The density increase in the cortex is usually diffuse but may be spotty, depending on the degree of fragmentation and lysis of the embolus. The NCCT may have a normal appearance, but usually the underlying white matter remains hypodense (Fig. 14-18).

Prominent enhancement develops following lysis of the embolus, usually appearing as a cortical gyral pattern (Fig. 14-18) with frequent involvement of the basal ganglia. The high reperfusion pressure potentiates spread of enhancement into the adjacent white matter (Fig. 14-21). Enhancement appears in most cases by the fifth day and frequently develops earlier, depending on the time it takes for clot lysis to occur. Enhancement is related to disturbance in the blood-brain barrier and, to a lesser extent, hyperemia. Kohlmeyer (1978), evaluating the relationships between CT and cerebral blood flow, found that enhancement was usually not associated with luxury perfusion unless the enhancement develops during the first 3 to 5 days after the stroke. These observations suggest that early enhancement, since it is associated with increased cerebral blood flow, may indicate embolic infarction after clot lysis. Enhancement and luxury perfusion are potentiated by high reperfusion pressure. Hayman et al. (1981) re-

cently described an ominous enhancement pattern in infarcts 9 to 28 hours old that were mainly embolic in origin. The enhancement appeared 1 to 3 hours after intravenous infusion of 80 g of iodine. The enhancement pattern consisted of a large, frequently wedge-shaped, nonhomogeneous zone of increased density which involved the cortex and extended down through the white matter to the ventricle (Fig. 14-22). Over half the patients with this pattern (four of seven) subsequently developed hemorrhagic infarcts and died. No other "double dose" CECT pattern could be associated with development of hemorrhagic infarction.

Brain swelling is frequently present when enhancement develops with embolic infarcts. This is because enhancement usually becomes evident between the second and fifth day, a time period when infarct brain swelling is maximal. This is in contrast to the general lack of mass effect at the time enhancement appears with atherosclerotic thrombotic infarcts at 10 to 14 days. Brain swelling with embolic infarcts may further increase after the appearance of enhancement, because the increased perfusion pressure resulting from clot lysis potentiates the formation of vasogenic edema (Olsson 1971). In the extreme case, hemorrhagic infarction may develop which further increases the degree of mass effect.

HEMORRHAGIC INFARCTION This is in most instances an adverse sequela of embolic infarction related to the effects of high-pressure reperfusion of severe ischemic brain. Fisher and Adams (1951) found that in 66 hemorrhagic infarcts, only three were not clearly caused by embolism. Jorgensen and Torbik (1964) observed that 80 percent of embolic infarcts were found at autopsy to be hemorrhagic. Angiography in combination with CT has confirmed the relationship between fragmentation and lysis of the embolus and hemorrhagic infarction (Irino 1977*b*; Davis 1975, 1977). In the report of Davis et al. (1977), three patients with hemorrhagic infarction all had clinical evidence of an embolic stroke, and in two, cerebral angiography documented the embolic occlusion before there was clinical or CT evidence of the hemorrhagic infarct. In one patient, a repeat cerebral angiogram at the time of neurologic dete-

Figure 14-20 Embolic infarction, conversion on NCCT of hypodense tissue to isodensity after reestablishment of antegrade circulation. **A.** NCCT on day 3 reveals cortical hypodensity in the posterior frontal region (arrow). NCCT on day 8 fails to demonstrate hypodensity. **B.** CECT on day 8 reveals cortical enhancement (arrow) in region of hypodensity in **A.** **C.** Lateral carotid angiogram on day 9 demonstrates embolic occlusion of posterior inferior (arrow) and parietal branches (arrowheads) of middle cerebral artery tributary. Avascular parietal region fills well on subsequent films from distal anterior cerebral artery branches. There is relatively normal antegrade circulation into region of CT abnormality in posterior frontal area (arrowheads) suggesting previous lysis of embolic fragment. Large ulcerated plaque at origin of internal carotid artery is probable source of emboli (**D**).

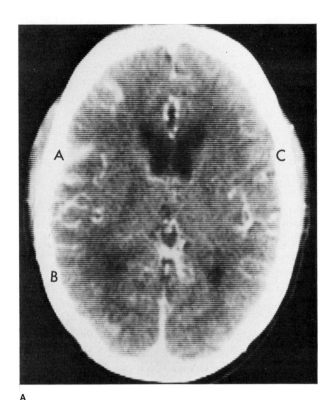

A

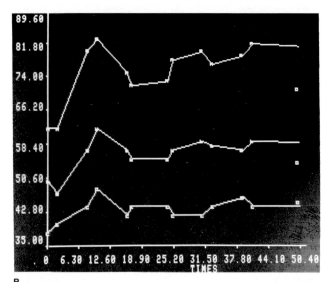

B

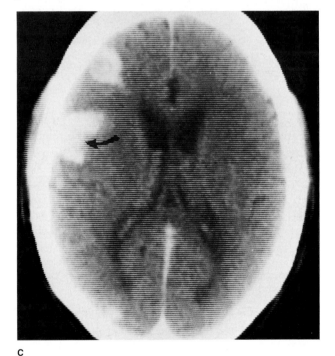

C

Figure 14-21 Hyperemic changes on rapid-sequence bolus injection CT. Probable embolic infarction at day 10. **A.** Rapid-sequence CT approximately 6 seconds after contrast bolus arrival at brain. Maximum vascular phase contrast density at this time. Highest cortical contrast density at location *A*, site of ischemic circulatory changes at day 2 (Fig. 14-9). Locations *B* and *C* over uninvolved cortical regions on previous CT. **B.** Time-density curves of locations, *A*, *B*, and *C* in **A**. Graph parameters are the same as in Figure 14-9*B*. Curve *A* (upper) demonstrates a more rapid and greater rise and a fall of contrast density than curves *B* (middle) and *C* (lower) during their first passage through the brain. Secondary density increase of curve *A* reflects tissue enhancement due to a defective blood-brain barrier and high tissue perfusion pressure. **C.** CT 30 minutes after **A**. Increased cortical enhancement (arrow) with spread of enhancement into adjacent white matter as evidenced by thickening of the cortical ribbon (compare with **A**) and obliteration of the intergyral white-matter hypodensity.

Figure 14-22 Enhancement on delayed high-contrast dose CT during the first day after the infarct. **A.** NCCT 20 hours after infarct reveals obliteration of the right sylvian fissure and ill-defined slight hypodensity in right posterior frontal region (arrow). **B.** Immediate high-contrast dose CT demonstrates absence of enhancement. **C.** Delayed high-dose CT 3 hours after **B**. Marked enhancement of the cortex in the right frontal region (short arrow) extending in a wedge-shaped fashion deep into the white matter in the middle and posterior-frontal region (large arrow). There is in addition enhancement in the region of the right basal ganglia. **D.** Autopsy section of brain 8 days later at same level as CT scans. There is hemorrhagic infarction in region of enhancement on delayed CT in **C** (arrows) and anemic infarction with small cortical petechial hemorrhage in nonenhanced region of adjacent middle cerebral artery territory. (*From Hayman LA et al. 1981.*)

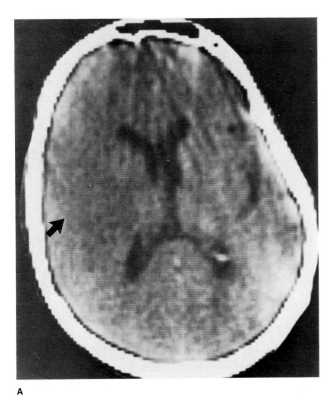

A

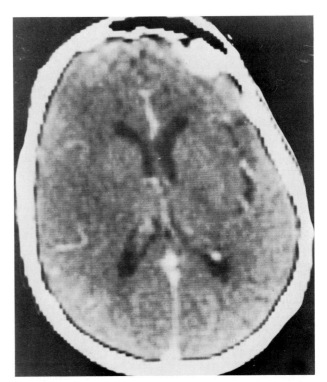

B

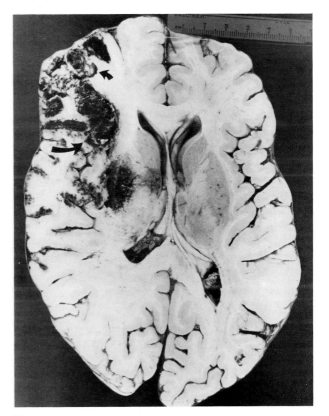

C

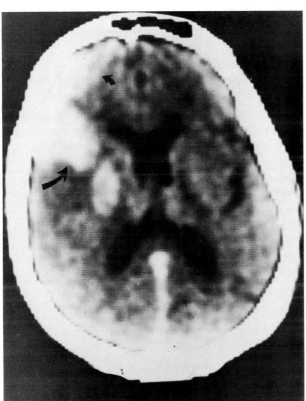

D

rioration and appearance of the hemorrhagic infarct on CT revealed lysis of a previously demonstrated embolic occlusion. Hemorrhagic infarction may also occur with atherosclerotic thrombotic infarcts in patients with coagulation disorders and in those on antithrombotic therapy (Wood 1958). The incidence of hemorrhagic infarction has been reported to range between 18 and 23 percent (Fisher 1951; Davis 1977; Hayman 1981).

Small areas of petechial hemorrhage are identified pathologically on the periphery of many otherwise bland infarcts, but in hemorrhagic infarcts the petechial hemorrhage is more marked and spread diffusely throughout, though predominantly in the cortex and deep gray matter (Adams 1968). It may involve only areas of cortex located in the depth of sulci. On occasion an area of frank hemorrhage develops from leakage of blood out of small arteries and capillaries into the perivascular spaces. Microscopically vessels may not show evidence of ischemic damage, which is usually very severe in the surrounding brain parenchyma.

Hemorrhagic infarct is more likely to develop when tissue necrosis is marked. In animal studies, prolonging the initial period of ischemia from 6 to 24 hours before reperfusion increases the incidence of hemorrhagic infarction from 40 to 60 percent (Kamijyo 1977). Increasing blood pressure (Laurent 1976) and the use of heparin (Wood 1958) have also been shown to result in hemorrhagic transformation of some infarcts produced by permanent arterial occlusions. Clinical experience with carotid endarterectomy has similarly shown that reestablishing increased perfusion pressure by surgical removal of the obstructing atheromatous plaque during the first several weeks after a recent infarct may cause conversion of an anemic into a hemorrhagic infarct.

In a serial CT study by Cronqvist (1976), the initial CT scan obtained during the first 5 days revealed only a low-density lesion within the brain in six out of seven patients who developed hemorrhagic infarcts. In one patient the initial scan at 2 days demonstrated hemorrhagic infarction. In the six with initial low-density lesions, hemorrhagic infarction became evident between 5 and 21 days after the onset of the stroke. In another study, Davis et al. (1977) reported that 10 of 12 stroke patients who developed secondary abrupt neurologic deterioration revealed hemorrhagic infarct on CT within 5 days of the initial stroke. Two of the patients had had earlier scans which showed no evidence of hemorrhage. Four developed the hemorrhagic infarct after 1 day, three after 2 days, one after 4 days, and two at 5 days.

The hemorrhagic infarct will in most instances reveal a very characteristic CT appearance, which can usually be readily differentiated from that of an intracerebral hematoma (Davis 1975). The hemorrhage primarily involves the cortex (Figs. 14-23, 14-24), either alone, as confluent petechiae, or with occasional secondary extension into the underlying white matter (Davis 1977). It may also involve the deep gray matter if the embolus initially arrests in the middle cerebral artery proximal to or at the origins of the lenticulostriate arteries. Cortical hemorrhage generally appears as a ribbon or bandlike region of slightly to moderately increased density. It has unsharp margins and assumes the wavy configuration of the cortical gyri. The surrounding white matter is hypodense, and its involvement is limited to the same vascular distribution as the region of hemorrhage. This pattern may be diffuse over a large region of the cortex or may be more localized to the depth of one or more sulci. The hemorrhage may be nonhomogeneous or speckled in appearance (Fig. 14-25). At times the petechial hemorrhage is mild and, because of volume averaging, may elevate the low density only up to the isodense range (Alcala 1978). If the hemorrhage extends into the white matter, it may resemble an intracerebral hematoma, from which differentiation may be difficult. An intracerebral hematoma is usually homogeneously dense, with a rounded to oval configuration and sharp, distinct borders. White-matter extension of hemorrhagic infarct, in contrast, may be wedge-shaped to rectangular and is not usually homogeneously dense; its border may be somewhat indistinct.

On CECT, hemorrhagic infarction will usually develop contrast enhancement in the already dense cortical and basal ganglia and, to a variable degree, in the surrounding isodense cortex (Fig. 14-25). The intracerebral hematoma does not show enhancement in the area of hemorrhage.

Clinical deterioration and increased mass effect

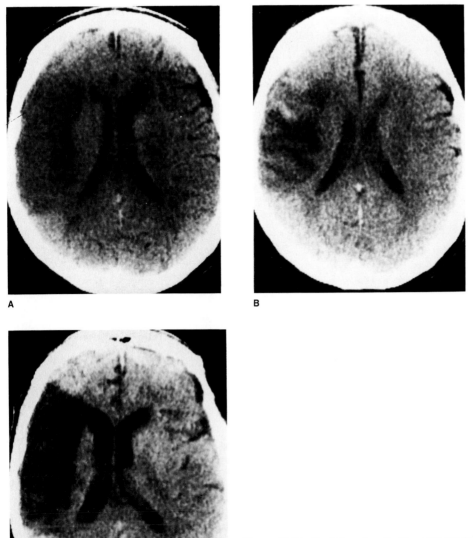

Figure 14-23 Evolution of cortical hemorrhagic infarct in 73-year-old female. **A.** NCCT 2 days after onset of stroke demonstrates well-defined hypodensity in right frontoparietal cortex. **B.** NCCT 10 days later shows mild cortical hemorrhage. **C.** NCCT 5 months later reveals encephalomalacia with ipsilateral ventriculography. DSA study disclosed R ICA occlusion and severe stenosis of L ICA.

usually occur when hemorrhagic infarction develops; they are related to the extravasated blood in the brain and the increase in vasogenic edema resulting from the higher perfusion pressure at the infarct after clot lysis.

Hemodynamic Infarction

Cerebral ischemic episodes may develop in patients with vasoocclusive disease when there are temporary alterations in circulatory dynamics (Denny-

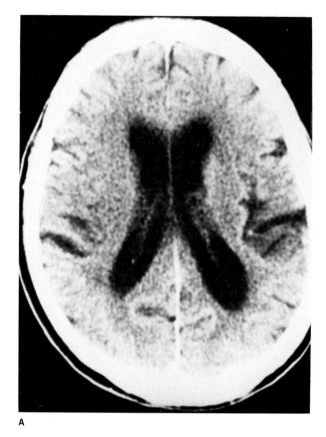

A

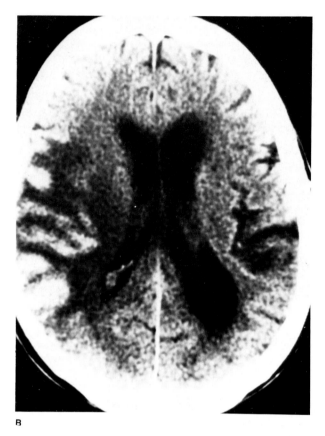

B

Figure 14-24 Hemorrhagic cortical infarct. **A.** NCCT, on admission, shows no discernible abnormality. **B.** NCCT, 2½ weeks later, exhibits cortical hemorrhage in typical gyral pattern with worsening of clinical status; 6 months and 18 months following, CTs (not shown) revealed an area of encephalomalacia with ipsilateral ventriculomegaly.

Brown 1960; Brierley 1976). This mainly occurs in older patients with hypertension or cardiac arrhythmias who have a fixed vascular lesion in an extra- or intracranial artery (Ruff 1981). The vascular lesion could be either a severe stenosis or an occlusion of long standing.

Cerebral blood-flow studies have demonstrated disturbed autoregulation in this group of patients (Kindt 1967); any decrease in perfusion pressure, therefore, may cause a proportional decrease in cerebral blood flow either focally or diffusely. Depending on the length of time the perfusion pressure is reduced and its severity, the patient may incur a transient ischemic attack, a reversible ischemic neurologic deficit, or an infarction. In many of these patients, the stroke occurs while they are asleep at night, probably brought about by a nocturnal reduction of blood pressure. In some hypertensive persons, a reduction in blood pressure, even to only a normotensive level, can result in severe focal cerebral ischemia in the brain already perfused through a stenosed artery or collateral circulation. Cardiac arrhythmias, which can reduce both cardiac output and blood pressure, may cause hemodynamic infarction. Not infrequently, when a patient is first examined after a stroke, blood pressure has returned to its usual level and the cardiac arrhythmia has cleared. Correction of the hemodynamic alteration reestablishes brain-perfusion pressure at its normal level and accounts for the early appearance

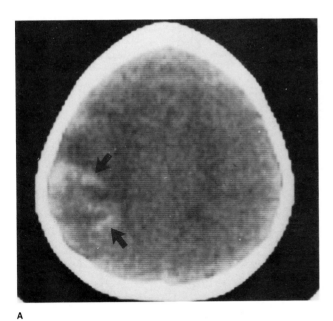

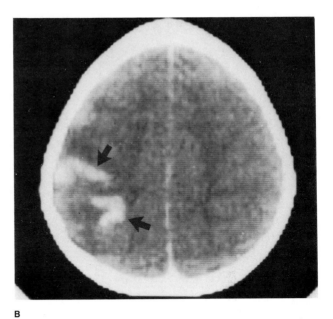

A

B

Figure 14-25 Contrast enhancement of cortical hemorrhagic infarct. **A.** NCCT: patchy gyriform cortical hemorrhagic involvement in the right superior posterior parietal region (arrows). Ischemic infarct hypodensity involving adjacent cortex and underlying white matter. **B.** CECT: enhancement in region of hemorrhagic cortical ribbon (arrows).

on angiography of luxury perfusion and abnormalities in the blood-brain barrier on CT (Fig. 14-26).

The regions of the brain most severely affected by hemodynamic infarction are the border zones, or watershed area (Romanul 1964; Brierley 1976), located at the junctions of the anterior, middle, and posterior cerebral artery circulations. Border zones are most vulnerable to ischemic injury from a generalized reduction in perfusion pressure, because they are the terminal areas of supply of each major artery and therefore have the lowest perfusion pressure in these vascular distributions. If significant occlusive disease develops in the large arteries at the base of the brain or extracranially, ischemic damage in the watershed region may develop from even a mild reduction in blood pressure, because the occlusive disease reduces distal perfusion pressure to a level at which autoregulation produces maximum vasodilatation. At this point no further compensation for additional pressure reduction is possible, particularly in the watershed zone, and ischemic injury occurs. The watershed region tends to shift into the territory of the involved vascular system. The parietal occipital border zone is the region most susceptible to hemodynamic ischemic injury, as it is the most peripheral region of the anterior, middle, and posterior cerebral arterial circulations to the cerebral hemispheres.

On CT, the cortical luxury-perfusion pattern in hemodynamic infarction is similar to that seen with embolic infarction after clot lysis but occurs earlier and in a different distribution. It is usually present when the patient is first seen during the initial 24 hours. NCCT will in most instances appear normal but may show slight density reduction in the white matter. This may only become evident in later scans or may not develop at all. The ischemic injury frequently remains localized to the cortex, which histologically reveals incomplete infarction, with the damage limited to neurons in the third or the fifth and sixth cortical layers, or both. This variety of infarction is frequently referred to as *laminar necrosis*. If the ischemic insult is severe, all layers of the cortex will be involved, along with the underlying white

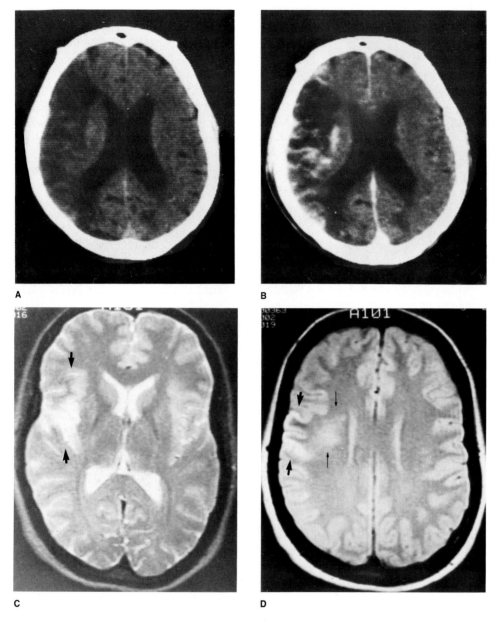

A

B

C

D

Figure 14-26 Middle cerebral artery territory infarct with gyral contrast enhancement on (**A**) NCCT and (**B**) CECT. Minimal, if any, mass effect on the lateral ventricle is noted in spite of extensive area of exuberant enhancement. These findings are unusual for brain tumor. **C** and **D.** MRIs (T_2-WI) in another case demonstrates ischemic infarction of the right frontoparietal cortex (arrows). Minimal subtle involvement of the adjacent white matter (small arrows) is also noted.

matter (Brierley 1976). On CECT, a cortical gyral blush develops, predominantly in the parietal-occipital watershed region (Fig. 14-26). Enhancement may persist for only a few days or may last for several weeks, depending on the severity of the initial ischemic damage.

Hemodynamic watershed infarction may on oc-

casion be hemorrhagic in nature (Brierley 1976). This may occur if the initial ischemia is very severe or the reperfusion pressure is high, as may develop with hypertensive disease.

The chronic change of incomplete (laminary) cortical infarction on CT is sulcal dilatation (Fig. 14-7). It generally becomes evident after 2 to 3 months in the region where the gyral enhancement pattern was demonstrated. In cases with more profound ischemia resulting in complete cortical infarction and white-matter involvement, the affected cortex, initially isodense, becomes hypodense during the next 4 to 6 weeks; the underlying white matter, which may originally have been slightly hypodense, becomes a more sharply demarcated region of hypodensity. The adjacent portion of the lateral ventricle usually dilates. Some surrounding sulci may also enlarge because of incomplete infarction in the bordering cortex.

Another CT pattern associated with hemodynamic infarction is hypodensity involving mainly the deep periventricular white matter. This alteration tends to occur when there is a long-standing carotid occlusion and chronic ischemia in the hemisphere from poor collateral circulation (Fig. 14-27). It is not

entirely clear why the white matter is preferentially involved in these circumstances. It is possible that with chronic ischemia there is a change in the blood-flow relationship between the cortex and white matter, with greater flow going to cortical areas. This might occur because of a more pronounced effect of autoregulatory vasodilatation in the cortical vascular bed, which is about four times greater than that in the white matter, and the potentially higher perfusion pressure in the cortical arterioles, which are closer to the supplying vessels on the brain surface. The combination of these two factors would tend to result in shunting of circulation away from the white matter. A reduction in arterial perfusion pressure might then cause a significant ischemia only in the white matter and not in the cortex.

This white-matter involvement is primarily located adjacent to the superior lateral border of the

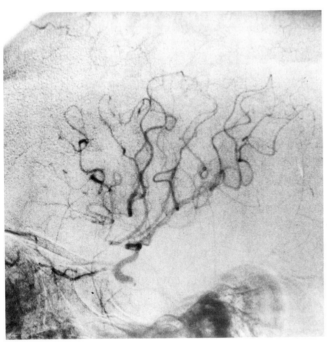

A

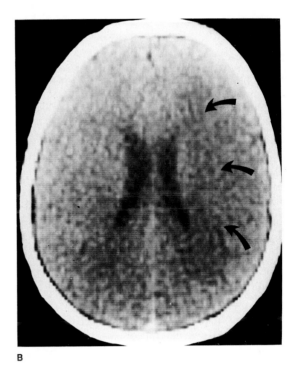

B

Figure 14-27 Deep watershed infarct. **A.** Lateral carotid angiogram, mid-arterial phase. Internal carotid artery completely occluded in neck at origin (not shown). Retrograde ophthalmic artery flow to intracranial carotid and middle cerebral arteries. Very slow filling and washout of middle cerebral artery branches. **B.** NCCT 3 days after stroke: poorly defined diffuse slight hypodensity in left periventricular white matter (arrows). (*Continued on p. 676.*)

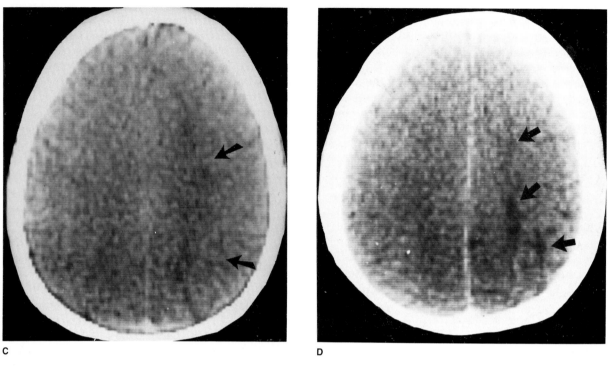

C   D

Figure 14-27 *(Cont.)*   **C.** NCCT, day 3, at supraventricular level: slight white-matter hypodensity on the left extends more superficially in parietal-occipital watershed region (arrows).   **D.** NCCT at 4 months: well-defined more hypodense region in left central white matter extending superficially in parietal-occipital watershed region (arrows).

lateral ventricle, in the region of the body and trigone (Fig. 14-27). This area is not only a terminal field of supply for the penetrating (ventriculopetal) transmedullary white-matter arteries originating on the brain surface but is also a deep watershed zone between these arteries and the short arterial branches radiating outward from the lateral ventricle (ventriculofugal tributaries) (De Reuck 1971). The ventriculofugal arteries originate from two sources. They are the terminal tributaries of the lenticulostriate artery branches which supply the lateral aspect of the caudate nucleus as well as tributaries of branches from the anterior choroidal and posterior lateral choroidal arteries which supply the ventricular wall.

A severe episode of hypotension or reduction in cardiac output, such as may occur following myocardial infarction or during surgery, can result in extensive bilateral cortical infarction with accentuation in the watershed distribution even in patients without preexisting vascular disease (Brierley 1976). White-matter involvement is not usual but may occur in cases with severe circulatory deficiency or, more commonly, if there is associated hypoxia (De Reuck 1978). In addition, the terminal territories of the lenticulostriate supply to the basal ganglia may also be affected. The main areas of basal ganglia involvement are the inferomedial portion of the head of the caudate nucleus, the upper and outer border of the head and body of the caudate nucleus, and the upper part of the anterior third of the putamen (Brierley 1976). The thalamus is usually not significantly affected. Watershed infarction may also occur in the cerebellum, in the boundary between the areas supplied by the superior cerebellar and posterior inferior cerebellar arteries. In the acute phase the graymatter regions may be isodense on NCCT and show enhancement on CECT. In the chronic stage, depending on the severity of the initial oligemia, the gray matter may demonstrate hypodense necrotic areas or diffuse atrophic change. White matter may become hypodense, particularly in the periventricular regions.

Intracerebral Arteriolar Disease

Occlusive disease of the intraparenchymal arterioles may be the sole or major vascular involvement in several disease entities. *Arteriolosclerosis* is the pathologic process mainly encountered in patients with long-standing hypertension. The long, penetrating lenticulostriate arteries and arterioles supplying the internal capsule and basal ganglia region are the ones most commonly involved with this disease process (Prineas 1966; Fisher 1979). To a lesser extent the penetrating arteries to the brainstem and cerebral white matter are affected. Pathologically, arteriolosclerosis resembles atherosclerosis of the larger arteries in that there may be fibroblastic intimal proliferation with increased collagen fibers, but in addition wall thickening and stenosis from hyalin deposition in the subintimal, medial, and outer layers of the arteries also occurs. Microaneurysms develop from wall weakening due to the hyalin degeneration (Russell 1963; Cole 1967) and may lead to thrombosis of the vessel or intracerebral hemorrhage, both of which are prevalent in hypertensive persons.

Amyloid or *congophilic angiopathy* is another type of small-vessel disease which occurs with increasing incidence in the elderly. It is reported to be present in 46 percent of those over 70 years of age (Vinters 1981). The disease, unlike arteriolosclerosis, affects only the intracortical arterioles and does not involve the penetrating arteries to the white matter, basal ganglia nuclei, brainstem, or cerebellum. The occipital and parietal cortex is most commonly involved. The disease is associated with Alzheimer's plaques in patients without a familial history of Alzheimer's disease. Dementia is commonly associated with amyloid angiopathy. Occasionally, intracerebral hemorrhage situated mainly in the cortex and superficial white matter and frequently associated with subarachnoid hemorrhage occurs, in contrast to hypertensive intracerebral hemorrhages, which are usually centered more deeply in the white matter and rarely involve the cortex or extend into the subarachnoid space (Wagle 1984; Gilles 1985).

Several varieties of collagen arteritis may affect the small intracerebral arteries, including polyarteritis nodosa, lupus erythematosus, and Wegener's granulomatosis. Granulomatous arteritis, infectious or allergic, primarily involves the intracerebral arterioles but may affect the larger surface arteries. Some forms of central nervous system infection, including viral meningoencephalitis, purulent meningitis, mucormycosis meningitis, and syphilitic angiitis, may have prominent intraparenchymal arterial involvement.

LACUNAR INFARCTS The arteriolosclerotic vascular disease process associated with the chronically hypertensive patient frequently produces small lacunar infarcts, most commonly located in the basal ganglia–internal capsule territory. These are in the distribution of the six to twelve lenticulostriate penetrating arteries which arise from the proximal anterior and middle cerebral arteries. Other arteries to this territory arise from the anterior choroidal artery. Severe neurologic deficit may develop from occlusion or significant stenosis of even one of these small penetrating vessels (Fisher 1965), which range in size at their origin from about 0.2 to 0.8 mm in diameter. The lacunar infarcts may be as small as 0.5 cm in maximum diameter or less or as large as 2.5 cm in maximum diameter. The variation in infarct size is determined by the site of lenticulostriate artery occlusion (origin or peripheral branch) and the caliber of the individual artery at its origin (Fisher 1979).

Lacunar infarcts assume a cylindrical to conical configuration and extend through a portion of the basal ganglia and internal capsule, often terminating in the periventricular white matter (Fig. 14-28). The location of the infarct in the basal ganglia depends on which striate artery is occluded (Manelfe 1981). When a middle cerebral artery lenticulostriate branch is occluded, the infarct may involve a greater or lesser portion of either the putamen along with the superior and periventricular part of the knee and posterior limb of the internal capsule and body

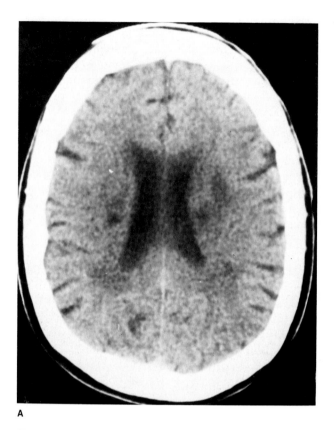

A

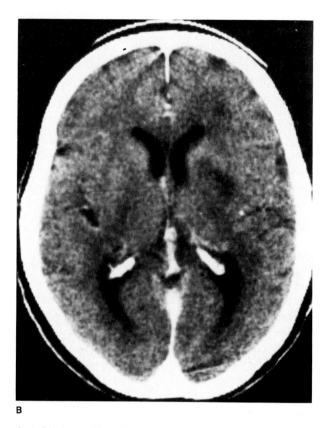

B

Figure 14-28 **A.** Old right paraventricular white matter infarct presents as a well-demarcated, discrete hypodense lesion. Recent left infarcts show slightly less hypodense and relatively poorly mar-ginated lesions with mild mass effect.   **B.** Acute infarction of left basal ganglia involving the globus pallidus and left frontal white matter.

of the caudate nucleus (Fig. 14-15), or the lateral aspects of the head of the caudate nucleus and anterior limb of the internal capsule. When the anterior cerebral striate artery (recurrent artery of Heubner) is involved, the medial inferior portion of both the head of the caudate nucleus and anterior limb of the internal capsule are affected. When anterior choroidal striate arteries are occluded, the infarct involves the globus pallidus, (Fig. 14-28), the inferior part of the knee and posterior limb of the internal capsule, and the retrolenticular capsular fibers. Less frequently, lacunar infarcts involve the thalamus. Brainstem lacunar infarcts are commonly observed pathologically but may escape detection on CT, especially in the early stage of small infarcts.

Larger lesions can be identified on CT (Fig. 14-29).

MRI clearly depicts anatomical details in the basal ganglia region and the brainstem (Fig. 14-30).

Depending on the size of the occluded lenticulostriate artery, the basal ganglia lacunar infarct may or may not be revealed in the acute phase by CT (Nelson 1980). Those less than 1 cm in size are usually not defined during the first week after the infarct but may become evident after 3 to 4 weeks when cystic encephalomalacic change has developed. Larger lesions are usually demonstrated by 48 hours, appearing as ill-defined oval regions of hypodensity with their longest dimension in the anterior posterior direction (Fig. 14-15). They lie within the confines of the basal ganglia and adjacent inter-

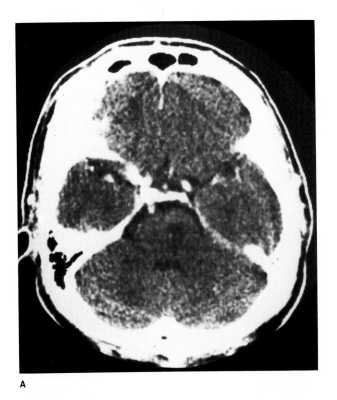

A

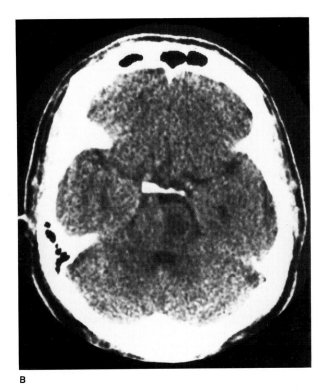

B

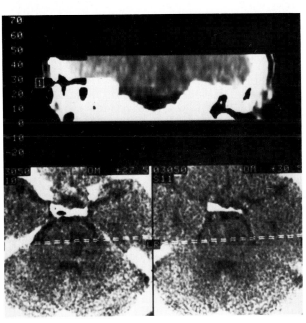

C

Figure 14-29 Acute brainstem infarcts. Acute left brainstem infarct with mild compression of the fourth ventricle (**A** and **B**). Coronal re-formation image (**C**) clarifies the exact location.

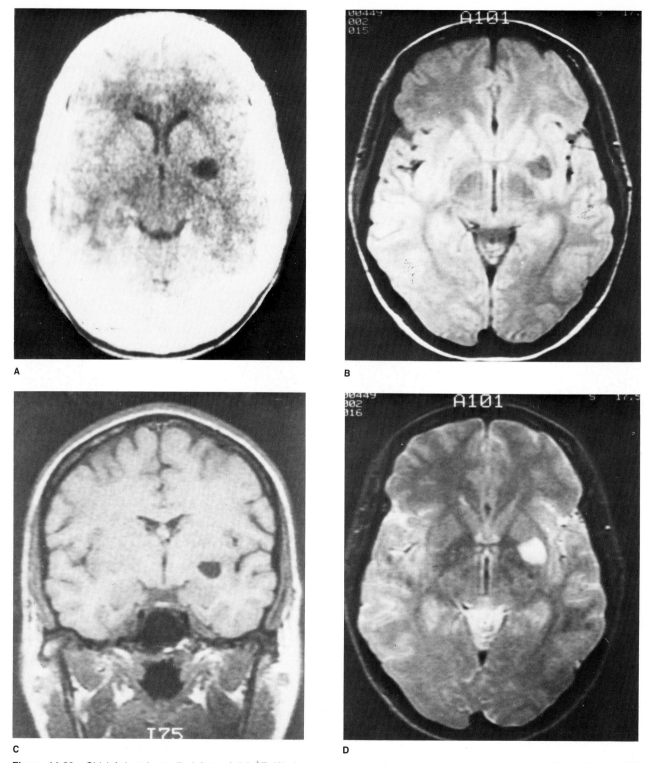

Figure 14-30 Old left basal ganglia infarct. Axial CT (**A**) demonstrates a well-demarcated hypointense lesion in the putamen. MRI: **B** (axial), **C** (coronal) T_1-WI, and **D** (axial) T_2-WI show abnormal signal intensity.

nal capsule. Comparison with the tissue density in the contralateral homologous basal ganglia region will aid in appreciating early, minimal, low-density change. Not infrequently the hypodense region involves only the most superior portion of the putamen and the white matter adjacent to the outer angle of the lateral ventricle (Fig. 14-28). Slight mass effect and contrast enhancement may develop at the appropriate times, that is, 3 to 5 days for mass effect and 7 to 10 days for enhancement (Fig. 14-13). After 3 to 4 weeks a more sharply defined and lower-density lesion becomes evident. Small lacunes not previously identified may be revealed, confined to a single CT section. Naturally, the thinner the CT section, the more likely it is that small lesions will be identified.

BINSWANGER'S DISEASE (SUBCORTICAL ARTERIOSCLEROTIC ENCEPHALOPATHY) At times the arteriolosclerotic vasculopathy of hypertension may predominantly involve the long, penetrating transmedullary arterioles which extend from the brain surface into the deep frontal and parietal white matter. The arteries to the basal ganglia are usually also affected. Progressive dementia is the cardinal clinical feature of this peculiar variety of hypertensive vascular disease. There is usually also a history, physical findings, and CT evidence of previous stroke.

The neuropathologic changes in Binswanger's disease consist of diffuse demyelination or focal areas of partial necrosis in the cerebral white matter (or both), mainly in the frontal and occipital lobes.

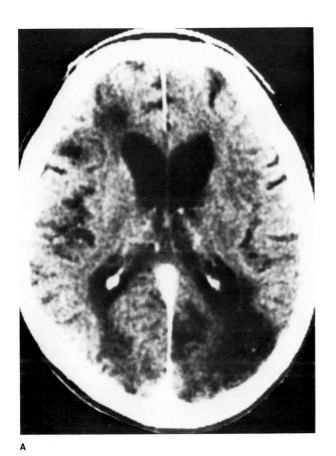

A

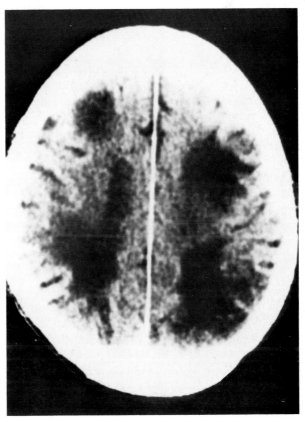

B

Figure 14-31 Binswanger's disease. Diffuse bilateral patchy white matter hypodensities with relative sparing of cortex.

Lacunar infarcts in the basal ganglia are frequently present. The white matter and basal ganglia arterioles are affected by arteriolosclerosis.

On CT, Binswanger's disease demonstrates either diffuse or patchy low-density areas in the white matter of the centrum semiovale and the frontal and occipital regions with prominent involvement of the periventricular area. The changes occur bilaterally but not always in a symmetrical pattern. One or more lacunar infarcts are usually evident in the basal ganglia–internal capsule region or thalamus (Fig. 14-31) (Rosenberg 1979; Zeumer 1980; Lotz 1986). MR findings are described in Chaps. 15 and 17.

Arteritis

Cerebral arteritis may involve the large arteries at the base of the brain, the convexity branches, the smaller intracerebral arterioles, or a combination of the three (Sole-Llenas 1978). Many of the disease processes causing arteritis characteristically involve arteries of only one size. Cranial arteritis may be primary or secondary. When primary, the disease process primarily involves the arteries; when secondary, the disease is primarily affecting the meninges or brain parenchyma and involves the arteries secondarily.

With *primary arteritis* the cerebral involvement may be just one of many manifestations of a systemic disorder, such as collagen disease, giant cell arteritis, sarcoidosis, or tertiary syphilis. Occasionally the intracranial arteritis is the sole manifestation at the time of one of these disease processes. Alternatively, primary arteritis may be caused by a disease process which affects mainly the brain arteries, such as granulomatous and chemical arteritis. Cerebral chemical arteritis may be caused by amphetamine and heroin abuse (Rumbaugh 1971), ergotamine, and anovulatory medication. There are undoubtedly other drugs and chemical agents which produce cerebral arteritis. In many cases the exact cause for a primary arteritis cannot be identified.

The CT alterations caused by primary cerebral arteritis are nonspecific and quite varied. Correlation of the CT findings with the clinical history, physical examination, age, and sex of the patient will greatly aid in arriving at the most appropriate diagnosis.

Cerebral arteritis develops with systemic lupus erythematosus (SLE) and occurs mainly in young women, who may manifest psychosis, mental alterations, seizures, or focal neurologic deficits (Johnson 1968; Glaser 1952, 1955; Bilaniuk 1977). Nervous-system involvement in SLE has been reported in 25 to 75 percent of cases (Johnson 1968), but arteritis is not common, being present in from 6 to 13 percent of cases (Ellis 1979). It primarily involves the small cerebral arteries. On CT the most frequent abnormality is enlargement of cortical sulci (Fig. 14-32) (Bilaniuk 1977). This change reflects arteritic involvement of the cortical arterioles, resulting in microinfarcts in this region (Johnson 1968). The small arteries supplying the basal ganglia–internal capsule region may also be involved causing either lacunar infarcts or intracerebral hemorrhage (Bilaniuk 1977; Ellis 1979). Arteritic involvement of the large arteries

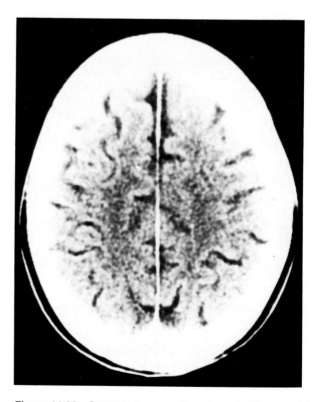

Figure 14-32   Systemic lupus erythematosus in 18-year-old female. Progressive mental deterioration with enlarged sulci for age.

at the base of the brain and the medium-sized arteries in the sylvian fissures and over the convexity on occasion may cause more typical cerebral hemispheric infarcts (Trevor 1972). Aisen (1985) reported three patterns of MR findings of SLE: large white-matter infarctions, microinfarctions of white matter, and gray-matter hyperintensity.

Granulomatous arteritis predominantly involves the small leptomeningeal and penetrating arteries and veins of less than 200 μm in diameter to the white matter. Occasionally the larger cerebral arteries are affected (Cravioto 1959; Nurick 1972; Rosenblum 1972). The CT manifestation of this involvement is a diffuse edematous-like, bilateral, white-matter low-density pattern (Fig. 14-33) (Faer 1977). Contrast enhancement is generally not seen with white-matter involvement (Faer 1977). There may also be focal low-density regions of the cortex and white matter representing more typical infarcts and reflecting arteritic involvement of large and medium-sized branches (Fig. 14-33). Contrast enhancement and mass effect develop with lesions in this location (Valvanis 1979).

In many cases of primary arteritis there is bilateral involvement, with multiple areas of infarction similar to those seen with emboli. Angiography is usually required to substantiate the diagnosis and will demonstrate multiple segmental regions of irregular narrowing in the secondary and tertiary peripheral branches of the main cerebral arteries (Fig. 14-33).

Secondary cerebral arteritis is caused by central nervous system inflammatory disease. Although the diagnosis can usually be readily established clinically and by cerebral spinal fluid examination, occasionally the appropriate clinical manifestations are not apparent and only the manifestations caused by the arteritis are evident. In these instances the CT may reveal alterations which will suggest the correct diagnosis. This situation may occur with the more indolent types of meningitis such as tuberculous and fungal.

Secondary arteritis, besides revealing CT alterations of ischemic disease, frequently reveals other abnormalities related to the subarachnoid inflammatory disease which are suggestive of this diagnosis. CECT may show enhancement of the subarachnoid spaces around the basal cisterns, in the sylvian fissure, over the convexity, or in a combination of these locations (Enzmann 1976; Bilaniuk 1978; Chu 1980). Hydrocephalus may develop from obstruction of the subarachnoid pathways, the ventricular outflow at the exit foramina of the fourth ventricle, or the aqueduct of Sylvius by inflammatory exudate and fibrosis (Sole-Llenas 1978).

Purulent meningitis causes a heavy inflammatory exudate which mainly accumulates around the base of the brain. Here it may produce arteritic involvement of the supraclinoid carotid (Leeds 1971), the proximal segments of the anterior and middle cerebral arteries, or the penetrating arteries to the basal ganglia and thalamic region (Cairns 1946). Bilateral or unilateral infarctions may develop in basal ganglia, cerebral hemisphere, or both.

With *Haemophilus influenzae* meningitis the purulent exudate may be around the base but is also located more peripherally over the brain surface, causing arteritis in the insula and convexity arteries (Leeds 1971). This may produce multiple small or large regions of infarction, which are more frequently located anteriorly in the frontal lobes (Cockrill 1978).

Tuberculous meningitis may involve both the basal and convexity subarachnoid spaces and can affect the arteries at either or both locations (Dastur 1966; Lehrer 1966; Leeds 1971). Depending on which region is primarily involved, the CT may reveal either a large infarct in one vascular territory or one or more small infarcts in several vascular territories (Chu 1980). Hydrocephalus may be a prominent feature with tuberculous meningitis (see Chap. 12).

Moyamoya Disease

Moyamoya disease is a condition of unknown etiology resulting in progressive occlusion of the terminal segment of the supraclinoid portion of the internal carotid artery and the proximal portions of the anterior and middle cerebral arteries. The proximal posterior cerebral arteries may also be affected. The disease usually develops in childhood and is most prevalent in the Japanese (Kudo 1968) but has been reported in other races as well (Taveras 1969).

In children the initial manifestations are usually

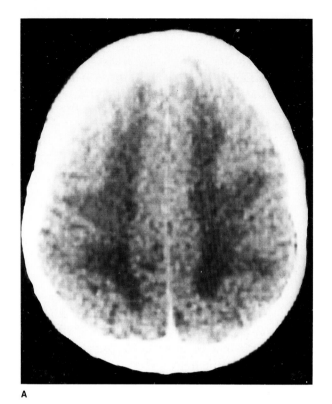

A

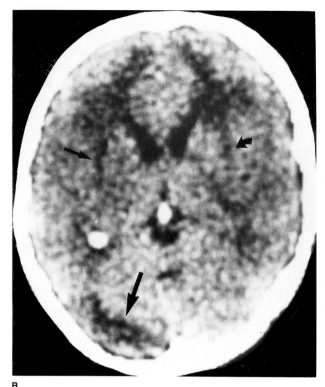

B

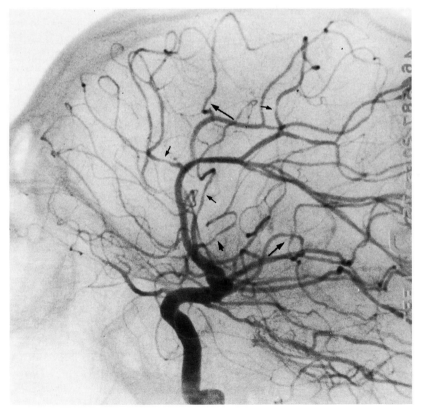

C

Figure 14-33 Granulomatous arteritis in 38-year-old male (biopsy confirmation). **A.** Diffuse bilateral white-matter hypodensity. **B.** Diffuse bilateral anterior frontal white-matter hypodensity. Focal infarct hypodensities at left posterior putamen (curved arrow), right occipital region (large arrow), and right occipital region (large arrow). **C.** Lateral carotid angiogram: multiple focal regions of peripheral arterial branch narrowing (arrows).

related to cerebral ischemia and include motor and sensory disturbance, involuntary movements, convulsions, headaches, and mental deterioration. In adults the disease usually presents with subarachnoid or intracerebral hemorrhage.

Angiography and pathologic examination reveal tapered partial-to-complete occlusions of the vessels about the internal carotid artery bifurcation bilaterally. Marked dilatation develops in the intraparenchymal arteries in the basal ganglia, upper brainstem, and thalamus, which provide collateral circulation to the middle and anterior cerebral arteries distal to their occlusions. This vascular dilatation is the so-called moyamoya blush (Fig. 14-34*A*), *moyamoya* meaning "puff of smoke" in Japanese. The collateral vessels arise from the internal carotid artery proximal to its occlusion and from the anterior choroidal, posterior communicating, and terminal basilar artery bifurcation (Nishimoto 1968; Suzuki 1969; Taveras 1969; Pecker 1973).

The CT scan may reveal nonspecific abnormalities related to focal and diffuse ischemia, such as multiple small areas of parenchymal hypodensity and evidence of cerebral atrophy consisting of dilatation of sulci, interhemispheric and sylvian fissures, and ventricles (Handa 1977). In adults and occasionally in children hemorrhage occurs which may be subarachnoid, basal ganglionic (Fig. 14-34*C*), or intraventricular. The hemorrhage is caused by rupture of a dilated collateral vessel which may develop pseudoaneurysms (Kodama 1978). Takahashi et al. (1980) recently reported a more characteristic abnormality consisting of irregular interrupted or tortuous curvilinear densities in the basal ganglia on CECT. These densities correspond to the location of the most prominent parenchymal collaterals on carotid angiography (Fig. 14-34*B*).

Complicated Migraine

The majority of patients with classical migraine have EEG abnormalities during the attack, usually most marked in the occipital region, and many of these patients develop focal neurologic changes at this time. It is postulated that during the prodromal phase vasospasm develops in some intracranial arteries, resulting in localized cerebral ischemia. This is sup-

ported by angiographic and cerebral blood-flow studies, which have shown vasospasm and decreased flow during the attack.

Abnormal CT scans have been noted during and sometimes shortly after the migraine attack in one-third to one-half of the patients (Mathew 1976; Hungerford 1976). The CT reveals focal low-density regions that do not enhance or cause mass effect. They are more commonly located posteriorly in the cerebral hemispheres (Fig. 14-35). The hypodensities will resolve completely on follow-up scans obtained after several weeks if the neurologic deficit clears.

Brainstem and Cerebellar Infarction

Fewer infarcts are detected by CT in the posterior fossa (Campbell 1978; Kingsley 1980), in part because of inherent computer artifacts in this region from the dense petrous ridges and the occipital bony crest which degrade the images. In addition, significant neurologic deficit may result from very small, critically located infarcts in the brainstem. These small lesions are frequently below the resolution capability of the CT scanner, especially during the acute phase of the infarct. MRI can be of help in this situation (Fox 1986). Follow-up scans at 3 months may reveal a higher percentage of infarcts because of the sharper demarcation and greater hypodensity of residual small cystic areas of necrosis. The fourth ventricle and brainstem cisterns may dilate in the chronic phase. In patients with a diffuse ischemic insult, degeneration in the cerebellar cortex may be a prominent abnormality (Brierley 1976). Large brainstem infarctions are more readily identifiable on CT, usually by 48 hours (Fig. 14-36).

Infarcts in the anterior and inferior portions of the cerebellum may be difficult to define, particularly in the acute phase, because of their proximity to the regions where bone artifacts are maximal. Superior cerebellar infarcts are more readily identified, but care must be taken to distinguish them from infarcts in the adjacent inferior occipital lobe on the opposite side of the tentorium (Fig. 14-36). In this situation, CECT will usually aid in determining the correct location by identifying the enhancing tentorium, especially in coronal views.

With a large cerebellar infarct, severe secondary

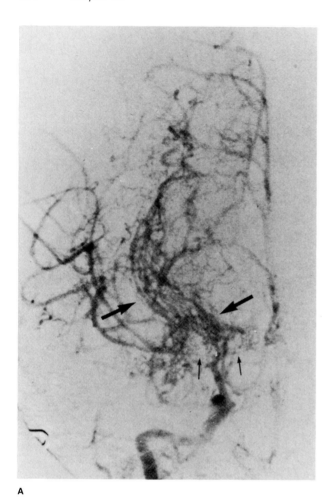

A

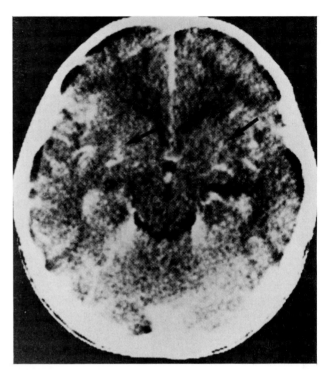

B

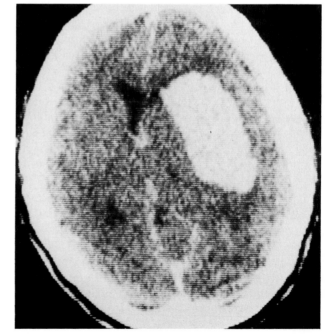

C

Figure 14-34   Moyamoya disease.   **A.** Frontal carotid angiogram: tapered occlusion of proximal segments of anterior and middle cerebral arteries (small arrows). Marked dilatation of lenticulostriate arteries representing the moyamoya blush (large arrows). **B.** CECT: prominent curvilinear and punctate vascular-like densities in lenticulostriate artery distribution (arrows). (*From Takahashi M, et al. 1980.*)   **C.** Moyamoya disease with large hematoma in basal ganglia on left. (*Courtesy of J. H. Suh, M.D., Severance Hospital, Seoul, Korea.*)

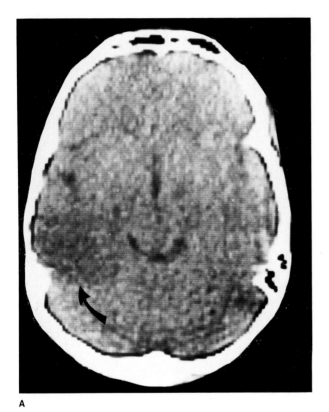
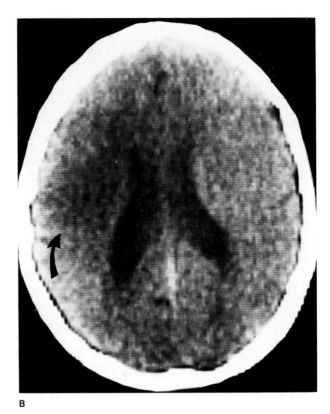

A   B

Figure 14-35   Complicated migraine: recurrent neurologic deficits associated with headaches.   **A.** Diffuse mild hypodensity in right posterior temporal region (arrow).   **B.** Diffuse hypodensity in right parietal and posterior frontal region (arrow). Moderate ventricular dilatation.

neurologic deficits may develop from brainstem compression secondary to cerebellar swelling and tonsillar herniation. The infarct edema usually becomes maximum between the third and fifth days. It may be difficult to distinguish between infarction and tumor at this time; the fourth ventricle will be displaced and the brainstem cisterns compressed in both situations. With infarction, however, the low density tends to remain localized within a vascular distribution and usually does not cross the vermis to the opposite side of the midline (Fig. 14-37). In addition, contrast enhancement is not present at this time with most infarctions but is frequently present with tumor. It is important to carefully evaluate for any early evidence of swelling due to infarction so as to alert the clinicians to the possibility of later severe developments; prognosis might then be favorably affected by early surgical decompression and removal of necrotic cerebellar tissue.

Follow-up CT scans after the first week that show contrast enhancement in the cerebellar folia suggest infarction in one or more branches of the vertebral and basilar arteries. After several months a sharply demarcated low-density region will usually become evident involving the cerebellar surface and extending into the white matter. Focal dilatation of the ipsilateral side of the fourth ventricle may also develop (Fig. 14-37).

Anoxic Ischemic Encephalopathy and Carbon Monoxide Poisoning

Individuals who suffer acute respiratory insufficiency such as may occur with allergic reaction, primary central respiratory failure, or overdose from central respiratory depressant drugs such as alcohol, narcotics, or barbiturates may develop either

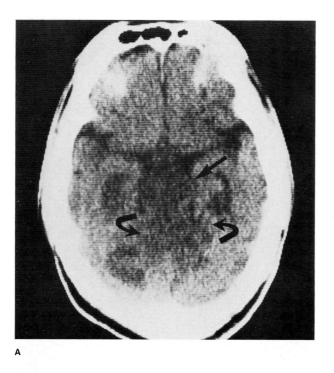

A

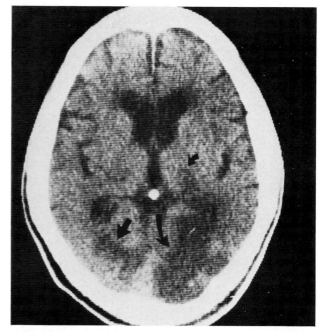

B

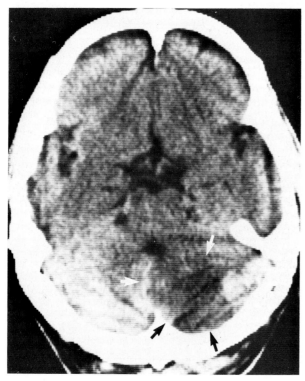

A

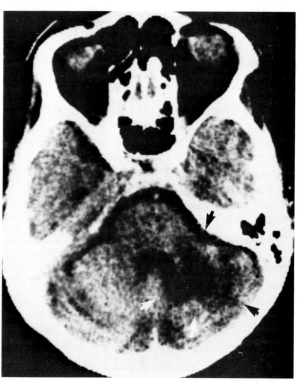

B

acute or delayed onset of brain damage. Carbon monoxide intoxication may cause similar clinical manifestations and brain pathologic alterations (Brucher 1967; Lapresle 1967; Ginsberg 1974, 1979). Anoxia or prolonged hypoxia usually results in hypotension and cardiac failure, adding cerebral ischemic insult to the hypoxemia, as may be seen in drowning victims (Murray 1984). Conversely, acute cardiac failure or hypotension may lead to respiratory failure (De Reuck 1978), possibly as a result of brainstem ischemia.

Clinically, most patients with anoxic ischemia present with coma (De Reuck 1978; Ginsberg 1979). Some never demonstrate any significant recovery, while others awaken and initially improve, only to have a delayed onset of progressive neurologic deterioration after a period of several weeks (Plum 1962; Ginsberg 1976, 1979). Pathologically the patients with irreversible acute brain injury reveal necrosis, which may affect predominantly either the gray or the white matter. The watershed region, particularly the periventricular white matter, is usually the most severely affected area (Brierley 1976; De Reuck 1978). The deep parts of the basal ganglia, which can also be considered a terminal field of supply, are also commonly involved (De Reuck 1971; Brierley 1976). The pathologic change that develops in those patients with delayed onset of hypoxic ischemic symptoms is progressive demyelination, with or without

zones of focal necrosis which is most severe in the periventricular region (Plum 1962; Ginsberg 1976, 1979). Rarely, the neuropathologic alterations are confined to the basal ganglia in patients with the delayed-onset hypoxic ischemic syndrome (Ginsberg 1979).

The CT in patients with unremitting neurologic deficits demonstrates by 24 to 48 hours low-density regions which may be situated in the basal ganglia, the watershed cortex and white matter, or the periventricular white matter (Fig. 14-38). Involved gray matter may be isodense during the acute phase, since reperfusion hyperemia during this period could counterbalance the basic hypoxic ischemic low-density tissue change. On CECT, diffuse enhancement in the watershed cortex may appear, indicating probably hyperemia with blood-brain-barrier abnormality (Fig. 14-39). If the patient survives the acute

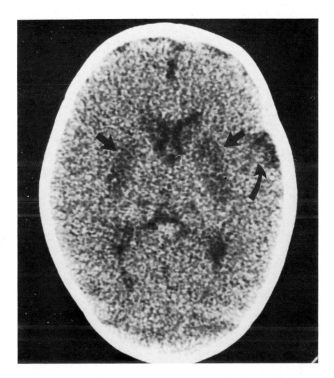

Figure 14-38 Respiratory arrest in 4-month-old child (crib anoxia), at 2 weeks. Hypodensity involving caudate and putamen bilaterally (arrows) and left anterior temporal (curved arrow) and frontal pole regions of the cortex.

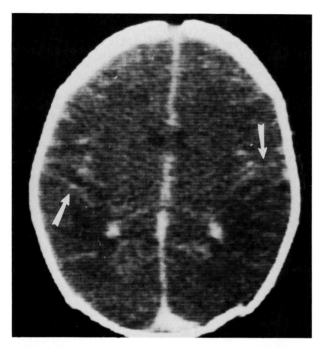

Figure 14-39 CECT: postanoxic cortical enhancement (arrows). Cortical ribbon isodense on NCCT. Diffuse white-matter hypodensity.

when circulation ceases both supra- and infratentorially. If the patient is kept alive by artificial measures, low density develops in all posterior fossa tissues. Once cerebral death occurs, the large arteries at the base of the brain (internal carotid, proximal anterior, and middle cerebral and basilar) and the large cerebral veins and sinuses (vein of Galen, superior sagittal, straight and transverse sinuses) are not visualized on CECT (Rangel 1978; Rappaport 1978). Rapid bolus contrast injection (40 ml in 5 seconds) or large bolus infusion (80 g iodine) more dramatically indicates the lack of vascular contrast filling. Although the CT findings may strongly indicate an absence of cerebral circulation, angiography is still needed for confirmation.

In those patients who manifest the biphasic clinical response to hypoxic ischemic insult with delayed onset of secondary neurologic deterioration, the CT obtained during the first 1 to 2 weeks may

phase, marked enlargement of the lateral ventricular system and cortical sulci will develop during the next few months, and previously isodense enhancing regions will become hypodense (Fig. 14-40).

In the most severe cases of anoxic ischemic insult, all the cortical, basal ganglia, and white-matter regions of the cerebrum may be involved and reveal diffuse hypodensity after a few days. Initially there is preservation of normal tissue density in the posterior fossa region. The lateral ventricles and basal cisterns are obliterated, reflecting the development of marked brain swelling and increased supratentorial intracranial pressure, which causes further ischemic insult by reducing perfusion pressure. Eventually this vicious circle causes cessation of blood flow in the supratentorial region. The vertebral-basilar circulation to the posterior fossa is similarly affected as the increased intracranial pressure is transmitted transtentorially. A state of cerebral death exists

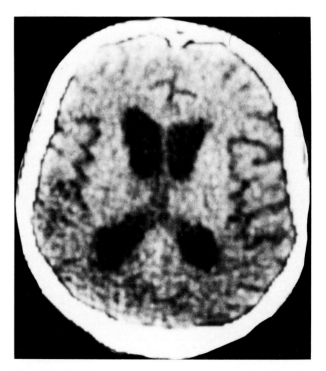

Figure 14-40 Chronic post-anoxic-ischemic changes. Six months after anoxic-ischemic insult: diffuse cortical and ventricular enlargement. Normal CT before episode of respiratory arrest.

be entirely normal. With the onset of neurologic deterioration after a period of 3 to 5 weeks, a mild, diffuse low density will appear in the white matter. Over the next 3 to 4 weeks the hypodensity becomes progressively more marked (Yagnik 1980). The hypodensity is most severe in the deep white-matter regions but extends in a pseudopod-like manner outward in the white-matter tracks between the involved cortical convolutions.

With acute *carbon monoxide* poisoning (a form of anemic hypoxia due to a reduction in the amount of circulating oxyhemoglobin) the prevalent CT abnormality appears to be bilateral hypodensity in the basal ganglia, most conspicuous in the region of the globus pallidus (Fig. 14-41). This was present in all nine of the patients reported by Kim et al. (1980). It was observed in four of five patients examined dur-

ing the first week, being present as early as the first day in two. Five of five patients examined after 6 weeks had bilateral basal ganglia involvement. Diffuse bilateral white-matter hypodensity developed in three of the nine patients. Only one of these patients had a relapsing clinical course with delayed onset of neurologic deterioration after recovery from initial coma. All the rest had severe original deficits, which showed little, if any, improvement.

In Miura's series (1985), the most common finding was symmetric and diffuse white matter (23/60) to be followed by a symmetric, bilateral, round hypodense lesion in the globus pallidus (18/60) with frequent extension to the internal capsules (Fig. 14-41). He stated that the prognosis depended on the severity of the cerebral white-matter changes and not on that of hypodense globus pallidus lesions.

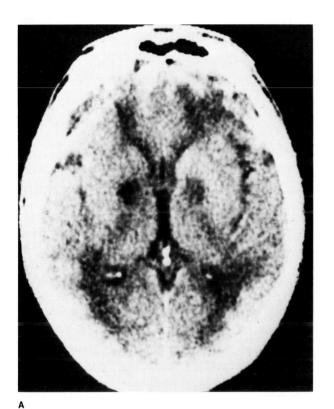

A

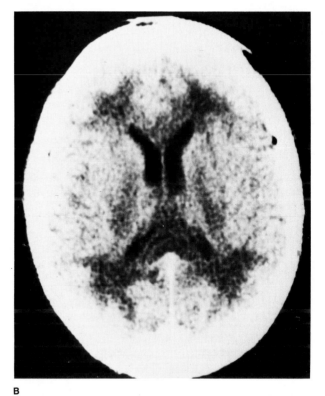

B

Figure 14-41 Acute carbon monoxide insult. **A.** Bilateral, symmetrical globus pallidus and diffuse white-matter hypodense lesions. **B.** Extension to the internal capsules and symmetricity of white-matter hypodensity are more apparent at higher level.

Hypertensive Encephalopathy

Those persons, particularly normotensive ones, who experience a rapid and sustained elevation in blood pressure may develop hypertensive encephalopathy (Ziegler 1965). This is manifested by severe headache, vomiting, convulsions, focal neurologic signs, and drowsiness or coma. Pathologically the brain demonstrates generalized edema, petechial hemorrhages, and patchy vessel-wall necrosis (Yates 1972). These changes are believed to occur because the normal limit of autoregulatory vasoconstriction has been exceeded (Lassen 1972). This breakthrough in the upper limits of autoregulation leads to increased cerebral blood flow and capillary perfusion pressure, and these hemodynamic alterations result in the pathologic abnormalities.

The CT appearance reflects the main pathologic change, diffuse edema. Generalized, well-demarcated, symmetrical hypodensity is present in the cerebral white matter (Kendall 1977), which may be more marked in the upper posterior parts of the cerebral hemispheres (Fig. 14-42) (Rail 1980), and is also noted in the posterior fossa (Weingarten 1985). Varying degrees of edema and mass effect on the ventricles and subarachnoid spaces are present. The degree and duration of blood pressure elevation correlate well with the severity of edema (Weingarten 1985). Follow-up scans demonstrate resolution of the hypodensity after the blood pressure is reduced for a period of time.

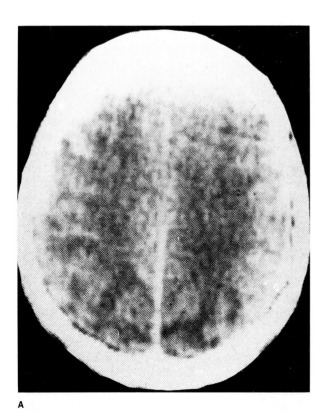

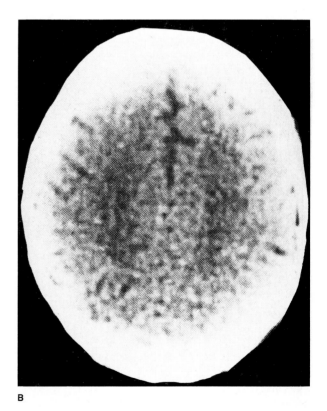

A

B

Figure 14-42 Hypertensive encephalopathy. **A.** CT at time of severe hypertension and symptoms: hypodensity throughout white matter most marked in the upper posterior portions of the cerebral hemispheres. **B.** CT 2 months after control of hypertension, with mild residual mental function deficits: resolution of white-matter hypodensity, moderate prominence of cortical sulci. (*From Rail DL 1980.*)

Cerebral Venous Thrombosis

Venous thrombosis in the brain may involve the major venous sinuses, superficial cortical veins, or deep venous system, or two or more of these regions may be affected simultaneously. There is a high incidence of grave morbidity and mortality with cerebral sinovenous occlusion (Kalberg 1967). To improve survival and reduce debilitating complications, early recognition and institution of appropriate therapy are essential.

The causes of cerebral venous thrombosis fall in two main categories—septic and aseptic. Septic sinovenous occlusion is the result of inflammatory vasculitis, which may be caused either by direct involvement of the cerebral veins from intracranial infections such as meningitis, encephalitis, and subdural and epidural empyema or by intracranial spread of paracranial infections along emissary and communicating veins from inflammatory disease in such areas as the mastoids, paranasal sinuses, face, and scalp (Rao 1981; Eick 1981).

The aseptic causes of venous sinus thrombosis are numerous (Buonanno 1978). They include pregnancy in the prepartum and postpartum periods, use of oral contraceptives, dehydration, rapid diuresis, polycythemia vera, sickle cell disease, sickle cell trait, leukemia, thrombocytopenia, disseminated intravascular coagulation, cryofibrinogenemia, malnutrition, acquired and congenital heart disease, head trauma, diabetes mellitus, collagen vascular disease, cerebral arterial occlusion, cerebral and dural arteriovenous malformations, carotid cavernous fistula, compression or invasion by intracranial tumor, and indirect effects of extracranial neoplasms and chronic inflammatory diseases (Merritt 1979). In addition, many cases are idiopathic.

The clinical manifestations are nonspecific and include headache, increased intracranial pressure, stroke, seizures, personality change, hallucinations, decreased mental function, diplopia, blurred vision, and coma (Merritt 1979). Patients with this disorder not infrequently are initially diagnosed as having "functional" problems or benign pseudotumor cerebri. The clinical symptomatology may develop over a relatively long period of time or be fulminant, with rapid progression to coma and death. The mortality rate has been reported to range from 40 percent to as high as 88 percent (Krayenbuhl 1954; Buonanno 1978).

The CT reveals a wide spectrum of abnormalities, which may change over the course of the disease. Some of the CT abnormalities are diagnostic for sinovenous occlusion, while others may be either strongly suggestive or nonspecific. The CT abnormalities may be present singly or in combination. If subsequent scans are obtained, additional abnormalities may be identified. Occasionally, no abnormality is present. Buonanno et al. (1978) reported that only 1 patient out of 11 with sinovenous occlusion had a normal-appearing CT.

A diagnostic CT abnormality which may be present during the first 1 to 2 weeks after the development of sinovenous occlusion is increased density on the NCCT within the region of a dural sinus or a superficial or deep vein (Wendling 1978; Buonanno 1978; Eick 1981). This hyperdensity on CT is due to formation of a recent blood clot and measures between 50 and 90 HU. It is best seen when the scan plane is perpendicular to the long axis of the thrombosed sinus or vein. Small thrombosed convexity veins situated immediately adjacent to the calvarium may be obscured by the overlying bony density. Fresh thrombus in the straight sinus region can usually be readily appreciated, since it is sufficiently removed from the skull table. Here it appears as an elongated oval or a bandlike density following the expected course of the straight sinus (Fig. 14-43). Likewise, recent thrombosis of the vein of Galen, which is situated just anterior and inferior to the beginning of the straight sinus, should be visualized (Fig. 14-43). Care must be taken not to confuse the thrombosed vein of Galen with a partially calcified pineal gland; the latter is located slightly anterior and inferior to the vein of Galen and immediately adjacent to the posterior third ventricle. A fresh thrombus within the superior sagittal sinus may be identified by its density on axial scans if the occlusion is in its posterior vertical portion. In this location the scan plane is relatively perpendicular to the sinus and, because of the large size of the sinus at this location, should

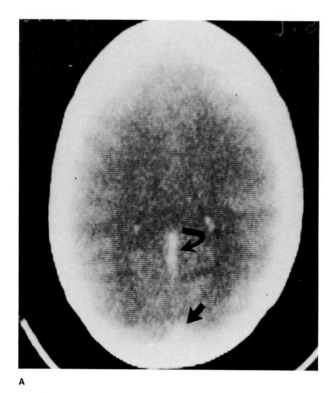

A

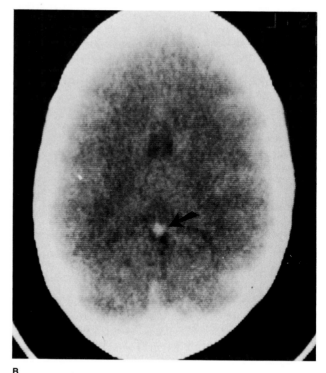

B

Figure 14-43   Venous thrombosis 3 days after onset of symptoms. Dense thrombus in straight sinus, superior sagittal sinus, and vein of Galen; diffuse brain swelling.   **A.** NCCT: band of increased density along course of straight sinus (curved arrow) and posterior aspect of superior sagittal sinus (straight arrow). Diffuse increased hypodensity throughout white matter with compressed lateral ventricles.   **B.** NCCT, section 1 cm below **A:** increased density of vein of Galen (arrow). Diffuse white-matter hypodensity with ventricular compression.

not be obscured by the overlying bone (Fig. 14-44). For occlusions more anteriorly situated in the horizontal portion of the superior sagittal sinus, coronal scans made perpendicular to its long axis are necessary. Occasionally the increased density of small thrombosed surface veins is evident if they are not located close to the calvarium—for example, those in sulci or in the sylvian cistern (Fig. 14-44).

Another diagnostic CT abnormality of venous sinus occlusion may appear on CECT, usually not becoming evident for at least a week or more after the development of sinus thrombosis, since it follows on the breakdown of the hemoglobin molecules in the clotted blood of the sinus, which then becomes isodense. The superior sagittal sinus, normally demonstrable on CECT as a homogeneous region of increased density, will reveal only enhance-

ment of its outer triangular margin; its central luminal area remains relatively hypodense—the "empty triangle" or "delta" sign (Fig. 14-45) (Buonanno 1978). This appearance represents absence of contrast flow into the sinus (the nonenhanced center) in that region. The enhancing outer triangle represents the normal enhancement of the dural walls of the sinus in combination with the added increased density from the collateral venous channels which develop in the dura (Vines 1971) and from the neovascularity which is probably appearing in the outer portion of the thrombus secondary to its organization. Both these processes may cause the sinus wall to appear thickened and to encroach on the lumen.

On the standard axial scan the delta sign will be identified mainly in those cases in which the sinus thrombosis involves the posterior third of the superior sagittal sinus, since this is the region where the scan plane is most perpendicular to the sinus. It may be necessary to utilize a high window setting to identify the delta sign, since the thickened enhanced wall of the sinus may obscure the central hypodensity when viewed at normal brain window settings (Zilkha 1980). On the axial scan the anterior third of the superior sagittal sinus is also perpendicular to the scan plane, and the delta sign may be seen with thrombosis in this location (Rao 1981). It may not be evident, however, because of the small size of the sinus in this region. To identify the delta sign in occlusion of the middle portion of the superior sagittal sinus, coronal scans are needed for perpendicular sections of this region. Buonanno et al. (1978) observed the delta sign in only 2 of 11 cases (18 percent) of sinovenous occlusion, whereas Rao et al. (1981) identified it in 8 of their 11 patients (72 percent). In addition, Rao observed the delta sign outside the usual location in the superior sagittal sinus in two cases. It was demonstrated as a

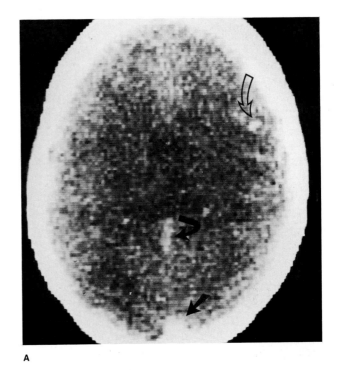

A

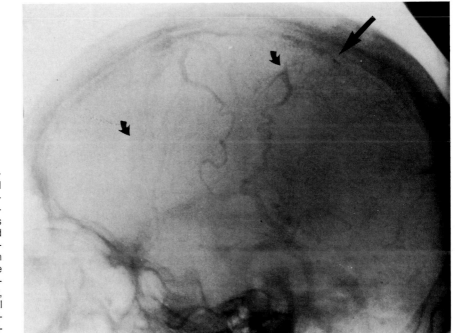

Figure 14-44 Venous thrombosis. Development of dense thrombus in cortical vein. **A** NCCT: same patient as in Figure 14-43 four days later. Persistent hyperdensity of superior sagittal sinus (straight arrow) and straight sinus (curved arrow). Nodular hyperdensity has appeared near brain surface on left (open arrow). **B.** Lateral carotid angiogram, late venous phase: occlusion of superior sagittal sinus (straight arrow), vein of Galen, and straight sinus (not filled), and cortical veins (curved arrows). Tortuous convexity veins provide collateral drainage inferiorly for the superior aspect of the brain.

B

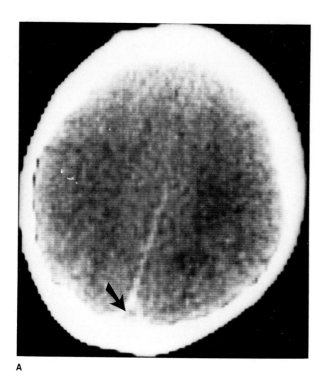

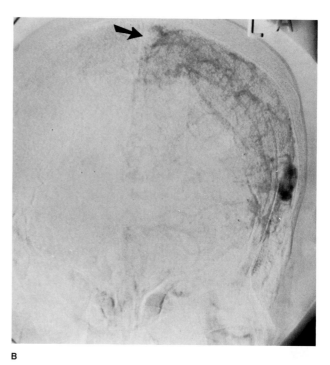

A

B

Figure 14-45 Venous thrombosis "delta" sign   **A.** CECT: no contrast density in central lumen of posterior aspect of superior sagittal sinus with thick enhancement of its walls (arrow).   **B.** Frontal carotid angiogram, venous phase: no contrast filling of superior sagittal sinus (arrow).

filling defect in the transverse sinus in one case and in the straight sinus in a second.

Another highly probable pathognomonic finding of venous thrombosis on CECT is visualization of punctate and streaklike hyperdensities within the deep white matter of the brain (Fig. 14-46) (Banna 1979). These have been postulated to represent engorgement and dilatation of transcerebral medullary veins, which serve as collateral channels between the cortical and deep venous systems. Angiographically, dilated medullary veins may be observed with occlusion of either the deep or the superficial venous systems (Gabrielsen 1969). To identify these dilated medullary veins on CT, scans with very high spatial resolution are needed.

CT abnormalities similar to those of arterial infarction frequently develop with sinovenous occlusion but usually have characteristics more indicative of venous than of arterial infarction. Since the major cerebral veins generally drain more than one arterial distribution, venous infarcts are not always strictly confined, as with arterial infarcts, to the territory of a single artery or to the watershed zone (Fig. 14-47). The involvement, particularly in the white matter, may extend asymmetrically, usually between the three main arterial regions. On NCCT the white matter is hypodense due to congestive edema and necrosis. The pattern of white-matter low density in venous infarcts usually appears different from that in arterial infarcts (Fig. 14-47). In venous infarction the white-matter hypodensity tends to have a rounded, ill-defined border, compared to the more sharply marginated wedge or rectangular shape of an arterial infarct. These differences are probably related to a greater degree of vasogenic edema in venous infarction caused by the high capillary pressure from back-pressure congestion. This factor also results in a greater mass effect on venous infarction for a lesion of comparable size.

With venous infarcts the cortex is usually iso-

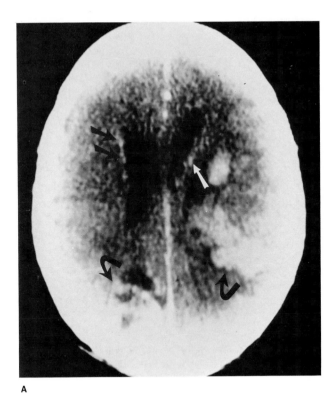

A

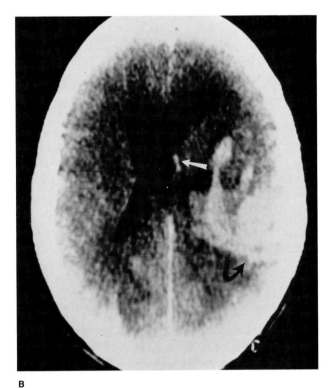

B

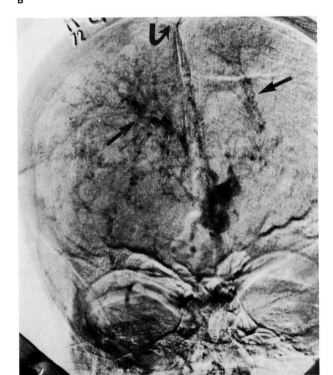

C

Figure 14-46 Venous thrombosis with dilated medullary veins.
A. and **B.** CECT: bilateral hemorrhagic venous infarcts (curved
arrows). Multiple punctate periventricular nodular densities (arrows) were not present before enhancement.   **C.** Frontal carotid
angiogram, venous phase: non-filling of superior sagittal sinus
(curved arrow) and superficial veins. Marked dilatation of medullary
veins (arrows) draining into deep venous system.

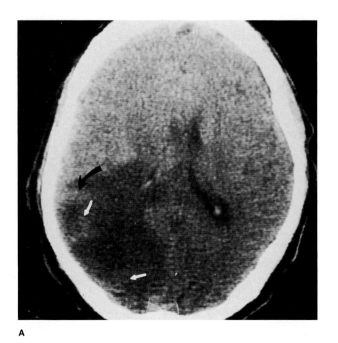

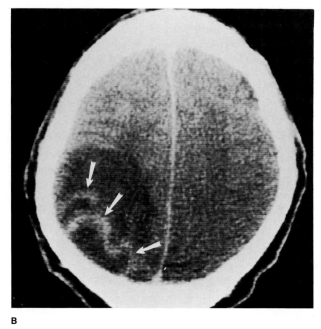

A

B

Figure 14-47   Venous infarct, mass effect, and enhancement. **A.** NCCT: large hypodensity involving right posterior temporal, parietal, and occipital regions. Hypodensity not confined to an arterial territory. Cortical density within infarct territory, although reduced, is more isodense than the white matter (arrows). Considerable compression of ipsilateral ventricle.   **B.** CECT at higher level: enhancement of cortical ribbon (arrows) centrally in posterior part of infarct.

dense to slightly hyperdense on NCCT because of congestive dilatation of the capillaries and petechial hemorrhages. On CECT a frequent cortical abnormality is an intense gyral enhancement pattern over and around the region of the venous infarction (Fig. 14-47). Prominent gyral enhancement may also occur in the absence of other evidence for venous infarction. The gyral enhancement is caused by capillary engorgement and breakdown of the blood-brain barrier related to high venous back pressure and its associated ischemic effects. Rao et al. (1981) observed gyral enhancement in 7 of 11 patients with venous infarcts. This is a considerably higher frequency than they found on review of the literature, where only 4 of 14 patients having CECT demonstrated gyral enhancement.

Intense enhancement, considerably greater than normal, may develop in the tentorium and falx. This probably reflects enlargement of dural venous collateral channels (Vines 1971) and increased dural capillary pressure, leading to a greater leakage of contrast into the dura. This enhancement has been observed most commonly in the tentorium, associated with thrombosis of the straight sinus (Buonanno 1978; Rao 1981).

Hemorrhage is also frequently associated with venous infarcts. The hemorrhage most commonly involves the cortex but may affect the white matter in the central and deep portions of the infarct (Fig. 14-46). Extensive low density in the white matter when the hemorrhage is first observed is related to the necrosis and edema caused by the venous infarction. The venous-infarction hemorrhage may assume a dense gyral pattern similar in appearance to that of arterial hemorrhagic infarction. Venous hemorrhages tend to be more bulky and less strictly confined to the cortical ribbon. In addition, the white-matter hypodensity and the hemorrhagic region may not be located within the territory of a single major cerebral artery as with arterial hemorrhagic infarction. At times the venous hemorrhage will be very bulky and extend deeply into the white matter, strongly resembling an arterial intracerebral hematoma. The venous hemorrhage may, however, reveal changes different from those occurring with an arterial hemispheric hematoma. With venous infarction the hematoma is not so sharply demarcated, and its density may be slightly nonhomogeneous. It is also more superficially located and is surrounded by a greater degree of hypodensity in the white matter, especially in its early stage.

Not infrequently, multiple separate regions of venous infarction may develop. A common pattern seen with multiple venous infarcts is bilateral involvement in the parasagittal high-convexity region of the brain. This may reveal bilateral hypodensities in the anterior cerebral territory, frequently extending beyond the watershed zone into the middle cerebral artery territory. Occasionally multiple venous hemorrhagic infarcts develop in this same distribution.

Nonspecific alterations that may develop with sinovenous thrombosis include small ventricles, mild, diffuse white-matter hypodensity which may be unilateral or bilateral, and obliteration of the basal cisterns (Fig. 14-43). These alterations reflect increased intracranial pressure from vasogenic edema caused by the increasing outflow resistance from venous obstruction.

CT may demonstrate nonfilling of a variable segment of the superior sagittal, straight, transverse, or sigmoid sinuses and/or obstruction of superficial convexity or deep veins (Figs. 14-44, 14-45). Thrombi may be identified within occluded or partially obstructed venous sinuses and cerebral veins. Enlargement and frequently corkscrew tortuosity of anastomotic collateral veins (Fig. 14-44) and medullary veins (Fig. 14-46) may be observed. Although the characteristic and highly specific CT findings frequently strongly suggest the diagnosis of sinovenous thrombosis, cerebral angiography is the definitive method for diagnosis and is indicated in questionable cases for confirmation (Krayenbuhl 1954; Gabrielsen 1969, 1981; Vines 1971). MRI has been extremely sensitive in detection of sinovenous thrombosis and underlying parenchymal alterations in the authors' experience (Fig. 14-48).

INTRACEREBRAL HEMORRHAGE

CT is the most accurate and reliable method for diagnosing intracerebral hematoma. The true incidence of this diagnosis has increased since the advent of CT. The density of freshly clotted blood on CT (55 to 95 HU) is significantly greater than that of brain tissue, permitting reliable identification of even very small intracerebral hematomas. Hemorrhages of 1 cm or possibly less in diameter can usually be diagnosed if technically good scans are obtained using collimators 0.8 cm or less in size (Fig. 14-49). Intracerebral hematomas may extend to the brain surface or rupture intraventricularly, resulting in secondary subarachnoid hemorrhage.

Aside from head trauma, the principal cause of intracerebral hematoma is hypertensive vascular disease. Rupture of a berry aneurysm and arteriovenous malformation are less frequent causes. Other etiologies include venous thrombosis, amyloid angiopathy, collagen vascular disease, anticoagulation therapy, primary and metastatic brain tumor, and prematurity in the neonate. Although hematomas from various causes may present a similar CT appearance, frequently the correct etiology may be suggested by consideration of the patient's age, the clinical history, and the location of the hematoma. Use of contrast may reveal associated specific enhancement characteristics which will indicate the diagnosis (Weisberg 1979). Hematomas caused by venous infarction have been discussed earlier in this chapter; those associated with trauma, aneurysm, arteriovenous malformation, and tumor are presented in other chapters in this book.

Hypertensive Hematoma

Intracerebral hematomas caused by hypertensive vascular disease tend to occur in older patients, usually those in their seventh decade. These hematomas are most commonly situated in the basal ganglia and internal capsule region. They predominantly involve the lateral portion of the putamen but also occur in the head of the caudate nucleus and the

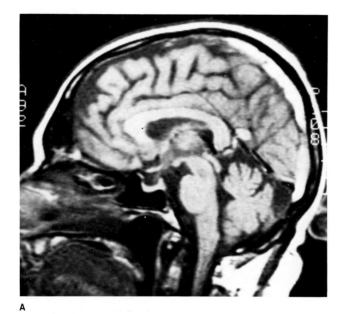

A

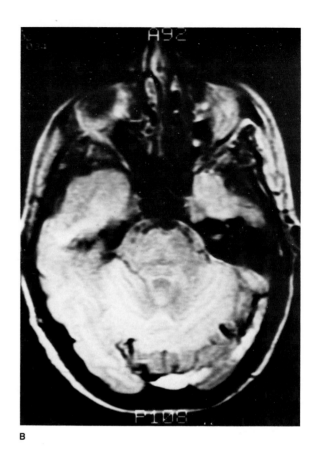

B

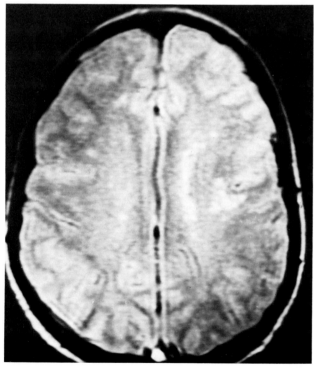

C

Figure 14-48   Venous thrombosis. MRI: **A** (sagittal T_1) and **B** (axial T_1) show hyperintense lesions along the sagittal, straight, and transverse sinuses. **C** (axial T_2) shows thrombosed sagittal sinus as hyperintense lesion on T_2 weighted image. Abnormal signal lesions are noted in the white matter of both hemispheres.

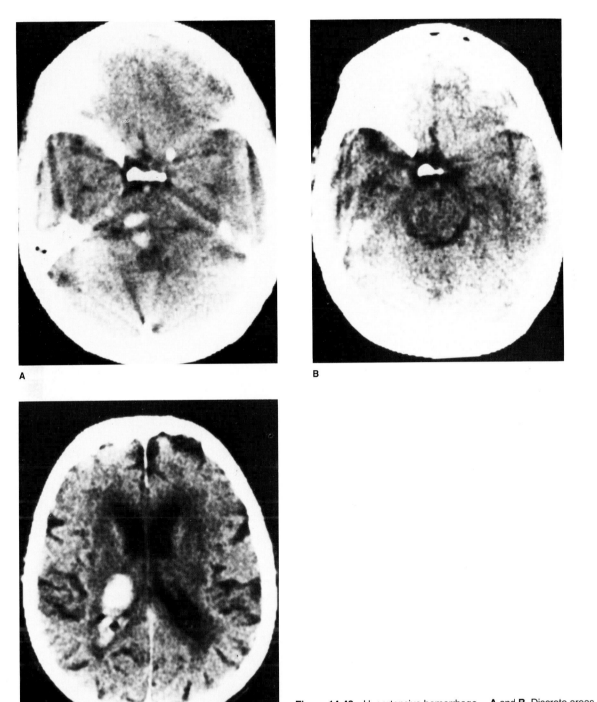

A

B

C

Figure 14-49   Hypertensive hemorrhage.   **A** and **B.** Discrete areas of hemorrhages in the brainstem (**A**); 3 weeks later (**B**) complete resorption is noted with small residual hypodense areas.   **C.** Another patient with hypertensive thalamic hemorrhage.

thalamus, brainstem, and cerebellum (Figs. 14-49, 14-50). They occasionally develop in the deep cerebral white matter in the parietal and posterior temporal occipital area (Cole 1967). Small hematomas may present clinically as a vasoocclusive stroke (Kinkel 1976). CT is then needed for appropriate diagnosis and management.

Larger basal ganglia-capsular hematomas not infrequently rupture into the lateral ventricle. Since the advent of CT, intraventricular rupture has been recognized as being much more common than previously believed. Small amounts of intraventricular bleeding do not significantly increase mortality. With large intraventricular rupture the prognosis becomes very grave (Fig. 14-50) (Weisberg 1979). Once it becomes intraventricular, a hemorrhage from any region can spread throughout the entire ventricular system and into the subarachnoid space.

Intracerebral hemorrhage frequently extends away from its site of origin into adjacent regions along white-matter tracts. Occasionally, the degree of spread may be so great that determining the primary site of hemorrhage is difficult. Basal ganglia–capsular hemorrhage may extend superiorly into the deep frontoparietal white matter via the internal capsule or inferiorly into the temporal lobe via the external capsule (Fig. 14-50C). Intraventricular rupture into the body of the lateral ventricle is frequent from this location. Thalamic hematomas may dissect inferiorly into the brainstem, laterally into the posterior limb of the internal capsule, or medially into the third ventricle. Superior extension into the lateral ventricle is not usual, probably because of the intervening subarachnoid space of the velum interpositum. Brainstem hematomas may extend superiorly into the thalamus or posteriorly either into the cerebellum through the cerebellar peduncles or directly into the fourth ventricle. Conversely, cerebellar hematomas can dissect anteriorly into the pons. Large cerebellar hematomas cause significant brainstem compression and tonsillar herniation and frequently require urgent surgical evacuation.

Hypertensive hematoma is believed by many to be caused by rupture of microaneurysms on the penetrating arteries. These aneurysms were first described by Charcot and Bouchard (1868) and are fre-

quently referred to by their names. Recent elegant microradiographic and histopathologic studies have reconfirmed their presence, their strong association with hypertension, and their prevalence at the usual sites of intracerebral hemorrhage, being most frequent in the basal ganglia–internal capsule region (Russell 1963; Cole 1967). They result from hyalin degeneration in the walls of the penetrating arteries, with loss of elastic fibers and smooth muscle in the intima and media. These microaneurysms are most often located at points of branching and are either fusiform or saccular dilatations ranging in size from 50 to 1000 μm (Kido 1978). They may occasionally be demonstrated with high-detail-magnification angiography and angiotomography (Goldberg 1973).

A fresh hematoma on NCCT appears as a homogeneously dense (55 to 90 HU), well-defined lesion with a rounded to oval configuration. The hemorrhage separates brain tissue rather than intermixing with it. A thin, well-defined low-density zone surrounding the hematoma can be observed as early as a few hours after the hemorrhage (Fig. 14-51). This early hypodense rim is probably caused by the clotting of the liquid hemorrhage with extrusion of the low-density plasma at the periphery of the hematoma. After 3 to 4 days, additional low density appears around the hematoma, spreading peripherally in the white matter. This is caused by compression ischemic necrosis of surrounding tissue and the development of edema related to clot lysis, with breakdown of the blood-brain barrier (Fig. 14-51) (Stehbens 1972; Grubb 1974; Laster 1978). Hematomas produce ventricular compression and, when large, considerable midline shift and brain herniation. Mass effect may increase during the third to seventh days from the development of edema. Steroid treatment, especially in nontraumatic hematomas, will usually control edema formation and therefore eliminate or considerably reduce the secondary increased mass effect both clinically and on CT.

A hematoma which is nonhomogeneously dense should lead the physician to consider hemorrhage occurring with tumor, inflammation, contusion, or arterial and venous infarction. In these situations the hemorrhage usually develops within the abnormal and necrotic tissue and, depending on the etiol-

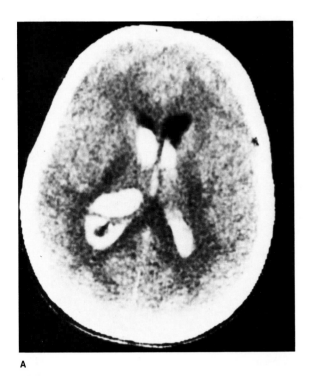

A

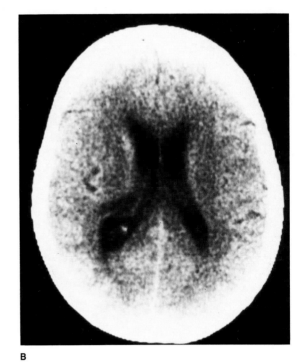

B

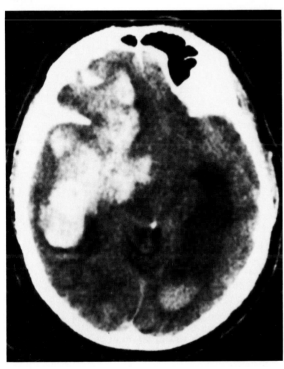

C

Figure 14-50 Hypertensive hemorrhage. **A** and **B.** Right thalamic hemorrhage (arrows) with rupture into the lateral ventricles (**A**). 6 months later (**B**) complete resorption of hemorrhage is noted with a small area of encephalomalacia. **C.** Right basal ganglia hemorrhage extends into the frontal and temporal lobes as well as the ventricles and upper midbrain.

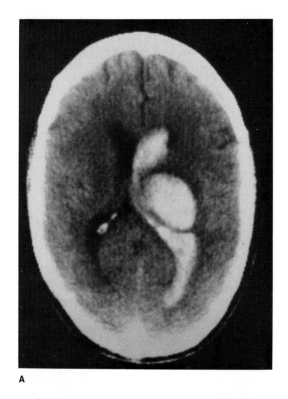

A

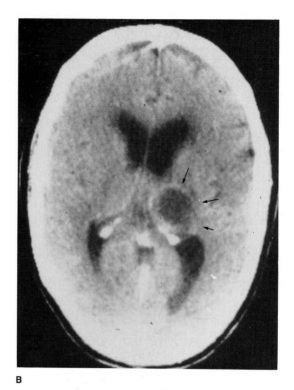

B

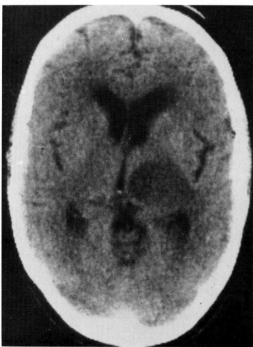

C

Figure 14-51   Evolution of hypertensive hematoma.   **A.** (NCCT) at day 1: left thalamic hematoma with thin rim of hypodensity around hematoma. Intraventricular hemorrhage is also present.   **B.** (CECT) at 6 weeks: peripheral ringlike enhancement (arrows) is associated with central hypodensity.   **C.** (NCCT) at 3 months: area of parenchymal hypodensity at the site of previous hematoma.

ogy, may appear either as a poorly marginated and patchy region of increased density, a nonhomogeneous region of hyperdensity centrally located in an area of hypodensity, or a complete or incomplete irregular ring of increased density around a low-density or isodense center with surrounding edema. CECT will frequently reveal abnormal enhancement associated with hemorrhages not caused by hypertensive vascular disease which will aid in their differentiation.

Dolinskas et al. (1977*a*) reported that hematomas show a decreasing peak density averaging 0.7 ± 0.31 EMI units per day (these values would be approximately double in Hounsfield units). Small hematomas tended to lose their density faster than the larger ones; hematomas of 2 cm or less reached isodensity on or before the nineteenth day after the bleeding, while larger hematomas frequently took 4 to 6 weeks to become isodense. The decreasing density of a hematoma is due to breakdown and absorption of the hemoglobin molecule. Hematomas lose their peripheral density rapidly and therefore show a progressive decrease in apparent size (Fig. 14-51). Dolinskas et al. (1977*a*) found a reduction in the visualized size of the hematoma averaging 0.65 ± 0.32 mm per day. Small hematomas showed this size reduction sooner than large ones. Although the visualized portion of the hematoma becomes smaller on CT, the actual size of the clot is not changing significantly at this time; it is merely becoming isodense, and this is reflected in a delay in the reduction of its mass effect. Mass effect may be prominent for as long as 4 weeks with a large hematoma. These authors also noted that the earliest visualized decrease in mass effect for hematomas of all sizes averaged 16.7 days after the bleeding. Smaller hematomas lost their mass effect faster than the larger ones. In addition it was found that mass effect did not increase unless an operation was performed or the hematoma was secondary to trauma.

Over the next 2 to 3 months the density of a hematoma becomes progressively lower. After passing through the isodense stage (Fig. 14-51) the hematoma becomes hypodense (Dolinskas 1977*a*; Laster 1978). At its end stage, which may vary between 3 and 6 months, depending on the initial size, a well-

defined low-density region, which may be considerably smaller than the original lesion, is present at the site of the original hematoma. With small hematomas a slitlike cystic area may be the residual change. Atrophic dilatation of the adjacent portion of the ventricular system occurs, as well as sulcal enlargement (Fig. 14-51). Rarely calcification develops at the hematoma site. The residual low density and the focal atrophic changes are pathologically related to the formation of a cystic encephalomalacic cavity containing a yellowish, high-protein fluid with vascular trabeculations. This region is surrounded by a variable degree of gliosis (Stehbens 1972).

Contrast enhancement usually develops around the periphery of a hematoma after 7 to 9 days (Zimmerman 1977; Laster 1978). The appearance of contrast enhancement corresponds to the time at which radionuclide studies become positive (Dolinskas 1977*b*). Pathologically there is ingrowth of capillary neovascularity at the margin of the hematoma by the end of the first week (Sugitani 1973; Zimmerman 1977). These newly formed capillaries, as in infarctions, have an abnormal blood-brain barrier which results in extravasation of contrast material around the hematoma (Molinari 1967; Di Chiro 1974).

The contrast enhancement appears as a ringlike density situated near the inner margin of the surrounding low-density zone and separated from the hematoma density by a thin isodense or hypodense zone (Fig. 14-51) (Dolinskas 1977*b*; Laster 1978). At the time when the hematoma is passing through its isodense stage, NCCT may show little abnormality except for possibly a slight residual mass effect. However, the ring contrast enhancement on CECT persists through the isodense period and into the first few months of the hypodense state (Fig. 14-51). The surrounding edema is clearing during the third to fourth weeks, and the ring enhancement then appears to surround an isodense or hypodense core, with normal surrounding brain tissue and no mass effect (Zimmerman 1977). The enhancing capsule becomes more intense and thicker over the next 4 to 6 weeks before beginning to fade. Pathologically at this stage there is a well-developed glial vascular capsule (Stehbens 1972; Laster 1978) which may be identified angiographically (Leeds 1973). The diameter of the enhancing ring decreases during the final hypodense stage as the gliotic capsule constricts around the absorbed hematoma. The CT appearance of the enhancing ring may easily be confused with that of a tumor or abscess. The lack of enhancement of the central region when the hematoma is isodense and the lack of surrounding edema and mass effect, particularly during the hypodense phase, tend to strongly favor a diagnosis of a resolving hematoma. In addition, with hemorrhagic tumors the enhancing rim is usually present on the initial scan during the first day, and it is thicker and irregular in shape (Gildersleve 1977).

Amyloid Angiopathy

Amyloid angiopathy is an infrequent cause of non-hypertensive massive spontaneous intracerebral hemorrhage in older persons. Over the age of 70, more than 40 percent of brains surveyed in one autopsy series demonstrated the presence of amyloid in the cerebral parenchymal blood vessels. Between the ages of 60 and 70 only about 12 percent of brains demonstrated amyloid change in the blood vessels. The disease affects only the arterioles of the cortex. This vascular disease has not been found in the white matter, basal ganglia, brainstem, or cerebellum. The cortical arterioles are most frequently involved in the parietal region (Vinters 1981).

The patients commonly have dementia, and pathologically Alzheimer's plaques may be found in association with the vascular lesions. The angiopathy, however, is often present in the absence of Alzheimer's changes or clinical dementia. The amyloid change is probably not related to a specific disease entity but rather is due to age-related change in the blood vessels.

The hemorrhage associated with amyloid angiopathy primarily involves the cortex with irregular borders, surrounding edema, and frequent extension into the adjacent portion of the brain (Wagle 1984) (Fig. 14-52). This is in contrast to the usual deep location of hypertensive hemorrhages, which only on occasion extend to the brain surface. As might be expected from its superficial origin, sub-

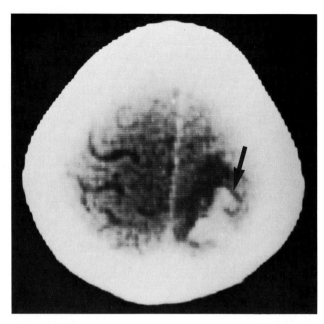

Figure 14-52 Superficial brain hemorrhage (arrow) in elderly individual with dementia suggesting amyloid angiopathy with hemorrhage.

arachnoid hemorrhage is commonly associated with the amyloid vasculopathy hemorrhage.

Hemorrhage in Premature Neonates

Intracerebral hemorrhage develops in 40 to 70 percent of neonates weighing less than 1500 g (Burstein 1979; Lee 1979). The hemorrhage is mild in about 25 percent. Intraventricular hemorrhage of varying degree develops in over 75 percent of such cases (Albright 1981). The hemorrhage is clinically unsuspected in the majority of these infants. Burstein et al. (1979) reported that 68 percent of surviving premature infants had unsuspected hemorrhage found on CT.

These neonatal hemorrhages originate in the germinal matrix, a loose meshwork of highly vascular tissue with little supporting stroma which contains primitive nerve cells (De Reuck 1977) and is located beneath the ependyma lining the lateral wall of the lateral ventricle. The germinal matrix is largest in the region of the head of the caudate nucleus. Its size is greatest between the twenty-fourth and thirty-second week of gestation, after which involution occurs. It is the source of nerve cells which migrate to the surface cortex during fetal development (Friede 1976). The exact cause of germinal-matrix hemorrhage is uncertain, but cerebral hypoxia related to neonatal respiratory distress, which is frequently associated with cardiac and vasomotor instability, is thought to predispose to this hemorrhage (Lou 1980). The hemorrhage usually develops during the first 4 days of life and is frequently not present at birth (Lee 1979).

The hemorrhages may range in degree from mild to very severe. They may be localized in one or several regions of the germinal matrix. The head of the caudate nucleus adjacent to the frontal horn is the site most frequently involved (Fig. 14-53) with hemorrhages, which may also originate from the region of the body and trigone of the lateral ventricle (Lee 1979). Varying degrees of intraventricular rupture occur in the majority of cases, being mild in about 25 percent (Fig. 14-53). Large brain hemorrhage or ventricular hemorrhage develops in about 25 percent of the cases and carries a grave prognosis (Burstein 1979).

Small intraventricular hemorrhages clear by 7 to 9 days; large ones take up to 2 weeks (Albright 1981), and parenchymal hemorrhages may take up to 3 weeks to resolve. The last frequently lead to porencephalic ventricular dilatation. Intraventricular hemorrhage results in hydrocephalus about one-third

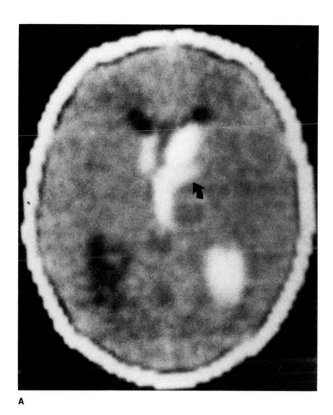

A

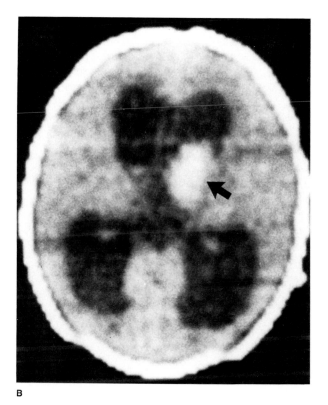

B

Figure 14-53 Large intraventricular rupture of germinal matrix hemorrhage with development of hydrocephalus. **A.** Extensive hemorrhage filling left lateral and third ventricles with small extension into right frontal horn. Site of hemorrhage appears to be sub-ependymal in the posterior portion of caudate nucleus head (arrow). **B.** Two weeks after **A:** Marked hydrocephalus has developed. Residual localized hematoma remains against the lateral wall at the posterior aspect of left frontal horn.

of the time. Burstein et al. (1979) reported that small intraventricular hemorrhages did not cause hydrocephalus, whereas 90 percent of large ones did. In contrast, Albright and Fellows (1981) observed that the size of the intraventricular hemorrhage did not correlate well with the subsequent development of hydrocephalus. In their series hydrocephalus was closely related to the ventricular size at the time of the initial hemorrhage; the larger the initial size of the ventricles, the greater was the probability for development of progressive hydrocephalus requiring shunting. Symptomatic hydrocephalus usually becomes evident between the first and the third week after birth.

Periventricular Leukomalacia

Periventricular hypodensity greater than would be expected with prematurity alone (Robinson 1966) has been observed in about 95 percent of premature neonates with intracerebral hemorrhage (Albright 1981). Serial CT scans on these infants have shown worsening of the periventricular hypodensity in 54 percent on scans obtained during the following several weeks. The areas of white-matter hypodensity become larger, with a progressively lower attenuation value. Subsequently, atrophic mild to severe ventricular and sulcal dilatation develops, depending on the maximum severity of periventricular hypodensity (Volpe 1966). The parenchymal hypodensity becomes less evident with the ventricular

enlargement, although there may be some persistence of hypodensity in the white matter. Pathologic studies have shown leukomalacia and white-matter coagulation necrosis, indicating that an anoxic ischemic insult to the brain is the most probable cause (de Reuck 1972). The hypodensity involves the frontal white matter alone in 45 percent, the frontal and parietal-occipital white matter together in 33 percent, the parietal-occipital white matter alone in eight percent, and the white matter diffusely in 15 percent of cases (Albright 1981). Its bilateral distribution in the white matter is frequently asymmetric.

Abnormal and progressive periventricular low density also develops in premature infants who have respiratory distress without intracerebral hemorrhage (Di Chiro 1978); a majority of these premature neonates develop this hypodensity (Albright 1981). Its distribution is similar to that seen in those infants with germinal-matrix hemorrhage. Caution must be exercised when calling periventricular hypodensity abnormal during the first 1 to 2 weeks post partum in premature infants, in whom the white matter is normally less dense than that of full-term infants because of less developed myelinization (Estrada 1980). In order to accurately evaluate these infants for possible periventricular leukomalacia, follow-up scans should be obtained in 4 to 6 weeks. The ultimate prognosis for surviving premature infants, both those with and those without intracerebral hemorrhage, appears most closely related to the degree and persistence of periventricular hypodensity and its subsequent atrophic consequences.

Bibliography

ADAMS RD, VANDER EECKEN HM: Vascular diseases of brain. *Ann Rev Med* **4**:213, 1953.

ADAMS RD and SIDMAN RL: *Introduction to Neuropathology*. New York, McGraw-Hill Book Company, 1968.

AEISEN AL, GABRIELSEN TO, MCCUNE WJ: MR imaging of systemic lupus erythematosus involving the brain. *Am J Neuroradiol* **6**:197–201, 1985.

ALBRIGHT L, FELLOWS R: Sequential CT scanning after neonatal intracerebral hemorrhage. *Am J Neuroradiol* **2**:133–137, 1981.

ALCALA H, GADO M, TORACK RM: The effect of size, histologic elements, and water content on the visualization of cerebral infarcts. *Arch Neurol* **35**:1–7, 1978.

ANDERSON DC, COSS DT, JACOBSON RL, MEYER MW: Tissue pertechnetate and iodinated contrast material in ischemic stroke. *Stroke* **11**:617–622, 1980.

BAKER HL JR, CAMPBELL JK, HOUSER OW et al: Early experience with the EMI scanner for study of the brain. *Radiology* **116**:327–333, 1975.

BANNA M, GROVES JT: Deep vascular congestion in dural venous thrombosis on computed tomography. *J Comput Assist Tomogr* **3**:539–541, 1979.

BILANIUK LT, PATEL S, ZIMMERMAN RA: Computed tomography of systemic lupus erythematosus. *Radiology* **124**:119–121, 1977.

BILANIUK LT, ZIMMERMAN RA, BROWN L, YOO HJ, GOLDBERG HI: Computed tomography in meningitis. *Neuroradiology* **16**:13–14, 1978.

BLAND WH: *Nuclear Medicine.* New York, McGraw-Hill Book Company, 1971, pp 262–267.

BRADAC GM, OBERSON R: CT and angiography in cases with occlusive disease of supratentorial cerebral vessels. *Neuroradiology* **19**:193–200, 1980.

BRIERLEY JB: Cerebral hypoxia, in Blackwood W, Corsellis JAN (eds): *Greenfield's Neuropathology.* London, Edward Arnold Ltd., 1976, pp 43–85.

BRUCHER JM: Neuropathological problems posed by carbon-monoxide poisoning and anoxia. *Prog Brain Res* **24**:75–100, 1967.

BUELL V, KAZNER E, RATH M, STEINHOFF H, KLEINHANS E, LANKSCH W: Sensitivity of computed tomography and serial scintigraphy in cerebrovascular disease. *Radiology* **131**:393, 1979.

BUONANNO FS, MOODY DM, BALL MR, LASTER DW: Computed cranial tomographic findings in cerebral sinovenous occlusion. *J Comput Assist Tomogr* **2**:281–290, 1978.

BURSTEIN J, PAPILE LA, BURSTEIN R: Intraventricular hemorrhage and hydrocephalus in premature newborns: A prospective study with CT. *Am J Roentgenol* **132**:631–635, 1979.

CAIRNS H, RUSSELL DS: Cerebral arteritis and phlebitis in pneumococcal meningitis. *J Pathol Bacteriol* **58**:649–665, 1946.

CAMPBELL JK, HOUSER OWN, STEVENS JC, WAHNER HW, BAKER HL, FOLGER WN: Computed tomography and radionuclide imaging in the evaluation of ischemic stroke. *Radiology* **126**:695–702, 1978.

CHARCOT JD, BOUCHARD C: Nouvelles recherches sur la pathogénie de l'hemorrhagie cérébrale. *Arch Physiol Norm Path (Paris)* **1**:110–127, 1868.

CHIU LC, CHRISTIE JH, SCHAPIRO RL: Nuclide imaging and computed tomography in cerebral vascular disease. *Semin Nucl Med* **7**:175–195, 1977.

CHU NS: Tuberculous meningitis: Computerized tomographic manifestations. *Arch Neurol* **37**:458–460, 1980.

COLE FM, YATES PO: The occurrence and significance of intracerebral microaneurysms. *J Pathol Bacteriol* **93**:393–411, 1967.

COCKRILL HH JR, DREISBACH J, LOWE B, YAM AUCHI T: Computed tomography in leptomeningeal infections. *Am J Roentgenol* **130**:511–515, 1978.

CRAVIOTO H, FEIGIN I: Noninfectious granulomatous angiitis with a predilection for the nervous system *Neurology* **9**:599–609, 1959.

CRONEVIST S, BRISMAR, J, KJELLIN K, SODERSTROM CE: Computer assisted axial tomography in cerebrovascular lesions. *Radiology* **118**:498, 1976.

CRONQVIST S, LAROCHE F: Transient hyperaemia in focal cerebral vascular lesions studied by angiography and regional cerebral blood flow measurements. *Br J Radiol* **40**:270–274, 1967.

CRONQVIST S: Regional cerebral blood flow and angiography in apoplexy. *Acta Radiol [Diagn] (Stockholm)* **7**:521–534, 1968.

DASTER DK, UDANI PM: The pathology and pathogenesis of tuberculous encephalopathy. *Acta Neuropathol (Berl)* **6:**311–326, 1966.

DAVIS KR, ACKERMAN RH, KISTLER JP, MOHR JP: Computed tomography of cerebral infarction: Hemorrhagic, contrast enhancement, and time of appearance. *Comput Tomogr* **1:**71–86, 1977.

DAVIS KR, TAVERAS JM, NEW PFJ, SCHNUR A, ROBERSON GH: Cerebral infarction diagnosis by computerized tomography: Analysis and evaluation of findings. *Am J Roentgenol* **124:**643–660, 1975.

DENNY-BROWN D: Recurrent cerebrovascular episodes. *Arch Neurol* **2:**194–210, 1960.

DE REUCK J: Arterial vascularisation and angioarchitecture of the nucleus caudatus in human brain. *Eur Neurol* **5:**130–136, 1971a.

DE REUCK JL, VANDER EECKEN HM: Periventricular leukomalacia in adults. *Arch Neurol* **35:**517–521, 1978.

DE REUCK J, CHATTA AS, RICHARDSON EP: Pathogenesis and evolution of periventricular leukomalacia in infancy. *Arch Neurol* **27:**229–236, 1972.

DE REUCK JL: The significance of the arterial angioarchitecture in perinatal cerebral damage. *Acta Neurol Belg* **77:**65–94, 1977.

DE REUCK, J: The human periventricular arterial blood supply and the anatomy of cerebral infarctions. *Eur Neurol* **5:**321–334, 1971b.

DI CHIRO G, ARIMITSU T, PELLOCK JM, LANDES RD: Periventricular leukomalacia related to neonatal anoxia: Recognition by computed tomography. *J Comput Assist Tomogr* **2:**352–355, 1978.

DI CHIRO G, TIMINS EL, JONES AE, JOHNSTON GS, HAMMOCK MK, SWANN SJ: Radionuclide scanning and microangiography of evolving and completed brain infarction: A correlative study in monkeys. *Neurology* **24:**418–423, 1974.

DOKINSKS CA, BILANIUK LT, ZIMMERMAN RA, KUHL DE: Computed tomography of intracerebral hematomas. I. Transmission CT observations on hematoma resolution. *Am J Roentgenol* **129:**681–688, 1977a.

DOKINSKAS CA, BILANIUK LT, ZIMMERMAN RA, KUHL DE, ALAVI A: Computed tomography of intracerebral hematomas: II. Radionuclide and transmission CT studies of the perihematoma region. *Am J Roentgenol* **129:**689–692, 1977b.

DUDLEY AW JR, LUNZER S, HEYMAN A: Localization of radioisotope (chlormerodrin He-203) in experimental cerebral infarction. *Stroke* **1:**143–148, 1970.

EICK JJ, MILLER KD, BELL KA, TUTTON RH: Computed tomography of deep cerebral venous thrombosis in children. *Radiology* **140:**399–402, 1981.

EISENBERG H, MORRISON JT, SULLIVAN P, FOOTE FM: Cerebrovascular accidents. *JAMA* **189:**883–888, 1964.

ELLIS GG, VERITY MA: Central nervous system involvement in systemic lupus erythematosus: A review of neuropathologic findings in 57 cases, 1955-1977. *Semin Arthritis Rheum* **8:**212–221, 1979.

ENZMANN DR, NORMAN D, MANI J, NEWTON H: Computed tomography of granulomatous basal arachnoiditis. *Radiology* **120:**341–344, 1976.

ESTRADA M, GAMMA TE, DYKEN PR: Periventricular low attenuations: A normal finding in computerized tomographic scans of neonates? *Arch Neurol* **37:**754–756, 1980.

FAER MJ, MEAD JH, LYNCH RD: Cerebral granulomatous angiitis: Case report and literature review. *Am J Roentgenol* **129:**463–467, 1977.

FERRIS EJ, SHAPIRO JH, SIMEONE FA: Arteriovenous shunting in cerebrovascular occlusive disease. *Am J Roentgenol Radium Ther Nucl Med* **98:**631–636, 1966.

FISHER CM, ADAMS RD: Observations on brain embolism with special reference to the mechanism of hemorrhagic infarction. *J Neuropathol Exp Neurol* **10:**92–94, 1951.

FISHER CM, CURRY HB: Pure motor hemiplegia of vascular origin. *Arch Neurol* **13**:30–44, 1965.

FISHER CM: Capsular infarcts: The underlying vascular lesion. *Arch Neurol* **36**:65–73, 1979.

FISHMAN RA: Brain edema. *N Engl J Med* **293**:706–711, 1975.

FOX AJ, BOGOUSSLAVSKY J, CAREY LS et al: MRI of small medullary infarctions. *Am J Neuroradiol* **7**:229–233, 1986.

FRIEDE RL: *Developmental Neuropathology*. New York, Springer, 1976, pp 1–37.

GABRIELSEN TO, HEINZ ER: Spontaneous aseptic thrombosis of the superior sagittal sinus and cerebral veins. *Am J Roentgenol Radium Ther Nucl Med* **107**:579–588, 1969.

GABRIELSEN TO, SEEGER JF, KNAKE JE, STILWILL EW: Radiology of cerebral vein occlusion without dural sinus occlusion. *Radiology* **140**:403–408, 1981.

GADO MH, PHELPS ME, COLEMAN RE: An extravascular component of contrast enhancement in cranial computed tomography. *Radiology* **117**:595–597, 1975.

GILDERSLEVE N, KOO AH, MCCONALD CJ: Metastastic tumor presenting as intracerebral hemorrhage. *Radiology* **124**:109–112, 1977.

GILLES C et al: Cerebral amyloid angiopathy as a cause of multiple cerebral hemorrhage. *Neurology* **34**:730–735, 1985.

GINSBERG MD, MYERS RE, MCDONAGH BF: Experimental carbon-monoxide encephalopathy in the primate: II. Clinical aspects, neuropathology, and physiological correlation. *Arch Neurol* **30**:209–216, 1974.

GINSBERG MD, HEDLEY-WHYTE TE, RICHARDSON EP JR: Hypoxic ischemic leukoencephalopathy in man. *Arch Neurol* **33**:5–14, 1976.

GINSBERG MD: Delayed neurological deterioration following hypoxia, in Fahn S et al (eds), *Advances in Neurology*. New York, Raven Press, 1979, pp 21–47.

GLASER GH: Lesions of CNS in disseminated lupus erythematosus. *Arch Neurol Psychiatr* **67**:745–753, 1952.

GLASER GH: Neurologic manifestion in collagen diseases. *Neurology* **5**:751–766, 1955.

GOLDBERG HI: Clinical cerebral microangiography—magnification angiography and angiotomography, in Hilal S (ed), *Symposium on Small Vessel Angiography*. St. Louis, C.V. Mosby Company, 1973, pp 219–237.

GOLDBERG HI: Wilkins R.H., and Regugachary SS (eds.): *Radiology of Ischemic Cerebrovascular Disease in Neurosurgery*. New York, McGraw-Hill, 1985, pp 1219–1236.

GRUBB RL, COXE WS: Central nervous system trauma: Cranial, in Eliasson SG, Prensky AL, Hardin WB (eds), *Neurological Pathophysiology*. New York, Oxford University Press, 1974, pp 292–309.

HAKIM AM, RYDER-COOKE A, MELANSON D: Sequential CT appearance of stroke. *Stroke* **14**:893–897, 1983.

HANDA J, HANDA H, NAKANO Y, OKUNO T: Computed tomography in moyamoya: Analysis of 16 cases. *Comput Axial Tomogr* **1**:165–174, 1977.

HAYMAN LA, EVANS RA, BASTION FO, HINCK VC: Delayed high dose contrast CT; Identifying patients at risk of massive hemorrhagic infarction. *Am J Neuroradiol* **2**:139–147, 1981.

HAYMAN LA, SAKAI F, MEYER JS, ARMSTRONG D, HINCK VC: Iodine-enhanced CT patterns after cerebral arterial embolization in baboons. *Am J Neuroradiol* **1**:233–238, 1980.

HEINZ ER, DUBOIS P, OSBORNE D et al: Dynamic computed tomography study of the brain. *J Comput Assist Tomogr* **3**:641–649, 1979.

HOEDT-RASMUSSEN K, SKINHOJ E, PAULSON O et al: Regional cerebral blood flow in acute apoplexy: The "luxury perfusion syndrome" of brain tissue. *Arch Neurol* **17**:271–281, 1967.

HUNGERFORD GD, DUBOULAY GH: CT in patients with severe migraine. *Neurol Neurosurg Psychiatr* **39**:990, 1976.

INQUE Y, TAKEMOTA K, MIYAMOTO T, YOSHIKAWA N, TANIGUCHI S, SAIWAI S, NISHIMURA Y, KOMATSU T: Sequential computed tomography scans in acute cerebral infarction. *Radiology* **135**:655–662, 1980.

IRINO T, MINAMI T, TANEDA M, HARA K: Brain edema and angiographical hyperemia in postrecanalized cerebral infarction. *Acta Neurol Scand* [Suppl] **64**:134–135, 1977*a*.

IRINO T, TANEDA M, MINAMI T: Angiographic manifestations in postrecanalized cerebral infarction. *Neurology* **17**:471–475, 1977*b*.

ITO U, OHNO K, TOMITA H, INABA Y: Cerebral changes during recirculation following temporary ischemia in mongolian gerbils, with special reference to blood brain barrier change, in Schmiedek P (ed), *Microsurgery for Stroke: Third Symposium*. New York, Springer, 1976, pp 29–38.

JOHNSON RT, RICHARDSON EP: The neurological manifestations of systemic lupus erythematosus: A clinical pathological study of 24 cases and review of literature. *Medicine* **47**:337–367, 1968.

JORGENSEN L, TORBIK A: Ischaemic cerebrovascular diseases in an autopsy series: II. Prevalency, location, pathogenesis and clinical course of cerebral infarcts. *J Neurol Sci* **9**:285–320, 1969.

KALBAG RM, WOOLF AL: *Cerebral Venous Thrombosis*, with Special Reference to Primary Aseptic Thrombosis. London, Oxford University Press, 1967, p. 237.

KAMIJYO Y, GARCIA JH, COOPER J: Temporary regional cerebral ischemia in the cat. *J Neuropathol Exp Neurol* **36**:338–350, 1977.

KASSIK AE, NILSSON L, SIESJO BK: Acid-base and lactate-pyruvate changes in brain and CSF in asphyxia and stagnant hypoxia. *Scand J Clin Lab Invest* **22** (suppl 102) **3**:6, 1968.

KENDALL BE, CLAVERIA LE, QUIROGA W: CAT in leukodystrophy and neuronal degeneration, in du Boulay GH, Moseley IF (eds): *Computerized Axial Tomography in Medical Practice*. New York, Springer-Verlag, 1977.

KIDO DK, GOMEZ DG, SANTOS-BUCH CA, CASTON TV, POTTS DG: Microradiographic study of cerebral and ocular aneurysms in hypertensive rabbits. *Neuroradiology* **15**:21–26, 1978.

KIM KS, WEINBERG PE, SUH JH, HO SU: Acute carbon monoxide poisoning: Computed tomography of the brain. *Am J Neuroradiol* **1**:399–402, 1980.

KINDT GW, YOUMANS JR, ALBRANDO O: Factors influencing the autoregulation of cerebral blood flow during hypotension and hypertension. *J Neurosurg* **26**:299–305, 1967.

KINGSLEY DPE, WRADUE E, DUBOULAY EPGH: Evaluation of computed tomography in vascular lesions of the vertebrobasilar territory. *J Neurol Neurosurg Psychiatr* **43**:193–197, 1980.

KINKEL WR, JACOBS L: Computerized axial transverse tomography in cerebrovascular disease. *Neurology* **26**:924–930, 1976.

KLATZO J: Pathophysiological aspects of brain edema, in Reulen HJ, Schurmann K (eds): *Steroids and Brain Edema*. New York, Springer-Verlag, 1972, pp 1–8.

KODAMA N, SUZUKI J: Moyamoya disease associated with aneurysm. *J Neurosurg* **58**:565–569, 1978.

KOHLMEYER K, GRASER C: Comparative studies of computed tomography and measurements of regional cerebral blood flow in stroke patients. *Neuroradiology* **16**:233–237, 1978.

KRAYENBUHL H: Cerebral venous thrombosis: The diagnostic value of cerebral angiography. *Schweiz Arch Neurol Psychiatr* **74**:261–287, 1954.

KUDO T: Spontaneous occlusion of the circle of Willis: A disease apparently confined to Japanese. *Neurology* **18**:485–496, 1968.

KURTZKE JF: Epidemiology of cerebrovascular disease, in *Cerebrovascular Survey Report*. National Institute of Neurological and Communicative Disorders and Stroke and National Heart and Lung Institute, Joint Council Subcommittee on Cerebrovascular Disease, 1980, pp 135–176.

LADURNER G, SAGER WD, ILIFF LD, LECHNER H: A correlation of clinical findings and CT in ischaemic cerebrovascular disease. *Eur Neurol* **18**:281–288, 1979.

LAPRESLE J, FARDEAU M: The central nervous system and carbonmonoxide poisoning: II. Anatomical study of brain lesions following intoxication with carbonmonoxide (22 cases). *Prog Brain Res* **24**:31–75, 1967.

LASSEN NA: The luxury-perfusion syndrome and its possible relation to acute metabolic acidosis localized within the brain. *Lancet* **2**:1113–1115, 1966.

LASSEN NA, AGNOLI A: The upper limit of autoregulation of cerebral blood flow in the pathogenesis of hypertensive encephalopathy. *Scand J Clin Lab Invest* **30**:113–115, 1972.

LASTER DW, MOODY DM, BALL MR: Resolving intracerebral hematoma: Alteration of the "ring sign" with steroids. *Am J Roentgenol* **130**:935–939, 1978.

LAURENT JP, MOLINARI GF, OAKLEY JC: Primate model of cerebral hematoma. *J Neuropathol Exp Neurol* **35**:560–568, 1976.

LEE KF, CHAMBERS RA, DIAMOND C, PARK CH, THOMPSON NL, SCHNAPF D, PRIPSTEIN S: Evaluation of cerebral infarction by computed tomography with special emphasis on microinfarction. *Neuroradiology* **16**:156–158, 1978.

LEE BCP, GRASSI AE, SCHECHNER S, AULD PAM: Neonatal intraventricular hemorrhage: A serial computed tomography study. *J Comput Assist Tomogr* **3**:483–490, 1979.

LEEDS NE, GOLDBERG HI: Angiographic manifestations in cerebral inflammatory disease. *Radiology* **98**:595–604, 1971.

LEEDS NE, GOLDBERG HI: Abnormal vascular patterns in benign intracranial lesions: Pseudotumors of the brain. *Am J Roentgenol* **118**:567–575, 1973.

LEHRER H: The angiographic triad in tuberculous meningitis. *Radiology* **87**:829–835, 1966.

LEWIS SE, HICKEY DC, PARKEY RW: Radionuclide brain imaging: Its role and relation to CT scanning. *Comput Tomogr* **2**:155–172, 1978.

LHERMITTE F, GAUTIER JC, DEROUSNE C: Nature of occlusion of the middle cerebral artery. *Neurology* **20**:82, 1970.

LOTZ PR, BALLINGER WE JR, QUISLING RG: Subcortical arteriosclerotic encephalopathy: CT spectrum and pathologic correlation. *Am J Neuroradiol* **7**:817–822, 1986.

LOU HC: Perinatal hypoxic-ischemic brain damage and intraventricular hemorrhage: A pathogenic model. *Arch Neurol* **37**:585–587, 1980.

MANELFE C, CLANET M, GIGUAD M, BONAFE A, GUIRAUD B, RASCOL A: Internal capsule: Normal anatomy and ischemic changes demonstrated by computed tomography. *Am J Neuroradiol* **2**:149–155, 1981.

MASDEU JC, BERHOOZ A-K, RUBINA FA: Evaluation of recent cerebral infarction by computerized tomography. *Arch Neurol* **34**:417–421, 1977.

MATHEW NT, MEYERS JS: Abnormal CT scans in migraine. *Headache* **16**:272, 1976.

MATSUMOTO N, WHISNANT JP, KURLAND LT, OKAZAKI H: Natural history of stroke in Rochester, Minn., 1955 through 1969: An extension of a previous study, 1945 through 1954. *Stroke* **4**:20–29, 1973.

MCCALL AJ, FLETCHER PHJ: Pathology, in Kutchinson EC, Ackason EJ (eds), *Strokes: Natural History, Pathology and Surgical Treatment*. Philadelphia, WB Saunders Company, 1975, pp 36–105.

MERRITT HH: *A Textbook of Neurology*, 6th ed. Philadelphia, Lea & Febiger, 1979, pp 40–45.

MIURA T, MITOMO M, KAWAI R, HARADA K: CT of the brain in acute carbon monoxide intoxication: characteristic features and prognosis. *Am J Neuroradiology* **6**:739–742, 1985.

MOHR JP, FISHER CM, ADAMS RD: Cerebrovascular diseases, in Isselbacher KJ, Adams RD, Braunwald E, Petersdorf RG, Wilson JD (eds) *Harrison's Principles of Internal Medicine*, 9th ed. McGraw-Hill Book Company, 1980, pp 1911–1942.

MOLINARI GF, PIRCHER F, HEYMAN A: Serial brain scanning using technetium 99m in patients with cerebral infarction. *Neurology* **17**:627, 1967.

MURRAY RR, KAPILA A et al: Cerebral CT in drowning victims. *Am J Neuroradiol* **5**:177–179, 1984.

MYER JS, DENNY-BROWN D: The cerebral collateral circulation: I. Factors influencing collateral blood flow. *Neurology* **7**:447–458, 1957.

NELSON RF, PULLICINO P, KENDALL BE, MARSHALL J: Computed tomography in patients presenting with lacunar syndromes. *Stroke* **11**:256–261, 1980.

NISHIMOTO A, TAKEUCHI S: Abnormal cerebrovascular network related to the internal carotid arteries. *J Neurosurg* **29**:255–260, 1968.

NORMAN D, AXEL L, BERNINGER WH, EDWARDS MS, CANN C, REDINGTON RW, COX E: Dynamic computed tomography of the brain: Techniques, data analysis, and applications. *Am J Neuroradiol* **2**:1–12, 1981.

NORTON GA, KISHORE PRS, LIN J: CT contrast enhancement in cerebral infarction. *Am J Roentgenol* **131**:881–885, 1978.

NURICK S, BLACKWOOD W, MAIR WGP: Giant cell granulomatous angiitis of the central nervous system. *Brain* **95**:133–142, 1972.

O'BRIEN MD, JORDAN MM, WALTZ AG: Ischemic cerebral edema and the blood-brain barrier: Distribution of pertechnetate, albumin, sodium, and antipyrine in brains of cats after occlusion of the middle cerebral artery. *Arch Neurol* **30**:461–465, 1974.

OLSSON Y, CROWELL RM, KLATZO I: The blood brain barrier to protein tracers in focal cerebral ischemia and infarction caused by occlusion of the middle cerebral artery. *Acta Neuropathol* **18**:89–102, 1971.

PAULSON OB, LASSEN NA, SKINHOJ E: Regional cerebral blood flow in apoplexy without arterial occlusion. *Neurology* **20**:125–138, 1970.

PECKER J, SIMON J, GUY G, HERRY JF: Nishimoto's disease: Significance of its angiographic appearances. *Neuroradiology* **5**:223–230, 1973.

PERRONE P, CANDELISE L, SCOTTI G, DE GRANDI C, SCIALFA G: CT evaluation in patients with transient ischemic attack: Correlation between clinical and angiographic findings. *Eur Neurol* **18**:217–221, 1979.

PITTS FW, HASKIN ME, RIGGS HE, GROFF RA: Tumor-strain in cerebrovascular disease. *J Neurosurg* **21**:298–300, 1964.

PLUM F, POSNER JB, HAIN RF: Delayed neurological deterioration after anoxia. *Arch Intern Med* **110**:18–25, 1962.

PRINEAS J, MARSHALL J: Hypertension and cerebral infarction. *Br Med J* **1**:l4–17, 1966.

PULLICINO P, KENDALL BE: Contrast enhancement in ischaemic lesions: I. Relationship to prognosis. *Neuroradiology* **19**:235–239, 1980.

RAIL DL, PERKIN GD: Computerized tomographic appearance of hypertensive encephalopathy. *Arch Neurol* **37**:310–311, 1980.

RANGEL RA: Computerized axial tomography in brain death. *Stroke* **9**:597–598, 1978.

RAO KCVG, KNIPP HC, WAGNER EJ: Computed tomographic findings in cerebral sinus and venous thrombosis. *Radiology* **140**:391–398, 1981.

RAPPAPORT ZH, BRINKER RA, ROVIT RL: Evaluation of brain death with contrast enhanced computerized cranial tomography. *Neurosurgery* **2**:230–232, 1978.

Report to the President: A National Program to Conquer Heart Disease, Cancer and Stroke. Washington, President's Commission on Heart Disease, Cancer and Stroke, 1964, 1965.

ROBINSON MA, TIZARD MA: The cerebral nervous system in the newborn. *Br Med Bull* **22:**49–55, 1966.

ROMANUL FCA, ABRAMOWICZ A: Changes in brain and pial vessels in arterial border zones. *Arch Neurol* **11:**40–65, 1964.

ROSENBLUM WI, HADFIELD MG: Granulomatous angiitis of the nervous system in cases of herpes zoster and lymphosarcoma. *Neurology* **22:**348–354, 1972.

ROSENBERG GA, KORNFELD M, STOVRING J, BICKNELL JM: Subcortical arteriosclerotic encephalopathy (Binswanger): Computerized tomography. *Neurology* **29:**1102–1106, 1979.

RUFF RL, TALMAN WT, PETITO F: Transient ischemic attacks associated with hypotension in hypertensive patients with carotid artery stenosis. *Stroke* **12:**353–355, 1981.

RUMBAUGH CL, BERGERON RT, FANG HCH, MCCORMICK R: Cerebral angiographic changes in drug abuse patients. *Radiology* **101:**335–344, 1971.

RUSSELF RWR: Observations on intracerebral aneurysms. *Brain* **86:**425–442, 1963.

SOIN JS, BURDINE JA: Acute cerebral vascular accident associated with hyperfusion. *Radiology* **118:**109–112, 1976.

SOLE-LLENAS J, PONS-TORTELLA E: Cerebral angiitis. *Neuroradiology* **15:**1-11, 1978.

STEPHENS WE: *Pathology of the Cerebral Blood Vessels.* St. Louis, C.V. Mosby Company, 1972, pp 291–323.

SUGITANI Y, NAKAMA M, YAMAGUCHI Y, IMAIZUMI M, NAKADA T, ABE H: Neovascularization and increased uptake of ^{99}m Tc in experimentally produced cerebral hematoma. *J Nucl Med* **14:**912–916, 1973.

SUZUKI J, TAKAKU A: Cerebrovascular "moyamoya" disease: Disease showing abnormal net-like vessels in base of brain. *Arch Neurol* **20:**88–299, 1969.

TABOADA D, ALONSO A, OLAGUE R, MULAS F, ANDREW V: Radiological diagnosis of periventricular and subcortical leukomalacia. *Neuroradiology* **20:**33–41, 1980.

TAKAHASHI M, SAITO Y, KONNO K: Intraventricular hemorrhage in childhood moyamoya disease. *J Comput Assist Tomogr* **4:**117–120, 1980.

TAVERAS JM: Multiple progressive intracranial arterial occlusion: A syndrome of children and young adults. *Am J Roentgenol Radium Ther Nucl Med* **106:**235–268, 1969.

TREVOR RP, SONDHEINER FK, FESSEL WJ et al: Angiographic demonstrations of major cerebral vessel occlusion in systemic lupus erythematosus. *Neuroradiology* **4:**202–207, 1972.

VALAVANIS A, FRIEDE R, SCHUBIGER O, HAYEK J: Cerebral granulomatous angiitis simulating brain tumor. *J Comput Assist Tomgr* **3:**536–538, 1979.

VALK J: *Computed Tomography and Cerebral Infarction:* New York, Raven Press, 1980, p. 56.

VINES FS, DAVIS DO: Clinical-radiological correlation in cerebral venous occlusive disease. *Radiology* **98:**9–22, 1971.

VINTERS HV, GILBERT JJ: Amyloid angiopathy: Its incidence and complications in the aging brain. *Stroke* **12:**118, 1981.

VOLPE JJ: Perinatal hypoxic ischemia brain injury. *Pediatr Clin North Am* **23:**383–397, 1976.

WAGLE WA, SMITH TW, WEINER M: Intracerebral hemorrhage caused by cerebral amyloid angiopathy—pathologic correlation. *Am J Neuroradiol* **5:** 171–176, 1984.

WALL SD, BRANDT-ZWADZKI M, JEFFREY RB, BARNES B: High frequency CT findings within 24 hours after cerebral infarction. *AJNR* **2:**553–557, 1981.

WEINGARTEN KL, ZIMMERMAN RD, PINTO RS, WHELAN MA: CT changes of hypertensive encephalopathy. *AJNR* **6**:395–398, 1985.

WEISBERG LA: Computerized tomography in intracranial hemorrhage. *Arch Neurol* **36**:422–426, 1979.

WEISBERG LA: Computerized tomographic enhancement patterns in cerebral infarction. *Arch Neurol* **37**:21, 1980.

WENDLING LR: Intracranial venous sinus thrombosis: Diagnosis suggested by computed tomography. *Am J Roentgenol* **130**:978–980, 1978.

WHISNANT JP, FITZGIBBONS JP, KURLAND LT, SAYRE GP: Natural history of stroke in Rochester, Minnesota, 1945 through 1954. *Stroke* **2**:11–21, 1971.

WING SD, NORMAN D, POLLOCK JA, NEWTON TH: Contrast enhancement of cerebral infarcts in computed tomography. *Radiology* **121**:89–92, 1976.

WOLFSON SK JR, GUR D, YONAS H: Latchaw RE (ed), *Cerebral Blood Flow Determination in CT of the Head, Neck and Spine.* Chicago, Year Book Medical Pub., 1985, pp 27–52.

WOOD MW, WAKIM KG, SAYRE, GP, MILLIKAN CH, WHISNANT JP: Relationship between anticoagulants and hemorrhagic cerebral infarction in experimental animals. *Arch Neurol Psychiatr* **79**:390–396, 1958.

YAGNIK P, GONZALEZ C: White matter involvement in anoxic encephalopathy in adults. *J Comput Assist Tomogr* **4**:788–790, 1980.

YAMAGUCHI T, WALTZ AG, OKAZAKI H: Hyperemia and ischemia in experimental cerebral infarction: Correlation of histopathology and regional blood flow. *Neurology* **21**:565–578, 1971.

YARNELL PR, EARNEST MP, SANDERS B, BURDICK D: The "hot stroke" and transient vascular occlusions. *Stroke* **6**:517–520, 1975.

YOCK DH JR, MARSHALL WH JR: Recent ischemic brain infarcts at computed tomography: Appearances pre- and postcontrast infusion. *Radiology* **117**:599–608, 1975.

YOCK DH JR: CT demonstration of cerebral emboli. *J Comput Assist Tomogr* **5**:190–196, 1981.

ZEUMER H, SCHONSKY B, STRUM KW: Predominant white matter involvement in subcortical arteriosclerotic encephalopathy (Binswanger disease). *J Comput Assist Tomogr* **4**:14–19, 1980.

ZILKHA A, DAIZ AS: Computed tomography in the diagnosis of superior sagittal sinus thrombosis. *J Comput Assist Tomogr* **4**:124–126, 1980.

ZIMMERMAN RD, LEEDS NE, NAIDICH TP: Ring blush with intracerebral hematoma. *Radiology* **122**:707–711, 1977.

ZIEGLER DK, ZOSA A, ZILELI T: Hypertensive encephalopathy. *Arch Neurol* **12**:472–478, 1965.

15

WHITE MATTER DISEASE OF THE BRAIN

Gordon E. Melville

Richard E. Fernandez

Pulla R.S. Kishore

Seungho Howard Lee

While many diseases affect the white matter of the brain, it has been the practice to set apart a group of diseases in which destruction of normal myelin or production of abnormal myelin is the prominent feature. Because almost any injury or disease of the central nervous system can cause destruction of myelin, this classification is somewhat arbitrary and inconsistent. In certain disorders such as anoxic encephalopathy, the sheaths of the nerve fibers in the deep white matter can be destroyed while the axis cylinders are spared.

The white matter disorders that will be discussed in this chapter are listed in Table 15-1. They are subdivided into those disorders within which there is breakdown of normal myelin, termed *myelinoclastic*, and those diseases involving either formation or maintenance of abnormal myelin, termed *dysmyelinating*.

CT is a well-established technique for studying white matter disease. Magnetic resonance imaging (MRI) is a new noninvasive technique which has shown greater sensitivity to white matter abnormalities (Young 1983). However, because of the rarity of many white matter diseases coupled with limited availability of MR facilities, the MRI experience in evaluating these patients is not extensive yet. Some patients may not be suitable for MRI because of the longer period of patient immobility that is required to avoid motion artifacts.

Identification of areas of abnormal enhancement following intravenous contrast administration does allow CT to identify areas of active blood-brain bar-

Table 15-1 White Matter Disease of the Brain

Myelinoclastic diseases
  Multiple sclerosis
  Progressive multifocal leukoencephalopathy
  Disseminated necrotizing leukoencephalopathy
  Acute disseminated encephalomyelitis
  Schilder's disease (diffuse sclerosis)
  Central pontine myelinolysis
  Marchiafava-Bignami disease
Dysmyelinating diseases
  Metachromatic leukodystrophy
  Spongy degeneration (Canavan's disease)
  Globoid cell leukodystrophy (Krabbe's disease)
  Alexander's disease
  Pelizaeus-Merzbacher disease
  Adrenoleukodystrophy

rier breakdown. At present, routine MRI is unable to distinguish areas of active blood-brain barrier breakdown from glial scarring. Currently investigational MR contrast agents such as paramagnetic species do allow identification of blood-brain barrier breakdown in a similar manner to contrast-enhanced CT.

The MRI signal intensity in different regions of the brain is highly dependent upon the local myelin content. Myelin contains a large lipid component which reduces the amount of free molecular water by hydrophobic effect (Young 1983; Norton 1981). Many protons in myelin are tightly bound within fatty acid chains and do not contribute significantly to regional signal-intensity differences. When breakdown of the myelin structure occurs, free molecular water may enter and provide increased mobile proton density, thereby increasing the MRI signal intensity. There is also prolongation of the T_1 and T_2 relaxation times. Many factors including iron concentration affect the T_1 and T_2 values and thereby alter the MRI signal intensity.

These factors and their effects upon signal intensity are discussed in greater detail in Chapters 1 and 17. Quantitative values for T_1 and T_2 permit assessment of brain maturity as the myelin content increases during childhood. Such quantitative assess-

ments may be of value in monitoring the effects of therapy upon white matter disease.

MYELINOCLASTIC DISEASES

These entities are acquired diseases having inflammatory characteristics. To this group of demyelinating diseases could also be added secondary demyelination of any etiology such as intoxication, anoxia, deficiency syndromes, cerebral infarct, brain abscess, and cerebral tumors, either primary or metastatic (Heinz 1979; Rubinstein 1978).

Multiple Sclerosis (MS)

MS is a chronic relapsing and remitting disease characterized clinically by protean manifestations that include motor weakness, paresthesias, impaired vision, diplopia, and bladder dysfunction. The diagnosis may be uncertain at onset. Remission and relapse and new areas of involvement increase the diagnostic accuracy. While the cause of this disease is unknown, there is evidence suggesting an autoimmune infectious (slow virus) etiology. The peak incidence is between 20 and 40 years of age, with no race or sex predilection. Paraclinical tests including evoked-response tests and urodynamic assessment along with cerebral spinal fluid analysis have provided support for the clinical diagnosis.

The lesions of MS consist of localized areas of myelin breakdown which occur most commonly in the deep hemispheric white matter and periventricular regions. Plaques of MS may also occur in other white matter areas including the cerebellum and spinal cord where the distribution is highly variable. Most plaques are small (less than 1.5 cm in diameter), but the size may vary greatly up to several centimeters in diameter. Large lesions with mass effect can occur and may cause diagnostic dilemma. Long-standing disease results in generalized atrophy of the cerebral hemispheres, corpus callosum, and cerebellum. Cortical and deep gray matter plaques are rare, consisting of less than 5 percent of total plaques (Brownell 1962). Pathologically, the lesions commonly progress to glial scarring (Schumacher 1965).

Before MRI was introduced, CT played a greater role in the diagnostic evaluation of the patient suspected of having MS (Aita 1978; Lebow 1978; Marano 1980; Morariu 1980). Old areas of glial scarring may be seen as well-defined hypodensities in the deep white matter and periventricular regions. In the acute phase, evolving plaques may show enhancement on CECT. An individual plaque may demonstrate a variety of enhancement patterns, described as homogeneous, diffuse, peripheral, edge, ring, and central (Marano 1980; Weisberg 1981; Wang 1983). Absence of associated subjacent edema and mass effect is noteworthy in most MS plaques (Fig. 15-1). Occasionally, CE plaques are associated with mass effect suggestive of brain tumors (Fig. 15-1*E* and *F*) (Wang 1983). The enhancement represents areas of blood-brain barrier breakdown which may become less apparent or disappear during steroid therapy (Sears 1978; Wang 1983). The posterior fossa and spinal cord lesions are considerably more difficult to identify by CT because of the inherent imaging limitations in those areas. Detection of plaques has been reported in 18 to 47 percent in various series (Glydensted 1976; Hershey 1979; Weinstein 1984; Sheldon 1985). High doses of intravenous contrast material and delayed scanning have modestly improved the detection rate (Spiegel 1985). In the face of long-standing disease, atrophy of the cerebral hemispheres (Fig. 15-1) and the cerebellum, especially the vermis, is common (Cala 1978). Nonetheless, CT is highly effective for identifying or excluding other disease abnormalities which can be confused with multiple sclerosis.

MRI is the most sensitive imaging procedure capable of detecting MS plaques, and it probably can replace CT in the diagnosis and follow-up of patients with MS (Sheldon 1985) and may be an acceptable tool for monitoring the progress of the disease and the response to therapy (Edwards 1986). In the authors' experience, MRI has largely replaced CT in the management of MS patients. In Sheldon's series, MRI was positive in 85 percent, paraclinical tests in 79 percent, CSF analysis in 74 percent, and CT in 25 percent. Even some plaques within the spinal cord can be imaged (Maravilla 1984; Sheldon 1985). A long thin (2- to 3-mm) lesion extending

along the inner surface of the corpus callosum has been observed in some patients (Simon 1986). At present, a single MRI evaluation cannot determine the activity of plaques, and serial examinations allow detection of increase in size and number of plaques which indicates active disease. Identification of active blood-brain barrier breakdown is possible only with investigational MR contrast agents or CECT.

The MS plaque appears as an area of hyperintensity on MR images with long TR. They vary in size and shape and are usually located along the paraventricular white matter (Fig. 15-2). The cerebral hemisphere was involved in all patients with definite MS and 44 percent had concomitant lesions in the posterior fossa (Sheldon 1985). Heavily T_2-weighted images (e.g., TR 2000/TE 120) may obscure some abnormalities by the contiguous hyperintense cerebral spinal fluid. MRI can be one of the most sensitive confirmatory examinations available at present, but about 15 percent of MS patients may have normal MRI even in the presence of definite clinical evidence (Sheldon 1985; Drayer 1986; Farlow 1986). Thalamic signal intensity on T_2-weighted images may be abnormally decreased in patients with severe or moderately severe MS. This change is most likely due to increased iron accumulation produced by metabolic dysfunction (Drayer 1986).

Correlation between the site of an MS plaque and the clinical symptoms has been inconsistent in both CT (Cala 1978; Reisner 1980) and MRI (Sheldon 1985). Small plaques within the brainstem and optic nerves are frequently not detectable even on T_2-weighted MR images. Another difficulty establishing clinical correlation results from demyelinated axons that continue to transmit pulses (Lebow 1978). Clinical remission most likely occurs when axons resume transmission which previously has been blocked at the time of acute demyelination. Remyelination can occur but to a limited degree (Prineas 1979). However, the duration of the disease appears to correlate with number of lesions, especially for those who had had the disease for 7 or more years (Sheldon 1985).

Difficulty can arise differentiating MS plaques from other causes of increased white matter signal intensity on MRI. Normally, punctate areas of high

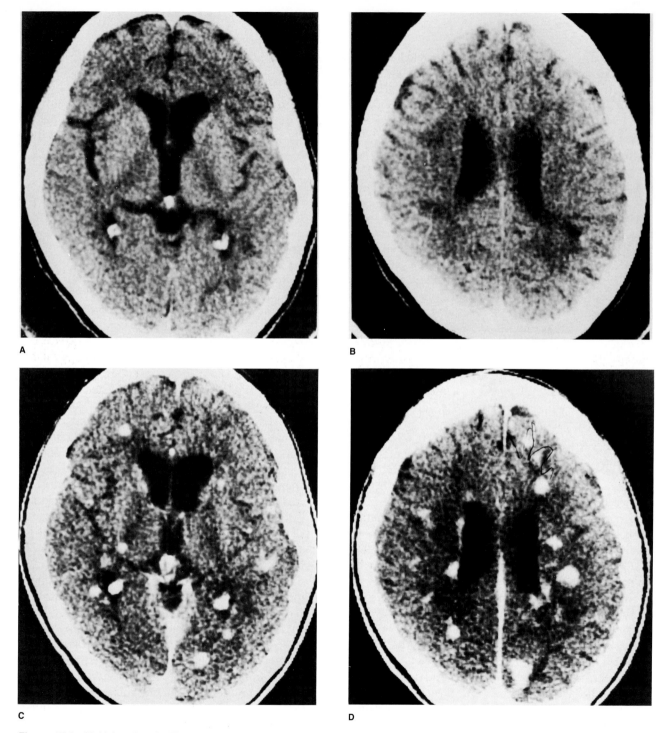

A

B

C

D

Figure 15-1 Multiple sclerosis. These images are of a 31-year-old female with a long history of known multiple sclerosis. **A** and **B.** NCCT images reveal diffuse central and cortical atrophy of both hemispheres. There are multiple areas of hypodensity in the white matter. **C** and **D.** CECT images disclose multiple contrast-enhancing plaques in the white matter, particularly in the per-iventricular region. A few of the hypodense areas do not show contrast enhancement, indicating old plaques. Dramatic improvement in clinical condition and almost complete disappearance of the multiple sclerosis plaques were noted after steroid therapy. Left frontal artifact is present. (*Continued on p. 721.*)

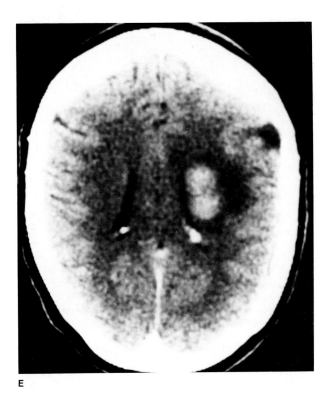

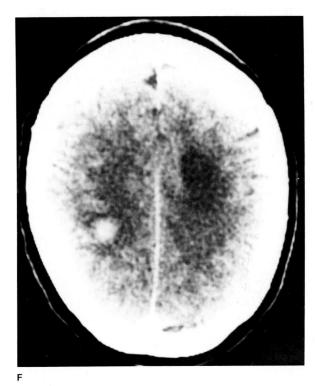

E

F

Figure 15-1 (*Cont.*) **E** and **F**: Unusual appearance of multiple sclerosis plaques with edema and mass effect around the CE plaques suggesting brain tumors.

signal intensity are identified in the white matter just anterior and lateral to both frontal horns. This finding is attributed to the loose network of axons with low myelin content and the greater flow of interstitial fluid in this region (Brant-Zawadzki 1985; Sze 1986). This should not be mistaken for an area of demyelination.

Focal and diffuse periventricular hyperintensity (PVH) on MRI is known to be associated with a variety of pathologic processes such as hydrocephalus, subcortical arteriosclerotic encephalopathy, radiation necrosis, systemic lupus erythematosus, MS and other white matter diseases, and also normal individuals (Bradley 1984; Zimmerman 1986). A thin rim of PVH may be seen in normal patients because of the slightly higher concentration of interstitial water at the ventricular lining that results from the normal flow of interstitial water into the lateral ventricles from the extracellular space (Rosenberg 1980). Zimmerman (1986) observed some degree of PVH in

93.5 percent of his 365 patients regardless of diagnosis. In our experience with 1.5T MR unit, we found that most patients do not have PVH although we agree that PVH may be seen in patients with no other evidence of intracranial pathology and is probably a nonspecific secondary phenomenon. This discrepancy could be due to different patient population, magnetic field size, and pulse sequences, requiring further analysis. Hydrocephalus produces diffuse PVH by transventricular absorption of CSF. This finding is more prominent on MRI than on CT. In severe hydrocephalus, the peripheral margins of PVH are irregular but blunted and do not extend to the gray-white matter junction. The PVH in severe demyelinating diseases has more sharply angled outer margins and usually does extend to the corticomedullary junction (Zimmerman 1986). In those patients with extensive multifocal white matter lesions produced by demyelination of ischemic disease, the PVH alone is indistinguishable from mild

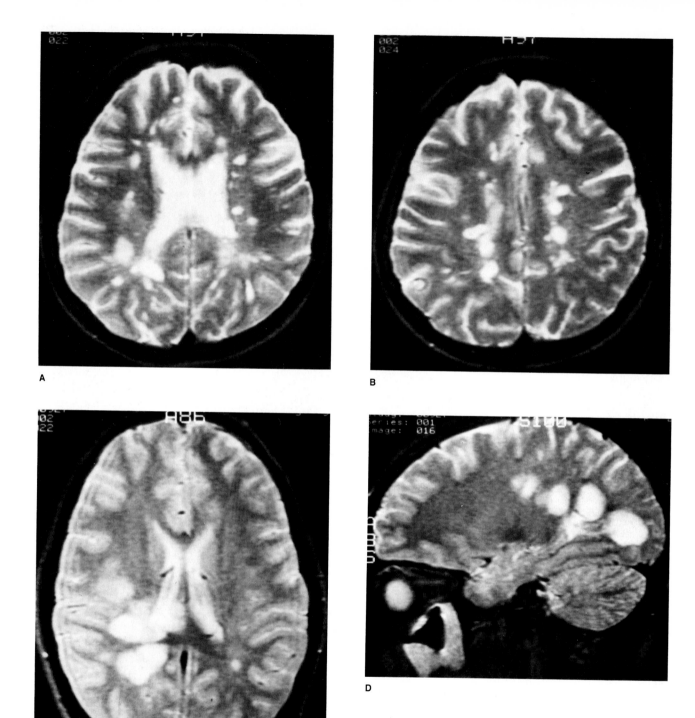

A

B

C

D

Figure 15-2 Multiple sclerosis on MRI. **A** and **B.** (T_2-WI) show multiple discrete periventricular hyperintense plaques. **C** and **D.** (T_2-WI) exhibit larger confluent plaques in the white matter on another patient.

to moderate periventricular edema resulting from hydrocephalus. The other white matter abnormalities usually allow differentiatation from the PVH in hydrocephalus, although both may coexist. The validity of these criteria should be further investigated.

Diffuse patchy white matter areas of hyperintensity on MRI are commonly found in 20 to 30 percent of patients over the age of 65 (Bradley 1984). Most of these areas are found within the deep hemispheric white matter and are generally not contiguous with the ventricles (Fig. 15-3). A recent report suggests that these foci probably represent areas of increased water content in the aging brain, most likely on an ischemic basis (Brant-Zawadski 1985). White matter experiences a lower regional perfusion than does gray matter. The white matter may be more vulnerable to decreases in perfusion with advancing age. Differentiation of these lesions from MS plaques can be difficult without clinical infor-

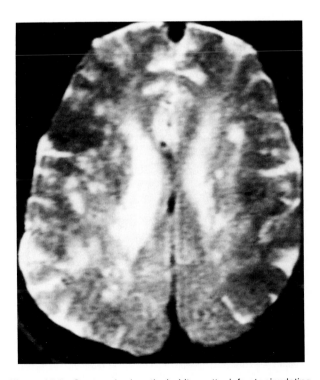

Figure 15-3 Scattered subcortical white matter infarcts simulating multiple sclerosis plaques on MRI (T$_2$-WI).

mation. The relationship of these lesions to diminished cognitive function and dementia is not consistent (Brant-Zawadski 1985).

Progressive Multifocal Leukoencephalopathy

Progressive multifocal leukoencephalopathy (PML) is a progressive disease of the central nervous system showing white matter involvement as a constant feature. The disease occurs usually in immunosuppressed patients (Post 1985; Levy 1985). The majority of these patients have either leukemia or lymphoma. It has also been reported in renal transplant recipients and in patients with tuberculosis, sarcoidosis, and macroglobulinemia (Carroll 1977; Lyon 1971; McCormick 1976). Only rarely was PML reported in patients with no known cause for immunosuppression (Richardson 1974). Papovavirus (JC, SV 40) has been isolated from the lesions of progressive multifocal leukoencephalopathy (Peters 1980). The usual clinical course is one of progression to coma, leading to death usually in 3 to 6 months after the onset of symptoms (Carroll 1977). The final diagnosis of progressive multifocal leukoencephalopathy depends on biopsy or postmortem examination (Peters 1980). Drug therapy has had varied success.

Pathological examination in PML demonstrates multifocal areas of demyelination with relative sparing of neurons. The mechanism for demyelination is considered by some to be a result of the death of oligodendroglia, the cells responsible for the sheath formation (Carroll 1977). The demyelinating lesions of PML appear to have a predilection for the subcortical white matter. Atrophy is a late occurrence in the disease.

Computed tomography plays an important role in the diagnosis of progressive multifocal leukoencephalopathy by suggesting the diagnosis as well as selecting sites for biopsy by revealing the characteristic low-density foci in the subcortical white matter (Carroll 1977; Wheelan 1983; Post 1985). The lesions are sharply marginated with a scalloped outer border (Fig.15-4). There appears to be a predilection for the parietooccipital region (Bosch 1976; Carroll 1977;

Post 1985). Follow-up examinations may show progressive enlargement of the demyelinating areas (Carroll 1977). Although rare, mass effect may be present (Cunningham 1977), as may contrast enhancement (Fig. 15-4*E, F, G*) (Heinz 1979).

MRI is a more sensitive technique for detection of white matter abnormalities caused by PML and other complications of the acquired immuno-deficiency syndrome (AIDS). While findings may be nonspecific, detection of an optimal biopsy site can be facilitated. Recently, direct brain involvement of LAV/HTLV-III virus known as AIDS dementia complex, a new clinical and pathological entity, presented diffuse atrophy and white matter and subcortical abnormalities on CT and MRI (see Chapter 12).

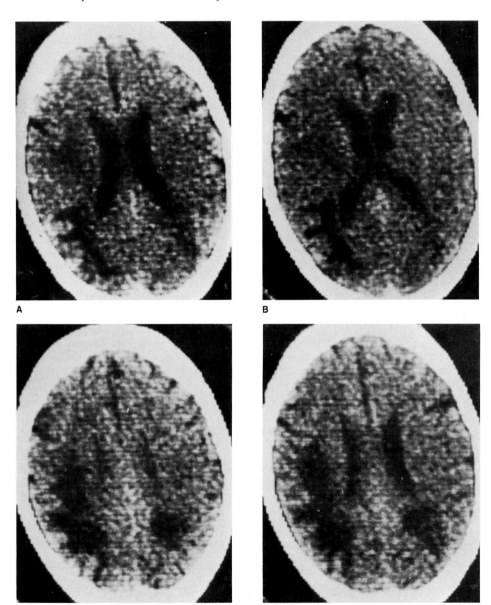

A

B

C

D

Figure 15-4   A, B, C, D. Progressive multifocal leukoencephalopathy. NCCTs of a 68-year-old man with a history of chronic lymphocytic leukemia reveal low-density zones (10–12 HU) in both hemispheres. Note the characteristic well-marginated medial aspect and scalloped outer border at junction of gray and white matter. No contrast enhancement was noted. *(Reproduced by permission from Carroll et al., 1977.)* *(Continued on p. 725.)*

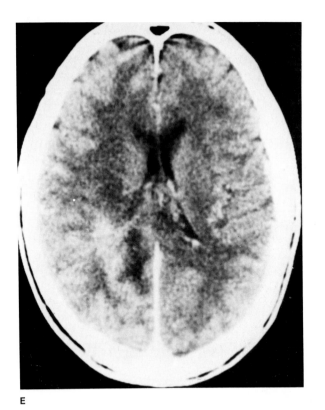

E

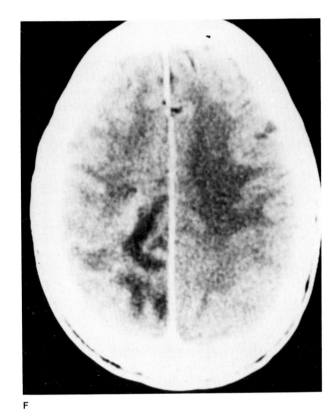

F

G

Figure 15-4 (*Cont.*)   Two AIDS patients with PML: **E** and **F** (CECT) show irregular parietooccipital lesion with enhancement.   **G** (CECT) reveals bilateral hypodense occipital periventricular lesions (arrows) with minimal enhancement. (*Courtesy of Dr. J.D. Post, University of Miami, Florida.*)

Disseminated Necrotizing Leukoencephalopathy

Disseminated necrotizing leukoencephalopathy is a disease affecting patients who have been treated with methotrexate, usually intrathecally for the prevention or treatment of meningeal leukemia or lymphoma as well as for the treatment of solid tumors (Allen 1978). In patients with leukemia or lymphoma who have been treated with systemic antitumor drugs, the central nervous system serves as a reservoir for tumor cells which are protected from the systemic drugs by the blood-brain barrier. To prevent relapse in these patients, radiation therapy and intrathecal administration of antitumor drugs have been undertaken (Aur 1972; Rubinstein 1975). Diffuse necrotizing leukoencephalopathy may occur following administration of systemic methotrexate without craniospinal irradiation (Allen 1978). The disease usually is clinically manifest as confusion, somnolence, spasticity, seizures, ataxia, and dementia and may lead to coma and death (Kay 1972; McIntosh 1973; Price 1975; De Vivo 1977).

Pathology of disseminated necrotizing leukoencephalopathy reveals multiple foci of coagulative necrosis of the white matter in a random manner which appears to extend by confluence and disseminates in the cerebral white matter (Rubinstein 1975, 1978). With progression of the disease, the demyelination may appear extensive and symmetrical (Rubinstein 1975). In the later phase of the disease, dystrophic calcification may occur in the basal ganglia or gray-white matter margin (Peylan-Ramu 1977).

Computed tomography can play an important role in necrotizing leukoencephalopathy because there has been some indication that the effects of this process may be partially reversible on discontinuation of the methotrexate therapy (Allen 1978; Pizzo 1976). Computed tomography in necrotizing leukoencephalopathy is to be distinguished from other changes seen in these patients such as dilatation of ventricular and subarachnoid spaces. These changes may be a result of cranial irradiation rather than those of necrotizing leukoencephalopathy (Peylan-Ramu 1978).

Computed tomography of necrotizing leukoencephalopathy demonstrates areas of hypodensity in the centrum semiovale and periventricular areas (Fig. 15-5) (Allen 1978; Peylan-Ramu 1977). On CECT there may be enhancement of the low-density lesions (Lane 1978). Mass effect may also be seen. When methotrexate is introduced via a reservoir in the ventricular system, necrotizing leukoencephalopathy may then be seen as a focal process at the tube tip, with edema and the appearance of a mass which may enhance following contrast administration and which may be confused with an abscess or other process (Bjorgen 1977). The intracerebral calcifications of necrotizing leukoencephalopathy have been demonstrated by CT (Mueller 1976; Peylan-Ramu 1977, 1978). No MR reports of this entity are known to us at this time.

Acute Disseminated Encephalomyelitis

Acute disseminated encephalomyelitis (ADE) is usually an explosive although sometimes subacute widespread central nervous system inflammatory condition which severely affects the white matter, leading to a marked neurologic impairment. The clinical outcome is varied, and the disease may be fatal, completely reversible, or may give permanent neurological disability (Schumacher 1965). There is no age or sex predilection. It is usually monophasic; however, a few recurrent cases have been reported (Poser 1978). The disease can be divided into four types on the basis of etiology (Oppenheimer 1976): (1) postinfectious (measles, vaccinia, or varicella); (2) spontaneous or during the course of a nonspecific respiratory infection; (3) allergic (postvaccination); and (4) fulminating (nearly always fatal and characterized by multiple punctate intracerebral hemorrhages). An immune complex etiology has been proposed for ADE (Reik 1980).

Pathologically, the lesions may be indistinguishable from those of multiple sclerosis while others may show a more typical pattern of perivascular extraadventitial demyelinization with microglial reaction following the course of the cerebral veins. The foci are not limited to the white matter of the cerebrum but are frequently seen in the cerebral cortex,

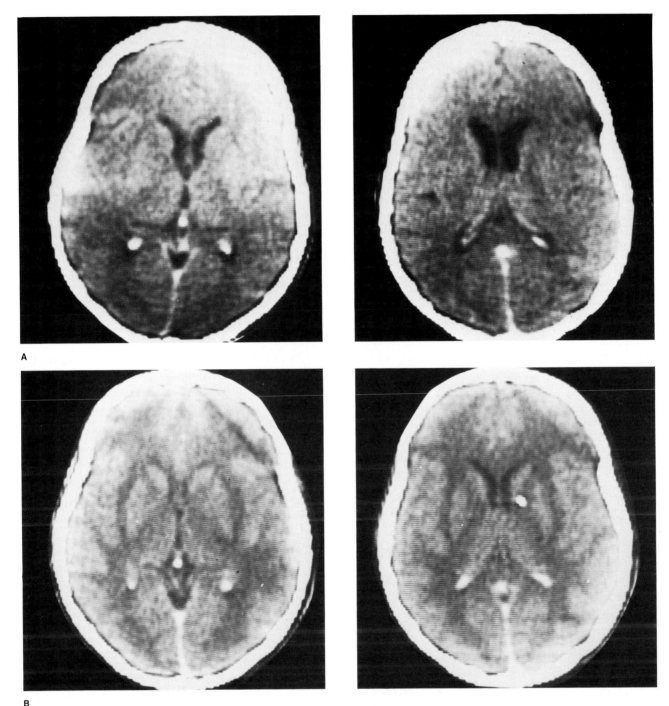

A

B

Figure 15-5   Disseminated necrotizing leukoencephalopathy. **A.** Initial CT of a patient on intrathecal methotrexate therapy reveals no gross abnormality.   **B.** CT images on the same patient performed 3 months later reveal diffuse low-density zones in both hemispheres.

cerebullum, basal ganglia, brainstem, and spinal cord as well (Oppenheimer 1976; Reik 1980; Schumacher 1965). Edema is a major component of the acute phase of the disease.

CT in ADE would show cerebral edema in the acute phase presenting as diffuse hypodensity within the hemispheric white matter (Adams 1985). Enhancement of the lesions is rare (Reich 1979; Valentine 1982). In the chronic stage CT would show variable amounts of white and gray matter loss with atrophy, depending on the severity and extent of involvement (Fig. 15-6). In our recent case of clini-

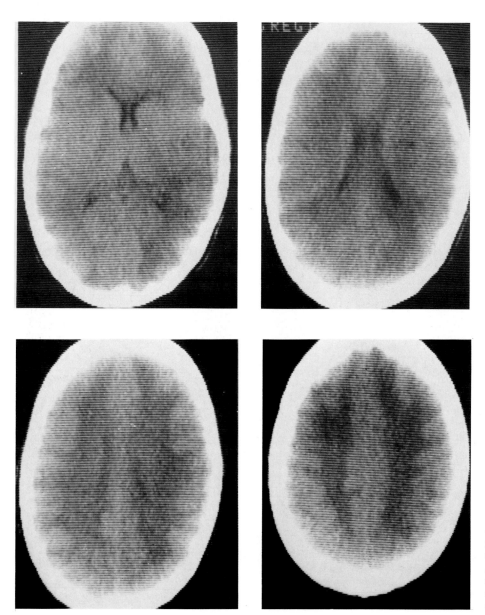

Figure 15-6 Acute disseminated encephalomyelitis. 18-year-old woman with bilateral hemispheric dysfunction and altered mental status. CT images reveal diffuse low-density zones in both hemispheres. Cerebrospinal fluid revealed markedly elevated gamma globulins with elevated rubella titers (1024:1).

cally evident ADE, T_2-weighted MRI showed diffuse punctate hyperintense lesions throughout the white matter and the basal ganglia 7 days after onset (Fig. 15-7).

It should be mentioned when considering ADE that there is another clinical entity known as *subacute sclerosing panencephalitis* which has been linked to the measles virus. Subacute sclerosing panencephalitis, unlike ADE, is a progressive disease showing at least two phases with the second phase characterized by periodic involuntary movements which may consist of jerking of the face, fingers, or limbs and may include torsion spasms of the trunk (Adams 1976). The CT appearance of subacute sclerosing panencephalitis has been described as showing no abnormality, cerebral atrophy either focal or diffuse, and low density areas of the basal ganglia as well as the white and gray matter (Duda 1980).

Schilder's Disease or Diffuse Sclerosis

The terms diffuse sclerosis and Schilder's disease have been applied to a wide variety of white matter diseases including hereditary metabolic leukodystrophies, adrenal leukodystrophy, and subacute viral encephalitis. If one separates these disorders, there is a characteristic group of cases that do correspond to Schilder's original description (Poser 1956, 1986). This disease is nonfamilial and occurs most frequently in children, with approximately 50 percent presenting before the age of 10. Dementia, homonymous hemianopsia, cortical blindness, cortical deafness, varying degrees of hemiplegia and quadriplegia are common clinical manifestations. Death usually occurs within a few months to years.

The characteristic lesion of diffuse sclerosis is a large, asymmetrical focus of myelin destruction that

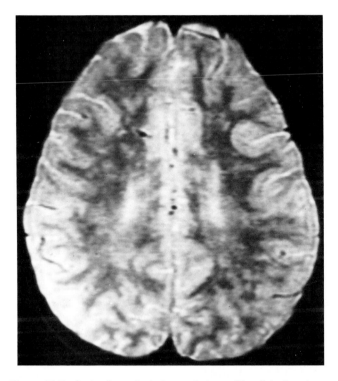

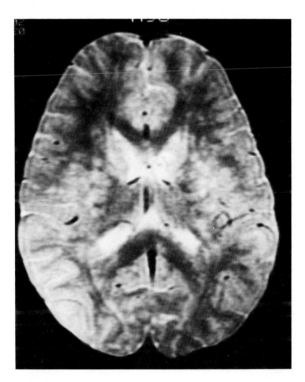

Figure 15-7 Acute disseminated encephalomyelitis, clinically evident in 6-year-old. MRI, 1 week after onset. Axial T_2 WIs show diffuse nonhomogeneous white matter and basal ganglia consisting of multiple punctate hyperintense signals.

often involves an entire lobe or hemisphere. Extension across the corpus callosum to involve the contralateral hemisphere may occur. Symmetrical disease has been found in some cases. Detailed pathologic study of the optic nerves, brainstem, and spinal cord reveals discrete lesions indistinguishable from MS. Many physicians consider that Schilder's

disease represents a form of progressive multiple sclerosis that occurs during childhood. The remitting and protracted symptom complex of MS that is commonly found in adults is quite rare in children.

The CT findings reflect the pathologic description above. CT identifies areas of hypodensity that correspond to the demyelination. This is most ap-

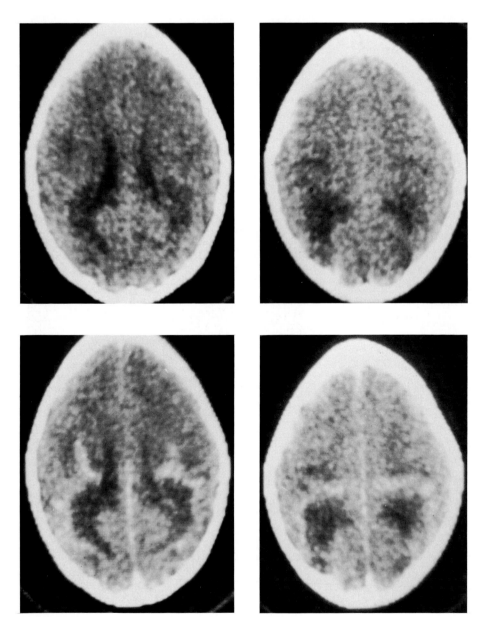

Figure 15-8 Schilder's disease. Noncontrast CT (*above*) and CECT (*below*) of a 6-year-old boy reveal periventricular hypodense zones that enhance markedly. These findings are consistent with an adrenoleukodystrophic form of Schilder's disease.

parent within the centrum semiovale. There may be mass effect. In the differential diagnosis, cerebral neoplasm is often a primary consideration. Enhancement can occur along the margin of the lesion (Fig. 15-8). The greater MRI sensitivity to white matter disease may allow detection of additional areas of involvement that are not apparent on CT, but to our knowledge, no MR report is available yet.

The *concentric sclerosis of Baló* is probably a variant of Schilder's disease. There are unique sharply demarcated alternating bands of destroyed and preserved myelin. There is a similar rapidly progressive clinical deterioration.

Central Pontine Myelinolysis

Adams (1959) first described the clinical and postmortem findings of this entity in four patients. The name, central pontine myelinolysis, precisely describes the anatomic localization of the disease and its key pathological finding: destruction of the myelin sheaths throughout the pons with relative sparing of the axis cylinders and preservation of the nerve cells of the pontine nuclei. Signs of inflammation are conspicuously absent, thereby allowing pathologic differentiation from MS and postinfectious encephalomyelitis. Many cases have presented during late chronic alcoholism, often associated with Wernicke disease and polyneuropathy. Quadriparesis, pseudobulbar palsy, and a "locked-in" state constitutes the major symptomatology of a well-developed lesion. Many cases go undetected, presumably because the pontine lesion is small and not suspected clinically. Variants of this syndrome are being discovered with increasing frequency. Brainstem evoked potential testing can confirm the pontine lesion.

Much attention has been focused upon the role of hyponatremia in the etiology of the disorder. All of Adams' patients and a series of 15 patients evaluated by Burcar (1977) had severe hyponatremia (less than 130 milliequivalents per liter). Laureno (1983) created a dog model of this disease wherein hyponatremia was produced by injections of vasopressin and intraperineal infusions of water. The dogs developed a rigid quadriparesis and showed at autopsy pontine lesions identical to those in the human disease. Presently, the lesion is thought to occur in association with a rapid rise in serum sodium in previously hyponatremic patients (Norenberg 1982; Sterns 1986). It can be difficult to determine whether severe brain damage associated with hyponatremia is secondary to the severity of hyponatremia or the speed of its correction (Arieff 1986). If respiratory arrest occurs, postanoxic encephalopathy may contribute to the neurologic injury.

On CT scan, a discrete area of hypodensity may be seen within the basis pontis (Hazratji 1983) (Fig. 15-9). Initially, this hypodensity may not be apparent, but may appear several days after the onset of

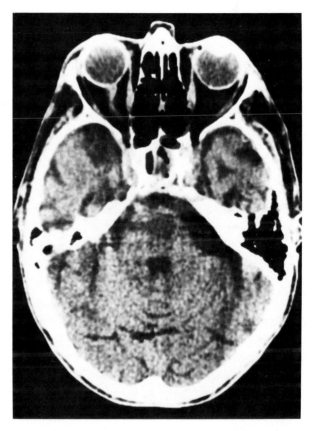

Figure 15-9 Central pontine myelinolysis. CT shows hypodensity in the pons representing central pontine myelinolysis. Note evidence of cerebellar atrophy.

the neurologic deterioration. Artifacts from the petrous bones frequently obscure detail in the brainstem on CT scans. Extension posteriorly into the medial lemnisci and up into the midbrain is uncommon, but extrapontine involvement of the anterior temporal lobe (Hazratji 1983) and the thalamic-putamenal region (Thompson 1981) has been reported on CT. An intact rim of myelin is preserved along the margin of the pons. Rarely other areas of demyelination may be seen in the internal capsule, thalamus, and cerebral cortex (Adams 1985).

A well-defined pontine lesion with prolonged relaxation times can be shown by MRI (DeWitt 1984). The lack of artifacts in the brainstem region on MRI should facilitate detection of these lesions. Differentiation from infarct, MS or encephalomyelitis can generally be made in conjunction with pertinent clinical information.

Marchiafava-Bignami Disease

This disease is characterized by clearly demarcated zones of demyelination within the corpus callosum. The first reported cases of this disease were Italian men who had a long history of alcoholism and frequently a high intake of red wine. Other investigators have identified the disease in multiple other nationalities and also in abstainers (Adams 1985). A nutritional etiology is suspected but the deficiency factor has not been identified. The mechanism of the selected white matter injury is also unknown.

Clinical features of the illness are variable and do not constitute a clear-cut syndrome. In many patients, the clinical picture is dominated by other alcohol effects, such as tremor, seizures, delirium tremens, and Wernicke's disease. The diagnosis is rarely made during life but can be suspected when an alcoholic presents with a frontal lobe syndrome.

During the acute phase of the disease, there is hypodensity of the corpus callosum on CT scan. Contrast enhancement in the corpus callosum has been reported. As the lesion progresses to glial scarring, the corpus callosum assumes an atrophic appearance. Accompanying cortical atrophy is common and frequently more pronounced in the frontal lobes (Rancurel 1982).

To our knowledge, there have been no reported cases of Marchiafava-Bignami disease studied by MRI.

DYSMYELINATING DISEASES

Dysmyelination was originally introduced to differentiate conditions in which normally formed myelin is destroyed (e.g., multiple sclerosis) from a group of diseases in which there appears to be abnormal myelin formation or maintenance (Poser 1957). The dysmyelinating diseases can be subdivided into those which are considered primarily white matter disease and those which, either additionally or primarily, affect gray matter, which would include Niemann-Pick disease, Gaucher's disease, and Tay-Sachs disease (Malone 1976; Poser 1978). Only those diseases that affect white matter primarily are discussed in this chapter.

This group of dysmyelinating diseases is made up largely of the leukodystrophies. These diseases are inherited diseases showing either autosomal recessive, autosomal dominant, or sex-linked recessive modes of inheritance. Specific enzyme deficiencies have been shown in two of the leukodystrophies, namely, globoid cell leukodystrophy and metachromatic leukodystrophy (Rubinstein 1978). While most authors feel that the pathological changes in leukodystrophy are secondary to a specific enzyme deficiency, this hypothesis has been questioned by others (Poser 1978). With the exception of metachromatic leukodystrophy and globoid cell leukodystrophy, the leukodystrophies do not affect the peripheral nervous system (Malone 1976). It is expected that MR will detect the white matter lesions earlier than CT, which may help in making the diagnosis promptly and facilitate precise selection of biopsy site. However, specificity of MR should be further investigated.

Metachromatic Leukodystrophy

Metachromatic leukodystrophy is a progressive autosomal recessive disorder which derives its name from the marked staining of metachromatic lipids. It may occur from the perinatal period (Feigin 1954) to advanced life. The oldest reported case is a man who became symptomatic for the first time at the age of 62 (Bosch 1978). The majority of the cases, however, present around the second year of life and become progressively worse with death by the third or fourth year. Occasional prolonged survival for several years has been reported (Malone 1976). The classic case is believed to have three clinical stages. The child is initially normal and then develops decreased truncal control, intellectual decline, and decreased responsiveness to the environment (Malone 1976). There is subsequent decline to an essentially unresponsive state with spasticity and "twitchlike" movements. In the late-onset type, there is a slower progression. The late juvenile and adult forms show dementia as a prominent feature, which may be the result of accumulation of sulfatides in neurons (Rubinstein 1978).

The role of CT in metachromatic leukodystrophy is to exclude other etiologies for the clinical findings.

The definitive diagnostic test as already noted is the demonstration of an aryl sulfatase A deficiency in the urine or serum. CT findings typically consist of diffuse symmetrical decrease in attenuation in the centrum semiovale (Fig. 15-10). Contrast enhancement or mass effect has not been reported (Buonanno 1978; Robertson 1977). Minimal ventricular dilatation suggesting atrophy has been described. A single case of late adult-onset type in which CT demonstrated normal attenuation of white matter has been described (Bosch 1978). Atrophy probably reflecting the patient's age was noted in this case.

Spongy Degeneration (Canavan's Disease)

Spongy degeneration is a disease of infancy demonstrating megalencephaly, blindness, initial hypotonia followed by spasticity, and progressive psychomotor deterioration with onset between the second and ninth months of life (Adornato 1972;

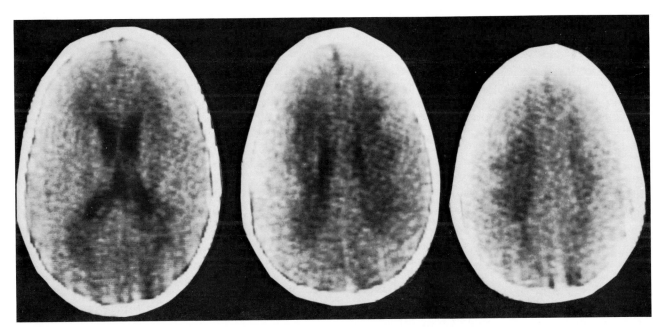

Figure 15-10 Metachromatic leukodystrophy. CT images of a 33-month-old girl reveal hypodense zones in the white matter without conforming to either lobar or vascular distribution. (*Reproduced by permission from Buonanno et al., 1978.*)

Crome 1976). Deafness has sometimes been noted. The disease is apparently transmitted as an autosomal recessive. Some authors feel that this leukodystrophy should no longer be considered as a single entity and that it actually represents a rather nonspecific manifestation of a large and diverse group of metabolic disturbances (Poser 1978).

Pathologically, there is considerable variation in the extent and location of the demyelination. Most severely affected is the centrum semiovale, where there is little evidence of myelin (Crome 1976; Poser 1978). Megalencephaly has been noted (Boltshauser 1976; Lane 1978). With the exception of Alexander's disease, spongy degeneration is the only degenerative neurologic syndrome in this age group which demonstrates megalencephaly.

Spongy degeneration is diagnosed by brain biopsy. Computed tomography assists in this diagnosis by demonstrating a marked decrease in the attenuation of the entire white matter in a symmetric fashion throughout both hemispheres (Fig. 15-11). Contrast enhancement is not reported.

Globoid Cell Leukodystrophy (Krabbe's Disease)

Globoid cell leukodystrophy is an autosomal recessive disorder causing progressive neurologic impairment. The disease receives its name from characteristic large multinucleated histiocytes (Crome 1976). The disease usually presents in the first year of life. Although late forms of the disease are known, globoid cell leukodystrophy occurs almost exclusively as an acute early infantile disorder. A subacute type with clinical similarities to metachromatic leukodystrophy is also known to occur. Two striking clinical features consisting of rapid spontaneous nystagmus and poikilothermia (sudden decrease and elevation of temperature) associated with globoid cell leukodystrophy should help to distinguish the two (Crome 1976; Malone 1976). The labile temperatures may cause confusion with sepsis. A specific enzyme deficiency of galactoside-β-galactosidase has been identified (Malone 1976; Suzuki 1970).

On pathological inspection the brain demon-

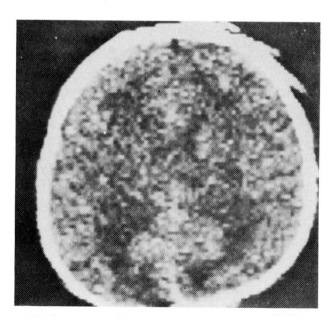

Figure 15-11 Spongy degeneration (Canavan's disease). CT images in a patient with spongy degeneration confirmed by brain biopsy reveal extensive areas of low attenuation in both hemi-

spheres. (*Reproduced by permission from Boltshauser and Isler, 1976.*)

strates widespread foci of disease in the centrum semiovale, cerebellum, and brainstem. There is severe or total lack of myelin in the white matter.

CT findings include a normal scan at an early stage, periventricular hypodensity in the intermediate phase, and atrophy at the late stage (Lane 1978; Barnes 1981; Kingsley 1981) (Fig. 15-12*A, B, C*). Kwan (1984) reported symmetrical hyperdensity in the cerebellum, brainstem, thalami, caudate nuclei, and corona radiata before and in conjunction with decreased attenuation of the white matter followed by atrophy at a later stage. In our proven case of a 6-year-old boy, the prominent CT finding was extensive white matter hypodensities throughout both hemispheres (Fig. 15-12*E* and *F*).

Alexander's Disease

Alexander's disease is a rare condition which is usually clinically manifest during the first year of life and shows gradual enlargement of the head, with progressive retardation, convulsions, and spasticity. All cases reported thus far have been sporadic (Crome 1976). A case occuring in an adult has been reported (Seil 1968).

On histologic examination of the brain, there is little stainable myelin. The characteristic feature of Alexander's disease is the presence of large numbers of Rosenthal bodies in a perivascular distribution (Holland 1980).

Computed tomography in Alexander's disease has been reported to show decreased attenuation of the cerebral white matter with relative sparing of subependymal regions. The findings are predominantly in the frontal lobes, and there may be dilatation of the lateral ventricles (Boltshauser 1978; Holland 1980). Apparent marked contrast enhancement of the caudate nuclei, anterior columns of the fornices, and periventricular areas were reported in a case where the white matter low density abutted these structures (Fig. 15-13) (Holland 1980). Megalencephaly, characteristic of this disease, may be evident on CT (see the section on spongy degeneration). While CT may show rather characteristic findings of megalencephaly and decreased white matter attenuation most pronounced in the frontal

lobes, the diagnosis of Alexander's disease at present still rests with brain biopsy. Needless to say, CT is extremely useful in making the diagnosis and as a guide to biopsy.

Pelizaeus-Merzbacher Disease

Pelizaeus-Merzbacher disease is a disease of the central white matter showing a very slow progression. There are apparently two types of this disease. One is a sex-linked recessive form presenting in early infancy. The second type appears later in childhood and seems to be transmitted by a dominant mode of inheritance and may present in later adulthood (Crome 1976; Malone 1976).

Pathological descriptions indicate a diffuse and symmetrical demyelination of the cerebral and cerebellar white matter as well as the brainstem and spinal cord with conspicuous residual "islands" of preserved or partially demyelinated fibers, which are considered the characteristic pathological finding of Pelizaeus-Merzbacher disease (Crome 1976; Malone 1976).

Computed tomography in a case of Pelizaeus-Merzbacher disease of long-standing duration and severe clinical involvement did not demonstrate any gross abnormality (Heinz 1979).

Adrenoleukodystrophy

Adrenoleukodystrophy is a sex-linked recessive disorder showing adrenal atrophy and cerebral demyelination. The disease occurs predominantly in males between the ages of 3 and 12 years. Adult cases have also been reported. Clinically the patients demonstrate abnormal behavior as well as disturbances of vision and gait. There may be asymmetry of clinical findings early in the disease. Adrenal insufficiency may not be apparent. The disease is progressive without remission. The diagnosis rests on adrenal biopsy findings. Brain biopsy at times may be misleading (Powell 1975; Schaumburg 1975). Steroid therapy appears to be ineffective in altering the course of the neurologic disease (Schaumburg 1975).

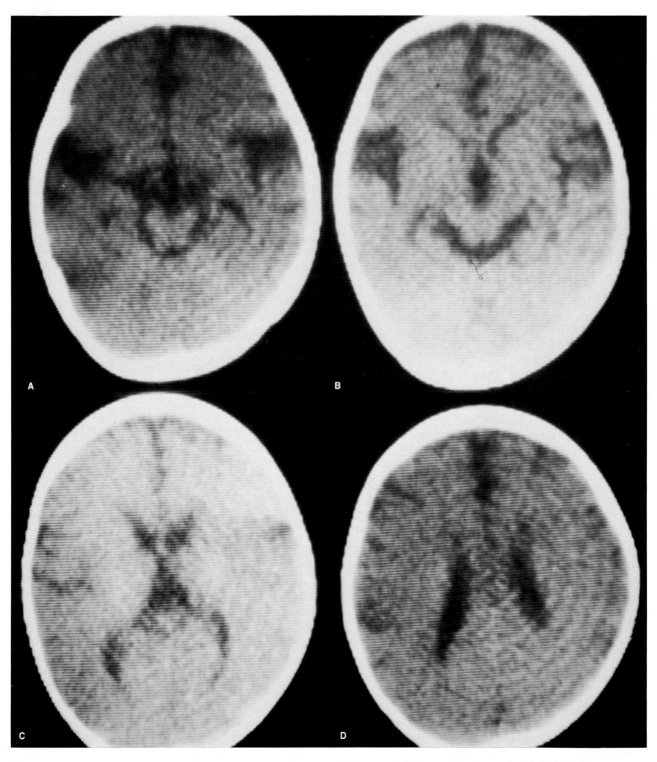

Figure 15-12   Globoid cell leukodystrophy (Krabbe's disease).   **A, B, C, D** (*above*). CT images in a 6-month-old child with biopsy-proven Krabbe's disease show evidence of enlarged subarachnoid spaces including sylvian fissures and lateral ventricles consistent with atrophy. (*Continued on p. 737.*)

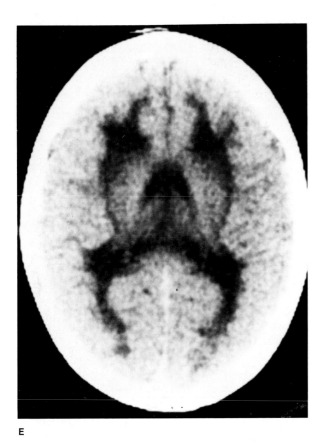

E

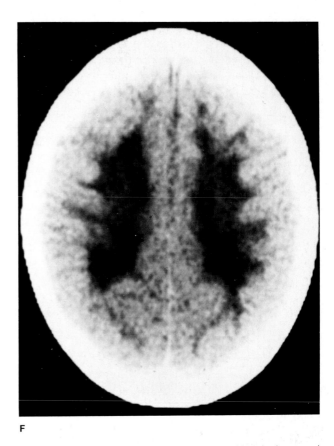

F

Figure 15-12 (*Cont.*) **E, F** (*above*). NCCT of Krabbe's disease in 6-year-old boy. Extensive white matter disease is evident by increased hypodensity in the paraventricular region and centrum semiovale. (*Case courtesy of Dr. J. Greenberg and D. Miller.*) CECT showed no appreciable enhancement.

Pathological inspection reveals demyelination of the subcortical white matter in the posterior cerebrum. The disease tends to be most severe in the parietal, occipital, and posterior temporal lobes. In the posterior cerebrum the disease is symmetric; however, when the frontal lobes are involved, it may be asymmetric. The disease appears to take a caudorostral direction of progression. The disease tends to extend across the splenium of the corpus callosum and be contiguous with the opposite hemisphere. Schaumburg et al. (1975) have identified three histologic zones. The first two zones contain macrophages and appear to be active areas of myelin destruction. The first two zones are most prominent along the frontal edge of the lesion. The third ap-

pears to be an inactive area of glial fibrosis. Dystrophic deposits of calcium may be identified.

Computed tomography demonstrates a striking correlation to the gross and microscopic findings in adrenoleukodystrophy (Fig. 15-14). Early in the disease there is bilateral symmetric decreased attenuation to the posterior cerebral white matter (Di Chiro 1980). There may be edge enhancement at the periphery of the lesion following contrast administration (Inoue 1983). Patients undergoing corticosteroid treatment may show decreased contrast enhancement (Eiben 1977). It is interesting to note that the maximal area of contrast enhancement along the anterior margin of the lesion corresponds to the histologic zones of active demyelination as described by Schaumburg. This correlation was described previously, and the zones of enhancement were considered to represent either Schaumburg's zone 1 (Quisling 1979) or Schaumburg's zones 1 and 2 (Greenberg 1977). The disease shows contiguity on CT across the splenium of the corpus callosum without involving the remainder of the corpus callosum. CT demonstrates progression in a caudorostral direction. The anterior edge of the lesion will show the most significant contrast enhancement and has been described as "serpiginous" (Lane 1978). As the disease progresses, there may be a decrease

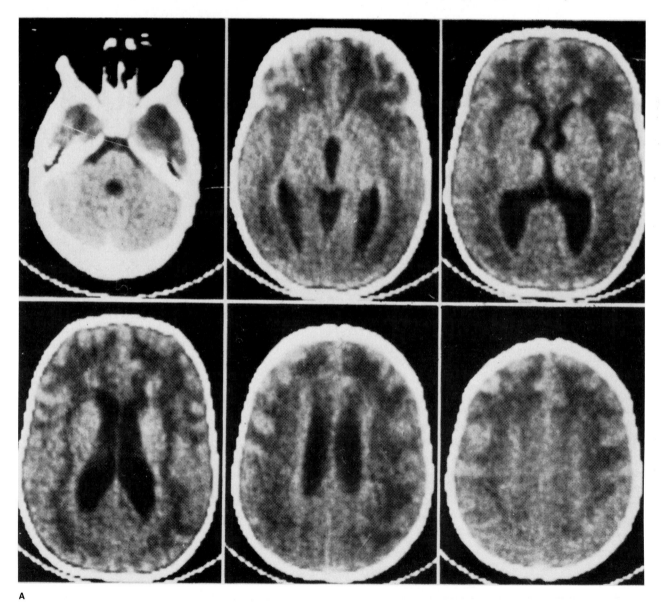

A

Figure 15-13 Alexander's disease. NCCT (**A**) and CECT (**B**) images reveal symmetrical low attenuation in deep white matter with more extensive changes in the frontal regions. Marked enhancement is seen in the caudate nuclei, anterior columns of fornices, and periventricular brain substance. (*Reproduced by permission from Holland and Kendall, 1980.*)

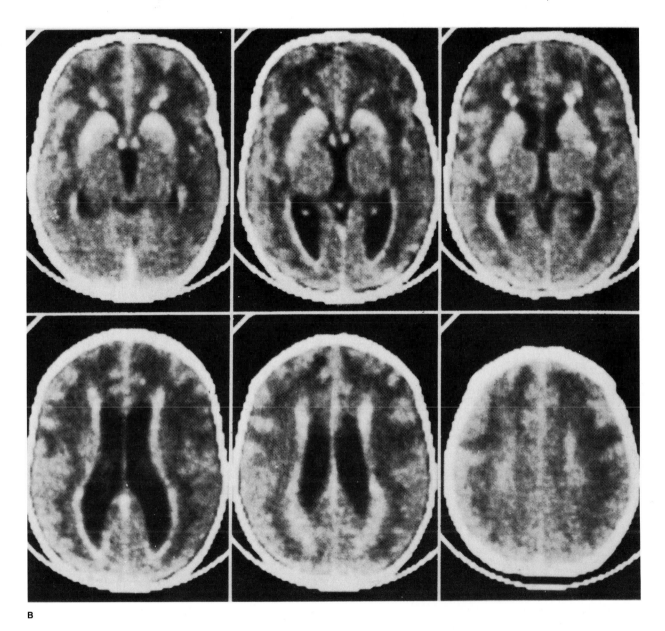

B

Figure 15-13 (*Cont.*)

in the degree of contrast enhancement. With involvement of the frontal lobes, the low-attenuation areas may become asymmetric. The disease eventually progresses to involve the cerebellum as well as the frontal lobes and there is extensive generalized cerebral atrophy (Greenberg 1977; Quisling 1979). The white matter may become so low in attenuation that it may appear indistinguishable from the conspicuously enlarged ventricles (Eiben 1977). Inoue (1983) reported calcification in the white matter along the trigones of the lateral ventricles and development of a mass effect during the active demyelinating period. Two cases of adrenoleukodystrophy are illustrated in Figure 15-14.

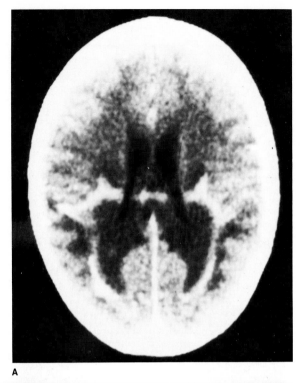

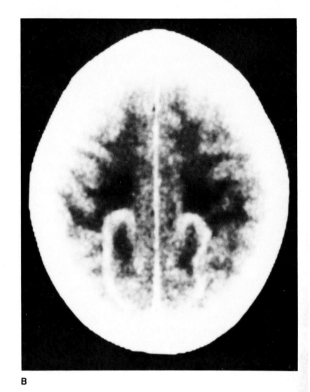

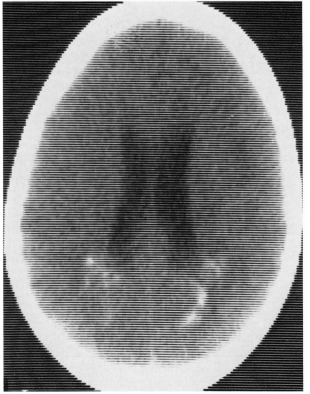

Figure 15-14 Andrenoleukodystrophy. CECT (**A** and **B**) shows peripheral enhancement of bilateral symmetrical hypodense posterior white matter. Note extension across the splenium of the corpus callosum in **A.** NCCT (not shown) demonstrated the same areas of periventricular hypodensity in both hemispheres posteriorly. **C.** CT image of a 10 year-old boy with known adrenoleukodystrophy shows areas of high density with Hounsfield numbers in the range of calcium in the previously demonstrated areas of low density. Dystrophic calcification in this area was confirmed at autopsy (see text).

Bibliography

ADAMS RD, VICTOR M, MANCALL EL: Central pontine myelinolysis. *Arch Neurol Psychiatry* **81**:154, 1959.

ADAMS RD, VICTOR M (eds): *Principles of Neurology*, 3d ed, New York, McGraw-Hill, 1985.

ADORNATO BT, O'BRIEN JS, LAMPERT PW, ROE TF, NEOSTEIN HB: Cerebral spongy degeneration of infancy: A biochemical and ultrastructural study of affected twins. *Neurology* **22**:202–210, 1972.

AITA JF, BENNETT DR, ANDERSON RE, ZITER F: Cranial CT appearance of acute multiple sclerosis. *Neurology* **28**:251–255, 1978.

ALLEN IV: Dysmyelinating diseases in Adams JH, Corsellis JAN, Duchen LW (eds), *Greenfield's Neuropathology*, 4th ed, New York, Wiley, pp 338–384.

ALLEN JC, THALER HT, DECK F, ROTTENBERG DA: Leukoencephalopathy following high dose intravenous methotrexate chemotherapy: Quantitative assessment of white matter attenuation using computed tomography. *Neuroradiology* **16**:44–47, 1978.

ARIEFF AI: Hyponatremia, convulsions, respiratory arrest and permanent brain damage after elective surgery in healthy women. *NEJM* **314**:1526–1535, 1986.

AUR RJA, SIMONE JV, HUSTU HO, VERZOSA MS: A comparative study of central nervous system irradiation and intensive chemotherapy early in remission of childhood acute lymphocytic leukemia. *Cancer* **29**:381–391, 1972.

BARNES D, ENZMANN D: The evolution of white matter disease as seen on CT. *Radiology* **138**:379–383, 1981.

BJORGEN JE, GOLD LHA: Computed tomographic appearance of methotrexate-inducing necrotizing leukoencephalopathy. *Radiology* **122**:377–378, 1977.

BOLTSHAUSER E, ISLER W: Computerized axial tomography in spongy degeneration. *Lancet* **1**:1123, 1976.

BOLTSHAUSER E, SPEISS H, ISLER W: Computed tomography in neurodegenerative disorders in childhood. *Neuroradiology* **16**:41–43, 1978.

BOSCH EP, HART MN: Late adult-onset metachromatic leukodystrophy. *Arch Neurol* **35**:475–477, 1978.

BOSCH EP, CANCILLA PA, CORNELL SH: Computerized tomography in progressive multifocal leukoencephalopathy. *Arch Neurol* **32**:216, 1976.

BRADLEY WG, WALUCH V, BRANT-ZAWADSKI M et al: Patchy, periventricular white matter lesions in the elderly common observation during NMR imaging. *Non-invasive Med Imaging* **1**:35–41, 1984.

BRANT-ZAWADSKI M, FEIN G, VAN DYKE C et al: MR imaging of the aging brain: patchy white-matter lesions and dementia. *AJNR* **6**:675–682, 1985.

BROWNELL B, HUGHES JT: The distribution of plaques in the cerebrum in multiple sclerosis. *J Neurol Neurosurg Psychiatry* **25**:315–320, 1962.

BUONANNO FS, BALL MR, LASTER DW, MOODY DM, MCLEAN WT: computed tomography in late-infantile metachromatic leukodystrophy. *Ann Neurol* **4**:43–46, 1978.

BURCAR PJ, NORENBERG MD, YARNELL PR: Hyponatremia and central pontine myelinolysis. *Neurology* **27**:223, 1977.

CALA LA, MASTAGLIA FL, BLACK JL: Computerized tomography of brain and optic nerve in multiple sclerosis. *J Neurol* **36**:411–426, 1978.

CARROLL BA, LANE B, NORMAN D, ENZMANN D: Diagnosis of progressive multifocal leukoencephalopathy by computed tomography. *Radiology* **122**:137–141, 1977.

COIN CG, HUCKS-FOLLISS A: Cervical computed tomography in multiple sclerosis with spinal cord involvement. *J Comput Assist Tomog* **3**:421–422, 1979.

CROME L, STERN J: Inborn lysosomal enzyme deficiencies, in Blackwood W, Corsellis JAN (eds): *Greenfield's Neuropathology*, Chicago, Year Book Medical Publishers, 1976, pp 541–557.

CUNNINGHAM ME, KISHORE PRS, RENGACHARY SS, PRESKORN S: Progressive multifocal leukoencephalopathy presenting as focal mass lesion in the brain. *Surg Neurol* 8:448–450, 1977.

DE VIVO DC, MALAS D, NELSON JS, LAND VJ: Leukoencephalopathy in childhood leukemia. *Neurology* 27:609–613, 1977.

DEWITT LD, BONAMO FS, KISTLER JP et al: Central pontine myelinolysis: Demonstration by nuclear magnetic resonance. *Neurology* 34:570–576, 1984.

DRAYER BP, HURWITZ B, HEINZ ER, DJANG W et al: High field MR imaging and multiple sclerosis decreased thalamic T_2 relaxation time. Presented at the 24th meeting of the ASNR, San Diego, 1986.

DUDA EE, HUTTENLOCHER PR, PATRONAS NJ: CT of subacute sclerosing panencephalitis. *AJNR* 1:35–38, 1980.

DUDA EE, HUTTENLOCHER PR, PATRONAS NT: CT of subacute sclerosing panencephalitis. *Am J Neuroradiol* 1:35–38, 1980.

EDWARDS MK, FARLOW MR, STEVENS JC: Multiple sclerosis: MRI and clinical correlation. *Am J Neuroradiol* 7:595–598, 1986.

EIBEN RM, DI CHIRO G: Computer assisted tomography in adrenoleukodystrophy. *J Comput Assist Tomogr* 1:308–314, 1977.

FARLOW MR, MARKAND ON, EDWARD MK, STEVENS JC, OLDRICH JK: Multiple sclerosis: Magnetic resonance imaging, evoked responses and spinal fluid electrophoresis. *Neurology* 36:828–831, 1986.

FEIGIN I: Diffuse cerebral sclerosis (metachromatic leukoencephalopathy). *Am J Pathol* 30:715, 1954.

GARRICK R, GOMEZ MR, HOUSER OW: Demyelination of the brain in tuberous sclerosis: Computed tomography evidence. *Mayo Clin Proc* 54:685–689, 1979.

GEBARSKI SS, ALLEN R, GEBARSKI KMS: Magnetic resonance imaging of white matter diseases excluding multiple sclerosis and ischemic leukoencephalopathy. Presented at the 23rd meeting of the ASNR, New Orleans, 1985.

GREENBERG HS, HALVERSON D, LANE B: CT scanning and diagnosis of adrenoleukodystrophy. *Neurology* 27:884–886, 1977.

HAUGHTON VM, HOCK, WILLIAMS AL et al: CT dictation of demyelinated plaques in multiple sclerosis. *AJR* 132:213–215, 1979.

HAZRATJI SMA, KIM RL, LEE SH, MARASIGAN AV: Evolution of pontine and extrapontine myelinolysis. *JCAT* 7:356–361, 1983.

HEINZ ER, DRAYER BP, HAENGGELI CA, PAINTER MJ, CROMRINE P: Computed tomography in white-matter disease. *Radiology* 130:371–378, 1979.

HOLLAND IM, KENDALL BE: Computed tomography in Alexander's disease. *Neuroradiology* 20:103–106, 1980.

INOUE Y, FUKUDA T, TAKASHIMA S et al: Adrenoleukodystrophy: New CT findings. *Am J Neuroradiol* 4:951–954, 1983.

JELLINGER K, SEIFELBERGER F: Pelizaeus-Merzbacher disease: Transitional form between classical and co-natal (Seitelberger) type. *Acta Neuropath (Berlin)* 14:108–117, 1969.

JOHNSON KP (ed): Neurovirology. *Neurologic Clinics*. Philadelphia, W. B. Saunders, 2 (May), 1984.

KAY HEM et al: Encephalopathy in acute leukemia associated with methotrexate therapy. *Arch Dis Childh* 47:344–354, 1972.

KINGSLEY DPE, KENDALL BE: Demyelinating and neurodegenerative disease in childhood. *J Neuroradiol* 8:243–255, 1981.

KWAN E, DRACE J, ENZMANN D: Specific CT findings in Krabbe disease. *Am J Neuroradiol* **5**:453–458, 1984.

LANE B, CARROLL BA, PEDLEY TA: Computerized cranial tomography in cerebral diseases of white matter. *Neurology* **28**:534–544, 1978.

LAURENO R: Central pontine myelinolysis following rapid correction of hyponatremia. *Ann Neurol* **13**:232, 1983.

LEBOW S, ANDERSON DC, MASTRI A et al: Acute multiple sclerosis with contrast-enhancing plaques. *Arch Neurol* **35**:435–439, 1978.

LEVY RM, BREDESEN DE, ROSENBLUM ML: Neurological manifestations of the acquired immunodeficiency syndrome (AIDS): Experience at UCSF and review of the literature. *J Neurosurg* **62**:475–495, 1985.

LYON LW, MCCORMICK WF, SCHOCHET SS: Progressive multifocal leukoencephalopathy. *Arch Intern Med* **128**:420–426, 1971.

MALONE MJ: The cerebral lipidoses. *Pediatr Clin North Am* **23**:303–326, 1976.

MALONE MJ, SZOKE MC, LOONEY GL: Globoid leukodystrophy: Clinical and enzymatic studies. *Arch Neurol* **32**:606–612, 1975.

MARANO GD, GOODWIN GA, KO JP: Atypical contrast enhancement in computerized tomography of demyelinating disease. *Arch Neurol* **37**:523–524, 1980.

MARAVILLA, KR, WEINREB JC, SUSS R, NUNUALLY RL: Magnetic resonance demonstration of multiple sclerosis plaques in the cervical cord. *AJNR* **5**:685–789, 1984.

MCCORMICK WF, SCHOCHET SS, SARLES HE, CALVERLEY JR: Progressive multifocal leukoencephalopathy in renal transplant recipients. *Arch Intern Med* **136**:829–834, 1976.

MCINTOSH S, ASPNES GT: Encephalopathy following CNS prophylaxis in childhood lymphoblastic leukemia. *Pediatrics* **52**:612–615, 1973.

MORARIU MA, WILKINS DE, PATEL S: Multiple sclerosis and serial computerized tomography: Delayed contrast enhancement of acute and early lesions. *Arch Neurol* **37**:189–190, 1980.

MUELLER S, BELL W, SEIBERT J: Cerebral calcifications associated with intrathecal methotrexate therapy in acute lymphocytic leukemia. *J Pediatr* **88**:650–653, 1976.

NORENBERG MD, LESLIE KO, ROBERTSON AS: Association between rise in serum sodium and central pontine myelinolysis. *Am Neurol* **11**:128–135, 1982.

NORENBERG MD: A hypothesis of osmotic endothelial injury: A pathogenetic mechanism of central pontine myelinolysis. *Arch Neurol* **40**:66–69, 1983.

NORTON WT: Formation, structure and biochemistry of myelin, in Siegel GJ, Albers R, Agranoff B W, Katzman R, eds. *Basic Neurochemistry*. Boston, Little, Brown, 1981, pp 63–93.

OPPENHEIMER DR: Demyelinating diseases, in Blackwood W, Corsellis JAN (eds): *Greenfield's Neuropathology*, Chicago, Year Book Medical Publishers, 1976, pp 487–495.

PEDERSON H, WULFF CH: Computed tomographic findings of early subacute sclerosing panencephalitis. *Neuroradiology* **23**:31–32, 1982.

PETERS ACB, VERSTEEG J, BOTS GTAM, BOOGERD W, VIELVOYE GT: Progressive multifocal leukoencephalopathy: Immunofluorescent demonstration of Simian virus 40 antigen in CSF cells and response to cyturabine therapy. *Arch Neurol* **37**:497–501, 1980.

PEYLAN-RAMU N, POPLACK DG, BLEI L, HERDT TR, VERMESS M, DI CHIRO G: Computer assisted tomography in methotrexate encephalopathy. *J Comput Assist Tomogr* **1**:216–221, 1977.

PEYLAN-RAMU N, POPLACK DG, PIZZO PH, ADORNATO BT, DI CHIRO G: Abnormal CT scans of the brain in asymptomatic children with acute lymphocytic leukemia after prophylactic treatment of the central nervous system with radiation and intrathecal chemotherapy. *New Engl J Med* **298**:815–818, 1978.

PIZZO PA, BLEYER WA, POPLACK DG, LEVENTHAL BG: Reversible dementia temporarily associated with intraventricular therapy with methotrexate in a child with acute myelogenous leukemia. *J Pediatr* **88**:131–133, 1976.

POSER CM, VON BOGAERT L: Natural history and evolution of the concept of Schilder's diffuse sclerosis. *Active Psychiatric Neurol Scand* **31**:285, 1956.

POSER C: Leukodystrophy as an example of dysmyelinating disease. *Proceedings of the Third International Congress of Neuropathology, Brussels,* Editions *Acta Medica Belgica,* 1957, pp 106–111.

POSER C: Dysmyelination revisited. *Arch Neurol* **35**:401–408, 1978.

POSER C, ROMAN G, EMERY S III: Recurrent disseminated vasculomyelinopathy. *Arch Neurol* **35**:166–170, 1978.

POSER CM, GOUTIERES F, CARPENTER MA, AICARDI J: Schilder's myelinoclastic diffuse sclerosis. *Pediatrics* **77**:107–112, 1986.

POST MJD, KURSUNOGHA SJ, HENSLEY GT, CHAN JC, MOSKOWITZ LB, HOFFMAN TA: Cranial CT in acquired immunodeficiency syndrome. *AJNR* **6**:743—754, 1985.

POWELL H, TINDALL R, SCHULTZ P, PAA D, O'BRIEN J, LAMPERT P: Adrenoleukodystrophy: Electron microscopic findings. *Arch Neurol* **32**:250–260, 1975.

PRICE RA, JAMIESON PA: The central nervous system in childhood leukemia: II. Subacute leukoencephalopathy. *Cancer* **35**:306—318, 1975.

PRINEAS JW, CONNELL F: Remyelination in multiple sclerosis, *Arch Neurol* **5**:22–31, 1979.

QUISLING RG, ANDRIOLA MR: Computed tomographic evaluation of the early phase of adrenoleukodystrophy. *Neuroradiology* **17**:285–288, 1979.

RANCUREL G, GARDEUR D, THIBIERGE M et al: Computed tomography of Marchiafava-Bignami disease. Presented at the Twelfth Neuroradiologram Symposium, Washington, D.C., Oct. 10–16, 1982.

REICH H, SHU REN L, GOLDBLATT D: Computerized tomography in acute leukoencephalopathy: A case report. *Neurology* **29**:255–258, 1979.

REIK L: Disseminated vasculomyelinopathy an immune complex disease. *Ann Neurol* **7**:291–296, 1980.

REISNER T, MAIDA E: Computerized tomography in multiple sclerosis. *Arch Neurol* **37**:475–477, 1980.

RICHARDSON EP: Our evolving understanding of progressive multifocal leukoencephalopathy. *Ann NY Acad Sci* **230**:358–364, 1974.

ROBERTSON WC, GOMEZ RC, REESE DF, OKAZAKI H: Computerized tomography in demyelinating disease of the young. *Neurology* **27**:838–842, 1977.

ROSENBERG GA, KYNER WT, ESTRADA E: Bulk flow of brain interstitial edema under normal and hyposmolar conditions. *Ann J Physiol* **238**:F42–F49, 1980.

RUBINSTEIN LJ, HERMAN MM, LONG TF, WILBUR JR: Disseminated necrotizing leukoencephalopathy: A complication of treated central nervous system leukemia and lymphoma. *Cancer* **35**:291–305, 1975.

SCHAUMBURG HH, POWERS JM, RAINE CS, SUZUKI K, RICHARDSON EP: Adrenoleukodystrophy: A clinical and pathological study of 17 cases. *Arch Neurol* **32**:577–591, 1975

SCHUMACHER GA: The demyelinating diseases, in Baker AB (ed): *Clinical Neurology,* New York, Harper and Row, 1965, pp 1226–1284.

SEARS ES, TINDALL RSA, ZARNOW H: Active multiple sclerosis. Enhanced computerized tomographic imaging of lesions and the effect of corticosteroids. *Arch Neurol* **35**:426–434, 1978.

SEIGEL RS, SEEGER JF, GABRIELSON TO, ALLEN RJ: Computed tomography in oculocraniosomatic disease (Kearns-Sayre syndrome). *Radiology* **130**:159–164, 1979.

SEIL FJ, SCHOCHET SS, EARLE KM: Alexander's disease in an adult: Report of a case. *Arch Neurol* **19**:494–502, 1968.

SHELDON JJ, SIDDHARTHAN R, TOBIAS J et al: MR Imaging of multiple sclerosis: comparison with clinical and CT examinations in 74 patients. *AJNR* **6**:683–690, 1985.

SIMON JH, SCHIFFER RB, RUDICK RA, HERADON RM: Corpus callosum atrophy and callosal-subcallosal periventricular lesions in multiple sclerosis. Presented at the 24th meeting of the ASNR, San Diego, 1986.

SMITH AS, WEINSTEIN MH, MODIC MT et al: MR with marked T2-weighted images: improved demonstration of brain lesions, tumor, and edema. *AJNR* **6**:691–697, 1985.

SPIEGEL SM, VIMALA FV, FOX AJ et al: CT of multiple sclerosis: reassessment of delayed scanning with high doses of contrast material. *AJNR* **6**:533, 1985.

STERNS RH, RIGGS JE, SCHOCHET SS: Osmotic demyelination syndrome following correction of hyponatremia. *NEJM* **314**:1535–1542, 1985.

SUZUKI K, SUZUKI Y: Globoid leukodystrophy (Krabbe disease) deficiency of galactocerebroside-beta-galactosidase. *Proc Natl Acad Sci (USA)* **66**:302–308, 1970.

SZE G, DE ARINAND SJ, BRANT-ZAWADSKI M et al: Foci of MRI signal (pseudolesions) anterior to the frontal horns: histologic correlations of a normal finding. *AJNR* **7**:381–387, 1986.

THOMPSON DS, HUTTON T, STEARS J et al: CT in the diagnosis of central and extrapontine myelinolysis. *Arch Neurol* **38**:243–246, 1981.

VALENTINE AR, KENDALL BE, HARDING BN: Computed tomography in acute hemorrhagic leukoencephalitis. *Neuroradiology* **22**:215–219, 1982.

VAN DER VELDEN M, BOTS GTAM, ENDTZ L: Cranial CT in multiple sclerosis showing a mass effect. *Surg Neurol* **12**:307–310, 1979.

WANG A-M, MORRIS JH, HICKEY WF et al: Unusual CT patterns of multiple sclerosis. *Am J Neuroradiol* **4**:47–50, 1983.

WEISBERG L: Contrast enhancement visualized by computerized tomography in acute multiple sclerosis. *J Comput Assist Tomogr* **5**:293–300, 1981.

WHEELAN MA, KRICHEFF II, HANDLER M et al: AIDS: CT manifestations. *Radiology* **149**:477–484, 1983.

YOUNG IR, HALL AS, PALLIG CA et al: NMR imaging of the brain in multiple sclerosis. *Lancet* **2**:1063–1066, 1981.

YOUNG IR, RANDALL CP, KAPLAN PW et al: Neuroimaging of white matter disease of the brain using spin-echo sequences *JCAT* **7**:290–294, 1983.

ZIMMERMAN RD, FLEMING CA, LEE BCP et al: Periventricular hyperintensity as seen by magnetic resonance: prevalence and significance *AJNR* **7**:13–20, 1986.

16

PITFALLS AND LIMITATIONS OF CT IN NEURODIAGNOSIS

Seungho Howard Lee

Stephen A. Kieffer

Despite initial skepticism in some quarters, the value and efficacy of computed tomography of the brain was quickly established. CT has emerged as the primary diagnostic screening modality for the *detection* of intracranial pathology. Accuracy of *localization* of structural abnormalities of the brain by CT often exceeds that which can be obtained by cerebral angiography or other invasive diagnostic procedure. Frequently CT can also provide information permitting *characterization* of the nature of the disease process.

Accumulated experience with CT scanning of the head indicates that even this remarkable diagnostic tool has its limitations. However, the limitations of CT are probably fewer in number and less in severity than those associated with any other neurological diagnostic modality.

TECHNICAL

Motion artifacts have been a severe problem for the radiologist from the earliest 4½-minute translate-rotate scanners up to the present fourth-generation stationary detector array units capable of scanning times of 2 seconds or less (Ter-Pogossian 1977). The severity of motion artifacts depends on the extent of displacement of the object being scanned. They are most prominent in regions of sharp gradients of x-ray attenuation. The artifacts due to intracranial metallic foreign bodies (e.g., vascular clips, metal plates, shunt catheters, bullet fragments) (Fig. 16-1) are particularly aggravated by motion. While the much shorter scan time of the newer CT units has reduced the likelihood of patient movement during

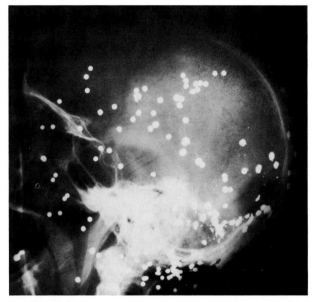

A

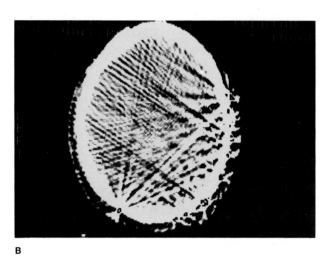

B

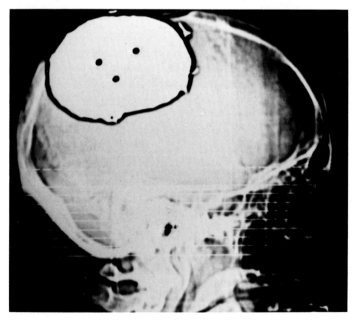

C

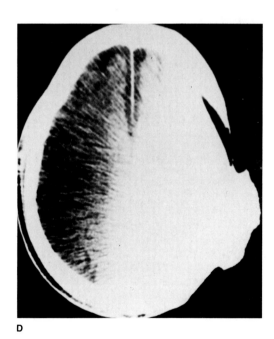

D

Figure 16-1   A, B. Metallic artifacts.   **A.** Lateral view of skull demonstrates numerous metallic pellets overlying the cranial vault and face.   **B.** CT image demonstrates multiple linear artifacts emanating from the metallic pellets in the scalp. Intracranial anat-omy cannot be recognized.   **C, D.** Metal plate artifacts: Lateral scout view (**C**) shows a large metal plate at the craniectomy site. CT (**D**) shows complete obscuration of left hemisphere due to artifacts, precluding any diagnostic possibility.

scanning, the severity of such artifacts, when they occur, has not been significantly altered.

Meticulous care in patient positioning is essential for successful and reliable CT scanning. Even slight degrees of *tilting of the head* can result in factitious abnormalities, notably apparent shifts of midline structures. An apparent mass in the floor of the body of one lateral ventricle may be simulated by the normal thalamus if the plane of section is slightly tilted (Fig. 16-2).

Despite considerable improvement in resolution, even the newer scanners have not solved the problems resulting from *beam hardening* due to absorption of "softer" incident radiation by areas of thick, dense bone (Brooks 1976). This is a particular problem in the posterior cranial fossa, where a narrow transverse hypodense stripe (the Hounsfield artifact) is frequently observed extending between the two petrous pyramids and obscuring definition of the pons and aqueduct (Fig. 16-3).

Small lesions with a diameter less than or approximating the thickness of the scan slice may not be accurately represented on the CT image. If the volume of the lesion does not occupy the entire thickness of the slice, the attenuation coefficient on the CT image will reflect averaging of the x-ray attenuation of the lesion and the surrounding normal tissue (*volume averaging*) (Dohrmann 1978). Volume averaging is also a problem at the margins of larger lesions. Reduction in scan slice thickness and in size of matrix pixels diminishes the impact of volume averaging on CT scan accuracy.

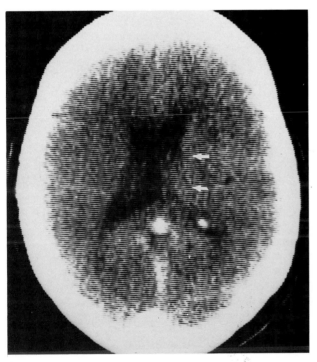

A

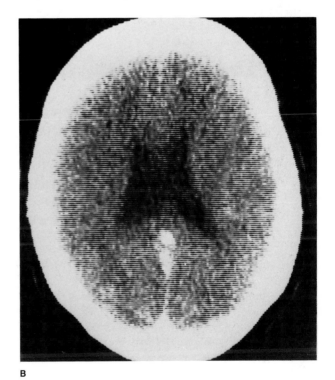

B

Figure 16-2 Tilting of head simulating a thalamic mass. **A.** Initial CT image suggests the presence of a mass in the body of the left lateral ventricle in a 52-year-old female (arrows). CT images at lower levels demonstrated asymmetry of structures at the skull base, indicating that the patient's head was tilted within the gantry. **B.** Following repositioning of the patient's head, a repeat CT image at the same level as in **A** shows no evidence of a mass in the left lateral ventricle.

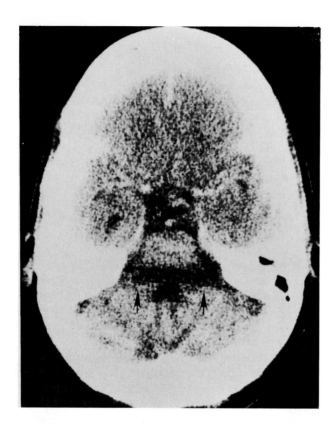

Figure 16-3 Beam-hardening (Hounsfield) artifact. A narrow transverse hypodense stripe extends between the two petrous pyramids (arrows) and obscures definition of the posterior aspect of the pons and the middle cerebellar peduncles.

Figure 16-4 (*Below*) Dermoid cyst: importance of varying center and window settings. **A.** On the initial CT image obtained with a low center level and a narrow window (usual settings for head CT studies), a round, fatty tumor with a partially calcified wall was considered to be a lipoma. **B.** A repeat CT image with a slightly higher center level and a much wider window demonstrates soft-tissue mass within the cyst (arrows). At surgery, a hair ball was found inside a dermoid cyst.

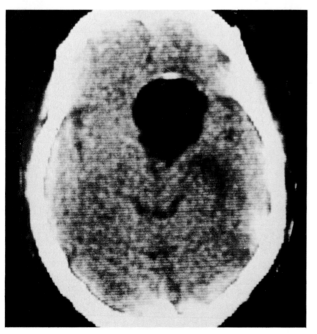

A

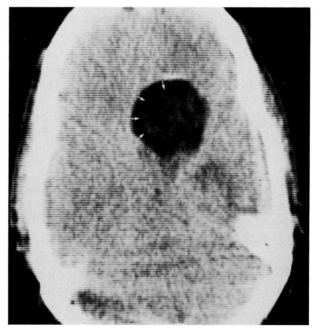

B

Failure to identify the fourth ventricle should not be lightly disregarded, particularly when the lateral and third ventricles are mildly enlarged. A mass lesion in or adjacent to the brainstem or cerebellum compressing the fourth ventricle could easily be overlooked (Gado 1977). Repeat scans in alternate planes or thinner section studies will usually demonstrate the elusive ventricle.

Proper *window and center settings* are important in elucidating subtle tissue-density differences (Fig. 16-4). Dense peripheral intracranial lesions may blend with the overlying calvarium and be overlooked. At conventional window and center settings, a thin bandlike acute subdural hematoma which does not produce a significant shift of midline structures could be missed. To precisely define such peripheral densities, a relatively high center setting (60 or 70 HU)

and wider window (200 to 400 HU) should be employed (Fig. 16-5).

Malfunction of a multiformat camera can give rise to nonhomogeneous artifactual density which may result in false positive finding (Fig. 16-6).

NORMAL VARIATIONS

A thorough understanding of the normal gross anatomy of the brain on CT studies and an awareness of common normal anatomic variations will reduce the likelihood of false positive diagnoses and thus obviate the need for invasive studies.

The *jugular tubercles* are rounded bony elevations

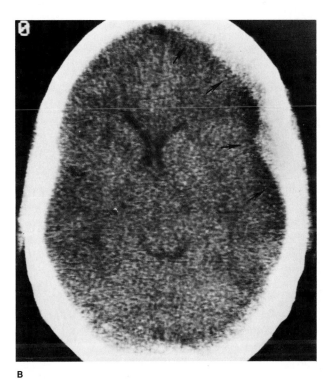

A

B

Figure 16-5 Acute subdural hematoma: importance of varying center and window settings.   **A.** A 55-year-old man was found somnolent and unresponsive following head trauma. CT image at usual center and window settings demonstrates a shift of the septum pellucidum to the right of the midline but no evident intra-

cerebral mass to account for the shift.   **B.** The same image as in **A** is viewed with a higher center level and a wider window. A crescentic band of increased density (acute subdural hematoma) is identified along the lateral margin of the left frontal and temporal lobes (arrows).

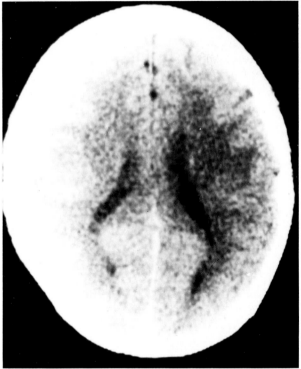

A

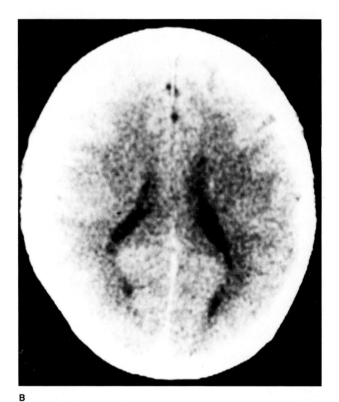

B

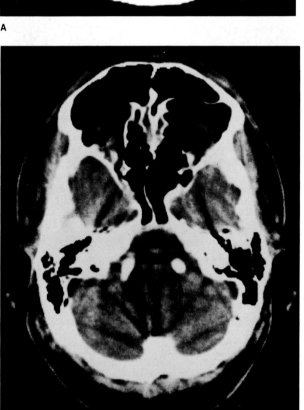

Figure 16-6   A, B. Artifact from multiformat camera. NCCT (**A**) shows diffuse hypodensity of the left white matter without mass effect or atrophy. The right side of the background was lighter than the left. Repeat filming (**B**) after camera adjustment demonstrates normal white-gray matter differentiation.

Figure 16-7   Jugular tubercles. Bilateral oblong bony densities are identified within the posterior fossa medial and inferior to the internal auditory meatus (arrows). A clear separation from the adjacent petrous temporal bones, with intervening normal brain tissue or subarachnoid cisterns, is an important finding in differentiating a jugular tubercle from a possible meningioma or other hyperdense or calcified tumor in this region.

arising from the inner surface of the occipital bone adjacent to the anterolateral margins of the foramen magnum on each side. The tubercles vary widely in size and shape and are often asymmetric. Axial CT sections through the posterior fossa often demonstrate one or both jugular tubercles as rounded densities located medial and just inferior to the internal auditory meatus. These densities can be confused with extraaxial mass lesions in the cerebellopontine angle (Fig. 16-7). Careful review of adjacent consecutive axial CT images in this region, repetition of axial scanning with reduced scan slice thickness, and obtaining scans in alternate planes (e.g., coronal) will usually clarify the situation.

The right *jugular foramen* is larger than the left in 50 to 70 percent of persons; this disparity is related to the size of the corresponding transverse and sigmoid sinuses. One jugular bulb may be hypoplastic while the opposite bulb is markedly enlarged, mimicking a tumor in the jugular foramen (Fig. 16-8).

A *large cisterna magna* may simulate a cystic lesion in the posterior cranial fossa (Leo 1979). The size of the cisterna magna varies widely in the normal population. It may normally extend up to the level of the internal occipital protuberance, and rarely it may protrude farther upward through a defect in the tentorium (Liliequist 1960). The adjacent occipital bone may be thinned. The absence of compression of the fourth ventricle usually permits a definitive diagnosis of an enlarged cisterna magna (Adam 1978) (Fig. 16-9).

The *inferior vermis* of the cerebellum occasionally appears quite dense on NCCT in normal persons. On CECT, the normal vermis often exhibits homogeneous opacification, appearing as a triangular or elliptical homogeneous density extending on axial

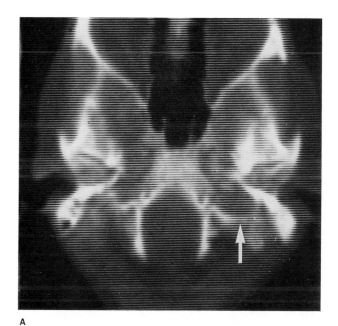

A

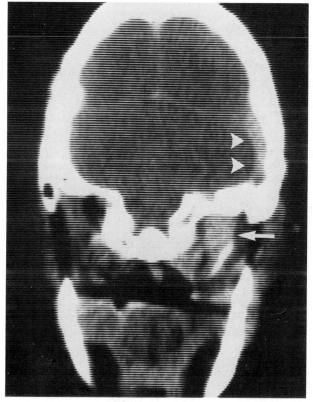

B

Figure 16-8 Large left jugular foramen. **A.** Axial CT image at the level of the foramen magnum shows the left jugular foramen (arrow) to be larger than its companion on the right. Note that the cortical margin of the foramen is intact. **B.** Coronal CECT demonstrates a large ipsilateral transverse sinus (arrowheads) and jugular bulb (arrow).

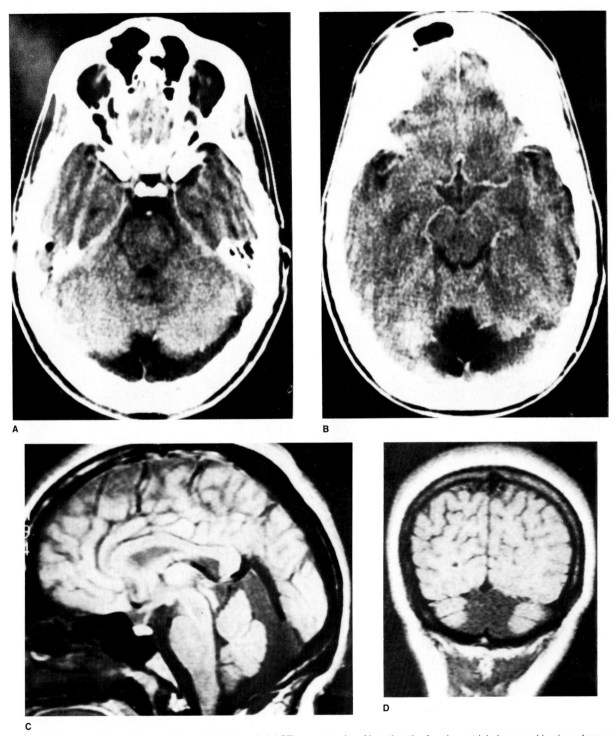

A

B

C

D

Figure 16-9 Large cisterna magna and vermian cistern. Axial CT images (**A** and **B**) demonstrate a sharply marginated triangular hypodensity between the posterior margin of the cerebellum and the inner table of the occipital bone, with superior and lateral ex- tension. Note that the fourth ventricle is normal in size, shape, and position. Sagittal (**C**) and coronal (**D**) MRI exhibits large cervico- medullary and vermian cisterns.

CT images from the posterior margin of the fourth ventricle to the cisterna magna (Kramer 1977). The increased density and prominent contrast enhancement may reflect the high concentration of cortical tissue surrounded by CSF spaces (Fig. 16-10). Differentiation from neoplasm or other pathologic condition is based on the lack of deformity or displacement of the adjacent fourth ventricle.

Physiological calcification of the basal ganglia is occasionally recognized on CT studies of the brain (Fig. 16-11). The calcification is typically located in the globus pallidus, is usually but not always bilateral, and usually occurs in persons above age 40 (Cohen 1980). Demonstration of basal ganglia calcification in a patient under age 40 may prompt a search for associated pathologic conditions (e.g., hypopara-

thyroidism, pseudohypoparathyroidism). Children with Down's syndrome may show early calcification of the basal ganglia.

Physiological calcification of the choroid plexuses in the bodies of the lateral ventricles (Fig. 16-12) is 5 to 15 times more commonly detected on CT studies, as compared with plain skull radiographs. Demonstration of calcification in the choroid plexus of the temporal horn or third ventricle suggests the presence of neurofibromatosis (Modic 1980).

Asymmetry of the frontal or occipital horns of the lateral ventricles is a common normal developmental variant (LeMay 1978). Coarctation of ependymal surfaces during fetal development may produce interruption or obliteration (either unilateral or bilateral) of these portions of the ventricular system

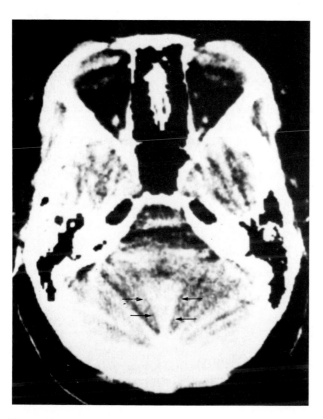

Figure 16-10   Normal inferior vermis. A triangular area of increased density extends posteriorly in the midline from the fourth ventricle toward the internal occipital crest (arrows) on this NCCT image. Note that the fourth ventricle is not displaced or compressed.

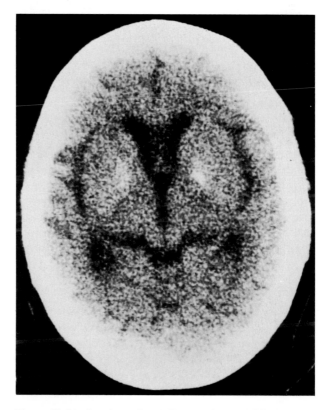

Figure 16-11   Basal ganglia calcification. On this NCCT image of a 42-year-old male, calcifications are noted in the region of the globus pallidus bilaterally.

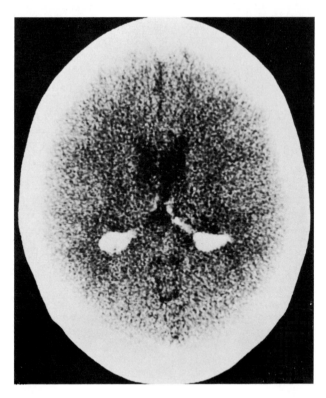

Figure 16-12 Physiological calcification of the choroid plexuses. Bilateral calcifications of the choroid plexus of the lateral ventricles are identified on this NCCT image. In this patient, calcification is heaviest in the glomera but also extends anteriorly to the region of the foramen of Monro.

(Fig. 16-13*A*). The lack of ventricular compression or displacement or of any focal parenchymal abnormality differentiates this normal variation from compression due to a mass lesion. Occipital horns can be asymmetrical owing to the calcar avis (Fig. 16-13*C*).

Other cerebral asymmetries may be demonstrated by CT (LeMay 1978). The left occipital pole is frequently wider and protrudes farther posteriorly than the right occipital pole; thus the calcified choroid plexus glomus of the left lateral ventricle often is located slightly posterior to the right glomus. The right frontal pole often protrudes slightly more anteriorly than the left, and the right frontal horn is frequently smaller than its companion on the left. These asymmetries are more common in right-handed persons; hemispheric asymmetry is less common and less striking in left-handed persons. The pineal gland often lies slightly to the left of the midline in normal persons.

Contrast enhancement of the *choroid plexus of the temporal horn* produces a crescentic density on the medial aspect of the temporal horn. In combination with the diverging bandlike blush of the adjacent contrast-enhanced tentorium, this forms an incomplete ringlike density which can simulate the CECT appearance of a medial temporal lobe tumor (Naidich 1977) but is usually bilateral and symmetrical and is not associated with any mass effect (Fig. 16-14).

The *falx cerebri* is commonly visualized as a long, thin band of slightly increased density in the region of the interhemispheric fissure in normal persons on NCCT (false falx sign) (Osborn 1980). This finding must be differentiated from the appearance of subarachnoid hemorrhage in the interhemispheric fissure (Dolinskas 1978)—the falx sign—which appears as a midline band of increased density extending into the paramedian cerebral sulci (Fig. 16-15) and is confirmatory of the presence of extracerebral blood (Osborn 1980).

Occasionally, prominent *dural veins* in the tentorial leaves present as multiple curvilinear densities on CECT, mimicking a bizarre appearance of a tumor or arteriovenous malformation (Fig. 16-16). These are more frequently observed in infants and children than in adults.

The *torcular Herophili* typically appears triangular on normal CECT studies and is located in close approximation to the occipital bone in the midline (Naidich 1977). However, variations in the location and configuration of this confluence of the dural venous sinuses are common. It may appear round or elongated and may lie as much as a centimeter anterior to the occipital bone or to one side of the midline (Fig. 16-17).

Prominent clinoid processes may mimic aneurysms at the circle of Willis. Careful analysis of NCCT and CECT with controlled window and center settings can be helpful in recognizing this potential problem (Fig. 16-18). Frequently, coronal CT is of value in ruling out aneurysms or small tumors.

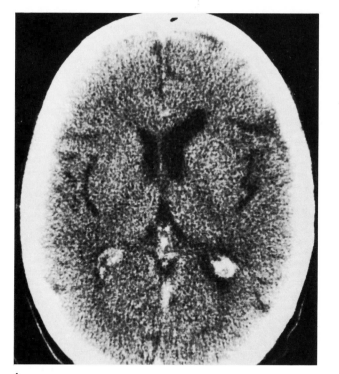

A

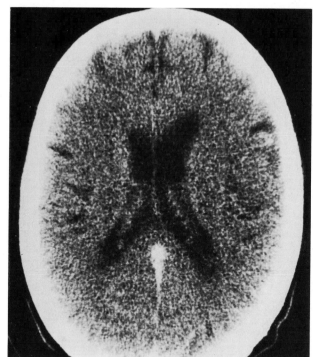

B

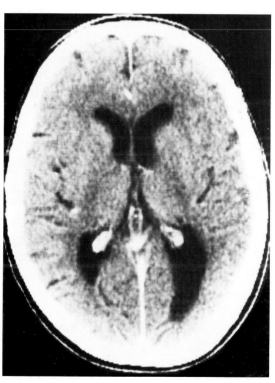

C

Figure 16-13 **A** and **B.** Asymmetry of the lateral ventricles. The left lateral ventricle is larger than its companion on the right in this right-handed person with normal mentation and function. The left frontal horn projects farther anteriorly than the right frontal horn. The sharp lateral angle of the right front horn suggests coaptation of its ependymal surfaces. Axial CT (**C**) shows asymmetrical occipital horns; the right occipital horn is shorter owing to the calcar avis.

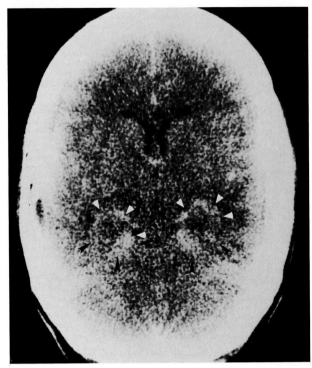

Figure 16-14 Incomplete density ring in medial temporal region. Bilateral symmetrical curvilinear contrast enhancement in the posteromedial temporal regions is due to a combination of the choroid plexuses of the temporal horns (arrowheads) and the anterolateral margins of the tentorium.

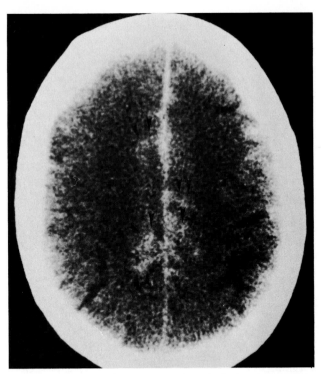

Figure 16-15 Subarachnoid hemorrhage in the interhemispheric fissure extending into the paramedian sulci. NCCT of a middle-aged man with a ruptured aneurysm shows a midline increased density in the interhemispheric fissure (subarachnoid hemorrhage) and its extension into the contiguous paramedian cortical sulci (arrowheads). The CT diagnosis of subarachnoid hemorrhage can be confirmed by the presence of free blood in the cortical sulci and other subarachnoid cisterns.

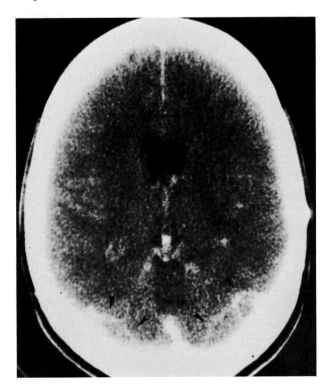

Figure 16-16 Prominent dural veins in the tentorium cerebelli. CECT shows multiple curvilinear densities (arrows) at the upper level of tentorial surfaces mimicking vascular malformation or an infarct of unusual appearance. These are normal dural veins frequently found in the normal pediatric age group.

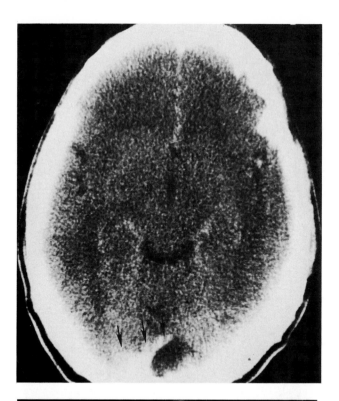

Figure 16-17 Torcular Herophili: normal variant. A thick, band-like, contrast-enhancing structure to the right of the midline (arrow) represents the opacified confluence of the dural venous sinuses, displaced from the midline by a superior extension of a large cisterna magna. Also note temporal "rings."

Figure 16-18 (*Below*) **A, B.** Prominent anterior clinoid processes mimicking aneurysms at the circle of Willis. Axial CECT (**A**) demonstrates two round hyperdense projections at the distal ends of both internal carotid arteries. NCCT (**B**) clarifies that they represent prominent anterior clinoid processes.

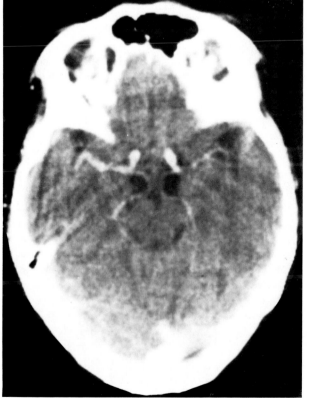

A

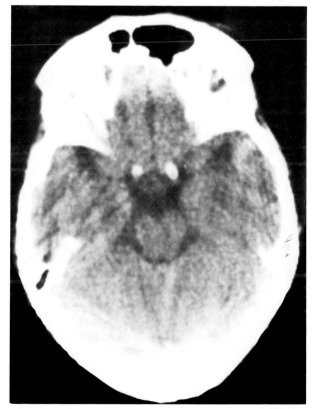

B

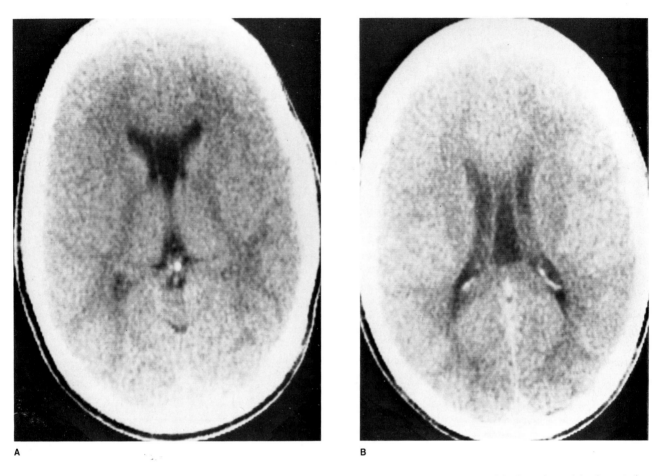

A   B

Figure 16-19   A. Cavum septi pellucidi between the frontal horns.   **B.** Cavum vergae between bodies of the lateral ventricles is posterior extension of the cavum septi pellucidi.

Cavum septi pellucidi is present between the frontal horns, and its posterior extension should be properly identified as a cavum vergae (Fig. 16-19).

LOCALIZATION

It is the accepted convention in CT scanning of the skull and brain to angle the gantry (and therefore the plane of CT section) slightly craniocaudad (about 10° to 15° with respect to the canthomeatal line) in order to include the volume of the brain in the smallest number of scans. Thus, "axial" CT images of the brain are really modified transaxial sections, and the anatomy visualized on these images differs considerably from true horizontal sections. Accurate surgical localization of intracranial lesions demonstrated on axial CT scans is often difficult, particularly when the lesion is small and situated superiorly in the high convexity; the absence of calvarial landmarks on the CT image and the angled plane of section contribute to this difficulty (Fig. 16-20). Solutions to this problem include the use of radiopaque external marking devices (Lee 1980) or the digital radiographic imaging mode (scout view) available in many of the newer CT scanning units.

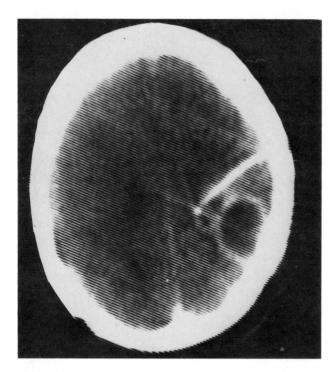

Figure 16-20 Parietal convexity abscesses. CT image obtained in the modified transaxial plane (angled craniocaudad approximately 15° with respect to the canthomeatal line) following surgery demonstrates an opaque cannula entering a daughter abscess. The position of the cannula is anterior to the major abscess cavity. Surgical localization of high-convexity masses may be difficult because of the absence of anatomic landmarks and the angulation of the plane of the CT image.

Differentiation of extra- from intracerebral masses on axial CT images is a frequent problem. Many extracerebral masses invaginate the underlying brain and thus simulate intracerebral lesions on CT. Notorious in this regard are meningiomas, cranial nerve neuromas, and large arterial aneurysms. Factors which may aid in establishing a lesion as extracerebral include demonstration of adjacent bone destruction, widening of adjacent subarachnoid spaces and cisterns, and continuity of the lesion with the falx or tentorium (Miller 1978). Rescanning in a modified coronal plane may also be helpful. Extracerebral masses displacing and compressing the adjacent brain produce inward buckling of the underlying white matter, while intracerebral tumors tend

to stretch the adjacent white matter (George 1980). However, if the CT findings do not permit clear differentiation of extra- from intracerebral mass, MRI or angiography may be of value.

Mass lesions in the region of the tentorial incisura may be supratentorial or infratentorial (that is, either above or below the tentorium). A clear understanding of normal tentorial anatomy on axial CT scans is invaluable in making this differentiation (Naidich 1977). The authors have found that images in the modified coronal plane are frequently of great help in this situation (Fig. 16-21). Also MRI in orthogonal planes may resolve localization difficulties on CT.

NONSPECIFICITY

Not long after the advent of CT scanning as a clinical modality, it was realized that intravenous injection of iodinated contrast media aided considerably in the discrimination of the various causes of intracranial masses. However, in the case of low-density lesions, cerebral edema is often a major contributor to both the apparent size and the low density of the mass. Edematous tissue does not exhibit contrast enhancement, but neither do many low-grade gliomas (Tans 1978). It is important to recognize that many infarcts provoke significant local edema and thus appear as space-occupying masses with ventricular compression and shift of midline structures (Davis 1975). Thus it may be very difficult to differentiate a cerebral infarct from a low-grade glioma on CT (Handa 1978); both lesions may appear as low-density masses without contrast enhancement. Clinical signs and history may be misleading, and often only follow-up CT studies a few weeks later will clarify the situation (Fig. 16-22).

However, many infarcts exhibit contrast enhancement, usually between 1 and 4 weeks after the acute ischemic episode (Wing 1976). This often appears as a gyral pattern of opacification in the area of infarction. This gyral enhancement pattern is also nonspecific; its persistence beyond 4 weeks post-

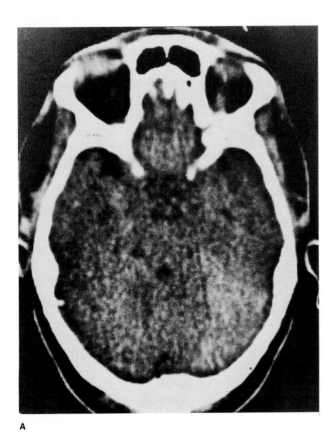

A

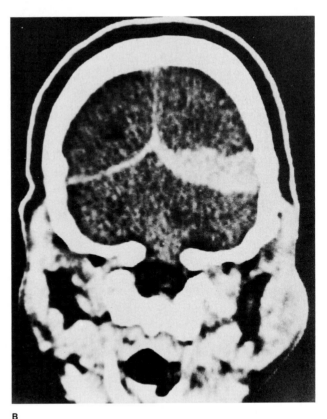

B

Figure 16-21 Tentorial en plaque meningioma. **A.** Transaxial CECT image demonstrates a large, well-marginated triangular area of increased density on the left posteriorly. On this image, it is not possible to be certain whether the lesion lies above the tentorium or in the posterior fossa. **B.** Coronal CECT image shows a ho-mogeneous contrast-enhancing mass which appears continuous with the superior aspect of the tentorium. Surgery confirmed the presence of an en plaque meningioma attached to the tentorium and growing into the supratentorial compartment.

ictus should suggest the possibility of an inflammatory or neoplastic process in the meninges and adjacent cerebral parenchyma (Fig. 16-23).

Round, well-marginated, hypodense (5 to 15 HU) lesions strongly suggest fluid-filled cysts. However, these are not always found, and both solid and microcystic masses may have a similar appearance (Latchaw 1977) (Fig. 16-24).

Intracerebral masses exhibiting significantly increased density on NCCT may represent tumor or hemorrhage. Glioma, metastatic carcinoma, and meningioma may all exhibit increased density on NCCT and may be difficult to differentiate from intracerebral hematoma. Hemorrhage within a tumor may further complicate this problem. Enhance-

ment of the periphery of the dense mass following intravenous injection of contrast medium is seen in many of these tumors (Russell 1980). When a dense mass on NCCT fails to show contrast enhancement,

Figure 16-23 Tuberculous meningoencephalitis simulating cerebral infarction. **A.** CECT image obtained 4 days after the sudden onset of ataxia, dysarthria, and right hemiparesis in a 45-year-old female. Note contrast enhancement of several gyri in the left frontoparietal convexity, with underlying white matter edema. The CT and clinical findings were interpreted as being compatible with a diagnosis of cerebral infarction. **B.** A follow-up CECT study 5 weeks later demonstrates persistent gyral enhancement with significant increase in white matter edema. The patient's condition had not improved. Surgical exploration revealed extensive meningoencephalitis; histologic examination confirmed a diagnosis of tuberculosis.

▶

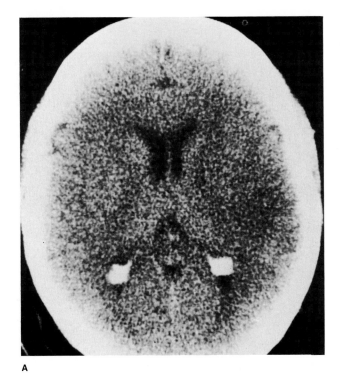

A

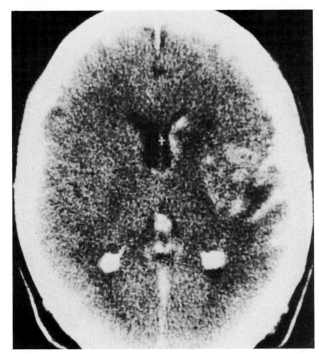

B

Figure 16-22 Evolution of recent infarction and CT distinction from low-grade glioma. **A.** CT within 2 days after ictus demonstrates a poorly defined area of hypodensity in the left temporoparietal lobe. No contrast enhancement was noted in the area, but mild mass effect was present on the same side. **B.** CECT, a week later, demonstrates extensive enhancement in the same area with no apparent shift of the midline or localized mass effect. A focal area of infarction in the head of the caudate nucleus on the left side is also visible. This rapid evolution of the contrast-enhancement pattern, which is gyral in configuration, and relative absence of mass effect are rather characteristic of a recent infarction rather than a low-grade glioma.

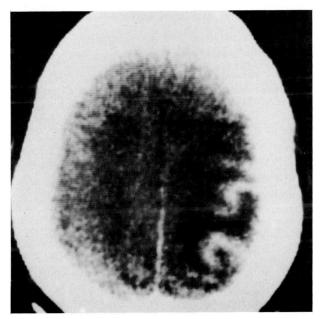

A

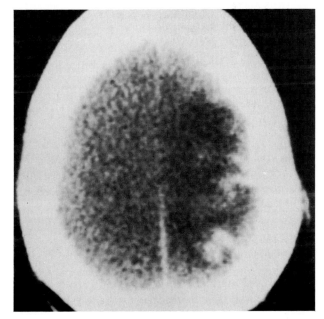

B

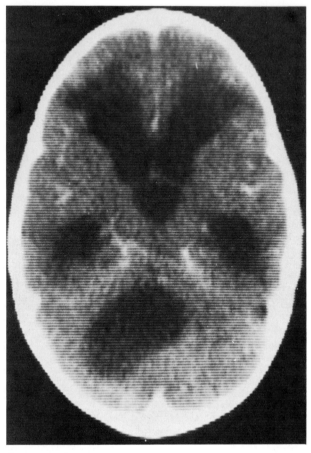

A

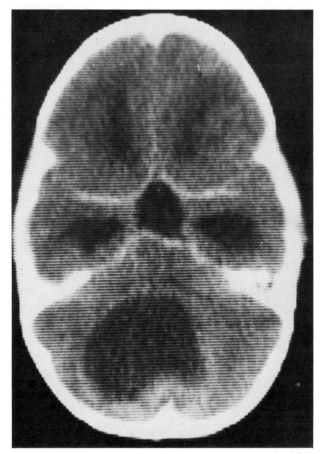

B

Figure 16-24 Microcystic astrocytoma of the cerebellum. NCCT (**A**) and CECT (**B**) images demonstrate a cystic-appearing hypodense (12 HU) mass in the right cerebellar hemisphere extending across the midline, with contrast enhancement of the margin of the "cyst." Exploration revealed a well-encapsulated solid mass.

Histologic examination showed the lesion to be composed of a myriad of microcysts, probably accounting for the low attenuation values. The tumor has compressed and obstructed the fourth ventricle. Note the markedly distended third and lateral ventricles, with periventricular hypodensity (interstitial edema) in both frontal regions.

serial studies may be necessary for differentiation of tumor from hematoma. One should be able to observe a significant decline in CT numbers of a hematoma within 10 to 14 days, as the packed red blood cells lyse and hemoglobin is broken down and absorbed (Davis K. 1977). Omission of serial follow-up studies in dense lesions presumed to be hematomas may prove tragic for the patient (Fig 16-25).

In the immediate postoperative period following resection of a space-occupying mass, the appearance in the former tumor site of a well-defined area of slightly increased density (40 to 50 HU) may suggest hemorrhage and lead to reoperation. The density of such masses is slightly less than an acute hematoma (usually in the range of 60 to 80 HU). This postoperative abnormality is due to Oxycel or Gelfoam strips laid in the tumor bed which become soaked with blood and tissue fluids (Fig. 16-26).

A *ring pattern* of peripheral rimlike contrast enhancement of a hypodense mass was originally presumed to be characteristic of a malignant neoplasm (glioblastoma or metastasis) with central coagulative

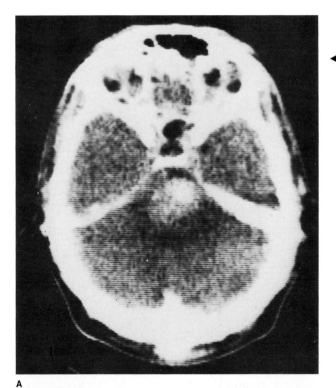

A

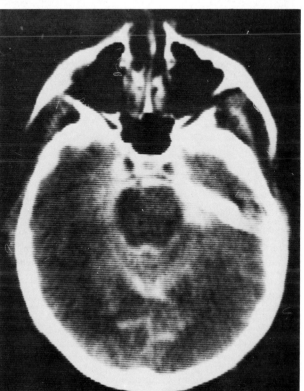

B

Figure 16-25 Hyperdense lesion in pons. **A.** NCCT image obtained following the sudden onset of left hemiparesis in a 58-year-old. A rounded, hyperdense lesion is noted in the left side of the pons, extending across the midline and posteriorly. In view of the patient's history, a diagnosis of pontine hematoma was suggested. However, serial CT studies over the ensuing 8 weeks showed no change in the size or density of the mass. **B.** Metrizimide CT cisternogram obtained 8 weeks after **A** shows asymmetry, with bulging of the left anterolateral margin of the pons. The hyperdense lesion is still evident on this higher center–wide window image. The patient subsequently died, and autopsy confirmed a diagnosis of pontine glioma.

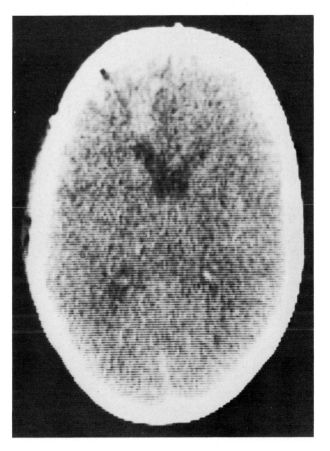

Figure 16-26 Surgical packing simulating postoperative hemorrhage. NCCT image demonstrates an irregularly marginated, slightly hyperdense (43 HU) lesion in the right anterior frontal region. There is no evident compression or displacement of the adjacent right frontal horn. The image was obtained 5 hours following the excision of a meningioma in the same location. Hemorrhage into the former tumor site was questioned, although the density of the lesion is less than what might be expected in an acute hematoma. Reexploration demonstrated no hematoma or other mass, only blood and serum-soaked strips of surgical packing.

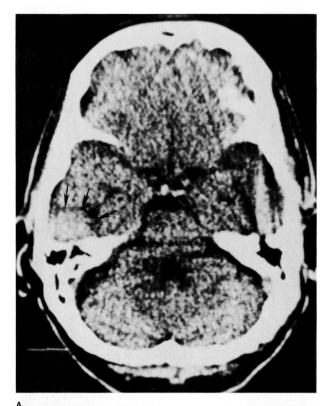

A

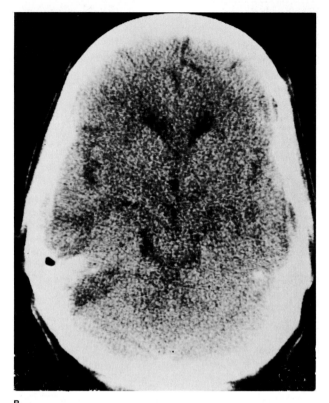

B

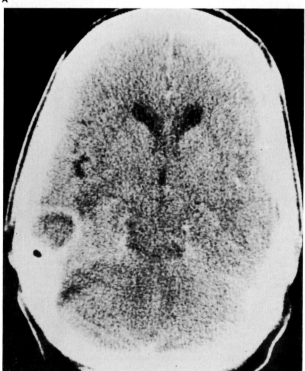

C

Figure 16-27 Ringlike contrast enhancement: intracerebral hematoma. **A.** NCCT image obtained shortly after patient fell out of a moving vehicle, striking the right side of his head on the pavement. A slightly hyperdense round mass is identified in the right temporal lobe laterally and inferiorly (arrows). A very thin peripheral hypodense rim around the anteromedial margin of the mass probably represents edema. **B.** Ten days later, an NCCT image shows significant diminution in size and density of the temporal lobe mass, consistent with a diagnosis of resolving intracerebral hematoma. The peripheral hypodense rim is now much wider (edema? gliosis?). **C.** CECT immediately following **B** shows smooth, uniform contrast enhancement of the peripheral hypodense rim due to gliosis and neovascularity (repair reaction).

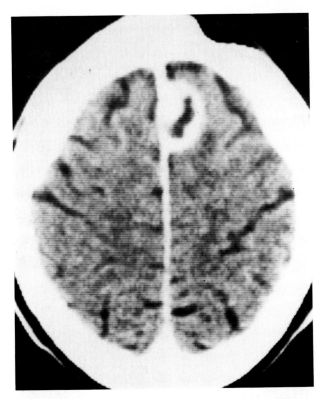

Figure 16-28 Postradiation necrosis. One year after radiation therapy following left frontal craniectomy for glioma, CECT shows a ringlike enhancement. Differential diagnosis from recurrent or residual tumor is extremely difficult. At surgery, no tumor was found.

Figure 16-29 (*Below*) Isodense subacute subdural hematoma. **A.** NCCT image in a 60-year-old man who presented with low-grade fever, recent personality change, and disorientation. Cerebral abscess was suspected clinically. There is compression of the right lateral ventricle, and the gyral pattern of the right frontoparietal cortex is displaced inward from the skull margin, separated by a thick homogeneous band which is virtually isodense with the cortex. A fluid level near the anterior margin of the band (arrow) probably represents a fluid level within the subdural hematoma. **B.** CECT image accentuates the interface between hematoma and cortex by demonstrating opacified veins on the convexity of the right hemisphere (arrows).

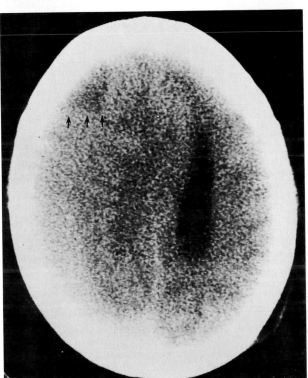

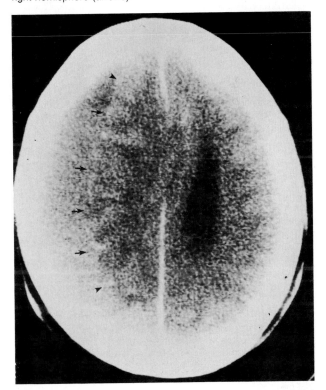

A

B

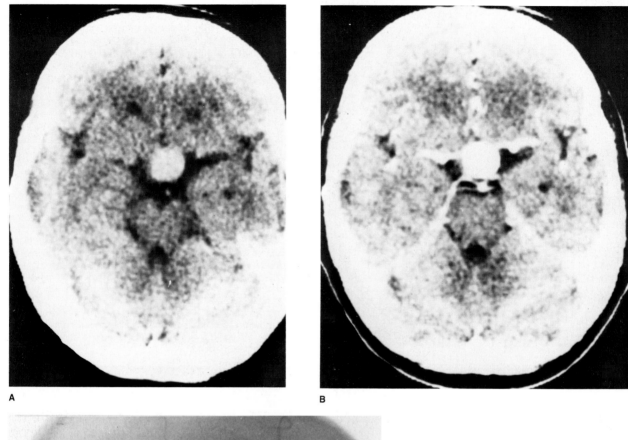

A

B

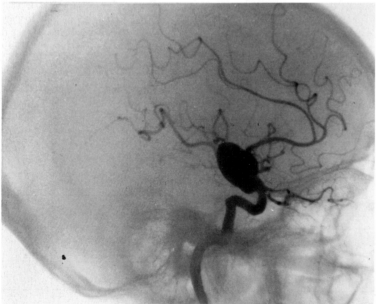

C

Figure 16-30   Internal carotid artery aneurysm. NCCT (**A**) presents as round hyperdense mass in the suprasellar region exhibiting homogeneous intense enhancement on CECT (**B**). Carotid angiogram demonstrates an aneurysm of the distal internal carotid artery projecting toward the midline.

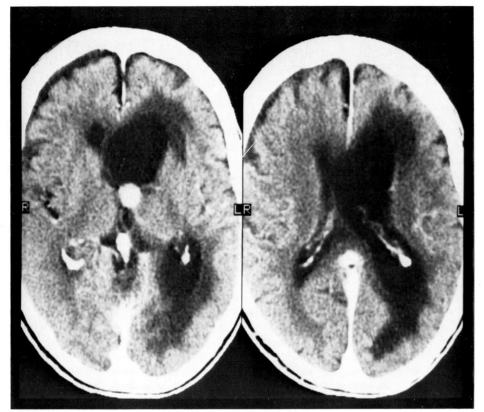

Figure 16-31 Basilar artery aneurysm. CECT (**A**) shows a small round enhancing lesion in the anterior third ventricular region. Left lateral ventriculomegaly is due to obstruction of ipsilateral foramen of Monro. Note unilateral periventricular hypodensity representing transventricular CSF absorption. Sagittal reformation image (**B**) shows its relationship to the third ventricle. Vertebral angiogram (**C**) reveals an aneurysm at the tip of the basilar artery (see also Fig. 6-27).

A   B

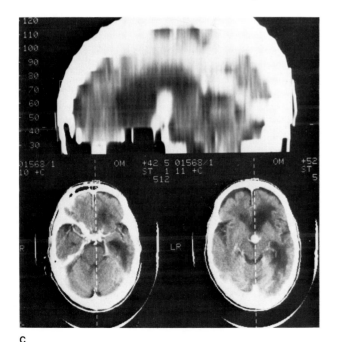

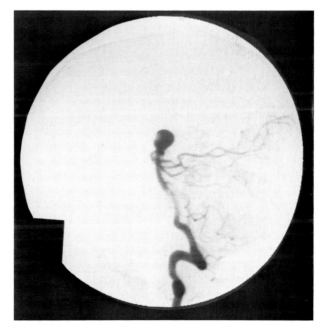

C   D

necrosis. It was quickly realized that intracerebral abscess often presented the same appearance on CT (Davis D. 1977; Whelan 1980). Some meningiomas contain foci of necrosis or cystic degeneration, which may produce a ring pattern on CECT (Russell 1980). A wide margin of low density surrounding the opacified ring and due to cerebral edema may be seen in all these lesions. However, serial follow-up studies in other disease processes have demonstrated that the ring sign is even less specific. In the process of resolution of an intracerebral hematoma (Zimmerman 1977) or a cerebral infarct (Wing 1976; Yock 1975), a ring of contrast enhancement may develop around the periphery of the resolving mass. Gliosis and neovascularity, typical components of the repair process, probably account for this pattern (Fig. 16-27).

Postradiation parenchymal change may present as a ring contrast enhancement mimicking closely recurrent or residual tumor (Fig 16-28).

It is well recognized that intracranial meningiomas frequently have the same density as adjacent normal brain and cannot be differentiated on CT studies without contrast injection (Davis D. 1977).

However, this pattern is also nonspecific. Extraaxial neuroma, carcinomatous metastasis, and intracerebral histiocytic lymphoma (Brant-Zawadzki 1978) may also be of the same density as the surrounding brain and may be defined only after contrast medium is administered intravenously. A subacute subdural hematoma (10 to 20 days after the acute bleeding) may also be indistinguishable from adjacent brain, due to partial resorption of protein from the hematoma; restudy after intravenous contrast injection may demonstrate marginal membrane formation (Davis K. 1977) or displaced surface veins on the inner aspect of the hematoma (Kim 1978). In all these lesions, the plain CT study usually gives some indication of a space-occupying mass, for example, compression or shift of portions of the ventricular system, which should alert the radiologist to the necessity for repeat study with intravenous contrast (Fig 16-29).

Differential diagnosis of midline lesions such as a suprasellar mass should include an aneurysm, and angiography should be considered prior to surgical intervention (Figs. 16-30, 16-31).

Bibliography

ADAM R, GREENBERG JO: The large cisterna magna. Neurosurgery **48**(2):109–192, 1978.

BRANT-ZAWADZKI M, ENZMANN DR: Computed tomographic brain scanning in patients with lymphoma. *Radiology* **129**:67–71, 1978.

BROOKS RA, DICHIRO G: Beam hardening in x-ray reconstructive tomography. *Phys Med Biol* **21**:390–398, 1976

COHEN CR, DUCHESNEAU P, WEINSTEIN MA: Calcification of the basal ganglia as visualized by CT. *Radiology* **134**:97–99, 1980.

DAVIS DO: CT in the diagnosis of supratentorial tumors. *Semin Roentgenol* **12**:97–108, 1977.

DAVIS KR, TAVERAS JM, NEW PFJ, SCHNUR JA, ROBERSON GH: Cerebral infarction diagnosed by computerized tomography analysis and evaluation of findings. *Am J Roentgenol* **124**:643–660, 1975.

DAVIS KR et al: Computed tomography in head trauma. *Semin Roentgenol* **12**:53–62, 1977.

DOHRMANN GJ, GEEHR RB, ROBINSON F: Small hemorrhages vs. small calcifications in brain tumors: Difficulty in differentiation by CT. *Surg Neurol* **10**:309–312, 1978.

DOLINSKAS CA, ZIMMERMAN RA, BILANIUK LT: A sign of subarachnoid bleeding on cranial computed tomograms of pediatric head trauma patients. *Radiology* **126**:409–411, 1978.

GADO M, HEUTE I, MIKHAEL M: Computerized tomography of infratentorial tumors. *Semin Roentgenol* **12**:109–120, 1977.

GEORGE AE, RUSSELL EJ, KRICHEFF II: White matter buckling: CT sign of extra-axial intracranial mass. *Am J Neuroradiol* **1**:425–430, 1980.

HANDA J, NAKANO Y, HANDA H: Computed tomography in the differential diagnosis of low-density intracranial lesions. *Surg Neurol* **10**:179–185, 1978.

KIM KS, HEMMATI M, WEINBERG PE: Computed tomography in isodense subdural hematoma. *Radiology* **128**:71–72, 1978.

KRAMER RA: Vermian pseudotumor: A potential pitfall of CT brain scanning with contrast enhancement. *Neuroradiology* **13**:229–230, 1977.

KUHNS, LR, SEEGER J: *Atlas of CT Variants.* Chicago, Year Book Medical Publishers, Inc., 1983.

LATCHAW RE et al: The monospecificity of absorption coefficients in the differentiation of solid tumors and cystic lesions. *Radiology* **125**:141–144, 1977.

LEE SH, VILLAFANA T: Localization of vertex lesions on cranial computed tomography. *Radiology* **134**:539–540, 1980.

LEMAY M, KIDO D: Asymmetries of the cerebral hemispheres on CT. *J Comput Assist Tomogr* **2**:471–476, 1978.

LEO JS, PINTO RS, HULVAT GF, EPSTEIN F, KRICHEFF II: Computed tomography of arachnoid cysts. *Radiology* **130**:675–680, 1979.

LILIEQUIST B, TOVI D, SCHISANO G: Developmental defects of the tentorium and cisterna magna. *Acta Psychiatr Neurol Scand* **35**:223–234, 1960.

MILLER EM, NEWTON TH: Extra-axial posterior fossa lesions simulating intra-axial lesions on CT. *Radiology* **127**:675–679, 1978.

MODIC MT et al: Calcification of the choroid plexus visualized by computed tomography. *Radiology* **135**:369–372, 1980.

NAIDICH TP et al: The normal contrast-enhanced computed axial tomogram of the brain. *J Comput Assist Tomogr* **1**:16–29, 1977.

NORMAN D et al: Quantitative aspects of computed tomography of the blood and cerebrospinal fluid. *Radiology* **123**:335–338, 1977.

OSBORN AG, ANDERSON RE, WING SD: The false falx sign. *Radiology* **134**:421–425, 1980.

RUSSELL EJ et al: Atypical computed tomographic features of intracranial meningioma. *Radiology* **135**:673–682, 1980.

TANS J, DE JONGH IE: Computed tomography of supratentorial astrocytoma. *Clin Neurol Neurosurg* **80**:156–168, 1978.

TER-POGOSSIAN MM: Computerized cranial tomography: Equipment and physics. *Semin Roentgenol* **12**:13–25, 1977.

WHELAN MA, HILAL SK: CT as a guide in the diagnosis and follow-up of brain abscesses. *Radiology* **135**:663–671, 1980.

WING SD et al: Contrast enhancement of cerebral infarcts in computed tomography. *Radiology* **121**:89–92, 1976.

YOCK DH, MARSHALL WH: Recent ischemic brain infarcts at computed tomography: Appearance pre- and post-contrast infusion. *Radiology* **117**:599–608, 1975.

YOCK DH JR: *CT of CNS Disease—A Teaching File.* Chicago, Year Book Medical Publishers, Inc., 1985.

ZIMMERMAN RA et al: Cranial computed tomography in diagnosis and management of acute head trauma. *Am J Roentgenol* **131**:27–34,1978.

ZIMMERMAN RD, LEEDS NE, NAIDICH TP: Ring blush associated with intracerebral hematoma. *Radiology* **122**:707–711, 1977.

17

CRANIAL MRI: CURRENT CLINICAL APPLICATIONS*

William G. Bradley, Jr.

Keith E. Kortman

INTRODUCTION

Like x-ray computed tomography (CT), magnetic resonance imaging (MRI) is a computer-based imaging modality which depicts anatomic sections in tomographic slices of varying thickness (Bradley 1983). In contrast to CT, which requires the use of ionizing radiation, MR is based on an interaction between radio waves and specific nuclei in the body in the presence of a strong magnetic field, with no demonstrable adverse effects on biologic tissues. In addition to providing precise anatomic detail with spatial resolution comparable with that of fourth-generation CT, MR also allows imaging in any of the three orthogonal planes (axial, sagittal, and co-ronal), with some systems allowing direct oblique imaging as well.

Human MR images were first published by the Nottingham group in 1980 (Holland 1980; Hawkes 1980). Since that time, there have been steady improvements in image quality and significant reductions in imaging time. After initial studies by the Hammersmith group in London (Young 1981; Bydder 1982), investigators at UCSF published studies comparing CT with MR (Crooks 1982; Brant-Zawadzki 1983, 1984a), clearly demonstrating the higher sensitivity of MR to pathologic intracranial processes.

* We thank Leslee Watson, Terry Andrues, and Jay Mericle for technical assistance, and Kaye Finley for manuscript preparation.

Since that time, several investigators have demonstrated the efficacy of MR in the evaluation of a wide range of intracranial pathologic processes, including neoplasms (Lee 1985*a*; Smith 1985; Zimmerman 1985; Lee 1985*b*; New 1985), demyelinating disease (Jackson 1985; Sheldon 1985), trauma (Han 1984*a*), and congenital abnormalities (Spinos 1985). In our studies comparing MR with CT in 400 consecutive cases of suspected CNS pathology, MR detected abnormalities which were not seen on CT in 30 percent of these cases (Bradley 1984*c*). MR has become established as the imaging modality of choice in the evaluation of a broad range of CNS abnormalities (Brant-Zawadzki 1984*b*) and is rapidly being implemented not only at university medical centers but also in community hospitals and free-standing clinics. This chapter deals with fundamental principles of MR image interpretation and provides insight into current clinical indications for MR in intracranial disorders.

FUNDAMENTALS OF MR IMAGE INTERPRETATION

The physical principles of nuclear magnetic resonance (NMR) imaging have been described previously (Bradley 1983), as have the fundamentals of MR image interpretation (Wehrli 1983, 1984; Bradley 1984*a*, 1985*a*). The following brief discussion is intended to assist the reader in the clinical discussion which follows.

Just as the CT number reflects a physical property (electron density) in x-ray computed tomography, so there are basic determinants of signal intensity in MR. Although the MR image could be simply considered to be a map of hydrogen density within the body, it is strongly influenced by two physical parameters which are unique to NMR: the magnetic relaxation times, T_1 and T_2.

To be more exact, NMR is concerned with the *nucleus* of the hydrogen atom. Hydrogen nuclei in the body are composed of single *protons* (positively charged particles) which spin. When charged par-

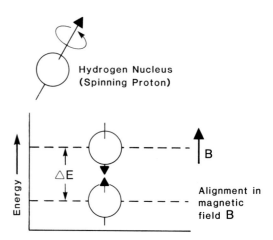

Figure 17-1 Alignment of hydrogen nucleus in presence of magnetic field. The hydrogen nucleus consists of a single proton: a positively charged particle which spins, generating a magnetic moment. When placed in a magnetic field, these magnetic moments tend to align parallel or antiparallel to the main magnetic field. The parallel protons have a lower relative energy level than those in the antiparallel configuration. The energy difference (ΔE) depends on the strength of the magnetic field and, in general, on the specific nucleus involved.

ticles spin, they generate small magnetic fields called *magnetic moments* and behave like bar magnets. When placed in a stronger magnetic field, they align in the north/south direction, much like compass needles in the earth's magnetic field (Fig. 17-1) (Bradley 1983). Unlike compass needles, the hydrogen nuclei can point either north (parallel to the field) or south (antiparallel). Immediately after they are placed in the magnetic field, there is an equal number of hydrogen nuclei pointing north and south so that the individual magnetic moments exactly cancel. Over the next second or so in biological substances, a redistribution occurs such that there is a slightly greater number of hydrogen nuclei pointing parallel with the field. The effect of this redistribution and the resulting inequality in the number of north- and south-pointing nuclei is to produce a physical characteristic called the *magnetization* which represents the overall magnetic effect of all the individual hydrogen nuclei (Fig. 17-2). It is the changing magnetization that is actually measured during NMR experiments in the chemistry laboratory or during clinical magnetic resonance imaging (MRI).

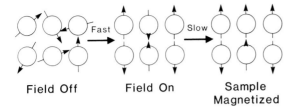

Figure 17-2 Magnetization. When the field is off (or the protons are outside the field), the protons point randomly. Almost immediately following placement within a magnetic field (or turning the magnetic field on) there is an equal number of protons in the parallel and antiparallel configurations; thus, the individual magnetic moments exactly cancel. Over the next few seconds or so, a realignment occurs such that a slightly greater number of protons point in the parallel direction, giving the tissue a bulk property called the magnetization. (The period of time required for magnetization to occur is characterized by the T_1 relaxation time.)

When magnetized hydrogen nuclei are exposed to certain radio waves, they can undergo a process known as *resonance* (Fig. 17-3). This occurs at only one radiofrequency (the resonant or "Larmor" frequency) which, for a given nucleus, is entirely determined by the local value of the magnetic field (Bradley 1983). The resonant frequency is directly proportional to the field strength; thus nuclei resonate at higher frequency in stronger magnetic fields.

When the body is exposed to radio waves at the Larmor frequency, resonance occurs and detectable radio waves are radiated by the body. (Radio waves are actually being continuously emitted whenever

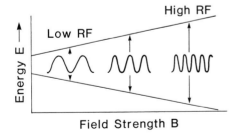

Figure 17-3 Variation of resonant radio frequency with field strength: In stronger magnetic fields, more energy is required to flip a proton from the parallel to antiparallel configuration. When this transition is caused by exposure to radio waves at the Larmor frequency, resonance occurs. Since the energy of a radio wave is directly proportional to its frequency, higher-frequency RF energy is required to cause resonance at higher fields compared with lower fields.

the body is in a magnetic field but they are out of phase and therefore not detectable as a signal but only as "noise.") The process of resonance causes the hydrogen nuclei to get into phase, i.e., to become "coherent," which allows them to be detected (Bradley 1983). The frequency of the signal emitted reflects the local strength of the magnetic field.

The local value of the magnetic field is determined by adding the fields from two different magnets: the main static field and the smaller gradient field (Fig. 17-3). The main static magnetic field is generated by a superconducting or permanent magnet or by a resistive electromagnet. It should not fluctuate over time and is not supposed to vary with position across the patient by more than 1 part in 10,000 to 100,000 (i.e., 10 to 100 parts per million). Resistive electromagnetic coils are used to provide spatial variation in the *net* magnetic field, creating a magnetic field *gradient*. The gradient coils and their fields can be activated and inactivated rapidly, changing the resonant frequency at each position in the patient at precisely specified times.

The net magnetic field is determined by adding the value of the static field (which can be mapped very precisely) to the value of any gradient fields which may be activated at that moment. Since the value of the gradient field at each position is also known quite precisely, the exact value of the *net* magnetic field can be specified at each point in the body. The specific frequencies comprising the signal detected by the receiving antenna are an indication of the specific positions of resonating protons in the body. To a first approximation, therefore, the intensity of the signal at a particular frequency indicates the *density* of resonating protons and the frequency indicates *position* (Bradley 1983). The apparent reradiation of radio waves which occurs following resonance has been compared with an acoustic echo. For this reason, the term *spin echo* (Hahn 1950) has been applied to one of the more common pulsing sequences and signals used in NMR spectroscopy and now in clinical MR imaging. Subsequent discussion of pulsing sequences and signals in this chapter will be limited to the spin echo.

The variable intensity of the spin-echo signal can be explained very simply as the result of a two-step

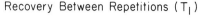

Recovery Between Repetitions (T$_1$)

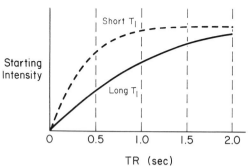

Figure 17-4 Recovery of magnetization between repetitions: The T$_1$ relaxation time is indicative of the rate of recovery of magnetization between repetitions. Substances with a short T$_1$ recover more rapidly than those with a long T$_1$. Given a long enough time between repetitions (TR), both substances will achieve an equilibrium magnetization (the plateau value) corresponding to the hydrogen density. (*From Bradley, 1984b.*)

process if only the magnitude of the signal is considered (Bradley 1985*a*). The first step is a recovery process (Fig. 17-4) and the second is a decay process (Fig. 17-5). Since the radiofrequency signal of magnetic resonance is much weaker (approximately 11 orders of magnitude) than its x-ray equivalent, it

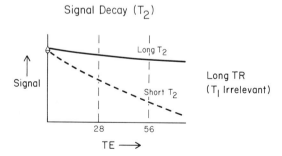

Signal Decay (T$_2$)

Figure 17-5 Signal decay due to T$_2$ relaxation: If a sufficiently long TR is allowed to achieve full magnetization, individual T$_1$ relaxation times become irrelevant. If proton density values are also assumed to be equal, two substances will start to decay from the maximum magnetization. A substance with a long T$_2$ will decay more slowly than one with a short T$_2$. The decay curves are "sampled" at the echo delay times (TE) when the spin echoes are obtained. The acquisition of spin-echo signals at 28 and 56 msec echo delay time is demonstrated. The T$_2$ relaxation time is indicative of the ability of the substance to maintain phase coherence. Substances with short T$_2$ relaxation times lose phase coherence and thus have lower signal intensity. (*From Bradley, 1984b.*)

must be repeated many times. The T$_1$ *relaxation time* is an indication of the rate of recovery of magnetization between repetitions. This is a first-order exponential time constant similar to that used for the generation of ^{99m}Tc in nuclear medicine. The amount of time allowed for this recovery to occur is one of the programmable sequence parameters, the repetition time TR. At the beginning of every time interval TR, a new pulsing sequence is initiated by a burst of radio waves called an RF (radiofrequency) pulse. Following this RF pulse, the intensity of the spin-echo signal decays over several hundred milliseconds in biological systems because of magnetic nonuniformities in the tissue. These nonuniformities cause the protons at slightly different positions to resonate at slightly different frequencies and to get out of phase, i.e., to "lose coherence." As phase coherence is lost, the net magnetization decays (Fig. 17-5). The rate of this decay is indicated by the second magnetic *relaxation time* T$_2$. The time allowed for the decay to occur is given by a second programmable sequence parameter, the echo delay time TE (Fig. 17-6). The intensity of the resultant signal reflects the influence of both TR/T$_1$ and TE/T$_2$. As shown in Fig. 17-7, the relative intensities of two tissues (brain and CSF) depend not only on their own T$_1$ and T$_2$ values but also on the programmed TR and TE times.

Multiple Spin Echo Sequence

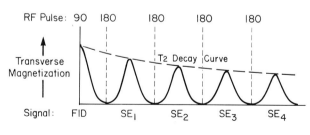

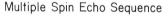

Echo Delay Time (TE)

Figure 17-6 Multiple spin-echo sequence. Following the 90° pulse, transverse magnetization decays according to the T$_2$ decay curve. When multiple 180° pulses are applied, multiple spin echoes can be generated, producing an "echo train." As shown in the diagram, later echoes in the multiple spin-echo sequence have decreased signal to noise relative to those acquired immediately following the 90° pulse.

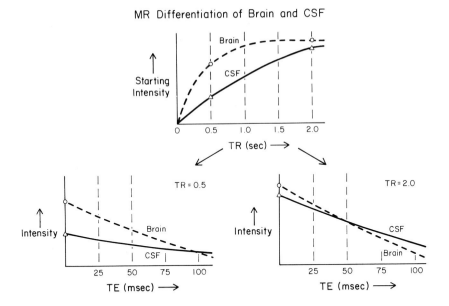

MR Differentiation of Brain and CSF

Figure 17-7 Variation in relative intensities of brain and CSF due to different combinations of TR and TE. The relative intensities of brain and CSF are determined both by their own magnetic relaxation times (T_1 and T_2) and by the programmable sequence parameter times (TR and TE). When TR = 0.5 sec, brain, having a shorter T_1, has recovered more signal than CSF. When TR = 2.0 sec, CSF catches up to brain and both start to decay from higher values of the magnetization. The rates of decay are determined by the relative T_2 relaxation times. Since CSF has a longer T_2 than brain, it will become isointense with brain at approximately 50 msec and will become more intense than brain at longer TE. (*From Bradley, 1984b.*)

Mathematically, the intensity of the spin-echo signal can be approximated (Crooks, 1982):

$$I = N(\text{H})f(v)\,(1 - e^{-\text{TR}/T_1})\,(e^{-\text{TE}/T_2})$$

where $N(\text{H})$ is the density of hydrogen nuclei and $f(v)$ is a function of flow. [The symbol e represents the base of the natural logarithm (Bradley 1983) and has a numerical value of approximately 2.7.] A stationary substance with a short T_1 and a long T_2 will have a stronger MR signal than a substance with a long T_1 and short T_2, assuming constant hydrogen density (Bradley 1985a). For this reason, fat (short T_1, long T_2) generally appears bright on MR while skeletal muscle (longer T_1 shorter T_2) appears relatively dark. Rapidly flowing blood generally appears dark (Hawkes 1980) because it does not remain in position long enough to acquire the appropriate RF pulses. Cortical bone and air also appear dark owing to low hydrogen density (Hawkes 1980).

Water is the most common source of hydrogen nuclei contributing to the MR signal. The local chemical environment of the water determines the T_1 and T_2 relaxation times (Hazelwood 1979; Fullerton 1984). The hydrogen nuclei in the water (and other) molecules are always in motion, vibrating, rotating, and translating at certain characteristic frequencies. The chemical environment and the size of the molecules determine these natural motional frequencies. How well these frequencies match the Larmor frequency (the operating radiofrequency of the MR imager) determines the T_1 relaxation time (Roberts 1959; Farrar 1971). Water in the bulk phase (like CSF) has intrinsic frequencies much higher than the resonant Larmor frequency because the water molecule is relatively small (Fullerton 1984). Such bulk phase water is inefficient at T_1 relaxation and thus has a long T_1 time. Much of the water in tissues, however, is found in hydration layers around proteins which slow the naturally rapid motions (Fig. 17-8). Hydration layer water has natural frequencies closer to the Larmor frequency and consequently has a shorter T_1 relaxation time (Fullerton 1984). To a first approximation, the relative proportion of "bulk phase" and "hydration layer" water determines the T_1 time of a tissue.

The T_2 relaxation time of a tissue is also determined by the specific frequencies of natural molecular motion. Most motions that cause T_1 relaxation also cause T_2 relaxation. Unlike T_1 relaxation, however, T_2 relaxation is accomplished most efficiently by static or slowly fluctuating internal fields. These

Molecular Environment of Water

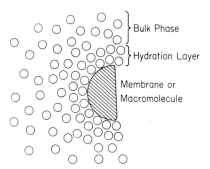

Figure 17-8 Molecular environment of water. Water molecules adjacent to membranes or macromolecules are held in hydration layers by attraction to hydrophilic side groups of component proteins. Several layers removed from the macromolecule, water is in the bulk phase where its intrinsic motions are very rapid because of its small size. Closer to the macromolecule, the water molecules are held in hydration layers by attraction to the charged side groups and thus move at a much slower frequency than those in the bulk phase. The water molecules closest to the macromolecule move at the slow tumbling frequency of the larger structure. The T_1 relaxation time of water in the bulk phase is long because the natural motional frequencies of this water are much higher than the Larmor frequencies used for MR imaging. Hydration layer water has motional frequencies closer to the Larmor frequency which is thus more efficient at T_1 relaxation and therefore has a shorter T_1 relaxation time.

fields are generally due to protons and other magnetic nuclei attached to large molecules. When static fields are present, the T_2 relaxation time is shortened. The more solidlike the tissue, the shorter the T_2; bulk phase water is very liquid and thus has a very long T_2 (Roberts 1959; Fullerton 1984).

The MR acquisition sequence can be varied to bring out the T_1 or T_2 differences between tissues, i.e., to increase the T_1 weighting or T_2 weighting of the MR image. T_1-weighted images (T_1-WI) are produced by short values of TR and TE; T_2-weighted images (T_2-WI) are produced by long values of TR and TE (Bradley 1985a). Short TR–short TE images may also be called "partial saturation" images. As shown in Figure 17-5, long TR values allow different tissues to recover equilibrium magnetization between repetitions, regardless of individual T_1 values. The equilibrium magnetization achieved at long TR reflects differences in proton density. Thus long

TR values demonstrate differences in proton density and minimize T_1 weighting. Conversely, short TR values enhance T_1 weighting. Long TE values enhance the difference in signal from tissues with different T_2 decay times, increasing the T_2 weighting. Short TE times allow less time for differential decay and thus have less T_2 weighting. When specifying the intensity of an object on an MR image, one must also specify the TR and TE of the MR pulsing sequence used. As shown in Fig. 17-9, CSF will appear dark on T_1-WI (owing to its long T_1 value), it will be isointense with brain on moderate T_2-WI, and it will appear bright on heavily T_2-WI (owing to its long T_2 value).

PATHOPHYSIOLOGY OF BRAIN EDEMA

Pathologic intracranial processes are recognized on MR by virtue of alterations of normal anatomy and signal intensity. The changes in intensity are often due to the presence of edema (Fig. 17-10), reflecting focal changes in brain water concentration and local molecular environment. In a simplified scheme described by Fishman, edema can be divided into three types: vasogenic, cytotoxic, and interstitial (Fishman 1975). *Vasogenic edema* results from a breakdown of the blood-brain barrier and leakage of a proteinaceous plasma filtrate into the extracellular space (Fig. 17-11). On CT, edema is depicted as an area of decreased attenuation but may be apparent only when the involved area is relatively extensive. Blood-brain barrier breakdown may also be manifested on CT by focal enhancement after intravenous administration of iodinated contrast material. Vasogenic edema causes prolongation of the T_2 relaxation time which is manifested as increased signal intensity on T_2-WI (Bradley 1984b). On MR, vasogenic edema is depicted with high conspicuity without the need to inject intravenous contrast material. The greater conspicuity of edema on T_2-WI allows much smaller lesions to be detected by MR than by unenhanced or even enhanced CT. Vaso-

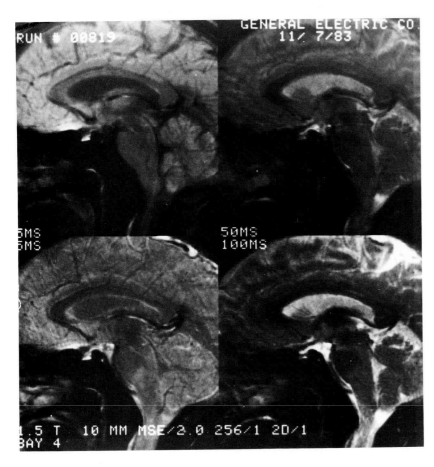

Figure 17-9 Intensity crossover of brain and CSF. The images shown were acquired with a TR of 2.0 sec and TE times varying from 25 to 100 msec. At 25 msec, the CSF is clearly lower in intensity than brain while at 50 to 75 msec, the two are isointense. At 100 msec TE, the CSF is clearly more intense than brain. Such images are referred to as "heavily T2-weighted." (*Images obtained at 1.5 tesla courtesy of Felix Wehrli, Ph.D., and General Electric.*)

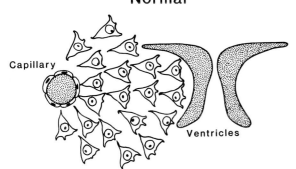

Figure 17-10 Schematic representation of normal blood-brain barrier, cells, and extracellular space. (*From Bradley, 1984b.*)

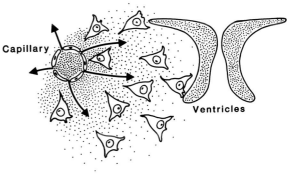

Figure 17-11 Schematic representation of vasogenic edema demonstrating blood-brain barrier breakdown and increased fluid in the extracellular space. (*From Bradley, 1984b.*)

genic edema is produced by a variety of pathologic processes, including primary and metastatic tumors, vaso-occlusive disease, hemorrhage, contusion, and inflammation (Bradley, 1984*b*). It is the most readily demonstrable form of cerebral edema, and preferentially involves the white matter, extending along white matter fiber tracts and generally sparing the more tightly integrated cortical gray matter (Reulen 1975).

Cytotoxic edema results in cellular swelling and is most often due to ischemia (Fig. 17-12). When the blood supply to a cell is decreased, the level of intracellular oxygen is decreased and oxidative phosphorylation ceases, leading to a reduction of ATP and failure of the sodium-potassium pump. Intracellular influx of sodium and water results in cellular swelling and a concomitant decrease in the volume of the extracellular space (Klatzo 1967). This results in loss of cellular function; however, cytostructure is largely maintained. Such an insult may be reversible if the oxygen supply to the cell is reestablished (Shaller 1980). In contrast to vasogenic edema, cytotoxic edema tends to involve cortical gray matter as well as subjacent white matter. It is often observed in the boundary zone of infarcts between the central areas of infarction and the surrounding normal brain. When present, cytotoxic edema may result in sharp margination of acute infarcts since the swollen cells

Interstitial Edema

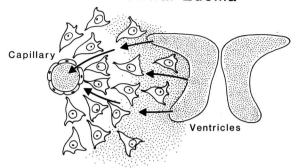

Figure 17-13 Schematic representation of interstitial edema. Increased intraventricular pressure forces the CSF transependymally into the periventricular tissues. (*From Bradley, 1984b.*)

at the periphery dam up the vasogenic edema produced centrally (Bradley 1984*b*).

Interstitial edema (Fig. 17-13) results from transependymal migration of CSF under a pressure gradient from the ventricles into the periventricular white matter (Fishman 1975). This results in a smooth and symmetric border of increased signal intensity surrounding the lateral ventricles on T_2-WI (Bradley 1984*b*). It has been observed not only in the various acute forms of obstructive and communicating hydrocephalus but also in patients with symptoms and shunt response consistent with the syndrome of "normal pressure hydrocephalus" (NPH) (Kortman 1986).

Cytotoxic Edema

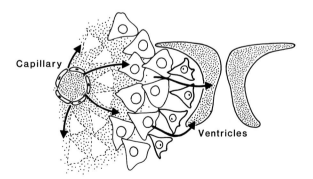

Figure 17-12 Schematic representation of cytotoxic edema. Cells at periphery of infarct are swollen, decreasing extracellular space and limiting diffusion of vasogenic edema produced centrally by blood-brain barrier breakdown. (*From Bradley, 1984b.*)

Neoplastic Abnormalities of the Brain

Intracranial neoplasia alters the T_1 and T_2 relaxation times of affected tissues and is recognized by the resultant change in normal signal intensity. Gliomas and most other intraaxial tumors typically produce marked alterations in signal intensity, most conspicuous on T_2-WI (Smith 1985; Brant-Zawadzki 1984*b*). Highly cellular lesions, such as meningiomas and neurofibromas, may be less conspicuous on MR than on CECT (Zimmerman 1985); with application of appropriate pulsing sequences and imaging planes, however, very few of these lesions should be missed by MR (Bucon 1985).

In many cases, tissue characterization can be accomplished with MR, as specific patterns of altered signal may indicate the presence of cyst formation, necrosis, hemorrhage, fatty tissue, or calcification (Bradley 1986c). Subacute hemorrhage (Bradley 1985b) and fatty tissue are characterized by hyperintensity reflecting short T_1 and relatively long T_2 relaxation times. Calcifications of sufficient size may be recognized as areas of hypointensity owing to the relatively low concentration of mobile protons. However, calcification is generally less conspicuous by MR than by CT (Tsuruda 1986). While the MR signal intensity may allow tissue characterization, other diagnostic criteria in MR are similar to those established for CT. These criteria include lesion location, number, size, mass effect, and amount of associated edema.

With respect to location, it is almost always possible to characterize the lesion as being either intraaxial or extraaxial in location. Extraaxial lesions

in the brain periphery produce displacement of superficial blood vessels and white matter (Fig. 17-14) (Bucon 1985). These structures are often more readily identified by MR than with CT, and distortion of these structures is easily recognized, provided that the appropriate imaging plane is utilized. Lesions at the skull base or vertex are best demonstrated in the coronal plane (Fig. 17-15), while midline lesions may be best evaluated in the sagittal plane (Fig. 17-16).

The presence of multiple intracranial masses is usually an indication of metastatic disease. Because of its greater sensitivity, MR may demonstrate several lesions when only one is evident on CT, markedly altering the diagnosis, prognosis, and therapy (Bradley 1984c; Brant-Zawadzki 1984b).

As with CT, the size of a lesion should be accurately determined and reported in conventional units. When possible, an attempt should be made to separate tumor from surrounding edema. As

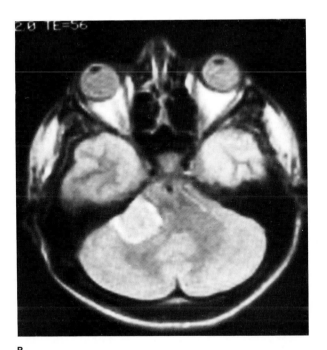

A

B

Figure 17-14 Acoustic neuroma. **A.** A slightly hyperintense rounded mass is seen within the right side of the posterior fossa. The mass is broad-based against the petrous bone. The cerebellar white matter is "buckled" medially, further evidence of the tumor's extraaxial location (TR = 2.0 sec, TE = 28 msec). **B.** On the second echo image, there is an increase in mass intensity relative to adjacent brain (TR = 2.0 sec, TE = 56 msec). (*Continued on p. 782.*)

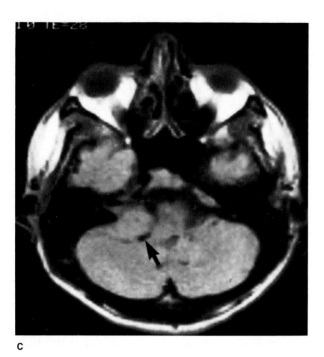

C

Figure 17-14 (*cont.*)   **C.** On a more T₁-WI (TR = 1.0 sec, TE = 28 msec), the mass is isointense with brain and can be seen extending into the internal auditory canal. A hypointense superficial blood vessel (arrow) has been medially displaced by the mass, confirming its extraaxial location.

edema has a longer T_2 and a shorter T_1 than tumor, the separation may be possible using heavily T_1- (Brant-Zawadzki 1984*a*) or T_2-weighted sequences (Smith 1985) (Figs. 17-17 and 17-18). In certain cases, tumor cannot be distinguished from edema (Bradley 1984*b*). In this circumstance CECT maintains an advantage over MR by virtue of its ability to demonstrate blood-brain barrier breakdown. Several paramagnetic intravenous contrast agents have been tested in animals, and one such substance, Gadolinium-DTPA, is currently undergoing clinical trials in Europe and the United States (Graif 1985; Claussen 1985; Bradley 1985*f*). It appears to be relatively nontoxic and is as effective as iodinated x-ray contrast material in demonstrating blood-brain barrier breakdown (Fig. 17-19).

Primary Intra-axial Neoplasms

Gliomas

Astrocytomas, ependymomas, and oligodendrogliomas all appear as conspicuous areas of hyperintensity on T_2-WI and as less apparent regions of hypointensity on T_1-WI (Brant-Zawadzki 1984*a*) (Fig.

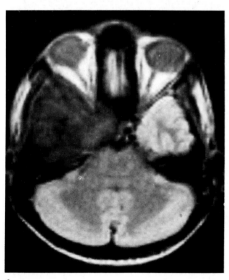

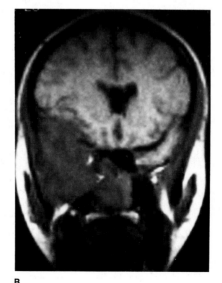

Figure 17-15   Chondrosarcoma of the skull base.   **A.** An axial image at the level of the petrous bones demonstrates a large hypointense mass filling the right temporal fossa and extending into the right petrous apex, the sphenoid sinus, and the lateral aspect of the right orbit (TR = 2.0 sec, TE = 28 msec).   **B.** A coronal image better demonstrates the cranio-caudad extent of the tumor and its relationship to the skull base (TR = 0.5 sec, TE = 28 msec).

A   B

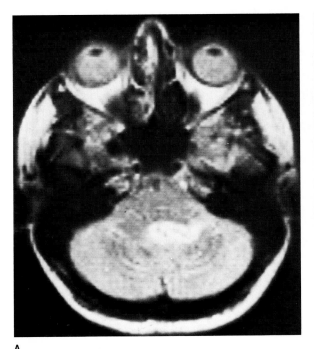

A

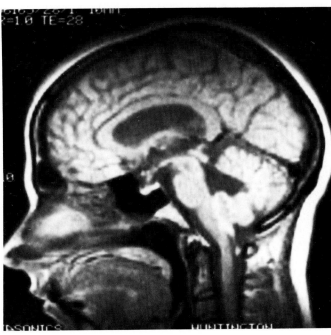

B

Figure 17-16 Fourth ventricular ependymoma. **A.** An axial T₂-WI (TR = 2.0 sec, TE = 56 msec) demonstrates a well-defined and hyperintense midline mass immediately posterior to the brainstem. **B.** The intraventricular location of the tumor is better ap-

preciated on the direct sagittal image. Note the dilatation of the ventricular system above the level of obstruction (TR = 1.0 sec, TE = 28 msec).

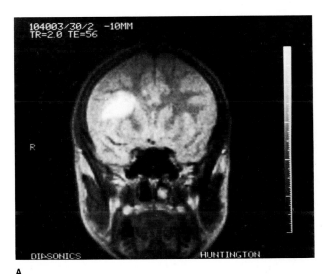

A

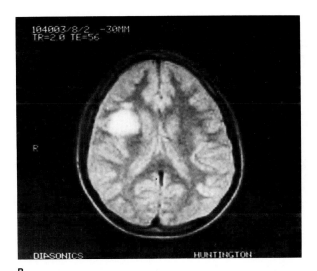

B

Figure 17-17 Astrocytoma. **A.** A coronal T₂-WI demonstrates a hyperintense lesion at the gray-white junction of the right frontal lobe. The lesion appears homogeneous; i.e., central tumor cannot

be separated from edema (TR = 2.0 sec, TE = 56 msec). **B.** Corresponding axial image with the same sequence parameters. (*Continued on p. 784.*)

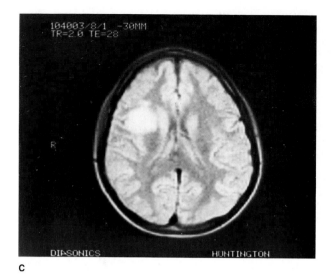

C

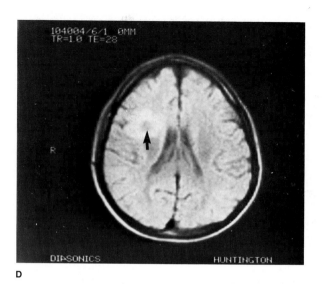

D

Figure 17-17 (*cont.*)   **C.** The first echo image also fails to separate tumor from edema (TR = 2.0 sec, TE = 28 msec).   **D.** On a more T$_1$-weighted (TR = 1.0 sec, TE = 28 msec) image, the central

tumor (arrow) can be identified as an area of slightly decreased signal intensity with respect to surrounding edema.

17-20). Tumoral calcification, when present, may be seen as foci of relative hypointensity, but is much less obvious than on CT (Tsuruda 1986). For this reason, a specific histologic diagnosis can seldom be made on the basis of MR findings alone at the present time.

Mass effect may be best appreciated on T$_1$-WI, which accentuates the contrast between brain parenchyma and adjacent CSF spaces (Lee 1985*a*). Tumor may be distinguished from surrounding edema by application of either heavily T$_1$- or T$_2$-WI (Smith 1985), or via administration of intravenous Gadoli-

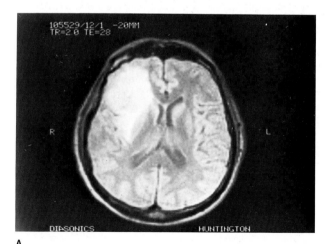

A

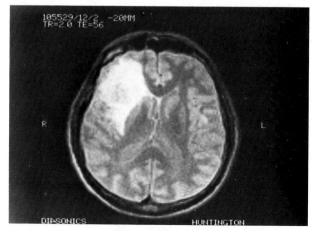

B

Figure 17-18   Intracranial metastasis.   **A.** A "balanced" (TR = 2.0 sec, TE = 28 msec) transaxial image demonstrates a hyperintense mass involving both gray and white matter in the right frontal lobe.   **B.** On a more T$_2$-weighted second echo image, the

tumor now appears as an area of slight hypointensity and can be differentiated from the surrounding higher-intensity edema (TR = 2.0 sec, TE = 56 msec).

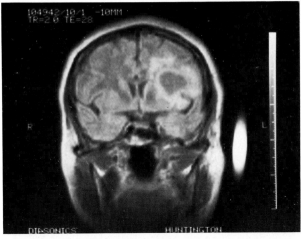

A

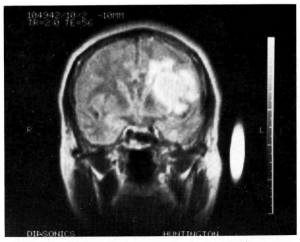

B

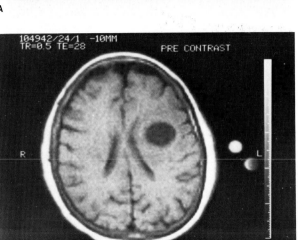

C

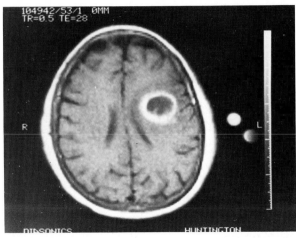

D

Figure 17-19 Glioblastoma multiforme. **A.** The coronal image demonstrates a slightly hypointense necrotic mass in the left frontal lobe. Note the surrounding high-intensity edema (TR = 2.0 sec, TE = 28 msec). **B.** On a more T$_2$-weighted second echo image, the necrotic center of the tumor is increased in signal intensity with respect to adjacent brain and is more difficult to distinguish from surrounding edema (TR = 2.0 sec, TE = 56 msec). **C.** On an axial T$_1$-WI the central tumor appears markedly hypointense. The surrounding edema is now inconspicuous (TR = 0.5 sec, TE = 28 msec). **D.** Following Gadolinium-DTPA administration, the rim of the tumor enhances markedly.

nium-DTPA (Graif 1985; Claussen 1985). Both mass effect and edema tend to be more pronounced in higher-grade tumors. Tumor extension across the midline through the corpus callosum is readily identified on direct coronal or sagittal MR images (Fig 17-21), and can thus be used to better distinguish tumors from nonneoplastic processes.

Optic Glioma

The intracranial extent of these tumors is well depicted by MR (Sobel 1985; Daniels 1984c) (Fig 17-22). T$_2$ prolongation results in hyperintensity on T$_2$-WI, typically involving the optic chiasm and extending to a variable degree along the optic nerves as well.

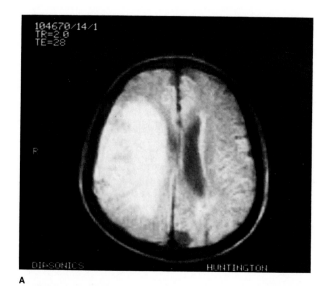

A

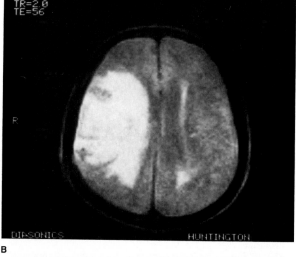

B

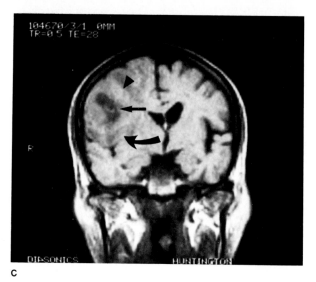

C

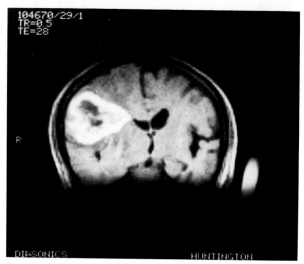

D

Figure 17-20   Glioblastoma multiforme.   **A.** This axial image demonstrates a hyperintense mass in the right frontal-parietal region. There is effacement and displacement of the adjacent lateral ventricle (TR = 2.0 sec, TE = 28 msec).   **B.** The conspicuity of the lesion is increased on the second echo image (TR = 2.0 sec, TE = 56 msec)   **C.** On a coronal T_1-WI (TR = 0.5 sec, TE = 28 msec) the periphery of the tumor (arrowhead) appears isointense with respect to brain, while an area of central necrosis (arrow) appears hypointense. Surrounding edema (curved arrow) also appears somewhat hypointense. Mass effect is more readily demonstrated on T_1-WI, and in this case is manifested by effacement of the cortical sulci, inferior displacement of sylvian fissure, and medial displacement and distortion of the right lateral ventricle (TR = 0.5 sec, TE = 28 msec).   **D.** Following intravenous administration of Gadolinium-DTPA, the mass enhances intensely (TR = 0.5 sec, TE = 28 msec).

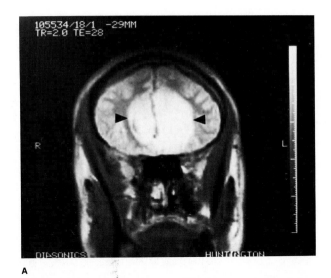

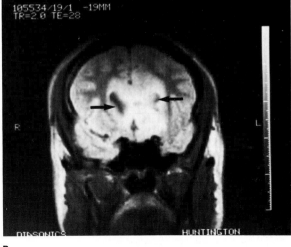

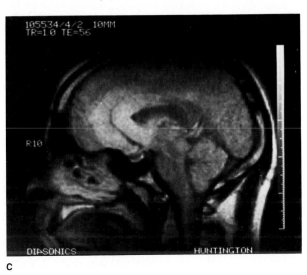

Figure 17-21 "Butterfly" glioma of the corpus callosum. **A.** This coronal image demonstrates a bifrontal hyperintense mass (arrowhead), extending to either side of the hypointense falx, which is displaced to the right. **B.** On a slightly more posterior section, the tumor can be seen extending above and below the hypointense frontal horns (arrows), indicating corpus callosum involvement (TR = 2.0 sec, TE = 28 msec). **C.** The direct sagittal image better demonstrates the enlargement of the anterior corpus callosum secondary to tumor involvement (TR = 1.0 sec, TE = 56 msec).

Posterior extension along the optic tracts is not unusual and is much more easily appreciated on MR than on contrast CT examination.

Brainstem Glioma

These lesions are particularly well evaluated by MR (Lee 1985b; Han 1984b). Tumor involvement of the brainstem is characterized by prolongation of T_1 and T_2 relaxation times. Associated mass effect is most easily appreciated on direct sagittal scanning, and is manifested by posterior displacement of the fourth ventricle and effacement of the ambient, pontine, and medullary cisterns (Fig. 17-23). Extension into the cervical cord is a common finding and is easily recognized by MR (Lee 1985c).

Cystic Astrocytoma

This lesion, although histologically similar to solid low-grade astrocytomas, may be considered as a separate entity based on the typical gross appear-

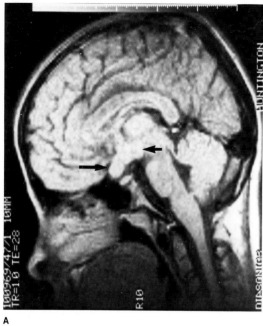

A

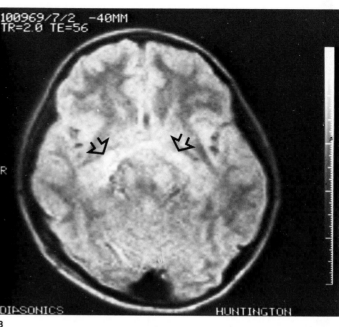

B

Figure 17-22   Optic glioma.   **A.** A direct sagittal image of this patient with neurofibromatosis reveals a lobulated mass involving the optic chiasm (short arrow) and extending along the optic nerve (long arrow) (TR = 1.0 sec, TE = 28 msec).   **B.** On a more T$_2$-WI (transaxial), the tumor can be seen extending along the optic tracts (open arrowheads) bilaterally (TR = 2.0 sec, TE = 56 msec).

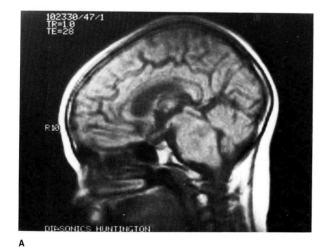

A

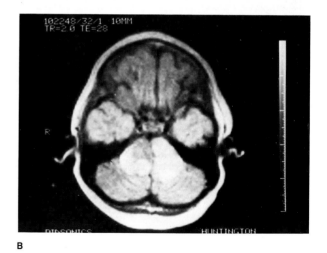

B

Figure 17-23   Pontine glioma.   **A.** A sagittal T$_1$-WI demonstrates a marked expansion of the pons, producing posterior displacement of the fourth ventricle and effacement of the prepontine cistern. Note the focal areas of hypointensity within the mass (TR = 1.0 sec, TE = 28 msec).   **B.** On the more T$_2$-WI (transaxial), T$_2$ prolongation is manifested as hyperintensity (TR = 2.0 sec, TE = 28 msec). (*Continued on p. 789.*) (*From Bradley, 1984b.*)

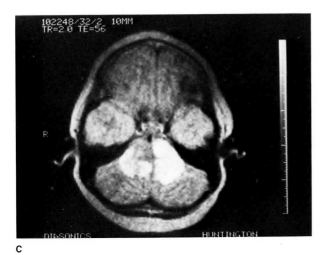

C

Figure 17-23 (*cont.*)   **C.** The increase in tumor intensity is more conspicuous on the second echo image (TR = 2.0 sec, TE = 56 msec).

ance (cystic with a mural nodule) and location (posterior fossa).

On MR the protein concentration of the cyst fluid determines its intensity (Fullerton 1984) (Fig. 17-24). The proteinaceous fluid in a neoplastic cyst can be distinguished from CSF by virtue of its shorter T_1, this shortening being due to a greater percentage of hydration layer water. Since the T_2 relaxation time remains prolonged in a fluid, the resulting MR intensity is greater than that of CSF. The tumor nodule may be distinguished from cyst fluid by virtue of its greater intensity, except on very heavily T_2-WI (Lee 1984). As with CT, it may be difficult to distinguish a cystic astrocytoma from a hemangioblastoma.

Medulloblastoma

As with other intracranial tumors, medulloblastomas may be identified by virtue of prolonged T_1 and

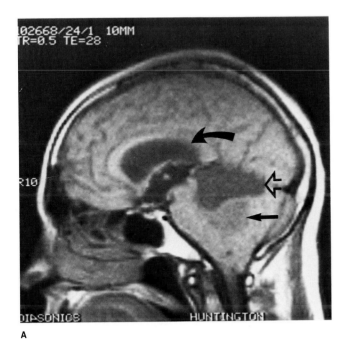

A

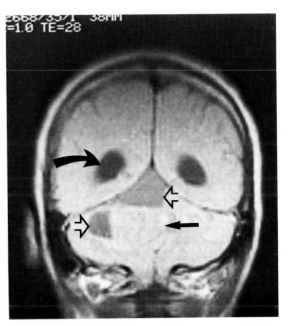

B

Figure 17-24   Cystic astrocytoma.   **A.** A heavily T_1-WI (sagittal) demonstrates a cystic and solid mass in the superior cerebellum. The solid component (arrow) is slightly hypointense with respect to brain, but more intense than cyst fluid (open arrowhead), which in turn is more intense than intraventricular CSF (curved arrow) (TR = 0.5 sec, TE = 28 msec).   **B.** On a slightly less T_1-WI (coronal), the solid tumor (arrow) is isointense with adjacent brain, but more intense than proteinaceous cyst fluid (open arrowheads). Intraventricular CSF (curved arrow) appears the least intense (TR = 1.0 sec, TE = 28 msec). (*Continued on p. 790.*)

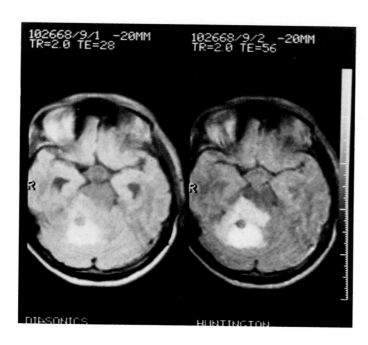

Figure 17-24 (*cont.*)   **C.** With increased T_2 weighting (TR = 2.0 sec, TE = 28 and 56 msec), the solid tumor becomes markedly hyperintense with respect to brain. Note central rounded area of hypointensity due to calcification. (*From Bradley, 1984b.*)

T_2 relaxation times. Direct sagittal imaging demonstrates anterosuperior displacement of the fourth ventricle, as these tumors typically arise from the posterior medullary velum of the inferior cerebellar vermis. Subarachnoid ("drop") metastases are a well-known complication and may be seen by MR without requiring intrathecal or subarachnoid contrast (Fig. 17-25).

Hemangioblastoma

On MR images (Fig. 17-26), cystic hemagioblastomas will appear as well-defined masses with prolonged T_2 relaxation times and T_1 times shorter than that of CSF. Thus the cyst fluid has greater hyperintensity than CSF. The mural nodule may be recognized as a peripheral focus of soft tissue intensity on T_1-weighted images. The cranio-caudal extent of the tumor is well depicted on direct sagittal images, as are additional lesions located within the spinal cord.

In view of the difficulty in distinguishing cystic hemangioblastomas from cystic astrocytomas on both MR and CT, cerebral angiography may still be re-quired, intense staining of the mural nodule being pathognomonic of hemangioblastoma.

Primary Intracranial Lymphoma

Premorbid diagnosis of this disease is often difficult, and thus primary intracranial lymphoma carries a poor prognosis. Early recognition and radiation therapy may result in partial or temporary resolution; therefore, the radiologist may play a key role in the early and timely diagnosis of such patients.

The tumor may be solitary or multifocal. Any site within the brain may be affected (Jack 1985), although it has been reported (Spillane 1982; Tadmor 1978) that there is a predilection for the periventricular white matter, basal ganglia, brainstem, and cerebellum. The tumor is identified by virtue of T_1 and T_2 prolongation, increasing intensity on T_2-WI. The extent of disease is better appreciated by MR than by CT. A relative lack of mass effect is quite characteristic of this disease (Jack 1985) (Fig. 17-27). Leptomeningeal involvement is manifested on MR by hyperintensity of the meninges on T_2-WI (Fig. 17-28).

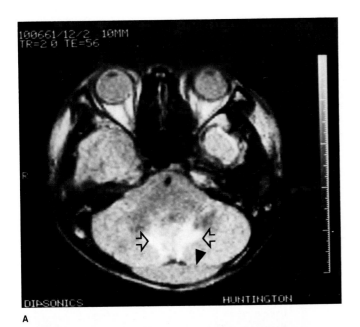

A

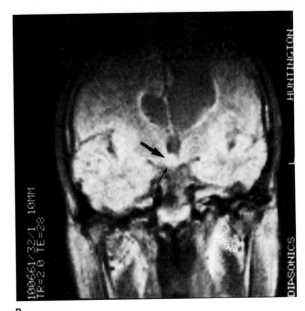

B

C

Figure 17-25 Medulloblastoma.   **A.** There is an irregular area of hyperintensity extending to either side of the cerebellar vermis (open arrowheads). The patient had previously undergone subtotal resection of a medulloblastoma. Note the isointense extraaxial fluid collection posterior to the cerebellum (curved arrow) (TR 2.0 sec, TE = 56 msec).   **B.** On a direct coronal image, a CSF mediated metastasis can be seen within the inferior aspect of the third ventricle (arrows). There is an area of porencephaly along the superior aspect of the left lateral ventricle, secondary to a previous attempted resection of this lesion (TR = 2.0 sec, TE = 28 msec). **C.** On a midsagittal section through the lumbosacral spine, a subtle rounded mass is seen posterior to the S_1 vertebral body (white arrow) (TR = 1.0 sec, TE = 28 msec).

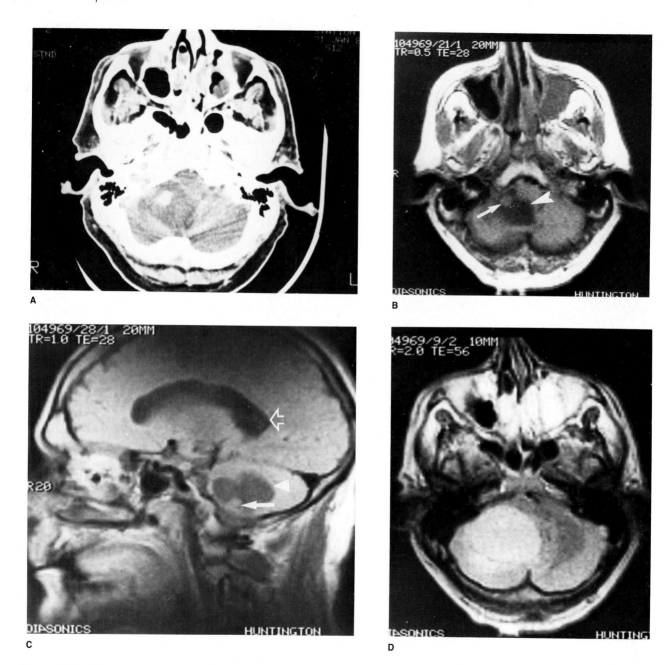

Figure 17-26   Hemangioblastoma.   **A.** A CECT through the posterior fossa demonstrates a right-sided cystic mass (arrowhead) with an enhancing mural nodule (arrow).   **B.** On a corresponding T_1-WI (axial MRI), the cyst fluid (arrowhead) appears hypointense, while the tumor nodule (arrow) is isointense with adjacent brain (TR = 0.5 sec, TE = 28 msec).   **C.** On a slightly less T_1-WI (sagittal), the tumor nodule can be seen within the inferior aspect of the cyst. The cyst fluid is slightly more intense than intraventricular CSF (open arrowhead) (TR = 1.0 sec, TE = 28 msec). **D.** On an (axial) T_2-WI, the intensity of the cyst fluid increases markedly (TR = 2.0 sec, TE = 56 msec).

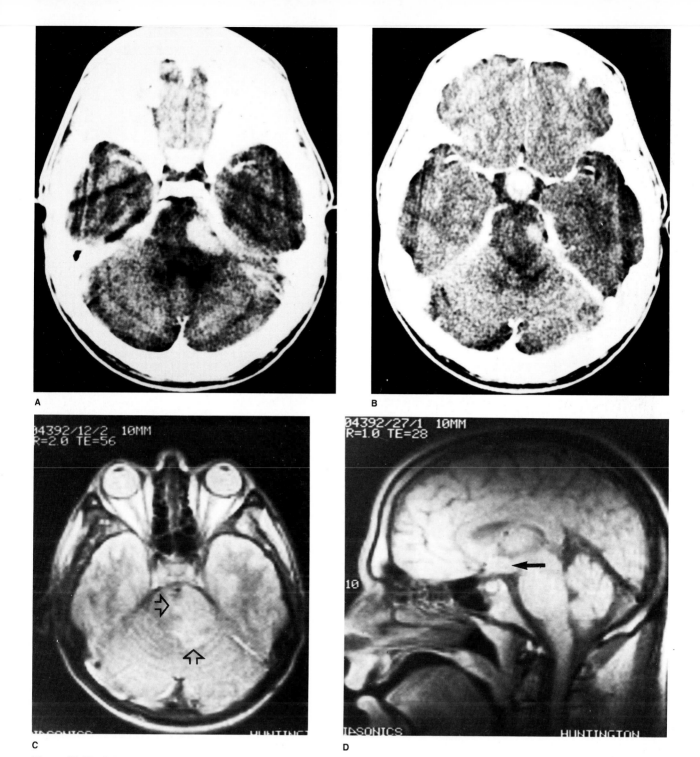

Figure 17-27 Primary intracranial lymphoma. **A.** A CECT at the level of the fourth ventricle demonstrates the enhancing mass along the lateral aspect of the midpons. **B.** On a slightly higher section, a second rounded enhancing lesion is seen within the suprasellar cistern. **C.** On a T$_2$-WI (axial MRI), the extent of pontine and cerebellar involvement by tumor is much more readily apparent (open arrowheads) (TR = 2.0 sec, TE = 56 msec). **D.** On a more T$_1$-WI (sagittal), the pons appears expanded. In addition, the hypothalamus (arrow) is also enlarged, accounting for the apparent suprasellar mass on CT. On the basis of these findings, a diagnosis of intracranial lymphoma was suggested, and later confirmed by biopsy (TR = 1.0 sec, TE = 28 msec).

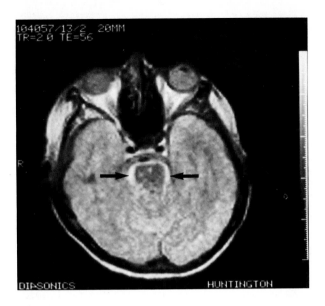

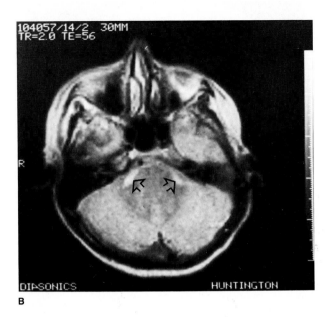

B

Figure 17-28 Leptomeningeal lymphoma: **A.** This elderly woman had undergone prior resection of the submandibular gland lymphoma, and now presented with multiple cranial nerve palsies. This axial T$_2$-WI demonstrated circumferential hyperintensity surrounding the midbrain (arrows) (TR = 2.0 sec, TE = 56 msec). **B.** At a slightly more inferior level, this hyperintensity can be seen extending into both cerebellar pontine angle cisterns (open arrowheads). Because of the distribution of the abnormalities, a diagnosis of leptomeningeal lymphoma was suggested and confirmed by CSF analysis.

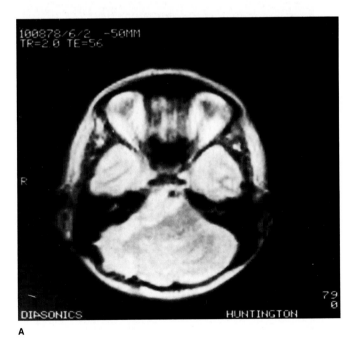

A

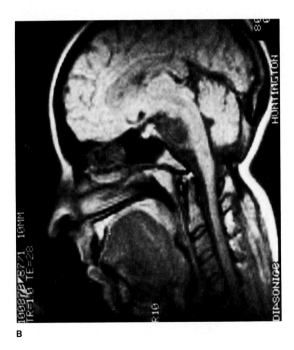

B

Figure 17-29 Epidermoid tumor. **A.** A transaxial T$_2$-WI demonstrates a hyperintense mass (arrowheads) anterior to the pons, surrounding the hypointensity basilar artery (TR = 2.0 sec, TE = 56 msec). **B.** On a sagittal T$_1$-WI the mass (arrowheads) is decreased in signal intensity, and can be seen invaginating the pons. Surgical excision revealed an epidermoid tumor (TR = 1.0 sec, TE = 28 msec).

Primary Extra-axial Neoplasms

Epidermoids, Dermoids, and Lipomas

These lesions result from inclusion of ectodermal and/or mesodermal elements during closure of the neural tube during the fifth to seventh week of gestation. *Epidermoids* often have a characteristic appearance on CT examination, presenting as hypodense lesions with irregular margins, relatively little mass effect, and no contrast enhancement. In the posterior fossa, streak artifacts may obscure the presence of small lesions and the full extent of larger ones. Prior to MR, CT metrizamide cisternography was effectively used to evaluate posterior fossa epidermoids, but carried the risk of spinal puncture and the side effects of intrathecal contrast material. The presence and extent of these lesions is readily appreciated on MR, particularly when sagittal and coronal images are utilized in addition to standard transaxial scans. These lesions are found to have prolongation of both the T_1 and T_2 relaxation times (Kortman 1986*b*) (Figs. 17-29, 17-30). The prolonged T_1 may be surprising, considering the high cholesterin content within these tumors. However, it should be noted that this cholesterin is in the solid, crystalline form which is MR-invisible (Kortman 1986*b*). Therefore, the typical appearance of these lesions is hypointense on T_1-WI and hyperintense on T_2-WI. Marked nonhomogeneity of signal intensity reflects the complex matrix and multiple interstices within the lesion, and results in a "cottage cheese" appearance closely simulating the gross pathology of this tumor. Cisternal infiltration and interdigitation, rather than focal expansion, is a characteristic finding.

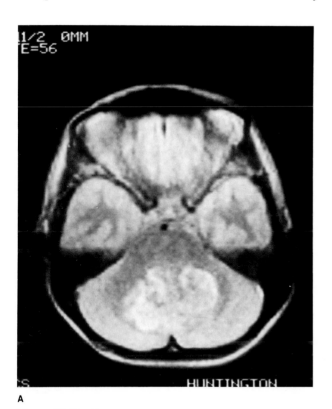

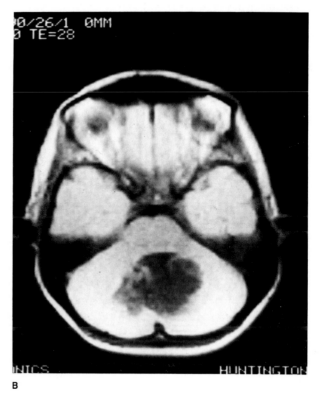

A   **B**

Figure 17-30 Fourth ventricular epidermoid tumor. **A.** This patient presented with mild but progressive ataxia. A transaxial T_2-WI demonstrates a heterogeneous hyperintensity mass posterior to the fourth ventricle (TR = 2.0 sec, TE = 56 msec). **B.** On a corresponding T_1-WI, the mass appears hypointense with respect to brain (TR = 1.0 sec, TE = 28 msec). (*Continued on p. 796.*)

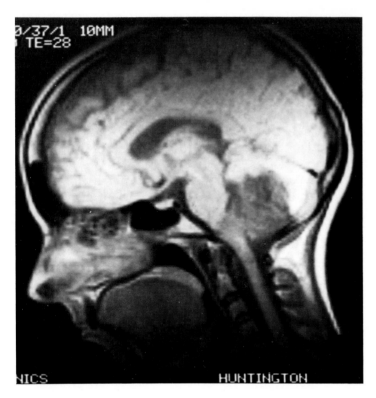

Figure 17-30 (*cont.*) **C.** On the sagittal image, hypointensity tumor can be seen extending into the vallecula. Note the absence of hydrocephalus, indicating a relative lack of obstruction. Diagnosis of epidermoid was confirmed at surgery (TR = 1.0 sec, TE = 28 msec).

Unlike epidermoids, *dermoids* are generally not solid at body temperature. The liquid cholesterin and protein content of the fluid result in significant T_1 shortening, and as a result, these lesions are hyperintense with respect to brain on all conventional pulsing sequences (Fig. 17-31). The cyst may also contain focal areas of hair, skin, and dental elements, and these appear as foci of hypointensity.

Lipomas contain mesodermal fatty elements. They occur most often near the midsagittal plane, frequently within the corpus callosum. Because of the short T_1 and long T_2 relaxation times of fat compared with brain, these lesions are relatively high in signal intensity on all pulsing sequences (Fig. 17-32). Associated anomalies, such as agenesis of the corpus callosum, myelomeningocele, and spinal dysraphism, are all well visualized on MR.

Pineal Region Tumors

The most common lesions in this area are dysgerminomas, teratomas, and other germ cell tumors (Ganti 1986). Tumors of pineal origin (pinealcytomas and pinealblastomas) and gliomas of the adjacent posterior hypothalamus or midbrain tectum are less often seen. On direct sagittal or coronal images, pineal tumors can usually be distinguished from parapineal lesions. Although tumors originating from the pineal gland differ histologically, distinction between tissue types is typically difficult with either CT or MR (Kilgore 1986) (Fig. 17-33). Identification of a second lesion along the hypothalamic axis (multiple midline tumor syndrome) suggests a diagnosis of dysgerminoma and may warrant a trial of radiation therapy without biopsy (Swischuk 1974).

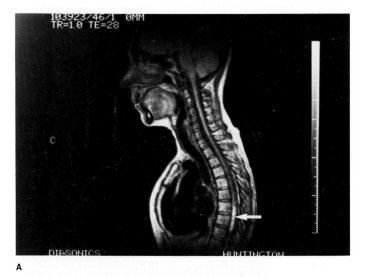

A

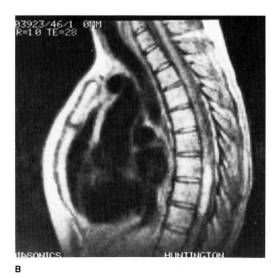

B

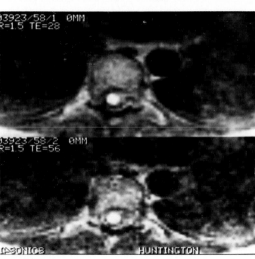

C

Figure 17-31 Intraspinal dermoid. **A.** Midline sagittal T_1-WI of the spine demonstrates a hyperintense intramedullary lesion at the T_{6-7} level (TR = 1.0 sec, TE = 28 msec). **B.** Slightly magnified image. **C.** On T_2-WI (axial), the lesion remains hyperintense. Excisional biopsy reveals an intramedullary dermoid tumor (TR = 2.0 sec, TE = 56 msec).

Arachnoid Cysts

As with CT, arachnoid cysts generally appear as extraaxial lesions of CSF intensity (Bradley 1984*b*) (Fig. 17-34). Marked increased intensity is indicative of a complication (i.e., infection or hemorrhage). Heterogeneity within the cyst is distinctly uncommon, and when seen should suggest the possibility of a solid lesion, such as an epidermoid or a cystic astrocytoma.

Meningiomas

In contrast to their typical appearance on enhanced CT exams, these lesions may be relatively inconspicuous on MR (Zimmerman 1985). Typically, mild prolongation of T_1 is manifested as decreased signal intensity on heavily T_1-WI. The T_2 relaxation time of meningiomas is characteristically slightly greater than normal brain but significantly less than that of edema or other intracranial neoplasms, such as

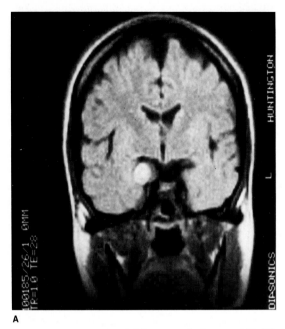

A

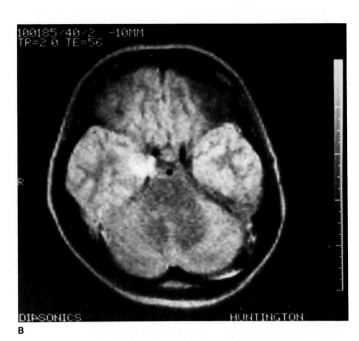

B

Figure 17-32 Intracranial lipoma. **A.** A coronal T_1-WI demonstrates a hyperintense lesion in the medial aspect of the right temporal fossa (TR = 1.0 sec, TE = 28 msec). **B.** The lesion remains hyperintense on a moderately T_2-WI (axial) (TR = 2.0 sec, TE = 56 msec). The lesion had a negative attenuation value on CT examination, and is presumed to be a lipoma.

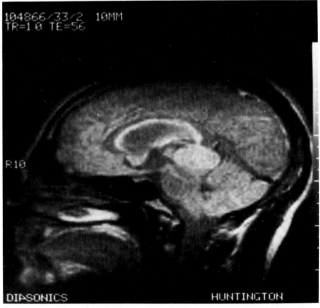

A

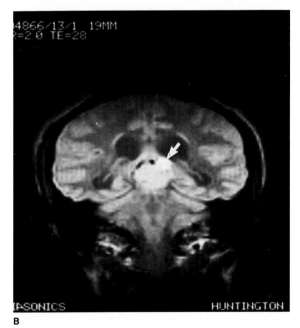

B

Figure 17-33 Pineal dysgerminoma. **A.** This young male presented with progressively worsening headaches. Paralysis of upgaze was noted on physical examination. A sagittal image demonstrates a rounded hyperintense mass in the supravermian/pineal region. The midbrain tectum and cerebral aqueduct are compressed anteroinferiorly. Apparent elongation of the head is due to a malfunctioning gradient coil power supply (TR = 1.0 sec, TE = 56 msec). **B.** On a corresponding coronal section, the bulk of the mass appears slightly hypointense with respect to surrounding brain. There is a more markedly hypointense exophytic component along the left supralateral aspect of the mass (arrow). This corresponds to an area of increased attenuation on CT examination, and proved to be an area of focal hemorrhage at the time of surgical inspection. Histologic diagnosis was dysgerminoma (TR = 2.0 sec, TE = 28 msec).

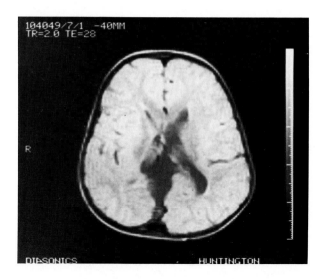 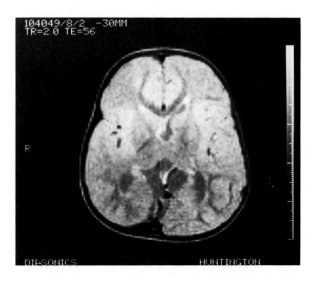

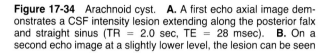

Figure 17-34 Arachnoid cyst. **A.** A first echo axial image demonstrates a CSF intensity lesion extending along the posterior falx and straight sinus (TR = 2.0 sec, TE = 28 msec). **B.** On a second echo image at a slightly lower level, the lesion can be seen extending into the supravermian cistern. The cyst is increased slightly in signal intensity but remains isointense with intraventricular CSF. Note hyperintense even echo rephasing of the basal veins around the cyst (TR = 2.0 sec, TE = 56 msec).

gliomas (Bucon 1985). As a result, most meningiomas are approximately isointense with brain on moderately T_1 or T_2-WI (Fig. 17-35). A densely calcified or fibrous meningioma may appear hypointense on all pulsing sequences, reflecting the relative lack of mobile protons and shorter T_2 of such tumors (Fig. 17-36).

Buckling of the white matter and displacement of cortical vascular structures may be better appreciated with MR than with CT, and may facilitate documentation of the extraaxial origin of the tumor (Fig. 17-37). However, adjacent bony changes in the calvarium or skull base are less well visualized with MR than by CT.

The distinction between enhancing parasellar meningiomas and aneurysms may be difficult by CT. On MR, however, there is a striking difference between the low intensity of flowing blood within an aneurysm and the soft-tissue intensity of a meningioma (Fig. 17-38). As might be expected, meningiomas enhance markedly and homogeneously after intravenous administration of paramagnetic contrast agents (Bydder 1985*a*) (Fig. 17-39).

Chordomas

On MR, these lesions appear as masses with prolonged T_1 and T_2 relaxation times, reflected as hyperintensity of T_2-weighted spin-echo images. Focal calcifications may be recognized as areas of hypointensity. Clival origin and erosion are best appreciated on T_1-weighted direct sagittal images, and are manifested by replacement of the hyperintense intraclival marrow by hypointense tumor (Fig. 17-40). Sagittal images also best delineate tumor extension anteriorly into the nasopharynx and posteriorly into the prepontine cistern.

Pituitary Adenomas

MR may be used effectively in the preoperative evaluation of macroadenomas, i.e., those tumors measuring greater than 1 cm in diameter (Wiener 1985). The ability to scan directly in either the sagittal or coronal plane is a distinct advantage of MR over CT, and allows accurate assessment of infra- and suprasellar tumor extension, as well as lateral

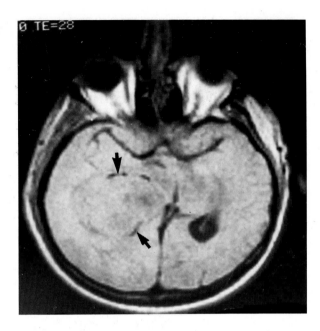
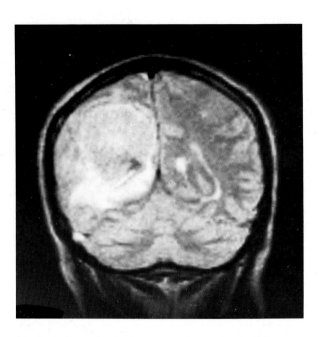

Figure 17-35 Intraventricular meningioma. **A.** On a T$_1$-weighted axial image, an isointense mass (arrows) can be seen in the region of the right ventricular trigone, and produces distortion of the adjacent basal cistern. Many areas of hypointensity can be seen along the periphery of the mass and may represent displaced blood vessels (TR = 1.0 sec, TE = 28 msec). **B.** On a coronal T$_2$-WI, the mass remains isointense with gray matter, while subjacent edema appears increased in signal intensity. The isointense appearance is typical of meningioma, and this diagnosis was confirmed at the time of surgery (TR = 2.0 sec, TE = 56 msec).

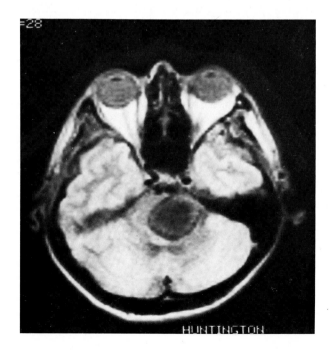

Figure 17-36 Calcified meningioma. This densely calcified lesion appeared hypointense on all pulsing sequences. Note the even more hypointense tumor capsule. The adjacent pons is markedly distorted, and the fourth ventricle is displaced posteriorly (TR = 2.0 sec, TE = 28 msec).   ▶

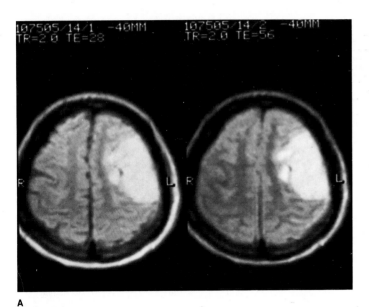

A

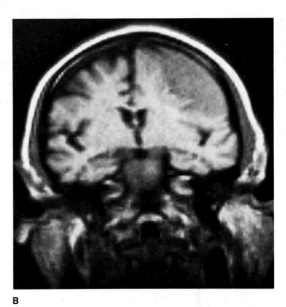

B

Figure 17-37 Meningioma. **A.** A transaxial section at the level of the lateral ventricles demonstrates a left frontoparietal isointense mass. The adjacent white matter is buckled medially, and displaced hypointense cortical vessels can be seen along the medial aspect of the tumor (TR = 2.0 sec, TE = 28 and 56 msec). **B.** The mass appears slightly hypointense on a more T_1-weighted coronal image (TR = 0.5 sec, TE = 28 msec).

extension into the cavernous sinuses (Fig. 17-41). Typically, pituitary adenomas are mildly hypointense with respect to brain on T_1-WI and hyperintense on T_2-WI. Increased intensity due to T_1 shortening has also been observed following treatment with Bromocriptine, presumably secondary to tumor necrosis and increased hydration layer water.

Microadenomas (those tumors which measure less than 1 cm in diameter) are poorly visualized on lower-field strength units without thin-section capability, presumably reflecting the limited spatial resolution of MR with respect to CT, and the relative lack of sensitivity of MR to subtle bone erosion. Also, a limited experience with high-resolution MR imaging utilizing 1.5T systems revealed variable MR signals and high failure rate in delineating the focal mass within the pituitary gland (Pojunas 1986). For this reason, patients presenting only with hormonal disturbance (e.g., amenorrhea and galactorrhea) and no clinical evidence of extrasellar tumor extension are best studied by CT (see Chapter 10).

An empty sella is easily recognized on MR as an area of CSF intensity extending below the expected level of the diaphragma sellae (Fig. 17-42). On direct coronal or sagittal images, often a small compressed pituitary gland can be seen within the sella.

Craniopharyngiomas

These are relatively common lesions which arise from epithelial rests from the vestigial craniopharyngeal duct. The tumors may be solid or cystic, and the latter variety contain an oily fluid composed of desquamated epithelial cells and cholesterol, similar to that seen in dermoid cysts.

On MR examination, these tumors appear as well-circumscribed suprasellar and occasionally intrasellar masses. Sufficient liquid cholesterol content will result in T_1 shortening (Fig. 17-43, 17-44), and in our experience this has been seen in greater than 50 percent of all craniopharyngiomas (Pusey 1986). Calcifications are often present, and although easily identified with CT, are poorly visualized with MR. As with pituitary tumors, direct sagittal and coronal images best depict the relationship of the mass to adjacent structures.

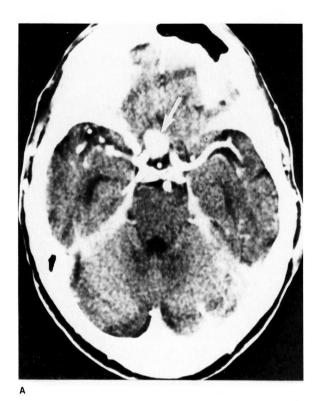

A

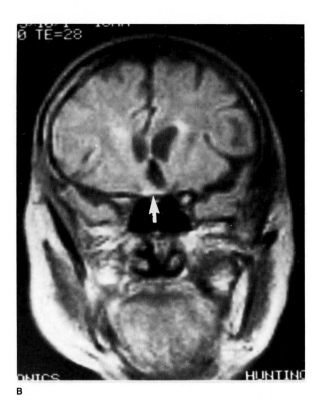

B

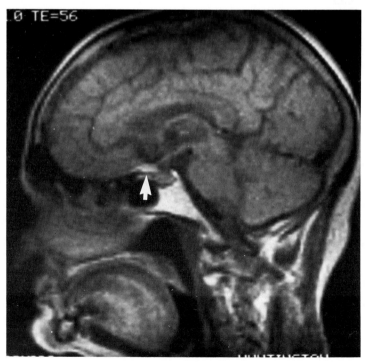

C

Figure 17-38 Parasellar meningioma. **A.** A CECT through the circle of Willis demonstrates an intense enhancing rounded lesion near the expected location of the anterior communicating artery. The differential diagnosis would include aneurysm and meningioma. **B.** A direct coronal MR image demonstrates leftward displacement of the inferior third ventricle by a thin hyperintense lesion extending along the planum sphenoidale (arrow) (TR = 2.0 sec, TE = 28 msec). **C.** A similar appearance is noted on a midline sagittal section. Note that the mass (arrow) is immediately subjacent to the hypointense anterior cerebral arteries. The lack of flow void within the lesion is inconsistent with the diagnosis of aneurysm, and thus a presumptive diagnosis of meningioma can be made (TR = 1.0 sec, TE = 56 msec).

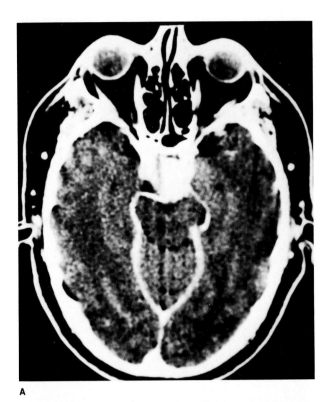

A

Figure 17-39 Diaphragma sella meningioma. **A.** A CECT demonstrates a hyperdense and enhancing suprasellar mass. **B.** On a T_1-WI (midline sagittal MR) the mass (arrows) appears isointense, and can be seen extending from the superior aspect of the sellar diaphram (TR = 0.5 sec, TE = 28 msec). **C.** Following administration of intravenous Gadolinium-DTPA, the tumor enhances markedly and homogeneously.

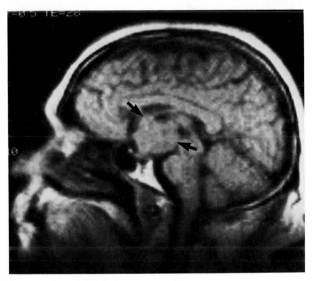

B

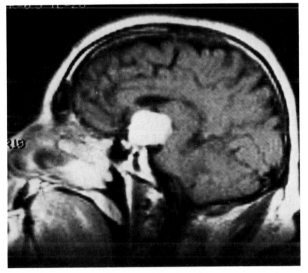

C

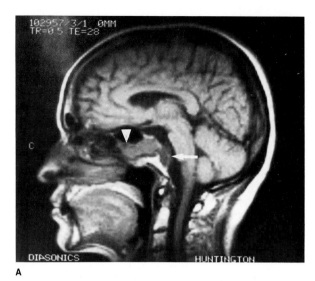

A

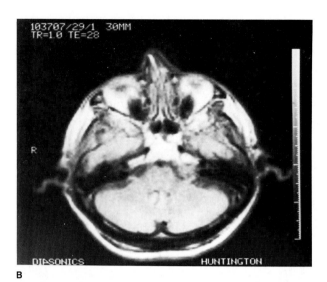

B

Figure 17-40 Clivus chordoma. **A.** This patient presented with bilateral sixth nerve palsies. A T$_1$-WI (midline sagittal) demonstrates a soft-tissue mass extending along the superior aspect of the clivus into the sphenoid sinus (arrowhead) and the prepontine cistern (arrow). The mass is readily distinguished from the normal clivus by virtue of the hyperintense marrow fat in the latter structure (TR = 0.5 sec, TE = 28 msec). **B.** On an axial T$_2$-WI, the mass appears hyperintense and somewhat heterogeneous. Transsphenoidal biopsy confirmed the diagnosis of chordoma (TR = 2.0 sec, TE = 56 msec).

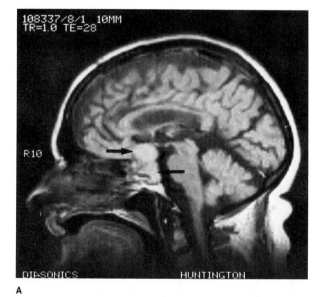

A

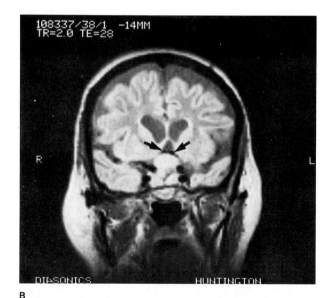

B

Figure 17-41 Pituitary adenoma. **A.** This patient presented with progressive bitemporal hemianopsia. A moderately T$_1$-WI (midline sagittal section) demonstrates an isointense lobulated intra- and suprasellar mass (arrows) extending to the anterior aspect of the hypothalamus. The optic chiasm and optic nerves cannot be distinguished as structures separate from the mass (TR = 1.0 sec, TE = 28 msec). **B.** On a more T$_2$-WI (coronal section), the mass appears slightly hyperintense. Superiorly, the mass can be seen displacing the paired hypointense anterior cerebral arteries (arrowheads). Laterally the tumor can be seen extending into both cavernous sinuses, insinuating between the inferior and superior segments of the intracavernous internal carotid arteries (TR = 2.0 sec, TE = 28 msec). (*Continued on p. 805.*)

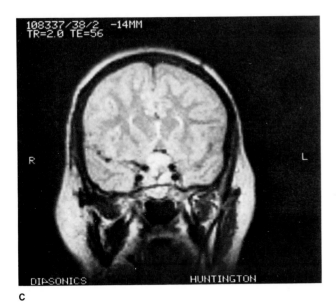

C

Figure 17-41 (*cont.*) **C.** The tumor appears more conspicuously intense on the second echo image (TR = 2.0 sec, TE = 56 msec).

Figure 17-42 Empty sella. A T$_1$-WI (midline sagittal) demonstrates a CSF intensity "lesion" producing expansion of the sella. Note the oblique course of the optic nerve above the sella.

Colloid Cysts

These lesions are recognized by their characteristic location in the anterior aspect of the third ventricle, and are thought to arise from elements of the ves-

tigeal paraphysis. They are composed of gelatinous material; they become symptomatic when they obstruct the lateral ventricles at the foramen of Monro. In our experience, the intensity of these lesions has varied significantly. While more often hyperintense

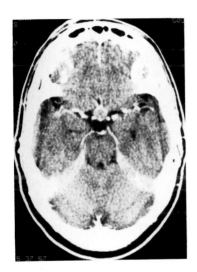

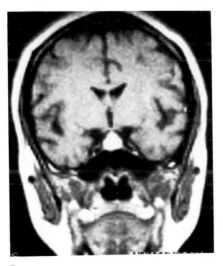

Figure 17-43 Craniopharyngioma. **A.** A CECT demonstrates a rounded mass in the suprasellar cistern with anterior rim calcification and/or enhancement. **B.** On a T$_1$-WI (coronal MR) the mass appears markedly hyperintense, indicating the presence of fat (cholesterol) or, less likely, subacute hemorrhage (TR = 0.5 sec, TE = 28 msec). (*Continued on p. 806.*)

A

B

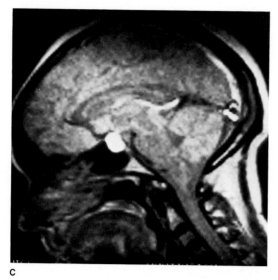

c

Figure 17-43 *(cont.)* **C.** On a more T$_2$-WI (sagittal section), the mass remains hyperintense with respect to the remainder of the brain (TR = 1.5 sec, TE = 56 msec). A cystic craniopharyngioma containing a moderate amount of cholesterol was found at the time of surgery.

on T$_2$-WI (Fig. 17-45), we have seen three hypointense lesions, the hypointensity becoming more pronounced with prolongation of echo delay times (Fig. 17-46). Such a pattern is indicative of T$_2$ shortening. This may be attributable to the presence of a paramagnetic material such as iron (in the form of hemosiderin) or copper. Conversely, the highly structured colloid matrix may in and of itself have a short T$_2$.

Neurinomas

Eighth nerve neurinomas, also referred to as acoustic schwannomas or neurolemomas, are among the most common of all primary intracranial tumors. Although larger lesions may be recognized on CT by virtue of gross mass effect or contrast enhancement, the majority of small lesions cannot be identified without intrathecal administration of either air or contrast. Acoustic neuromas are well demonstrated

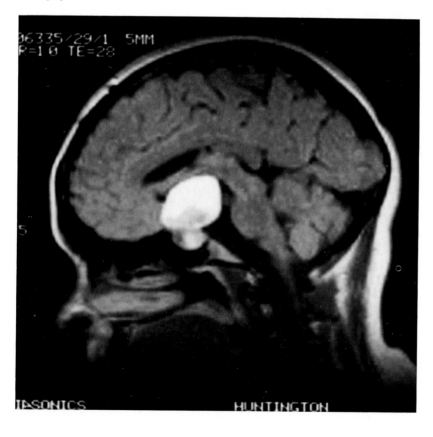

Figure 17-44 Craniopharyngioma. **A.** A larger and more heterogeneous hyperintense intra- and suprasellar mass is graphically demonstrated on this T$_1$-WI (sagittal section: TR = 1.0 sec, TE = 28 msec). *(Continued on p. 807.)*

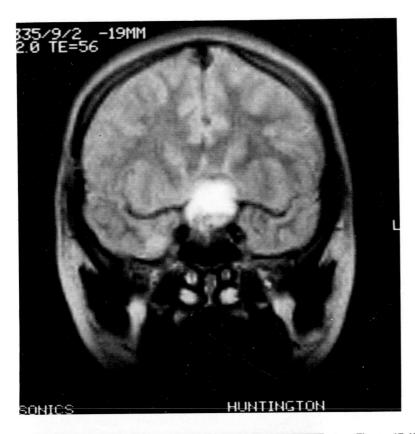

Figure 17-44 (*cont.*)   **B.** The hyperintense appearance persists on a T$_2$-WI (coronal section) (TR = 2.0 sec, TE = 56 msec).

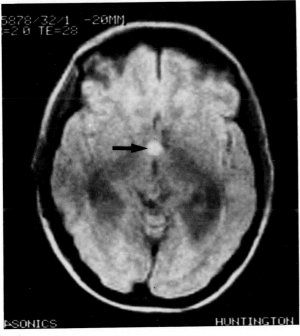

Figure 17-45   Colloid cyst. This elderly female presented with acute obstructive hydrocephalus. NCCT and CECT demonstrated only ventricular dilatation (not shown). The axial MR image demonstrates a conspicuous hyperintense rounded mass (arrow) in the anterior aspect of the third ventricle. The location is typical of a colloid cyst, and this diagnosis was confirmed at surgery (TR = 2.0 sec, TE = 28 msec).

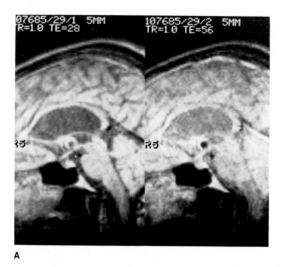

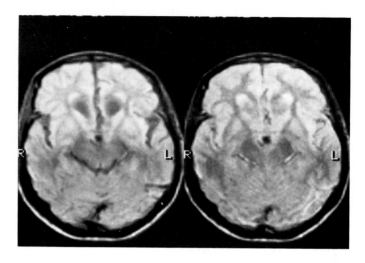

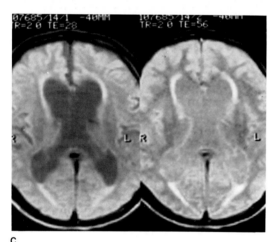

Figure 17-46 Colloid cyst. **A.** Midline sagittal images demonstrate a rounded mass (arrow) in the anterior aspect of the third ventricle. The center of the lesion is hypointense, and becomes more markedly hypointense on the second echo image (TR = 1.0 sec, TE = 28 and 56 msec). **B.** More T$_2$-WI (transaxial) verify T$_2$ shortening within the mass, most likely due to hemosiderin deposition (TR = 2.0 sec, TE = 28 and 56 msec). **C.** On a slightly more superior section, obstructive hydrocephalus is evidenced by lateral ventricular dilatation and a smooth and confluent hyperintense periventricular rim of interstitial edema.

by thin-slice contiguous T$_2$-weighted axial MR images (New 1985; Daniels 1985a; Mikhael 1985). They typically are seen extending from the porus acousticus into the cerebellopontine angle (Fig. 17-47). Extension of the tumor into the internal auditory canal will result in focal thickening of the eighth nerve bundle, and totally intracanalicular lesions may be readily identified (Fig. 17-48). The T$_2$ relaxation time of these tumors is prolonged. As a result they appear as hyperintense masses on T$_2$-WI. Early experience with Gadolinium-DTPA has demonstrated dense, homogeneous enhancement, allowing the sensitive detection of tumors only a few millimeters

in diameter (Curati 1986). Neuromas involving other cranial nerves most often have intensity patterns similar to acoustic tumors, appearing at characteristic locations near the base of the brain (Fig. 17-49).

Intracranial Metastases

Because of the high sensitivity of MR, it is currently the modality of choice in the evaluation of suspected intracranial metastatic disease (Bradley 1984c; Brant-Zawadzki 1984b). Its sensitivity is significantly greater than that of CT, such that lesions may be demonstrated in patients with normal CT scans (Fig.

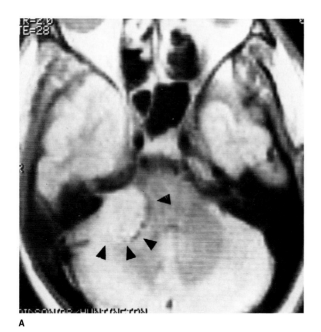

A

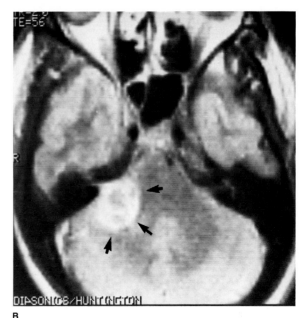

B

Figure 17-47 Acoustic neuroma. **A.** There is a rounded and slightly hyperintense mass (arrowheads) in the cerebellar pontine angle extending into the internal auditory canal. Note the hypointense rim of the tumor, typical of extraaxial lesions (TR = 2.0 sec,

TE = 28 msec). **B.** On a more T_2-WI (second echo), the mass appears well markedly hyperintense. Heterogeneity within the lesion is most likely secondary to central tumor necrosis (TR = 2.0 sec, TE = 56 msec).

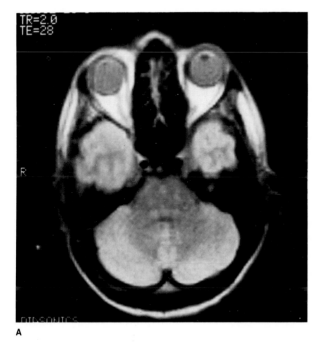

A

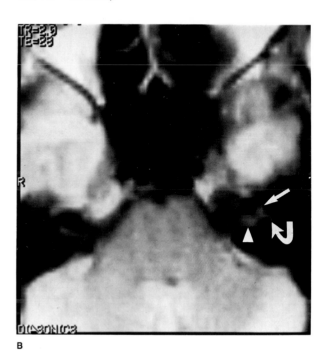

B

Figure 17-48 Intracanalicular acoustic neuroma. **A.** This patient presented with left-sided sensorineural hearing loss. There is a 3-mm bulbous mass in the lateral aspect of the left internal auditory canal, a surgically confirmed acoustic neuroma (TR = 2.0 sec, TE

= 28 msec). **B.** A slightly magnified image. Note relation of tumor (arrowhead) to cochlea (arrow) and superior semicircular canal (curved arrow).

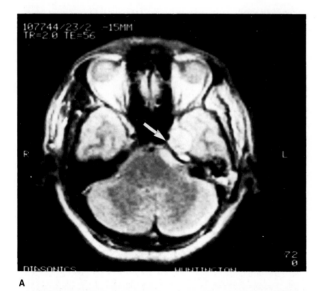

A

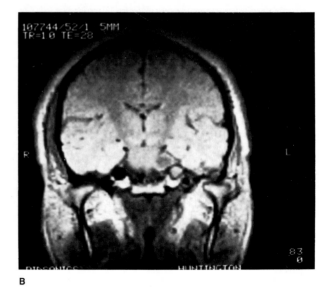

B

Figure 17-49 Trigeminal neuroma. **A.** A hyperintense mass is seen extending from the posterior aspect of the cavernous sinus into the region of Meckel's cave (arrow) (TR = 2.0 sec, TE = 56 msec). **B.** The relationship of this lesion, now hypointense, to the adjacent brainstem is accurately demonstrated on this direct coronal image (TR = 1.0 sec, TE = 28 msec). **C.** On a more inferior axial section, there is conspicuous fatty atrophy of the left-sided muscles of mastication, indicative of fifth nerve involvement. This lesion proved to be a fifth nerve neuroma (TR = 2.0 sec, TE = 56 msec).

C

17-50). Similarly, MR may be able to demonstrate multiple abnormalities when only a solitary lesion is seen on CT, and thus markedly alter the differential diagnosis and treatment.

Intraaxial metastases will appear as hyperintense lesions on T_2-WI, with varying degrees of surrounding edema and associated mass effect. Although the T_1 relaxation time of metastases is typically prolonged, T_1 shortening may be seen in hemorrhagic metastases. In addition, the paramagnetic effects of melanin may produce T_1 shortening in melanoma metastases (Gomori 1986).

For the purposes of biopsy planning, tumor may often be separated from edema by use of either heavily T_1- or T_2-weighted (Smith 1985) pulsing sequences. Alternatively, enhancement with Gadolinium-DTPA (Graif 1985; Claussen 1985) may demonstrate tumor location and contrast (Fig. 17-51).

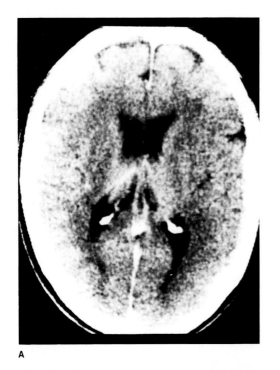

A

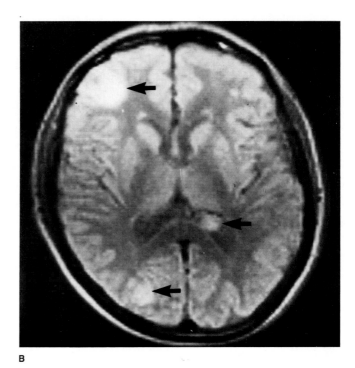

B

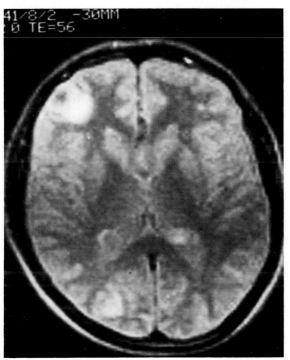

C

Figure 17-50 Intracranial metastases. This 57-year-old man presented with a progressive decline in mental status. **A.** CECT demonstrated no abnormalities. **B.** A corresponding MR image demonstrates three discrete regions of increased signal intensity (arrows) (TR = 2.0 sec, TE = 56 msec). **C.** These lesions are more conspicuous on the T_2-WI. The findings are consistent with metastatic disease. A subsequent chest x-ray revealed a bronchogenic carcinoma.

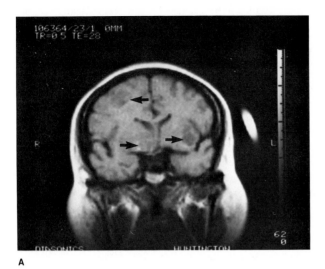

A

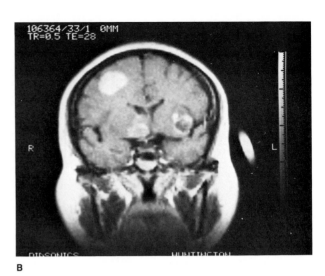

B

Figure 17-51 Enhancing metastases. **A.** This 60-year-old woman had a history of a primary breast carcinoma. A T_1-weighted (TR = 0.5 sec, TE = 28 msec) coronal image demonstrates several foci of slightly decreased signal intensity in both cerebral hemi- spheres (arrows). **B.** After the intravenous administration of Ga- dolinium-DTPA, each of these lesions enhances to a variable de- gree. Biopsy confirmed the impression of metastases.

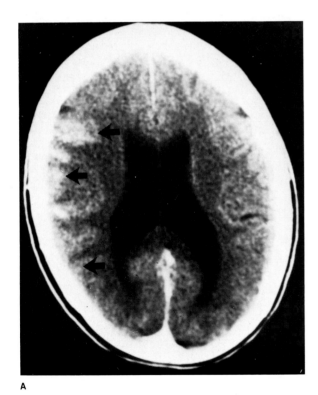

A

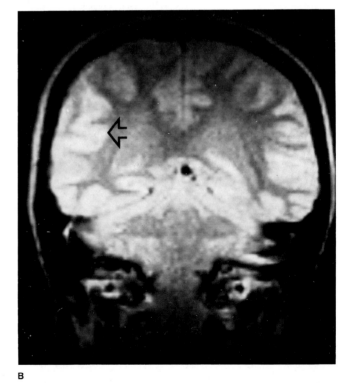

B

Figure 17-52 Carcinomatous meningitis. This 36-year-old woman presented with adult-onset seizures. **A.** CECT demonstrated asymmetric enhancement of the right hemispheric sulci and ad- jacent subarachnoid space. **B.** A coronal T_2-WI (TR = 2.0 sec, TE = 56 msec) demonstrates asymmetric hyperintensity over the same distribution (open arrow). Melanoma cells were found on the CSF analysis.

Carcinomatous meningitis may result in hyperintensity of the meninges and subjacent gyri (Fig. 17-52). Resultant obstructive hydrocephalus will produce a confluent symmetric pattern of periventricular hyperintensity, and this diagnosis may be suggested prior to development of marked ventricular dilatation.

Calvarial metastases are best demonstrated by CT but may result in alterations of signal intensity within the diploic space and the inner and outer tables. At the skull base, MR maintains some advantage over CT, in that the soft-tissue component of metastatic lesions is easily recognized on direct coronal or sagittal images (Fig. 17-53).

Non-neoplastic Abnormalities of the Brain

Ischemia-Infarction

In the setting of cerebral infarction, CT may be utilized to verify the presence of a lesion, to determine the presence of hemorrhage, or to demonstrate abnormalities other than infarcts (e.g., tumor or abscess) which may simulate vaso-occlusive disease clinically. MR offers some advantages over CT in infarct imaging, the most significant being its greater sensitivity. In acute cerebral infarction, the CT may be normal or demonstrate only mild mass effect. MR consistently demonstrates prolongation of the T_1 and T_2 relaxation times, these changes being apparent in animal models within a few hours of vascular occlusion (Buonanno 1982; Levy 1983; Bryan 1983; Brant-Zawadzki 1986). Preliminary animal and human clinical studies have shown that sodium MR imaging may be more sensitive than proton MRI in the detection of early ischemia (Hilal 1983, 1985).

Within one or two days of a stroke, blood-brain barrier breakdown will result in vasogenic edema, making the diagnosis more readily apparent by CT (Wall 1982). Subacute infarcts remain conspicuous on moderately T_2-weighted MR examinations. Swollen cells (cytotoxic edema) at the infarct periphery are thought to "dam up" central vasogenic edema, producing relatively sharp margins (Bradley 1984*b*) (Fig. 17-54). In a manner similar to CECT,

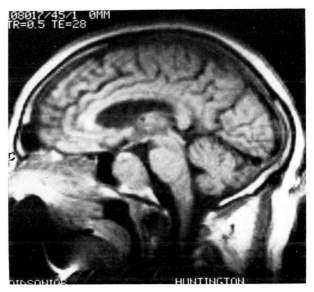

A

B

Figure 17-53 Skull base metastases. This elderly individual presented with progressive sixth cranial nerve palsy. **A.** A transaxial T_2-WI demonstrates an isointense mass near the region of the sella (arrow) (TR = 2.0 sec, TE = 56 msec). **B.** A more T_1-WI (midsagittal) shows a soft-tissue mass eroding the superior aspect of the clivus (TR = 0.5 sec, TE = 28 msec). (*Continued on p. 814.*)

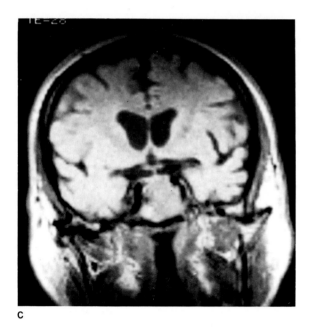

C

Figure 17-53 (*cont.*)   **C.** The lesion is also well demonstrated on coronal section (TR = 1.0 sec, TE = 28 msec). The patient had known metastatic prostate carcinoma.

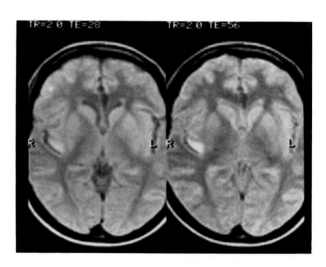

Figure 17-54   Acute insular infarct. Sharp peripheral margins of this high-intensity lesion are due to central vasogenic edema confined by peripheral, swollen, cytotoxic cells (TR = 2.0 sec, TE = 28 and 56 msec).

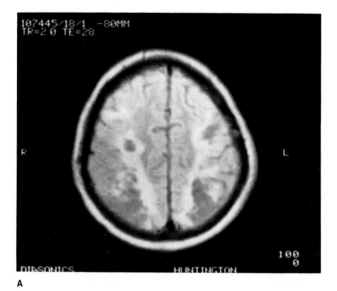

A

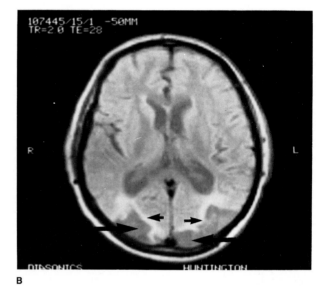

B

Figure 17-55   Chronic watershed infarcts. This patient suffered an episode of prolonged hypoperfusion during cardiac bypass surgery.   **A.** An axial mildly T$_2$-WI demonstrates symmetric areas of CSF intensity (arrows) in the occipital lobes, bridging the vascular distribution of the posterior and middle cerebral arteries. These areas are bordered areas of increased signal intensity (arrowheads) (TR = 2.0 sec, TE = 28 msec).   **B.** Similar lesions were seen at a slightly more cephalad level.

MR with Gadolinium-DTPA may be used to directly demonstrate loss of blood-brain barrier integrity.

Chronic infarcts produce local atrophy and encephalomalacia on CT, both manifested as areas of hypodensity similar to CSF. Regions of the brain which show only hypodensity on CT can frequently be separated into two components on MR: those which behave more like CSF, and those which behave more like edematous or gliotic brain (Flannigan 1986) (Fig.17-55). This reflects the changing molecular environment of water during the evolution of an infarct (Flannigan 1986). The center of the infarct is replaced by large cysts and has a higher ratio of water to solid tissue ("macrocystic encephalomalacia") (Bradley 1986c) such that the water is largely in the bulk phase and behaves like CSF (Fullerton 1984). The periphery of the infarct may appear more like edema or gliosis where the water is in hydration layers in small cystic spaces ("microcystic encephalomalacia").

Small infarcts along the brain convexity are seen on moderately T_2-WI (Fig. 17-56) which enhance the contrast between isointense brain and CSF and the more intense infarct. Heavily T_1-WIs may show an area of focal sulcal enlargement but are relatively insensitive to small parenchymal foci with T_1 prolongation. On heavily T_2-WIs, the peripheral parenchymal lesion may be difficult to distinguish from adjacent CSF, as both will appear bright. Lacunar infarcts in the basal ganglia and the periventricular white matter show hyperintensity on T_2-WIs due to the prolonged T_2 relaxation time (Fig. 17-57). Lesions in the periventricular region are much more obvious on MR than on CT (Fig. 17-58). Poor conspicuity and partial volume artifacts from the adjacent ventricular CSF make diagnosis of hypodense lesions difficult by CT. On moderately T_2-weighted MR images, the infarcts appear bright while the CSF is isointense with brain (Bradley 1985a). The ability to confidently image the periventricular region with MR has allowed demonstration of a much higher incidence of deep white matter infarction than was previously suspected (Bradley 1984d; Kortman 1986c). Small lesions in the periventricular region, while abnormal, are commonly seen in the asymptomatic elderly (Kortman 1986c). When these changes are

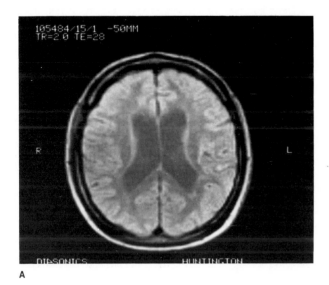

A

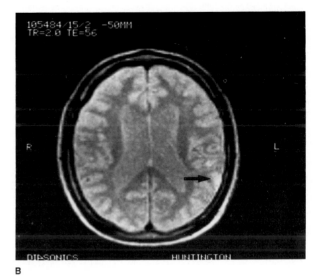

B

Figure 17-56 Small cortical infarct. This patient presented with acute onset of fluent aphasia three weeks previously. **A.** A mildly T_2-WI (axial TR = 2.0 sec, TE = 28 msec) at the level of the lateral ventricles is unremarkable. **B.** A more T_2-WI (second echo) demonstrates a small wedge-shaped area of hyperintensity in the left temporoparietal cortex (arrow), corresponding to Wernicke's region.

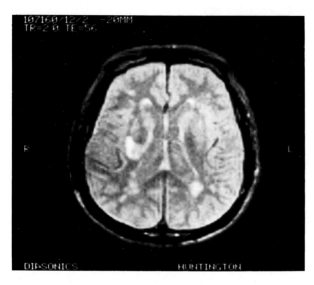

Figure 17-57   Internal capsule lacunar infarct. This hypertensive patient presented with acute onset of left hemiparesis. A high-intensity lacunar infarct is identified in the posterior limb of the right internal capsule, extending laterally to involve the posterior putamen and external capsule (TR = 2.0 sec, TE = 56 msec).

mild, they are usually not associated with clinical symptoms. More pronounced changes may be seen (Bradley 1984*d*) in patients with risk factors for cerebrovascular disease (especially hypertension). In conjunction with well-defined clinical and histologic criteria, deep white matter and basal ganglia infarcts have been described in subcortical arteriosclerotic encephalopathy, "Binswanger's" disease. Whether the MR findings in isolation represent a forme fruste of this disease is a matter of some controversy. Similar but typically more confluent periventricular hyperintensity lesions may be seen following radiation therapy (Fig. 17-59) and are presumed secondary to a combination of focal demyelination and a vasculitis of the perforating arteries supplying this region, the latter resulting in focal ischemia and/or infarction (Bradley 1984*d*).

Infarcts in the vertebrobasilar distribution in the brainstem and cerebellum are diagnosed on the basis of increased MR intensity in the appropriate anatomic distribution and clinical setting (Fig.17-60).

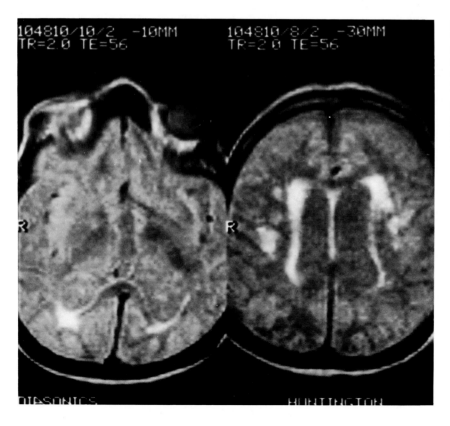

Figure 17-58   Deep white matter infarcts. This patient had a history of longstanding and poorly controlled hypertension. Multiple focal and confluent areas of hyperintensity are seen involving the periventricular white matter bilaterally. Involved areas represent a border zone between thalamostriate and deep cortical perforating arteries, and the hyperintensity changes are attributed to arteriosclerotic ischemia and/or infarction.

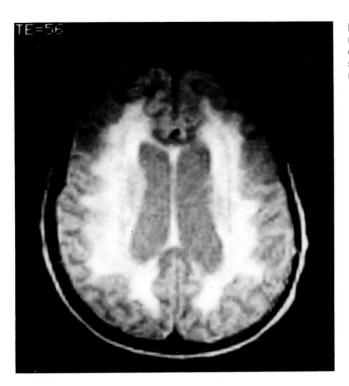

Figure 17-59 Postirradiation change. This patient had previously received cranial irradiation (5000 rads for metastatic oat cell carcinoma). Confluent and irregular but symmetric hyperintense lesions surround the lateral ventricles (TR = 2.0 sec, TE = 56 msec).

Such lesions are much better seen by MR than CT (Bradley 1984c). In such cases, slow flow may be diagnosed in the basilar artery (Bradley 1985a) by virtue of high intraluminal intensity (Fig. 17-60c) on even-numbered spin-echo images, e.g., "even-echo rephasing" (Waluch 1984). It should be noted that high intraluminal signal may also be seen on the first and second echoes in normal vessels with slow inflow, due to "flow-related enhancement" on or near the entry surface of a multislice imaging volume (Bradley 1985c).

Demyelinating Disease

MR has proven effective in the evaluation of demyelinating disorders such as multiple sclerosis (MS), largely by virtue of its great sensitivity to focal alterations of brain water content. The reported sensitivity of MR in patients with definite MS by clinical criteria is 85 percent (Sheldon 1985). In our experience with over 800 patients with MS, the sensitivity has been greater than 95 percent.

The combination of myelin loss and inflamma-

tion produces focal areas of increased water content and prolongation of the T_1 and T_2 relaxation times (Jackson 1985; Sheldon 1985), these changes being most conspicuous as hyperintense foci on T_2-weighted spin-echo images (Fig. 17-61). The plaques are typically discrete and most pronounced in the periventricular white matter. The majority of lesions are 5 to 10 mm in diameter, but patients with acute or fulminant disease may have larger lesions, occasionally with mass effect. Chronic MS may result in conglomerate lesions which appear as confluent and irregular high intensity bordering the lateral ventricles. Plaques may also be seen in the brainstem and cervical cord, as well as the cerebellar white matter and basal ganglia.

Periventricular hyperintensity has been described in non-MS patients, including those with hypertension and elderly (but otherwise normal) individuals (Bradley 1984d; Brant-Zawadzki 1985). Diagnostic difficulties may be encountered when MS is suspected in these patients, since 10 percent of all patients with MS present after age 60. A distinction may often be made on the basis of lesion distribution.

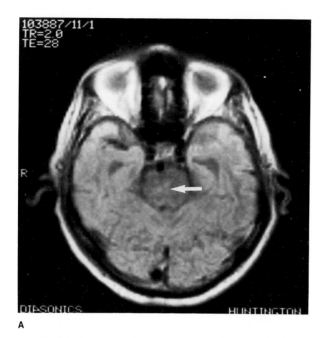

A

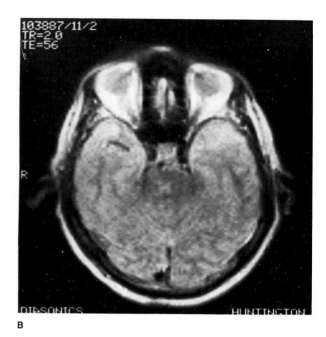

B

C

Figure 17-60 Vertebrobasilar infarcts. **A.** This patient presented with vertebrobasilar insufficiency. On the first echo axial image (TR = 2.0 sec, TE = 28 msec), multiple hyperintense infarcts were seen within the brainstem (arrow). **B.** On the second echo image, these lesions become more conspicuous (TR = 2.0 sec, TE = 56 msec). **C.** Hyperintensity is seen on the second echo image within the vertebral artery (arrowhead), indicating slow flow within this structure ("even echo rephasing").

MS plaques are typically more discrete in the centrum semiovale with periventricular distribution, as compared with the more confluent pattern of deep white matter infarction or age-related changes closer to the corticomedullary junction. Confluent

MS plaques, when present, tend to be most pronounced along the lateral aspect of the atria and occipital horns. Brainstem and cervical cord lesions are seen much more often in MS patients than in elderly or hypertensive individuals (Kortman 1986*d*).

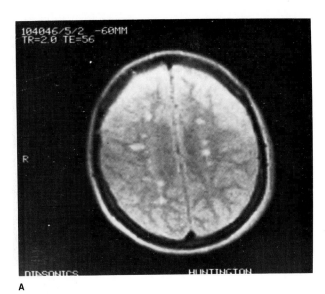

A

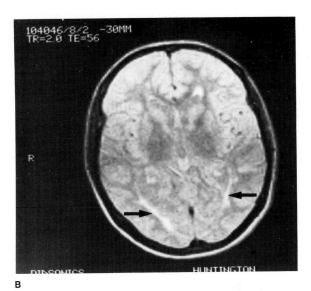

B

Figure 17-61 Multiple sclerosis. **A.** Multiple foci of hyperintensity are seen throughout the periventricular white matter bilaterally (TR = 2.0 sec, TE = 56 msec). **B.** At a slightly lower level, confluent high intensity is seen along the lateral aspect of the atria and occipital horns (arrows).

MR is useful in the evaluation of other myelinating disorders (Young 1983*a*), including the leukodystrophies (Fig. 17-62) and viral leukoencephalopathies (Fig. 17-63). As previously mentioned, white matter abnormalities are frequently seen in patients who have undergone prior cranial irradiation, secondary to a combination of focal demyelination and vasculopathy/infarction (Dooms 1986).

Brainstem Lesions without Mass Effect

Pathologic processes within the posterior fossa can be accurately localized and characterized with MR to a degree never before possible with CT. This is due to a number of factors, including high contrast and spatial resolution, lack of bony artifacts, and the ability to image in any orthogonal plane.

Within the brainstem, specific white matter tracts and nuclei can be identified as discrete structures by virtue of their location and signal intensity (Flannigan 1985). Specifically, the red nuclei, substantia nigra, cerebral peduncles, corticospinal tracts, and medial leminisci are demonstrated routinely on moderately T_2-weighted spin-echo images (Fig. 17-64). Thin sections in appropriate projections allow depiction of most of the cranial nerves at their

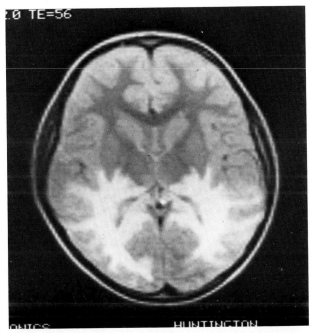

Figure 17-62 Adrenoleukodystrophy. This 6-year-old male presented with a progressive decline in mental status and adrenal insufficiency. A younger male sibling was similarly affected. A transaxial T_2-WI at the level of lateral ventricles demonstrates diffuse and symmetric hyperintensity involving the periventricular white matter with a striking posterior distribution, typical of adrenoleukodystrophy.

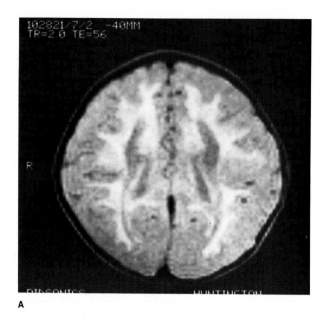

A

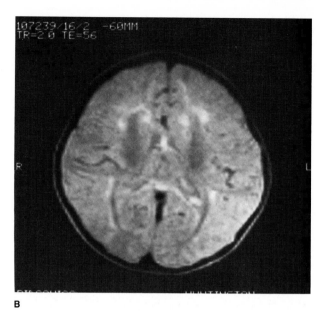

B

Figure 17-63 Postviral leukoencephalopathy: This patient presented with progressive neurologic dysfunction. **A.** A transaxial T_2-WI demonstrates diffuse and irregular hyperintensity involving the periventricular white matter (TR = 2.0 sec, TE = 56 msec).

B. Two years following the first examination, the patient was much improved clinically. The follow-up MR examination demonstrates a significant but subtotal resolution of the white matter abnormalities.

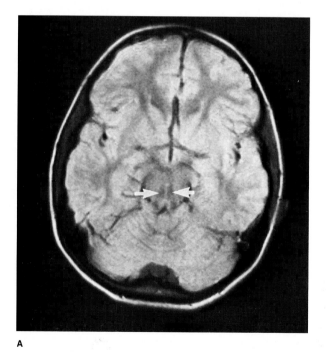

A

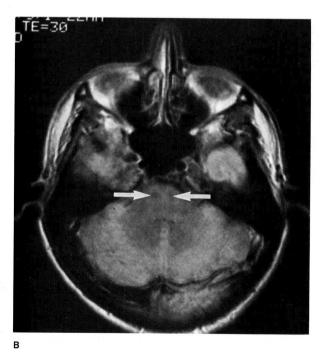

B

Figure 17-64 Normal brainstem structures. **A.** Red nuclei (arrows) seen as low-intensity paired structures in midbrain. Low intensity reflects high density of myelinated fibers running through

these nuclei. At higher fields, low intensity also reflects ferritin deposition in older normal individuals. **B.** Corticospinal tracts (arrows) appear dark on T_2-WI due to presence of myelin.

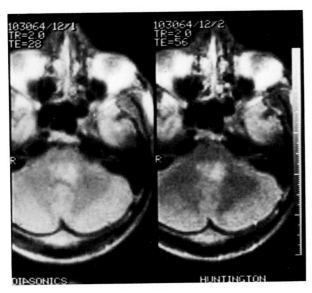

Figure 17-65 Pontine glioma. This patient presented with cranial nerve palsies, and physical examination revealed an intranuclear ophthalmoplegia. A hyperintense mass can be seen immediately anterior to the fourth ventricle in the expected position of the medial longitudinal fasciculus (TR = 2.0 sec, TE = 28 and 56 msec).

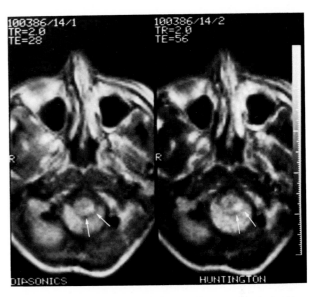

Figure 17-66 Brainstem infarct. This patient presented with a Wallenberg (lateral medullary) syndrome. A small hyperintense infarct is seen in the left lateral aspect of the medulla (arrows) (TR = 2.0 sec, TE = 28 and 56 msec).

origin. The location of other brainstem structures may be inferred from their relationship to these and other landmarks, including the cerebral aqueduct and fourth ventricle.

A working knowledge of the location and function of brainstem structures allows a more accurate correlation between MR findings and clinical presentation (Flannigan 1985) (Figs. 17-65, 17-66). Focal MR abnormalities, though conspicuous, may not be specific. For example, it may be difficult to distinguish between a brainstem MS plaque and a vertebrobasilar infarct. In these cases, consideration of findings outside the posterior fossa may be helpful. Obviously, clinical correlation is essential.

Hemorrhage

In the circulation, hemoglobin exists in the oxy and deoxy forms (Wintrobe 1981) which have relaxation times similar to normal brain (Bradley 1986a). Acute hemorrhage within the brain or in an extraaxial location may thus be detected only on the basis of

mass effect or associated vasogenic edema (Bradley 1986a) (Fig. 17-67). At higher fields, acute hematomas (intraparenchymal or subdural) may have a hypointense appearance (Gomori 1985). This is due to T_2 shortening from the magnetic heterogeneity of the magnetically susceptible deoxyhemoglobin within intact red blood cells. This T_2 shortening effect has been said to increase with the square of the magnetic field strength (Gomori 1985).

After a period of several days, hemoglobin undergoes oxidative denaturation, forming methemoglobin, which is paramagnetic (Bradley 1985b). The short T_1 of methemoglobin gives subacute hemorrhage hyperintensity on MR (Fig. 17-68). Continued oxidation over a period of months results in the formation of hemichromes, which are not paramagnetic (Bradley 1985b). Before oxidative denaturation occurs, a blood-brain barrier defect may be present in parenchymal hematomas, resulting in vasogenic edema. Thus T_2-WI are more sensitive than T_1-WI in the MR evaluation of early intracranial hemorrhage (Bradley 1986a; Gomori 1985). CT, however,

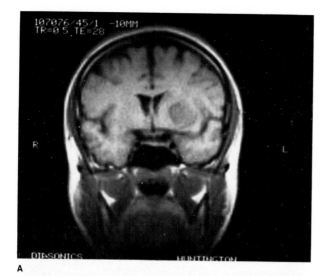

A

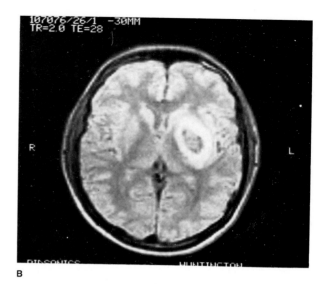

B

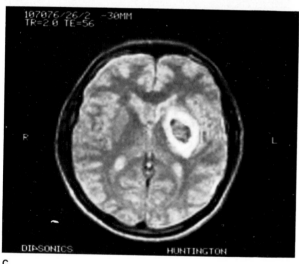

C

Figure 17-67 Acute basal ganglia hemorrhage. **A.** A coronal T₁-WI demonstrates a rounded hypointense lesion in the left basal ganglia. Note the absence of T_1 shortening, i.e., methemoglobin effect. Mild mass effect is manifested by distortion of the adjacent frontal horn (TR = 0.5 sec, TE = 28 msec). **B.** A more T₂-WI (axial) demonstrates an isointense hematoma with a hyperintense rim of surrounding edema (TR = 2.0 sec, TE = 28 msec). **C.** On the second echo image, the hematoma becomes slightly less intense, while the edema is more intense (TR = 2.0 sec, TE = 56 msec).

is more specific than MR and thus should be considered the preferred imaging modality for the evaluation of *acute* intracranial hemorrhage (Bradley 1985*b*; 1986*a*; De LaPaz 1984).

Acute subarachnoid hemorrhage is also more difficult to demonstrate on MR than CT because of only minimal shortening of the T_1 relaxation time of CSF by blood proteins (Bradley 1985*b*). A week following subarachnoid hemorrhage, methemoglobin is formed, making the appearance much more obvious (Bradley 1985*b*) (Fig. 17-69).

Subdural hematomas are well seen (Fig. 17-70) on axial or direct coronal images (Bradley 1984*c*; Young 1983*b*; Sipponen 1984). Small extraaxial collections at the vertex or along the tentorium can be missed on axial CT but are easily seen on direct coronal MR. In addition, subacute subdural hematomas are easily distinguished from chronic subdural collections (Sipponen 1984) by virtue of their different T_1 relaxation times (Bradley 1984*b*). A shortened T_1 relaxation time reflects the presence of methemoglobin in subacute subdural hematomas,

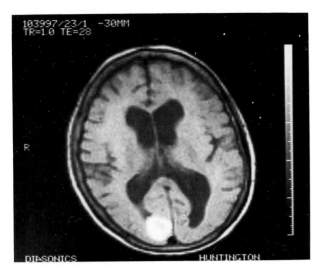

Figure 17-68 Subacute intracranial hemorrhage. An occipital hematoma is seen as an area of hyperintensity on this T_1-WI. T_1 shortening is attributed to the presence of paramagnetic methemoglobin (TR = 1.0 sec, TE = 28 msec).

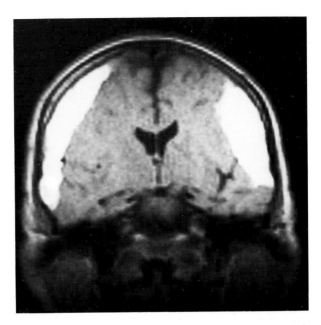

Figure 17-70 Subdural hematomas. Bilateral hyperintense subdural hematomas are graphically demonstrated on this coronal T_1-WI. T_1 shortening is attributed to the presence of methemoglobin (TR = 0.5 sec, TE = 28 msec).

while continued oxidative denaturation leading to formation of nonparamagnetic hemichromes results in T_1 prolongation and decreased intensity of chronic subdural collections (Bradley 1986a).

Hydrocephalus

If the intraventricular pressure is elevated owing to obstruction of normal CSF absorption pathways, CSF passes transependymally into the periventricular white matter (Fishman 1975). In its new environment, the CSF becomes interstitial edema. The water is organized into hydration layers around the proteins in the myelin, resulting in shortening of the T_1 relaxation time (Fullerton 1984). Its presence is

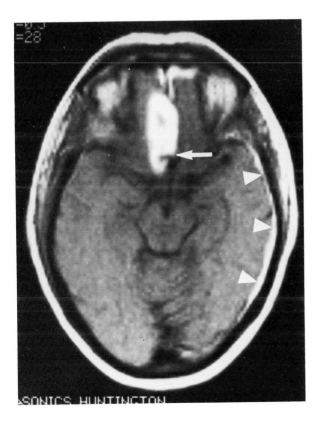

◀ **Figure 17-69** Subacute subarachnoid hemorrhage. This patient had an anterior communicating artery aneurysm which had ruptured one week prior to this exam. An inferior frontal hematoma is seen adjacent to the aneurysm (arrow). Subarachnoid hemorrhage is seen extendng over the frontal pole and the lateral aspect of the temporal lobe (arrowheads) (TR = 0.5 sec, TE = 28 msec).

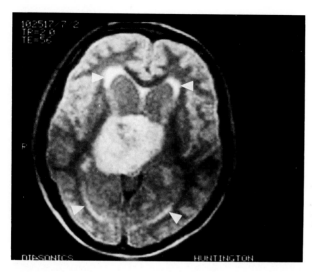

Figure 17-71   Obstructive hydrocephalus. A hyperintense thalamic glioma has produced obstructive hydrocephalus at the foramen of Monro. The lateral ventricles are dilated and surrounded by a smooth rim of symmetric hyperintensity (arrowheads), indicating the presence of interstitial edema (TR = 2.0 sec, TE = 56 msec).

recognized on MR images by a smooth border of increased intensity surrounding the lateral ventricles on T_2-weighted images (Fig. 17-71).

The finding of interstitial edema is useful in dis-

tinguishing patients with elevated CSF pressure from those with compensated hydrocephalus (Bradley 1984*b*) (Fig. 17-72). When the site of obstruction is from the foramen of Monro to the foramina of Luschka or Magendie, it can be readily identified on midsagittal sections.

Dementia

MR is particularly useful in evaluating demented patients. Unlike CT, MR can distinguish several causes of dementia associated with ventricular dilatation (Kortman 1986*a*; Bradley 1984*d*). More important, MR may be able to identify those patients who are amenable to treatment (Kortman 1986*a*). Patients presenting with the clinical triad of dementia, gait disturbance, and incontinence who also have dilated ventricles may be considered to have *normal pressure hydrocephalus* (NPH). Patients with appropriate clinical findings and with a smooth border of hyperintensity surrounding the ventricles (Fig. 17-73) have the best chance of responding to ventriculoperitoneal (VP) shunting. The hyperintense border is similar to that seen in obstructive and acute communicating forms of (elevated-pressure) hydrocephalus and is thought to represent either (1) in-

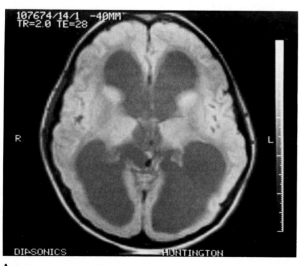

A

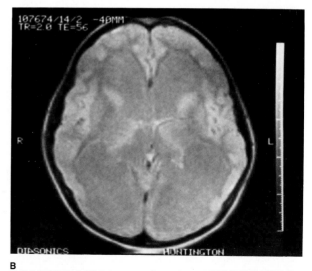

B

Figure 17-72   Compensated obstructive hydrocephalus.   **A.** The lateral and third ventricles are severely dilated (TR = 2.0 sec, TE = 28 msec).   **B.** On the second-echo image, there is no evidence of periventricular interstitial edema (TR = 2.0 sec, TE = 56 msec). (*Continued on p. 825.*)

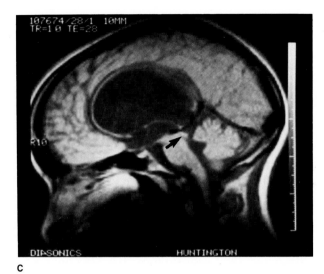

C

Figure 17-72 (*cont.*)   **C.** On a midsagittal T$_1$-WI, the cerebral aqueduct appears significantly narrowed (arrow), and this most likely represents the site of obstruction.

terstitial edema due to transependymal migration of CSF into the weakened periventricular tissues or (2) demyelination due to the previous interstitial edema (Fishman 1975). Irregular or numerous focal peri-

ventricular lesions (Fig. 17-74) are an indication of deep white matter infarction which may either co-exist with, or result from, ventricular enlargement in patients with NPH (Kortman 1986a). The two entities can be difficult to distinguish clinically, particularly if the stepwise progression characteristic of multi-infarct dementia is not appreciated. Regardless of the etiology, patients with dilated ventricles and *no* evidence of white matter infarction are much more likely to respond to VP shunting than those *with* patchy periventricular abnormalities (Kortman 1986a). Recently, marked signal loss (Fig. 17-75) has been observed in the aqueduct in patients with NPH (Bradley 1986b). Although the "aqueductal flow void" can be seen in normals as well, it is more marked in NPH and is thought to reflect the greater pulsatile motion of CSF through the aqueduct in these patients with decreased ventricular compliance (Bradley 1986b).

Huntington's disease is manifested by atrophy of the caudate head and secondary enlargement of the frontal horns. In our experience, MR is less sensitive than positron emission tomography (PET) which demonstrates hypometabolic areas prior to atrophy;

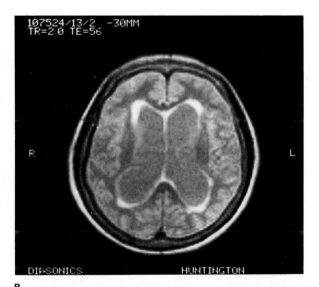

A

Figure 17-73 Normal pressure hydrocephalus. This elderly patient presented with the clinical triad of dementia, gait disturbance, and urinary incontinence.   **A.** On the first-echo axial image, the lateral ventricles appear mildly dilated, while the cortical sulci are less prominent than usual (TR = 2.0 sec, TE = 28 msec).

B

B. The second-echo image demonstrates a rim of surrounding periventricular hyperintensity similar to that seen in obstructive hydrocephalus. Note the absence of focal hyperintense abnormalities within the periventricular white matter. The patient responded well to ventricular shunting.

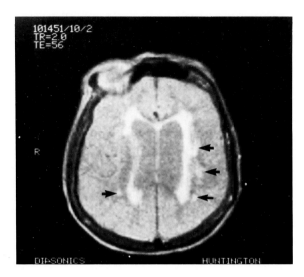

Figure 17-74 Multi-infarct dementia. This patient also presented with memory loss and gait disturbance. Note the more irregular pattern of confluent periventricular hyperintense, as well as the presence of multiple focal lesions (arrowheads) within the periventricular white matter.

MR is equivalent to CT in the diagnosis of Huntington's disease (Simmonas 1986).

Alzheimer's disease remains a diagnosis of exclusion, manifested by generalized atrophy. There are no focal findings on MR specifically suggestive of this entity to our knowledge.

Vascular Abnormalities

Intraluminal blood has a variable appearance on MR imaging, depending on its velocity and direction of flow (Bradley 1985c, 1984e). Rapidly flowing blood generally is associated with loss of intraluminal signal (Bradley 1984e) which facilitates the diagnosis of arteriovenous malformations (Young 1983c; Lee 1985d) (Fig. 17-76) and aneurysms (Worthington 1983) (Fig. 17-77). Angiographically occult vascular malformation may escape detection on MR when only focal calcification and subtle enhancement are present on CT (Lemme-Plaghos 1986). In aneurysms, mural thrombus can be distinguished from the patent lumen (Worthington 1983). Edema or gliosis and hemorrhage associated with an AVM can be demonstrated. Lack of first-echo dephasing and second-echo rephasing can be used to diagnose dural sinus thrombosis (see Chapters 12 and 14).

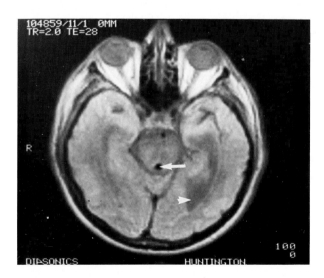

Figure 17-75 Aqueductal flow void sign in NPH. Marked signal loss (arrow) is noted in the aqueduct due to pulsatile flow of CSF. Compare with intensity of CSF in lateral ventricle (arrowhead).

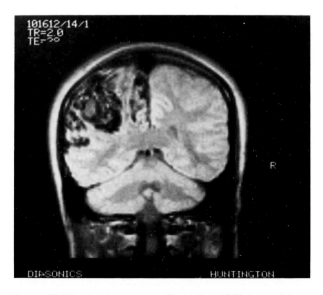

Figure 17-76 Arteriovenous malformation. Multiple serpiginous areas of hypointensity are seen in the deep and superficial portions of the right cerebral cortex and basal ganglia. The hypointensity of these structures is attributed to signal void from flowing blood, and is typical of vascular malformations (TR = 2.0 sec, TE = 28 msec).

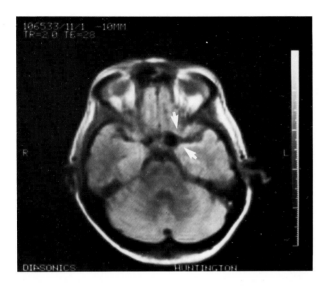

Figure 17-77 Intracranial aneurysm. A flow-related focal hypointense signal is seen in the left suprasellar cistern (arrows). Arteriography confirmed the presence of an aneurysm at ICA bifurcation.

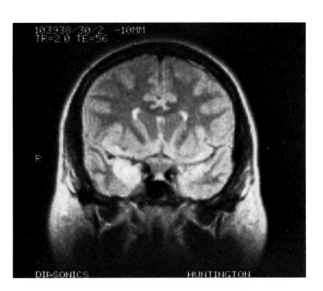

Figure 17-78 Cerebritis. This 21-year-old male presented with progressively worsening seizures. On serial scans over a 6-month period, the patient developed a hyperintense lesion involving the right temporal lobe, associated with minimal if any mass effect. Biopsy revealed chronic and acute inflammatory changes, with no evidence of tumor (TR = 2.0 sec, TE = 56 msec).

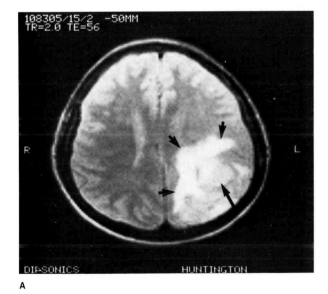

A

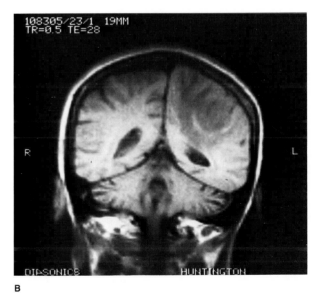

B

Figure 17-79 Intracerebral abscess. **A.** On an axial T_2-WI, a rounded mass (arrow) with extensive surrounding edema (arrowheads) is seen in the left parietal lobe (TR = 2.0 sec, TE = 56 msec). **B.** On a coronal T_1-WI, the mass is decreased in signal intensity (TR = 0.5 sec, TE = 28 msec). The patient had a history of a left parietal lobe infarct and had undergone a recent dental procedure. This lesion resolved with antibiotic therapy.

Slowly flowing blood may be diagnosed using a multiecho sequence where the intensity is greater on even echoes due to a rephasing phenomenon (Waluch 1984). Thus the intraluminal intensity of a venous angioma may be greater on the second-echo image than on the first (Bradley 1984*b*).

Inflammation

The efficacy of MR in the evaluation of intracranial inflammatory disease reflects its high sensitivity to focal alterations in brain water content (Scott 1985; Kortman 1986*e*). As with other processes, such changes are most conspicuous as hyperintense abnormalities on T_2-WIs and are more readily appreciated by MR than by CT, particularly in the posterior fossa.

The appearance of focal cerebritis (Fig. 17-78) or abscess (Fig. 17-79) is nonspecific. When associated with mass effect, solitary lesions may resemble gliomas, while multiple lesions cannot be reliably differentiated from metastases. Clinical information (including CSF analysis) may be helpful in distinguishing these processes. However, in some cases, biopsy may be needed to determine diagnosis and appropriate therapy.

During the acute phase of cerebral granulomatous infections, both the inflammatory nidus and reactive edema are readily demonstrated by MRI (Fig. 17-80). Evolution to the chronic phase often results in intraparenchymal calcifications, which may serve to characterize these diseases on CT examination (Kortman 1986*e*). Such calcifications are poorly appreciated by MR (Holland 1985; Tsuruda 1986). Intraventricular cysticercotic cysts may be appreciated on MR exam as areas of increased signal intensity relative to CSF (Fig. 17-81), precluding the need for CT metrizamide ventriculography.

Immunosuppressed patients, particularly those with AIDS, are subject to intracranial infestation with a number of pathogens, including toxoplasmosis, fungal agents, and Papova viruses (see Chapter 12). On MR examination, these processes cannot be reliably differentiated from each other, from other in-

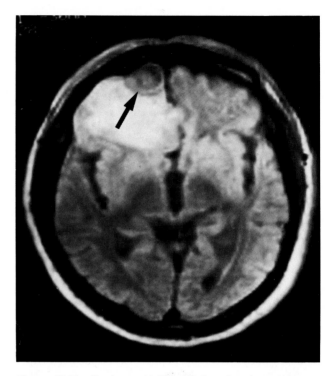

Figure 17-80 Cysticercosis. This Mexican-American male presented with headache and seizure. An axial image at the level of the third ventricle demonstrates a rounded hypertense lesion in the right frontal pole (arrow), with extensive surrounding edema. Biopsy revealed an intraparenchymal cysticercotic cyst with acute inflammatory changes (TR = 2.0 sec, TE = 28 msec).

fectious processes, or from lymphoma (Post 1986). In such cases, MR is useful for biopsy planning (Fig. 17-82) and may be utilized to monitor response to therapy.

Meningeal inflammation may be manifested as alteration of signal intensity over the surface of the brain (Bradley 1984*b*) (Fig. 17-83). Reactive subdural effusions are transudative and low in protein content, resembling CSF in signal intensity. Extraaxial empyemas have relatively short T_1 times and prolonged T_2 times, appearing hyperintense with respect to CSF on mild to moderately T_2-weighted images.

Active intracranial inflammation often produces alterations in mental status. Motion by affected pa-

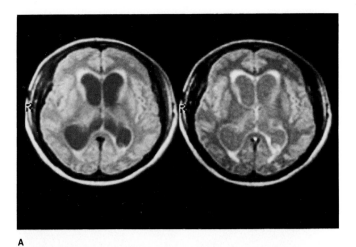

A

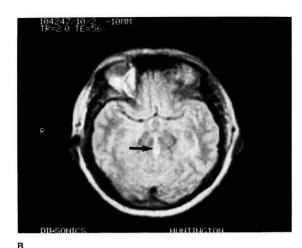

B

C

Figure 17-81 Intraventricular cysticercosis: This middle-aged Mexican-American woman presented with worsening headaches. **A.** An axial section of the level of the lateral ventricles demonstrates symmetric ventricular dilatation with surrounding periventricular high intensity consistent with interstitial edema (TR = 2.0 sec, TE = 28 and 56 msec).   **B.** At a lower level, a linear band of hyperintensity is seen coursing over the midbrain (arrow). **C.** A midsagittal section shows that this lesion lies within the cerebral aqueduct (arrowhead). CSF cysticercosis titers were elevated. The intraaqueductal lesion is presumed to be a cysticercotic cyst.

tients results in image degradation, and such individuals may therefore be more effectively evaluated by CT.

Developmental Anomalies

The marked gray-white differentiation present on MR images allows determination of the normal course of myelination and alterations of that process (Byd-

der 1985*b*). Agenesis and partial agenesis of the corpus callosum is easily evaluated (Fig. 17-84). Chiari malformations (Spinos 1985) and other abnormalities which involve the craniovertebral junction are also well seen on direct sagittal images (Fig. 17-84), as are associated anomalies such as myelomeningoceles and encephaloceles (Fig. 17-85). Associated hydrocephalus is also well seen. Dandy-Walker cysts are readily evaluated (Fig. 17-86) (see Chapter 4).

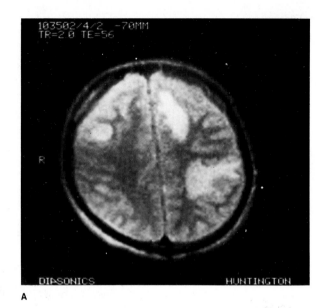

A

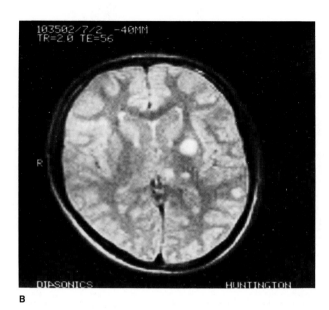

B

Figure 17-82   Toxoplasmosis: This AIDS patient presented with progressive decline in mental status and seizures.   **A.** An axial section at the supraventricular level demonstrates irregular hyperintense lesions involving the white matter and gray-white junction bilaterally (TR = 2.0 sec, TE = 56 msec).   **B.** At a lower level, rounded lesions are seen in the basal ganglia as well. Biopsy revealed toxoplasmosis.

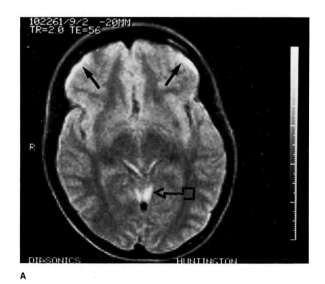

A

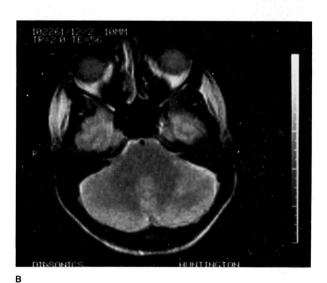

B

Figure 17-83   Meningitis.   **A.** An axial T_2-WI demonstrates abnormal areas of hyperintensity over both frontal convexities (arrows) and in the supravermian cistern (open arrow) (TR = 2.0 sec, TE = 56 msec).   **B.** Similar changes are noted in the prepontine and cerebellopontine angle cisterns. The patient suffered from chronic meningitis.

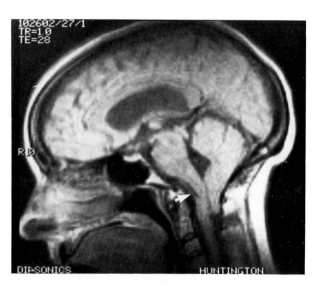

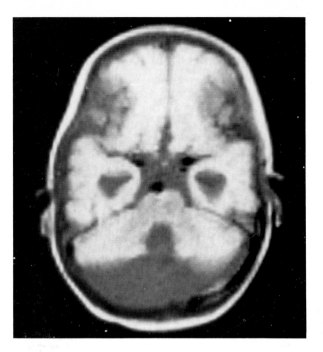

Figure 17-84 Chiari I malformation. This midsagittal image demonstrates abnormal elongation and inferior extension of the cerebellar tonsils below the level of the foramen magnum. There is mild buckling at the cervical-medullary junction (arrowhead). The ventricular system is slightly dilated secondary to obstructive hydrocephalus. No discernible corpus callosum is present.

Figure 17-86 Dandy-Walker malformation. There is a large CSF collection in the posterior aspect of the posterior fossa. This communicates widely with the fourth ventricle (arrow), with no intervening vermis tissue.

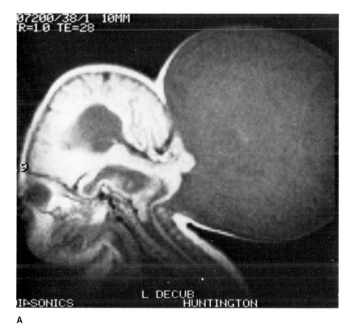

A

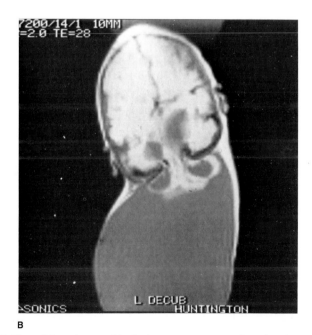

B

Figure 17-85 Occipital encephalocele. **A.** This midline sagittal image demonstrates a large occipital encephalocele associated with a complex Chiari malformation (TR = 1.0 sec, TE = 28 msec).

B. The axial section graphically demonstrates protrusion of occipital lobes and cerebellar structures through the occipital defects (TR = 2.0 sec, TE = 28 msec).

FUTURE PERSPECTIVES IN MR OF THE CENTRAL NERVOUS SYSTEM

As MR imaging technology continues to evolve, images with high signal to noise, submillimeter spatial resolution, and slice thickness of a few millimeters will be acquired in less and less time. Surface coil imaging coupled with different field strength systems will permit the rapid acquisition of very high resolution images (i.e., less than .5 mm) in the orbit (Daniels 1984a), cavernous sinus (Daniels 1985b), and internal auditory canal (Daniels 1984b, 1985a).

The ability to obtain nonorthogonal images in oblique planes will increase the utility of MR in the evaluation of not only the orbit but also the spine (Daniels 1986). Sequences which allow variable degrees of axial angulation at different disc levels in a single multislice acquisition have already been demonstrated in the evaluation of the lumbar spine (Flannigan 1986b). The ability to obtain images which are angled in two planes—relatively not only to the axial but also to the coronal or sagittal planes—will be useful in the evaluation of the cervical neural foramina.

Although synthesized images have been produced since clinical MR imaging was first demonstrated, these have been degraded by patient motion between the acquisition of short and long TR multiecho sequences. As imaging times are reduced and as software improves, image synthesis may become more useful in the clinical setting (Bobman 1985).

MR is currently limited by motion artifact in traumatized, demented, or otherwise uncooperative patients. In such instances, CT is currently preferred by virtue of its ability to acquire single-slice images within a few seconds. Fast MR scanning techniques with similar acquisition times have been recently demonstrated (Matthaei 1986) and are expected to be available for clinical use within the next year. Although these techniques are likely to be more routinely applied in the upper abdomen where respiratory motion has continued to be a source of difficulty, it is expected that such sequences will also be useful in the setting of head trauma.

MR is currently at a disadvantage relative to CT by not having a generally available intravenous contrast agent. Although MR is sensitive to the vasogenic edema produced by such blood-brain barrier breakdown, intravenous contrast may still be required prior to stereotactic biopsy to distinguish enhancing portions of the tumor from necrotic portions or edema. Gadolinium-DTPA has already been demonstrated to be useful in this setting in early clinical trials in Europe and the United States. Gadolinium has been shown to be particularly useful in the evaluation of meningiomas (Bydder 1985a) and acoustic neuromas (Curati 1986) which enhance densely as expected from prior experience with CT. The use of Gadolinium in one early collaborative study increased the detection of metastatic disease by 15 percent (Bradley 1985f). Whether Gadolinium-DTPA will be used as ubiquitously as iodinated contrast is currently used for CT remains to be seen. At the time of this writing, the best estimate for general availability for Gadolinium-DTPA is mid-1987. Although other paramagnetic contrast agents (e.g., nitroxide stable free radicals, paramagnetically tagged monoclonal antibodies, and ferrite particles) have been evaluated in animal models, none yet has been used clinically.

The sensitivity of magnetic resonance to the presence of low concentrations of paramagnetic ferritin has already been demonstrated in normals, particularly on the higher field units which are more sensitive to the magnetic susceptibility effects of such substances. Preliminary work has demonstrated abnormal patterns of ferritin deposition in the basal ganglia and cortex in various demented states (Drayer 1985). Should the detection of abnormal ferritin deposition be shown to have widespread clinical utility, such detection is best accomplished at high field or using "gradient echoes" (which are sensitive to magnetic susceptibility effects) at low field.

The recent early work on the motion of CSF within the ventricles (Bradley 1985d) as well as within the intracranial and intraspinal (Bradley 1986b) subarachnoid spaces suggests that there will be continued research in the use of cardiac-gated, velocity-sensitive sequences in the analysis of CSF flow in disease states. One could envision obtaining CSF flow profiles through the ventricular system for use in the preoperative evaluation of patients with suspected normal pressure hydrocephalus. Sensitivity to CSF motion in the spine may not only furnish information on CSF flow dynamics but also facilitate demonstration of pathology.

Imaging of other elements such as sodium is currently at a very early stage of development but shows great clinical potential. Using a very short echo technique, Hilal et al. (1986) have shown preliminary data which suggest the ability to distinguish intra- and extracellular sodium. If this capacity is substantiated with further work, sodium imaging may be proven to be useful in the separation of tumor and edema and possibly in the distinction of radiation necrosis from recurrent tumor (Hilal 1986), both of which currently can only be done by the pathologist.

MR spectroscopy results in the measurement of different chemical species of the same atomic nucleus. ^{31}P spectroscopy permits quantitation of the high-energy phosphate metabolites such as phosphocreatine and ATP as well as their breakdown products, including inorganic phosphate. pH can be measured from the chemical shift of the inorganic phosphate peak. Proton spectroscopy permits visualization of water and fat as separate peaks and, using various water suppression techniques, the visualization of lactate and other species which may be present in lower concentration. A substantial effort has already been devoted to the use of spectroscopy in the early diagnosis of cerebral ischemia, which, at the time of this writing, has meager results. This unfortunately raises doubts as to the ultimate clinical utility of MR spectroscopy in the evaluation of stroke. Spectroscopy may be useful, however, in the characterization of neoplasia and in the individualized planning of chemotherapy and radiation therapy (Bradley 1985e).

Bibliography

BOBMAN SA, RIEDERER SJ, LEE JN et al: Cerebral magnetic resonance image synthesis. *AJNR* 6(2):265–270, 1985.

BRADLEY WG, CROOKS LE, NEWTON TH: Physical principles of NMR. In Newton TH, Potts DG, eds. *Modern Neuroradiology: Advanced Imaging Techniques*. Vol. II, San Francisco, Clavadel Press, 1983.

BRADLEY WG: Effect of magnetic relaxation times on magnetic resonance image interpretation. *Noninvasive Med Imaging* 1:193–204, 1984a.

BRADLEY WG: NMR imaging of the central nervous system. *Neurol Res* 6:91–106, 1984b.

BRADLEY WG, WALUCH V, YADLEY RA, WYCOFF RR: Comparison of CT and NMR in 400 cases of suspected disease of the brain and cervical cord. *Radiology* 152:695–702, 1984c.

BRADLEY WG, WALUCH V, BRANT-ZAWADZKI M et al: Patchy periventricular white matter lesions in the elderly: a common observation during NMR imaging. *Noninvasive Med Imaging* 1:35–41, 1984d.

BRADLEY WG, WALUCH V, KAI K et al: The appearance of rapidly flowing blood on magnetic resonance images. *AJR* 143:1167–1174, 1984e.

BRADLEY WG: Fundamentals of MR image interpretation. In Bradley WG, Adey WR, Hasso AN. *Magnetic Resonance Imaging of the Brain, Head, and Neck: A Text Atlas*. Rockville, Maryland, Aspen, 1985a.

BRADLEY WG, SCHMIDT PC: Effect of methemoglobin formation on the MRI appearance of subarachnoid hemorrhage. *Radiology* 165:99–103, 1985b.

BRADLEY WG, WALUCH V: Blood flow: magnetic resonance imaging. *Radiology* **154**:443–450, 1985*c*.

BRADLEY WG, KORTMAN KE, BURGOYNE B: Effect of pulsatile flow on CSF intensity in MR imaging of the brain (SS). *Radiology* **157**(P):125, 1985*d*.

BRADLEY WG: Notes and impressions: third annual meeting of Society of Magnetic Resonance in Medicine. *J Comput Assist Tomogr* **9**(1):220–224, 1985*e*.

BRADLEY WG, BRANT-ZAWADZKI M, BRASCH RC et al: Initial clinical experience with Gd-DPTA in North America: MR contrast enhancement of brain tumors (SS). *Radiology* **157**(P):125, 1985*f*.

BRADLEY WG: MRI of intracranial hemorrhage. In Partain CL, Price RR, Patton JA, Kulkarni MV, James AE, eds. *Magnetic Resonance Imaging*, 2d ed. Philadelphia, Pennsylvania, WB Saunders Co, (in press), 1986*a*.

BRADLEY WG, KORTMAN KE, BURGOYNE B: MR of flowing CSF in normal and hydrocephalic states. *Radiology* **159**:611–616, 1986*b*.

BRADLEY WG: Tissue characterization on MR images. In Brant-Zawadzki M, ed. *Magnetic Resonance in the Central Nervous System*. New York, Raven Press, in press, 1986*c*.

BRANT-ZAWADZKI M, DAVIS PL, CROOKS LE et al: NMR demonstration of cerebral abnormalities: comparison with CT. *AJR* **140**:847–854, 1983.

BRANT-ZAWADZKI M, BADAMI JP, MILLS CM et al: Primary intracranial tumor imaging: a comparison of magnetic resonance and CT. *Radiology* **150**:435–440, 1984*a*.

BRANT-ZAWADZKI M, NORMAN D, NEWTON TH et al: Magnetic resonance of the brain: the optimal screening technique. *Radiology* **152**:71–77, 1984*b*.

BRANT-ZAWADZKI M, FEIN G, VAN DYKE C, KIERNAN R, DAVENPORT L, DE GROOT J: MR imaging of the aging brain: patchy white-matter lesions and dementia. *AJNR* **6**(5):675–682, 1985.

BRANT-ZAWADZKI M, PEREIRA B, WEINSTEIN P et al: MR imaging of acute experimental ischemia in cats. *AJNR* **7**(1):7–12, 1986.

BRYAN RN, WILLCOTT MR, SCHNEIDERS NJ, ROSE JE: NMR evaluation of stroke in the rat. *AJNR* **4**:242–244, 1983.

BUCON KA, BRADLEY WG, KORTMAN KE: MR of meningiomas with and without paramagnetic contrast (SS). *Radiology* **157**(P):125, 1985.

BUONANNO FD, PYKETT IL, KISTLER JP et al: Cranial anatomy and detection of ischemic stroke in the cat by nuclear magnetic resonance imaging. *Radiology* **142**:187–193, 1982.

BYDDER GM, STEINER RE, YOUNG IR: Clinical NMR imaging of the brain: 140 cases. *AJR* **189**:215–236, 1982.

BYDDER GM, KINGSLEY DPE, BROWN J, NIENDORF HP, YOUNG IR: MR imaging of meningiomas including studies with and without Gadolinium-DTPA. *J Comput Assist Tomogr* **9**(4):690–697, 1985*a*.

BYDDER GM, YOUNG IR: MR imaging: clinical use of the inversion recovery sequence. *J Comput Assist Tomogr* **9**(4):659–675, 1985*b*.

CLAUSSEN C, LANIADO M, SCHORNER W et al: Gadolinium-DPTA in MR imaging of glioblastomas and intracranial metastases. *AJNR* **6**(5):669–674, 1985.

CROOKS LE, ARAKAWA M, HOENNINGER J et al: Nuclear magnetic resonance whole body imager operating at 3.5 gauss. *Radiology* **143**:169–181, 1982.

CURATI WL, GRAIF M, KINGSLEY DPE, NIENDORF HP, YOUNG IR: Acoustic neuromas: Gd-DTPA enhancement in MR imaging. *Radiology* **158**:447–451, 1986.

DANIELS DL, HERFKENS R, GAGER WE et al: Magnetic resonance imaging of the optic nerves and chiasm. *Radiology* **152**:79–83, 1984*a*.

DANIELS DL, HERFKENS R, KOEHLER PR, MILLEN SJ, SHAFFER KW, WILLIAMS AL, HAUGHTON VM: Magnetic resonance imaging of the internal auditory canal. *Radiology* **151**:105, 1984*b*.

DANIELS DL, SCHENCK JF, FOSTER T et al: Surface-coil magnetic resonance imaging of the internal auditory canal. *AJNR* **6**(4):487–490, 1985*a*.

DANIELS DL, PECH P, MARK L et al: Magnetic resonance imaging of the cavernous sinus. *AJNR* **6**:187, 1985*b*.

DANIELS DL, KNEELAND JB, KILGORE DP et al: Surface coil magnetic resonance imaging of cervical disc disease: the direct 45 degree oblique view. Presented at annual meeting of the ASNR, San Diego, California, Jan. 19–23, 1986.

DELAPAZ RL, NEW PFJ, BUONANNO FS et al: NMR imaging of intracranial hemorrhage. *J Comput Assist Tomogr* **8**:599–607, 1984.

DOOMS GC, HECHT S, BRANT-ZAWADZKI M, BERTHIAUME Y, NORMAN D, NEWTON TH: Brain radiation lesions: MR imaging. *Radiology* **158**:149–155, 1986.

DRAYER BP, BURGER P, PAYNE C, PERICAK-VANCE M et al: MR mapping of brain iron: II basal ganglia disorders (SS). *Radiology* **157**(P): 290, 1985.

FARRAR TC, BECKER ED: *Pulse and Fourier Transform NMR: Introduction to Theory and Methods.* New York, Academic Press, 1971.

FISHMAN RA: Brain edema. *N Eng J Med* **293**:706, 1975.

FLANNIGAN BD, BRADLEY WG, MAZZIOTTA JC et al: Magnetic resonance imaging of the brainstem: normal structure and basic functional anatomy. *Radiology* **154**:375–383, 1985.

FLANNIGAN BD, BRADLEY WG, KORTMAN KE, LIU A: MRI of cerebral infarction. In Rossi DR, Gerard G, eds. *Seminars in Neurology.* New York, Woodbury, in press, 1986*a*.

FLANNIGAN BD, WINTER J, BRADLEY WG: MRI appearance of the lumbar neural foramina, normal anatomy and pathology. Presented at annual meeting of the ASNR, San Diego, California, Jan. 19–23, 1986*b*.

FULLERTON GD, CAMERON IL, ORD VA: Frequency dependence of magnetic resonance spin-lattice relaxation of protons in biological materials. *Radiology* **151**:135–138, 1984.

GANTI SR, HILAL SK, STEIN BM, SILVER AJ, MAWAD M, SANE P: CT of pineal region tumors. *AJNR* **7**(1):97–104, 1986.

GOMORI JM, GROSSMAN RI, GOLDBERG M, ZIMMERMAN RA, BILANIUK LT: Intracranial hematomas: imaging by high field MR. *Radiology* **157**:87–92, 1985.

GOMORI JM, GROSSMAN RI, SHIELDS JA et al: Choroidal melanomas: correlation of NMR spectroscopy and MR imaging. *Radiology* **158**:443–445, 1986.

GRAIF M, BYDDER GM, STEINER RE, NIENDORF P, THOMAS DGT, YOUNG IR: Contrast-enhanced MR imaging of malignant brain tumors. *AJNR* **6**:855–862, 1985.

HAHN EL: Spin echoes. *Phys Rev* **80**:580–594, 1950.

HAN JS, KAUFMAN B, ALFIDI RJ et al: Head trauma evaluated by magnetic resonance and computed tomography: a comparison. *Radiology* **150**:71–77, 1984*a*.

HAN JS, BONSTELLE T, KAUFMAN B et al: Magnetic resonance imaging in the evaluation of the brainstem. *Radiology* **150**:705–712, 1984*b*.

HAWKES RC, HOLLAND GN, MOORE WS, WORTHINGTON BS: Nuclear magnetic resonance (NMR) tomography of the brain: a preliminary clinical assessment with demonstration of pathology. *J Comput Assist Tomogr* **4**:577–586, 1980.

HAZELWOOD CF: A view of the significance and understanding of the physical properties of cell-associated water, in Drost-Hansen W, Clegg J, eds. *Cell Associated Water.* New York, Academic Press, 1979.

HILAL SK, MAUDSLEY AA, SIMON HE et al: In vivo NMR imaging of tissue sodium in the intact cat before and after acute cerebral stroke. *AJNR* **4**:245–249, 1983.

HILAL SK, MAUDSLEY AA, RA JB et al: In vivo NMR imaging of sodium-23 in the human head. *J Comput Assist Tomogr* **9**(1):1–7, 1985.

HILAL SK, RA JB, SILVER AJ, MUN IK, OH CH: Selective imaging of intracellular sodium in brain tumors. Presented at annual meeting of the ASNR, San Diego, California, Jan. 19–23, 1986.

HOLLAND GN, HAWKES RC, MOORE WS: Nuclear magnetic resonance (NMR) tomography of the brain: coronal and sagittal sections. *J Comput Assist Tomogr* **4**:429–433, 1980.

HOLLAND BA, KUCHARCYSK W, BRANT-ZAWADZKI M, NORMAN D, HAAS DK, HARPER PS: MR imaging of calcified intracranial lesions. *Radiology* **157**:353–356, 1985.

JACK CR JR, REESE DF, SCHEITHAUER BW: Radiographic findings in 32 cases of primary CNS lymphoma. *AJNR* **6**:(1):899–904, 1985.

JACKSON JA, LEAKE DR, SCHNEIDERS NJ et al: Magnetic resonance imaging in multiple sclerosis: results in 32 cases. *AJNR* **6**(2):171–177, 1985.

KILGORE DP, STROTHER CM, STRASHAK RJ, HAUGHTON VM: Pineal germinoma: MR imaging. *Radiology* **158**:435–438, 1986.

KLATZO I, SEITELBERGER F (eds): *Brain Edema.* New York, Springer Verlag, 1967.

KORTMAN KE, BRADLEY WG: MR of normal pressure hydrocephalus. *AJNR,* submitted, 1986*a*.

KORTMAN KE, VAN DALSEM W, BRADLEY WG: MRI of intracranial epidermoid tumors. *Radiology,* submitted, 1986*b*.

KORTMAN KE, BRADLEY WG, RAUCH RA, POTEAT H, HOLSHOUSER B: Periventricular high intensity in MRI of the brain: incidence, pattern, and significance. *Radiology,* submitted, 1986*c*.

KORTMAN KE, BRADLEY WG, RAUCH RA et al: Multiple sclerosis versus cerebral vascular disease: differentiation by MRI. *Radiology,* submitted, 1986*d*.

KORTMAN KE, BRADLEY WG: MR imaging in CNS inflammatory disease. In Partain CL, Price RR, Patton JA, Kulkarni MV, James AE, eds., *Magnetic Resonance Imaging,* 2d ed. Philadelphia, Pennsylvania, WB Saunders Co, (in press), 1986*e*.

LEE BCP, KNEELAND JB, DECK MDF, CAHILL PT: Posterior fossa lesions: magnetic resonance imaging. *Radiology* **153**:137–143, 1984.

LEE BCP, KNEELAND JB, CAHILL PT, DECK MDE: MR recognition of supratentorial tumors. *AJNR* **6**(6) 871–878, 1985*a*.

LEE BCP, KNEELAND JB, WALKER RW et al: MR imaging of brainstem tumors. *AJNR* **6**(2):159–164, 1985*b*.

LEE BCP, DECK MDF, KNEELAND JB, CAHILL PT: MR imaging of the craniocervical junction. *AJNR* **6**(2):209–214, 1985*c*.

LEE BCP, HERZBERG L, ZIMMERMAN RD, DECK MDF: MR imaging of cerebral vascular malformations. *AJNR* **6**(6):863–870, 1985*d*.

LEMME-PLAGHOS L, KUCHARCZYK W, BRANDT-ZAWADZKI M et al: MR imaging of angiographically occult vascular malformations. *AJNR* **7**:217–222, 1986.

LEVY RM, MANO I, BRITO A. HOSOBUCHI Y: NMR imaging of acute experimental cerebral ischemia: time course and pharmacologic manipulations. *AJNR* **4**:238–241, 1983.

MATTHAEI D, FRAHM J, HAASE A, MERBOLDT KD, HANICKE W: Flash and steam MR imaging in neuroradiology. Presented at annual meeting of the ASNR, San Diego, California, Jan. 19–23, 1986.

MIKHAEL MA, CIRIC IS, WOLFF AP: Differentiation of cerebellopontine angle neuromas and meningiomas with MR imaging. *J Comput Assist Tomogr* **9**(5):852–586, 1985.

NEW PFJ, BACHOW TB, WISMER GL, ROSEN BR, BRADY TJ: MR imaging of the acoustic nerves and small acoustic neuromas at 0.6 T: prospective study. *AJNR* **6**(2):165–171, 1985.

POJUNAS KW, DANIELS DL, WILLIAMS AL, HAUGHTON VM: MR imaging of prolactin secreting microadenomas *AJNR* 7:209–213, 1986.

POST MJD, SHELDON JJ, HENSLEY GT et al: Central nervous system disease in acquired immunodeficiency syndrome: prospective correlation using CT, MR imaging, and pathologic studies. *Radiology* **158**:141–148, 1986.

PUSEY E, KORTMAN KE, FLANNIGAN BD, TSURUDA JS, BRADLEY WG: MR of craniopharyngioma. *Radiology*, submitted, 1986.

REULEN HJ et al: Role of pressure gradients and bulk flow in dynamics of vasogenic brain edema. *J Neurosurg* 46:24, 1977; **293**:706, 1975.

ROBERTS JD: *Nuclear Magnetic Resonance: Applications to Organic Chemistry.* New York, McGraw-Hill, 1959.

SCOTT JA, AUGUSTYN GT, GILMOR RL, MEALEY J JR, OLSON EW: Magnetic resonance imaging of a venous angioma. *AJNR* 6(2):284–286, 1985.

SHALLER CA, JACQUES DB, SHELDEN CH: The pathophysiology of stroke: a review with molecular considerations. *Surg Neurol* **14**:433–443, 1980.

SHELDON JJ, SIDDHARTHAN R, TOBIAS J, SHEREMATA WA, SOILA K, VIAMONTE M JR: MR imaging of multiple sclerosis: comparison with clinical and CT examinations in 74 patients. *AJNR* 6(5):683–691, 1985.

SIMMONAS JT PASTAKIA B, CHASE TN, SHULTS CW: Magnetic resonance imaging in Huntington disease. *AJNR* 7(1):25–28, 1986.

SIPPONEN JT, SEPPONEN RE, SIVULA A: Chronic subdural hematoma: demonstration by magnetic resonance. *Radiology* **150**:79–85, 1984.

SMITH AS, WEINSTEIN MA, MODIC MT et al: Magnetic resonance with marked T2-weighted images: improved demonstration of brain lesions, tumor, and edema. *AJNR* 6(5):691–698, 1985.

SOBEL DF, KELLY W, KJOS BO, CHAR D, BRANT-ZAWADZKI M, NORMAN D: MR imaging of orbital and ocular disease. *AJNR* 6(2):259–264, 1985.

SPILLANE JA, KENDALL BE, MOSELEY IF: Cerebral lymphoma: clinical radiological correlation. *J Neurol Neurosurg Psychiatry* 45:199–208, 1982.

SPINOS E, LASTER DW, MOODY DM, BALL MR, WITCOFSKI RL, KELLY DK JR: MR evaluation of Chiari I malformations at 0.15 T. *AJNR* 6(2):203–209, 1985.

SWISCHUK LE, BRYAN RN: Double midline intracranial atypical teratomas: a recognizable neuroendocrinologic syndrome. *Am J Roentgenol* 122:517–524, 1974.

TADMOR R, DAVIS KR, ROBERSON GH, KLEINMAN GM: Computed tomography in primary malignant lymphoma of the brain. *J Comput Assist Tomogr* 2:135–140, 1978.

TSURUDA JS, BRADLEY WG, KORTMAN KE, KWONG L: MR detection of intracranial calcification. *AJNR*, submitted, 1986.

WALL SD, BRANT-ZAWADZKI M, JEFFREY RD, BARNES B: High frequency CT findings within 24 hours after cerebral infarction. *AJR* **138**:307–311, 1982.

WALUCH V, BRADLEY WG: NMR even echo rephasing in slow laminar flow. *J Comput Assist Tomogr* 8:594–598, 1984.

WEHRLI FW, MACFALL J, NEWTON TH: Parameters determining the appearance of NMR images. *Modern Neuroradiology: Advanced Imaging Techniques.* Vol. II, San Francisco, Clavadel Press, 1983.

WEHRLI FW, MACFALL JR, SHUTTS D et al: Mechanism of contrast in NMR imaging. *J Comput Assist Tomogr* 8(3):369–380, 1984.

WIENER SN, RZESZOTARSKI MS, DROEGE RT, PEARLSTEIN AE, SHAFRON M: Measurement of pituitary gland height with MR imaging. *AJNR* 6(5):717–722, 1985.

WINTROBE MM (ed.): *Clinical Hematology*. Philadelphia, Pennsylvania, Lea & Febiger, 1981.

WORTHINGTON BS, KEAN DM, HAWKES RC et al: NMR imaging in the recognition of giant intracranial aneurysms. *AJNR* **48**:35–836, 1983.

YOUNG IR, BURL M, CLARKE GJ et al: Magnetic resonance properties of hydrogen: imaging the posterior fossa. *AJR* **137**:895–901, 1981.

YOUNG IR, RANDELL CP, KAPLAN PW et al: Nuclear magnetic resonance (NMR) imaging in white matter disease of the brain using spin-echo sequences. *J Comput Assist Tomogr* **7**(2):290–294, 1983*a*.

YOUNG IR, BYDDER GM, HALL AS, STEINER RE et al: Extracerebral collections: recognition by NMR imaging. *AJNR* **4**:833–834, 1983*b*.

YOUNG IR, BYDDER GM, HALL AS et al: NMR imaging in the diagnosis and management of intracranial angiomas. *AJNR* **4**:837–838, 1983*c*.

ZIMMERMAN RD, FLEMING CA, SAINT-LOUIS LA et al: Magnetic resonance imaging of meningiomas. *AJNR* **6**(2):149–158, 1985.

Index

Index